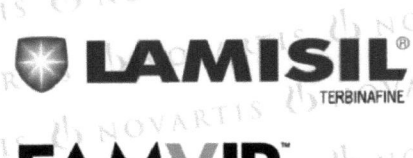

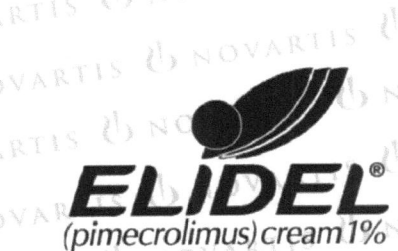

Springer
Berlin
Heidelberg
New York
Hong Kong
London
Milan
Paris
Tokyo

A.D. Katsambas · T.M. Lotti
(Eds.)

European Handbook of Dermatological Treatments

Second Edition

With 63 Figures and 157 Tables

Springer

Professor Andreas D. Katsambas
University of Athens
'A. Sygros' Hospital
Department of Dermatology
5, I. Dragoumi Street
161 21 Athens
Greece

Professor Torello M. Lotti
University Unit Allergology
Professional and
Environmental Dermatology
University of Florence
Via Alfani 37
50 121 Florence
Italy

ISBN 978-3-642-05657-4

Cataloging-in-Publication Data applied for

A catalog record for this book is available from the Library of Congress.

Bibliographic information published by Die Deutsche Bibliothek
Die Deutsche Bibliothek lists this publication in the Deutsche Nationalbibliografie; detailed bibliographic data is available in the Internet at http://dnb.ddb.de

Springer-Verlag Berlin Heidelberg New York
a member of BertelsmannSpringer
Science + Business Media GmbH

http://www.springer.de

Printed in Germany

Cover design: E. Kirchner, Heidelberg

Printed on acid-free paper
24/3150/PF – 5 4 3 2 1 0

Contents

Methods

Drugs

List of Contributors

S. Albert, *Assistant Professor, Department of Dermatology, Kasturba Medical College, Manipal, India*

A. Andreassi, *Istituto di Scienze Dermatologiche, Univ. Degli Studi – Policlinico Le Scotte, Viale Bracci, 53100 Siena, Italy*

L. Andreassi, *Professor of Dermatology, Direttore Istituto di Scienze Dermatologiche, Univ. Degli Studi – Policlinico Le Scotte, Viale Bracci, 53100 Siena, Italy*

C. Antoniou, *Associate Professor in Dermatology, University of Athens, "A Sygros Hospital", 5, I Dragoumi St, Kesariani 16121, Athens, Greece*

G. Avgerinou, *Department of Dermatology, University of Athens, "A Sygros Hospital", 5, I Dragoumi St, Kesariani 16121, Athens, Greece*

M. Balabanova, *Department of Dermatology, Alexander's Medical University Hospital, 1, Saint G. Sofiski St, Sofia BG-1431, Bulgaria*

B.-R. Balda, *Department of Dermatology & Allergology, Zentralklinikum Augsburg, Stenglinstraße 2, D-86156 Augsburg, Germany*

F. Bardazzi, *Department of Dermatology, Faculty of Medicine, University of Bologna, Via Massarenti 1, 40138 Bologna, Italy*

S. Belaich, *Department of Dermatology, Bichat Hôpital, Assistance Publique Hôpitaux de Paris, 46 rue Henri Huchard, 75018 Paris, France*

B. Bianchi, *Istituto di Scienze Dermatologiche, Univ. Degli Studi – Policlinico Le Scotte, Viale Bracci, 53100 Siena, Italy*

M.M. Black, *St. John's Institute of Dermatology, Basement, Block 7, St Thomas' Hospital, Lambeth Palace Road, London, SE1 7EH, U.K.*

B. Bonnekoh, *Department of Dermatology and Venereology, Otto-von-Guericke-University, Leipziger Str. 44, D-39120 Magdeburg, Germany*

J.D. Bos, *Department of Dermatology, Academic Medical Centre, University of Amsterdam, PO Box 22700, Meibergdreef 9, 1100 DE Amsterdam, The Netherlands*

F.M. Brandao, *Department of Dermatology, Hospital Garcia de Orta, Av. Torrado Silva, 2800 Almada, Portugal*

B. Brazzini, *Dipartimento di Scienze Derm, Universita degli studi di Firenze, Via Degli Alfani 37, I-50121 Firenze, Italy*

S. Brenner, *Department of Dermatology, Tel Aviv – Sourasky Medical Centre, Tel Aviv, Israel*

H.R. Bruckbauer, *Dermatologist and Allergologist, Marktplatz 7B, D-85375, Neufahrn, Germany*

F.M. Camacho-Martínez, *Universidad de Sevilla, Departamento de Dermatología, Avda. República Argentina 22, 5 D, Sevilla, Spain*

J.G. Camarasa (deceased), *Department of Dermatology, Hospital del Mar. IMIM, Universittat Autonoma de Barcelona, Passeig Maritim 25-29, 08003 Barcelona, Spain*

M.J. Camilleri, *Mayo Clinic, Rochester, MN, USA*

N. Cammarota, *Istituto di Scienze Dermatologiche, Univ. Degli Studio di Siena – Policlinico Le Scotte, Viale Bracci, 53100 Siena, Italy*

G. Campanile, *Dipartimento di Scienze Derm, Universita degli studi di Firenze, Via Degli Alfani 37, I-50121 Firenze, Italy*

P. Cappugi, *Department of Dermatological Science, University of Florence, Via degli Alfani 37, 50121 Florence, Italy*

R. Caputo, *Institute of Dermatological Sciences, IRCCS, University of Milan, Via Pace 9, I-20122 Milan, Italy*

P. Carli, *Dipartimento di Scienze Derm, Universita degli studi di Firenze, Via Degli Alfani 37, I-50121 Firenze, Italy*

G.W. Cherry, *Oxford Wound Healing Institute, Department of Dermatology, Churchill Hospital, Old Road, Headington, Oxford, OX3 7LJ, U.K.*

A. Claudy, *Service de Dermatologie, Hôpital Universitaire, Hôpital Edouard Herriot, Place d'Arsanval, F-69437 Lyon Cedex 03, France*

F. Coelho, *Superiori Technician Pharmacy, Centro de Dermatologia Medico-Cirurgica, ARS de Lisboa e Vale do Tejo, l, Rua Jose Estevao 135, 1150 Lisboa, Portugal*

C. Comacchi, *Dipartimento di Scienze Derm, Universita degli studi di Firenze, Via Degli Alfani 37, I-50121 Firenze, Italy*

N.M. Craven, *Section of Dermatology, University of Manchester, "Hope Hospital", Manchester, M6 8HD, U.K.*

B. Crickx, *Department of Dermatology, Bichat Hôpital, Assistance Publique Hôpitaux de Paris, 46 rue Henri Huchard, 75018 Paris, France*

W.J. Cunliffe, *Skin Research Centre, The General Infirmary at Leeds, Great George St, Leeds, LS1 3EX, U.K.*

I. Danopoulou, *Department of Dermatology, University of Athens, "A Sygros Hospital", 5, I Dragoumi St, Kesariani 16121, Athens, Greece*

R. Dawber, *Department of Dermatology, Churchill Hospital, Old Road, Headington, Oxford, OX3 7LJ, U.K.*

H. Degreef, *Universitaire Ziekenhuizen, Leuven Dermatologie, UZ St. Rafael, Kapucijnenvuer 33, B-3000 Leuven, Belgium*

V. De Giorgi, *Department of Dermatology, Universita degli studi di Firenze, Via Degli Alfani 37, I-50121 Firenze, Italy*

F.B. de Waard-van der Spek, *Department of Dermato-Venereology, University Hospital Rotterdam – Dijkzigt/Sophia, Molewaterplein 60, 3015 GJ Rotterdam, The Netherlands*

E. Del Bianco, *Department of Dermatological Science, University of Florence, Via degli Alfani 37, 50121 Florence, Italy*

A. Dompmartin, *Department of Dermatology, Center Hospitalier Universitaire Caen, Avenue Georges Clemenceau, 14033 Caen Cedex, France*

L. Dubertret, *Department of Dermatology, Hôpital Saint-Louis, 1 Avenue Claude Vellefaux, 75475, Paris Cedex 10, France*

J. Faergemann, *Associate Professor, Department of Dermatology, Sahlgrenska University Hospital, S-41345 Gothenburg, Sweden*

J. Ferguson, *Consultant Dermatologist, Photobiology Unit, University Department of Dermatology, Ninewells Hospital and Medical School, Dundee, DD1 9SY, U.K.*

B. Flageul, *Department of Dermatology, Hôpital Saint-Louis, 1 Avenue Claude Vellefaux, 75475, Paris Cedex 10, France*

D. Freedman, *Department of Medicine, University College, Dublin, and St James' Hospital, Dublin, Ireland*

M.L. Gantcheva, *Department of Dermatology, Alexander's Medical University Hospital, 1, Saint G. Sofiski St, Sofia BG-1431, Bulgaria*

X.-H. Gao, *Department of Dermatology, No.1 Hospital of China Medical University, Shenyang, China 110001*

B.C. Gee, *Department of Dermatology, Queen's Medical Centre, Nottinghan, NG7 2UH, U.K.*

S. Georgala, *Department of Dermatology, University of Athens, "A Sygros Hospital", 5, I Dragoumi St, Kesariani 16121, Athens, Greece*

I. Ghersetich, *Department of Dermatology, Universita degli studi di Firenze, Via Degli Alfani 37, I-50121 Firenze, Italy*

H. Giamarellou, *Professor of Internal Medicine, Infectious Diseases Specialist, Fourth Department of Internal Medicine, Sismanoglion General Hospital, 15126 Maroussi, Attikis, Athens, Greece*

A. Giannetti, *Department of Dermatology, University of Modena, 71 Del Pozzo str. 41100, Modena, Italy*

B. Giannotti, *Dipartimento di Scienze Derm, Universita degli studi di Firenze, Via Degli Alfani 37, I-50121 Firenze, Italy*

A. Giménez-Arnau, *Department of Dermatology, Hospital del Mar. IMIM, Universitdad Autonoma de Barcelona, Passeig Maritim 25-29, 08003 Barcelona, Spain*

H. Gollnick, *Department of Dermatology and Venereology, Otto-von-Guericke-University, Leipziger Str. 44, D-39120 Magdeburg, Germany*

C. Gooptu, *ICRF Cancer Medicine Research Unit, St. James' University Hospital, Beckett Street, Leeds, LS9 7TF, U.K.*

A. Górkiewicz-Petkow, *Department of Dermatology, Warsaw School of Medicine, Koszykowa 82A, 02-008 Warsaw, Poland*

C.E.M. Griffiths, *Section of Dermatology, University of Manchester, "Hope Hospital", Manchester, M6 8HD, U.K.*

E.M. Grosshans, *Head of the Dermatological Clinic, Faculté de Médecine, 1, Place de l'hôpital, F-67091 Strasbourg Cedex, France*

M. Ali Gurer, *Department of Dermatology, 11 kat, Gazi University School of Medicine, 06510 Besevler, Ankara, Turkey*

J.P. Hachem, *Akademisch Ziekenhuis Vrije Universiteit Brussel, Department of Dermatology, 101, Laarbeeklaan, B-1090 Brussels, Belgium*

E. Haneke, *Professor of Dermatology, Inst. Dermatol Klinikk Bunæs, Løkkeåsveien 3, 1337 Sandvika, Norway*

R. Happle, *Department of Dermatology, Philipp University of Marburg, Deutschhausstraße 9, D-35033 Marburg, Germany*

K.E. Harman, *St. John's Institute of Dermatology, Basement, Block 7, St Thomas' Hospital, Lambeth Palace Road, London, SE1 7EH, U.K.*

U.-F. Haustein, *Department of Dermatology, University of Leipzig, Stephanstraße 11, 04103 Leipzig, Germany*

G. Hautmann, *Specialist in Dermatology and Venereology, Dipartimento di Scienze Derm, Universita degli studi di Firenze, Via Degli Alfani 37, I-50121 Firenze, Italy*

J.L.M. Hawk, *Department of Environmental Dermatology, Guy's, King's and Thomas' School of Medicine, St John's Institute of Dermatology, St Thomas' Hospital, Lambeth Palace Road, London, SE1 7EH, U.K.*

R.J. Hay, *Faculty of Medicine and Health Sciences, Queen's University Belfast, Whitla Medical Building, 97 Lisburn Road, Belfast, BT9 7BL, U.K.*

J. Hercogova, *Department of Dermatology and Venereology, Charles University 2nd Medical School, Motol University Hospital, V úvalu 84, 150 06 Prague 5, Czech Republic*

C. Herrero, *Servei de Dermatologia, Hospital Clinic, Facultat de Medicina, Universidad de Barcelona, c/ Villarroel 17017, E-08036 Barcelona, Spain*

R. Husak, *Klinik und Poliklinik fur Dermatologie, Universitatsklinikum Benjamin Franklin der FU Berlin, Fabeckstr. 60-62, 14195 Berlin, Germany*

D. Ioannides, *Assistant Professor of Dermatology, Department of Dermatology and Venereology, Aristotle University Medical School, 3 PP Germanou Street, 54622 Salonika, Greece*

S. Jablonska, *Department of Dermatology, Warsaw School of Medicine, Koszykowa 82A, 02-008 Warsaw, Poland*

M. Jeanmougin, *Policlinique de Dermatology, Hospital St Louis, 1 Avenue Claude Vellefaux, 75475 Paris, Cedex 10, France*

D. Kalogeromitros, *Department of Dermatology, University of Athens, "A Sygros Hospital", 5, I Dragoumi St, Kesariani 16121, Athens, Greece*

L. Kanerva, *Finnish Institute of Occupational Health, Topeliuksenkatu 41 aA, FIN-00250 Helsinki, Finland*

S. Karl, *Dermatologist and Allergologist Marktplatz 7B, D-85375 Neufahrn, Germany*

A.C. Katoulis, *Department of Dermatology and Venereology, University of Athens, "A Sygros Hospital", 5, I Dragoumi St, Kesariani 16121, Athens, Greece*

A.D. Katsambas, *University of Athens, 'A. Sygros' Hospital, Department of Dermatology, 5, I. Dragoumi Street, 16121 Athens, Greece*

J.C. Katsantonis, *Department of Dermatology, Faculty of Medicine, University of Crete, Heraklion 71110, Crete, Greece*

A. Katsarou, *Department of Dermatology, University of Athens, "A Sygros Hospital", 5, I Dragoumi St, Kesariani 16121, Athens, Greece*

A. Kobza Black, *St John's Institute of Dermatology, Lambeth Palace Road, London, SE1 7EH, U.K.*

E. Koumantaki-Mathioudaki, *Department of Dermatology and Venereology, University of Athens, "A Sygros Hospital", 5, I Dragoumi St, Kesariani 16121, Athens, Greece*

S. Kroon, *Department of Dermatology and Venereology, Helse Stavanger, SiR, University of Bergen, Pb 8100, 4068 Stavanger, Norway*

J.M. Labareda, *Centro de Dermatologia Medico-Cirurgica, ARS de Lisboa e Vale do Tejo, l, Rua Jose Estevao 135, 1150 Lisboa, Portugal*

G. Laskaris, *Head, Oral Medicine Clinic, Department of Dermatology, University of Athens, "A Sygros Hospital", 5, I Dragoumi St, Kesariani 16121, Athens, Greece*

A.I. Lauerma, *Skin and Allergy Hospital Helsinki, University Central Hospital, Meilahdentie 2, 00250 Helsinki, Finland*

F. Lawlor, *Newham Dermatology Unit, St Andrew's Hospital, London, E3 3NT, U.K., and St John's Institute of Dermatology, St Thomas' Hospital, London, SE17 EH, U.K.*

M. Lecha, *Servei de Dermatologia, Hospital Clinic, Facultat de Medicina, Universidad de Barcelona, c/ Villarroel 17017, E-08036 Barcelona, Spain*

M. le Maître, *1 Avenue de 6 Juin, F-14000 Caen, France*

G. Leigheb, *Dermatology Clinic, Via Pansa 4, I-28100 Novara, Italy*

L. Leite, *Calcada da Ajuda 82-1, Lisboa, Portugal*

C. Ligeron, *Service de Dermatologie, Centre Hospitalier Caremeau, 30900 Nimes, France*

T.M. Lotti, *Dipartimento di Scienze Dermatologiche, Universita degli Studi di Firenze, Via Degli Alfani 37, I-50121 Firenze, Italy*

M.N. Manoussakis, *Department of Pathophysiology, School of Medicine, National University of Athens, 75 Mikras Asias St, 11527 Athens, Greece*

L. Marini, *SDC Studio Dermo Chirurgico, Via Pio Riego Gambini 35, 34138 Trieste, Italy*

J.M. Mascaró, *Departmento de Dermatologia, Hospital Clinico, Universidad de Barcelona, Casanova, 143, 08036, Barcelona, Spain*

J.M. Mascaró Jr, *Departmento de Dermatologia, Hospital Clinico, Universidad de Barcelona, Casanova, 143, 08036, Barcelona, Spain*

A. Mastrolorenzo, *Dipartimento di Scienze Derm, Universita degli studi di Firenze, Via Degli Alfani 37, I-50121 Firenze, Italy*

L.M. Medenica, *Department of Dermatology and Venereology Clinical Centre of Serbia, School of Medicine, University of Belgrade, 2 Pasterova St, 11000 Belgrade, Yugoslavia*

G. Menchini, *Istituto di Scienze Dermatologiche, Univ. Degli Studi – Policlinico Le Scotte, Viale Bracci, 53100 Siena, Italy*

L. Meunier, *Centrum Gruene Gentechnik, Staatliche Lehr- und Forschungsanstalt, Breitenweg 71, 67435, Neustadt an der Weinstrasse, Germany*

J. Meynadier, *Service de Dermatologie, Hopital st. Eloi, 2 Avenue Berlin Sans, F-34295 Montpellier Cedex 5, France*

M.V. Milinković, *Department of Dermatology and Venereology, Clinical Centre of Serbia, School of Medicine, University of Belgrade, 2 Pasterova St, 11000 Belgrade, Yugoslavia, and Harvard Skin Disease Research Center, Brigham and Women's Hospital, Department of Dermatology, Harvard Institutes of Medicine, 77 Avenue Louis Pasteur, Boston, MA 02115, USA*

A. Minas, *Department of Dermatology, Aristotle University Medical School, 124 Delphon Street, 54643 Salonika, Greece*

G. Monfrecola, *Department of Patologia Sistemica Section of Dermatology, Università di Napoli 'Federico II', Via S. Pansini 5, 80131 Napoli, Italy*

M. Monti, *Istituto Clinico Humanitas, Unit of Dermatology, University of Milan, Via Manzani 56, I-20089 Rozzano, Milan, Italy*

S. Motta, *Istituto Clinico Humanitas, Unit of Dermatology, University of Milan, Via Manzani 56, I-20089 Rozzano, Milan, Italy*

H.M. Moutsopoulos, *Department of Pathophysiology, School of Medicine, National University of Athens, 75 Mikras Asias St, 11527 Athens, Greece*

G.M. Murphy, *National Photobiology Unit, Beaumont Hospital, Dublin 9, Ireland*

G. Muscarella, *Department of Dermatological Science, University of Florence, Via degli Alfani 37, 50121 Florence, Italy*

M.D. Njoo, *Department of Dermatology, Academic Medical Centre, University of Amsterdam, PO Box 22700, Meibergdreef 9, 1100 DE Amsterdam, The Netherlands*

M. Onder, *Department of Dermatology, Gazi University School of Medicine, 06510 Besevler, Ankara, Turkey*

A.P. Oranje, *Department of Dermatology, University Hospital Rotterdam – Dijkzigt/Sophia, Molewaterplein 60, 3015 GJ Rotterdam, The Netherlands*

C.E. Orfanos, *Klinik und Poliklinik fur Dermatologie, Universitatsklinikum Benjamin Franklin der FU Berlin, Fabeckstr. 60-62, 14195 Berlin, Germany*

J.-P. Ortonne, *Department of Dermatology, University of Nice, Hopital de l'Archet 2, 151, route St-Antoine de Ginestiere, F-06202 Nice, Cedex 3, France*

D. Ozalla, *Servei de Dermatologia, Hospital Clinic, Facultat de Medicina, Universidad de Barcelona, c/ Villarroel 17017, E-08036 Barcelona, Spain*

J.L. Pace, *59 Marquis Scicluna St, Naxxar NXR 03, Malta*

E. Panconesi, *Specialist in Dermatology and Venereology, Dipartimento di Dermatologia, Universita degli studi di Firenze, Via Degli Alfani 37, I-50121 Firenze, Italy*

M. Paradisi, *"San Gallicano" Institute, Rome, Italy*

S. Petraglia, *Catholic University, Dept of Dermatology, L.go A. Gemelli 8, 00168 Rome, Italy*

A. Picoto, *Centro de Dermatologia Medico-Cirurgica, ARS de Lisboa e Vale do Tejo, l, Rua Jose Estevao 135, 1150 Lisboa, Portugal*

G.E. Piérard, *Department of Dermatopathology, CHV Sart Tilman, B-4000 Liège, Belgium*

C. Piérard-Franchimont, *Department of Dermatopathology, CHV Sart Tilman, B-4000 Liège, Belgium*

B.M. Piraccini, *Department of Dermatology, University of Bologna, Via Massarenti 1, 40138 Bologna, Italy*

G. Posteraro, *Department of Patologia Sistemica Section of Dermatology, Università di Napoli 'Federico II', Via Pansini 5, 80131 Napoli, Italy*

F.C. Powell, *Regional Centre of Dermatology, Mater Miseraecordia Hospital, Eccles Street, Dublin-7, Ireland*

E.M. Procaccini, *Department of Dermatology, Universita "Federico II" de Napoli, Via S. Pansini 5, 80131 Napoli, Italy*

A.A. Ramelet, *2 Place Benjamin-Constant, CH-1003 Lausanne, Switzerland*

L. Rauch, *Department of Dermatology-Hautklinik, Moorenstrasse 5, 40225 Düsseldorf, Germany*

A. Rebora, *Department of Dermatology, University of Genoa, Genoa, Italy*

J. Revuz, *Service de Dermatologie, Henri Mondor Hospital, 51, Ave du Marechal de Lattre de Tassigny, F-94010 Creteil Cedex, France*

D. Rigopoulos, *Department of Dermatology, University of Athens, "A Sygros Hospital", 5, I Dragoumi St, Kesariani 16121, Athens, Greece*

J. Ring, *Department of Dermatology and Allergy Biederstein, Technical University Munich, Biedersteinerstraße 29, D-80802 Munich, Germany*

D. Roseeuw, *Akademisch Ziekenhuis Vrije Universiteit Brussel, Department of Dermatology, 101, Laarbeeklaan, B-1090 Brussels, Belgium*

E. Ruocco, *Department of Dermatology, School of Medicine and Surgery, Second University of Naples, Via S. Pansini 5, 80131 Napoli, Italy*

V. Ruocco, *Head, Department of Dermatology, School of Medicine & Surgery, Second University of Naples, Via S. Pansini 5, 80131 Napoli, Italy*

L. Rusciani, *Department of Dermatology, Catholic University of Sacred Heart, Largo A. Gemelli 8, 00168 Rome, Italy*

T. Ruzicka, *Department of Dermatology-Hautklinik, Moorenstraße 5, 40225 Düsseldorf, Germany*

P. Santoianni, *Department of Dermatology, Universita "Federico II" de Napoli, Via S. Pansini 5, 80131 Napoli, Italy*

J.H. Saurat, *Clinique & Policlinique de Dermatologie, Hôpital Universitaire, CH-1211 Geneva 14, Switzerland*

M. Souli, *Fourth Department of Internal Medicine, Athens University School of Medicine, Sismanoglio General Hospital, 1 Sismanogliou Str., 15126 Maroussi, Attikis, Athens, Greece*

H. Starz, *Department of Dermatology and Allergology, Klinikum Augsburg, Stenglinstraße 2, D-86156 Augsburg, Germany*

N.G. Stavrianeas, *Department of Dermatology, University of Athens, "A Sygros Hospital", 5, I Dragoumi St, Kesariani 16121, Athens, Greece*

P.G. Stavropoulos, *Second Department of Dermatology, University of Athens, "A Sygros Hospital", 5, I Dragoumi St, Kesariani 16121, Athens, Greece*

M.P. Stefanidou, *Department of Dermatology, Heraklion University General Hospital, Heraklion, Crete, Greece*

L. Stransky, *Unit of Contact Dermatitis and Occupational Diseases of the Skin, Medical University, Alexander's Medical University Hospital, 1, Saint g. Sofiski St, Sofia BG-1431, Bulgaria*

A.J. Stratigos, *Department of Dermatology, University of Athens, "A Sygros Hospital", 5, I Dragoumi St, Kesariani 16121, Athens, Greece*

J.D. Stratigos, *Department of Dermatology, University of Athens, "A Sygros Hospital", 5, I Dragoumi St, Kesariani 16121, Athens, Greece*

R. Themido, *Centro de Dermatologia Medico-Cirurgica, ARS de Lisboa e Vale do Tejo, l, Rua Jose Estevao 135, 1150 Lisboa, Portugal*

K. Thestrup-Pedersen, *University of Aarhus, Department of Dermatology, Marselisborg Hospital, DK-8000 Aarhus C, Denmark*

A.D. Tosca, *Department of Dermatology, Heraklion University General Hospital of Crete, Heraklion, 71110 Crete, Greece*

A. Tosti, *Department of Dermatology, University of Bologna, Via Massarenti 1, 40138 Bologna, Italy*

N. Tsankov, *Department of Dermatology, Alexander's Medical University Hospital, 1, Saint g. Sofiski St, Sofia BG-1431, Bulgaria*

E. Tsoureli-Nikita, *Istituto di Scienze Dermatologiche, Univ. Degli Studi – Policlinico Le Scotte, Viale Bracci, 53100 Siena, Italy*

A.G. Tzioufas, *Department of Pathophysiology, School of Medicine, National University of Athens, 75 Mikras Asias St, 11527 Athens, Greece*

E.J.M. Van Leent, *Department of Dermatology, Academic Medical Centre, University of Amsterdam, PO Box 22700, Meibergdreef 9, 1100 DE Amsterdam, The Netherlands*

W.A. van Vloten, *Department of Dermatology, University Medical Centre Utrecht, PO Box 85500, 3508 GA Utrecht, The Netherlands*

A.E. Vareltzidis, *Department of Dermatology, University of Athens, "A Sygros Hospital", 5, I Dragoumi St, Kesariani 16121, Athens, Greece*

C. Varotti, *Department of Dermatology, University of Bologna, Via Massarenti 1, 40138 Bologna, Italy*

S. Veraldi, *Institute of Dermatological Sciences, IRCCS, University of Milan, Via Pace 9, I-20122 Milan, Italy*

P.G. Vlachoyiannopoulos, *Department of Pathophysiology, School of Medicine, National University of Athens, 75 Mikras Asias St, 11527 Athens, Greece*

H.-J. Vogt, *Department of Dermatology and Allergy Biederstein, Technical University Munich, Biedersteinerstraße 29, D-80802 Munich, Germany*

N.P.J. Walker, *Department of Dermatology, Churchill Hospital, Old Road, Headington, Oxford, OX3 7LJ, U.K.*

M.A. Waugh, *Genito Urinary Medicine Department, The General Infirmary at Leeds, Great George St, Leeds, LS1 3EX, U.K.*

W. Westerhof, *Netherlands Institute for Pigmentary Disorders/AMC IWO gebouw, Meibergdreef 35, 1105 AZ Amsterdam, The Netherlands*

F. Wojnarowska, *Department of Dermatology, Churchill Hospital, Old Road, Headington, Oxford, OX3 7LJ, U.K.*

Ch.C. Zouboulis, *Klinik und Poliklinik für Dermatologie, Universitätsklinikum Benjamin Franklin der FU Berlin, Fabeckstr. 60-62, 14195 Berlin, Germany*

Preface

This handbook presents the combined work of many prominent dermatologists from throughout Europe, based on their profound knowledge and clinical experience in various fields of dermatology. The purpose of this manual is to provide an easy to use guide that describes not only the many dermatological diseases diagnosed today, but also the analogous drugs and methods of treatment available. Hence, as indicated in the title, dermatologists and non-dermatologists will find its contents to be most useful and concise.

The manual is divided into three main sections: Diseases, Methods, and Drugs. The first part of the handbook defines each disease with brief information on its etiology and pathophysiology. This is followed by a short account of diagnostic procedures and an extensive discussion of treatment and therapy. The authors have not only presented classic and modern approaches to treatment, but also provided their personal recommendations on the bases of their expertise. The middle section describes up-to-date methods and the possible use of therapeutic equipment for diagnosis and treatment. The final section provides an alternative approach, indicating where medication and drugs could be an appropriate choice in the treatment of dermatological diseases.

This second edition of the *European Handbook of Dermatological Treatments* has been minimally revised and retains the exact form of the previous publication.

The response received from the initial publication was enthusiastic and the book was widely accepted. It has been a great pleasure to provide this handbook to fellow colleagues and new dermatologists in the continuing endeavour to treat dermatological and cutaneous diseases.

We wish to express our gratitude to all the distinguished colleagues who contributed towards this venture.

Andreas Katsambas, Torello Lotti
2003

Diseases

Acne

W.J. Cunliffe

Definition and epidemiology

Acne vulgaris is the most common disease involving the pilosebaceous unit. It is rarely misdiagnosed. It occurs at the site where there are sebaceous follicles and thus occurs predominantly on the face, back and chest. It occurs in all races and affects both sexes. The onset of acne is usually in early adolescence and affects up to 80% of all individuals. The milder physiological acne, which affects many adolescents, will last for 4 or 5 years, but the more clinical varieties will last for 12, and sometimes even 40 or 50 years.

Aetiology and pathophysiology

There are four major features involved in the production of acne:

- increased sebum production
- ductal hypercornification
- colonization of the duct with *Propionibacterium acnes*
- inflammation.

The increased grease production (seborrhoea) is due in most patients to an end-organ hyperresponse of the pilosebaceous unit to normal level of hormones. Comedogenesis is a very complex issue involving androgen and cytokine control of the ductal keratinocytes. Certain components of sebum are also comedogenic. Contrary to the bulk of published literature, most patients are not hormonal misfits.

There is no correlation between absolute numbers of *P. acnes* on the surface of the skin and acne severity but colonization of the duct with *P. acnes* is probably related to inflammation in many instances. Eventually, as the inflammation extends, duct rupture will occur and if the inflammation is extensive enough, this may result in the development of scars.

Clinical characteristics

The features of acne include seborrhoea, non-inflamed lesions (microcomedones, whiteheads, blackheads, macrocomedones), inflamed lesions (papules, superficial pustules), deep inflammatory lesions (nodules, deep pustules) predominantly on the face, back and chest. If the inflammation is severe enough scarring will follow. Scarring is associated with loss of tissue such as ice-pick scars and atrophic macular scars, or excessive collagen formation resulting in hypertrophic or keloid scars.

Sunshine tends to improve acne, but there is often a flare premenstrually and excessive sweating can also aggravate acne. Food does not influence the disease process. Times of stress will aggravate acne, probably due more to a patient interfering with the spots. However, acne can be associated with a marked impairment of the psychological and social well-being of the patient, and sometimes these effects are disproportionate to the physical appearance or the severity of the disease.

Diagnosis (laboratory investigations)

Acne is rarely misdiagnosed and usually does not require investigations such as a skin biopsy. However, in difficult patients swabbing the skin for *P. acnes*, in order to look for antibiotic resistance, can be useful.

Differential diagnosis

- Gram-negative folliculitis: rapid onset of many pustules, particularly around the nose and mouth.
- Rosacea: telangiectasia and absence of comedones.
- Drug-induced acne: monomorphic eruption.

- Acné excorié: papular lesions exacerbated by picking at lesions.

Treatment

General therapeutic guidelines

Treatment procedures involve patient discussion, acne assessment and appropriate prescribing based on the history, acne severity, lesion type and the psychological effects of the disease.

The cause of the acne should be discussed as should the goals and outcome of therapy.

- Patient leaflets are essential.
- The patient should be told that in mild cases the acne will last for 4–6 years but in severe cases the natural history could be in excess of 12 years.
- The patient should be informed that if the acne does not respond well to a reasonable trial of oral antibiotics, and appropriate topical therapy, then oral isotretinoin will usually be prescribed. With non-oral isotretinoin therapies, there is little improvement after 1 month of therapy; at 2 months there should be a 20% improvement, rising to 60% at 6 months and 80% at 8 months.

Choice of therapy

Patients with mild acne usually receive topical therapy; patients with moderate acne receive oral and topical therapies; patients with severe acne ideally should receive oral isotretinoin. The severity assessment should include not just the extent of the inflammatory and comedonal lesions but also the presence of scarring, the psychological effects of the disease and the lack of success with previous treatment.

Recommended therapies

Physical treatment

These are not often required and therefore can easily be forgotten and include the following.

- Use of a comedo extractor to remove the large blackheads.
- Gentle cautery, under the eutectic mixture of local anaesthetics (EMLA) to treat macrocomedones.
- Aspiration of larger 'cysts'/nodules. Treat with triamcinolone (this applies to cysts or nodules of less than 14 days duration).
- Cryotherapy to 'cysts'/nodules of greater than 14 days duration. Two 20-s freeze–thaw cycles may be required.
- α-hydroxy acids are used more in southern than northern Europe. Clinical trials are needed to help assess the benefit of this therapy.

Topical treatment

The most widely used topical therapies are benzoyl peroxide, antibiotics, azelaic acid, and retinoids as monotherapy or in combination; benozyl peroxide is available in concentrations of 2.5, 5 and 10% either alone or with a combination of sulphur, imidazole, hydroxyquinolone, glycolic acid or zinc lactate. Topical antibiotics include tetracycline, erythromycin and clindamycin. They are used in concentrations of 1–4% usually in a cream or lotion base. Combination antibiotics include erythromycin with zinc or with benzoyl peroxide. Azelaic acid is also useful in inflammatory acne. Topical tetracycline is probably the least effective topical antibiotic and combination of antibiotics with zinc or benzoyl peroxide are marginally better than single therapies.

Patients with predominantly non-inflamed lesions require topical retinoids or azelaic acid. Retinoic acid (vitamin A acid) is available in 0.01–0.05% concentrations as either a gel or a cream. A second-generation retinoid, 0.05% topical isotretinoin, is similar in efficacy to benzoyl peroxide and topical tretinoin. A third-generation retinoid, adapalene, has a greater benefit/risk ratio than tretinoin and is the only retinoid which has a significant anti-inflammatory action. More recently, in the States, tazorotene gel (0.05% or 0.1%), a new retinoid, is available. Topical therapy should be prescribed alone for mild acne, in conjunction with appropriate oral acne therapy for moderate acne and as a maintenance therapy after oral therapy has stopped. It is also important to stress to the patient that topical therapy must, if appropriate, be applied to the trunk and to the whole of the site prone to acne. Most patients should receive a topical retinoid since the microcomedone is the precursor of most acne lesions. Since most retinoids can be used daily, then an antimicrobial can be prescribed at the other end of the day in most patients with papulopustular acne.

There is an alarming increase in resistance of *P. acnes* to antibiotics. In 2001, 67% of patients sent to a special acne clinics in Leeds, UK, had antibiotic-resistant *P. acnes*. Most frequently, resistance is to erythromycin and clindamycin; less often, resistance to tetracycline and doxycycline is exhibited. Multiple resistance is seen in 18% of patients. Resistance to minocycline is rare (<2%). It is likely that of all topical therapies, topical benzoyl peroxide and a combination of erythromycin and benzoyl peroxide are associated with the least resistance. Physicians should also avoid prescribing dissimilar oral and topical antibiotics. With benzoyl peroxide alone, *P. acnes* exhibits less resistance. Azelaic acid and topical retinoids are not antibiotics and therefore not associated with resistance.

Potent steroids such as clobestal propionate (Dermovate), applied twice daily for 5 days, can dramatically reduce the inflammation of a severely inflamed nodule.

Our conclusion is that topical therapies alone or in combination should be used on their own in patients with mild acne. Retinoids are the choice for treatment of most acne patients. In appropriate cases a topical retinoid can be used in the evening and an anti-microbial agent in the morning. Topical therapies should also be used in conjunction with oral antibiotics in patients with moderate and severe acne and as a maintenance treatment after cessation of oral therapy.

Side-effects of topical agents

Many topical preparations produce a mild primary irritant dermatitis and the patient must be warned, so that treatment is not stopped prematurely. If a primary irritant reaction occurs, then the product should not be used for a few days and the dermatitis treated with moisturisers or a weak steroid cream for a few days. Thereafter the acne preparation can be restarted at a reduced frequency of application. Significant systemic absorption of topical retinoids does not occur. Nevertheless, it is prudent to stop retinoid therapy should a female patient become pregnant.

Oral therapy

Antibiotics

Worldwide antibiotics are the most widely prescribed oral therapy. Tetracyclines (tetracycline, oxytetracycline, doxycycline, lymecycline and minocycline) are the antibiotics of choice but erythromycin is preferable in the female who is or might become pregnant or is breastfeeding. Trimethoprim (400–600 mg/day) which is similar in efficacy to tetracycline can be reserved as a third-line antibiotic.

Not all patients respond in the same way; it is clear that young males with marked seborrhoea and truncal acne respond less well than females with facial acne. Patients who require antibiotics should initially be given 1 g/day of tetracycline. The major disadvantage of tetracycline is the need to take the tablet with water (not milk) half an hour before food: otherwise there is reduced absorption. Thus, with the more expensive lymecycline (408 mg/day), minocycline

(100 mg/day) or doxycycline (100 mg/day), which are better absorbed, there is enhanced patient compliance.

Oral therapy should be given for a minimum of 6 months in combination with topical therapy. If after 3 months there is no improvement, then alternative therapy is necessary. In non-responding patients, minocycline (100 mg) is better than tetracycline. Retrospective studies have shown that 200 mg of minocycline is better than the average dose of 100 mg in patients not responding to this dose. Doxycycline and minocycline are equally effective, provided *P. acnes* are not resistant to doxycycline.

Oral therapy is required in the following group of patients: those with moderate and moderate/severe acne, patients who are significantly depressed, even if the acne is mild, and dysmorphophobic patients, patients with scarring; those with postinflammatory pigmentation also should receive oral therapy sooner than later. Patients with acne fulminans and those with Gram-negative folliculitis may also benefit from oral antibiotics. However, in the latter two groups, oral isotretinoin is preferred. If isotretinoin is not available trimethoprim is the preferred antibiotic for Gram-negative folliculitis.

Side-effects of oral antibiotics

Oral tetracycline and erythromycin are both very safe. Gastrointestinal effects, especially colic and diarrhoea may occur in 5% of patients, but are easily controlled with a combination of diphenoxylate hydrochloride and atropine sulphate (Lomotil). Vaginal candidiasis occurs in 6% of women but is rarely a problem; it is important to treat the patient and her partner with appropriate anticandida therapy.

Uncommon complications of oral therapy include:

- onycholysis (with doxycycline)
- oesophagitis with ulceration (with doxycycline)
- fixed drug eruptions
- photosensitivity, including porphyria-like cutaneous changes, especially with the longer-acting tetracyclines
- a phototoxic rash in 3% of patients (doxycycline)
- widespread drug eruptions are rare except with trimethoprim where the incidence is 5%.

Tetracyclines, especially minocycline, may produce benign intracranial hypertension which presents with headache, loss of concentration and sometimes papilloedema, and quickly disappears on stopping therapy. This side-effect is dose-dependent and the patient should be warned of this potential problem.

Minocycline produces a blue–black pigmentation in the skin that is dose-dependent and presents in four ways:

- in inflamed acne lesions
- in scars (acne and non-acne)
- more rarely as a generalized dark-grey discoloration
- in the sclera, nails and oral mucosa.

Recent reports of serious systemic minocycline-induced side-effects have prompted much debate. Serious side-effects are very rare and include hypersensitivity syndrome reactions (including pulmonary eosinophilia) and serum sickness-like reactions occur characterized by fever, malaise, arthralgia ± major organ involvement, polyarthritis of the small joints and hepatitis. In such patients serology for systemic lupus erythematosus (SLE) may be positive; thus minocycline should be avoided in patients with a personal or family history of SLE.

Blood tests for liver function, ANA and pANCA are recommended 6 monthly in patients on minocycline.

Hormones

Various hormonal regimes exist for reducing sebaceous production. These regimes are indicated usually where standard antibiotic regimes have failed, and where concomitant menorrhoea control, contraception and acne therapy are required. Topical therapy should be prescribed alongside hormonal regimes. Hormonal regimes include prednisolone plus oestrogen, antiandrogens and spironolactone.

Antiandrogens are a logical approach to the treatment of acne as they suppress sebum production to an extent, depending on the drug and dose prescribed. An oral contraceptive (Dianette), which is a combination of 2 mg cyproterone acetate (CPA) and 35 μg ethinyl oestradiol, ameliorates acne. In women, the side-effects of CPA with oestrogen are no different from those of conventional contraceptive pills, apart from a possible slight risk of weight gain.

Dianette should be stopped once the disease is under control but recurrence is common and so the question of it being represcribed should be carefully discussed with the GP. The risk of DVT needs to be shared with the patient. Since Dianette reduces sebum production only by about 30%, it is likely that it acts by an additional mechanism, such as direct effect on comedogenesis, which is also androgen-mediated. In resistant disease the clinical benefit of Dianette can be enhanced by giving 50 or 100 mg CPA from the fifth to 14th day of the cycle. At this dosage, the reduction in sebum suppression is 67%. Spironolactone is an effective treatment for females over 30 years of age. Its effects are dose-dependent and is usually prescribed at a dose of 100–200 mg for 6 months. The main side-effects are menstrual irregularity, occasional fluid retention and, rarely, melasma.

Isotretinoin and steroids

Oral isotretinoin (Roaccutane) revolutionized the treatment of acne when it was introduced.

Which patients should receive isotretinoin?

Ideally any patient with severe disease should immediately be considered for isotretinoin. There are convincing data which indicate that isotretinoin should also be prescribed for patients with moderate acne who are failing to respond to conventional therapy, for whatever the reason. I recommend such therapy after three courses of conventional therapy have been tried.

Age should not be a barrier to the prescribing of isotretinoin, irrespective of the acne severity. Oral isotretinoin should be prescribed for paediatric acne patients if there are sufficient clinical indications.

Most patients with significant systemic disease can be treated with oral isotretinoin but it is prudent to start with very small doses and link with the appropriate physician.

Isotretinoin in the treatment of acne variants

These diseases are very rare and represent a small but essential indication for oral isotretinoin. This group includes patients with:

- acne fulminans
- rosacea fulminans
- Gram-negative folliculitis
- acne conglobata.

While patients with acne fulminans and rosacea fulminans respond to oral isotretinoin, the best response is obtained by starting treatment with a course of prednisone, 0.5–1.0 mg/kg for 4–6 weeks. Usually the steroids can be reduced gradually over the following 2 weeks and isotretinoin can be introduced at a dosage of 0.5 mg/kg. This can be increased gradually to 1 mg/kg per day according to the response.

Patients with acne conglobata and Gram-negative folliculitis usually do not require oral steroids and can be started immediately on oral isotretinoin at a dose of 0.5–1 mg/kg per day.

Recommended doses and duration of isotretinoin therapy

Most patients receive a dose within the range of 0.5–1 mg/kg per day. There are variations in the way treatment is started. Most physicians usually begin at 0.5 mg/kg per day and increase to 1.0 mg/kg per day, but in some centres patients are begun at 1.0 mg/kg. Published data indicate that an optimal benefit is achieved at the higher dose. The majority of physicians, whether they start on a higher or lower dose, will adjust the dose according to the response and the presence or absence of side-effects.

Ninety-five per cent of patients who receive a dose of 1.0 mg/kg are virtually clear of their acne by 16 weeks. Thirteen per cent are clear by 5 or 6 months, and 3% require a longer course.

What are the reasons for a slow response?

Analysis of slow responders to isotretinoin shows that the cause is due to the presence of macrocomedones in 70%, nodular acne in 15% and unknown in about 5%, and in 10% the reason is not clear. Rarely there may be a significant hormonal problem such as polycystic ovarian syndrome or late-onset congenital adrenal hyperplasia. It may be necessary to stretch the skin to detect the macrocomedones. These must be located prior to starting isotretinoin therapy and cauterized minimally.

Side-effects of isotretinoin

Isotretinoin is very teratogenic and pregnancy is completely contraindicated during therapy and for 4 weeks post-therapy.

Many side-effects of oral isotretinoin are predictable and do not interfere with the patient's management. They are tolerated by modification of the dose and/or additional symptomatic therapy.

Uncommonly oral isotretinoin will produce mood swings, depression and, in exceptional cases, suicide. This like other side-effects needs to be shared with the patient, family, friends and other relevant physicians.

An acne flare early in the course of isotretinoin occurs in 6% of subjects. In half of these it is clinically important. Risk factors for this flare include the presence of macrocomedones in two-thirds and nodules in almost a third of patients. Should a patient flare badly, then oral prednisolone should be given in a dose of 0.5–1 mg/kg per day over a period of 2–3 weeks and the dose slowly decreased over the next 6 weeks. When the acne flares, the isotretinoin should, depending on the extent of flare, either be stopped or reduced to a dosage of 0.25 mg/kg per day. If stopped, then the drug can be reintroduced slowly at a dose of 0.25 mg/kg per day and then increased or decreased as necessary.

The mucocutaneous side-effects can usually be well controlled by the use of moisturisers and lip salves but occasionally a retinoid dermatitis or a severe retinoid cheilitis occurs, which is often complicated by secondary infection with *Staphylococcus aureus*. If there is impetiginization, then oral antistaphylococcal therapy such as flucloxacillin and/or topical mupirocin 2% ointment may be required. A nasal preparation of mupirocin can be used to eradicate nasal carriage of staphylococci.

Significant systemic effects are uncommon and mainly consist of headaches, which rarely may be an early feature of benign intracranial hypertension and arthralgia. Systemic side-effects are usually well controlled by dose reduction and non-steroidal anti-inflammatories or aspirin.

Laboratory tests probably need not be repeated if after the baseline test and at 6 weeks there is no problem, except in groups at risk, such as diabetics and patients with known familial hypertriglyceridaemia.

Thus, since many excellent treatments are available there is really no justification for patients with acne to scar.

Further reading

Bottomley WW, Cunliffe WJ. Oral trimethoprim as a third-line antibiotic in the management of acne vulgaris. *Dermatology* 1993; 187: 193–6.

Chalker DK, Lesher JL, Smith JG *et al.* Efficacy of topical isotretinoin 0.05% gel in acne vulgaris. Results of a multicenter, double-blind investigation. *J Am Acad Dermatol* 1987; 17: 251–4.

Cunliffe WJ, Clayden AD, Gould D *et al.* Acne vulgaris—its aetiology and treatment. *Rev Clin Exp Dermatol* 1981; 6: 461–9.

Cunliffe WJ, Van der Kerkhof PCM, Caputo R *et al.* Roaccutane treatment guidelines, results of an international survey. *Dermatology* 1994; 351–7.

Eady EA, Jones CE, Tipper, JL, Cove JH, Cunliffe, WJ, Layton AM. Antibiotic resistant propionibacteria in acne: need for policies to modify antibiotic usage. *Br Med J* 1993; 306: 555–6.

Goulden V, Glass D, Cunliffe WJ. Safety of long term high dose minocycline in the treatment of acne. *Br J Dermatol* 1996; 134: 693–5.

Goulden V, Layton AM, Cunliffe WJ. Current indications for isotretinoin as a treatment for acne vulgaris. *Dermatology* 1995; 190: 284–7.

Hammerstein J, Cupceancu B. Behandlung des Hirsutismus mit Cyproteronacetat. *Dtsch Med Wochenschr* 1969; 94: 829–34.

Katsambas A. Why and when the treatment of acne fails. What to do. *Dermatology* 1998; 196: 158–61.

Lyons RE. Comparative effectiveness of benzoyl peroxide and tretinoin in acne vulgaris. *Int J Dermatol* 1978; 17: 246–51.

Ross JI, Carnegie E, Snelling AM *et al.* Prevalence of antibiotic resistant propionibacteria on the skin of acne patients from six European countries. *JEADV* 2001; 15 (Suppl. 2): 135.

Schaefer H. Penetration and percutaneous absorption of topical retinoids. *Rev Skin Pharmacol* 1993; 6: 17–23.

Seukeran DC, Eady AE, Cunliffe WJ. Benefit–risk assessment of acne therapies. *Lancet* 1997; 349: 1251.

Shalita A, Weiss JS, Chalker DK *et al.* A comparison of the efficacy and safety of adapalene gel 0.1% and tretinoin gel 0.025% in the treatment of acne vulgaris: a multicenter trial. *J Am Acad Dermatol* 1996; 34: 482–5.

Strauss JS, Rapini RP, Shalita AR *et al.* Isotretinoin therapy for acne: results of a multicenter dose–response study. *J Am Acad Dermatol* 1984; 10: 490–6.

Actinic keratosis

F.M. Camacho-Martínez

Synonyms

Solar keratosis: a more specific term because 'solar' indicates that the keratosis is produced by rays of the sun, unlike 'actinic' which is non-specific referring to rays of any kind. In several countries, it is also known as 'keratosis senilis'.

Definition and epidemiology

Actinic keratosis (AK) is a circumscribed cutaneous neoplasm presenting chromosomal abnormalities which occurs primarily on sun-exposed skin surfaces in fair-skinned individuals in the form of horny papules. Currently, Ackerman considers that AK is not a premalignant lesion but a real 'malignant neoplasm' from the very beginning. It should be considered a superficial squamous cell carcinoma in the same form, as there are superficial basal cell carcinomas. Some have stated clearly and emphatically their belief that AKs are on continuum and may or may not become malignant. Yantsos proposed a change in nomenclature to refer to AKs as keratinocytic intraepidermal neoplasia (KIN) with three grades of evolution that range from AKs to SCCs.

AK appears on the skin of persons with phototype I to III who have received too much actinic radiation in a short time (acute AK) or throughout their lives (chronic AK) due to professional activity (e.g. sailors, farmers, drivers). It is almost certain that, sooner or later, 100% of these persons will present with AK. Of the remaining people who have been exposed to the sun, it is unpredictable what percentage will develop AK.

AK is most frequent in sunny countries, e.g. Australia, parts of the USA (such as California), southern Europe (e.g. Italy, France, Spain), and so on.

If we agree that AK is a premalignant lesion, the risk of developing squamous cell carcinoma has been estimated to be in the range of 6–10% over 10 years.

Aetiology and pathophysiology

These neoplasms are extremely common on sun-exposed skin of middle-aged and elderly fair-skinned individuals who live in sunny climates. They can be a consequence of prolonged exposure to solar radiation. Occasionally they may also result from exposure to X-radiation and to ultraviolet (UV) light from artificial sources. This latter cause is very important because many people, commonly young women, receive excessive amounts of this radiation, from tanning beds.

The p53 chromosomal mutation, found in over 90% of human cutaneous squamous cell carcinomas, is also found in AK, including renal transplant recipients—this may occur as an early step in transplant-associated skin carcinogenesis. UVB radiation can modify the genetic material of keratinoblasts and fibroblasts, which can modify epidermodermic interrelations and produce a clone of abnormal cells. For some time these may stay in the epidermis but, sooner or later and in unpredictable percentages, they will invade the dermis.

The UVB radiation is directly related to the presence of AK on skin phototypes I to III. The ozone layer in the stratosphere is a natural filter for UVB radiation, but as its thickness decreases it allows more UVB to reach the earth's surface. Depletion of the ozone layer is another aetiological factor contributing to the incidence of AK.

There are other cocarcinogenic factors that must be taken into account. For example, prior therapy with methotrexate might put patients treated with psoralen and UVA (PUVA) at risk of developing skin cancer.

Clinical features and course

A dry and hyperpigmented photoageing skin that exhibits 'dermatoheliosis',—previously named 'chronic actinic degeneration' or 'solar degeneration'—begins to develop multiple 1–2-mm rough lesions. They have irregular edges, are slightly elevated but frequently are easier to visualize. They may be flesh-coloured or rosy, erythematous with telangiectasias or deeply pigmentated. Generally, the hyperkeratotic surface is formed by yellow or brown adherent scales, but when these are pulled up they reveal some slight horny downward proliferation inside the follicular pores. The pull-up manoeuvre of the hyperkeratotic scales produce, in the majority of cases, small painful erosions and minimal haemorrhage. We currently consider three types of AKs in accordance with its quantity of hyperkeratosis: grade 1, easily seen and slightly palpable; grade 2, well developed and easily palpable; and grade 3, hyperkeratotic lesion.

Common locations for the lesion are the skin surfaces exposed to the sun such as the face, mainly forehead, cheeks, nose and ears, back of the hands, forearm and occasionally, shoulders and scalp in men with premature baldness. AK on the head and neck are thin, whereas those on the back of the hands or on the forearms are often thicker.

The normal course of development for AK is for hard horny proliferations known as 'verrucous keratosis' to grow. In these circumstances, it is easier to display the deep invasion. Although there are authors who have communicated that AK commonly undergoes spontaneous regression, there is no proof of this.

Diagnosis

Usually, the diagnosis of AK is possible on the basis of the clinical appearance. Sometimes biopsy may be performed. The cells of the stratum malpighii present a chaotic arrangement. Some of these cells present pleomorphism and anaplasia of their nuclei and others present individual dyskeratosis with formation of corps ronds and grains. As the cytological features of the neoplastic cells of AK are indistinguishable from those of thicker squamous cell carcinomas, this justifies the theory of Ackerman that these two conditions, despite their different names, are really one and the same.

Histology reveals seven possible patterns.

1 Hypertrophic, characterized by pronounced hyperkeratosis intermingled with areas of parakeratosis. The epidermis is thickened in some areas which shows irregular downward proliferation limited to the uppermost dermis.
2 Atrophic, with slight hyperkeratosis and the epidermis on the whole is atrophic. The basal cell layer shows atypical cells with large hyperchromatic nuclei that lie close together and these cells may proliferate into the dermis as buds and duct-like structures.
3 Bowenoid, indistinguishable from that of Bowen's disease or carcinoma *in situ*.
4 Acantholytic or 'Darier type', with intercellular clefts or lacunae as resulting from anaplastic changes in the lowermost epidermis that produce dyskeratotic cells without intercellular bridges. Within suprabasal clefts or lacunae, a few acantholytic cells may be observed. This form of AK has been reviewed by Ackerman as a miniature type of pseudoglandular squamous cell carcinoma and provides evidence to support his theory that AK and squamous cell carcinoma are synonymous.
5 Epidermolytic, with granular degeneration or epidermolytic hyperkeratosis.
6 Lichenoid, with a dense band-like dermal infiltrate close to the epidermis which damage the basal cell layer

producing degenerate basal cells known as hyaline or colloid bodies.
7 Hyperpigmented, with accumulation of the melanin within basal cells and melanophages.

Differential diagnosis

- Solar lentigo: uniformly dark brown, macular, irregular outline.
- Seborrhoeic keratosis: verrucous surface, soft and friable consistency, also located on the trunk.
- Discoid lupus erythematosus: discoid patches with adherent thick scales and follicular plugging. In older lesions, atrophic scarring and hyperkeratosis at the periphery.
- Verrucous naevi: present at birth or appear in early childhood.
- Warty dyskeratoma: elevated papule with a keratotic umbilicated centre, occasionally found on skin not exposed to the sun.
- Keratoacanthoma: firm dome-shapped nodule, 1–2 mm in diameter, centre with a horn-filled crater, involutes spontaneously.
- Basal cell carcinoma: small telangiectatic vessels on its surface, pearly rolled border.

Treatment

General therapeutic guidelines

Irrespective of whether we accept that AK is a squamous cell carcinoma, the AK must be treated and removed using one of several different methods of therapy selected by the dermatologist.

Surgical treatments

Radiosurgery

The original techniques in electrosurgery (electrodesiccation, electrocoagulation) after curettage has been replaced by machines that use radiofrequency waves. This enables AK to be removed easily under anaesthetic.

Cryosurgery

Currently only liquid nitrogen is used to destroy AK. It is an easy method that permits removal of AK without the need for anaesthesia. It is possible to use cryoprobes of different sizes. When the AK has developed fully, it is preferable to first perform curettage and then to use a cryoprobe. When the patient presents with multiple AK, it is better to use a cryospray in a centrifugal or paintbrush pattern.

Dermabrasion

Dermabrasion is a method that is useful for treating multiple AK. Diamond fraises or wire brushes with a range between 800 and 33 000 revolutions per minute are used. It has the inconvenience that the patient must stay in hospital at least 1 week. It is well known that only this technique treats AK successfully and provides long-term prophylaxis.

Laser

Carbon dioxide (CO_2) laser skin resurfacing is being used with increasing frequency in dermatological practice. The ultrapulse CO_2 laser, introduced in 1990, is an excellent and probably the most suitable instrument for removing keratoses; it is relatively easy to use. The results are better and the operative time for full-face resurfacing is markedly reduced when using the new computer pattern generator (CPG), a new computer scanning device, in conjunction with the ultrapulse laser. It is the election treatment when multiple AK does not respond to other medical treatments.

Surgical extirpation

This procedure should be considered only when the AK is a firm horny papule with the possibility of invading deeper. The chosen technique must be governed by the location of the AK but commonly it is sufficient to remove the neoplasm and then perform a direct suture. When the AK is large, it may be useful to use a local flap to close the defect. Exceptionally, a graft will be necessary.

Medical treatments

5-fluorouracil (5-FU)

This is the oldest medical treatment for the removal of AK, especially when the patient has multiple AK. The usual regimen is twice daily application of a 5% cream for 3 weeks, however longer treatment (5–6 weeks) is preferred for a higher cure rate. Nevertheless since too many patients have discomfort with this technique it is not used so often now.

Medium-depth chemical peel

This is an excellent treatment for multiple AK. The medium-depth chemical peel may be achieved both with Jessner's solution and 35% trichloracetic acid. The patient treated with medium-deep chemical peel should be checked annually or every 1.5 years for reappearance of AK and retreated as appropriate. 70% trichloracetic acid instead of radiosurgery for individual AK can be used and then anaesthesia is not necessary.

Oral retinoids

Topical tretinoin alone is only partially effective in the treatment of AK even after 1 year of daily applications. Oral retinoids such as isotretinoin (13-*cis*-retinoic acid) and acitretin have an antitumour effect being useful both as prophylaxis and in therapy. Recently, a combination of low-dose oral isotretinoin and topical 5-FU was found effective in drastically reducing the number of AK and preventing the appearance of new ones.

Interferon-α_{2b}

Based on its antiproliferative and antitumour properties, interferon-α_{2b} has been used on AK and was found to clear 92% of treated lesions when used intralesionally at a dose of 500 000 IU three times per week for 3 weeks.

Photodynamic therapy (PDT) (topical 5-aminolevulinic acid or ALA)

PDT using topical ALA has been demonstrated to be useful in the treatment of various superficial cutaneous malignant neoplasms such as basal cell carcinomas, Bowen disease and AK. The mechanism of action of the ALA, when it is applied topically on the skin is dependent upon the accumulation of the endogenous photosensitizer protoporphyrin IX (PpIX) in epidermal cells of the lesion. Then, the PpIX is activated by the application of red or green light, resulting in a tissue-specific phototoxic effect. A recent study using topical concentrations of ALA (10%, 20% and 30%) vs. vehicle control using visible red light delivered by laser for the photodynamic therapy was performed to evaluate the safety and clinical efficacy in this treatment of AK. The results confirmed for the authors that PDT using topical ALA is an effective treatment of typical AK. Lesions on the face and scalp are more effectively treated than lesions on the trunk and extremities. While the non-hypertrophic AK had an excellent response, the hypertrophic AK did not respond effectively, probably due to an ineffective penetration of ALA and a consecutive insufficient production of PpIX. We currently know that non-hypertrophic AK grade 1 and 2 maximally improve with 30% ALA. The complete response rate of AKs located on the head and neck was significantly higher (93%) in comparison with keratoses on the trunk and extremities (45%), and on forearms and hands (51%) at the dose of 50 J/cm^2. Topical ALA-PDT is non-invasive and leaves patients with excellent cosmetic results, being most efficient to treat widespread AKs. In the most recently published article, Varma *et al.* have applied 5-ALA for 4–6 h on several AK, and after this, each AK was irradiated with 105 J/cm^2 of incoherent red light centred on 640 nm, demonstrating that all AK responded well to PDT, being especially efficacious to treat multiple lesions amounting to a 'field change', and also lesions up to 10 cm in diameter within an acceptable treatment time. Thus far, PDT failed to become established as a routine treatment for small AK not being superior to conventional therapies as cryotherapy, curettage, 5-FU or surgery.

Imiquimod 5% cream

Recently, imiquimod has been added to the therapeutic treatment possibilities. Excellent results have been achieved, but it is necessary to give clear instructions to the patients about its use in order to avoid local reactions such as erosions, induration or ulceration, and subjective systemic adverse side-effects such as headache, fever, nausea, diarrhoea, arthralgia or pain.

Photoprotection

Photoprotection must always be recommended. In the past, the Federal Drug Administration recommended that sunscreens had a sun protection factor (SPF) of 15 to block the erythema response in persons with phototypes I to III. Recent studies have demonstrated that an SPF of no less than 30 is necessary to prevent immunosuppression and therefore sun avoidance is highly recommended. Broad-spectrum sunscreens (SPF 30) should be applied to all exposed skin before sun exposure. Clothes and hats must also be recommended. Currently, three points must be considered to prevent sunburn and its consequences: (a) habits, avoiding sun from 11 a.m. to 4 p.m.; (b) sun protection with clothes, hats and glasses; and (c) sunscreens of high SPF well distributed on the skin. Men exhibit a significantly higher frequency of sunburn because generally they have less knowledge concerning sun safety information and skin cancer, and they employ fewer sun-protective measures than women. To all patients with dermatoheliosis, whether with AK or not, 30 mg of β-carotene in the morning is recommended.

Further reading

Ackerman AB. Respect at last for solar keratosis. *Dermatopathology: Pract Conceptual* 1997; 3: 101–3.

Alvanopoulos K *et al.* Photodynamic therapy of superficial basal cell carcinoma using 5-aminolevulinic acid and 517-nm light. *J Eur Acad Dermatol Venereol* 1997; 9: 134–6.

Beutner KR, Geisse JK, Helman D, Fox TL, Ginkel A, Owens ML. Therapeutic response of basal cell carcinoma to the immune response modifier imiquimod 5% cream. *J Am Acad Dermatol* 1999; 41: 1002–7.

Camacho F. Queratomas actínicos. In: Ledo A, ed. *Avances en Terapéutica Dermatológica.* Madrid: Gaceta Dermatologica Ed, 1988: 259–60.

Camacho F. Precancer epitelial cutáneo-mucoso. In: Armijo M, Camacho F, eds. *Dermatología,* 2nd edn. Madrid: Grupo Aula Médica Ed, 1997: 403–17.

Camacho FM. Chronic radiation dermatitis: what's new in management? Editorial. *J Eur Acad Dermatol Venereol* 2000; 14: 246–7.

Camacho F, Dulanto F. Colgajos locales. In: Camacho F, Dulanto F, eds. *Cirugía Dermatologica.* Madrid: Grupo Ala Médica Ed, 1995: 167–89.

Camacho F, García-Hernández MJ, Pérez-Bernal AM. Modelación cutánea (resurfacing). Concepto y fundamentos. In: Cisneros JL, eds. *Laser y Fuentes de Luz Pulsada Intensa en Dermatología y Dermocosmética.* Madrid: Grupo Aula Médica Ed, 2000: 205–16.

Ceburkov O, Golnick H. Photodynamic therapy in dermatology. *Eur J Dermatol* 2000; 10: 568–76.

Diffey BL. Sun protection with clothing. Editorial comments. *Br J Dermatol* 2001; 144: 449–50.

Edwards L. The interferons. *Dermatol Clin* 2001; 19: 139–46.

Ferrándiz C, Fuente MJ, Fernández-Figueras MT, Bielsa I, Just M. p53 immunohistochemical expression in early posttransplant-associated malignant and premalignant cutaneous lesions. *Dermatol Surg* 1999; 25: 97–101.

Haller JC, Cairnduff F, Slack G *et al.* Routine double treatments of superficial basal cell carcinomas using aminolaevulinic acid-based photodynamic therapy. *Br J Dermatol* 2000; 143: 1270–4.

Kalka K, Merk H, Mukhtar H. Photodynamic therapy in dermatology. *J Am Acad Dermatol* 2000; 42: 389–413.

Persaud AN, Shamuelova E, Sherer D *et al.* Clinical effect of imiquimod 5% cream in the treatment of actinic keratosis. *J Am Acad Dermatol* 2002; 47: 553–6.

Sander CA, Pfeiffer Ch, Kligman AM, Plewig G. Chemotherapy for disseminated actinic keratoses with 5-fluorouracil and isotretinoin. *J Am Acad Dermatol* 1997; 36: 236–8.

Varma S, Wilson H, Kurwa HA *et al.* Bowen's disease, solar keratoses and superficial basal cell carcinomas treated by photodynamic therapy using a large-field incoherent light source. *Br J Dermatol* 2001; 144: 567–74.

Witheiler DD, Lawrence N, Cox SE, Cruz Ch, Cockerell CJ, Freemen RG. Long-term efficacy and safety of Jessner's solution and 35% trichloroacetic acid vs 5% fluorouracil in the treatment of widespread facial actinic keratosis. *Dermatol Surg* 1997; 23: 191–6.

Yantsos V. Continuous spectrum between actinic keratoses and SCC, analogous to CIN (cervical intraepithelial neoplasia). *Semin Cutan Med Surg* 1999; 18: 3–14.

Adamantiades–Behçet's disease

Ch.C. Zouboulis

Synonyms

Behçet's disease, Behçet's syndrome.

Definition and epidemiology

Adamantiades–Behçet's disease is a relapsing multisystemic inflammatory disorder of unknown aetiology, classified as systemic vasculitis and characterized by recurrent oral and genital ulcers, cutaneous lesions and uveitis. It exhibits a worldwide occurrence with varying prevalence, presenting endemically in the eastern Mediterranean and in Middle and Far Eastern countries and is rare among inhabitants of north European countries, in central and southern Africa, in the Americas and in Australia. A prevalence of 80–370 patients per 100 000 inhabitants has been reported in Turkey, 2–30 patients per 100 000 inhabitants in the rest of the Asian continent (Japan 14–30/100 000; Iran 17/100 000; China 14/100 000) and 0.1–2.5 patients per 100 000 inhabitants in Europe and the USA.

The disease usually occurs around the third decade of life, however, early and late onsets (first year of life to 72 years) have been reported. The juvenile disease rates 2–21% in different ethnic groups. In the endemic areas a preponderance of the male gender has previously been observed but currently epidemiological studies have shown that—with the exception of Arabic populations—both genders are equally affected. Familial occurrence has been reported in 1–18% of the patients, mostly of Turkish, Israeli and Korean origin, and is increased in patients with juvenile disease.

Aetiology and pathophysiology

Although the disease had been described as early as in the 5th century BC by Hippocrates, its aetiology remains unknown and its pathogenesis is not fully understood. Linked intrinsic and extrinsic factors are thought to contribute to the development of the disease. The major involvement of certain ethnic groups and the wide variation of the prevalence of the disease in the same ethnic group in association with the geographical area of residence indicate environmental triggering of a genetically determined disorder. The spreading of the endemic areas along the old silk route and associated immunogenetic data support the hypothesis that the disease was carried over through the immigration of old nomadic tribes. Transmission is solely vertical since the disease is not contagious. Genetic factors have been investigated and a significant link of HLA-B51 (relative risk of ≥ 3 except in India and the USA), especially of HLA-B5101 which is one of the three HLA-B51 alleles, to the disease has been well known. However, none of the functional correlates of the disease appear to be restricted by HLA-B51. Recently, the role of the genes encoding tumour necrosis factor (TNF), transporter in antigen processing proteins and MICA (major histocompatibility class I chain related gene A) has been emphasized.

At least four extrinsic pathogenetic candidates have been identified, including autoimmunity or cross-reactivity between microbial and oral mucosal antigens, herpes simplex virus infection affecting the immune responses and certain streptococcal infection (*Streptococcus sanguis*). A common factor linking some of the possible pathogenetic agents is microbial stress or heat shock proteins, which cross-react with host tissues and elicit significant T-cell responses. A possible polarization of T lymphocytes towards the T-helper type 1 (Th1) phenotype has been suggested by recent observations in experimental uveoretinitis and by preliminary data in humans. Neutrophils may also play a role in the pathogenesis of the disease, as they are attracted by macrophage- and endothelial cell-released cytokines and chemokines (especially interleukin-8) at the site of the lesions, and thus contribute to tissue damage and self-maintenance of inflammation. The chronic local inflammation process together with platelet and serum factors lead to enhanced coagulation and thrombosis.

Clinical characteristics and course

The disease runs a characteristic course of exacerbation and remission. Mucosal and skin lesions consist of the onset feature in 70–95% of the patients whereas oral aphthous ulcers are the most common onset lesions worldwide (47–86%). It takes 1 to 8 years to develop the complete clinical picture, and the activity of the disease gradually abates after a few years. Serious morbidity can occur due to blindness (20–40% of the patients) and the sequelae of central nervous system lesions. The disease can occasionally be fatal (0–6%) due to vascular complications (arterial occlusion, arterial aneurysm rupture, pulmonary vasculitis), involvement of the central nervous system and bowel perforation. Male gender, vascular onset of the disease, and HLA-B51 positivity are markers of severe prognosis.

Oral aphthous ulcers (92–100%), genital ulcerations (57–93%), skin lesions (38–99%), ocular lesions (29–100%) and arthropathy (16–84%) are the most frequent clinical features; sterile pustules (28–66%) and erythema nodosum (15–78%) are the most commonly encountered skin lesions. A brief summary of the clinical manifestations is shown in Table 1. The pathergy test (skin hypersensitivity: a papule or pustule formed 48 h after a sterile needle puncture) varies widely (6–71%) in different populations.

Two major clinical forms are recognized: the *mucocutaneous type* of the disease with recurrent aphthous ulcers, genital ulcerations, skin lesions including superficial thrombophlebitis and/or arthropathy and the *systemic type* mainly characterized by the presence of ocular lesions, central nervous system involvement, vascular or gastrointestinal manifestations.

Diagnosis

Diagnosis is still based on clinical signs only, and especially on the classical triad: recurrent aphthous ulcers, genital

Table 1 Clinical findings in Adamantiades–Behçet's disease

Lesions	Prevalence (%)	Characteristics
Oral aphthous ulcers	92–100	Minor, major or herpetiform
Genital ulcerations	57–91	Most common on scrotum, penis and vulva
Skin lesions	38–99	Papules/sterile pustules, erythema nodosum, thrombophlebitis, skin ulcerations
Ocular lesions	29–100	Anterior/posterior uveitis, retinal vasculitis
Arthropathy/arthritis	16–84	Non-deforming, seronegative mono-/polyarthritis
Neurological features	2–44	Benign intracranial hypertension, multiple inflammatory lesions, pyramidal involvement
Vascular involvement	2–37	Arterial aneurysms, venous thrombosis
Gastrointestinal features	1–60	Intestinal ulcerations
Prostatitis–epididymitis (male)	0–28	Sterile inflammation
Chest disease	0–17	Pulmonary vasculitis, arterial aneurysms
Kidney involvement	0–10	Glomerulonephritis
Cardiac disease	0–7	Pericarditis, sterile endocarditis
Ear involvement		Inner ear involvement

Table 2 Classification criteria for Adamantiades–Behçet's disease

After the criteria of the International Study Group for Behçet's disease		
Recurrent oral aphthous ulcers (at least 3 times per year) plus two of:		
Recurrent genital ulcerations		
Ocular lesions (uveitis, iritis, retinitis)		
Skin lesions (erythema nodosum, folliculitis, sterile pustules, aphthous ulcerations)		
Positive pathergy test		
After the criteria of the Behçet's Syndrome Research Committee of Japan		
Complete syndrome: all four major criteria, i.e. recurrent oral aphthous ulcers, skin lesions, ocular lesions, and recurrent genital ulcerations present		
Incomplete syndrome: three of four major criteria or two major and two minor (arthralgia, gastrointestinal involvement, epididymitis, vascular manifestation, CNS manifestation) present		
After the Iranian criteria of the 'Classification and Regression Tree'		
Diagnosis in the presence of one of the following combinations of signs:		
– Recurrent oral aphthous ulcers	+	recurrent genital ulcerations
– Recurrent oral aphthous ulcers	+	hypopyoniritis, uveitis
– Recurrent oral aphthous ulcers	+	positive pathergy test + papules and pustules and/or erythema nodosum and/or superficial thrombophlebitis
– Hypopyoniritis, uveitis	+	positive pathergy test
– Hypopyoniritis, uveitis	+	recurrent genital ulcerations

ulcerations and iritis/uveitis. No diagnostic laboratory examination exists. Efforts for performing accurate diagnosis have led to the proposal of several sets of clinical criteria. Among them three sets of criteria are mostly used (Table 2).

Differential diagnosis

- Oculomucocutaneous syndromes: erythema exudativum multiforme and variants (Stevens–Johnson syndrome, ectodermosis erosiva pluriorificialis Fiessinger–Rendu, dermatostomatitis Baader, mucocutaneous-ocular syndrome Fuchs), Vogt–Koyanagi–Harada syndrome, systemic lupus erythematosus, secondary syphilis.
- Bipolar aphthosis/mucocutaneous syndromes: bipolar acute aphthosis Neumann, viral infections (herpes, coxsackie, echo), pemphigus vulgaris, secondary syphilis.
- Articulomucocutaneous syndromes: Reiter's disease, mouth and genital ulcers with inflamed cartilage (MAGIC) syndrome, *Yersinia* infection, bowel-associated dermatitis–arthritis syndrome (pustular) psoriasis arthropathica.
- Gastrointestinal–mucocutaneous syndromes: colitis ulcerosa, Crohn's disease, pyostomatitis and pyodermatitis vegetans, tuberculosis.
- Aphthous oral ulcers: recurrent oral aphthosis, herpes simplex infection.
- Genital ulcerations: ulcus vulvae acutum Lipschütz, herpes simplex infection, primary syphilis.
- Uveitis: uveitis of other aetiology.
- Arthritis: spondylitis, juvenile rheumatoid arthritis, Bechterew's disease.
- Central nervous system manifestation: multiple sclerosis.
- Chest disease: lung sarcoidosis.

Treatment

General therapeutic guidelines

Because no drug addresses all the features of Adamantiades–Behçet's disease, therapy is adapted to individual clinical manifestations (Tables 3 and 4).

Recommended therapies

Treatment of the mucocutaneous type

In mild forms of the mucocutaneous type disease initial therapeutic measures consist of:

Table 3 Activity spectrum of different regimens on recurrent oral aphthous ulcers

Treatment	Pain amelioration	Decrease of duration	Prevention of appearance of new lesions
Dietary measures	+	–	–
SLS-free mouth hygiene	+	+	–
Topical treatment			
Anaesthetics	+	–	–
Caustic therapy	+	+/–	–
Antiseptics/antiphlogistics	+	+	–
Corticosteroids	+	+	–
5-Aminosalicylic acid	+	+	–
Tetracycline	+	+	–
Systemic treatment			
Colchicine	+	+/–	–
DADPS	+	+/–	–
Corticosteroids	+	+	–
Pentoxifylline	+	+	+/–
Methotrexate	+	+	+/–
Interferon-α	+	+	+
Ciclosporin A	+	+	+
Thalidomide	+	+	+

Table 4 Activity spectrum of different compounds on the manifestations of Adamantiades–Behçet's disease

	Muco-cutaneous	Ocular lesions	Neuro-logical in-volvement	Vascular in-volvement	Arthropathy/ Arthritis	Gastro-intestinal lesions
Topical treatment	+	+	–	–	+	+[1]
Colchicine	+	–	–	–	–	–
Pentoxifylline	+	–	–	–	–	–
DADPS	+	–	–	–	–	–
Thalidomide	+[2]	–	–	–	–	–
Non-steroidal anti-inflammatory agents	+[3]	–	–	–	+	+[4]
Sulfazalazine	–	+	–	–	+/–	+
Corticosteroids	+	+	+	+	+	–[5]
Interferon-α	+	+	–	+	+	+
Ciclosporin A	+	+	–	+	–	–
Methotrexate	+	+	+	+	+	–
Azathioprine	+	+	–	+	–	–[5]
Other immunosuppressives	–	+	+[6]	–	–	–
Anticoagulants	–	–	–	+/–	–	–

[1]Surgery.
[2]Worsening of erythema nodosum lesions reported.
[3]Skin lesions.
[4]Sulphasalazine.
[5]Deterioration.
[6]Chlorambucil/cyclophosphamide.

- mild diet
- avoidance of hard, spicy or salty nutrients and chemicals such as are present in toast breads, nuts, oranges, lemons, tomatoes, spices (pepper, paprika, curry), alcohol- or CO_2-containing drinks, mouthwashes, toothpastes.

Topical treatment of the aphthous oral ulcers includes:

- caustic solutions (silver nitrate 1–2%, tinctura myrrhae 5–10% w/v, H_2O_2

0.5%, methyl violet 0.5%) 1–2 times/day
- topical antiseptic and anti-inflammatory preparations amlexanox 5% in oral paste, hexetidine 1%, chlorhexidine 1–2% mouthwash solutions, benzydamine, camomile extracts), as well as tetracycline mouthwash (as glycerine solution 250 mg/5 mL glycerine) 2 min 4–6 times/day (contraindicated in pregnancy)
- topical corticosteroids (triamcinolone mucosal ointment, dexamethasone mucosal paste, betamethasone pastilles) 4 times/day or during the night (ointment/paste) or intrafocal infiltrations with triamcinolone suspension 0.1–0.5 mL per lesion
- topical anaesthetics [lidocaine (lignocaine) 2–5%, mepivacaine 1.5%, tetracaine 0.5–1% gels or mucosal ointments) 2–3 times/day (contraindicated in allergy)]
- topical aminosalicylic acid (5% cream) 3 times/day (has been shown to reduce the duration of acne lesions and the pain intensity).

A close association of smoking with a decrease of recurrences of oral aphthous ulcers has been described.

For the topical treatment of genital ulcers and skin lesions corticosteroid and antiseptic creams can be applied for a short period of time (7 days). Painful genital ulcerations can be managed by topical anaesthetics in cream. Corticosteroid injections (triamcinolone 0.1–0.5 mL/lesion) can be focally applied in recalcitrant ulcerations.

In severe forms of the mucocutaneous type of the disease an additional systemic treatment is required. The following agents have been proven to be beneficial.

- Corticosteroids (prednisolone, initial dose 30–60 mg/day p.o. for at least 4 weeks) can be administered as monotherapy or in combination with colchicine (1–2 mg/day p.o), diaminodiphenyl sulphone (DADPS; 100–150 mg/day p.o), interferon-α (IFN-α; 3–12 million IU 3 times per week s.c.) or azathioprine (initial dose 100 mg/day p.o.). Monotherapy with the non-steroidal agent to prevent the development of new aphthous ulcers should follow.
- Non-steroidal anti-inflammatory drugs, like indometacine (100 mg/day p.o. over 3 months) can be effective occasionally on the mucocutaneous lesions.
- Pentoxifylline (300 mg 1–3 times/day p.o.) or oxypentifylline (400 mg 3 times/day p.o.) treatment for 4 weeks induced a remission of recurrent aphthous oral ulcers in two-thirds of patients in open studies. However, recurrences occurred in all patients after discontinuation of treatment. Pentoxifylline (600 mg/day p.o.) has also been described as alternative treatments for mucocutaneous and ocular lesions in few patients with Adamantiades–Behçet's disease. The compound decreases superoxide production by neutrophils.
- Colchicine (0.5–2 mg/day p.o.) can be used as a second-line alternative, especially for the treatment of cutaneous lesions, such as erythema nodosum, and of oral aphthous ulcers. It inhibits the enhanced chemotactic activity of neutrophils. Oligospermia and gastrointestinal complaints are known adverse effects of colchicine (contraindicated in pregnancy). Interestingly, the compound has been shown to be more effective in female than in male patients.
- DADPS (100–150 mg/day p.o.) also inhibits the enhanced chemotactic activity of neutrophils and can be used as an alternative compound to colchicine. Quick relapses have been observed after discontinuation of the DADPS treatment. Intermittent treatment with ascorbic acid (vitamin C;

500 mg/day) is advisable to prevent increased methaemoglobin serum levels.

- IFN-α was introduced in the treatment of Adamantiades–Behçet's disease 10 years ago because of its antiviral activity, its ability to augment *in vitro* the decreased activity of patients' natural killer cells and its capacity to inhibit neovascular proliferation. IFN-α has been shown to inhibit interleukin (IL)-8 (serum levels are increased in active disease) synthesis and secretion by human microvascular endothelial cells. Eighty-five of 99 patients with mucocutaneous symptoms (86%), 29 of 32 patients with uveitis (91%), and 61 of 65 patients with arthropathy and/or arthritis (94%) reported in 19 open studies and case reports exhibited a partial or complete response. The maximum response of mucocutaneous and ocular symptoms occurred within 1–4 months after the initiation of therapy. Discontinuation of treatment resulted in relapses in a considerable number of patients, especially those with uveitis and arthropathy/arthritis. The symptoms responded again after reintroduction of the drug. Mild side-effects were generally recorded, mainly transient flu-like symptoms and reversible mild leukopenia. After an initial treatment with 9 million IU 3 times/week s.c. followed by a low-dose IFN-α scheme (3–6 million IU 3 times/week s.c.) should be administered, since they are as effective as high doses with fewer side-effects. The efficacy of the regimen should be controlled after a 6-month treatment period. Recurrences of up to 40% have been observed immediately or up to 6 months after discontinuation of treatment.
- Ciclosporin A (3 mg/kg body weight/day p.o.) is capable of markedly ameliorating mucocutaneous lesions, however, it has to be kept as a reserve medication because of its significant long-term adverse effects.
- Methotrexate (7.5–20 mg once a week p.o. over 4 weeks) is able of inducing an improvement of severe mucocutaneous involvement (contraindicated in pregnancy, lactation, severe bone marrow depression, liver dysfunction, acute infections, gastrointestinal ulcers, kidney insufficiency).
- Thalidomide (100–300 mg/day p.o., optimal dose 100 mg/day at the evening for 2 months) has recently been approved for the treatment of men, and sterilized as well as postmenopausal women with Adamantiades–Behçet's disease in the USA. The drug (contraindicated in pregnancy due to teratogenicity, peripheral neuropathy) was shown to selectively inhibit TNF-α synthesis by monocytes. In a randomized, double-blind, placebo-controlled study with 63 patients, a remission of oral and genital ulcers and folliculitis was detected in 24% of the patients over 8 weeks. During the 6-month treatment 30% of the patients remained free of lesions. Discontinuation of the treatment results in recurrence of the aphthous lesions, therefore a maintenance treatment with 50 mg/day to 50 mg twice a week is required. Peripheral neuropathy with acral paraesthesia was found clinically in 6% and electrophysiologically in 22% of the patients who received thalidomide 100–300 mg/day over 6 months. Central nervous system signs with sleepiness and headaches as well as xerostomia and constipation can occur.

Treatment of the systemic type

Treatment of the systemic type of the disease is dependent on the diseased organ(s) (Table 4). Evaluation of the therapeutic success is complicated through the relapsing–remitting character of the disease and the small number of controlled studies performed. Controlled studies only involved colchicine, levamisole, azathioprine, ciclosporin A, thalidomide (for aphthous lesions) and penicillin. In addition, there are large studies of uncontrolled treatments with chlorambucil, cyclophosphamide, IFN-α and tacrolimus. There are widely different procedures concerning the treatment of the disease, however, Yazici and Barnes (1991) have defined aspects of treatment with consensus of opinion among international experts (Table 5). Since the most active pharmaceutical compounds are linked to severe adverse effects, the adequate drug has to be chosen according to the leading feature and/or the manifestation with worse prognosis.

Eye involvement

- High-dose corticosteroids (methylprednisolone 0.5–1.0 g or prednisolone 1 mg/kg body weight as pulsed short infusion/day) are able to improve the acute eye disease but do not prevent recurrences and do not influence the natural course of uveitis.
- Ciclosporin A (5–6 mg/kg body weight/day in 2 daily doses p.o., maintenance dose 3 mg/kg body weight/day) has been demonstrated to be effective in controlling the acute inflammatory eye disease. It has a more rapid action than azathioprine and it has been shown to be superior to colchicine and cyclophosphamide in halting the progression of the ocular disease for the initial 6 months of treatment (contraindicated in lactation, renal insufficiency). However, this beneficial effect diminishes with time. Because of its severe adverse events (especially nephrotoxicity) a close control of the treatment with evaluation of the serum levels (therapeutic levels: 50–150 ng/mL monoclonal ciclosporin A) is required. Ciclosporin A doses can be reduced in a combined regimen with corticosteroids (prednisolone 0.2–0.4 mg/kg/day p.o) in order to decrease toxicity.
- IFN-α (9 million IU 3–5 times/week s.c.) has been found beneficial in 29 of 32 patients with uveitis (91%) of a recent meta-analysis study as well as in 90% of the patients in two small open studies. Even patients who have been non-responders or moderate responders to ciclosporin A experienced a positive development of their eye disease under IFN-α.
- Azathioprine (100–150 mg/day or 1.0–2.5 mg/kg body weight/day) was demonstrated to be effective in maintaining visual acuity and preventing the development of new eye lesions. However, it is not the treatment of choice in established bilateral ocular involvement. Its adverse effects are those of immunosuppressive drugs (contraindicated in pregnancy, severe liver disease, bone marrow depression, severe infection, children).

The following immunosuppressive drugs (with or without corticosteroids) are active on ocular inflammation without influencing the prognosis of eye disease

- chlorambucil (0.1 mg/kg body weight/day p.o.)
- cyclophosphamide (maximal 2 mg/kg body weight/day p.o. until leukopenia occurs followed by 50 mg/day or pulsed 500 mg once a week i.v. plus

Table 5 Aspects of treatment with consensus of opinion ≥ 70% (modified from Yazici & Barnes, 1991)

- Steroids are beneficial in disabling oral and/or genital ulcerations and in retinal vasculitis
- High-dose steroids are beneficial in the treatment of central nervous system involvement (increased intracranial pressure, pyramidocerebellar syndrome)
- Non-steroidal anti-inflammatory agents are effective in controlling the inflammatory arthritis
- Colchicine is beneficial in treating erythema nodosum
- In ocular manifestation immune suppressive drugs followed by ciclosporin A have to be administered; no systemic treatment is required for eye disease that has been quiescent for more than 2 years

mesna 200 mg—contraindicated in haemorrhagic cystitis)
- methotrexate (7.5–20 mg once a week i.v.).

Patients with uveitis have to be treated early with azathioprine because of an expected better prognosis. The occasional patient with mild anterior uveitis has to be initially treated with topical mydriatics and local corticosteroid eye drops to prevent development of synechiae. Complaints due to permanent structural eye changes can be improved by surgery, including lens extraction and vitrectomy.

Nervous system involvement

Treatments of choice are the corticosteroids (prednisolone 1.5 mg/kg body weight/day p.o. or pulsed i.v. in acute stages). Therapy has to be performed over several months with gradual reduction of dosage (contraindicated in diabetes mellitus, steroid-induced psychoses). Chlorambucil or cyclophosphamide represent second-line alternative regimens. Occasionally, conventional antiepileptic treatment is also required.

Vascular disease

Combined use of corticosteroids (prednisolone 100–250 mg/day) with immunosuppressive drugs (e.g. azathioprine 200 mg/day) is required, like in other vasculitides. Aneurysms of small arteries can be embolized, defects of large arteries have to be surgically repaired. Because of the common occurrence of a pulmonary vasculitis and thrombophlebitis (Hughes–Stovin syndrome) the monotherapy with anticoagulants is not advisable. Heparin infusion and acetyl salicylic acid (100–250 mg/day) are the treatment of acute thrombophlebitis; heparin and fibrinolytics (streptokinase) is the treatment of acute phlebothrombosis of the large veins. Long-term treatment drugs are coumarin or warfarin. Anticoagulants and ciclosporin A can prevent further thromboembolic complications. We have had good experience with chlorambucil (0.1 mg/kg body weight/day p.o. initial dose) which seems to exhibit a morbostatic effect on vascular disease, especially progressive vessel thrombosis.

Gastrointestinal manifestation

Sulphasalazine (2–4 g/day) is the treatment of choice for ulcerations of the gastrointestinal tract. Acute bowel perforation has to be surgically treated.

Joint involvement

Arthralgia and mild arthritis can be efficiently treated with non-steroidal anti-inflammatory agents (e.g. indometacine 100 mg/day, and the newer cycloxygenase 2 inhibitors, e.g. rofecoxibe 12.5–25 mg/day p.o.) or corticosteroids (methylprednisolone 4 mg/day). Severe arthritis improves by intra-articular corticosteroid injections. Colchicine is also beneficial for arthropathy in Adamantiades–Behçet's disease.

Experimental treatments

Topical treatment

- Toothpastes and mouthwash solutions including triclosan (0.1%) have been shown to reduce the number of aphthous oral ulcers in a small double-blind study with 30 patients. Triclosan is an antiseptic substance with anti-inflammatory and analgesic properties.
- A toothpaste with the enzymes amyloglucosidase and glucoseoxidase (Zendium) did reduce the recurrence of aphthous oral ulcers and pain in a double-blind study with 33 patients. Fifty-five per cent of the patients experienced a full remission of their aphthous oral ulcers during the 6-month treatment and a 3-month post-treatment period.
- The use of a sodium lauryl sulphate (SLS)-free toothpaste led to a reduction of the recurrences of aphthous oral

ulcers in a study with 30 patients. Although further studies could not confirm this effect, it is advisable to avoid products with SLS in topical mouth hygiene and treatment of patients with aphthous oral ulcers.

- Topical sucralfate (suspension 20 mL/day over 4 months) has been shown to be effective on aphthous oral ulcers in a randomized, double-blind placebo-controlled study.
- The topical application of diclofenac 3% in hyaluronan 2.5% reduced pain in a randomized study with 60 patients with aphthous oral ulcers. The preparation showed a stronger analgetic activity than lidocaine 3% gel.
- The topical treatment of aphthous oral ulcers with doxymycine in isobutylcanoacrylate led to stronger reduction of pain than placebo in a randomized study with 31 patients.
- Ciclosporin A (500 mg solution for mouthwash 3 times a day over 2 months) has been shown to be effective as a topical immunosuppressive drug.
- Topical application of prostaglandin E2 (0.3 mg gel twice a day over 10 days) exhibited a significant reduction of the number of new lesions, however, no beneficial effect could be detected regarding the healing speed of existing aphthous ulcers and pain compared to placebo.

Systemic treatment

- Like pentoxifylline, rebamipide (300 mg/day), another inhibitor of superoxide production by neutrophils, has been currently described to improve oral aphthous lesions in a few patients.
- Minocycline (100 mg/day) was shown significantly to reduce genital ulcerations and skin lesions (erythema nodosum, perifolliculitis) but not oral aphthous ulcers in 13 patients with Adamantiades–Behçet's disease in a period of 3 months. Minocycline was shown to reduce IL-1β and IL-6 overproduction in patients' peripheral blood mononuclear cells *in vitro* but not that of IL-8.
- Sulfasalazine (1.5–3 g/day) in combination with medium-dose corticosteroids (0.5 mg/kg body weight/day) have been shown in an open study with 35 patients to be effective in anterior and/or posterior uveitis without retinal involvement. Improvement occurred 1–2 months after initiation of treatment.
- The effect of tacrolimus (FK506) on refractory uveitis associated with Adamantiades–Behcet's disease was investigated in an open study with 41 patients (0.05–0.2 mg/kg body weight/day p.o.). The improvement rate was increased dose-dependently up to 0.15 mg/kg initial dose. The final improvement rate of ocular lesions was 75% and the frequency of ocular attacks was significantly reduced. In eight of 12 patients (67%) in whom ciclosporin A treatment had failed, ocular lesions improved by tacrolimus. Main adverse reactions were renal impairment, neurological symptoms, gastrointestinal symptoms, hypomagnesaemia, hyperkalaemia and hyperglycaemia. Most of the adverse effects were dose-dependent and disappeared or ameliorated after dose reduction or withdrawal of the drug. Serum level is recommended to maintain between 15 and 25 ng/mL during the early days of treatment. On the basis of the efficacy and safety results it is recommended to use an initial daily dose of 0.15 mg/kg body weight/day.
- Treatment with monoclonal TNF-α antibody (i.v. infusion once monthly over 6 months) has been shown to be effective in severe ocular involvement (five patients) and chronically active gastrointestinal and extraintestinal lesions (one patient). TNF-α is believed to play a pivotal role in Th1-mediated disease.

- Purified bovine retinal S antigen (30 mg p.o.) was administered in a patient with a 12-year history of ocular Adamantiades–Behçet's disease three times a week with subsequent decrease to once a week. Inflammatory ocular episodes significantly decreased over the period of over 2 years despite the discontinuation of ciclosporin A and prednisolone. A randomized, masked study looking at the effect of feeding retinal antigens to uveitis patients is ongoing.
- Plasmapheresis as an acute measure has improved the disease in a number of patients. There are indications that the method can improve the acuity of the disease and increase the recurrence-free intervals.

The indication spectrum of the different agents engaged in the treatment of Adamantiades–Behçet's disease are shown in Table 5. It is noticeable that discontinuation of the majority of the active compounds prior to the natural remission of the disease results to an acute or subacute exacerbation.

Further reading

Alpsoy E, Er H, Durusoy C, Yilmaz E. The use of sucralfate suspension in the treatment of oral and genital ulceration of Behçet's disease. *Arch Dermatol* 1999; 135: 529–32.

Avci O, Gürler N, Günes AT. Efficacy of cyclosporine on mucocutaneous manifestations of Behçet's disease. *J Am Acad Dermatol* 1997; 36: 796–7.

Bang D. Treatment of Behcet's disease. *Yonsei Med J* 1997; 38: 401–10.

Binnie WH, Curro FA, Khandwala A, Van Inwegan RG. Amlexanox oral paste. A novel treatment that accelerates the healing of aphthous ulcers. *Compend Contin Educ Dent* 1997; 18: 1116–24.

Calderon P, Anzilotti M, Phelps R. Thalidomide in dermatology. New indications for an old drug. *Int J Dermatol* 1997; 36: 881–7.

Calgüneri M, Kiraz S, Ertenli I, Benekli M, Karaarslan Y, Çelik I. The effect of prophylactic penicillin treatment on the course of arthritis episodes in patients with Behcet's disease. A randomized clinical trial. *Arthritis Rheum* 1996; 39: 2062–5.

Chahine L, Sempson N, Wagoner C. The effect of sodium lauryl sulfate on recurrent aphthous ulcers: a clinical study. *Compend Contin Educ Dent* 1997; 18: 1238–40.

Chandrasekhar J, Liem AA, Cox NH, Paterson AW. Oxypentifylline in the management of recurrent aphthous oral ulcers: an open clinical trial. *Oral Surg Oral Med Oral Pathol Oral Radiol Endod* 1999; 87: 564–7.

de Wazières B, Gil H, Magy N, Berthier S. Vuitton DA, Dupond JL. Traitement de L'aphthose récurrente par thalidomide à faible dose. Étude pilote chez 17 patients. *Rev Méd Int* 1999; 20: 567–70.

Ehrlich GE. Behçet's disease: an update. *Comp Ther* 1999; 25: 216–20.

Fridh G, Koch G. Effect of a mouth rinse containing amyloglucosidase and glucose oxidase on recurrent aphthous ulcers in children and adolescents. *Swed Dent J* 1999; 23: 49–57.

Gardner-Medwin JMM, Smith NJ, Powell RJ. Clinical experience with thalidomide in the management of severe oral and genital ulceration in conditions such as Behçet's disease: use of neurophysiological studies to detect thalidomide neuropathy. *Ann Rheum Dis* 1994; 53: 828–32.

Ghate JV, Jorizzo JL. Behçet's disease and complex aphthosis. *J Am Acad Dermatol* 1999; 40: 1–18.

Hamuryudan V, Mat C, Saip S *et al.* Thalidomide in the treatment of the mucocutaneous lesions of the Behçet syndrome. A randomized, double-blind, placebo-controlled trial. *Ann Intern Med* 1998; 128: 443–50.

Hassard PV, Binder SW, Nelson V, Vasiliauskas EA. Anti-tumor necrosis factor monoclonal antibody therapy for gastrointestinal Behcet's disease: a case report. *Gastroenterology* 2001; 120: 995–9.

Healy CM, Paterson M, Joyston-Bechal S, Williams DM, Thornhill MH. The effect of a sodium lauryl sulfate-free dentifrice on patients with recurrent oral ulceration. *Oral Dis* 1999; 5: 39–43.

Hornstein OP. Aphthen und aphthoide Läsionen der Mundschleimhaut. *Hals-Nasen-Ohren-Arzt* 1998; 46: 102–11.

International Study Group for Behçet's disease. Criteria for diagnosis of Behçet's disease. *Lancet* 1990; 335: 1078–80.

Jorizzo JL, Schmalstieg FC, Solomon AR Jr *et al.* Thalidomide effects in Behçet's syndrome and pustular vasculitis. *Arch Intern Med* 1986; 146: 878–81.

Jorizzo JL, White WL, Wise CM, Zanolli MD, Sherertz EF. Low-dose weekly methotrexate for unusual neutrophilic vascular reactions. cutaneous polyarteriitis nodosa and Behçet's disease. *J Am Acad Dermatol* 1991; 24: 973–8.

Kaklamani VG, Vaiopoulos G, Kaklamanis PG. Behçet's disease. *Sem Arthritis Rheum* 1998; 27: 197–217.

Kotake S, Higashi K, Yoshikawa K, Sasamoto Y, Okamoto T, Matsuda H. Central nervous system symptoms in patients with Behcet disease receiving cyclosporine therapy. *Ophthalmology* 1999; 106: 586–9.

Kötter I, Eckstein AK, Stübiger N, Zierhut M. Treatment of ocular symptoms of Behçet's disease with interferon α_{2a}: a pilot study. *Br J Ophthalmol* 1998; 82: 488–94.

Mochizuki M. Immunotherapy for Behcet's disease. *Int Rev Immunol* 1997; 14: 49–66.

Oyama N, Inoue M, Matsui T, Nuhei Y, Nishibu A, Kaneko F. Minocycline effects on the clinical symptoms in correlation with cytokines produced by peripheral blood mononuclear cells stimulated with streptococcal antigens in Behçet's disease. In: Hamza M, ed. *Behçet's Disease*. Tunis: Publications Adhoua, 1997: 481–6.

Özyazgan Y, Hizli N, Mat C *et al.* Azathioprine in Behcet's syndrome. effects on long-term prognosis. *Arthritis Rheum* 1997; 40: 769–74.

Rogers RS III. Recurrent aphthous stomatitis in the diagnosis of Behçet's disease. *Yonsei Med J* 1997; 38: 370–9.

Sakane T, Takeno M. Novel approaches to Behcet's disease. *Expert Opin Invest Drugs* 2000; 9: 1993–2005.

Sakane T, Takeno M, Suzuki N, Inaba G. Behçet's disease. *N Engl J Med* 1999; 341: 1284–91.

Samangooci SH, Mehryar M, Hakim SM, Safamanesk S. Clinical trial of sulfasalazine for treatment of uveitis Behçet's disease. In: Hamza M, ed. *Behçet's Disease*. Tunis: Publications Adhoua, 1997: 466–70.

Saxen MA, Ambrosius WT, Rehemtula al-KF Russell AL, Eckert GJ. Sustained relief of oral aphthous ulcer pain from topical diclofenac in hyaluronan: a randomized, double-blind clinical trial. *Oral Surg Oral Med Oral Pathol Oral Radiol Endod* 1997; 84: 356–61.

Stadler R, Bratzke B, Orfanos CE. Therapeutischer Einsatz von alpha-Interferon bei metastasierendem malignen Melanom, disseminiertem Kaposi-Sarkom und schwerem Morbus Behçet. *Hautarzt* 1987; 38: 453–60.

Tanaka C, Matsuda T, Yukinari Y *et al.* The beneficial effect of rebamipide on recurrent aphthous ulcers in Behçet's disease. In: Hamza M, ed. *Behçet's Disease*. Tunis: Publications Adhoua, 1997: 477–80.

Treudler R, Orfanos CE, Zouboulis CC. Twenty eight cases of juvenile-onset Adamantiades–Behçet's disease in Germany. *Dermatology* 1999; 199: 15–19.

Yasui K, Ohta K, Kobayashi M, Aizawa T, Komiyama A. Successful treatment of Behçet's disease with pentoxifylline. *Ann Intern Med* 1996; 124: 891–3.

Yazici H. Thalidomide in the treatment of the mucocutaneous lesions of the Behçet syndrome. A randomized, double-blind, placebo-controlled trial. *Ann Intern Med* 1998; 128: 443–50.

Yazici H, Barnes CG. Practical treatment recommendations for pharmacotherapy of Behçet's syndrome. *Drugs* 1991; 42: 796–804.

Yazici H, Yurdakul S, Hamuryudan V. The management of Behçet's syndrome: how are we doing? *Clin Exp Rheumato* 1999; 17: 145–7.

Zouboulis CC. Morbus Adamantiades–Behçet: Klinische und experimentelle Befunde von 53 Patienten aus dem Berliner Raum. Habilitationsschrift. Berlin: Freie Universität Berlin, 1995.

Zouboulis CC. Morbus Adamantiades–Behçet in Deutschland: Historischer Rückblick und aktueller Kenntnisstand. *Z Hautkr* 1996; 71: 491–501.

Zouboulis CC. Adamantiades–Behçet's disease. In: Katsambas AD, Lotti T, eds. *European Handbook of Dermatological Treatments*. Berlin: Springer: 1999, 21–30.

Zouboulis CC. Epidemiology of Adamantiades–Behçet's disease. *Ann Med Int* 1999; 150: 488–98.

Zouboulis CC, Katsantonis J, Ketteler R *et al.* Adamantiades–Behçet's disease. Interleukin-8 is increased in serum of patients with active oral and neurological manifestations and is secreted by small vessel endothelial cells. *Arch Dermatol Res* 2000; 292: 279–84.

Zouboulis CC, Kötter I, Djawari D *et al.* Epidemiological features of Adamantiades–Behçet's disease in Germany and in Europe. *Yonsei Med J* 1997; 38: 411–22.

Zouboulis CC, Orfanos CE. Treatment of Adamantiades–Behçet's disease with systemic interferon alfa. *Arch Dermatol* 1998; 134: 1010–16.

Zouboulis CC, Treudler R, Orfanos CE. Morbus Adamantiades–Behçet. therapeutischer Einsatz von systemischen rekombinantem Interferon-alpha-2a. *Hautarzt* 1993; 44: 440–5.

Alopecia areata

R. Happle

Definition and epidemiology

Alopecia areata is a non-scarring form of hair loss that usually begins with round patches. It can involve any hair-bearing area of the body and is characterized histopathologically by peribulbar lymphocytic infiltrates. Cases of mild involvement show a marked tendency to spontaneous regrowth of hair. With the exception of androgenetic hair loss, alopecia areata is by far the most frequently occurring form of hair loss.

Rationale of the following guidelines

The care for alopecia areata is still a difficult task for every dermatologist. When we consider the theoretical and practical requirements of evidence-based medicine, it seems mandatory to ask the following questions: Which measures are necessary in the diagnosis and treatment of alopecia areata? Which additional measures are desirable? Which approaches are unnecessary? Which measures are obsolete?

The guidelines as proposed in this chapter are derived from a 25-year experience in the management of alopecia areata. They differ considerably from the opinions published by American authors who advocate a rather broad therapeutic armamentarium, including minoxidil and anthralin, for this disorder. Indeed, it is amazing how many ineffective methods are recommended, reflecting the marked tendency of mild alopecia areata for a spontaneous improvement. The reader should be warned that, when screening articles on the management of alopecia areata, a swampy and unsafe area is being entered. For example, an article may be found claiming that, according to the rules of evidence-based medicine, aromatherapy is very effective. Every dermatologist should try to find their own way through this bewildering jungle of facts and fallacies. The present author cannot guarantee that his statements are free from error. Some physicians may even ask themselves whether in the management of alopecia areata the truth is very helpful. However, without an appropriate discrimination between a valid response and placebo effects, no true progress in the treatment of this disease will be achieved.

Necessary diagnostic measures

In general, a 'spot' diagnosis of alopecia areata can be established by any competent and experienced physician on the basis of the characteristic signs and symptoms, and the case history. In this way, various meaningless and expensive laboratory investigations can be avoided. In very rare cases of doubt (approximately 1 in 400 cases), a scalp biopsy may be helpful in order to confirm or to exclude the diagnosis.

Unnecessary diagnostic measures

In this disease, all laboratory examinations of bodily fluids such as red blood cell count, white blood cell count, sedimentation rate, determination of liver enzymes or renal parameters, hormone analysis, analysis of environmental poisons in blood or urine, determination of zinc levels or other trace elements, and determination of lymphocyte markers are unnecessary, because no conclusion can be drawn with regard to diagnosis or therapy.

A trichogram (hair root analysis) is likewise unnecessary. A simple pluck test performed with the fingers, especially at the margins of bald patches, yields far better information regarding the short-term prognosis.

Furthermore, all of the *diagnostic* measures performed in the field of psychiatry or psychotherapy, including psychoanalysis and psychosomatic approaches, are unnecessary. A sound evaluation of the advantages and disadvantages of such concepts leads to a 'zero position'. For the practical purpose of diagnosis and treatment, there is so far no evidence that there is any causal relationship between psychological problems or stressful life events and the development or aggravation of alopecia areata. The numerous studies claiming such relationship are unconvincing when the strict rules of evidence-based medicine are applied. It should be noted, however, that this view only applies to the practical situation of a given patient. Further intensive research in this field should be neither discouraged nor devalued.

Necessary therapeutic measures

Appropriate information on the course and prognosis of alopecia areata is needed. The patient should be informed that a spontaneous remission is always possible. In mild forms characterized by some round patches there is an 80% probability that spontaneous regrowth will occur within a period of 1 or 2 years. In cases of more extensive or total hair loss the prognosis is considerably less favourable, but a spontaneous regrowth of hair is never excluded. From this information the patient should learn to discriminate between reasonable and unnecessary therapeutic options.

The patient should be informed that there are not many effective therapeutic modalities (Fig. 1). The most effective treatment is topical immunotherapy. Although this mode of treatment is presently far more prevalent in Europe than in the USA, it is so far confined in general to some dermatological centres.

Guidelines for topical immunotherapy

Topical immunotherapy consists of repeated applications of a potent contact allergen to the scalp. Currently used substances are diphencyprone (diphenylcyclopropenone, DCP) and squaric acid dibutylester (SADBE). The rate of response is the same with both contact allergens.

A major practical problem is the fact that toxicological investigation of diphencyprone in animal experiments has so far not been completed. We know that the substance is not mutagenic in the Ames test and not teratogenic in mice and chickens. Furthermore, it does not show a toxic effect in the hen's egg test. More data, however, are needed in order to regard the drug as safe for routine use in alopecia areata. This situation implies that hitherto unknown adverse effects cannot be completely excluded. The same is true for SADBE.

Patients must be informed about this risk and must sign an informed consent. For safety reasons we do not treat children below the age of 10 years. Other authors, however, have reported good results obtained in children below this age. Women of childbearing age should take contraceptive measures. The risk of a teratogenic effect, however, is very low according to present knowledge. Hence, if a woman becomes pregnant during topical immunotherapy, the treatment should be discontinued immediately but there is no reason to give the advice to discontinue the pregnancy.

During treatment, we propose for formal reasons to monitor every 3 months the blood cell count and the parameters of liver and kidney function.

Practical management

Sensitization is performed with a 2% solution of diphencyprone applied to a 5×5 cm region on the crown. Many patients develop an eczematous response within 10 days, without any elicitation. Apparently, small amounts of the substance remaining in the scalp skin are sufficient to elicit a response in the sensitized patient. On the other hand, absence of an

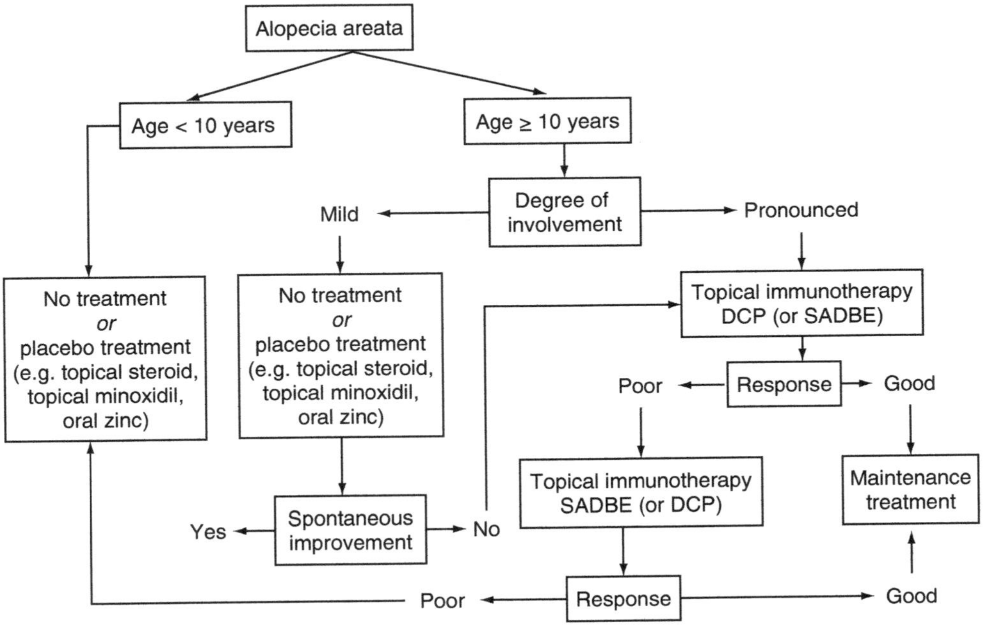

Figure 1 Algorithm for the treatment of alopecia areata

eczematous response does not mean that sensitization has failed. One single application of a 2% solution results in sensitization of 99% of individuals.

Two weeks after sensitization, elicitation is started with a 0.001% solution. However, this elicitation is only performed if no eczema is visible. Otherwise, the elicitation is delayed, and the dosage is lowered according to the severity of the initial response.

With weekly applications of the drug we try to find a concentration that results in slight erythema and itching lasting for 2 or 3 days without major blistering or oozing. For this purpose we are using 11 different concentrations:

2%
1%
0.5%
0.1%
0.05%
0.01%
0.001%
0.0001%
0.00001%
0.000001%
0.0000001%

When SADBE is used instead of DCP, the range of different concentrations is the same.

Initially we are treating one side of the scalp only. The untreated side serves as a control in order to recognize a possible spontaneous remission (Fig. 2). It is important to realize that the intensity of response to a given dosage may vary considerably during the first weeks of treatment. After a period of about 12 weeks, the degree of eczematous response becomes stable. This 'tuning' of the eczematous response is the key to success.

After a unilateral response in terms of improved hair growth has been noted, treatment is continued bilaterally. When full regrowth has been obtained, the intervals of application may be increased to 2 or 3 weeks. If hair loss is observed during this period, weekly applications of the contact allergen are resumed. The patient

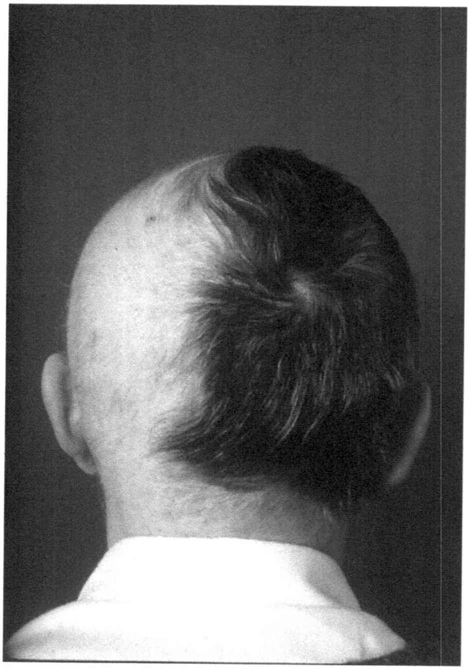

Figure 2 Topical immunotherapy of alopecia areata totalis with diphencyprone: result of 16-week unilateral treatment. The untreated side served as a control.

should be aware that this is a maintenance treatment although the therapy may be tentatively discontinued after 2 years of continuous hair growth.

In many patients, four or even more different concentrations of the drug have to be used in order to maintain an appropriate eczematous response. A fine modulation of the eczema may be performed by increasing the number of swabs from one to two during a given application. However, a new swab should always be used for the procedure, in order to avoid contamination of the solution with scalp material.

Treatment of the eyebrows is likewise possible but should only be started when the stage of a stable concentration has been reached. The eyebrows should be treated either with a lower concentration or by gentle rubbing with a swab that has been initially used on the scalp. It is important to realize that smaller amounts of the contact allergen are needed in the eyebrow region.

Which rate of response can be expected?

In cases of extensive or total alopecia areata, a complete hair regrowth can be expected in about 50%. The remaining patients either fail to produce any hair regrowth or show an unsatisfactory response. When no unilateral hair regrowth is observed within a period of 6 months, we advise discontinuing the treatment because a satisfactory response becomes highly unlikely. In the successfully treated patients, a unilateral response is usually seen within the first 3 months of treatment.

Side-effects

The patient should be appropriately informed of the following possible side-effects. Redness and itching of the scalp as well as swelling of the regional lymph nodes should be considered a desired effect inherent in the therapeutic mechanism. However, a severe eczematous reaction cannot entirely be excluded. If the patient cannot tolerate it, topical steroid treatment should be avoided because it would interfere with the therapeutic response. In cases of severe contact eczema, however, topical or even systemic corticosteroids may be given. Dissemination of eczema after topical application may occur in some patients and may cause discontinuation of treatment.

An important side-effect is the development of pigmentary disturbances in terms of hyperpigmentation or vitiligo-like hypopigmentation that may sometimes be intermingled in the form of 'dyschromia in confetti'. The risk of such side-effects is particularly high in more darkly pigmented individuals. According to our experience, such pigmentary disturbances are reversible to a large degree, but may constitute a considerable burden, especially when the patient fails to show hair regrowth.

Shift from DCP to SADBE

About 10% of patients treated with diphencyprone develop immunological unresponsiveness during the course of treatment. In such patients a change from diphencyprone to SADBE should be considered. According to our experience, many patients who failed to show a satisfactory response to diphencyprone could be successfully treated with SADBE.

Psoralen and ultraviolet A (PUVA) treatment

PUVA treatment with oral application of 8-methoxypsoralen can be categorized as effective but its practical applicability is rather limited because the UV light can no longer reach the scalp when hair is regrowing. The same is true for the 'PUVA-turban' treatment.

Local injections of corticosteroids

In exceptional cases of recalcitrant circumscribed bald patches, local injections of corticosteroids may be considered. However, in cases of more pronounced involvement this therapeutic approach is worthless.

Advice regarding prosthetic camouflage

In cases of extensive or total alopecia areata the question of applying a wig should be discussed with the patient. It is important to realize that wigs made of artificial hair appropriately fulfil the cosmetic requirements. Moreover, cleaning of a wig made of artificial hair is much easier. On the other hand, wigs made of genuine hair are more durable. For economic reasons it seems unjustified to demand that the health plan should take over the costs for wigs made of human hair for all patients with alopecia areata.

Additional desirable measures

From a psychological point of view, it is important that the dermatologist shows commitment and offers the option of regular appointments. In this way the patient will not feel left alone with his problems, and he will learn to cope adequately with this disease which often tends to run a chronic course. In exceptional cases, however, the psychological support that can be given by a dermatologist may be insufficient, and in such cases the help of a specialized psychologist should be considered. It is important, however, that the physician and the patient himself both understand the aim of such psychological help. Such interviews cannot be offered with the aim to elucidate the 'cause' or 'meaning' of alopecia areata, or to induce regrowth of hair. Rather, the rationale of any psychosomatic approach is to offer support in coping with a cosmetically devastating disease. Dermatologists should be aware that many psychologists erroneously believe that their specialized knowledge and skills enable them to induce hair regrowth in alopecia areata. In reality, such psychosomatic approaches do not inhibit a spontaneous remission of alopecia areata.

Most dermatologists tend to perform one of the various forms of placebo treatment such as topical application of corticosteroids, anthralin or minoxidil. In view of the marked tendency of alopecia areata to spontaneous remission, such placebo treatment may be sometimes considered, especially in children. Any placebo treatment, however, should fulfil the following criteria: the treatment should not be expensive and the method should not be associated with major side-effects (e.g. topical hydrocortisone is preferable to more potent steroids that exert adverse effects without inducing hair regrowth).

Unnecessary therapeutic measures

According to the author's experience, the following therapeutic measures are ineffective and therefore unjustified. The superfluous therapeutic measures can be divided into systemic and topical approaches. However, some of the approaches categorized as unnecessary may be considered for the purpose of placebo treatment.

Unnecessary systemic approaches

There is so far no drug that can reasonably be given for systemic treatment of alopecia areata. The substances that have been tried until now are either ineffective or obsolete. Ineffective systemic treatments include the application of dapsone, gelatin, immunoglobulins, isoprinosine, thymopentin, vitamins and zinc or other trace elements. Clinical studies claiming effectiveness of one of these drugs are unconvincing when the criteria of evidence-based medicine are applied.

Furthermore, the various approaches of so-called alternative medicine such as acupuncture, autohaemotherapy, bioresonance method, Chinese herbs, homeopathy, as well as testing and treating of 'amalgam intoxication' or other forms of 'environmental poisoning', are unnecessary. These methods are not compatible with the criteria of rational thinking.

Unnecessary topical approaches

Ineffective topical approaches include treatment with anthralin, ciclosporin A, minoxidil or phenol, as well as aromatherapy. The same is true for all over-the-counter hair lotions.

Topical tacrolimus, although shown to be effective in murine models of alopecia areata is ineffective in the human disorder when applied in the presently available vehicle. Topical photodynamic therapy with 5-aminolaevulinic acid is likewise ineffective.

Topical treatment with corticosteroids is unnecessary because the effect is too weak. Repeated applications under occlusion can induce minimal hair regrowth. However, this response is only of theoretical and never of practical importance.

Obsolete therapeutic measures

Systemic application of corticosteroids as presently recommended by some authors is considered obsolete because the expected therapeutic effect does not outweigh the dangerous side-effects. Because of these inevitable adverse effects, the drug has to be discontinued after a very short period of time, rendering this treatment practically worthless.

Systemic application of ciclosporin A is likewise considered obsolete because of the well-known side-effects of long-term application of this drug.

Some of the above-mentioned unnecessary approaches could likewise be classified as obsolete. For example, topical treatment with anthralin is associated with troublesome skin irritation that is not acceptable in view of the ineffectiveness of the drug. Similarly, oral dapsone treatment may result in methaemoglobinaemia, and this risk is not acceptable because the effectiveness of the drug has never been proven.

Conclusion

In the diagnosis and treatment of alopecia areata, all medical measures should be evaluated according to the criteria of rational thinking. If this rule is followed, considerable financial costs can be avoided.

The diagnosis of alopecia areata can be made on the basis of the clinical features and the case history. In exceptional cases, a scalp biopsy may be helpful. For the purpose of an aetiological evaluation in clinical pratice, all other laboratory investigations as well as psychological or psychosomatic approaches are inconclusive and therefore unnecessary.

When performing a placebo treatment such as topical application of steroids, minoxidil or anthralin, physicians should be aware of the epistemological pitfalls of this approach. They will see 'good results' and tend to believe in such treatment although, in fact, these results simply show that the given drug could not inhibit a spontaneous hair regrowth.

With the exception of topical immunotherapy, there is so far no other effective and practically applicable method available (Fig. 1). PUVA treatment or local injection of corticosteroids may be considered in exceptional cases, but the rate of response to those therapeutic modalities is rather limited.

More specific and more effective therapeutic approaches will hopefully be developed in the near future.

Further reading

Abel E, Munro DD. Intralesional treatment of alopecia areata with triamcinolone acetonide by jet injector. *Br J Dermatol* 1972; 88: 55–8.

Behrens-Williams S, Leiter U, Schiener R, Weidmann M, Peter RU, Kerscher M. The PUVA-turban as a new option of applying a dilute psoralen solution selectively to the scalp of patients with alopecia areata. *J Am Acad Dermatol* 2001; 44: 248–52.

Bernard P, Arnoult-Coudoux E. Pelade: Stratégie de prise en charge. *Ann Dermatol Venereol* 2001; 128: 177–9.

Bissonnette R, Shapiro J, Zeng H, McLean DI, Lui H. Topical photodynamic therapy with 5-aminolaevulinic acid does not induce hair regrowth in patients with extensive alopecia areata. *Br J Dermatol* 2000; 143: 1032–5.

Charuwichitratana S, Wattanakrai P, Tanrattanakorn S. Randomized double-blind placebo-controlled trial in the treatment of alopecia areata with 0.25% desoximetasone cream. *Arch Dermatol* 2000; 136: 1276–7.

Cotellessa C, Peris K, Caracciolo E, Mordenti C, Chimenti S. The use of topical diphenylcyclopropenone for the treatment of extensive alopecia areata. *J Am Acad Dermatol* 2001; 44: 73–6.

Drake LA, Ceilly RI, Comelison RL *et al.* Guidelines of care for alopecia areata. *J Am Acad Dermatol* 1992; 26: 247–50.

Ead RD. Oral zinc sulfate in alopecia areata – a double blind trial. *Br J Dermatol* 1981; 104: 484.

Freyschmidt-Paul P, Hoffmann R, Levin E, Sundberg JP, Happle R, McElwee KJ. Current and potential agents for the treatment of alopecia areata. *Curr Pharm Des* 2001; 7: 213–30.

Galbraight GM, Thiers BH, Jensen J, Hoehler F. A randomized double-blind study of inosiplex therapy in patients with alopecia totalis. *J Am Acad Dermatol* 1987; 16: 977–83.

Gordon PM, Aldridge RD, McVittie E, Hunter JAA. Topical diphencyprone for alopecia areata. evaluation of 48 cases after 30 months' follow up. *Br J Dermatol* 1996; 134: 869–71.

Happle R, Kalveram KJ, Büchner U *et al.* Contact allergy as a therapeutic tool for alopecia areata. application of squaric acid dibutylester. *Dermatologica* 1980; 161: 289–97.

Happle R, van der Steen PHM. Der kreisrunde Haarausfall oder das Denken im Kreis. *Z Hautkr* 1997; 72: 564–9.

Hatzis JK, Gourgiotou K, Tosca A, Varelzidis A, Stratigos J. Vitiligo as a reaction to topical treatment with diphencyprone. *Dermatologica* 1988; 177: 146–8.

Hay IC, Jamieson M, Ormerod AD. Randomized trial of aromatherapy: successful treatment for alopecia areata. *Arch Dermatol* 1998; 134: 1349–52.

Healy E, Rogers S. PUVA treatment for alopecia areata—does it work? A retrospective review of 102 cases. *Br J Dermatol* 1993; 129: 42–4.

Henderson CA, Ilchyshyn A. Vitiligo complicating diphencyprone sensitization therapy for alopecia universalis. *Br J Dermatol* 1995; 133: 492–500.

Hoffmann R, Happle R. The therapeutic role of contact sensitization in alopecia areata: what, how, and why? *Am J Contact Dermatitis* 1995; 6: 228–31.

Hoffmann R, Happle R. Alopecia areata: Aktuelles über Ätiologie, Pathogenese, Klinik und Therapie. *Z Hautkr* 1996; 71: 528–41.

Madani S, Shapiro J. Alopecia areata update. *J Am Acad Dermatol* 2000; 42: 549–66.

McDonald-Hull S, Pepall L, Cunliffe WJ. Alopecia areata in children: response to treatment with diphencyprone. *Br J Dermatol* 1991; 125: 164–8.

Perret CM, Steijlen PM, Happle R. Erythema multiforme-like eruptions. A rare side effect of topical immunotherapy with diphenylcyclopropenone. *Dermatologica* 1990; 180: 5–7.

Price VH. Treatment of hair loss. *N Engl J Med* 1999; 341: 964–73.

Reinhold U, Buttgereit F. Hochdosis-Steroid-Pulstherapie: Gibt es Indikationen in der Dermatologie? *Hautarzt* 2000; 10: 738–45.

Schulz A, Hamm H, Weiglein U, Axt M, Bröcker EB. Dexamethasone pulse therapy in severe long-standing alopecia areata: a treatment failure. *Eur J Dermatol* 1996; 6: 26–9.

Seiter S, Ugurel S, Tilgen W, Reinhold U. High-dose pulse corticosteroid therapy in the treatment of severe alopecia areata. *Dermatology* 2001; 202: 230–4.

Sharma VK, Muralidhar S. Treatment of widespread alopecia areata in young patients with monthly oral corticosteroid pulse. *Pediatr Dermatol* 1998; 15: 313–17.

Thiers BH. Topical tacrolimus: treatment failure in a patient with alopecia areata. *Arch Dermatol* 2000; 136: 124.

Tosti A, Manuzzi P, Gasponi A. Thymopentin in the treatment of severe alopecia areata. *Dermatologica* 1988; 177: 170–4.

Van Baar HMJ, van der Vleuten CJM, van de Kerkhof PCM. Dapsone versus topical immunotherapy in alopecia areata. *Br J Dermatol* 1995; 133: 270–4.

Van der Steen PHM, Boezeman J, Duller P, Happle R. Can alopecia areata be triggered by emotional stress? An uncontrolled evaluation of 178 patients with extensive hair loss. *Acta Derm Venereol* 1992; 72: 279–80.

Van der Steen PHM, Happle R. 'Dyschromia in confetti' as a side effect of topical immunotherapy in alopecia areata. *Arch Dermatol* 1992; 128: 518–20.

Van der Steen PHM, Happle R. Immunological treatment of alopecia areata including the use of diphencyprone. *J Dermatol Treat* 1992; 3: 35–40.

Van der Steen PHM, van Baar HJM, Perret CM, Happle R. Treatment of alopecia areata with diphenylcyclopropenone. *J Am Acad Dermatol* 1991; 24: 253–7.

Androgenic alopecia

C. Piérard-Franchimont and G. E. Piérard

Synonyms

Androgenic alopecia is also known as androgenetic alopecia to indicate the influence of both genetic background and androgens in this condition. Male pattern baldness, common baldness and androgen-dependent alopecia are also used although women can also be affected. Seborrhoeic alopecia is a former name coined by Sabouraud to insist on the oily aspect of the scalp and hair which is so common in these patients.

Definition and epidemiology

Androgenic alopecia is at least in part hereditary. It depends on the androgen impact on hairs at specific sites of the scalp. The result is a progressive shortening of the hair cycle with miniaturization of the hair follicle. It represents a physiological process in men. In women the same is true although it may be secondary to hormonal imbalance.

The prevalence of androgenic alopecia has not been really defined. In Caucasian men it may reach 25% at the age of 25 years. The percentage increases with age, androgenic alopecia affects about half of the quinquagenarians. In women the prevalence is much lower although it has been reported that about 30% of them could show signs of androgenic alopecia after menopause.

Aetiology and pathophysiology

Androgenic alopecia is a multifactorial condition where genetic factors determine a peculiar sensibility to androgens and probably to some inflammatory influences. Dihydrotestosterone (DHT) is the main androgen influencing hair growth and size. It is synthesized locally through the activity of the two isoenzymes 5α-reductase types I and II.

There is also histological evidence that inflammation is present abutted to the infra-infundibulum and isthmus, at a site where follicular stem cells are believed to be located. The inflammatory cell infiltrate rich in memory T lymphocytes and dermal dendrocytes might affect the regulation of the hair cycle. Such a process is likely triggered by the intrafollicular microflora.

Increased hair shedding is followed by progressive balding. Affected hairs become thinner and shorter with a reduced anagen phase duration and altered time to teloptosis (hair shedding). The ratio of terminal to vellus hair decreases with the severity of alopecia down to 2 : 1 and even less in severe cases.

Clinical characteristics and course

There are distinct patterns of hair loss in androgenic alopecia affecting men and women. The male pattern begins with recession of the frontotemporal hairline, followed by thinning on the vertex. It may begin as early as the late teens. The time over which the hair loss progresses is extremely variable.

Women often present a more diffuse pattern of hair loss which usually predominates on the vertex. Usually the frontal hairline does not recede as in men. The female pattern may accompany signs of hyperandrogeny such as seborrhoea, acne, hirsutism, dysmenorrhoea and sterility. In these cases, the clinical presentation may be similar to the hair pattern seen in men.

Part of the concern in subjects suffering from androgenic alopecia is their current appearance but a major worry is what might happen in the years beyond.

Diagnosis

The diagnosis of androgenic alopecia relies primarily on the clinical examination. In the earliest stage of evolution, trichograms or phototrichograms performed on the frontal and vertex areas can reveal an increased proportion of telogen hairs. Terminal vs. vellus hair densities are also useful parameters. The histological and immunohistochemical assessments of skin biopsies are useful for research purpose only.

Hormonal screening may be informative in some cases. In young women who deny intake of anabolic drugs, corticosteroids and some progestatives, a biological check-up is recommended including dosages of total and free testosterone, Δ4-androstenedione and dehydroepiandrosterone sulphate (DHEAS). In rare cases, search for abnormal values of prolactin, follicle-stimulating hormone (FSH), luteinizing hormone (LH) and 17-OH progesterone may be useful. Levels of sex hormone-binding globulin (SHBG) and insulin-like growth factor-1 (IGF-1) may determine hair patterning in man.

Differential diagnosis

Diffuse alopecia areata and discrete cicatricial alopecia of the vertex may be difficult to distinguish from androgenic alopecia. However, miniature hairs are very typical for the latter condition. In women, chronic telogen effluvium is a self-limiting sustained moult corresponding to hair shedding without progressive balding. Diffuse alopecia related to drugs, hyposideraemia and abnormal thyroid function should be ruled out. It should be stressed that any intercurrent hair shedding irrespective of its origin may reveal or amplify the pattern of a previously unrecognized androgenic alopecia.

Treatment

General therapeutic guidelines

The treatment of androgenic alopecia aiming at hair regrowth is medical and/or surgical. It may be beneficial in preventing excessive hair shedding and in maintaining hair density and fullness. The drawback to the current medications is that they only work for about as long as they are used. Cosmetic products are also on the market, but most of them show little or no evidence for efficacy in hair regrowth. However, some cosmetic procedures may be beneficial in subjects with thinned hair, in giving the impression of thicker and more numerous hair. In any case, the basic aim of topical treatments is to limit hair shedding and to retard hair loss without expecting much improvement in the hair mass in less than 1 year. Conversely, surgical treatments provide immediate benefit in the aspect of hair density without, however, modifying the alopecia evolution. It is inferred that genuine hair growth modulators are indicated in early evolving androgenic alopecia in men, in the diffuse hair loss pattern in women, and as an adjunct to surgical procedures. The appropriate choice of therapy should be decided on only after discussion with the patient indicating the advantages and disadvantages of the various methods affording varying degrees of improvement in the hair density. The main therapeutic drawback is that results are usually far less impressive than the majority of patients want and could reasonably hope for. In general, the younger the patient, the less satisfactory a limited goal will be to him.

Most men are more aware of frontal hair loss rather than loss on the vertex, which they seldom see. Unfortunately, the response of the frontal margin to genuine hair regrowth compounds is less dramatic than on the crown of the head. Managing disappointment remains unfortunately a large part of caring for anyone with androgenic alopecia. Ensuring reasonable expectations at the outset is important. Indeed, regrowth of very fine hairs is of limited cosmetic value.

Recommended therapies

Surgical treatments

Concealment and surgery are the only procedures correcting the clinical aspect of androgenic alopecia within a short period of time. The current progress in hair loss should be assessed thoroughly before the intervention. In addition, the prognosis of an eventual relentless extent of the alopecia should be established as accurately as possible. Hair grafts (7–30 hairs), minigrafts (3–6 hairs) and micrografts (1–2 hairs) are the basic surgical approaches to correct androgenic alopecia. In cases of broad areas of baldness, alopecia reduction with or without scalp expansion can be performed prior to any transplanting or between sessions. Flap transpositions are also possible.

Hormonal medications

Most hormonal treatments which might improve androgenic alopecia are contraindicated in men. Oestroprogestatives are useful in women showing signs of hyperandrogeny. They may be offered in absence of hormonal pathology to young women requesting oral contraception. Similarly, hormone replacement therapy may appear adequate in some menopausal women. The goal of hormonal therapies in female androgenic alopecia is to slow down the progression of hair loss. Target hair follicles are no longer abated in their growth cycle, but miniaturized follicules which have been previously established do not enlarge with a new hormonal balance alone. When present, the response to treatment is slow. Hair shedding appears reduced but many patients return after some period of hormonal therapy expressing disappointment because alopecia is still present.

Oral contraceptives

Oral contraception acts on the hypothalamopituitary axis and reduces the androgen secretion by ovaries. Oestrogens also cause an increase in SHBG synthesis and a reduction in free testosterone. To be active in androgenic alopecia, oestrogen dosage should not be as low as in the contraceptive pills. The new progestogen derivatives (gestodene, norgestimate, desogestrel) are most appropriate because they do not cause significant androgen effects. Oestrogen–progesterone combinations, present in contraceptives, have limited benefit in controlling the development of androgenic alopecia when these compounds are used alone. The beneficial effect of oestrogen–progestogen combinations present in contraceptives is weak on the evolution of androgenic alopecia when these compounds are used alone. Very new contraceptive pills contain progestational derivatives such as drospirenone with antiandrogenic properties whose effect on hair follicle remain to be established. Dienogest is another compound with antiandrogenic activity.

Cyproterone acetate

Cyproterone acetate is an antiandrogen which is a powerful gonadotrophin inhibitor. It decreases the glandular androgen biosynthesis and acts also by competitive inhibition with DHT on its cytosolic receptor in target peripheral cells.

Cyproterone acetate is available in three dosages: 2, 10 and 50 mg. It is given in combination with cyclical therapy with an oestrogen (i.e. 0.035 mg ethinyloestradiol) or with a low-dose standard birth control pill. The reverse sequential regimen of taking the drug from day 5 to day 14 in conjunction with an oestrogen or birth control pill from day 5 to day 25 is the usual form of treatment. The efficacy of cyproterone acetate (up to 100 mg daily) with cyclical oestrogen therapy is unpredictable on androgenic alopecia in women. About 10% of patients require the drug to be discontinued due to intolerable side-effects (headache, nausea, depression, and so on).

Hormone replacement therapy
In menopausal women, the androgen levels are often low as are those of the other sexual hormones. Hormone replacement therapy using an oestrogen in combination with a non-androgenic progestogen can be proposed. Low-dose cyproterone acetate (1 mg) is also available in association with an oestrogen. Generally, hormone replacement therapy, given at menopause, provides an ancillary means for the management of androgenic alopecia.

Finasteride
Finasteride is a potent specific inhibitor of the 5α-reductase type II. It is used orally for the treatment of androgenic alopecia in men at the dosage of 1 mg o.d. At this dosage, it has been shown to lower DHT levels in the scalp and in the blood. Several studies have shown the efficacy of a 12-month treatment with finasteride in mild to moderate vertex alopecia in about 40% of men. The response of the frontal hairline is not so good. Continuous administration is necessary to maintain the benefit. Finasteride is usually well tolerated and adverse side-effects on sexual function (decreased libido, decreased ejaculation volume, erectile dysfunction) are globally estimated at 3.8% vs. 2.1% for placebo. Some other rare side-effects such as gynaecomastia have also been reported. Dosage of the prostate-specific antigen (PSA) used for monitoring prostatic hypertrophy is lowered during the treatment. Finasteride is contraindicated in women who are or may become pregnant. In postmenopausal women with androgenic alopecia, finasteride 1 mg o.d. taken over 12 months did not show efficacy.

Finasteride as a topical treatment using 0.005% and 0.05% solution remains so far disappointing.

Spironolactone
Spironolactone is an aldosterone antagonist. It inhibits partially the ovarian production of androgens and the 5α-reductase activity as well. It also competes for the androgen receptors in the hair follicles. Spironolactone is prescribed in dosages of 25 mg, two to four times a day to achieve total daily dosages ranging from 50 to 200 mg. Its efficacy on androgenic alopecia is unpredictable and it may take over 6 months before any appreciable improvement becomes noticeable. Spironolactone works best as an adjunct to oestrogen–progestogen therapy. However, its unwanted side-effects limit its use.

Non-hormonal medications

Minoxidil
Topical 2% minoxidil lotion is a well-established treatment for androgenic alopecia. Although the drug increases blood flow to the skin, it is its active metabolite minoxidil sulphate which directly stimulates follicular target cells probably acting as a potassium channel opener. However, the exact way by which minoxidil stimulates hair follicle remains hypothetical.

At a 2% concentration, it is recommended that 1 mg is applied twice daily. The best results are obtained in early androgenic alopecia in man and, as alone or in combination with hormonal treatment in woman. In good responders, a decrease in hair loss begins to be perceived after 3–5 months of treatment. The efficacy culminates after 1 year when a plateau effect is reached. The improvement is lost when treatment is stopped for 3–4 months.

Minoxidil is generally well tolerated. However, pruritus with or without erythema and desquamation can occur. These signs may be attributed to the reactivation of seborrhoeic dermatitis, to irritation or to contact allergic dermatitis to minoxidil, propyleneglycol or alcohol. Hypertrichosis of the temporal areas and cheeks may develop in sensitive women. This regresses within a few months once treatment has been stopped. Headaches and dizziness have been reported, but cardiovascular effects are apparently absent. However, a cautionary note should be given to patients with cardiopathy and those with hypertension taking oral guanethidine derivates or minoxidil. The same applies to patients suffering from a scalp dermatitis which might increase the drug resorption. Minoxidil should not be prescribed during pregnancy and breast feeding.

The minoxidil effect on androgenic alopecia is dose-dependent. The efficacy of a 5% formulation appears greater than with 2%, but secondary side-effects are apparently not more frequent. The 5% topical solution is only indicated in men having not responded to a 4-month treatment with the 2% formulation. The 5% topical solution is not indicated in woman because of the risk of facial hypertrichosis. The association between minoxidil and retinoic acid has been proposed to increase efficacy but the local tolerance is impaired and the risk of significant resorption is increased.

Alternative and experimental treatments

Antiandrogen therapy

Cimetidine

Cimetidine is a histamine H_2-receptor antagonist which has no direct hormonal activity. This molecule has, however, antiandrogenic properties acting as a peripheral blocker at the receptor level in the hair follicles. Cimetidine, prescribed at the dosage of 300 mg five times a day, has been effective in androgenic alopecia in women when used as an adjunct to a specific androgen suppressive therapy. Cimetidine has however, no recognized indication in androgenic alopecia.

Flutamide

The antiandrogen flutamide has been used for hirsutism. Its effect on androgenic alopecia in women has never been evaluated. This drug is not licensed for the treatment of androgenic alopecia.

Progesterone

Topical applications of a 0.5% progesterone formulation has no proven effect on androgenic alopecia although the drug aims at inhibiting the 5α-reductase activity. Moreover, antiandrogenic activity of orally administered progesterone is negligible at therapeutic dosage.

Zinc

Zinc is a 'secondary' inhibitor of 5α-reductase. It was proposed as a topical treatment in association with ancillary supplementations. No efficacy has been proven so far in androgenic alopecia.

Topical antimicrobials

The rationale for using some antimicrobial formulations for treating androgenic alopecia depends on clinical and histological observations. Patients with androgenic alopecia who also have superimposed seborrhoeic dermatitis often exhibit an increased hair loss. The skin surface and hair infundibula harbour a dense microflora enriched in *Malassezia ovalis* and various bacteria species. As a result, the inflammatory cell reaction adjacent to the hair follicles is enhanced. In such circumstances, a ketoconazole 2% shampoo and a lotion containing piroctone–olamine and trichlosan have shown some efficacy in limiting the hair loss and improving the hair density appearance.

Antifibrosing compound

Recently, the 2,4-diamino-pyrimidin-3-oxide, which is a minoxidil-related compound, was introduced with the claim that it has an antifibrosing action. Accordingly, it should facilitate the deep insertion of the anagen follicle into the skin. While, the results from preliminary trials are encouraging, we await for these to be substantiated by large-scale clinical studies.

Herbal preparation

A 7.5% herbal preparation (extract of fennel, polygonum, mentha, chamomile, thuja and hibiscus in a water-based cream) was reported to be effective in male pattern alopecia. The underlying mechanism is not biologically explained.

Ancillary supplementations

Some vitamins (A, B_5, B_6, H) and various amino acids (cystine, cysteine, methionine), have been advocated for the treatment of androgenic alopecia. In this context, their efficacy has never been demonstrated.

Shaping the future

New compounds are on the horizon. They are type I inhibitors and other type II inhibitors of 5α-reductase. Type I 5α-reductase is present in the sebaceous gland and at a lesser extent in the hair follicle. Its role in androgenic alopecia cannot be denied, even if the type II isoenzyme appears to predominate in hair follicle. Inhibiting both isoenzymes might be beneficial and new compounds with potent dual inhibitory activity are under development. Molecules acting as androgen receptor blockers including the topically active antiandrogen RU-58841 are another promising therapeutic approach. However, no current topical compound with antiandrogenic activity has brought satisfactory results. There is a need to search for more effective drug delivery systems following topical application of these compounds. Targeting more precisely the pilosebaceous unit is a fascinating goal for the future of hair loss and alopecia management.

Further reading

Amichai B, Grunwald MH, Sobel R. 5α-reductase inhibitors—a new hope in dermatology? *Int J Dermatol* 1997; 36: 182–4.

Barth JH. Should men still go bald gracefully? *Lancet* 2000; 355: 161–2.

Greenberg JH, Katz M. Treatment of androgenetic alopecia with a 7.5% herbal preparation. *J Dermatol Treat* 1996; 7: 159–62.

Guarrera M, Rebora A. Anagen hairs may fail to replace telogen hairs in early androgenetic female alopecia. *Dermatology* 1996; 192: 28–31.

Kaufman KD, Olsen EA, Whiting D *et al.* Finasteride in the treatment of men with androgenetic alopecia. *J Am Acad Dermatol* 1998; 39: 578–89.

Leyden J, Dunlap F, Miller B *et al.* Finasteride in the treatment of man with frontal male pattern hair loss. *J Am Acad Dermatol* 1999; 40: 930–7.

Mahé YF, Buan B, Bernard BA. A minoxidil-related compound lacking a C6 substitution still exhibit strong anti-lysyl hydroxylase activity in vitro. *Skin Pharmacol* 1996; 9: 177–83.

Mahé YF, Michelet JF, Billoni N *et al.* Androgenetic alopecia and microinflammation. *Int J Dermatol* 2000; 39: 576–84.

Mazzarella F, Loconsole F, Commisa A, Mastrolonardo M, Vena GA. Topical finasteride in the treatment of androgenic alopecia. Preliminary evaluations after 16 month therapy course. *J Dermatol Treat* 1997; 8: 189–92.

Niiyama S, Kojima K, Hamada T, Happle R, Hoffmann R. The novel drug CS891 inhibits 5α-reductase activity in freshly isolated dermal papilla of human hair follicles. *Eur J Dermatol* 2000; 10: 593–5.

Piérard GE, Piérard-Franchimont C, Nikkels-Tassoudji N, Nikkels AF, Saint Léger D. Improvement in the inflammatory aspect of androgenetic alopecia. A pilot study with an antimicrobial lotion. *J Dermatol Treat* 1996; 7: 153–7.

Piérard-Franchimont C, De Doncker P, Wallace R, Cauwenbergh G, Piérard GE. Ketoconazole shampoo: effect of long term use in male pattern alopecia. *Dermatology* 1998; 196: 474–7.

Price VH. Treatment of hair loss. *N Engl J Med* 1999; 341: 964–73.

Price VH, Menefee E, Strauss PC. Changes in hair weight and hair count in men with androgenetic alopecia, after application of 5% and 2% topical minoxidil, placebo, or no treatment. *J Am Acad Dermatol* 1999; 41: 717–21.

Price V, Roberts JL, Hordinsky M *et al*. Lack of efficacy of finasteride in post menopausal women with androgenetic alopecia. *J Am Acad Dermatol* 2000; 43: 768–76.

Rongioletti F, Guarrera M, Rebora A. Physiopathologie de l'alopécie androgénétique. *Ann Dermatol Venereol* 1998; 125: 33–7.

Sasson M, Shupack JL, Stiller MJ. Status of medical treatment for androgenetic alopecia. *Int J Dermatol* 1993; 32: 701–6.

Sawaya ME, Price VH. Different levels of 5α-reductase type I and II, aromatase and androgen receptor in hair follicles of women and men with androgenetic alopecia. *J Invest Dermatol* 1997; 109: 296–300.

Shaw JC. Spironolactone in dermatologic therapy. *J Am Acad Dermatol* 1991; 24: 236–43.

Sufki H, Stoudemayer T, Kligman AM, Murphy GF. Quantitative and ultrastructural analysis at inflammatory infiltrates in male pattern alopecia. *Acta Derm Venereol* 1999; 79: 347–50.

Unger WP. What's new in hair replacement surgery? *Dermatol Clin* 1996; 14 (4): 783–802.

Antiphospholipid syndrome

P.G. Vlachoyiannopoulos and H.M. Moutsopoulos

Definition and epidemiology

Antiphospholipid (anticardiolipin) syndrome (APS) is a chronic disorder associated with recurrent venous and/or arterial thrombosis, recurrent abortions, thrombocytopenia and/or autoimmune haemolytic anaemia and positive results are obtained from tests for antiphospholipid (aPL) antibodies and/or lupus anticoagulant (LA). The disease can occur alone (primary APS) or in association with other systemic autoimmune diseases, especially systemic lupus erythematosus (SLE) (secondary APS).

Less than one-third of patients with SLE possess aPL antibodies and one-third of them develop APS. Nearly one-third of new cases with strokes under the age of 50, 15% of all episodes of deep vein thrombosis, and nearly 10% of women with recurrent fetal losses may have APS.

Aetiology and pathophysiology

The disease-related features are linked to the prethrombotic (or thrombogenic) effects of aPL antibodies. Why these antibodies are produced is unknown. The thrombogenic aPL antibodies recognize phospholipids usually in complex with a plasma inhibitor of coagulation known as β_2-glycoprotein I (β_2-GPI). However, it is not well known whether the potential antithrombotic effect of β_2-GPI is clinically significant.

Therefore a number of pleotropic effects of aPL antibodies on the clotting cascade have been considered: (a) direct injury of the endothelium and/or reduction of prostacyclin production; (b) activation of the endothelium to a procoagulant stage, by inducing transient expression of adhesion molecules and tissue factor (TF), which triggers the initiation of the exogenous coagulation cascade; (c) platelet activation; and (d) inhibition of the function of various phospholipid-binding proteins which control coagulation (such as protein C, protein S, antithrombin III or annexin V).

Clinical characteristics and course

Thrombosis of veins and/or arteries of any size may occur. Features related to vein thrombosis are the following.

- deep or superficial vein thrombosis, usually of the lower extremities
- pulmonary emboli/pulmonary infarcts
- nephrotic syndrome due to thrombosis of both renal arteries
- Budd–Chiari syndrome and ascites due to hepatic vein thrombosis
- thrombosis of the inferior vena cava
- pulmonary hypertension due to microthrombi in the pulmonary arterioles.

Features related to arterial thrombosis are:

- cerebral infarctions which are expressed either as strokes, as multi-infarct dementia, or episodes of transient confusion
- myocardial infarctions
- peripheral gangrene
- bowel infarction with clinical features of peritonitis
- scotomas due to ophthalmic artery occlusion
- kidney dysfunction due to occlusion of large-, medium- or small-sized renal arteries, expressed as tubulointerstitial or glomerular dysfunction.

Skin infarcts

The most characteristic clinical sign from the skin is a persistent cyanotic mottling of the skin, affecting the extremities and the trunk which is known as livedo reticularis.

It is accentuated by cold exposure but it occurs also at usual environmental temperatures; it is related to vasospasm. Skin infarcts expressed as subepidermal nodules associated with the erythematous appearance of the above skin and skin ulcers derived from infarcts of small- and medium-sized arteries. Peripheral gangrene is the result of thrombosis in medium- and large-sized arteries. Non-palpable purpura may occur because of thrombocytopenia.

Pregnancy loss, especially in the second trimester, as well as giving birth to still-born or premature babies are also associated with the syndrome.

Diagnosis

To establish the diagnosis the patient should fullfil at least two criteria (one clinical and one laboratory) from the following:

1 Clinical
   - arterial or venous thrombosis
   - unexplained fetal loss.
2 Laboratory
   - lupus anticoagulant
   - immunoglobulin G (IgG) and/or IgM anticardiolipin (aCL) antibodies.

Antibodies to phospholipids are usually detected in enzyme-linked immunosorbent assays (ELISAs) using as antigen the phospholipid cardiolipin (aCL antibodies). It has been shown that cardiolipin is simply a factor stabilizing on to the ELISA plates the real antigen recognized by the aPL antibodies; this antigen is the α_2-GPI as well as other phospholipid-binding proteins, which exist in abundance in the human serum under testing, as well as in the bovine serum used as the 'blocking factor' in the aCL ELISA. Recently, specific anti-α_2-GPI ELISA assays have been proposed to detect specific anti-α_2-GPI antibodies; a high anti-α_2-GPI serum reactivity obtained by such assays rather associated with APS than the aCL reactivity. The LA test measures the activity of aPL antibodies to inhibit *in vitro* the conversion of prothrombin to thrombin having as a result the prolongation of the partial thromboplastin time (PTT); the result is not corrected by adding normal plasma. A prolonged PTT is a measure of LA activity of the serum. Other tests to measure LA activity are the kaolin clotting time or the Russel viper venom time. Antibodies of the type of LA recognize mainly prothrombin.

Differential diagnosis

Two per cent of the general population, 50% of the elderly population, 6% of pregnant women, 8% of psychiatric patients, 30% of psychiatric patients taking phenothiazines, 60% of patients with acquired immune deficiency syndrome (AIDS), and various percentages of patients with bacterial or viral infections possess aCL antibodies. These antibodies are not usually thrombogenic. On the other hand, even among APS patients, levels of aCL antibodies may be negative for long periods or for a short period preceding thrombosis. Therefore other causes of thrombosis or ischaemia should be excluded either in the absence or presence of aCL antibodies (Table 1).

Other causes of thrombocytopenia should be excluded (Table 2).

Other causes of Coombs' positive haemolytic anaemia should be excluded (Table 3).

Treatment

General therapeutic guidelines

Agents inducing thrombosis should be eliminated. High cholesterol levels should be treated initially by diet and where this fails, with cholesterol-lowering drugs. The patient's weight should be as close to the ideal weight as possible. Oestrogen-containing pills should be avoided. Smoking should be discontinued. Diabetes should be treated appropriately. If the patient undergoes surgery it

Table 1 Other causes of thrombosis and ischaemia to be excluded

Atherosclerosis	Older age, aortic valve calcifications, hypercholesterolaemia, diabetes mellitus
Systemic vasculitis	Inflammatory vasculitis lesions in biopsy specimens from affected organs
Cardiac valve vegetations, endocarditis	Cardiac ultrasound, blood cultures positive
Cardiac myxoma	Cardiac ultrasound, surgical repair, biopsy
Protein C and S deficiency	Very low levels of proteins C and S (*Note*: reduction of proteins C and S levels occurs in APS and SLE patients with aPL antibodies, but not as impressive as it is in primary protein C and protein S deficiency)
Burger's disease	Usually men, heavy smokers. Biopsy: thrombangiitis obliterans
Homocystinuria	Dislocated optic lenses for homozygotes, mental retardation, ill-defined behavioural changes. The cyanide–nitroprusside test is a simple way to demonstrate increased excretion of sulfhydryl-containing compounds in urine
Nephrotic syndrome	24-h urine protein > 3 g (*Note*: the nephrotic syndrome may be the cause, but also the result of thrombosis)
Malignancy	Search for malignancy of the lung, stomach, pancreas
Thrombotic thrombocytopenic purpura (TTP)	Haemolytic anaemia, fragmented and nucleated red blood cells, thrombocytopenia fever, central nervous system disease from mental disorientation to coma and renal dysfunction. The PTT is usually normal (*Note*: haemolytic anaemia and thrombocytopenia, as well as TTP itself may be features of APS)

Table 2 Other causes of thrombocytopenia to be excluded

Idiopathic thrombocytopenic purpura (ITP)	Antibodies to platelets; large numbers of megacaryocytes in bone marrow (*Note*: ITP can be a feature of APS)
Systemic lupus erythematosus (SLE)	The APS can be a feature of SLE (secondary APS). The therapy is not different. Antinuclear antibodies and antibodies to double-stranded DNA favour the diagnosis of SLE
Leukaemias	Peripheral blood smear and bone marrow examination

Table 3 Other causes of Coombs' positive haemolytic anaemia to be excluded

SLE	As described earlier
Advanced Hodgkin's disease	Histological diagnosis
Drugs	α-methyldopa: Usually Coombs' positive, but not clinically significant anaemia
	Penicillin-type antibiotics History
	Quinidine type drugs History

is imperative to prescribe a prophylactic dose of heparin, 5000 units twice daily as long as the patient is unable to walk. In case of APS secondary to other systemic autoimmune diseases, the primary disease should be under control.

Recommended therapies

Treatment and prevention of venous thrombotic events

Initial management is 5000 units bolus i.v. followed by 1000–1200 units per hour;

continuous infusion is preferable. The PTT is not a suitable test to evaluate the intensity of therapy, because PTT is prolonged in APS patients. In this case, heparin plasma levels can be obtained. When these levels reach 0.4 units/mL, usually in 1 or 2 days after initial treatment, warfarin therapy can be initiated. This should be given for 2–3 days in parallel with heparin and alone thereafter. The dose of warfarin is individualized with the following aim: the prothrombin time (PT) of the patient should be as high as to obtain an international normalized ratio (INR) higher than 2.9. The INR is calculated as the ratio: PT (patient)/mean normal PT. Mean normal PT is the PT obtained by different laboratories examining normal plasmas providing that these laboratories used thromboplastin reagents, having the same international sensitivity index (ISI) value. Thrombotic recurrences have occurred even at INR 2.5; on the other hand, the risk for haemorrhage increases at INR values above 3. Therefore some authors recommend an intensity of treatment with INR values between 2.6 and 3.0, while others favour higher intensity treatments (INR above 3.0). Treatment of patients with APS for preventing thrombotic recurrences should be for life.

Treatment and prevention of arterial thrombotic events

Initially treatment with heparin is recommended for venous thrombotic events. When heparin plasma levels reach 0.4 units/mL, warfarin is initiated with an intensity of INR 2.9–3.5. Some authors add aspirin 325 mg daily and the combination has been slightly more effective than warfarin alone in preventing thrombotic recurrences, while the risk of haemorrhage did not increase. Treatment should continue for idefinite periods.

Treatment of skin manifestations

Livedo reticularis alone does not require treatment. It is, however, a sign strongly related to the syndrome. Patients with skin infarcts, transient ischaemic attacks or abdominal pain should be carefully evaluated for APS because early vigorous treatment is imperative. Skin infarcts, skin ulcers and gangrene should be treated with intensive antithrombotic treatment.

Treatment of thrombocytopenia

Mild thrombocytopenia (platelet counts 50 000–150 000 per mm^3) does not require therapy. For platelet counts between 20 000 and 50 000 per mm^3 there is a higher risk for development of severe thrombocytopenia and we recommend prednisolone 10 mg/day and azathioprine 100–150 mg/day. To initiate azathioprine treatment 50 mg/day azathioprine is given for 1 week and complete blood count and platelet count are obtained. If haematocrit and white blood cell count are within normal limits increasing of the azathioprine dose to 100 mg and later to 150 mg daily is recommended.

In case of severe thrombocytopenia with purpura and/or haemorrhage 1 g of methylprednisolone i.v. for 3 days is recommended, followed by 60 mg of prednisolone per day and tapering according to the clinical setting. If the pulses of methylprednisolone are ineffective, i.v. pulses of immunoglobulin at a dose of 0.4 g/kg per day for 5 days should be given. In case of no response i.v. pulses of cyclosphophamide 0.25 g/m^2 per month are recommended. Patients with severe thrombocytopenia unresponsive to the previous measures may need splenectomy.

Treatment of pregnant women with APS to prevent fetal loss

Prednisolone 10 mg daily with heparin 5000 units s.c. twice daily with 80 mg of aspirin significantly reduced fetal losses. The group of women with prenisolone, however, is characterized by a higher prevalence of premature infants. Patients receiving heparin should also receive vitamin D (0.25 μg $1,1(OH)_2D_3$/daily) and calcium (500 mg daily).

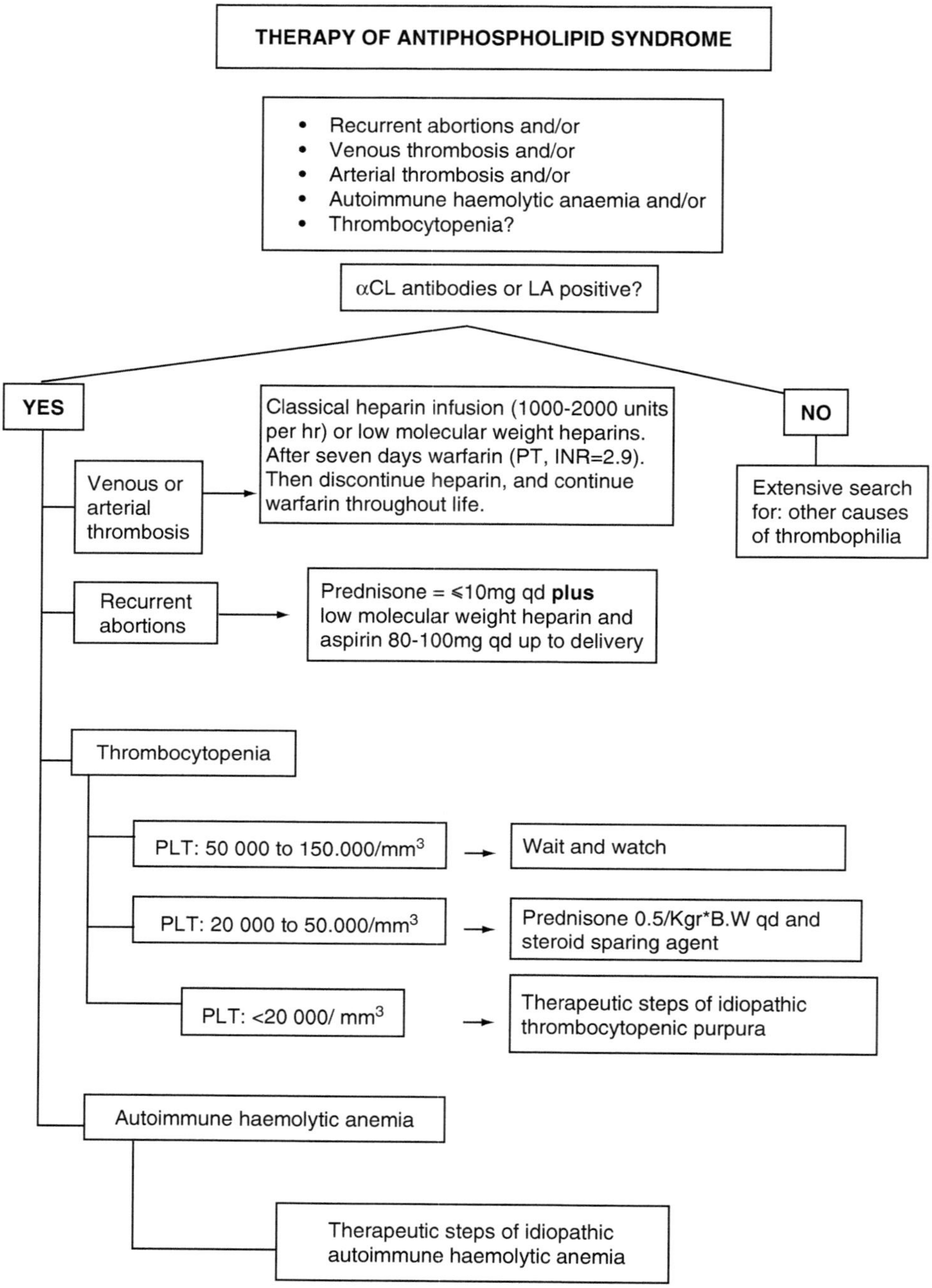
THERAPY OF ANTIPHOSPHOLIPID SYNDROME
• Recurrent abortions and/or
• Venous thrombosis and/or
• Arterial thrombosis and/or
• Autoimmune haemolytic anaemia and/or
• Thrombocytopenia?
αCL antibodies or LA positive?
YES
NO
Extensive search for: other causes of thrombophilia
Venous or arterial thrombosis
Classical heparin infusion (1000-2000 units per hr) or low molecular weight heparins. After seven days warfarin (PT, INR=2.9). Then discontinue heparin, and continue warfarin throughout life.
Recurrent abortions
Prednisone = ≤10mg qd **plus** low molecular weight heparin and aspirin 80-100mg qd up to delivery
Thrombocytopenia
PLT: 50 000 to 150.000/mm³
Wait and watch
PLT: 20 000 to 50.000/mm³
Prednisone 0.5/Kgr*B.W qd and steroid sparing agent
PLT: <20 000/ mm³
Therapeutic steps of idiopathic thrombocytopenic purpura
Autoimmune haemolytic anemia
Therapeutic steps of idiopathic autoimmune haemolytic anemia

Alternative and experimental treatments

Intravenous immunoglobulin therapy

Although it is recognized as one of the therapeutic strategies for the thrombocytopenia it remains an experimental treatment for preventing fetal loss. Immunoglobulin pulses in a dose of 0.4 g/kg per day for 4–5 days per month for the duration of pregancy is recommended. Aspirin 80 mg daily with or without heparin is administered as previously described.

Azathioprine and cyclophosphamide

Helpful in treating thrombocytopenia; there is no evidence that these immunosuppressive agents can prevent thrombotic recurrences. Some authors recommend such therapies in addition to a complete antithrombotic therapy, if thrombotic recurrences still occur, despite the antithrombotic regimens.

Further reading

Boumpas DJ, Basez S, Klippel JH, Balow E. Intermittent cyclophosphamide for the treatment of autoimmune thrombocytopenia in systemic lupus erythematosus. *Ann Intern Med* 1990; 112: 674–7.

Choi CW, Kim BS, Seo JH *et al*. Response to high-dose intravenous immune globulin as a valuable factor predicting the effect of splenectomy in chronic idiopathic thrombocytopenic purpura patients. *Am J Hematol* 2001; 66: 197–202.

Harris EN. Management of the antiphospholipid syndrome. In: van de Putte LBA, Furst DE, Williams HJ, van Riel PLCM, eds. *Therapy of Systemic Rheumatic Disorders*. New York: Marcel Dekker, 1997: 629–56.

Laskin CA, Bombardieri C, Hannah M *et al*. Prednisone and aspirin in women with autoantibodies and unexplained recurrent fetal loss. *N Engl J Med* 1997; 337: 148–52.

Rosove MH, Brewer PMC. Antiphospholipid thrombosis: clinical course after the first thrombotic event in 70 patients. *Ann Intern Med* 1992; 17: 303–8.

Vlachoyiannopoulos PG, Tsiakou E, Chalevelakis G, Raptis SA, Moutsopoulos HM. Antiphospholipid syndrome. Clinical and therapeutic aspects. *Lupus* 1993; 3: 91–6.

Aphthous stomatitis

G. Laskaris

Definition and epidemiology

Recurrent aphthous stomatitis (RAS) or recurrent aphthous ulcers (RAU) are painful oral ulcerations that characteristically recur at intervals ranging from days to months or even years. They represent the most common lesion of the oral mucosa with an overall prevalence; ranging from 15 to 30%. Females are more commonly affected than males and although they may begin at any age, they usually start during the second and third decades of life. Familial occurrence is common and about 30–40% of the patients with RAS have another affected family member.

Aetiology and pathophysiology

Although RAS is one of the oldest oral diseases known from the time of Hippocrates, its aetiology still remains unclear. Many predisposing factors have been incriminated such as genetics, trauma, food hypersensitivities, stress, infections (*Streptococcus sanguis* and *S. mitis*, herpes simplex virus-1 (HSV-1), varicella-zoster virus (VZV), cytomegalovirus), systemic factors (Behçet's disease), gastrointestinal disorders, some nutritional deficiencies, cyclic neutropenia, blood deficiencies, Sweet's syndrome, human immunodeficiency virus (HIV) infection, hormonal changes, immunological disorders and others. Although these predisposing factors may play a role in the developments of RAS, the disease is idiopathic and its aetiology is unknown. Accumulated data support the concept that the pathophysiology is immunologically mediated and that the cell-mediated immune response is dysregulated.

In addition several reports show a negative association between RAS and smoking.

Clinical characteristics and course

The main clinical features of RAS are the recurrence of painful oral ulcerations at intervals ranging from days to weeks or even months. The prodromal stage is variable and is usually characterized by discomfort and occasionally erythema of 1–3 days duration. This stage is soon followed by a painful oral ulcer.

The lesions are usually confined to movable non-keratinized or poorly keratinized oral mucosa, e.g. the buccal mucosa, the labial mucosa, tongue, floor of the mouth, soft palate and uvula. Occasionally the attached gingiva and the hard palate may also be involved. The lesions usually begin in childhood or adolescence and have a slight predilection for females. Clinicians should keep in mind that RAS may be associated with the following systemic disorders:

- Behçet's disease
- Sweet's syndrome
- FAPA syndrome
- Crohn's disease
- ulcerative colitis
- coeliac disease
- HIV infection
- malabsorption syndromes
- haematinic deficiencies
- neutropenias.

Based on clinical criteria, recurrent aphthae are classified into three forms: minor, major and herpertiform ulcers.

Minor RAS

This is the most common form of the disease. It is clinically characterized by a shallow oval and painful ulcer 2–6 mm in diameter. The ulcer is covered by a yellow–white necrotic membrane and is surrounded by an erythematous halo. Ulcers may be single or multiple (2–6); they persist for 6–10 days, heal with no evidence of scarring and recur usually at 1–5-month intervals.

Major RAS

This is much less commonly encountered and represents the severe form of RAS. The ulcers are deep, extremely painful, 1–2 cm in diameter and their number varies from one to three. They last approximately 3–6 weeks and occasionally leave a scar on healing and often recur, at 1–3-month intervals.

Herpetiform ulcers

These belong to the least common variety of RAS. The lesions present as multiple (10–100 or more), shallow ulcers, 1–3 mm in diameter and characteristically tend to occur in clusters. The ulcers persist for 1–2 weeks, often recur over a period of 1–3 years and are more commonly seen in females. The onset is at an older age than the other forms of RAS.

Diagnosis

The diagnosis of all three forms of aphthous stomatitis is based exclusively on clinical criteria, as there is no specific diagnostic test, unless there is an underlying systemic disease.

Differential diagnosis

See Table 1.

Treatment

General therapeutic guidelines

- It is important in managing RAS to rule out aphthous-like ulcers associated with systemic diseases. The great majority of patients with RAS are healthy individuals without a history or signs of a systemic disease.
- Successful therapy for RAS requires a correct diagnosis and control of the contributing aetiological factors.
- A wide spectrum of therapeutic regimes or agents have been suggested, but the management of RAS is unsatisfactory, as there is no cure and all attempts are palliative.
- The goal of treatment should be (a) elimination of pain and discomfort; (b) shortening of the course; and (c) avoidance of recurrence.

Recommended therapies

Control of possible contributing aetiological factors

Patients should be encouraged to keep a food diary in an attempt to identify a potential precipitating link with the onset of aphthous ulcers. Patients should avoid minor trauma of the oral mucosa. Stress and female sex hormonal changes should also be controlled. A gluten-free diet may be useful in controlling lesions even in the absence of coeliac disease.

Topical measures

Topical medications may reduce pain and shorten the course, but they do not prevent recurrence.

Topical anaesthetics such as 2% viscous lidocaine (lignocaine), benzocaine and benzydamine hydrochloride may reduce pain only for a short time. Recently, 5% amlexanox oral paste, 3% diclofenac in 2.5% hyaluronan have also been used to reduce pain. Topical tetracyclines have been used with partial success. A 250-mg capsule is dissolved in 30 mL of water. Then 5 mL of the solution is used to rinse the lesion four to six times a day. This is repeated for 3–5 days. Many other anti-inflammatory and antimicrobial agents (chlorhexidine, Listerine) have also been used with unsatisfactory results. The best of the topical treatments is 0.1% triamcinolone acetonide in an oral adhesive base (Orabase) or fluocinonide gel (Lidex gel) or clobetasol propionate gel 0.05% (Temovate) applied to the ulcer three to six times a day for 4–6 days. Intralesional injection of triamcinolone accetonide retard or betamethasone dipropionate and sodium phosphate retard may be successfully used only in major aphthous ulcers.

Table 1 The differential diagnosis of aphthous stomatitis

Traumatic ulcer	History, clinical features, histopathological examination
Primary and secondary herpetic stomatitis	History, clinical features, serum viral antibody tests, viral cultures
Hand, foot and mouth disease	Clinical evaluation, viral cultures
Herpangina	Clinical evaluation, viral cultures
Erythema multiforme	Clinical features, histopathological examination
Pemphigus	Clinical features, histopathological examination, direct and indirect immunofluorescence
Pemphigoid	Clinical features, histopathological examination, direct and indirect immunofluorescent tests
Syphilis	Clinical evaluation, microbiology, serological tests
Behçet's disease	Clinical features, histopathological examination, HLA antigens
Crohn's disease	Clinical evaluation, histopathological examination
Ulcerative colitis	Clinical evaluation, histopathological examination
Cyclic neutropenia	Clinical evaluation, repeated determination of neutrophils in the peripheral blood

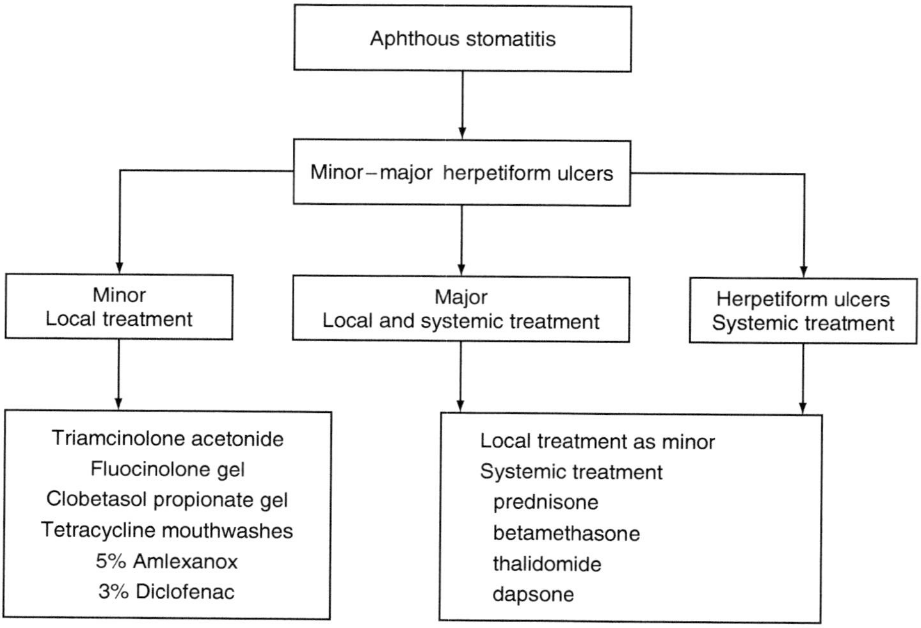

Systemic measures

Systemic corticosteroids (prednisone, betamethasone) in an average dose of 20–30 mg or 2–3 mg, respectively, for 4–8 days is very helpful for major ulcers or herpetiform ulcers. In cases of repeated episodes and when new ulcers occur before the previous ones have healed, systemic medications may prove useful in preventing new lesions.

In my experience 20 mg predisone or 2 mg betamethasone for 10–15 days and then an injection of betamethasone dipropionate and sodium phosphate retard every 2 weeks for a period of 2 months may significantly increase the time intervals between recurrence. Long-term systemic corticosteroid is contraindicated because of its side-effects.

In severe cases with a high recurrence rate and in HIV-infected patients, thalidomide 100–300 mg/day for 2–3 months may result in complete remission of the ulcers for a long time. However teratogenesis and polyneuropathy preclude the routine use of thalidomide.

Clinicians should know that safe prophylaxis of RAS recurrence for a long time is not available.

Alternative and experimental treatments

In severe cases, many other systemic medications have been used with ambiguous results. These include:

- dapsone 25–50 mg/day for several weeks
- levamisole hydrochloride
- azathioprine
- colchicine
- interferon-α
- ciclosporin
- pentoxifilline
- aciclovir
- etretinate.

Further reading

Ball SC, Sepkowitz KA, Jacobs JL. Thalidomide for treatment of oral aphthous ulcers in patients with human immunodeficiency virus: case report and review. *Am J Gastroenterol* 1997; 92: 169–70.

Brown RS, Bottomley WK. Combination immunosuppressant and topical steroid therapy for treatment of recurrent major aphthae. *Oral Surg Oral Med Oral Pathol* 1990; 69: 42–4.

Haeyrinen-Immonen R, Sorsa T, Pettilae J *et al.* Effect of tetracycline on collagenase activity in patients with recurrent aphthous ulcers. *J Oral Pathol Med* 1994; 23: 269–72.

Laskaris G. *Color Atlas of Oral Diseases*, 2nd edn. Stuttgart: Thieme, 1994: 177–8.

Laskaris G. Advances in the classification and treatment of recurrent aphthous ulcers. *Balk J Stomatol* 1999; 3: 83–4.

Paterson DL, Georghiou PR, Allworth AM, Kemp RJ. Thalidomide as treatment of refractory aphthous ulceration related to human immunodeficiency virus infection. *Clin Infect Dis* 1995; 20: 250–4.

Porter SR, Scully C. Aphthous stomatitis—an overview of aetiopathogenesis and management. *Clin Exp Dermatol* 1991; 16: 235–43.

Rees TD, Binnie WH. Recurrent aphthous stomatitis. *Dermatol Clin* 1996; 14: 243–56.

Vincent SD, Lilly GE. Clinical, historic and therapeutic features of aphthous stomatitis. *Oral Surg Oral Med Oral Pathol* 1992; 74: 79–86.

Woo SB, Sonis ST. Recurrent aphthous ulcers. a review of diagnosis and treatment. *J Am Dermatol Acad* 1996; 127: 1202–13.

Apocrine miliaria

H.R. Bruckbauer and H.-J. Vogt

Definition and epidemiology

This is a chronic papulous disorder of the apocrine glands appearing especially in young women between puberty and menopause. Remissions during pregnancy have been observed.

Aetiology and pathophysiology

Apocrine miliaria is characterized by intraepidermal occlusion of the excretion ducts of the apocrine glands. As a result, apocrine anhidrosis and intraepidermal rupture of sweat retention vesicles can be found.

Clinical characteristics and course

At the sites of apocrine glands (axillary, genital, anal, periumbilical, perimamillary) pruritic, erythematous papules occur on the follicles, depending on the activity of the glands. Typical are apocrine anhidrosis and provocation of pruritus after emotional, physical or pharmacological (epinephrine (adrenaline) 0.1 mg intradermal) stress. Subsequently cysts, lichenification and impetiginization can be observed. Hair growth in the affected regions is often sparse. Histology shows distal occlusion of the ducts of apocrine glands with intraepidermal vesiculation (apocrine sweat retention vesicle) and non-specific inflammatory infiltration.

Apocrine miliaria is a chronic disease with a rarely remitting course during pregnancy. Premenstrual deterioration can be noted; postmenopausal regression can be expected.

Diagnosis

The diagnosis is based on the typical clinical characteristics and the restricted distribution of eruption to apocrine areas with follicular and parafollicular orientation of the papules. Histopathological findings confirm the diagnosis; transverse histological sections can be helpful.

Differential diagnosis

This includes dyskeratosis follicularis (Darier's disease), acanthosis nigricans, lichen planus, syringomas and pseudo-Fox–Fordyce disease (induced by zirconium- or aluminium-containing deodorants). These can usually be distinguished by the history, typical distribution and histology. Ectopic apocrine glands sometimes may cause diagnostic problems.

Treatment

The treatment of apocrine miliaria is difficult. Topical glucocorticoids show limited success. They are effective when they are administered intralesionally (triamcinolone acetonide crystalline suspension) or systemically (high doses necessary and relapse must be expected when therapy is stopped).

Topical antibiotic and antiseptic solutions help prevent superinfections.

Good effects could be observed with topical vitamin A acid (tretinoin) 0.1% in cream. It shows good antipruritic effects and normalizes the hair growth, but shows only minor effects on the papules.

Oral contraceptives show good effects in apocrine miliaria of women, especially when oestrogen–progesterone combinations are applied. Relapse is to be expected when the drug is stopped.

In treatment-resistant cases plastic surgical ablation with skin transplantation should be considered.

Further reading

Braun-Falco O, Plewig G, Wolf HH. *Dermatologie und Venerologie,* 4th edn. Berlin: Springer, 1996.

Feng E, Janniger CK. Miliaria. *Cutis* 1995; 55: 213–16.

Henning DR, Griffin TB, Maibach HI. Studies on changes in skin surface bacteria induced

miliaria and associated hypohidrosis. *Acta Dermatovener (Stockh)* 1972; 52: 371–5.
Hölzle E, Kligman AG. The pathogenesis of miliaria rubra. *Br J Dermatol* 1978; 99: 117.
Kirk JF, Wilson BB, Chun W, Cooper P. Miliaria profunda. *J Am Acad Dermatol* 1996; 35: 854–6.
Mayser P, Gründer K, Nilles M, Schill W-B. Morbus Fox-Fordyce (Apokrine Miliaria). *Hautarzt* 1993; 44: 309–11.
Mowald CM, McGinley KJ, Foglia A, Leyden JJ. The role of extracellular polysaccharide substance produced by *Staphylococcus epidermidis* in miliaria. *J Am Acad Dermatol* 1995; 33: 729–33.
Orfanos CE, Garbe C. *Therapie der Hautkrankheiten.* Berlin: Springer, 1995.
Shelley WB, Levy EJ. Apocrine sweat retention in man. II. Fox-Fordyce disease (apocrine miliaria). *Arch Dermatol* 1956; 73: 38–49.
Shuster S. Duct disruption, a new explanation of Miliaria. *Acta Derm Venereol (Stockh)* 1997; 77: 1–3.
Stashower LM, Krivda MS, Turiansky LG. Fox-Fordyce disease: diagnosis with transverse histologic sections. *J Am Acad Dermatol* 2000; 42: 89–91.

Atopic dermatitis

E.J.M. Van Leent and J.D. Bos

Synonyms

Atopic eczema, neurodermatitis, prurigo Besnier.

Definition and epidemiology

Atopic dermatitis is a chronic, itching skin disease with a relapsing course. It forms part of the atopic syndrome, also known as atopy. Other clinical manifestations of atopy are allergic rhinitis (hay fever), allergic (extrinsic) asthma, certain gastrointestinal allergies and allergic conjunctivitis. Associated disorders include anaphylaxis, urticaria and dyshidrotic eczema, as well as a variety of other symptoms and signs known as the minor criteria of Hanifin and Rajka.

Clinical and laboratory criteria have been developed for the definition of atopic dermatitis. The most widely used are those of Hanifin and Rajka as listed later in this chapter. Recently, the millennium criteria for the diagnosis of atopic eczema were defined as outlined in Table 1.

In the millenium criteria, emphasis is given to the presence of allergen-specific immunoglobulin E (IgE) in the patient. When present, the patient has truly atopic eczema (also known as extrinsic atopic eczema) and recommendation of allergen avoidance makes sense. When allergen-specific IgE cannot be detected, the diagnosis of intrinsic atopic dermatitis is sometimes used, but we prefer to designate such patients as having atopiform dermatitis. They have no atopy and allergen avoidance does not make sense.

It is to be predicted that in the future, when a more precise knowledge of the multigenic background of atopy and atopic dermatitis has surfaced, genetic criteria will replace both immunological and clinical criteria. Atopic dermatitis is one of the most common skin diseases with a lifetime prevalence of up to 30%. Its incidence is increasing in Western countries. The highest incidence is among children. When one or two parents have atopic dermatitis, the prevalence in children is 6% and 81%, respectively.

Aetiology and pathophysiology

Atopic dermatitis is a common disease entity forming part of a syndrome called atopy. A major immunological abnormality is the skewing, within the secondary immune organs (lymphoid tissues) of T-helper cell type 0 (Th0) cells towards Th2 lymphocytes, upon allergenic challenge. As a result, Th2 cells dominate the central responses, and through their specific cytokine secretion profile, induce B cells to produce allergen-specific IgE. These molecules are secreted into the circulation and will then sensitize different organs, by binding via FCϵRI receptors on mast cells and dendritic cells (including Langerhans' cells). Allergenic challenge of a particular organ then leads to local allergic responses such as atopic dermatitis.

Table 1 The millenium criteria for the diagnosis of atopic dermatitis

1 Mandatory criteria: presence of allergen-specific IgE:
- historical, actual or expected (in very young children)
- in peripheral blood (RAST, ELISA) or in skin (intracutaneous challenge)

2 Principal criteria (two of three present):
- typical distribution and morphology of eczema lesions: infant, childhood or adult type
- if distribution is not typical, exclude other entity (dyshidrotic eczema, contact dermatitis, contact urticaria)
- pruritus
- chronic or chronically relapsing course

Within involved skin, a complex interplay between Th1 cells, Th2 cells, dendritic cells and mast cells leads to inflammation, and atopic allergens are thought to play a role. Dendritic cells facilitate antigen processing (antigen focusing), by trapping of allergens through FCeRI receptor-bound IgE. A major question open for research is whether this induction of immune responses and inflammation is indeed by nanoquantities of allergens present in skin, or that there is cross-reactivity with endogenous autoantigens that share epitope specificity with atopic allergens. It is clear that allergic reactions in particular to aeroallergens may play a role in the pathogenesis of the disease. On the other hand there are exogenous triggering factors like irritants, stress, pollutants and foods.

The atopy syndrome thus may be seen as a Th2 disease, while atopic dermatitis may be seen as the resulting IgE-mediated skin disorder. However, there are a number of patients (10% in some studies), who have atopic dermatitis clinically (and fulfilling the Hanifin and Rajka criteria), but allergen-specific IgE cannot be demonstrated in them. Some investigators therefore assume that IgE is not central in atopic dermatitis immunopathogenesis. In these allergen-specific IgE-negative patients, there is atopy-specific Th2 polarization, but the Th2 cells do not produce sufficient amounts of interleukin-4 (IL-4) and/or IL-13, cytokines responsible for the IgM–IgE shift in B cells, although they do produce IL-5 and do not produce interferon-γ (IFN-γ), making them Th2 cells of a special subset.

Another explanation for the lack of discernible allergen-specific IgE in a limited subset of patients might be that we do not know the allergens in these patients that are responsible for the disease. Thus, there is no substrate for further testing and detecting allergen-specific IgE. Finally, it may be that these patients have no atopy at all, and have a disease clinically similar to atopic dermatitis. Analogous to psoriasis and psoriasiform dermatitis, one might diagnose these patients as having atopiform dermatitis, as stated above.

Clinical characteristics and course

Atopic dermatitis is an itching, inflammatory skin disorder which usually starts in early childhood. The infant phase usually starts during the third month and is characterized by dry red scaling areas on the cheeks and chin, sparing the perioral and paranasal region. More severe cases show generalized papulation, redness, scaling, vesicles and crusts. The nappy area is usually spared. Exudative lesions typical of the infant phase are not as common in the childhood phase. The childhood phase is characterized by inflammation in flexural areas with depigmentation and the first signs of lichenification. The intense itch initiates the itch–scratch cycle. Marks of the adult phase are flexural inflammation, hand and/or foot dermatitis, inflammation around the eyes and lichenification of the anogenital area.

The dermatitis improves in most children. At the age of 18 months 50% of the patients have their disease completely resolved. Unfavourable prognostic factors are:

- persistent dry or itchy skin
- widespread dermatitis
- associated allergic rhinitis
- family history of atopic dermatitis
- asthma
- early age of onset and female sex.

Most patients are in remission by the age of 30. In a few patients the disease becomes a lifelong chronic disease with periods of exacerbation and remission often related to the seasons.

Diagnosis

Since there are no laboratory tests available to confirm the diagnosis, this is made clinically, for which diagnostic features were published in 1980 by Hanifan and

Rajka. These are generally used for clinical research. Major criteria include:

- pruritus
- flexural lichenification
- chronically relapsing course
- a personal or family history of atopy.

There are 23 minor criteria, the most relevant of which are:

- xerosis
- ichthyosis
- immediate skin test reactivity
- elevated serum IgE
- early age of onset
- tendency for developing cutaneous infections
- tendency for developing non-specific hand or foot dermatitis
- Dennie–Morgan infraorbital fold
- keratoconus
- anterior subcapsular cataracts
- orbital darkening
- facial pallor/erythema
- pityriasis alba
- itch when sweating
- intolerance to wool and lipid solvents
- perifollicular accentuation
- food intolerance
- the influence of emotional factors
- white dermographism/delayed blanch.

To fulfil the criteria, the patient must have three or more of the major and three or more of the minor criteria. Additional features identified in patients are scaling of the scalp and infra-auricular fissures.

The presence of atopic syndrome can be confirmed by serum testing (i.e. radioallergosorbent test or RAST) or by intracutaneous challenge, looking for allergen-specific IgE antibodies to:

- house dust
- house dust mite
- pollen (tree/grass/weed)
- animal dander (cat/dog)
- moulds.

If atopy is not confirmed (in up to 10% of the patients with the clinical diagnosis according to the criteria of Hanifin and Rajka) by this test (or by the use of a skin-prick test) the test should be repeated at a later point in time. This is especially applicable in small children.

Differential diagnosis

These are outlined in Table 2.

Treatment

General therapeutic guidelines

Elimination of triggering factors

The most important aeroallergens in atopy are:

- house dust
- house dust mite
- pollen (tree/grass/weed)
- animal dander (cat/dog)
- moulds.

It is generally believed that they should be avoided. In fact for house dust mite allergens, elimination has indeed been proved to have a beneficial effect on the course of atopic dermatitis. Contact with these allergens is prevented by use of dust mite proof (Goretex) covers for mattresses and pillows, wet-mopping floors and avoiding rugs (especially in bedrooms).

Several investigators emphasize the aetiological role of food allergens in atopic dermatitis and note improvement after an elimination diet. Common food allergens implicated in atopic dermatitis are:

- milk
- egg whites
- peanuts
- soybeans
- tree nuts
- fish
- shellfish
- wheat.

It is accepted that with increasing age, the importance of food allergens rapidly decreases. The frequency of positive reactions to aeroallergens increases with age whereas the frequency of positive reactions to food allergens decreases with age.

Irritants like wool, soaps, perfumes, make-up, prolonged hot showers, high

Table 2 Overview of differentiating features in other skin diseases*

Type of disease	Diagnosis	Differentiating features
Inflammatory	Seborrhoeic eczema	Seborrhoeic areas No excoriated lesions on the extremities
	Nummular eczema	Disseminated Coin-shaped Sharply demarcated
	Contact dermatitis	No improvement with appropriate treatment
	Photocontact and photoallergic dermatitis	Photo-distribution
	Lichen simplex chronicus	Circumscribed, Usually limited to single area
	Psoriasis	Sharply demarcated Very scaly Biopsy
Infectious	Dermatomycosis	KOH examination
	Scabies	Interdigital or genital burrow Search for a mite
	HIV-associated dermatoses	Immunosuppression
Immunological or infiltrative	Wiskott–Aldrich syndrome	Thrombocytopenia
	Hyper-IgE syndrome	Recurrent bacterial infections
	Hypogammaglobulinaemia	Boys Laboratory γ-globulin
	Bruton's type X-linked agammaglobulinaemia	Purpura Telangiectasia Fine sparse hairs
	Severe combined immunodeficiency (SCID)	Pyoderma, candidiasis—present from birth
	Cutaneous T-cell lymphoma (CTCL)	Clinical presentation
	Cutaneous lymphomas (Hodgkin) lymphadenopathy	Fever, weight loss
Genetic	Ectodermal dysplasia	Anhidrosis Dental or hair abnormalities
	Netherton's syndrome	Bamboo hairs
	Phenylketonuria	Pyogenic infections Laboratory phenylalanine
	Ataxia telangiectasia	Ataxia Telangiectasia Pigmentation abnormalities
	Hurler's syndrome	Ivory-white nodules or ridges

*Modified from V.S. Beltrani.

temperature and low humidity can all contribute to the severity of atopic dermatitis and should be avoided. Stress anxiety can be a triggering factor, as well as depression, because it may reduce the threshold for pruritus. To reduce the scratch behaviour the help of a psychologist can be useful.

Indifferent therapies

Emollients for preserving and restoring the stratum corneum barrier should be used together with other topical treatments, and are to be continued long after topical corticosteroids have been stopped. Only in case of impetiginization are emollients contraindicated. Petroleum jelly is very effective. For practical reasons we recommend a combination of white petrolatum with liquid paraffin in equal parts. They are to be prescribed in large amounts. When the occlusive effect is too pronounced, emollients can cause folliculitis. This is a good reason to reduce the amount of grease in the emollient and replace it with 10–50% cream. Immediate lubrication after a bath is very effective. Bath-oils can be used here, and in the shower.

Topical antimicrobials

Ketoconazole shampoo and topical miconazol do not enhance the improvement of conventional therapy, compared to placebo. To decrease the bacterial load of the skin, chlorhexidin or iodide solutions can be used topically. This is recommended for patients with recurrent bacterial infection of the skin. In general, many clinicians assume that exacerbations of atopic dermatitis are the result of bacterial superinfections, mainly due to *Staphylococcus aureus*. Thus, fucidin has become a standard in many countries. With this topical antibiotic, that can be combined with corticosteroids, the bacterial load is brought down and secondary infection and impetiginization are minimized. Another approach is by adding antiseptics to the bathing water in mineral bathing oils. Benzalkonium chloride is used for this purpose.

Diet

The role of diet and food allergy/intolerance in the management of atopic dermatitis is controversial. For pregnant or nursing women at risk, a hypoallergenic diet can reduce the prevalence of atopic dermatitis in their high-risk infants. The use of diet in such a situation may decrease the incidence of allergic diseases from 40% to 14%. Hypoallergenic diets are also recommended for children in their first months to years. Because sensitivity to food tends to wane with age, consideration can be given to reintroducing eliminated foods to the diet, with the exception of peanuts. For the hypoallergenetic diet, elimination of milk and egg whites, and to a lesser extent peanuts, soybeans, tree nuts, fish, shellfish and wheat, are often recommended.

Treatment failure

Reasons for failure to respond to adequate therapy are: poor patient compliance, allergic contact dermatitis to a topical medicine or vehiculum, the simultaneous occurrence of asthma or hay fever, inadequate sedation and continued emotional stress.

Recommended therapies

Topical therapies

Before corticosteroids were introduced in the late 1950s, coal tar ointment was the most frequently used therapy. Tar is effective but does not work quickly. Nowadays coal tar preparations are used to save topical corticosteroids for the times when the dermatitis is exacerbated. Besides cosmetic distress tar can enhance the appearance of sunburn. Tar shampoos are often beneficial for scalp involvement.

Topical antihistamines, non-steroidal anti-inflammatory drugs (NSAIDs)

Examples of these include doxepin, sodium cromoglycate, bisacodyl or bufexamac, and are not recommended because they do not work topically (NSAIDs) or they tend to sensitize the skin and result in allergic contact dermatitis (topical antihistamines).

Topical steroids

A large variety of topical steroids are available. The potency of these corticosteroids ranges from mild to very potent. In addition, the vehiculum may differ, which is of limited influence on therapeutic efficacy. Most steroid preparations are available as lotion, cream, fatty-cream and ointment. In special cases it is possible to choose different ointments and/or creams as a base for the steroid, if the pharmacist is willing to cooperate. This is very helpful in the case of an allergy to ingredients of the vehiculum.

There are different grading systems for the potency of the steroids. An overview is given in Table 3.

To prevent tachyphylaxis, side-effects and rebound phenomena, it is better to use a potent steroid intermittently or in the short term, followed by a less potent preparation or the alternate use with emollients. It is recommended to use topical steroids once daily in combination with at least once daily application of emollients. In the first weeks corticosteroids are to be used every day; after the acute phase an alternate use is recommended. In this pulse therapy the topical steroid is used for 4 to 5 consecutive days a week, while during the other 2 to 3 days only emollients, or tar preparations, are recommended. The patient should be instructed not to stop the treatment too early, a few days or up to 1 week after the redness of the skin has disappeared will be sufficient.

Wet wraps

Wet wraps are used for short periods during acute exacerbations. They can be used as occlusion after topical therapy, to enhance the absorption. It is also protective to persistent scratching, and decreases the itch by cooling the skin.

Table 3 Topical corticosteroids

Mild
Hydrocortisone acetate
Moderately potent
Alclometasone dipropionate
Clobetason butyrate
Fluocinolone acetonide
Fluocortin butylester
Flumetason pivalate
Triamcinolone acetonide
Potent
Amcinonide
Betamethasone valerate/dipropionate/benzoate
Budesonide
Desoximethasone
Diflucortolone valerate
Fluocinonide
Fluticasone
Very potent
Beclomethasone dipropionate
Clobetasol propionate

Systemic therapies

Antihistamines are used to reduce self-inflicted damage to the skin. The relief of itching may be minor; the sedating/calming effect can give a more comfortable sleep. Therefore the sedating antihistamines are more effective in comparison to newer non-sedating antihistamines. Sedating antihistamines should be avoided in young children under 1 year of age. In pregnancy, it is said that promethazine is safe.

Antibiotics are also of benefit when there is no clear impetiginization, probably by reducing the bacterial load of the skin. It is recommended to start with clarithromycin twice daily (2dd) 250 mg or erythromycin four times daily (4dd) 250–500 mg for 1 week (or equivalent doses in children: erythromycin 50 mg/kg per day, clarithromycin 7.5 mg/kg per day). If necessary this can be continued for some weeks; if desired half of the dose can be tried.

Systemic use of ciclosporin (CsA) has been proven to be effective but its use is restricted to severe cases only. After double checking the serum creatinine a starting dose of 3 mg/kg per day is advised, and a maximum of 5 mg/kg per day should be adhered to. After control is achieved, the dose should be slowly reduced. Controls of blood pressure and serum creatinine must be performed at a regular (6-weekly) intervals. Trough levels can be measured, for example in cases where a response is expected but not apparent.

The use of a short course of oral prednisolone, for example in a dose of 20 mg twice daily (adult dose), is occasionally needed to control difficult cases. The main problem with short courses is the rebound effect, shortly after the medication is discontinued. Other disadvantages are the loss of patient compliance towards topical steroids and the association with the development of atopic cataracts.

Phototherapy and photochemotherapy

Many patients are convinced of the benefit of exposure to sunlight. This has resulted in the development of different ultraviolet (UV) schedules for the management of this inflammatory skin disease. In addition to UVA, PUVA, UVA + UVB, and UVB, UVA1 (wavelength 340–400 nm) has been recently developed as a promising alternative for atopic dermatitis.

Studies have indicated that UVB radiation (295–315 nm) is not suitable for acute exacerbations and is thus restricted to chronic cases. Combinations of UVB with UVA (300–400 nm) are more effective than UVB alone and the result can be improved by increasing the UVA portion. Systemic photochemotherapy, PUVA, is more effective but is associated with a number of side-effects such as the rebound effect and an increased risk of developing skin cancer.

Hospitalization and day-care centres

Patients with severe, generalized inflammation who do not respond to treatment or flare soon after the use of topical steroids or appear erythrodermic are candidates for hospitalization. By hospitalization the patient is protected from allergens and stressors. There is an almost guaranteed compliance, and education can be more effective. Time-consuming or difficult treatments can be done, and different therapies can be combined. The admission period can also be used for identifying potential allergens correctly.

Treatment of complications

Bacterial infections

Impetiginization. Because of the high rate of colonization with *Staphylococcus aureus* in patients with atopic dermatitis, infection of the skin is frequent in these patients. Even a good treatment cannot prevent recolonization when the dermatitis is in remission. The bacterial load of the skin also gives rise to superantigen exposure which is associated with worsening of the dermatitis. Superantigens themselves are unlikely to be directly responsible in view of their molecular weight, but it may be that they are rubbed into the epidermis by scratching. Topical cleansing products with chlorhexidin or iodine are available for treatment. Topical antibiotics such as 2% mupirocine ointment or 2% sodium fusidate ointment may also be considered. Impetiginization can be treated well with systemic antibiotics. It is preferable to choose the antibiotic knowing the results of a bacterial sensitivity test. For a blinded start, 1 week clarithromycin 2dd 250 mg or erythromycin 4dd 250–500 mg (adult doses) are recommended. In cases of known allergy or insensitivity to these macrolides, 1 week flucloxacilline 3dd 500 mg or azitromycine 2dd 250 mg (adult doses) are recommended.

Viral infections

Eczema herpeticum (Kaposi's varicelliform eruption). Patients with atopic dermatitis are susceptible to the spread of cutaneous (not systemic) herpes simplex infection. The spread of herpes simplex is enhanced by the damaged stratum corneum barrier. Typical for atopic dermatitis is the spread from a small area to a more extensive area or to an area elsewhere on the body. Especially in the first 48 h an antiviral treatment such as valaciclovir 3dd 100 mg for 7 days, or aciclovir 5dd 800 mg for 5 days can be useful. For severe cases (i.e. fever), hospitalization for intravenous treatment with aciclovir 5 mg/kg every 8 h for 5 days is to be considered. In cases of neuralgia analgesics such as paracetamol 500 mg or paracetamol–codeine 500/20 mg up to 6 times a day (maximum adult dose) can give relief.

Warts and molluscum contagiosum
Patients with atopic dermatitis who contract warts are relatively recalcitrant to treatment, but their treatment does not differ from that in non-atopics.

Dermatomycosis
In particular *Trichophyton rubrum* can be treated with antifungal agents, but creams like ketoconazole can be drying and irritating.

Cheiro/podo pompholyx
In the acute phase, the hands and/or feet should be soaked three or four times a day in Burow's solution (aluminium acetate 10%) or zinc sulphate ointment may be applied. The soaks can be stopped after a few days, when the eruption subsides. A zinc cream or oily calamine lotion can be substituted; in the chronic phase topical steroids are useful. In case of secondary bacterial infection flucloxacillin (adult dose 3dd 500 mg) can be used.

Alternative and experimental treatments

Experimental therapies
Essential fatty acids have been found in increased levels in lesional skin of atopic dermatitis patients, with normal values in unlesional skin. In addition abnormalities in the fatty acid composition in breast milk of mothers with affected children have been found. It has been suggested that a deficiency of these fatty acids plays a role in the pathogenesis of atopic dermatitis. Dietary supplementation with evening primrose oil and marine fish oil did not demonstrate any significant clinical improvement in double-blind, placebo-controlled trials.

Chinese herbs have non-steroidal anti-inflammatory activities, some of them have in addition also steroid like, antihistaminic or immunosuppressive activity. This herbal therapy seems to target the inflammatory character of the disease. Positive results have been reported, but its potential hepatotoxicity has to be studied. Other problems are a guaranteed constant quality of supply and unpalatability.

Because airborne allergens such as *Dermatophagoides pteronyssinus* seem to play an important role in atopic dermatitis as a triggering factor, allergen desensitization with extracts of these allergens have been published. Some investigators reported positive results in unblinded uncontrolled studies while others reported no alleviation after desensitization in a placebo-controlled, double-blind study. The major limitation of this treatment is the complicated procedure of preparing specific immune complexes.

Atopic patients have a reduced IFN-γ production, leading to an overproduction of IgE. This suggest that IFN-γ may be effective in the treatment of atopic dermatitis. Subcutaneous injection of IFN-γ is effective in nearly half of the patients, achieving 50% improvement. A major disadvantage is its high cost.

Thymic factors have been tried in atopic dermatitis. Intramuscular thymostimulin (TP-1) achieved no significant difference to placebo; subcutaneous thymopentin (TP-5) achieved a small improvement in combination with topical steroids and oral antihistamines.

Patients with atopic dermatitis are predisposed to cutaneous infections, often with *Staphylococcus aureus*. This is a well-known triggering factor. Topical γ-globulin (IgG) preparations have been used with specific antimicrobial antibodies with neutralizing and opsonizing activity. Improvement was reported, but double-blind placebo-controlled studies are not available.

In atopic dermatitis patients phosphodiesterase activity in mononuclear leucocytes has been reported to be increased. Phosphodiesterase inhibitors are used experimentally as therapy in atopic dermatitis. However these agents are not yet clinically available.

Imminent new therapies

Tacrolimus (FK506) and pimecrolimus (SDZ ASM 981) are new macrolide-type inflammatory cytokine inhibitors, with a mechanism of action similar to CsA. In contrast to CsA, they are effective in the topical treatment of atopic dermatitis, due to their relatively small size. Both compounds are highly effective against itch, one of the most prominent problems of patients with atopic dermatitis. In contrast to topical corticosteroids, these compounds seems to have a more favourable side-effect profile. This might be of importance for patients suffering from:

1 The local side-effects of corticosteroids:
   - atrophy
   - telangiectasia
   - striae or tachyphylaxis.
2 Systemic side-effects: adrenal suppression.

Burning of the skin or a feeling of warmth is a frequently reported side-effect of these new compounds. This is only a minor problem, disappearing after a few days. These topical inflammatory cytokine inhibitors are, as with corticosteroids, contraindicated for use in infected skin.

In children, extra precautions are to be considered when using topical corticosteroids. Growth retardation is a major issue and in severe cases where long periods of corticosteroid application is necessary, keeping growth curves should be part of the patient follow-up.

Further reading

Akdis CA, Akdis M, Simon D *et al.* T cells and T cell-derived cytokines as pathogenic factors in the nonallergic form of atopic dermatitis. *J Invest Dermatol* 1999; 13: 628–34.

Atherton DJ. Diet and atopic eczema. *Clin Allergy* 1988; 18: 215–28.

Beltrani VS. The clinical manifestations of atopic dermatitis. In: Leung DYM, ed. *Atopic Dermatitis: from Pathogenesis to Treatment.* Berlin: Springer, 1996: 1–39.

Bos JD, Kapsenberg ML, Sillevis Smitt JH. Pathogenesis of atopic eczema. *Lancet* 1994; 343: 1338–41.

Bos JD, Meinardi MMHM. The 500 Dalton rule for the skin penetration of chemical compounds and drugs. *Exp Dermatol* 2000; 9: 165–9.

Bos JD, Van Leent EJM, Sillevis Smitt JH. The millennium criteria for the diagnosis of atopic dermatitis. *Exp Dermatol* 1998; 7: 132–8.

Forrest S, Dunn K, Elliott K *et al.* Identifying genes predisposing to atopic eczema. *J Allergy Clin Immunol* 1999; 104: 1066–70.

Goerz G, Lehmann P, Ruzicka T, Ring J, Przybilla B, eds. *Handbook of Atopic Eczema.* Berlin: Springer, 1991.

Hanifin JM, Rajka G. Diagnostic features of atopic dermatitis. *Acta Derm Venereol (Stockh) Supplement* 1980; 92: 44–7.

Kay J, Gawkrodger DJ, Mortimer MJ, Jaron AG. The prevalence of childhood atopic eczema in a general population. *J Am Acad Dermatol* 1994; 30: 35–9.

Krutmann J, Czech W, Diepgen T, Niedner R, Kapp A, Schöpf E. High-dose UVA1 therapy in the treatment of patients with atopic dermatitis. *J Am Acad Dermatol* 1992; 26: 225–30.

Nakagawa H, Ethoh T, Ishibashi Y *et al.* Tacrolimus ointment for atopic dermatitis. *Lancet* 1994; 344: 883.

Przybilla B, Eberlein-König B, Ruëff F. Practical management of atopic eczema. *Lancet* 1994; 343: 1342–6.

Ruzicka T, Bieber T, Schöpf E *et al.* A short-term trial of tacrolimus ointment for atopic dermatitis. *N Engl J Med* 1997; 337: 816–21.

Snowden JM, Berth-Jones J, Ross JS *et al.* Double-blind, controlled, crossover study of cyclosporin in adults with severe refractory atopic dermatitis. *Lancet* 1991; 338: 137–40.

Van Leent EJM, Gräber M, Thurston M, Wagenaar A, Spuls PI, Bos JD. Effectiveness of the ascomycin macrolactam SDZ ASM 981 in the topical treatment of atopic dermatitis. *Arch Dermatol* 1998; 134: 805–9.

Williams HC. Is the prevalence of atopic dermatitis increasing? *Clin Exp Dermatol* 1992; 17: 385–91.

Balanitis

D. Freedman

Definition and epidemiology

- Balanitis: inflammation of the glans penis.
- Balanoposthitis: inflammation of the foreskin and surface of the underlying glans penis. Frequently occurs with a tight or not easily retracted foreskin or phimosis. Usually a more acute and extensive local inflammation than simple balanitis.
- Posthitis: inflammation of the preputial mucosa.

The term 'balanitis' is often used to include all of the above. The condition is common in infancy when the prepuce is adherent and non-retractable, as well as subject to moisture and contamination from urine and faeces.

It is very common in adulthood in circumstances of poor hygiene and accumulation of subprepuce secretions. It is equally frequent with overzealous and even obsessive washing, causing irritation. *Candida* balanitis is associated with diabetics. Sexual transmission is not well described in the literature, but most physicians have clinical experience of balanitis occurring postcoitus with a woman who has either candidal or bacterial vaginosis. This may be an indicator of sexual risk taking, and as such warrants a full sexually transmitted disease (STD) screen, unless risk is specifically denied.

Essentially, diagnosis is anatomical, but there are multiple causes.

Aetiology and pathophysiology

The blind subpreputial sac results in a warm moist environment, with an accumulation of desquamated cells and smegma, an ideal culture medium. The epithelium of the glans penis is protected and covered, so that it remains moist, non-keratinized, thin and sensitive. In some respects the male preputial sac is the equivalent of the vagina, with a similar polymicrobial ecology and a similar susceptibility to overgrowth of microorganisms normally present to produce symptomatic conditions, and a similar predisposition to recurrence of these conditions.

Most commonly, balanitis is a simple intertrigo with no specific aetiological agent. The majority of cases are mild and may have mechanical or irritant associations. With infective causes, a more acute inflammatory reaction may be seen, such as with infection/overgrowth of *Candida* or anaerobes. Many dermatological conditions affect the genital epithelium, where their clinical features may be atypical due to the different nature of the epithelium.

Sexual transmission has been described with both candidal and anaerobic infections, but it is thought to be infrequent. Partner treatment does not markedly influence the risk of recurrence.

Clinical characteristics and course

Clinical presentation is variable and is frequently inversely related to guilt and anxiety. The anxious or guilty patient may present with symptoms of non-specific irritation, itching or burning of the glans or prepuce and little or no findings at all. Often there is just a minimal red spotty rash on the glans. Other patients may present with an obvious red inflamed glans and prepuce, erosive ulcers and an offensive subpreputial discharge: amine odour indicates anaerobic overgrowth. Inguinal adenopathy is rarely present with simple balanitis and its presence should indicate consideration of a wider differential diagnosis, including the need to exclude STDs and carcinoma.

In the many symptomatic cases, the course will be episodic with recurrences, unless specific care is taken to reverse the predisposing factors.

Diagnosis

In simple balanitis, diagnosis is clinical and tested by response to simple measures.

Microscopy of the subpreputial secretions may reveal *Candida* or anaerobes which may indicate the same condition in the sexual partner(s). Potassium hydroxide preparation is useful in the identification of *Candida*; Gram stain will be more specific for anaerobes. Culture will identify bacterial causes, although one must be careful not to attribute the cause to commensals.

The presence of ulceration, adenopathy or a positive sexual risk history should prompt a full screen for STDs. Samples from ulcerated lesions should be examined by dark ground microscopy to eliminate syphilis, and cultured for herpes virus. Consideration should be given to chancroid, lymphogranuloma venerium and granuloma inguinale. A high degree of suspicion should be maintained for squamous cell carcinoma of the penis and any persisting or suspicious lesions biopsied. The skin of the glans penis and prepuce may be affected by a wide variety of dermatological conditions, the more important of which are considered in the differential diagnosis provided in Table 1. The presentation and appearance of these conditions is modified in the soft non-keratinized skin. In case of persisting lesions, or if in any doubt, biopsy.

Differential diagnosis

As an area of skin, the prepuce and glans penis is subject to abrasion, trauma, infection and the entire gamut of dermatological conditions, including cancer and precancer (Table 1).

Treatment

General therapeutic guidelines

The principle is to change the micro ecosystem of the subpreputial sac to one which will not readily become superinfected by *Candida*, anaerobes or other bacteria. Exposure and drying of the skin encourages keratinization and further enhancement of resistance to infection, abrasion and trauma.

Recommended therapies

The vast majority of cases respond to simple measures such as:

- retraction of the foreskin
- saline baths
- simple drying powder.

Retraction of the foreskin

Advising patients to change their habits of a lifetime and maintain retraction of the foreskin requires considerable persuasion. Most find it uncomfortable and oversensitive initially and it takes about 3–4 weeks for the hypersensitivity to settle down as keratinization occurs. Once this has been achieved, few wish to revert to their previous mode of wearing the foreskin down.

Some men cannot achieve retraction because of a tight prepuce: application of an emollient cream and stretching over a period of time may allow the desired effect to be achieved. Retraction may not be maintained by others because of a natural tendency of the prepuce to slip down. Use of a thin narrow surgical tape (Micropore® 12.5 mm, 3M®) along the shaft of the penis may retain the prepuce back for a sufficient time for keratinization to occur.

Patients must be warned to guard against paraphimos on retraction of the foreskin. This may occur at night, with erotic dreams, when patients may awake with an acute paraphimosis.

On occasions circumcision is warranted for persisting irritation.

Table 1 Differential diagnosis of common or important conditions

Condition	Clinical Features	Diagnosis
Sexually transmitted		
Herpes genitalis (classical)	Vesicles, sores, crusts - painful	Viral culture
Syphilis		Dark ground microscopy serology (>3/12)
- Primary	Ulcers(s) – painless	
- Secondary	Condylomata lata Multiple circinate lesions	
Chancroid	Painful ulcer(s) Adenopathy	Culture / P.C.R.
Lymphogranuloma venereum	Painful shallow ulcer(s) adenopathy	Culture / clinical
Granuloma inguinale	Beefy lesions – painless	Microscopy biopsy
Gonorrhoea	Acute ulcers and pustules, acute infection of glands & ducts, i.e. Tysonilis, Cowpers duct	Microscopy culture
Trichomonas	Acute erosive lesions	Microscopy (wet prep)
Human papilloma virus	Asymptomatic patchy variable macula, hypoaesthesia – pruritis chronic / recurrent	Aceto-white lesions (5% acetic acid stupes) confirm by biopsy HPV typing
Infections: potential of sexual transmission		
Candida infection	Short incubation, burning, itching – acute pain, variable erythema – dry glazed small papules and pustules coalesce to form erosive patches	Microscopy KOH preparation 'adhesive tape' sample
Candida hypersensitivity	Transient post-coital erythema and burning	History check partner
Gardnerella	Mild symptoms Macular erythema 'Fishy' odour	Clinical culture
Anaerobic erosive balanitis (*Bacteroides* spp.)	Tender ulcers, odour	Microscopy mixed spirochetes bacteria ++
Group B haemolytic streptococci	Erythema – purulent discharge, cellulitis	Culture
Infections: sexual transmission unlikely		
Group A haemolytic streptococci	Pre-pubertal erythematous, moist	Culture
Staphylococcus aureus	Pre-pubertal boys (toxic shock syndrome)	Culture
Pityriasis versicolor	Discreet fine scaling hypopigmented areas	Fluoresce with 'woods' light
Herpes zoster	Pain++ grouped blisters	Clinical dermatome distribution serology
Specific balanitides		
Lichen sclerosis et atrophicus	Atrophic white papules or plaques. Phimosis, burning, pruritis, hypoaesthesia, sexual dysfunction	Sclerotic white ring at tip of prepuce
	Lesions progress to sclerotic/ atrophic white/ivory/blue flat topped papules. Progressive chronic course	Biopsy
	Fibrosis – obliteration of anatomical features. Meatal stenosis	
Plasma cell balanitis	Solitary glazed-smooth red-orange plaque *'cayenne pepper'*	Biopsy

(*continued*)

Table 1 (*Continued*)

Condition	Clinical Features	Diagnosis
Localized balanitides		
Fixed drug eruption	Well demarcated erythematous areas bullous – occasionally ulcerated	History recur at same site on re-exposure to drug
Allergic and contact dermatitis	Intense pruritis / burning, marked odema, rapid onset	History patch testing
Trauma	Direct accidental: burn/scald/ frostbite – suction/vacuum devices, zipper entrapment, sexually induced pubic hair friction, bites, instrumentation, masturbation	History
Implantation	Studs, rings, balls etc.	Clinical
Manifestation of systemic / generalized disease		
Psoriasis	Well demarcated erythematous plaques without scale (inverse pattern)	Other stigmata of psoriasis family history biopsy
Behçet's syndrome	Ulcers	Extra genital lesions biopsy pathergy test
Aphthosis ulcers	Painful, solitary halo of erythema	Outrule other causes of genital ulcers – especially Behçet's
Circinate balanitis	Moist plaque with irregular ragged border – geographic (circumcised – dry scaling)	Other clinical features of Reiter's syndrome HLA B27+ve (80%)
Sebhorraeic dermatitis	Mild erythema and scaling	Clinical
Lichen planus	Polygonal violaceous flat-topped papules Lacy erosive ulcers	Clinical
Erythema multiforme	Erythematous papules vesicles – ulcers	Clinical
Pemphigus	Vegetating plaques	Biopsy
Neoplasia		
Erythroplasia of Queyrat	Plaques: glazed – velvety slightly raised sharp margins	Biopsy
Penile carcinoma	Pruritis / burning papillary / flat ulcer with rolled edge	Biopsy
Verrucous carcinoma (Buschke – Loewenstein)	Exophytic lesions infiltrative	Biopsy
Extra mammary Paget's disease	Plaques red-brown raised, scaly	Biopsy

Saline baths

These appear to help to dry out the skin, encourage keratinization, and may have a mild fungistatic/bacteristatic effect. Essentially, a tablespoon (20 mL) of ordinary domestic table salt in a warm bath of water; or more convenient for frequent daily use, a pinch of salt in a tumbler glass or small jar. The penis and subpreputial area should be dried gently, by patting, rather than any rough or abrasive action. Care should be taken not to use too much salt, or the skin will become 'pickled' or irritated, which would be quite counterproductive.

If retraction is not possible initially, one can wash out the subpreputial space with warm saline by the use of a small syringe to irrigate the area.

Simple drying powder

Application of a simple drying powder to the subpreputial space can assist in maintaining dryness. A simple talc may be used, or one with a mild antiseptic as commonly used for infants (calcium undecylenate 10% powder). Care should be taken to ensure that there is no hypersensitivity to the talc or other constituents.

Alternative treatments

Antifungals and steroids

Antifungal creams are very commonly prescribed. In my experience I have found them only to be useful in providing short-term symptomatic relief. Recurrence occurs shortly after discontinuation of usage. There is danger of hypersensitivity to these agents and their vehicles. Antifungal/antibacterial powders have produced better results as they dry out the area. They are particularly useful in acute erosive balanitis, with secondary bacterial infection. Miconazole powder, used three to four times a day, is one such agent.

Local corticosteroid applications should only be used where there is a specific dermatitis, as they would only weaken the skin and may mask an infection.

These simple measures should be tried initially, and given sufficient time for patient compliance to be established and for them to show effect. With persisting balanitis, much stronger consideration must be given to the differential diagnosis, taking special care to exclude an STD, dermatosis or a precancer/cancer. At this stage biopsy becomes mandatory.

Screening for STDs

This is mandatory in all cases where a history of potential acquisition has been obtained, and is useful reassurance in the majority of other cases. Many patients who present with balanitis have an underlying anxiety regarding STDs and this must be firmly addressed.

Further reading

Edwards S. Balanitis and balinoposthitis: a review. *Genitourin Med* 1996; 72: 155–9.

English JC, Laws RA, Keough GC, Wilde JL, Poley JP, Elston DM. Dermatoses of the glans penis and prepuce. *J Am Acad Dermatol* 1997; 37: 1–24.

Johnson RA. Diseases and disorders of the anogenitalia of males. In: Fitzpatrick TB, Eisen AZ, Wolf K, Freedberg IM, Austin FK, eds. *Dermatology in General Medicine*, 4th edn. New York: McGraw Hill, 1993.

Schoen EJ. The status of circumcision of newborns. *N Engl Med J* 1990; 322: 1308.

Basal cell carcinoma

D. Roseeuw, A.D. Katsambas and J.P. Hachem

Definition and synonyms

Basal cell carcinoma (BCC), is a slow-growing locally invasive epidermal tumour and metastases are extremely rare. BCC, the most common malignancy among Caucasians, is also known as basalioma, basal cell epithelioma, basal cell cancer, rodent ulcer, rodent cancer and non-Malpighian epithelioma.

The term 'basal cell' refers to the histological resemblance of the tumour cells to those of the basal cells of the epidermis and its appendages. The term 'carcinoma' refers to the growth of a tumour that may result in significant local destruction and disfigurement if not treated adequately.

Epidemiology

Seventy-five per cent of all skin carcinoma are BCCs. The majority of patients are between the ages of 40 and 80 years old. Slightly more than half of all patients are men with a known history of sun exposure.

The prevalence of BCC increases with solar or ultraviolet (UV) light exposure and is found to mostly occur in white individuals with photo types I and II. Photodamaged skin is the predilection site for BCCs. While 85% of all BCCs appear on the head and neck area the frequency of carcinoma affecting the nose is around 30%.

It has been observed that UV light cannot be the only cause of BCC. Many do not develop on sites of maximum solar exposure. Sites commonly spared from photodamage, such as eyelids, inner canthus, retro-auricular skin, back, forearms and even the vulva have been described as potential areas for BCC occurrence.

BCC may also occur on sites of traumatic injuries, such as scars from burns or smallpox vaccination. Multiple BCCs may develop on the skin of patients having taken arsenic salts.

The incidence of BCC varies according to sun exposure and climate. In the USA the annual incidence of 730 per 100 000 inhabitants per year was reported.

In Australia the incidence is 1000–2000 per 100 000 inhabitants per year (1–2%) and one European study showed an incidence of 132 per 100 000 inhabitants per year. However, epidemiological data collected from populations living under temperate climatic conditions reveal an increased incidence of BCC. In Australia a 5% increase per year has been indicated and a study done in a temperate climate in Switzerland has shown a steady increase of 2.6% per year from 1976 to 1990.

Aetiology and pathogenesis

Several hypotheses have been proposed as to the origin of BCC. It has been suggested that a pluripotent cell, like a primary epithelial germ cell or an adult progenitor epithelial cell may lead to most BCCs. Currently, it is postulated that a slow cycling stem cell, with great proliferative potential, can occasionally form transient amplifying cells, which further multiply before terminal differentiation can occur.

It is thought that stem cells are localized in protected, well-vascularized and highly nerved anatomical sites, such as the connection between the musculus arrector pili and the outer root sheath. BCCs are considered to originate from these cells.

One argument suggests that tumour formation induced by topical carcinogens is dependent on the hair cycle—topical carcinogens can be accumulated at levels 10 times in the telogenic phase than in the anagenic phase.

Clinical characteristics and course

The concept of 'low-risk' and 'high-risk' BCC has been described in order to allow the clinician to choose the most appropriate form of treatment. Factors determining these risk factors are: tumour size, type and site, definition of tumour margins, histological type and growth pattern, recurrent tumours and finally immunocompromised patients (Table 1).

Primary BCC

BCC grows slowly, is painless and frequently ignored by the patient. If metastases are rare, local invasion could be destructive when tumours are neglected. In such cases, the tumour may infiltrate in depth through the different tissue layers into the cranial cavity or along the embryological fusion planes, provoking important morbidity or eventually a fatal outcome.

Clinical variants of BCC have been described. The five most frequent clinical subtypes are: superficial, noduloulcerative (rodent ulcer), pigmented, cystic, morphoeic and metatypical (basosquamous). The main characteristics of the clinical subtypes are given in Table 2.

Diagnosis of the clinical variants is of great importance as the choice of treatment modality depends on the clinical type of the BCC.

Special attention should be paid to the basosquamous and metatypical type of BCC. Initially, their clinical aspect does not differ much from other BCCs. However it grows fast, has a destructive capacity and produces metastases.

Metatypical BCCs share uncharacteristic pathological features. These lesions frequently show a morphoeic aspect, and an intermediate histological pattern between squamous cell and BCC.

Table 1 Low- and high-risk BCC

	Low-risk BCC	High-risk BCC
Type	Superficial Nodular	Morphoeic, Metatypical
Localization		Mid-face Ear region
Size	< 2 cm	> 2 cm
Histology	Non-basosquamous	Basosquamous
Course	Primary	Recurrent
Immunity	Normal	Compromised

Recurrent BCC and the risk of developing another BCC

Some BCCs have a high potential to recur and to be destructive. Reported recurrence rates vary from 30% to 60%.

Analysis of recurrent BCCs is difficult. Several factors implying tumour

Table 2 Main characteristics of clinical BCC subtypes

Clinical subtypes	Localization	Growth	Lesion	Colour	Surface
Solid or nodular	Face	Slow	Nodule	Skin translucent	Telangiectasia
Rodent ulcer	Face	Faster	Central ulcer rolled border	Translucent necrotic, red	Telangiectasia
Pigmented	Face	Slow	Nodule	Brown	Telangiectasia
Adenocystic	Face	Slow	Lobulated cyst + rolled edge	Erythymatous/ +squamous Translucent	Telangiectasia
Superficial	Trunk Limbs	Slow	Plaque pearly border	Red scaly	Well defined
Morphoeic	Face	Slow	Scar-like plaque	Yellowish	Undefined telangiectasia
Metatypical or basosquamous	Face	Rapid	Plaque+ metastases	Yellowish	Undefined

conditions and type of previous treatment play a role in their development.

Factors influencing the recurrence rate of BCCs are: localization in the midfacial or ear region, neglected chronic BCCs, lesions greater than 2 cm in diameter, aggressive morphoeic and basosquamous types, recurrent BCCs and the form of the chosen treatment.

Five-year recurrence has been shown to be increased for the non-microscopically orientated histological surgery (MOHS, also known as Mohs' surgery after Dr Frederic Mohs), i.e. surgical excision, electrosurgery, cryotherapy and radiation therapy, from 9% for primary BCCs to 20% for recurrent lesions. Recurrent rates for MOHS surgery increased from 1% for primary tumours to 5.6% for recurrent BCCs.

In the literature, a recurrence rate as high as 40% has been found when recurrent BCCs were treated with curettage and electrodessication.

Based on the above-mentioned studies it is recommended that MOHS, which has the highest cure rate, is the treatment of choice for recurrent BCC.

A long follow-up period of treated BCCs is advised to exclude recurrences.

Diagnosis

The diagnosis can be established by the anamnesis, the clinical appearance and the skin biopsy or following definitive surgery. A long-standing, slow-growing and painless tumour should be suspected for BCC.

A simple and efficient technique is cytological examination of the lesion. Scraped cells are smeared onto a slide and fixed. After appropriate staining, clumps of malignant basal cells can be identified.

Treatment

General therapeutic guidelines

Many therapeutic modalities and strategies have been developed for the management of BCCs. Treatment consists of total destruction or removal of the carcinoma by various methods. However, considering the frequency, variability, facial localization and progressive growth resulting in destruction of vital organs, not one therapy is ideally suited to treat all BCCs efficiently.

The most frequently used modalities for the treatment of BCC include: simple surgical excision, MOHS surgery, curettage and electrodesiccation (electrosurgery), cryosurgery, radiation therapy and combined methods. A multidisciplinary approach between dermatologists, dermato-surgeons and radiotherapists, is therefore the key element optimal for a successful treatment (Fig. 1).

In order to select the best method available to treat a specific BCC, the clinician should be able to determine the risk values as described in Table 1. Even if MOHS surgery is believed to be the state-of-the-art therapeutic method, other techniques could be considered if micrographic surgery is contraindicated or unfeasible.

In general, when the physician selects a treatment modality, the decision will depend on several 'criteria' namely, the tumour, the patient, his skills, the previous treatments and the financial aspects. Factors related to the tumour, such as the clinical type, anatomical localization, primary or recurrent lesions, single or multiple lesions, size, depth, duration and growth speed of the tumour, determination possibilities of the margins and cell type should be considered (Table 3).

Recommended therapies

Excision surgery

This form of treatment is most common among dermatologists and surgeons. The primary objective of this procedure is to remove all tumour cells.

Excision surgery is a recommended choice of treatment if certain clinical conditions are fulfilled. These conditions are related to the type, diameter,

Table 3 Factors related to therapeutic decision

Tumour characteristics
Clinical type
Anatomical localization
Primary or recurrent
Size and depth
Margin determination
Histological type
Single or multiple
Duration
Growth
Previous treatments
Experience of physician
Patient
Age
General health
Sun-damaged skin
Psychological status
Possibilities of care at home
Financial aspects

anatomical site and are summarized in Table 4.

The major advantages of excision surgery include: the rapid healing time, a good to excellent cosmetic result and the microscopic examination of the resection tissue.

Certain contraindications and disadvantages of excision surgery in the treatment of skin cancer may exist. For instance, allergy to local anaesthesia is seldom but could be circumvented by a general anaesthesia. For patients on anticoagulants, the risk of bleeding during operation and postoperatively may exclude excision surgery. Also patients with multiple skin cancers may present surgical problems when adequate margins have to be taken for cure and when different wounds have to be closed.

It is not indicated to close the surgical wound with tissue flaps or grafts if the margins of resection are not clear. Tumour recurrences may spread laterally and deeply under such flaps or grafts before there are any clinical signs of the recurrent cancer.

If reconstruction is necessary or highly desirable after BCC excision, margins of resection should be checked and the primary choice of surgical procedure should be the MOHS technique.

When using excision surgery, the orientation of the excision and the size of the final wound are often determined by the lesion size, skin tension lines and lesion localization. When possible a simple fusiform excision is performed and haemostasis achieved before wound closure. Excessive cauterization of superficial and deep dermal capillary plexuses must be avoided to improve scar formation. Often, the way to close the defect becomes obvious when the lesion is removed and the wound edges are undermined. Generally, incisions are preferably closed in a layered fashion.

On the face of elderly individuals, excess tissue is available and allows closure of rather large defects with simple suture techniques or flaps. However reconstructive surgery may become necessary.

Pressure dressings and skin closure bandages provide extra support. Wound healing is accelerated by a 24-h impermeable wound dressing. Wound infection

Table 4 Recommendation criteria for excision surgery in BCC

Nodular and superficial BCCs with well-defined borders
Well-defined primary small BCCs of less than 2 cm diameter which can be effectively excised with a safety margin of 4 mm. In these cases success rate of 95% is obtained
In anatomical areas such as the cheeks, neck, trunk, arms and legs where primary closure is possible after an adequate margin is obtained
In anatomical areas such as the legs or feet if no complete primary closure is possible, but a quick healing time is desired
After total removal of the BCC, the cosmetic result, quick healing and minimal morbidity are a prerequisite

after simple excision skin surgery is uncommon and postoperative antibiotherapy is not required.

The micrographic orientated histological or microscopically controlled surgery: MOHS

The MOHS technique was first described by Dr Mohs in 1930 and has since undergone many modifications. This technique has the advantage that the BCC is excised completely while as much normal tissue as possible is preserved. The margins of the excised tumour are microscopically examined in horizontal sections and mapped. Indications for micrographic surgery are listed in Table 5.

In addition, because of its tissue-sparing properties, MOHS surgery is often performed in delicate regions around the eyes, nose, lips and ears to preserve normal anatomy and prevent disfigurement.

The different Mohs techniques offer a 98% chance for complete removal of a primary BCC without recurrence. For recurrent BCCs the chance of complete removal is 95%.

Curettage and electrodesiccation (electrosurgery)

Dermatologists treat many BCCs with curettage and electrodesiccation because it is easy to perform in the office and it requires a minimum of equipment. However, it has its limitations and to avoid high recurrence rates of 40% as reported in the literature, there must be strict application of the indication rules.

The indications and advantages of electrosurgery are based upon the restricted technical possibilities, the knowledge of the type of BCC, the recurrence rates and the localization of the lesion. Table 6 summarizes the indications and contraindications of electrosurgery in BCC.

The main disadvantages of electrosurgery are related to the fact that there is no specimen for histological study to determine if the margins are clear. It is a blind method and cure rate depends on the clinical judgement of the physician to decide on the extent of the tissue destruction.

There is a risk of damage to underlying vital structures such as nerves, blood vessels and tendons during operation.

Postoperatively, an open wound is left which must heal by secondary intention with a risk of infection. The use of topical antibiotic preparations up to the first 3 days or so may be advised. Then, if no infection occurs, hydrocolloid dressings are favoured to stimulate healing. The risk of bleeding postoperatively occurs rarely, but results from inadequate electrocoagulation, or when the coagulum separates. The cosmetic aspect of the scar after electrosurgery is more noticeable than after suture closure.

Curettage and electrodesiccation requires local anaesthesia. With the curette, the soft and visible cancer tissues are removed until adjacent firm normal tissue is left. A security margin of 2–4 mm is also curetted. After each curettage, haemostasis by electrodesiccation is done. A minimum of two or three levels of curet-

Table 5 Indications for micrographic surgery in BCC

Large tumour (larger than 2 cm)
Previously treated lesions (recurrent BCCs)
BCC in young adults
Tumours with indistinct margins such as morphoeic BCC
Localization of a tumour in the facial H-zone (preauricular, around eyes, nose and lips), which is an area of high recurrence
Localization of BCC on or adjacent to a critical functional or cosmetic structure
BCC with aggressive histological growth pattern on biopsy

Table 6 Indications and contraindications of electrosurgery in BCC

Indications
Primary BCC
13 mm or less with very well-defined clinical borders
In localities other than the H-zone of the face
Contraindications
Lesions greater than 13 mm in diameter
Lesions around the eyes, nostrils, ears, upper lip and scalp (high-risk mid-facial areas and along embryonal fusion lines)
Deeply ulcerated lesion extending in dermis or fat
Morphoeic BCCs with poorly defined clinical borders
Recurrent BCCs
Patients with cardiac pacemakers

tage is necessary to remove the BCC thoroughly.

However, if the dermis is very thin, such as on the eyelid, or if the tumour penetrates the dermis and the subcutaneous fat, or if it has invaded scar tissue, it is impossible to evaluate whether the BCC has been totally removed. Thus, multiple microscopic foci of tumour cells may still remain.

Iatrogenic multifocal lesions can occur in 50% of recurrent BCCs treated with electrosurgery. Therefore, recurrent lesions should not be treated with electrosurgery but with MOHS surgery.

For primary BCCs, if electrosurgery is applied and done according to the indications and with precision and skill, the recurrence rates are comparable with those of surgery or radiotherapy.

Cryosurgery

Cryosurgery is a well-established therapeutic modality for BCC. Frequency of recurrence after performing cryosurgery has been recently estimated to 9%, approximately similar to excision, radiotherapy or electrosurgery modalities.

Freezing with liquid nitrogen is performed in well-defined nodular or superficial types of BCC of 3 mm or less in depth and smaller than 2 cm in diameter. Multiple BCCs such as in the basal cell naevus syndrome are also an adequate indication. Under these conditions very high success rates of up to 99% are reported.

Anatomical regions where surgery may induce both cosmesis and functional impairments, namely on the forehead, temporal region, nose, ears and dorsum of hand, are areas of predilection for the use of cryosurgery. In areas where keloids or hypertrophic scars are likely to form, cryosurgery is advisable. Elderly patients on anticoagulant therapy and/or with pacemakers may benefit from this technique. Patients refusing invasive therapies or unable to attend hospital facilities may be more likely to accept cryosurgery. Morphoeic BCCs, those occurring in high recurrent zones (H-zones) or extending into the subcutaneous tissues should not be treated with cryotherapy. Cryoglobulinaemia, cryofibrinogenaemia, cold agglutinins, Raynaud's phenomenon and other autoimmune diseases are contraindications for the use of cryosurgery.

The main disadvantage of cryosurgery is the open wound that must heal by secondary intention, requiring 3–10 weeks, depending on the size and localization of the BCC. Large superficial lesions on the trunk and lower leg heal very slowly. Other techniques giving improved results at these sites are preferred. Cryosurgery does not provide tissue for histopathological testing, and cure is highly dependent upon the physician's evaluation and experience in removing the entire BCC.

Liquid nitrogen is applied with a spray apparatus. It can also be administered by cryoprobes in a closed system. The extent of cell damage is determined by the rate of temperature fall, the coldest temperature reached, the length of time the cells are exposed to freezing temperature between 0°C to −50°C, the rate of thaw and the concentration of solutes.

For cutaneous cancers the currently recommended temperature is between −50°C and −60°C, measured at the base of the tumour.

Cryotherapy of skin cancers leaves a wound that is swollen, painful and weepy for 3–4 weeks. They often heal with an acceptable scar and sometimes leave hypopigmentation. In general, the cosmetic results are usually acceptable but seem inferior to excision surgery.

With cryotherapy as with any other procedure, experience and precision is necessary to achieve high cure rates. To obtain cure of BCCs, it is safer to use repeated freeze–thaw cycles and to treat the BCC with an adequate margin of 0.5–0.7 cm. Two successive freeze–thaw cycles give in common types of BCC cure rates equivalent to radiotherapy and surgical excision. Single freeze–thaw cycles have been reported to be adequate only for truncal superficial BCCs.

Radiation therapy

For many dermatologists, radiotherapy remains a second choice of treatment. Many population-based control studies suggest an evidence-based relation between the increased incidence of BCC and therapeutic ionizing radiations. Yet, radiotherapy is used for the treatment of BCC. A comparative study using surgical techniques and radiotherapy has shown that postoperative complications were higher after radiotherapy and the final cosmetic results after 4 years of follow-up were rated significantly better with surgery than with radiotherapy. On the contrary, for radiotherapists the treatment cure rate of BCC was 90.73% after the fifth year of follow-up and the cosmetic results were evaluated to be 'good' or 'acceptable' in 84% of the treated lesions.

After histological confirmation, either soft X-rays or fast electrons can be used. Radioprotection of organs such as the sexual organs, eyes, thyroid, hairy skin, teeth, bone and cartilage, should be performed during therapy.

Dose fractionation electron beam schedules using fraction sizes less than 4 Gy may reduce the risk of necrosis and ulceration, particularly for field sizes superior to 5 cm^2. Well-fractionated electron beam therapy improves cosmetic results than the large fraction superficial X-ray therapy and is more efficient for the treatment of large tumours. However in contrast to X-ray electron therapy is expensive.

A comparison of late cosmetic results following fractionated superficial X-ray therapy and gold grain brachytherapy Elastoplast mould (EPM) techniques for treating BCC showed that EPM was more appropriate. Mould radiotherapy for BCC of the head and neck region is easy to perform and a suitable method since it is adapted to the changing contour of the region.

It is important to take a margin of 5 mm around the tumour since it is very often more extended than seen clinically. When the margins are poorly defined, a larger radiation field of 10 mm is used. Recurrences can only be avoided in this way.

Choosing ionizing radiations for the treatment of BCC depends on different parameters. The anatomical location of the lesions where the cosmetic and the functional issues are important could be decisional for the treatment modality. Lesions smaller than 4 cm can be removed surgically in the head and neck regions. Radiotherapy, on the other hand, constitutes a tissue-sparing method around the eyes, nose and ears for larger BCCs and is obviously less advantageous for lesions of the trunk and extremities because these areas have tendencies to develop telangiectases and postinflammatory pigmentation disorders. Radiotherapy is more indicated in the elderly patient with advanced cancers or on anticoagulant therapy, and should be avoided below the age of 40 in order to minimize the additive deleterious effects of solar radiation. It is as well performed in recurrent BCC after surgical resection. However, Mohs surgery avoids recurrences and if used primarily after skin biopsy, ionizing radiation is not needed. Carcinomatous tissues buried by flap techniques, both Mohs surgery and radiotherapy, are potentially achievable. Patients prone to keloids respond satisfactorily to radiotherapy. Ionizing radiations are also performed for the palliative treatment of xeroderma pigmenstosum-related malignancy.

Recurrent BCC previously treated with radiotherapy are not eligible for retreatment by radiation. This may provoke ulcerations due to dose accumulation and increased skin cancer aggressiveness. Cure rates following retreatment are also very low. Ionizing radiations are to be avoided in BCCs secondary to radiodermitis or occurring in osteomyelitis, chronic ulcers and burn scars.

Advantages of radiotherapy are numerous. The radiation field can be adapted to the required area of treatment with preservation of uninvolved tissues. Tumour margins can be adapted as needed, usually 0.5–1 cm on each side of the lesion. Radiation therapy does not require anaesthesia or hospitalization, and is painless.

Whereas surgical scars tend to improve over time, skin treated with ionizing radiation may worsen in some patients especially on areas exposed to solar radiation. Chronic radiodermitis may develop with atrophy, sclerosis, telangiectases and hypo- or hyperpigmentation. Due to the secondary effects on skin appendages, areas of alopecia may arise from radiotherapy. All these factors, together with the high cost of certain technologies and the requirement of well-trained experienced physicians, represent practical disadvantages for the use of radiotherapy.

Alternative and experimental treatments

Certain extensive BCCs or multiple cancers such as naevus BCC syndrome or xeroderma pigmentosum cannot be treated with the classical modalities described here. Alternative forms of treatment working through biological pathways may be required.

Topical treatment

Local chemotherapy has been used for the treatment of various premalignant and malignant lesions, sometimes with success but frequently with limitations in efficacy and safety. To treat small and superficial BCCs compounds such as podophyllin, methotrexate, colchicine analogues and 5-fluorouracil (5-FU) have been used.

5-FU

Topical 5-FU from 5% to 20% is used on a daily basis for 3 to 4 weeks in the treatment of actinic keratosis, Bowen's disease and small superficial BCCs.

The cure rate from topical application of 5-FU in the treatment of BCCs is low (60–78%) and is followed by a high recurrence rate. Contact dermatitis, local discomfort and phototoxic reactions may occur. Efforts have been made to facilitate the penetration of 5-FU by adding an appropriate carrier such as phosphatidyl choline which is able to carry small water-soluble molecules, nucleotides, across skin lipid barriers.

Nevertheless, intralesional 5-FU is reported to be efficient in the treatment of keratoacanthomas and nodular BCCs. Intralesional injections of 5-FU are easy to administer, even in facial localities or surfaces where excision would be difficult. Improved results were reported by Miller with an intralesional drug delivery system consisting of 5-FU with epinephrine (adrenaline) in an aqueous gel system with purified bovine collagen used as a biodegradable carrier matrix. Complete response rate was 91% in well-defined, 6–15 mm large, not invasive BCCs of the trunk and limbs.

This way of treatment is therefore recommended if the patient refuses surgical intervention or if surgery is contraindicated.

The major disadvantages of intralesional injections of 5-FU is that it is a 'blind' procedure. However, biopsies taken for follow-up may resolve this problem. A life-threatening toxicity in cancer patients with decreased dihydropyrimidine dehydrogenase deficiency has been reported with topical 5-FU. Dihydropyrimidine dehydrogenase is the initial rate-limiting enzyme in pyrimidine catabolism and may be decreased in cancer patients. An increased risk for severe toxicity including diarrhoea, stomatitis, mucositis, myelosuppression, neurotoxicity and, in some cases, death have been reported with topical 5-FU.

How intralesional 5-FU induces regression of cutaneous tumours is unknown. It has been speculated that this drug inhibits the DNA synthesis in rapidly proliferating tumour cells.

Interferon (IFN)

IFNs have an antineoplastic action because they inhibit cellular growth and modulate cellular function. IFN-α appears to have much more effect on BCCs than IFN-β or -γ. One study has reported on 52 BCC patients treated with IFN more than 10 years ago, and 58 more than 5 years ago, with two recurrences only. In another trial, only two of 13 BCC patients required surgery due to insufficient improvement.

IFN therapy may be recommended for patients who refuse surgery, have a non-resectable or large BCC for which other treatments are not indicated, are impossible, dangerous or cosmetically risky. Although there is limited evidence it has been reported that intralesional IFN-α_{2b} (or IFN-β_{2a}) therapy for BCC cured 80–86% of small uncomplicated noduloulcerative or superficial BCCs after 16–20 weeks of follow-up. The recommended dose is $13.5.10^6$ IU three times a week to be spread over 3 weeks. After each session of IFN many patients experience transient flu-like symptoms.

While the mechanism of regresion after IFN injection remains unknown, it is most likely that BCC regresses by committing suicide through apoptosis induction.

Taking into consideration the side-effects of this treatment after each administration, the relatively low cure rate, and the high cost of the drug, it is best to consider this form of therapy as an experimental one.

Polyethylene-glycol modified interleukin-2 (PEG-IL-2)

IL-2 is produced by activated T lymphocytes and has been used in the treatment of skin melanoma and non-skin cancers such as renal cell carcinoma. It has been recently administered perilesionally to BCC in an open label, uncontrolled pilot study. Injection doses ranged from 3000 to 1200000 IU in one to four weekly administrations. Total response was observed in 66% of the treated cases. IL-2 seems therefore an encouraging approach and future investigations including larger numbers of patients is needed.

Imiquimod

Imiquimod is a cytokine and IFN inducer. It also appears to modulate Langerhans' cell function by enhancing its migration from the skin to regional lymph nodes. Imiquimod 5% cream has been approved for the treatment of external and perianal warts and recent data suggest its efficacy in the treatment of BCC. In one study, BCC cleared in 100% of the patients dosed twice daily, once daily and 3 times weekly for a period of 8 weeks. Local inflammatory reactions were observed at tumour sites, and could be avoided by declining dosage frequency. A five times weekly dosage, for a period of 6 weeks, seems like a possible alternative between the induction of adverse effect and therapeutic efficacy. The value of imiquimod has been established in non-aggressive skin types of BCC namely nodular and superficial types and no data concerning more aggressive BCCs are available. Carefully selected patients could benefit from this new and promising therapy where surgical morbidity in terms of cosmetic result is high. Patients suffering from multiple lesions such as BCC naevus syndrome or xeroderma pigmentosum syndrome are eligible for topical treatment of imiquimod.

Tazarotene

Generally, topical retinoids have proven to be inefficient in the treatment of psoriasis. However, tazarotene is effective and safe for the topical therapy of plaque psoriasis. This new-generation retinoid regulates differentiation and proliferation of keratinocytes. Tazarotene is currently undergoing clinical trials for the treatment of BCC.

Preliminary results have been reported as promising and 53% of the treated BCC cleared after 6 months of treatment using 0.1 tazarotene gel once daily. Longer-term follow-up for larger numbers of patients will be necessary to evaluate this approach further.

Systemic chemotherapy

BCCs are considered to be relatively insensitive to cytotoxic drugs. Systemic methotrexate, 5-FU, vinblastine and bleomycin have been used with poor results.

Recently, several reports indicated that BCC are sensitive to platinum-containing regimens. Treatment of 3–6 courses of cisplatinum in cycles of 3–4 weeks are suggested. If no favourable response is obtained after two courses, treatment should be discontinued.

Combination with other treatments may be considered. Systemic chemotherapy with platinum alone or in combination with other treatment modalities may be indicated in BCC refractory to standard treatment, in cases with advanced lesions making surgery or radiotherapy mutilating or in patients with metastatic BCC.

Retinoids

The mechanisms by which retinoids influence BCC development is not well understood but probably implicate the binding of the molecule to its nuclear receptor enhancing gene expression for cytodifferentiation and growth regulation. Chemically induced BCC tumours in rats, injected biweekly with retinol, have a two-to-threefold reduction in DNA synthesis.

Several studies show a significant reduction or complete regression of the tumours when high doses of 3–4 mg/kg per day were given orally. However recurrent lesions appeared a few months after discontinuation of the drug.

The promising role of retinoids is undoubtedly the chemopreventive effect. High-dose isotretinoin is effective in the prevention of primary cancers in patients suffering from BCC naevus syndrome and xeroderma pigmentosum. However when treatment was discontinued, incidence rose again, implying a lifelong prophylaxis with associated side-effects.

In conclusion retinoids are minimally effective as a chemotherapeutic agent. Trials involving retinoids for the treatment of patients with multiple BCCs have been promising. Yet, side-effects and the necessity for continued long-term therapy may limit their usefulness.

New insights in retinoid research includes combining therapeutics, retinoids/IFN, gene therapy to alter retinoid receptor expression and combining agents able to modulate signal transduction pathways.

Photodynamic therapy (PDT)

In recent years photodynamic cancer therapy has provoked much interest. This new technique for treating BCCs involves irradiation with a light source after local or systemic administration of a photosensitizing agent, a haematoporphyrin derivative.

One frequently used haematoporphyrin is 5-aminolaevulinic acid (5-ALA), the first metabolite of heambiosynthesis. A light source of 630 nm, is focused on the patient to activate the photosensitizer, which results in necrosis of the tumour.

PDT with systemic administration of photosensitizers is interesting because studies reported partial to complete eradication of BCC in 44–82% of cases.

In addition systemic administration has an important disadvantage, namely the accumulation of the photosensitizers and their metabolites resulting in prolonged (1–6 months) skin photosensitivity. Therefore topical application of photosensitizing agents is more convenient to use.

PDT with topical application of photosensitizer has been used to treat BCCs, with remission of up to 96% of superficial lesions. No photosensitivity was observed. However during irradiation, patients experience a severe burn sensation and pain, in particular when performed on the face.

The efficacy of topical PDT is limited to superficial and early tumours.

In superficial BCCs PDT may be a good treatment replacing standard treatments. PDT is also a tissue-saving method with cosmetic advantages—it leaves very discrete scars.

PDT is a treatment that should be considered in patients with multiple BCCs, superficial lesions localized to keloid-prone areas such as the chest, shoulders and back, and where conventional treatment produces large open wounds which have to be transplanted. Combining partial surgical techniques such as debulking techniques followed by PDT for nodular BCC showed 92% of complete response on clinical and histopathological examination.

The disadvantage of PDT is the insufficient penetration of PDT resulting in the lesion healing on the surface with tumour cells still intact underneath. To detect these cancer cells it is important to biopsy at regular intervals. It should be noted that PDT is ineffective for pigmented BCC because melanin absorbs the photoactivating of porphyrin. BCCs thicker than 2 mm or recurrent lesions are not indicated for this treatment.

Conclusion

Epidemiological statistics worldwide show that the incidence of BCCs and SCCs is increasing at an alarming rate.

Skin carcinomas can be controlled reasonably well.

However, we consider that all skin cancers should be removed totally using the treatment modalities giving the highest cure rate. All studies in the literature show that the highest cure rates are obtained with histologically controlled surgery of the margins of the skin carcinomas. Therefore many BCCs (and all SCCs) should be treated by one of the microscopic-orientated histological surgical techniques. It would be of much greater benefit to the patient and to the financial situation of health-care insurers if MOHS technique is used at first on high-risk primary lesions than later on the lesions that have recurred or metastasized.

Table 7 Major guidelines for mode of treatment of BCC to obtain the higest cure rate

	BCC											Patient's condition	
Mode of treatment	Type	Well-defined border	Anatomy/ locality	Primary	Recurrent	Size + depth (*small,	large)	Safety margins to take	Single	Multiple	Previous treatment	Indication	Contra-indication
Excision	Nodular superficial	+	Moveable	+		+		+	+			Quick healing	Allergy to anticoagulation
MOHS	Morphoea aggressive		H-zone functional zone	+	++	+		–			+	Young	
Electrosurgery		+	In H-zone	+	–	+	–	+			If electrosurgery or cryosurgery		Pacemaker
Cryosurgery	Nodular superficial	+	Nose, ears, forehead, hands, keloid zone	+	–	+	–	+		+		Pacemaker anticoagulation allergy	Cryoglobulinaemia Cold agglutination Autoimmune disease
Radiation	No morphoea not if preceding disease	+	Head, neck		–	–	+	+		+	If radiation	> 60 years	
Intralesional 5-FU		+	Trunk, limbs			+				+			
Retinoids						+	+			++			
PDT	Superficial		Keloid zone	+			+			+			

*small: < 2 cm diameter and < 3–4 mm depth; large: > 2 cm diameter and > 4 mm depth or into deep dermis or fat.

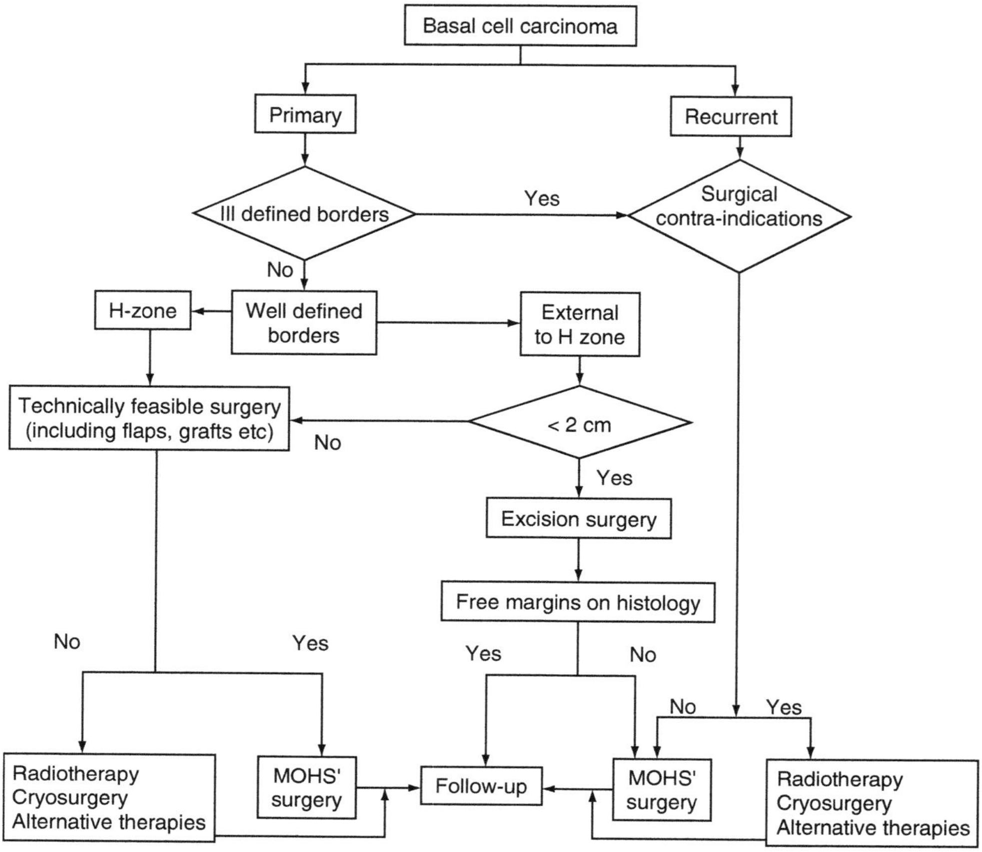

Figure 1 Decision-making algorithm for the appropriate treatment of basal cell carcinoma

If MOHS surgery is not possible, a very careful and thorough selection of the treatment modality should be done according to the indication criteria.

Table 7 summarizes the most important criteria to be considered in making the best choice of treatment to obtain the highest cure rates for BCCs.

Further reading

Bernardeau K, Derancourt C, Cambie M *et al*. Cryosurgery of basal cell carcinoma: a study of 358 patients. *Ann Dermatol Venereol* 2000; 127: 175–9.

Berridge JK, Morgan DA. A comparison of late cosmetic results following two different radiotherapy techniques for treating basal cell carcinoma. *Clin Oncol (R Coll Radiol)* 1997; 9: 400–2.

Beutner KR, Geisse JK, Helman D, Fox TL, Ginkel A, Owens ML. Therapeutic response of basal cell carcinoma to the immune response modifier imiquimod 5% cream. *J Am Acad Dermatol* 1999; 41: 1002–7.

Buechner SA, Wernli M, Harr T, Hahn S, Itin P, Erb P. Regression of basal cell carcinoma by intralesional interferon-alpha treatment is mediated by CD95 (Apo-1/Fas) -CD95 ligand-induced suicide. *J Clin Invest* 1997; 100: 2691–6.

Caccialanza M, Piccinno R, Beretta M, Gnecchi L. Results and side effects of dermatologic radiotherapy: a retrospective study of irradiated cutaneous epithelial neoplasms. *J Am Acad Dermatol* 1999; 41: 589–94.

Dogan B, Harmanyeri Y, Baloglu H, Oztek I. Intralesional alfa-2a interferon therapy for basal cell carcinoma. *Cancer Lett* 1995; 91: 215–19.

Duvic M, Asano AT, Hager C, Mays S. The pathogenesis of psoriasis and the mechanism of action of tazarotene. *J Am Acad Dermatol* 1998; 39: S129–S132.

Griep C, Davelaar J, Scholten AN, Chin A, Leer JW. Electron beam therapy is not inferior to superficial X-ray therapy in the treatment of skin carcinoma. *Int J Radiat Oncol Biol Phys* 1995; 32: 1347–50.

Ikic D, Padovan I, Pipic N *et al.* Interferon reduces recurrences of basal cell and squamous cell cancers. *Int J Dermatol* 1995; 34: 58–60.

Johnson MR, Hageboutros A, Wang K, High L, Smith JB, Diasio RB. Life-threatening toxicity in a dihydropyrimidine dehydrogenase-deficient patient after treatment with topical 5-fluorouracil. *Clin Cancer Res* 1999; 5: 2006–11.

Kagy MK, Amonette R. The use of imiquimod 5% cream for the treatment of superficial basal cell carcinomas in a basal cell nevus syndrome patient. *Dermatol Surg* 2000; 26: 577–8.

Kaplan B, Moy RL. Effect of perilesional injections of PEG-interleukin-2 on basal cell carcinoma. *Dermatol Surg* 2000; 26: 1037–40.

Kuflike EG, Gage AA. The five year cure rate achieved by cryosurgery for cancer. *J Am Acad Dermatol* 1991; 24: 1002–4.

Levine N. Role of retinoids in skin cancer treatment and prevention. *J Am Acad Dermatol* 1998; 39: S62–6.

Miller BH, Shavin JS, Cognetta A *et al.* Nonsurgical treatment of basal cell carcinomas with interlesional 5-fluorouracil/epinephrine infectable gel. *J Am Acad Dermatol* 1997; 36: 72–7.

Moeholt K, Aagaard H, Pfeiffer P, Hansen O. Platinum based cytotoxic therapy in basal cell carcinoma. *Acta Oncol* 1996; 35: 677–82.

Peck GL, DiGiovanna JJ, Sarnoff DS *et al.* Treatment and prevention of basal cell carcinoma with oral isotretinoin. *J Am Acad Dermatol* 1988; 19: 176–85.

Peris K, Fargnoli MC, Chimenti S. Preliminary observations on the use of topical tazarotene to treat basal-cell carcinoma. *N Engl J Med* 1999; 341: 1767–8.

Petit JY, Avril MF, Margulis A *et al.* Evaluation of cosmetic results of a randomized trial comparing surgery and radiotherapy in the treatment of basal cell carcinoma of the face. *Plast Reconstr Surg* 2000; 105: 2544–51.

Reymann F. Treatment of basal cell carcinoma of the skin with 5-fluorouracil ointment. A 10-year follow-up study. *Dermatologica* 1979; 158: 368–72.

Romagosa R, Saap L, Givens M *et al.* A pilot study to evaluate the treatment of basal cell carcinoma with 5-fluorouracil using phosphatidyl choline as a transepidermal carrier. *Dermatol Surg* 2000; 26: 338–40.

Rowe DE, Carroll RJ, Day CL Jr. Long-term recurrence rates in previously untreated primary basal cell carcinoma: implications for patient follow-up. *J Dermatol Surg Oncol* 1989; 15: 315–28.

Rowe DE, Carroll RJ, Day CL Jr. Mohs surgery is the treatment of choice for recurrent (previously treated) basal cell carcinoma. *J Dermatol Surg Oncol* 1989; 15: 424–31.

Sakata K, Aoki Y, Kumakura Y *et al.* Radiation therapy for patients with xeroderma pigmentosum. *Radiat Med* 1996; 14: 87–90.

Silverman MK, Kopf AW, Bart RS, Grin CM, Levenstein MS. Recurrence rates of treated basal cell carcinomas. Part 3: Surgical excision. *J Dermatol Surg Oncol* 1992; 18: 471–6.

Suhge d'Aubermont PC, Bennett RG. Failure of curettage and electrodesiccation for removal of basal cell carcinoma. *Arch Dermatol* 1984; 120: 1456–60.

Thissen MR, Nieman FH, Ideler AH, Berretty PJ, Neumann HA. Cosmetic results of cryosurgery versus surgical excision for primary uncomplicated basal cell carcinomas of the head and neck. *Dermatol Surg* 2000; 26: 759–64.

Thissen MR, Schroeter CA, Neumann HA. Photodynamic therapy with delta-aminolaevulinic acid for nodular basal cell carcinomas using a prior debulking technique. *Br J Dermatol* 2000; 142: 338–9.

Wagner RF, Cottel WI. Multifocal recurrent basal cell carcinoma following primary tumour treatment by electrodesiccation and curettage. *J Am Acad Dermatol* 1987; 17: 1047–9.

Weinstein GD, Krueger GG, Lowe NJ *et al.* Tazarotene gel, a new retinoid, for topical therapy of psoriasis: vehicle-controlled study of safety, efficacy, and duration of therapeutic effect. *Am Acad Dermatol* 1997; 37: 85–92.

Wennberg AM, Lindholm LE, Alpsten M, Larkö O. Treatment of surperficial basal cell carcinomas using topically applied delta-aminolaevulinic acid and a filtered xenon lamp. *Arch Dermatol Res* 1996; 288: 561–4.

Bowen's disease

G. Avgerinou

Definition and epidemiology

Bowen's disease is a persistent, progressive non-elevated, red scaly or crusted plaque which is due to an intraepidermal carcinoma and is potentially malignant.

John T. Bowen first described the entity bearing his name in 1912. From that time Bowen's disease has been identified as squamous cell carcinoma *in situ*.

Bowen's disease occurs predominantly in the elderly population (mean age in the sixth, seventh or eighth decade).

The male to female ratio is roughly equal varying from 1.2 to 0.8 : 1, depending on the study.

Aetiology and pathophysiology

A number of aetiological factors have been implicated in the development of Bowen's disease. Genetic and subtle defects in DNA repair may also play a role. As with the non-melanoma skin cancers, the sun-exposed distribution of Bowen's disease implicates ultraviolet light as one factor. Human papillomavirus (HPV) have been well detected, by both *in situ* hybridization and polymerase chain reaction (PCR) in lesions of Bowen's disease. Chemical carcinogens among these are the inorganic arsenicals. These may be obtained from a variety of sources, including formerly used medications, and occupational chemicals such as Fowler's solution, used in the past in the treatment of psoriasis.

Clinical characteristics

Lesions of Bowen's disease typically appear as isolated, well-demarcated, scaly plaques—persistent, discrete and irregular in shape. Erythematous and scaly or crusted lesions may resemble psoriasis or dermatitis.

The lesions occur equally on covered and exposed skin surfaces, with half of all lesions occurring on the head.

The lesions may occur anywhere on the skin surface or on mucosal membranes. Mucosal surfaces affected include the oral cavity, anogenitalia and conjuctivae.

Diagnosis

Diagnosis is based on the physical examination and biopsy. Skin biopsy is the most important diagnostic tool, and is usually required.

The epidermis shows full-thickness dysplasia (carcinoma *in situ*), which characteristically involves the entire epidermis. The keratinocytes show loss of polarity, atypia and mitoses, producing a 'wind-blown' appearance. There is marked acanthosis, with complete disorganization of the epidermal architecture. The upper dermis shows an infiltrate of lymphocytes, histiocytes and plasma cells.

Histological differentiation of Bowen's disease includes Paget's disease, melanoma, pseudoepitheliomatosus hyperplasia, podophyllin-induced alterations of genital warts, bowenoid papulosis and Borst-Jadassohn epithelioma.

Differential diagnosis

See Table 1.

Treatment

General therapeutic guidelines

Avoidance of the sun is highly recommended. Broad-spectrum sunscreen (SPF 15 or greater) should be applied.

Recommended therapies

Excisional surgery

The therapy of choice for Bowen's disease is surgical excision. Margin of 5 mm are advisable with a depth down to

Table 1 Differential diagnosis of Bowen's disease

Pigmented BCC	When the scalp is removed and the edge stretched the thread-like margin will reveal telangiectasia
Eczema	Pruritus—symmetrical—wide spreading improvement when steroids are applied—mostly relapsing
Verruca vulgaris	Simple or multiple keratotic papules Kobner phenomenon—multiple lesions—papillomatous—predominantly hands/feet—no crust
Pigment actinic keratosis	Superficial verrucous plaque which appears to be stuck on the epidermis—marginated rough scales—sun-exposed skin
Seborrhoeic keratosis	Well-demarcated—smooth greasy scales—slight pigmentation—pasted on appearance

subcutaneous fat to ensure removal of a possible invasive lesion.

Topical chemotherapeutic agents

A non-invasive alternative therapy includes application of the topical chemotherapeutic agent 5-fluorouracil, which may be used in conjuction with dinitrochlorobenzene (DNCB), a topical sensitizer. However, these therapies may be impractical for patients with numerous or large lesions in anatomically difficult areas.

Radiotherapy

This is another alternative to surgery. However, if used, it must be in full tumour doses.

Cryotherapy

This has been used widely as effective therapy, with few recurrences and adverse reactions.

Photodynamic therapy (PDT)

PDT may be used as adjuvant therapy for difficult lesions. PDT, also known as photochemotherapy or photoradiation therapy, is effective for many forms of malignant tumours including skin cancers.

Topical PDT with endogenous porphyrins consists of irradiation of the tumour with visible light after the application of exogenous 5-aminolevulinic acid (ALA).

Photoactivation of photosensitizing porphyrins, which selectively accumulate in malignant cells, leads to the release of cytotoxic substances and causes tumour destruction with minimal damage to surrounding normal tissue. When PDT is given systemically, the porphyrin compounds haematoporphyrin derivative (HPD), or a mixture of its active components (commercially known as Photofrin II) lead to generalized serious phototoxic reactions in the skin. This is the main reason that PDT by intravenous injection of porphyrins is not used much more widely.

Recently, Kennedy & Pottier described a novel method of topical PDT, and showed favourable results in the treatment of Bowen's disease.

Topical application of sensitizers, especially ALA, in aqueous solution passes through abnormal keratin and is metabolized by the tumour cells to photosensitizing concentrations of porphyrin. Subsequent exposure to photoactivation selectively destroys skin cancers.

PDT has many advantages:

1 There is no systemic toxicity or interaction with other medications.
2 It is tissue sparing and leaves the skin surrounding the tumour intact.
3 Good cosmetic results.
4 No anaesthesia required.
5 Several sites can be treated simultaneously.
6 It can be used repeatedly for the treatment of the same or new lesions.
7 It does not exclude the use of other modalities.
8 Treatment is possible on an outpatient basis.
9 It can be used as adjuvant therapy

The main clinical disadvantage of PDT is patient photosensitivity. This requires sun avoidance and/or sun protection for 4–6 weeks. Another side-effect of PDT is the development of moderate pain in some patients. Because the drug is retained longer in the liver, spleen and kidneys it should be avoided in patients with severe liver or kidney disease.

The tumour shows complete remission and up to 12 months after treatment there are no clinical or histological sign. Cosmetic results are good.

Other alternative therapies that have been used are electrodessication, curettage and laser ablation with ND:YAG or CO_2 lasers and hypothermic treatment.

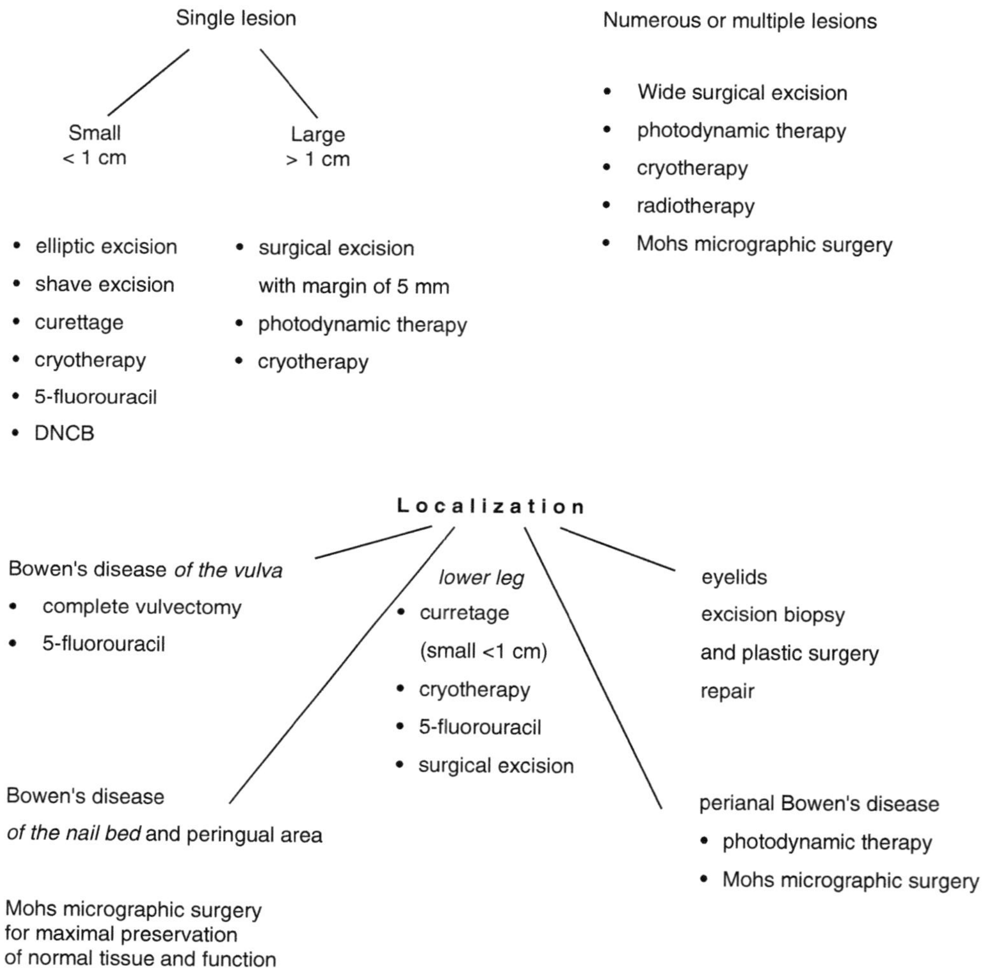

Figure 1 Therapeutic algorithm of Bowen's disease

Further reading

Alvanopoulos K *et al.* Photodynamic therapy of superficial basal cell carcinoma using 5-aminolevulinic acid and 514-nm light. *JEADV* 1997; 9: 134–6.

Antoniou C *et al.* Aminolevulinic acid—topical photodynamic therapy in skin cancers and solar keratoses. *Skin cancer* 1996; 11: 81–4.

Avgerinou G. Bowen's disease. *European Handbook of Dermatological Treatments*. Berlin-Heidelberg: Springer-Verlag, 1999: 89–91.

Cox NM, Syson P. Wound healing on the lower leg after radiotherapy or cryotherapy of Bowen's disease and other malignant skin lesions. *Br J Dermatol* 1995; 133: 60–5.

Cullin A *et al.* Photodynamic therapy for large or multiple patches of Bowen's disease and basal cell carcinoma. *Arch Dermatol* 2001; 137: 319–24.

Kennedy JC, Pottier RH. Endogenous protoporphyrin IX, a clinical useful photosensitizer for photodynamic therapy. *J Photochem Photobiol* 1987; 14: 275–92.

Krenden OP, Herzog V, Acherman C, Scuppisser JD, Spichtin HP, Tondelli P. 11 cases of anal Bowen's disease. *Schweiz Med Wochenchz* 1996; 126: 1536–40.

Mang J, Cooper H, Wilson BD, Stoll HL. Photodynamic therapy in the treatment of Bowen's disease. *J Am Dermatol* 1992; 27: 979–82.

Masataro H, Akira K. Hyperthermic treatment of Bowen's disease with disposable chemical pocket warmers: a report of 8 cases. *J Am Acad Dermatol, Tokyo Osaka, Japan* 2000; 43: 1070–5.

Morton CA, Whitechurst C, Moseley H, McCoil JH, Moore JV, Mackie RM. Comparison of photodynamic therapy with cryotherapy in the treatment of Bowen's disease. *Br J Dermatol* 1996; 135: 766–71.

Niyom T. Treatment of Bowen's disease of the digit with carbon dioxide laser. *J Am Acad Dermatol* 2000; 43: 1080–3.

San P, McMarlin SC, Sperling CC, Katz B. Bowen's disease of the nail bed and peringual area: a clinicopathologic analysis of seven cases. *Arch Dermatol* 1994; 130 (2): 204–9.

Svanberg K, Andersson T, Killander D, Wang I, Stenram V. Photodynamic therapy of non-melanoma, malignant tumors of the skin using topical delta-amino levulinic acid sensitization and laser irradiation. *Br J Dermatol* 1994; 130: 743–51.

Bullous pemphigoid

A.G. Vareltzidis and
P.G. Stavropoulos

Definition and epidemiology

Bullous pemphigoid (BP) is an acquired, non-scarring, subepidermal blistering disease, usually occurring in the elderly, characterized by large tense blisters. Women and men are equally affected and no racial or geographical predilection is recognized. There is no known specific HLA correlation. BP has been reported in association with a variety of autoimmune diseases, including systemic lupus erythematosus, diabetes mellitus, lichen planus, rheumatoid arthritis, Hashimoto thyroiditis, pemphigus vulgaris and psoriasis. There have been many reports of BP associated with malignancy, although there is much controversy over this association.

Aetiology and pathophysiology

BP is an autoimmune skin disease and the cause of the autoantibody production remains obscure. The target antigens are the hemidesmosomal BP antigens with molecular weights of 230 and 180 kDa (BPAG1 and BPAG2, respectively). Antibody binding to BP antigen is postulated to be the initial step in blister formulation. Fixation of immunoglobulin G (IgG) to the basement membrane zone activates the complement cascade (mainly C3, C5a), which causes chemotaxis of leucocytes and degranulation of mast cells. Eosinophils and neutrophilis are recruited by mast cells produced factors to the basement membrane zone, where they release tissue-destructive enzymes (proteases) resulting in dermal–epidermal separation. Several drugs have been associated with the onset of BP including frusemide, sulphasalasine, penicillamine and captopril. Local irritation and damage to the skin have all been implicated in the induction of the disease. Ultraviolet (UV) light or psoralen and UVA (PUVA) and other physical agents including thermal burns, wounds, skin grafts and radiotherapy have been reported to induce BP in normal skin.

Clinical characteristics and course

Urticarial and figured erythemas are common prodromal eruptions in BP. Subsequently, large tense blisters arise with a base of normal or erythematous skin. Grouping may be present, and lower abdomen, inner thighs, groin, axillae and flexural aspects of the forearms and the legs are sites of predilection for the lesions. However, localized forms of BP are not uncommon. Pemphigoid nodularis, vegetans and dyshidrosiform represent some clinical variants of 'classical' BP. Nikolsky's sign is negative and mucosal lesions are usually clinically insignificant, consisting of small tense bullae in the oropharynx. The natural history of BP is that of persistent disease with eventual remission occurring within 5 years in the majority of patients. Prognosis is considered fair, but BP is a potentially fatal disease particularly in the elderly, where health may already be fragile.

Diagnosis

A subepidermal split containing eosinophils and a mixed dermal infiltrate of numerous eosinophils, some neutrophils and lymphocytes, is found in biopsy specimens. IgG and/or C3 are deposited along the basement membrane zone in virtually all active cases of BP (direct immunofluorescence) and about 70–80% of patients are found to have circulating IgG to the basement membrane zone of normal stratified squamous epithelia (indirect immunofluorescence). In occasional cases these diagnostic techniques will require supplementation with the so-called 'split-skin'

Table 1 Differential diagnosis of bullous pemphigoid

Pemphigoid gestationis	Rare disease of pregnancy and postpartum period
Cicatrical pemphigoid	Scarring autoimmune bullous disease primarily affecting mucosal surfaces
Epidermolysis bullosa acquisita	Trauma-induced blisters healing with scars, different target antigen
Dermatitis herpetiformis	Young adults, pruritic papules and vesicles symmetrically distributed over extensor surfaces. Enteropathy (80% of cases). HLA-B8-DR3
Linear IgA dermatosis	Younger age group, linear IgA deposition at basement membrane zone (direct immunofluorescence)
Erythema multiforme (bullous)	Typical distribution of lesions, different immunofluorescence findings
Bullous systemic lupus erythematosus	Lesions distributed on sun-exposed areas, subepidermal blisters with neutrophils, different immunofluorescence findings
Other disorders	Porphyria cutanea tarda, drug reactions, insect bite reaction, bullous lichen planus, etc.

technique, immunoelectron microscopy, immunoblotting and immunoprecipitation.

Differential diagnosis

See Table 1.

Treatment

General therapeutic guidelines

- Treatment can be divided into three phases: initial control, consolidation and withdrawal. The first objective is stopping or significantly reducing new blister formation. Therapy is introduced and adjusted upwards as required and slowly reduced to the lowest possible level while maintaining a low level of disease activity. Complete withdrawal of therapy is carried out if possible.
- The severity of disease, age of patient and presence of underlying disease (diabetes mellitus, hypertension, peptic ulceration, osteoporosis, malignancy) must be considered in determining therapeutic agents and doses.
- Localized disease may initially be managed with local potent steroids and adjunctive topical measures.
- Moderate (20–60 lesions) to severe (more than 60 lesions) disease will usually require systemic steroids in moderate doses alone or in combination with immunosuppressives, dapsone or tetracyclines.
- Severe therapy-resistant disease requires systemic steroids in higher doses and immunosuppressives, ciclosporin, plasmapheresis or γ-globulin therapy as adjunctive agents.
- Immunosuppressive agents, due to their delayed onset of action (4–8 weeks), can be started at the same time as systemic steroids. Thus, steroids are used to achieve initial control then tapered at the time when the immunosuppressives are taking effect.

Recommended therapies

Supportive care and adjuvant therapy

Supportive care is essential in cases in which widespread skin denudation and immobility render the patient susceptible to fluid loss, electrolyte imbalance, infection and thromboembolic events. A bed that spreads pressure is useful in severe disease. The blisters caused by widespread cutaneous and mucosal erosive disease may require frequent oral analgesics, and sedating antihistamines are frequently given in the initial stages of BP to reduce pruritus. Diluted saline or potassium permanganate compresses and baths assist in keeping the lesions clean. Cimetidine (400 mg twice daily) may be administered to prevent peptic ulceration in ill patients and those receiving systemic steroids. Calcium supplementations and vitamin D (50 000 U once or twice weekly) may be used to reduce the risk of osteoporotic complications in patients receiving systemic corticosteroids.

Topical therapy

Topical steroids may constitute adequate therapy in localized or moderate BP, and they are also extremely useful adjuvants to systemic therapy when disease is more severe. Potent topical steroids (clobetasol propionate 0.05% twice daily) are usually required initially, with tapering to lower potency agents. Triamcinolone acetonide 3.10 mg/mL may be injected weekly to resistant lesions. In the event of secondary infection, topical antibacterial agents may be safely applied. Soothing bland emollients seem to help when applied to lesional skin. Oral hygiene should be maintained with antiseptic mouthwashes before, after and between meals. A soft diet including pureed food and liquid protein supplements is best during active disease. Severe pain may be treated with topical anaesthesia (lidocaine (lignocaine) 2% viscous solution) particularly before meals. Tetracycline mouthwashes (250 mg dissolved in 50 mL of water) may be used to treat oral mucosa infections.

Systemic corticosteroids

These are the most useful drugs in the treatment of BP, rapidly inducing remission in the majority of patients. Our experience and most large series show that the majority of patients with generalized disease are controlled with 40–80 mg daily of prednisone or prednisolone and it is only rarely necessary to exceed 100 mg daily. Healing of existing lesions and cessation of new blister formation reflects a positive response to therapy. Once the disease is under control, the steroid dose should be tapered slowly and eventually changed to an alternate-day regimen to minimize the steroid side-effects. Corticosteroid pulse therapy, in which patients are given 1 g of methylprednisolone intravenously for 3 consecutive days, may be given for resistant disease. Oral steroids must then be given as maintenance therapy. However, caution must be recommended in utilizing this type of therapy, particularly concerning the effects of prolonged systemic steroid therapy which are numerous: diabetes mellitus, hypertension, gastrointestinal bleeding, osteoporosis, cataracts and increased susceptibility to bacterial, fungal and viral infections. Appropriate monitoring includes urinalysis for glucose, fluid imbalance, blood pressure and body weight. Routine biochemistry may be done at weekly or twice weekly intervals in the first instance, dropping to monthly thereafter. Osteoporosis profile tests and ophthalmological examination for cataracts should be performed as a baseline and thereafter every 6 months, particularly in postmenopausal women.

Immunosuppressive agents

Azathioprine

This drug is most commonly employed in combination with steroids and sometimes for maintenance following steroid withdrawal. The usual dose is 50–100 mg daily. After 3–4 weeks of azathioprine use, the steroid maintenance dose may be significantly reduced and in some instances discontinued. Side-effects of azathioprine include dose dependent bone marrow depression, idiopathic hepatitis, increased susceptibility to infection, teratogenicity and increased risk of internal and cutaneous liver function tests and urinalysis. The full blood count, renal and liver function tests are repeated weekly for 8 weeks and then monthly.

Cyclophosphamide

Cyclophosphamide appears to be an effective steroid-sparing agent. The drug may be given initially in doses of 100–200 mg daily and 3 weeks later in maintenance doses of 100 mg daily. A pulsed steroid cyclophosphamide regimen is effective in severe cases of BP, permitting low cumulative steroid doses. Dexamethasone 100 mg i.v. given on 3 consecutive days, with the addition on day 1 of cyclophosphamide 500 mg to the infusion. Cyclophosphamide 50 mg is given per day between pulses. The pulses are initially repeated every 2 weeks, reducing to every 10 weeks in combination with ongoing oral cyclophosphamide over a period of 6 months. Side-effects include nausea and vomiting, bone marrow depression, haemorrhagic cystitis and increased risk of malignancy. Monitoring is as for azathioprine, with the addition of urinalysis weekly for the first 8–12 weeks, and every 2 weeks thereafter. Cardiac monitoring is required during pulse therapy.

Chlorambucil

Chlorambucil has been used as a steroid-sparing agent in the treatment of BP with excellent results. However, its use is not recommended except in special cases because of concern about the induction of haematological malignancy (acute myeloid leukaemia). The drug is initially given at 0.1 mg/kg per day in combination with prednisolone 40–60 mg/day. The chlorambucil dose is reduced over 6 weeks to a maintenance dose of 2 mg daily. Prednisolone is gradually withdrawn over a 4-month period, chlorambucil being discontinued some weeks later. There is a 50% reduction in the cumulative dose of prednisolone. Side-effects include bone marrow suppression, which can be severe, often resulting in transient dose-related thrombocytopenia. Appropriate monitoring is with baseline and weekly blood counts. Haematological malignancies may be related to a cumulative dose of 1 g or more of the drug.

Ciclosporin

Ciclosporin is used in the treatment of BP at doses of 5–8 mg/kg per day as a single agent or of 5 mg/kg per day in combination with steroids. According to our experience, combined therapy has a significant steroid-sparing effect and induces remission of BP in all patients, with monotherapy being less successful. The side-effects include hypertension, renal dysfunction, raised lipids, hypertrichosis, gum hyperplasia, susceptibility to infection and increased risk of malignancy. Baseline blood pressure should be recorded, and the laboratory investigations required include complete blood picture, urea, serum creatinine, creatinine clearance, liver function tests, fasting lipids and urinalysis. Serum creatinine should be repeated every 2 weeks for the first month with all the other previously mentioned laboratory parameters.

Dapsone and sulphonamides

BP may respond well to dapsone or the sulphonamides (sulfapyridine and sulfamethoxypyridazine) either alone or in combination with other agents. Dapsone is started at 50 mg daily and increased to 100 mg daily after 5–7 days if no response is apparent. Response is rapid, within 2 weeks. Dapsone may be used in combination with topical steroids or may be added (150–300 mg daily) to prednisolone or azathioprine therapy achieving adequate control of disease activity and permitting a reduction in the steroid dose. Younger patients showing neutrophil predominance on biopsy respond well to 2–4 g daily of sulfapyridine. Although these are not drugs of first choice for BP, they may be useful in the management of patients in whom corticosteroids are contraindicated or not tolerated. Side-effects include dose-related haemolysis and methaemoglobulinaemia, cutaneous hypersensitivity reactions, peripheral neuropathy, hepatic damage and renal failure. Monitoring should be with baseline tests and electrolytes. Glucose-6-phosphate dehydrogenase deficiency must be excluded prior to commencing therapy. Estimation of methaemoglobinaemia is obtained as clinically indicated.

Alternative and experimental treatment

Antibiotics/niacinamide

The combination of tetracycline 500 mg four times daily or minocycline 100 mg twice daily and niacinamide 500 mg twice daily is efficacious in some BP patients. Erythromycin 500 mg four times daily alone is also successfully used. Side-effects include gastrointestinal symptoms, photosensitivity, headache, benign intracranial hypertension, hyperpigmentation (minocycline) and candidosis.

Plasmapheresis

Plasmapheresis is used as an adjuvant to corticosteroids in the treatment of BP, showing a steroid-sparing effect. Prednisolone is administrered in combination with eight large-volume plasma exchanges over 4 weeks. In our experience a higher mean daily steroid dose is required to control disease activity when steroids are given alone (1 mg/kg) than with the dual therapy (0.6 mg/kg). The mild side-effects of fever, chills and hypertension, are relatively common. However, the potential difficulties include maintaining venous access, a bleeding tendency, electrolyte imbalances, allergic reactions to foreign proteins, pulmonary oedema and septicaemia. Deaths may also occur. Frequent observation of vital signs and cardiac monitoring are required during the procedure. It is suggested that weekly full blood examination, electrolytes, coagulation studies and liver function tests are carried out.

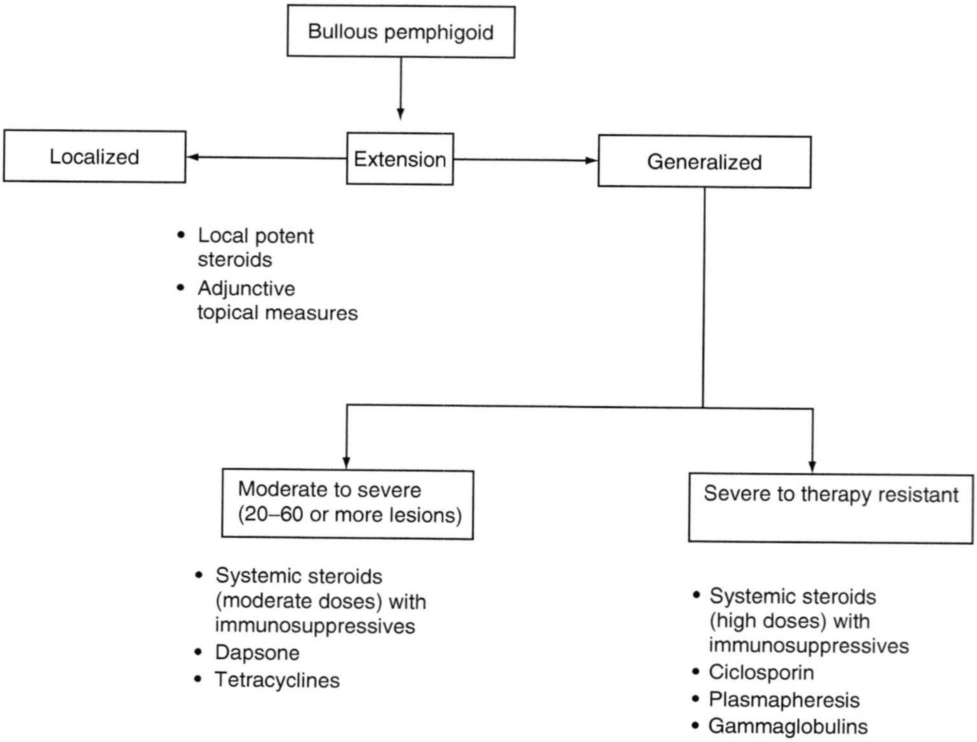

Gammaglobulins

Gammaglobulins given alone in a dose of 100–400 mg/kg for 5 consecutive days do not appear to be more than temporarily effective in the treatment of BP. The possible steroid-sparing effect awaits further investigation. Mycophenolate mofetil, a newly developed immunosuppressive agent, has recently been used as an effective, well tolerated, steroid-sparing agent in BD. Methorexate may also be useful as monotherapy in elderly patients with BD.

The recent production of recombinant forms of autoantigens recognized by B and T cells from patients with various forms of BP suggests that it may be possible to develop antigen-specific forms of immunotherapy for this disease. Alternatively, production of blocking of toxin-conjugated peptides that either impair of eliminate antigen-specific T cells driving to autoantibody production in these patients, represent another immunotherapeutic approach. Besides, the application of growth-enhancing cytokines might be used to speed healing of existing lesions.

Further reading

Bouscarat F *et al*. Treatment of bullous pemphigoid with dapsone: Retrospective study of thirty six cases. *J Am Acad Dermatol* 1996; 34: 683–7.

Engineer L, Ahmed AR. Role of intravenous immunoglobulin in the treatment of bullous pemphigoid. *J Am Acad Dermatol* 2001; 44: 83–8.

Fine JD. Management of acquired bullous skin diseases. *N Engl J Med* 1995; 333: 1475–81.

Grundmann-Kollmann M, Korting HC *et al*. Mycophenolate mofetil: A new therapeutic option in the treatment of blistering autoimmune diseases. *J Am Acad Dermatol* 1999; 40: 957–61.

Heilborn JD, Stahle-Bäckdahl *et al*. Low-dose oral pulse methotrexate as monotherapy in elderly patients with bullous pemphigoid. *J Am Acad Dermatol* 1999; 40: 741–9.

Huilgol SC, Black MM. Management of immunobullous diseases. I. Pemphigoid. *Clin Exp Dermatol* 1995; 20: 189–201.

Katsambas A. Quality of life in dermatology and the European Academy of Dermatology. *JEADV* 1994; 3: 211–14.

Kirtsching G, Wonjarowska F. Autoimmune blistering diseases. An update of diagnostic and investigations. *Clin Exp Dermatol* 1994; 19: 97–112.

Kolbach DN *et al*. Bullous pemphigoid successfully controlled by tetracycline and nicotinamide. *Br J Dermatol* 1995; 133: 88–92.

Korman NJ. Bullous pemphigoid. *Dermatol Clin* 1993; 11: 483–98.

Milligan H, Hutchinson PE. The use of chlorambucil in the treatment of bullous pemphigoid. *J Am Acad Dermatol* 1990; 22: 796–801.

Ronjeau JC, Morel P, Malle E. Plasma exchange in bullous pemphigoid. *Lancet* 1984; II: 486–9.

Schmidt E, Obe K, Brocker EB, Zillikens D. Serum levels of autoantibodies to BP 180 correlate with disease activity in patients with bullous pemphigoid. *Arch Dermatol* 2000; 136: 174–8.

Schmidt E, Zillikens D. Autoimmune and inherited subepidermal blistering diseases. Advances in the clinic and the laboratory. *Adv Dermatol* 2000; 16: 113–57.

Scott JE, Ahmed AR. The blistering diseases. *Med Clin North Am* 1998; 82: 1239–83.

Taylor G, Venning V, Wonjarowska F, Welsch K. Bullous pemphigoid and autoimmunity. *J Am Acad Dermatol* 1993; 29: 181–4.

Yancey KB, Egan CA. Pemphigoid. Clinical, histology, immunopathologic, and therapeutic considerations. *JAMA* 2000; 19: 284 (3): 350–6.

Candidiasis

D. Rigopoulos

Synonyms

Candidosis, moniliasis, thrush.

Definition

The term candidiasis refers to infections caused mainly by the classic opportunistic pathogen *Candida albicans*, or occasionally by other species of *Candida*, such as *C. tropicalis*, *C. guilliermondii*, *C. parapsilosis*, *C. krusei*, *C. stellatoidea*, *C. pseudotropicalis* and *C. glabrata*. These various yeast species differ in their potential to invade and colonize epithelial and epidermal sites, *C. albicans* being the species with the greatest such potential. Infections of the skin, nails and mucous membranes are the most often encoutered *Candida* infections.

Aetiology and pathophysiology

C. albicans, which is part of the normal human flora, is a dimorphic organism, developing in different morphological forms, such as yeasts, hyphae and pseudohyphae. This development is dependent on local conditions. Different predisposing factors exist, which lead to different types of candidiasis. Immunosuppression or leucopenia usually lead to systemic candidiasis, which is rare. Endocrinopathies (hypoparathyroidism, hypothyroidism, diabetes mellitus), iron or zinc deficiencies and inherited defects of immunity lead to chronic mucocutaneous candidiasis, which is also rare. Diabetes, pregnancy, antibiotic therapy, high humidity, immersion in water and oral contraceptive drugs lead to localized cutaneous candidiasis, which is the commonest type of disease. These predisposing factors are extremely important in the management of candidiasis patients, since the reversal of these factors is of great significance and part of the treatment protocol.

Clinical characteristics and course

Oral candidiasis

This disease is most commonly seen in infants and the elderly (associated with denture plates). The lesions may be situated on the mucosal surfaces or the tongue or at the corner of the mouth. One or more whitish, sharply defined, adherent plaques are the characteristic signs of the condition. If these plaques are wiped off an underlying erythematous base is seen. Erosion or ulceration are occasional complications.

In some cases, patients present with erythema, soreness, marked pain, atrophic mucous membranes and lack of whitish plaques (acute atrophic oral candidiasis).

Hyperplastic plaques on the cheek or the tongue that are not easily removed, especially in men who are smokers and over the age of 30, constitute a condition known as *Candida* leukoplakia (chronic hyperplastic candidiasis).

Median thomboid glossitis is another condition associated with candidiasis and presents with erythema of the tongue surface in absence of papillae, pain and tenderness.

Chronic atrophic candidiasis (denture stomatitis) affects nearly 25% of all denture wearers, and sometimes children with orthodontic appliances. The condition is characterized by bright red dusky erythema of the palate and gums, with atrophy of the epithelium and sometimes oedema.

Angular cheilitis (perlèche) occurs at the corner of the mouth and it is not always associated with *Candida*. The area is moist, red and fissured, and the symptoms include pain.

Superficial cutaneous candidiasis (*Candida* intertrigo)

Any occluded skin-fold, especially in hot and humid weather, may become moist and macerated, favouring the development of candidiasis. Erythema and moist exudation deep in the fold are the characteristic symptoms at the beginning. Erythema with well-defined borders, though not razor sharp as in tinea cruris, subcorneal pustule, satellite pustular papular lesions, itching and soreness make up the typical clinical pictures as the condition progresses.

Candida balanitis

Although *Candida* balanitis (which is seen mostly in uncircumcised men) is usually acquired from a sexual partner with vulgovaginitis, the possible oral and anal origins of the disease should not be forgotten. In mild cases erythema and tiny papules predominate and are seen after intercourse; in more severe cases, the entire glans can be involved, and soreness may prevent sexual intercourse as it becomes painful.

Vaginal candidiasis

It has been estimated that 75% of all adult women will suffer from vaginal candidiasis at some time during their lives. There are two types of the disease, the occasional and the recurrent. In the case of occasional vaginal candidiasis, *C. albicans* is the commonest causative yeast, accounting for over 80% of isolates. The predisposing factors are: antibiotics (which alter the normal vaginal flora), peak production of oestrogen before menstruation or use of high-oestrogen contraceptives (increase of glycogen, a nutrient source of *C. albicans*), pregnancy (increased levels or circulating oestrogen and progesterone raise the glycogen content of vaginal epithelial cells), immunosuppressive drugs, increased sugar levels of the urine and vaginal secretions and synthetic or tight-fitting clothes (they create a warm and moist environment). The condition presents with itching, soreness, erythema and a thick, creamy-white discharge. Vaginal candidiasis is recurrent in 10–20% of patients, and the male partner may play a part in reinfection (50% of male partners carry, the same strain of *Candida* on the penis or in the mouth). Symptoms are the same as in occasional vulvovaginitis, and only in chronic cases does the vaginal mucosa become glazed and atrophic.

Candida paronychia

This is a chronic condition found mainly in those who frequently immerse their hands in water (housewives, chefs, etc.) The nail fold is red and swollen; thick white pus may be discharged and the patient complains of pain. Nail dystrophy, with onycholysis and nail plate discoloration, is also found.

Candida onychomycosis

C. albicans infection of the nail may be seen secondary to chronic paronychia or onycholysis. The nail plate is opaque, brownish-green in colour and altered in shape. There may be nail plate changes secondary to the inflammation of the nail fold.

Chronic mucocutaneous candidiasis

This is an immunodeficiency disease, which is characterized by persistent candidiasis of mucous membranes, skin and nails. The infection may vary from mild, localized, persistent lesions to a severe, generalized condition. The disease usually starts in infancy and is often associated with endocrinopathy (mainly Addison's disease and hypoparathyroidism) A few late-onset cases are associated with thymic tumours; *Candida* granulomas may appear on the scalp and face.

Diagnosis

Diagnosis is based on the clinical examination, the history and is usually confirmed by laboratory examination (direct microscopy and culture).

Direct microscopy

Skin scrapings are examined microscopically for yeasts, pseudohyphae or hyphae, after the addition of 10% KOH solution to the slide preparation.

Culture

Swabs from suspected areas are cultured on Sabouraud's agar. *C. albicans* is a fast grower; colonies mature in 1–3 days (with the exception of nail clipping cultures, which must be kept for at least 7 days). Other *Candida* species may require longer to mature.

Differential diagnosis

See Table 1.

Treatment

General therapeutic guidelines

- Removal of underlying predisposing factors.
- Denture hygiene and frequent mouth toilet plus abstention from smoking will help those suffering from oral candidiasis.
- Infected skin folds should be kept dry, and if possible separated.
- Patients with chronic paronychia should keep their hands warm and dry.
- In most cases of *Candida* infection topical treatment alone is sufficient.
- Consideration should always be given to reduction of the *Candida* reservoir in the mouth and gut.

Recommended therapies

Antifungal drugs belonging to the polyene and azole families are the ones used in the treatment of *Candida* infections. A morpholine antifungal agent, amorolfine, is also active.

Topical therapeutic agents

These drugs are used in the form of creams, solution, suspensions, vaginal suppositories, lacquers, shampoos and powders.

The members of the polyene family are topical amphotericin B, nystatin and natamycin, while the azole family provides the imidazole derivatives miconazole, ketoconazole, econazole, omoconazole, tioconazole and clotrimazole for use in these conditions.

Amorofline is also used in the form of cream or nail lacquer.

The use of topical preparations is effective in the majority of *Candida* infections, but their use is restricted by the extent of the area involved. Side-effects are minimal; when used topically, there is some risk of resistance, except in the case of nystatin. Importantly,

Table 1 Differential diagnosis of candidiasis

Leukoplakia	Does not clear with prolonged anti-*Candida* therapy
Flexural psoriasis	Histology, microbiology
Bacterial intertrigo	Microbiology
Tinea	Microbiology, sharp edges
Seborrhoeic dermatitis	Microbiology
Hailey–Hailey disease	Histology
Flexural Darier's disease	Histology
Trichmonas vaginitis	Watery brown discharge, microbiology
Contact dermatitis of the vagina	Microbiology, history
Herpes simplex of the penis	Anti-HSV antibody-positive (IgM), history
Psoriasis of the penis	Chronic psoriasis-plaques in other body areas
Erythroplasia	Chonic, persistent, more dusky colour
Napkin dermatitis	The skin deep in the fold is free of symptoms
Bacterial paronychia	Microbiology, acute onset

they lack interaction with other classes of drug.

The topical formulations (except amorolfine nail lacquer) should be used one to three times daily, and application should continue for at least 1 week after clinical resolution of the disease, to allow reconstitution of the stratum corneum.

The type of formulation selected for treatment depends on the site and the symptoms of the disease (for dry lesions, lotions or creams are preferable, for wet lesions powders, for oral lesions suspensions, for vaginal lesions pessaries and for nail lesions lacquers).

Systemic antifungal agents

For systemic candidiasis or extensive skin disease in immunosuppressed patients, and when there are frequent relapses after topical treatment, high patient compliance is needed. The triazoles intraconazole and fluconazole and the imidazole ketoconazole are used for systemic treatment. The major disadvantages of these drugs are the potential toxicity (ketoconazole) and the development of both clinical and microbiologically proven resistance (fluconazole). Another serious disadvantage of these antifungals is their interaction with other drugs.

The chief side-effects of ketoconazole are nausea, pruritus, transient elevations in liver enzymes and significant liver toxicity, which can lead to death.

The incidence of adverse events is higher for long-term itraconazole therapy (16.2%) than for short-term administration (7.0%). The side-effects observed with itraconazole are not severe and mainly take the form of gastrointestinal disturbances (nausea, epigastraglia and diarrhoea).

The most frequent side-effects of fluconazone are gastrointestinal symptoms and rash.

Use of the azoles is not recommended in pregnancy. Azole resistance is a substantial problem. It is found in patients with AIDS, in intensive care units and in leukaemia patients. It is manifested in two ways. Firstly by the replacement of susceptible *Candida* isolates with resistant *Candida* spp., such as *C. glabrata* and *C. krusei*. Secondly by the *in situ* development of resistance in a certain isolate. The problem of the resistance is focused chiefly on fluconazole, although cross-resistance to the other azoles is common.

Some of the drugs with which ketoconazole interacts are agents which decrease gastric acidity—rifampicin, aciclovir, coumarins, ciclosporin, phenytoin, terfenadine and astemizole. Fluconazole is reported to interact with amphotericin B, coumarins, ciclosporin, phenytoin, oestradiol, cimetidine, astemizole, terfenadine, sulphonylureas and thiazides, among others.

Itraconazole interacts mainly with ciclosporin, food, digoxin, phenytoin, rifampicin, H_2-antagonists, terfenadine and astemizole.

Treatment of clinical forms

Oral candidiasis and perlèche

The main treatment agents are topical nystatin suspension and miconazole oral gel. For more persistent disease oral antifungals are used: ketoconazole 200 mg daily for 1–2 weeks, fluconazole 50–100 mg daily for 1 week, or itraconazole 100 mg daily for 1–3 weeks. Fluconazole is reported to be effective with a single 150-mg dose. Perlèche is treated with topical antifungal creams.

Cutaneous candidiasis

Topical antifungal preparations are used, with excellent results. For widespread disease oral antifungal drugs are used: itraconazole 200 mg daily for 1 week or fluconazole 50–100 mg for 1–3 weeks. A dose of 150 mg fluconazole once a week for 2 weeks has also proven to be very effective in the treatment of cutaneous candidiasis.

Candida balanitis

Topical treatment has proven sufficient in treating this condition. Fluconazole in a single 150-mg dose is effective in more resistant cases.

Vaginal candidiasis

Topical treatment generally results in a good mycotic and clinical cure rate. Owing to common relapses and complaints from patients that intravaginal products are messy and often leak, oral treatment is prescribed. Cases of occasional vulvovaginitis are treated with fluconazole orally in a single dose of 150 mg, ketoconazole 200 mg daily for 5 days or itraconazole 400 mg in a single dose. Recurrent vulvovaginitis is treated with a single dose of 150 mg fluconazole, given on day 21 of each menstrual cycle for 6–12 months. Clotrimazole as a 500-mg vaginal pessary once a week has proven efficient in suppressing relapses of recurrent vaginitis.

Candida paronychia

This condition requires prolonged topical treatment. The hands should be kept warm and dry.

Candida onychomycosis

Topical treatment with the ordinary polyene or azole antifungal drugs is not effective, as these drugs are not absorbed from the nail plate. For mild *Candida* onychomycosis of the hands involving not more than 60% of the entire nail plate, amorolfine nail lacquer is used once a week for 6 months. For more severe onychomycosis of the hands, itraconazole is used in a pulsed regimen of 400 mg daily for 1 week. This scheme is repeated for 3 months.

For mild onychomycosis of the feet, amorolfine nail lacquer once weekly for 12 months and for more severe cases itraconazole pulse therapy with 400 mg daily for 1 week. This scheme is repeated for 4 months.

Fluconazole is used in a dose of 150 mg weekly for 6 months for hand onychomycosis and for up to 9 months for foot onychomycosis.

Chronic mucocutaneous candidiasis

A combination of antifungal drugs and immunological reconstruction is needed in the treatment strategy for this condition. A restoration of T-cell function is attempted by using transfer factor, of thymosin, or by grafting compatible lymphocytes from blood or marrow, or fetal thymic tissue.

The antifungal drugs most commonly used are ketoconazole, fluconazole and itraconazole, which are used for some years. The main problems encountered with use of these drugs are the growing problems of infection with *Candida* that has become resistant and hepatotoxicity with long-term use of ketoconazole.

Further reading

Come JA, Dismukes WE. Oral azole drugs as systemic antifungal therapy. *N Engl J Med* 1994; 330 (4): 263–72.

Hay RJ. Antifungal therapy of yeast infections. *J Am Acad Dermatol* 1994; 31: S6–S9.

Runeman B, Faergeman J. Experimental *Candida albicans* lesions in healthy humans. *Acta Derm Venereol* 2000; 8: 421–4.

Sentandreu M, Elorza MV, Sentandreu R, Fouri WA. Cloning and characterization of PRAI, a gene encoding a novel Ph regulated antigen of *Candida albicans*. *J Bacteriol* 1998; 180: 282–9.

Sobel JD. Controversial aspects in the management of vulvovaginal candidiasis. *J Am Acad Dermatol* 1994; 31: S10–S13.

Suchil P, Montero Gei F, Robles M *et al.* Once-weekly oral doses of fluconazole 150 mg in the treatment of tinea corporis/cruris and cutaneous candidiasis. *Clin Exp Dermatol* 1992; 17: 397–401.

Troke PF. Fluconazole. Its properties and efficacy in vaginal candidiasis. *Curr Prob Dermatol* 1996; 24: 203–8.

Yosipovitch G, Maibach HI. Skin surface pH: a protective acid mantle. *Cosmetic Toiletries* 1996; 111: 101–2.

Chronic actinic dermatitis

G.M. Murphy

Definition

Chronic actinic dermatitis (CAD) is an uncommon photosensitive disorder which occurs predominantly in elderly men. CAD is characterized by chronic eczema which is usually severe, accentuated in light-exposed sites, persists all year but is worse in summertime. CAD is associated with abnormal responses to ultraviolet (UV) radiation on testing with broad band or monochromator sources.

Aetiology

CAD is usually classified as an idiopathic photodermatosis, however, there is some evidence that the cellular infiltrate and adhesion molecule expression pattern induced in response to UV radiation resembles that of a delayed hypersensitivity reaction, probably to a cutaneous UV-induced antigen. The antigen has not been identified, but potential candidates include cellular DNA or other cellular constituents. The action spectrum for CAD is the same shape as that for human erythema, implying that the same chromophores may be implicated, but the mechanism of reduced threshold responsiveness has not been delineated. Patients exhibit very readily allergic reactions of the delayed type to a wide number of allergens, not necessarily photoallergens, thus the immune response appears to be heightened, and inappropriate. It therefore would appear sensible to consider CAD as an immunological disturbance of the autoimmune type.

Clinical features

Most patients with CAD are elderly men, often in the 7–8th decade. Ten per cent of patients are female. A history of endogenous eczema frequently precedes CAD, perhaps mild hand eczema or patchy eczema on the body. Patients develop facial eczema first, often mild in the summer but after 1–3 years symptoms become persistent, severe and the typical features of CAD emerge. Features suggestive of CAD include eczema which occurs on light-exposed sites: face, neck, 'V' of chest, dorsa of hands, with a sharp cut off at the cuff and collar lines. Key sites may be spared, including the submental area, the postauricular triangle, the eyelids, the depths of the nasolabial folds or other furrows on the face, and the finger webs. These sites are in shadow, thus receive less UV, but with severe CAD these clinical signs may be obscured and patients may also be erythrodermic. Many patients with CAD do not notice an association with sun exposure, though exacerbation over the summer months may be evident. Patients with CAD are very uncomfortable, relentless itching may lead to insomnia and severe depression. At times the clinical picture is so severe that cutaneous lymphoma is considered. Vitiligo-like depigmentation may be observed in affected skin.

Diagnostic criteria

The clinical picture may hint at the diagnosis of CAD. However, the gold standard for diagnosis of this disorder remains the demonstration of abnormally reduced responsiveness to UV. This is usually on the basis of monochromator testing. Patients are tested to a range of narrow band UV wavelengths, throughout the terrestrial solar spectrum, such as 300, 320, 340, 370 and 400 nm. The range of normal responses for the test wavelengths must be known within the population: CAD patients may exhibit reduced responses within the UVB (300–315 nm) range, or UVB and UVA (315–400 nm) or with severe disease UVB, UVA and visible light (400–800 nm). Biopsy of a UV-irradiated site shows eczematous features within a few days. Histology from clinically affected skin shows a dense, deep dermal lymphohistiocytic infiltrate with eczematous features in the epidermis. The lymphocytic infiltrate may be so dense that the diagnosis of cutaneous lymphoma is considered, particularly as such patients have Sézary type cells in the infiltrate, and even circulating Sézary cells. Thus the old term actinic reticuloid for these patients is retained but it is now known that this represents a severe form of CAD and there is no connection with progression to malignancy.

Other tests which must be carried out in these patients include patch and photopatch tests to the Standard European series of contact allergens, and photopatch tests to a series of photoallergens, the most relevant of which now appear to be sunscreens. Patients with CAD usually (70%) have allergic reactions to one or more of a number of allergens, the most commonly found include fragrance, balsalm of Peru, colophony, sesquiterpene lactone mix, cobalt, chromate and rubber. Sunscreen allergy is not uncommon, the level of exposure determines the allergen frequency. Gardeners and those in rural areas often show allergy to the Compositae, daisy-like plants, such as crysanthemums, or weeds such as feverfew which are ubiquitous in northern Europe. Allergen patterns would be expected to vary in keeping with exposure in different populations and countries.

It is prudent to rule out other autoimmune disorders such as lupus erythematosus by checking antinuclear and anti-Ro antibodies. This would be particularly relevant if PUVA desensitization were considered as treatment. It might at times be relevant to consider dermatomyositis and direct immunofluorescence of skin together with RNP and anti-Jo1 antibodies might be indicated clinically.

Differential diagnosis

Airborne allergic contact dermatitis should be considered in the differential diagnosis and patch testing with relevant allergens is necessary to rule this out. Allergic contact dermatitis may also simulate CAD: steroid allergy should be excluded. Photoallergic contact dermatitis may simulate or aggravate CAD. Photoaggravated endogenous eczema, either atopic or seborrhoeic eczema, where light tests are normal, may be a source of confusion, with the caveat that in the early stages of CAD the light tests may also be normal. Drug-induced photosensitivity may simulate CAD exactly, the action spectrum for drug-induced photosensitivity however, resides mostly in UVA wavelengths, so UVA photosensitivity in the absence of UVB photosensitivity, though not absolute, is a pointer towards a drug-induced cause.

Lupus erythematosus and dermatomyositis are usually clinically distinguishable, but occasional patients may require skin biopsy and autoantibody tests for confirmation. Cutaneous lymphoma may be considered with the gross infiltration and histological appearance of the skin biopsy. Light testing is very helpful and demonstrates severe photosensitivity usually throughout the UV spectrum and visible light region in these patients. Erythrodermic patients may be confused with all other causes of erythroderma, including eczema, psoriasis, drug-induced and lymphoma.

Treatment

General measures

Explanation of the nature of the disorder to patients represents the key to its optimal management. Simple patient information leaflets outlining the nature of UV radiation, the times of day when UV is most intense and the methods of UV avoidance are most important. Patients are very relieved to be given a reason for their problem, and benefit greatly by discussion of ways of minimizing UV exposure. Admission to hospital and treatment in a room from which UV has been excluded is a very effective short-term measure. Fluorescent lighting emits significant quantities of UVA sufficient to cause disease flares. Tungsten bulbs are much less liable to lead to clinical problems. UV-excluding film, which may be applied to window glass is extremely helpful and commercially available. One of my patients designed a hat with a brim where UV opaque film surrounds his face so that he could continue his work as a farmer. As soon as he showed this to other CAD patients, the idea was instantly copied. The hat was cool, practical and cheap, and most importantly allowed him to carry out his work in comfort.

Avoidance of allergens is important, particularly plants in the Compositae class. Education of patients as to which plants are relevant in their environment may present a challenge to dermatologists not versed in botany. It is very helpful to have pictures of the relevant plants.

Sunscreens of high SPF 30–60, of the inert type from the point of view of allergy are preferred. UV absorbers of the chemical kind are increasingly implicated as allergens or photoallergens in CAD patients. Microfine titanium dioxide and zinc oxide are not associated with allergy. New techniques of dispersing these sunscreens in a base give a cosmetically acceptable product. The sunscreen should be applied gently and not rubbed well into the skin, as this reduces its photoprotective effect by disturbing the dispersion of particles. New sunscreens are constantly being developed, but the allergenic potential of new chemicals remains unclear until they have been used widely and for sufficient time periods. It may be that compounds such as Mexoryl SX, Mexoryl XL and Tinasorb, which give good UVA protection, do not readily cause allergy, but this remains to be determined. Fragrance-free products should be used.

Specific therapy

Potent topical steroids or topical Tacrolimus 0.1% may give symptomatic relief, particularly when used in conjunction with the above measures. Most patients with CAD need more effective treatment. Systemic steroids give only marginal benefits and unacceptable long-term side-effects. PUVA desensitization is an effective treatment for patients with CAD who are not too severely affected, but have disease which significantly hampers their behaviour. The principle underlying this is to render patients tolerant to UV so that they may then take advantage of natural tolerance from the sun. Occasional patients are able to render themselves tolerant with natural sunlight, but this is exceptional. Most patients are extremely photosensitive, and require starting doses of $0.01\,J/cm^2$ with 70% dose increments, twice or three times weekly as tolerated. Most flare on reaching $0.5\,J/cm^2$ or higher and require prednisolone 40–60 mg daily to enable higher dosage to be given. It is often difficult for both patient and dermatologist to get through the treatment-induced flares, and it may take 3–6 weeks of unpleasant symptoms for the patient to achieve tolerance. The usual end dose achieved during this treatment period is $3.5\,J/cm^2$. Once patients have managed to endure the desensitization procedure, ambient sunlight becomes tolerable. Patients are encouraged to go out in sunlight, ideally at midday, for short periods of time without sunblocks to perpetuate the achieved tolerance. Many patients are able to achieve normal tolerance to sunlight and some become tanned and evidently able to withstand very considerable UV exposure. Others only achieve minimal tolerance and require ongoing PUVA treatment on a once weekly basis over the summer months. Patients with severe CAD prove difficult to desensitize, the steroid side-effects may prove unacceptable or intolerable.

Azathioprine is an immunosuppressive agent which has been shown to be highly effective in CAD. There are difficulties with the drug. Some patients develop severe gastrointestinal symptoms or hepatotoxic reactions. Careful monitoring of patients is therefore required, and the drug is best avoided in those with gastritis or symptoms of dyspepsia. Generally if the drug is started in low dosage 50 mg daily for a week and increased to therapeutic levels, usually 1.5 mg/kg, side-effects may be minimized. Lymphopenia may occur also and all patients should have monthly assessment of blood count, and liver function tests while treated. Most patients improve within a 3–month period, and may go into remission after 6 months of treatment. The drug may be discontinued then and restarted if the patients relapse. Occasional patients go into longstanding remission. Most require retreatment on an annual basis.

Ciclosporin is an alternative drug, and in my experience less effective and associated with less prolonged improvement. Most patients require high doses of 5–7 mg/kg to achieve comparable results to azathioprine. Patients with CAD are elderly, often have poor renal function, hypertension and other medical problems, thus the potential side-effects of ciclosporin must be balanced against the need for efficacy. Danazol has been used and in occasional patients shown some efficacy. All patients treated with potent systemic medication need careful monitoring for long-term side-effects.

Mycophenolate mofetil is a further agent with success in CAD, its main side-effect is nausea and gastrointestinal upset, lymphopenia may occur, but it is effective; one patient being weaned off ciclosporin to mycophenolate developed shingles. The immunosuppressive effects of these agents therefore need to be appreciated from the point of view of predisposing to infection, and long-term risk possibly to lymphoma. The risks and benefits of immunosuppression therefore must be considered in each individual case, especially when one is using treatments off licence.

Further reading

Bilsland D, Ferguson. J. Contact allergy to sunscreen chemicals in photosensitivity dermatitis/actinic reticuloid syndrome (PD/AR) and polymorphic light eruption. *Contact Dermatitis* 1993; 29: 70–3.

Hindson C, Downey A, Sinclair S, Cominos B. PUVA therapy of chronic actinic dermatitis: a 5 year follow-up. *Br J Dermatol* 1990.

Humbert P, Drobacheff C, Vigan M, Quencez E, Laurent R, Agache P. Chronic actinic dermatitis responding to danazol. *Br J Dermatol* 1991; 124: 195–7.

Lenane P, Shudell E, Collins S, Murphy GM. Mycophenolate mofetil an additional potent immunomodulatory agent in dermatological disease. *Br J Dermatol* 1999; Suppl. 55 (141): 71.

Murphy GM, Maurice PD, Norris PG, Morris RW, Hawk JLM. Azathioprine treatment in chronic actinic dermatitis. A double–blind controlled trial with monitoring of exposure to ultraviolet radiation. *Br J Dermatol* 1989; 121: 639–46.

Murphy GM, White IR, Hawk JL. Allergic airborne contact dermatitis to Compositae with photosensitivity—chronic actinic dermatitis in evolution. *Photoderm Photoimmunol Photomed* 1990; 7: 38–9.

Peter RU, Ruzicka T. Cyclosporin A in the treatment of inflammatory dermatoses. *Hautarzt* 1992; 43: 687–9.

Ross JS, du Peloux Menage H, Hawk JL, White IR. Sesquiterpene lactone contact sensitivity: clinical patterns of Compositae dermatitis and relationships to chronic actinic dermatitis. *Contact Dermatitis* 1993; 29: 84–7.

Von den Driesch P, Fartasch M, Hornstein OP. Chronic actinic dermatitis with vitiligo-like depigmentation. *Clin Exp Dermatol* 1992; 17: 38–43.

Cicatricial alopecia

A. Tosti and B.M. Piraccini

Definition and introduction

A large number of scalp disorders may destroy the hair follicles and result in cicatricial alopecia (Table 1). These include diseases that primarily affect the hair follicles as well as diseases that affect the dermis and secondarily cause follicular destruction.

Once established, cicatricial alopecia is a permanent condition that cannot be reversed by treatment. For this reason, it is very important to diagnose the hair or scalp disorders that may produce cicatricial alopecia as soon as possible in order to start a specific treatment and avoid diffuse follicular destruction.

The differential diagnosis between the diseases that cause cicatricial alopecia requires a pathological examination, since the clinical features are usually not diagnostic. A scalp biopsy is therefore mandatory in all cases of cicatricial alopecia. The site of biopsy is crucial for the diagnosis. The biopsy should in fact be taken from scalp areas that show inflammatory signs, since biopsies taken from atrophic scalp areas are not diagnostic, only revealing follicular or dermal fibrosis.

Table 1 Causes of cicatricial alopecia

Follicular diseases
- lichen planopilaris
- discoid lupus erythematosus
- keratosis follicularis spinulosa decalvans
- folliculitis decalvans
- traction alopecia

Dermal fibrosis
- localized scleroderma
- radiodermatitis
- pemphigoid
- chemical or physical injuries

The aim of treatment is to avoid further scarring and it is necessary to explain clearly to the patient that the hair that has been lost will not grow again. Surgical treatment of cicatricial alopecia includes excision of the scarring area after tissue expansion or hair transplantation. The latter technique is complicated by the poor recipient conditions due to the reduced blood perfusion present in scar tissue that may impair graft survival. The possibility that grafting may precipitate relapses through a Koebner phenomenon in lichen planopilaris should also be considered. The Er:YAG laser has recently been successfully utilized for hair transplantation in cicatricial alopecia.

This chapter discusses optimal management and treatment of some inflammatory scalp disorders that commonly cause cicatricial alopecia.

Lichen planopilaris

Synonym: pseudopelade—Brocq pseudoarea.

Lichen planopilaris is the most common cause of cicatricial alopecia.

Patients usually seek medical advice because they have noticed one or several patches of hair loss. A certain degree of itching is frequently reported. The clinical examination reveals a variable number of poorly circumscribed bald patches. The scalp of these alopecic areas may look normal, have an atrophic appearance or show some degree of follicular keratosis.

The diagnosis of lichen planopilaris derives from a careful examination of the scalp that surrounds the patches, where the hair follicles show perifollicular erythema and acuminated keratotic plugs. The pull test from these areas typically reveals anagen hairs.

Clinical variants of lichen planopilaris include 'frontal fibrosing alopecia' and 'fibrosing alopecia in a pattern distribution', which are characterized by the fact that the lichenoid infiltrate does not affect the hair follicles randomly, but selectively involves the frontal hairline in frontal fibrosing alopecia or the androgen-dependent miniaturized follicles of the crown in fibrosing alopecia in a pattern distribution. In the latter condition the immunological reaction specifically targets the miniaturized follicles for destruction. A case of lichen planopilaris selectively involving the follicles of a scalp epidermal naevus has been described. The authors suggest that the immunological privilege of the hair follicles may be disrupted by microorganisms colonizing the follicles.

Biopsy is mandatory for the diagnosis and should include some papular lesions. Never take the biopsy from a bald area because this is not useful. Transverse sections are necessary in order to detect active disease that is often restricted to a few follicles. Direct immunofluorescence can also help the diagnosis.

Treatment

Treatment results in complete remission of disease in about one-third of patients. Partial remission is obtained in another third, while the disease progresses despite treatment in the remaining patients.

Systemic treatment

1. Steroids represent the treatment of choice. We utilize intramuscular triamcinolone acetonide at the dosage 0.5–1 mg/kg per month. Steroids are gradually tapered when active lesions disappear. This may require 6–12 months.
2. Azathioprine 100 mg/day is useful in association with systemic steroids in severe cases.
3. Systemic ciclosporin 3 mg/kg per day is in our experience not effective.
4. Finasteride 1 mg/day in men or oral antiandrogens (ciproterone acetate) in women can be prescribed in fibrosing alopecia in a pattern distribution, where miniaturized follicles are selectively affected by the disease.

Intralesional steroids

Triamcinolone acetonide (5 mg/mL sterile saline solution) can be injected using a 30-gauge needle. Lesions are injected up to 3–4 times every 2–3 weeks. This treatment is applicable when the disease is limited to a circumscribed area. Intralesional steroids may induce permanent atrophy when the same scalp area is repeatedly injected. This is common in lichen planopilaris, where recurrent lesions tend to develop in close proximity.

Topical treatment

1. Topical 2% or 5% minoxidil may prevent fibrosis and is useful in association with systemic steroids.
2. High-potency topical steroids can be prescribed in association with systemic treatment. However, they may aggravate skin atrophy.
3. Topical tar is not effective.

Discoid lupus erythematosus

Diagnosis of discoid lupus erythematosus is strongly suggested by the presence of erythema, follicular hyperkeratosis, atrophy and telangiectasia. The patient complains of one or several patches of hair loss. The bald scalp areas may show the typical inflammatory signs of discoid lupus erythematosus or be atrophic with minimal inflammation. The pull test from active lesions reveals anagen hairs.

The biopsy should be taken from an inflamed area. Direct immunofluorescence is useful for the diagnosis.

All patients with discoid lupus erythematosus should be examined for systemic lupus erythematosus.

Treatment

Discoid lupus erythematosus usually responds to treatment.

Systemic treatment

1 Antimalaria drugs are the treatment of choice. Hydroxychloroquine (400 mg/day) or chloroquine (200 mg/day) can be prescribed alone or in association with systemic steroids. Treatment lasts for at least 3 months and is then tapered to the lowest effective dose.
2 Systemic steroids: initial dosages should be 40–60 mg/day of oral prednisone or 0.5–1 mg/month of intramuscular triamcinolone acetonide. Steroids are gradually tapered when active lesions disappear. This may require 3–6 months.
3 Thalidomide (100–300 mg/day) is a possible alternative.

Intralesional steroids

Triamcinolone acetonide (5 mg/mL sterile saline solution) can be useful in localized lesions.

Topical treatment

1 Topical steroids (class I–II) can be utilized when the disease is circumscribed to a small area of the scalp. They are usually scarcely effective.
2 Topical 2% or 5% minoxidil may prevent fibrosis and can be prescribed in association with systemic steroids.

General measures

Patients should wear a hat to avoid sun exposure.

Folliculitis decalvans

This term is utilized to include a spectrum of scalp disorders characterized by painful acute inflammatory changes with or without pustules. Relapsing inflammatory episodes result in cicatricial alopecia and tufted folliculitis.

Although *Staphylococcus aureus* may frequently be isolated from the pustules, folliculitis decalvans is not an infective condition, but possibly represents an abnormal host response against staphylococcal antigens or toxins.

The pathology reveals an acute folliculitis with a perifollicular infiltrate.

Treatment

Although the inflammatory scalp lesions usually subside with treatment, the condition has a chronic course with frequent relapses.

Systemic treatment

1 Oral antibiotics are the treatment of choice. Antibiotics mostly used are: erythromycin 1 g/day, clarithromycin 500 mg/day, cephalosporins or tetracyclines (minocycline 100 mg/day or hydroxytetracycline 200 mg/day). All of these are usually effective in arresting the inflammatory process, but relapses are common as soon as the treatment is interrupted. Combination therapy with fusidic acid 1500 mg/day for 3 weeks and zinc sulphate 400 mg/day resulted in permanent remission in three patients. The association of rifampicin 300 mg and clindamycin 300 mg both orally twice daily for 10 weeks is probably the most effective treatment. This may be due to the fact that rifampicin is an effective antistaphylococcal agent but has also immunomodulatory properties. This regimen produces long-term remissions in most patients. The association is required to avoid development of rifampicin resistance that is common when using this antibiotic alone.
2 Isotretinoin 0.5–1 mg/kg per day actually worsens the scalp inflammation in most cases.
3 A short course of systemic and topical steroids can be utilized to suppress inflammation in association with oral antibiotics.

Topical treatment

Shampoos containing antibacterial agents or 2% ketoconazole may be helpful in preventing relapses.

Shaving of the scalp may improve the disease.

Keratosis follicularis spinulosa decalvans (KFSD)

This inherited condition usually becomes evident in infancy. The gene for KFSD could be mapped to Xp21.13–p22.2. The clinical diagnosis is suggested by the presence of follicular keratotic papules and pustules involving the scalp. Follicular papules are also evident on the eyebrows and cheeks. Alopecia, which is more prominent in the vertex, usually develops after puberty.

Its severity varies considerably in different patients.

Treatment

In most patients the disease does not respond to treatment.

Systemic treatment

1 Acitretin (0.5–0.75 mg/kg per day) may be effective in some cases. Isotretinoin 1 mg/kg per day is usually not effective.
2 Dapsone 100 mg/day can be tried in patients who do not respond to retinoids.
3 Oral antibiotics (tetracyclines, macrolides or rifampicin) as for folliculitis decalvans are rarely effective.

Topical treatment

Topical steroids and keratolytics may partially improve the symptoms.

Brocq pseudoarea

Brocq pseudoarea is not a separate entity, but represents the cicatricial outcome of lichen planopilaris. The scalp presents multiple irregular bald atrophic areas, but no signs of inflammation.

Involvement of the beard area has also been reported.

Patients with this diagnosis may fall into two possible categories:

- patients in whom the disease has already spontaneously remitted
- patients in whom the biopsy has been wrongly taken from an atrophic area.

Treatment

No treatment is available.

Table 2 Scarring alopecia: suggested therapies

Lichen planopilaris	Systemic steroids + topical minoxidil Azathioprine + systemic steroids + topical minoxidil
Fibrosing alopecia in a pattern distribution	Finasteride + systemic steroids
DLE	Hydroxychloroquine Hydroxychloroquine + systemic steroids
Folliculitis decalvans	Rifampicin + clindamycin Tetracyclines Clarithromycin
KFSD	Retinoids Dapsone Tetracyclines
Localized scleroderma	Oral calcitriol Penicillin

Localized scleroderma

Localized scleroderma of the scalp presents as a slowly progressing irregular patch of hair loss. The skin often shows a certain degree of erythema or pigmentation in the absence of follicular keratosis or scaling. The patch is often not completely bald, but presents some vellus or intermediate hairs.

Severe atrophy with involvement of the hypodermis and muscles is a feature of frontoparietal linear scleroderma ('en coup de sabre').

Treatment

Localized scleroderma usually resolves spontaneously in a few years.

Systemic treatment

1 Systemic calcitriol at the dosage of 0.50–0.75 mg/day is effective in localized scleroderma of the scalp including frontoparietal linear scleroderma.

Topical treatment

1 Topical 2% or 5% minoxidil.
2 Calcipotriol lotion may be effective.

Further reading

Blaszczyk M, Krysicka Janniger K, Jablonska S. Childhood scleroderma and its peculiarities. *Cutis* 1996; 58: 141–4.

Camacho Martinez F, Garcia-Hernandez MJ, Mazuecos Blanca J. Postmenopausal frontal fibrosing alopecia. *Br J Dermatol* 1999; 140: 1181–2.

Duteille F, Le Fourn B, Hepner Lavergne D, Pannier M. The limitation of primary excision of cicatricial alopecia: a report of 63 patients. *Ann Plast Surg* 2000; 45: 145–9.

Kossard S, Lee MS, Wilkinson B. Postmenopausal frontal fibrosing alopecia. a variant of lichen planopilaris. *J Am Acad Dermatol* 1997; 36: 59–66.

Kunte C, Loeser C, Wolff H. Folliculitis spinulosa decalvans: successful therapy with dapsone. *J Am Acad Dermatol* 1997; 39: 891–993.

Madani S, Trotter MJ, Shapiro J. Pseudopelade of Broq in beard area. *J Am Acad Dermatol* 2000; 42: 895–6.

Michelet J-F, Commo S, Billoni N, Mahé YF, Bernard BA. Activation of cytoprotective prostaglandin synthase-1 by minoxidil as a possible explanation for its hair growth-stimulating effect. *J Invest Dermatol* 1997; 108: 250–9.

Piraccini BM, Vincenzi C, Lorenzi S, Jorizzo M, Tosti A. Oral calcitriol in the treatment of scleroderma 'en coupe de sabre'. *J Dermatol Treat* 2000; 11: 207–8.

Podda M, Spieth K, Kaufmann R. Er:YAG laser-assisted hair transplantation in cicatricial alopecia. *Dermatol Surg* 2000; 26: 1010–14.

Powell JJ, Dawber RPR. Successful treatment regime for folliculitis decalvans despite uncertainty of all aetiological factors. *Br J Dermatol* 2001; 144: 428–9.

Powell JJ, Dawber RPR, Gatter K. Folliculitis decalvans including tufted folliculitis. Clinical, histological and therapeutic findings. *Br J Dermatol* 1999; 140: 328–33.

Smith KJ, Crittenden J, Skelton H. Lichen planopilaris-like changes arising within an epidermal nevus. Does this case suggest clues to the etiology of lichen planopilaris? *J Cutan Med Surg* 2000; 4: 30–5.

Sperling LC, Solomon AR. Whiting DA. A new look at scarring alopecia. *Arch Dermatol* 2000; 136: 235–41.

Sperling LC, Whiting DA, Solomon AR. In reply. *Arch Dermatol* 2001; 137: 373–4.

Walker JL, Smith HR, Lun K, Griffiths WA. Improvement of folliculitis decalvans following shaving of the scalp. *Br J Dermatol* 2000; 142: 1245–6.

Wilson CL, Burge SM, Dean D, Dawber RPR. Scarring alopecia in discoid lupus erythematosus. *Br J Dermatol* 1992; 126: 307–14.

Zinkernagel MS, Trueb RM. Fibrosing alopecia in a pattern distribution. *Arch Dermatol* 2000; 136: 205–11.

Contact dermatitis

L. Kanerva and A.I. Lauerma

Definitions

The terms eczema and dermatitis are often used synonymously. Contact dermatitis is used to describe an inflammation of the skin caused by contact with exogenous substances. By definition, a contact dermatitis is morphologically a dermatitis, i.e. an inflammation of the epidermis with histological evidence of spongiosis. The polymorphic pattern of skin inflammation is characterized by erythema, oedema, vesiculation and pruritus. Less acute eczema and chronic eczema are characterized by scales, thickening and lichenification. Contact dermatitis may be caused by irritants, allergens and light-aggravated factors (Table 1).

Epidemiology

Contact dermatitis is often located on the hands. In fact, contact dermatitis is one of the most common dermatoses of the hands. The point prevalence of eczema, including other types of eczema than contact dermatitis, varies in various studies between 1% and 10%. The diagnosis accounts for about 10% of all visits to the dermatologist and for more than 90% of all occupational skin diseases. The point prevalence studies show that eczema was less common in earlier studies than in more recent ones, indicating an increase of eczema in the population over time. Very few studies have addressed the epidemiology of allergic contact dermatitis. In a Danish report 15.2% of a non-selected population had at least one allergic patch test reaction (Table 2).

Table 1 Classification of skin contact reactions

Irritant contact dermatitis
• acute (toxic) irritant contact dermtitis
• irritant reaction
• cumulative irritant/insult contact dermatitis
Allergic contact dermatitis
Phototoxic, photoallergic and light-aggravated contact dermatitis
Immediate-type reactions
• immunological contact urticaria
• protein contact dermatitis
• non-immunological contact urticaria (NICU)

Aetiology and pathophysiology

Allergic contact dermatitis

The immunology of allergic contact dermatitis is complex. It has three stages: (a) the formation of protein–hapten conjugates; (b) the recognition of conjugated antigen; and (c) the proliferation and dissemination of sensitized lymphocytes. Further contact with the allergen leads to development of T-lymphocyte mediated dermatitis at the site of skin contact. Most allergens in contact dermatitis are reactive chemicals (haptens) with low molecular weight (less than 1000 Da). They conjugate with skin proteins to form 'complete antigens' before they are able to sensitize. Examples of sensitizing haptens are given in Table 2.

Irritant contact dermatitis

Irritant contact dermatitis ranges from slight dryness, redness or chapping to an acute caustic burn.

Acute irritant contact dermatitis may be caused by accidental exposure to strong irritants such as acids, alkalis, etc. Repeated cumulative dermatitis results from a series of repeated and damaging insults to the skin. Friction, microtrauma, low humidity, heat, cold, solvents, degreasing agents such as soap and detergent may contribute to cumulative irritant dermatitis. The face, the scrotum and back of the hands are more permeable than skin elsewhere and therefore more vulnerable to the effects of irritants. There may be significant differences in the absorption and diffusion characteris-

Table 2 Patch test results of the standard series at Finnish university hospitals in 2012 patients in 1994. The results are compared to a Danish study of an unselected population

Allergen	Type of allergen/exposure	% in Finnish study ($n = 2012$)	% in Danish study ($n = 567$)
Nickel sulphate	Metal, alloys	22.5	6.7
Neomycin sulphate	Topical antibiotic	7.2	0
Fragrance mix	Perfumes	6.6	1.1
Bacitracin	Topical antibiotic	5.1	ND
Cobalt chloride	Metal, alloys	4.2	1.1
Balsam of Peru	Fragrances	4.0	1.1
Colophony	Resin	3.9	0.7
Tixocortol pivalate	Corticosteroid	3.5	ND
Formaldehyde	Antimicrobial	3.1	ND
Budesonide	Corticosteroid	2.6	ND
Kathon CG	Antimicrobial	2.6	0.7
Thiuram mix	Rubber chemical	2.6	0.5
Potassium dichromate	Metal, cement, leather	1.9	0.5
p-Phenylenediamine	Rubber chemical, dyes	1.9	0
Toluenesulfonamide-formaldehyde resin	Nail lacquers	1.5	ND
Quinoline-mix	Antimicrobial	1.0	0.4
p-*t*-Butyl-phenolformaldehyde resin	Resin, shoes, glues	1.0	1.1
Cetostearol	Emulsifier, creams, cosmetics	1.0	ND
Wool alcohols	Ointment base	1.0	0.2
Chlorhexidine gluconate	Antimicrobial	0.9	ND
Mercapto mix	Rubber chemical	0.9	0.4
Mercaptobenzothiazole	Rubber chemical	0.8	0.2
Black rubber mix	Rubber chemical	0.7	0.2
Epoxy resin	Plastics	0.6	0.5
Quaternium 15	Antimicrobial	0.6	0.2
Propylene glycol	Vehicle in cosmetic bases	0.4	ND
Sesquiterpene lactone mix	Plant (Compositae) allergen	0.4	ND
Sorbitan sesquioleate	Emulsifier in creams	0.3	ND
Parabens (mix)	Antimicrobials	0.2	0.4
Caine mix	Local anaesthetic	ND	0
Ethylenediamine	Stabilizer in steroid creams	ND	0.2
Carba mix	Rubber chemical	ND	0.4
Thimerosal	Antimicrobial	ND	3.4

tics of different types of chemicals. The main barrier to water transport through the skin is attributable to intercellular lipids in the horny layer and to high molecular proteins of the corneocyte.

Most agents may be irritant if applied for a sufficient time and in sufficient concentrations. Irritants induce damage by denaturing keratin, removing horny layer lipids and altering the water-holding capacity of the skin. Individual susceptibility varies greatly. Strong irritants induce a clinical reaction in all individuals whereas mild irritants cause dermatitis only in susceptible individuals with 'sensitive skin'. Atopics and those with fair skin seem to be more easily irritated. Nearly 80% of those with chronic disability dermatitis may be atopics. Recently healed eczema increases the susceptibility to irritant dermatitis. Elderly people may have a reduced inflammatory response.

Cumulative irritant dermatitis most often affects thin exposed skin, e.g. the backs of the hands and the webs of the fingers. Chronic irritant dermatitis is due to the summation of various adverse factors, which would not themselves cause irritant dermatitis. Occupations with a high risk of cumulative risk irritant dermatitis are given in Table 3.

Contact urticaria

Two types of contact urticaria can be distinguished: immune and non-immune types. Immune-type contact urticaria is immunoglobulin E (IgE)-mediated and more common in atopics. IgE-mediated reactions may be based on an effect on mast cells/basophils, or possibly mediated via Langerhans' cells (protein contact dermatitis).

Clinical characteristics and course

A contact dermatitis is morphologically a dermatitis, i.e. an inflammation of the epidermis with histological evidence of spongiosis. The polymorphic pattern of skin inflammation is characterized by erythema, oedema, vesiculation and pruritis. Less acute eczema and chronic eczema are characterized by scale thickening and lichenification. Irritant contact dermatitis ranges from slight dryness, redness or chapping to an acute caustic burn.

The prognosis of contact dermatitis is worse for atopics and also for those allergic to certain allergens, particularly chromate and nickel. Hand dermatitis in general has a poor prognosis.

Diagnosis

The diagnosis is based on clinical examinations and patch testing. The most frequent sensitizers have been compiled to a 'standard series' comprising 20–30 allergens (Table 2). The allergens are commercially available in 20–30 series (Table 4). Allergens and allergy frequencies are given in Table 2.

Irritant contact dermatitis

A diagnosis of acute or chronic irritant contact dermatitis is based on an accurate history of exposure to the suspected irri-

Table 3 Occupations and the most important causes of irritant contact dermatitis

Occupations with a high risk of irritant contact dermatitis
- catering
- cleaning
- construction work
- dairy farming
- dental work
- engineering
- gardening
- hairdressing
- housework
- motor mechanics
- nursing

The most important causes of irritant contact dermatitis
- water
- skin cleansers
- detergents and solvents
- acids and alkalis
- cutting oils
- chemicals, e.g. peroxides, reducing agents
- physical and mechanical factors
- biological agents

Table 4 Commercially available patch and photopatch test series from Chemotechnique Diagnostics AB (Malmö, Sweden) or Hermal Chemie (Trolab, Reinbeck, Germany)

A	Patch test series
1	Standard series (European standard)
2	Antimicrobials, preservatives series
3	Bakery series
4	Corticosteroid series
5	Cosmetic series
6	Dental screening series
7	Epoxy series
8	Fragance series
9	Hairdressing series
10	Isocyanate series
11	Local anaesthetics series
12	Medicament series
13	Metal compounds series
14	Methacrylate and acrylate series
15	Oil and cooling fluid series
16	Organic dyes series
17	Pesticides series
18	Photographic chemicals series
19	Plants, woods series
20	Plastics and glues series
21	Rubber chemicals series
22	Shoe series
23	Sunscreen series
24	Textile colours and finishes series
25	Vehicles, emulsifiers series
B	Photopatch test series

tant that is consistent with the clinical appearance, distribution and course of eruption, since there is no reliable confirmatory test for irritation. Patch testing is mandatory to exclude allergic contact dermatitis.

Allergic contact dermatitis

The cause of allergic contact dermatitis is verified by patch tests. Although patch testing is an inexact biological assay, it is the clinician's only tool in the diagnosis.

Contact urticaria/protein contact dermatitis

The diagnosis of contact urticaria and protein contact dermatitis is confirmed by skin prick tests and use tests. The most important *in vitro* test is the radioallergosorbent test (RAST).

Differential diagnosis

Other exogenous and endogenous eczemas should be excluded. Non-eczematous contact dermatitis includes erythema multiforme-like eruptions (from, for example, exotic tropical wood species, laboratory chemicals, and topical medications); purpuric contact dermatitis from textile fabrics, antioxidants and other chemicals; pigmented contact dermatitis from optical whiteners in washing powders and from azo dyes; lichenoid contact dermatitis from contact with film developers; acneiform eruptions from cosmetics and chemicals; contact granulomas from, for example, talc, zirconium and beryllium; contact psoriasis from pressure, friction and trauma; and contact lymphangiitis from solvents entering abrasions and producing chemical lymphangiitis.

Treatment

General therapeutic guidelines

Treatment is based on an accurate diagnosis. Exposure to all possible irritant factors such as mechanical factors and chemicals including water, aggressive cleansing materials, shampoos, acids, alkalis, solvents (nail polish remover, paint thinner, etc.), soluble oils, bleaches, raw meat, fresh vegetables, etc. should be avoided as much as possible.

A wide variety of local treatment modalities are available (Table 5). Only mild cleansers should be used. Frequent application of emollient hand creams is helpful in preventing chapping and dryness. Cotton-lined plastic gloves should be used for dish-washing or when handling potential irritants. Gloves for use in an industrial setting should be chosen with care because many solvents and chemicals penetrate gloves with time.

The essential principles in the management of acute eczema are rest, protection and bland applications, explanation, reassurance and sedation. Rest should be complete or local according to the severity and extent of the eczema. An affected leg

Table 5 Principles of local therapy of contact dermatitis

Therapeutic agent	Acute	Subacute	Chronic	Prophylactic
Wet dressings	++	±	–	–
Creams, lotions	++	+	±	–
Pastes	–	+	++	–
Emollients	±	±	+	+
Corticosteroids, local	±	++	++	–
Immunosuppressants, local	±	+	++	–
Tar, ichthammol, etc.	–	±	++	–
Polythene occlusion	–	+	++	±
Paste bandage occlusion	–	+	++	–
Intralesional steroids	–	±	++	–

should be elevated or well supported and affected hands should be used as little as is practicable. Paste bandages are of special value in occluding areas which are frequently rubbed, as in many lower leg eczemas, and may help to break the itch/scratch vicious circle. All dressings should be firmly applied but be light and comfortable. In extremely acute eczema a sling is useful, and complete bed rest is advisable for severe eczema of the feet or widespread eczema of the limbs or trunk.

Topical applications should be bland. Wet dressings, aqueous cream or zinc cream are soothing. Irritant contact dermatitis is often a chronic eczematous process, especially if the hands are involved. The vehicle must contain enough fatty substances to hydrate the skin. The proportion of water and other drying ingredients should be as low as feasible. White petrolatum may be of particular value. Non-irritating fatty substances hydrate the skin and restore the barrier function. Cleaning and bathing need not be routinely forbidden, and may be comforting. Bath oils and after-cleansing emollients may be helpful. Treatment should not be stopped until healing is complete, and the patient should be warned that his or her skin will be extremely vulnerable for some weeks.

Recommended therapies

Topical therapy

Topical corticosteroids

Topical corticosteroids are generally used to speed the resolution. Hydrocortisone and mild corticosteroids are usually preferred for the face and genital areas, but the potent ones may be required, although medium-strength preparations are often adequate. Corticosteroids under polythene occlusion may be helpful in subacute eczema.

Topical corticosteroids are frequently used in the treatment of allergic contact dermatitis, but in irritant contact dermatitis, their efficacy has not been thoroughly established. Topical corticosteroids suppress the inflammation, but make the epidermis thinner and more vulnerable to trauma. Barrier function may be impaired. Therefore topical corticoids should be used with caution.

Interestingly, the use of topical corticosteroids can be an important cause of persistence of contact eczema because of allergy from corticosteroids. Cross-sensitivity among certain groups of corticosteroids is common and needs to be taken into consideration in treatments. Betametasone-17-valerate and monometasone furoate are rare sensitizers, and may be used if contact allergy to corticosteroid ointments is suspected, and patch testing cannot be performed.

Topical immunosuppressants

Recently two new topical agents have been discovered for treatment of contact dermatitis and other inflammatory skin diseases, i.e. tacrolimus and pimecrolimus. These drugs share the mechanism of action of ciclosporin, but while ciclosporin is not effective topically, tacrolimus and pimecrolimus are.

It has been shown that tacrolimus is effective in prevention of the elicitation phase of allergic contact dermatitis. Additionally, large-scale studies have been performed for atopic dermatitis, a condition sharing many pathophysiological attributes to contact dermatitis, such as the presence of inflammatory cell infiltrates in the skin. These studies have shown that tacrolimus has a relatively good safety profile with minor irritation as the most usual complication. Cases of severe herpes simplex infections have been reported, but in initial double-blind studies did not show higher incidence of herpes simplex with tacrolimus than with placebo cream. A greater concern is the possibility of increased incidence of lymphoma, as two patients were diagnosed with this during initial studies. Also, a mouse model for carcinogenesis has shown significantly higher incidence of lymphoma with tacrolimus than with placebo. Therefore, in at least paediatric patients lymph node status should be checked before starting tacrolimus cream. Tacrolimus has already been accepted for topical use in the USA and Japan. The main advantage of topical tacrolimus as compared to topical corticosteroids is the lack of atrophogenity. Its high cost remains a problem for its wider use.

Pimecrolimus is a derivative of ascomycin and it shares the mechanisms of action and efficacy/safety profiles of tacrolimus. Comparative studies between pimecrolimus and tacrolimus are missing.

Antimicrobials

Where secondary infection is thought likely to occur, antibacterial agents may be combined. When infection is present, antibiotics, such as erythromycin or cephalosporins will usually be given orally.

Antipruritic measures

Itching will be reduced by appropriate topical applications and may be helped by the antihistamine hydroxyzine. Hypnotics may be used to ensure sleep.

Tar

Tar (e.g. pix lithantracis 3–5% in an ointment) is known for its antieczematous effects. Cotton gloves can be worn to limit the inconvenience of the smell and colour of the tar.

Natural moisturising factor (NMF)

Sodium pyrrolidone carboxylic acid, sodium calcium lactate, amino acids, urea and a sugar–protein complex, derived from the protein filaggrin and called collectively NMF, keep the corneocyte hydrated under low relative humidity. Skin hydration and consequently skin barrier function may improve by applying an ointment with a substitute for NMF like urea or lactate.

Barrier cream

Barrier creams may facilitate cleaning but do not generally afford protection. Thus far barrier creams have not been proven useful.

Systemic therapy

Systemic corticosteroid therapy

Severe acute contact dermatitis may be treated with a 14–21-day course of oral corticosteroids. The initial dose is 30–50 mg of prednisolone, depending on the severity, taken daily after breakfast. This dose is decreased by 10 mg/day every 2–3 days to 20 mg/day and then decreased by 5 mg/day every 2–3 days. Oral therapy must be continued for at least 2 weeks to avoid relapses.

Ciclosporin

Ciclosporin has been used in the management of many inflammatory and non-inflammatory dermatoses. Its efficacy has been established especially in psoriasis and atopic dermatitis. Successful treatment of patients with severe allergic contact dermatitis or hand dermatitis has been reported. Granlund and co-workers found ciclosporin at 3 mg/kg per day as effective as topical betametasone-17, 21-dipropionate cream in the treatment of chronic hand eczema. Relapses occurred to the same extent in both groups. Ciclosporin is nephrotoxic, may cause hypertension and its long-term safety remains unclear. Therefore the risk : benefit ratio should always be considered before initiation of ciclosporin therapy, and the patient should be carefully followed for such adverse effects.

Azathioprine

In chronic contact dermatitis, e.g. from chromate, patients may not respond to potent topical steroids or allergen avoidance. In these recalcitrant cases azathioprine may be helpful. Lear and English reported successful treatment with 0.2 mg/kg azathioprine. They considered azathioprine to be cheaper and to have less side-effects than ciclosporin.

Antihistamines

Antihistamines are used mainly for their antipruritic effects in contact dermatitis. The classic H1-receptor antihistamines block H1-receptors causing sedation. Newer H1-receptor antagonists (terfenadine, loratadine, astemizole, cetirizine, ebastine) do not block central H1-receptors, and cause less sedation but have lower antipruritic effects, and their use in contact dermatitis is limited.

Doxepin

Eczematous dermatitis is commonly characterized by intense pruritus. Current treatment modalities are directed at reducing the cutaneous inflammatory response and thereby providing relief from pruritus. A recent new treatment by doxepin has shown promise; topical application of doxepin has been claimed to provide significant antipruritic activity with a favourable safety profile, suggesting a role of doxepin cream in the symptomatic treatment of pruritus associated with dermatitis. On the other hand, topical doxepin may elicit allergic contact dermatitis.

Pentoxiphylline

Pentoxiphylline (400 mg × 3) may reduce patch test reactivity because it influences the elicitation of contact dermatitis, but its role in therapy is not clear.

Phototherapy

Both ultraviolet (UV) B and psoralen and UVA (PUVA) phototherapy may be helpful in contact dermatitis. Data on the value of phototherapy in irritant contact dermatitis of the hands are scarce. UVB causes less photodamage than PUVA, but PUVA therapy has been shown to be superior to UVB in the treatment of chronic palmar eczema. Psoralens may be given orally (8-methoxypsoralen, 5-methoxypsoralen) or topically (cream or liquid; 8-methoxypsoralen or, trioxalen). The same treatment schedules as in psoriasis are used. PUVA therapy may also be used to suppress non-immunological immediate contact reactions.

Grenz rays

The use of Grenz rays (borderline rays, ultrasoft X-rays, Bucky rays) as an adjunct to topical therapy has been shown to be of benefit in treating chronic hand eczema. The suggested dosage has been 3 Gy (300 rad) of Grenz rays on six occasions at intervals of 1 week. This treatment schedule resulted in a significantly better response 5–10 weeks after the start of therapy compared with controls receiving topical corticosteroids throughout the study.

Future perspectives

New ligands of the steroid hormone superfamily, which have profound effects on epidermal growth and inflammation, may be developed, specifically facilitating adaptation to irritant stimuli or epidermal repair of irritated skin. Topical immunosuppressants with similar action than oral ciclosporin have been investigated. Tacrolimus (FK506) seems to share the efficacy and most of the adverse effects of ciclosporin when used systematically, presumably because of its similar intracellular actions. Unlike ciclosporin, tacrolimus is efficacious topically. Similarly, other medications affecting the afferent or efferent limb of allergic contact dermatitis are being evaluated.

Neuropeptides intervene as neurogenic modulators of inflammatory reaction and therefore participate in skin diseases, including contact dermatitis. Accordingly, topical neuropeptide agonists probably represent a new approach to the therapy of contact dermatitis in the near future.

New treatment modalities may focus on the improvement of the skin barrier function either by replenishing a lack of lipids, by restoring an altered lipid composition, both quantitatively and qualitatively, or by inhibition of the degradation of lipids in the intercellular space. Topical treatment with components of the normal intercellular domain (e.g. ceramides) may help to restore the highly ordered multilayered structure.

Treatment of contact urticaria

Contact urticaria and anaphylaxis that may sometimes occur following contact with natural rubber gloves has been shown to be an IgE-mediated response to rubber latex. Prophylactic treatment is avoidance of the responsible allergen (usually protein) and measures which help to restore the skin barrier. Oral antihistamines also help. Non-immune contact urticaria is an inflammatory response that is non-allergic in origin, and which may occur in atopics as well as in non-atopics. Some chemicals such as cinnamic aldehyde, cinnamic acid, methyl nicotinate, diethyl fumarate, benzoic acid and dimethyl sulphoxide may trigger this response in susceptible individuals. Non-immune contact urticaria is mostly blocked by corticosteroids and non-steroidal anti-inflammatories, although some chemicals have other mechanisms. Contact urticaria from natural rubber latex may be life-threatening or very mild, and present simply as discomfort when gloves are worn. Individuals allergic to latex may use plastic undergloves, vinyl gloves or non-latex (Elastyren) gloves.

Nickel allergy and dietary factors

Nickel allergy has become an epidemic in the industrialized world. Most women are sensitized either by ear piercing or by inexpensive metal jewellery. Nickel sensitivity tends to persist and may be an important factor in chronic eczema, including housewives' hand dermatitis. Manufacturers should be encouraged to use some of the safer nickel-containing alloys in jewellery and clothing accessories. Legislation in this regard has recently been passed in Denmark, and will soon become universal throughout the European Union.

Dietary factors

Some patients with nickel sensitivity experience chronic relapsing, vesicular hand eczema. Some of these patients may react to oral challenge with nickel (2.5 or 5 mg) or cobalt (1 mg). In these patients, a low-nickel diet may be helpful. A similar situation occurs with balsams and spices. Otherwise, foods probably have a low incidence of causing eczematous-type reactions in adults. The normal response is urticarial. Ingestion of allergens to which a patient is sensitive may lead not only to flares of vesicular hand eczema but also to urticaria, toxic erythemas, erythema multiforme-like reactions, and to other patterns of dermatitis, i.e. systemic contact dermatitis.

Children may more often have 'systemic allergic contact dermatitis' from foods, i.e. they display an allergic patch test reaction to foods, and dietary restrictions, e.g. avoiding cow milk, may be helpful.

Nappy dermatitis and treatment of dermatitis in children

Nappy dermatitis

Dampness, maceration, faecal enzymes, chemicals, increased pH from bacterial breakdown of urea, and other irritants may lead to nappy dermatitis in infants. Most cases can be cleared with frequent nappy changes, use of superabsorbent disposable nappies and a low-potency topical corticosteroid. Regular mild cleansing, use of emollient/silicone barrier creams and frequent changing of nappies have been shown to be helpful. If the eruption lasts for more than 3 days, addition of an antifungal agent may help to resolve the condition. Microbiological studies should be carried out to exclude significant secondary infection. Recalcitrant nappy dermatitis may signify other disorders, e.g. psoriasis. Prolonged use of fluorinated corticosteroids in the occluded nappy area may produce granulomatous lesions that subside when topical corticosteroid treatment is stopped.

Other contact dermatoses

Mild contact dermatitis is treated similarly as in adults. In severe, widespread contact dermatitis, systemic corticosteroid therapy may be indicated. The initial doses of corticosteroid are given for 3 days and then reduced over 2 weeks to avoid a rebound effect. To control pruritus, antihistamine (hydroxizine) may be given three times daily.

Management of other types of contact dermatitis

The management of specific types of contact dermatitis includes management of hydrofluoric acid burns, chromate sensitivity, cosmetic intolerance, atopic dermatitis, hairdressers, dental personnel and their patients (e.g. prostheses and fillings), formaldehyde sensitivity, chronic actinic dermatitis, frictional contact dermatitis, dermatitis from carbonless copy paper, and eyelid dermatitis.

Further reading

Dooms-Goossens A, Lepoittevin J-P. Studies on the contact allergenic potential of monomethasone furoate: a clinical and molecular study. *Eur J Dermatol* 1996; 6: 339–40.

Drake LA, Millikan LE. The antipruritic effect of 5% doxepin cream in patients with eczematous dermatitis. Doxepin Study Group. *Arch Dermatol* 1995; 131: 1403–8.

Funk JO, Maibach HI. Horizons in pharmacologic intervention in allergic contact dermatitis. *J Am Acad Dermatol* 1994; 31: 999–1014.

Granlund H, Erkko P, Eriksson E, Reitamo S. Comparison of ciclosporine and topical betamethasone-17,21-dipropionate in the treatment of severe chronic hand eczema. *Acta Derm-Venereol (Stockh)* 1996; 76: 371–6.

Guin J. Treatment of contact dermatitis. In: Guin JD, ed. *Practical Contact Dermatitis. A Handbook for the Practitioner.* McGraw-Hill, 1995: 673–86.

Katsarou-Katsari A, Armenaka M, Katsenis K, Papageorgiou M, Katsambas A, Bareltzidis A. Contact allergens in patients with leg ulcers. *JEADV* 1998; 11: 9–12.

Lauerma AI, Granlund H, Reitamo S. Use of newer immunosuppressive agents in dermatology. *Biodrugs* 1997; 8: 96–106.

Lauerma AI, Maibach HI, Granlund H, Erkko P, Kartamaa M, Stubb S. Inhibition of contact allergy reactions by topical FK506. *Lancet* 1992; 340: 556.

Lear JT, English JSC. Severe and chronic allergic contact dermatitis responding to azathioprine therapy. *J Dermatol Treat* 1996; 7: 109–10.

Lindelöf B, Wrangsjö K, Lidén S. A double-blind study of Grenz ray therapy in chronic eczema of the hands. *Br J Dermatol* 1987; 117: 77–80.

Lubbe J, Pournaras CC, Saurat JH. Eczema herpeticum during treatment of atopic dermatitis with 0.1% tacrolimus ointment. *Dermatology* 2000; 201: 249–51.

Mrowietz U. Macrolide immunosuppressants. *Eur J Dermatol* 1999; 9: 346–51.

Nielsen HH, Menné T. Allergic contact dermatitis in an unselected Danish population. *Acta Derm-Venereol, Stockh* 1992; 72: 456–60.

Rietschel RL, Fowler JF Jr. *Fisher's Contact Dermatitis.* Baltimore: Williams & Wilkins, 1995.

Rosen K, Mobacken H, Swanbeck G. Chronic eczematous dermatitis of the hands: a comparison of PUVA and UVB treatment. *Acta Derm-Venereol (Stockh)* 1987; 67: 48–54.

Ruzicka T, Bieber T, Schopf E *et al.* A short-term trial of tacrolimus ointment for atopic dermatitis. European Tacrolimus Multicenter Atopic Dermatitis Study Group. *N Engl J Med* 1997; 337: 816–21.

Cutaneous vasculitis

T.M. Lotti, C. Comacchi and I. Ghersetich

The vasculitic disorders are usually characterized by palpable purpura. This clinical condition of dermatological interest is mainly related to 'cutaneous necrotizing vasculitis' (CNV), characterized by angiocentric segmental inflammation, endothelial cell swelling and fibrinoid necrosis of blood vessel walls.

Although blood vessels of any size may be affected in systemic vasculitis, CNV usually occurs in the small venules (postcapillary venules), being characterized by the histological pattern of both a leukocytoclastic form, with a presumed immune complex-mediated pathogenesis, and a lymphomonocytic form in which a cell-mediated pathogenesis is proposed.

More recent data also seem to suggest the participation of a secondary cell-mediated immune response in the late phase of the leukocytoclastic form.

CNV can be idiopathic or associated with drugs, infection or underlying systemic disease (Tables 1–3). The disorder occurs equally in both sexes and at all ages, approximately 10% of the cases occurring in children.

Clinical features

Palpable purpura is the major clinical presentation of CNV, while erythematous macules, wheals, papules, blisters, large palpable nodules, ecchymoses, pustules, haemorrhagic vesicles, ulcers and a net-like skin (livedo reticularis) are less common manifestations. Lesions are often distributed symmetrically and may occur anywhere but are most commonly found on the lower legs (particularly if the patient is standing)—elevated hydrostatic pressure and tortuosity of the vessels may provoke more distorted and turbulent flow patterns, and increase viscosity leading to increased vasopermeability and to possible tissue deposition of circulating immune complexes. The mucous membranes are only rarely involved (petechiae, haemorrhagic blisters, ulcers). In the skin, the lesions may be moderately itchy or painful (especially in those chronic or recurrent episodes preceded by fever, myalgia, joint pain, headache and malaise). Usually, the lesions persist from 1 to 4 weeks and resolve with residual scarring and hyperpigmentation. Recently the Koebner phenomenon has been reported as an unusual cutaneous manifestation of immune complex-mediated CNV. The disease is often self-limited and confined to the skin, but visceral lesions (renal, gastrointestinal, pericardial, neurological and rheumatological) may occur.

Table 1 Cutaneous necrotizing vasculitis: precipitating agents

Viral infections: hepatitis A virus, hepatitis B virus, hepatitis C virus, herpes simplex, influenza virus
Bacterial infections: β-haemolytic *Streptococcus* group A, *Staphylococcus aureus, Mycobacterium leprae*
Fungal infections: *Candida albicans*
Protozoan infections: *Plasmodium malariae*
Helminth infections: *Schistosoma haematobium, Schistosoma mansoni, Onchocerca volvulus*
Drugs: insulin, penicillin, hydantoins, streptomycin, aminosalicylic acid, sulphonamides, thiazides, phenothiazines, vitamins, phenylbutazone, quinine, streptokinase, tamoxifen, anti-influenza vaccine, oral contraceptive, serum
Chemicals: insecticides, petroleum products
Foodstuff allergens: milk proteins, gluten

Table 2 Cutaneous necrotizing vasculitis: association with coexistent diseases

CNV associated with lymphoproliferative disorders:
Hodgkin's disease
Mycosis fungoides
Lymphosarcoma
Adult T-cell leukaemia
Multiple myeloma
CNV associated with solid tumours
Lung cancer
Colon carcinoma
Renal
Prostate
Head and neck cancer
Breast cancer
CNV associated with chronic diseases
Systemic lupus erythematous
Sjögren's syndrome
Rheumatoid arthritis
Behçet's disease
Hyperglobulinaemic states
Cryoglobulinaemia
Bowel bypass syndrome
Ulcerative colitis
Cystic fibrosis
Primary biliary cirrhosis
Human immunodeficiency virus seropositivity and acquired immunodeficiency syndrome

Table 3 Idiopathic cutaneous necrotizing vasculitis

Schönlein–Henoch purpura
Urticarial vasculitis
Erythema elevatum diutinium
Nodular vasculitis
Livedoid vasculitis
Atrophie blanche
Cutaneous polyarteritis nodosa

Evaluation should include a thorough history and physical examination with attention to possible aetiological agents, ingestants, infections and associated symptomatology (Table 4).

In patients with CNV a laboratory screening is always required for confirmation of the diagnosis and pathogenesis and to determine the extent of systemic vasculitis involvement and/or the existence of underlying associated diseases. Laboratory evaluation includes histopathological and immunofluorescence studies of skin lesions, blood and urinalysis.

Table 4 Evaluation of the patient with cutaneous necrotizing vasculitis

History
Infections?
Drugs?
Chemicals?
Foodstuffs allergens?
Underlying systemic disease?
Systemic symptoms?
Physical examination
Histopathological evaluation
Skin biopsy
Muscle biopsy
Renal biopsy
Rectal biopsy
Lung biopsy
Laboratory studies
Complete blood count
Urinalysis
Hepatitis surface antigen
Rheumatoid factor
Circulating immune complexes
Complement components
Antinuclear antibodies
Antiphospholipid antibodies
Cryoglobulins
Antineutrophil cytoplasmic antibody
Antistreptolysin antibodies
Chest roentgenogram

In the leukocytoclastic form, direct immunofluorescence may show immunoglobulins, complement components, and fibrin deposits in and around the blood vessels. Immunoglobulin G (IgG) rather than IgM are more likely to be present when there is an underlying collagen vascular disease, and IgA may be indicative of Schönlein–Henoch purpura. Decreased levels of complement components are often noted in leukocytoclastic CNV associated with rheumatoid arthritis (C1, C4, C2), systemic lupus erythematosus (C1q, C4, C2, C3, factor B, C9), cryoglobulinaemia and Sjögren's syndrome. Circulating immune complexes, rheumatoid factor; antinuclear antibodies, antiphospholipid antibodies and cryoglobulins can be detected with antistreptolysin antibodies and hepatitis B (C and A) surface antigens.

Urine analysis may reveal proteinuria, haematuria and cylindruria caused by possible renal involvement.

Also, in patients in whom systemic vasculitic syndromes have been considered, tests such as the antineutrophil cytoplasmic antibody (p-ANCA and/or c-ANCA) may be diagnostically helpful. ANCAs have been demonstrated in Wegener's granulomatosis, Churg–Strauss syndrome, pulmonary renal syndrome, microscopic polyarteritis nodosa, the leukocytoclastic form of CNV and idiopathic glomerulonephritis. The sensitivity of ANCAs to this group of diseases is high when there is renal involvement. The titre of ANCAs is not correlated with the severity of vasculitis, but the disappearance of ANCAs is associated with absence of disease activity. Elevated ANCA levels may precede a relapse. Patients have only one or other of the two types of ANCA antibodies. c-ANCA are sensitive and specific for active Wegener's granulomatosis and are found in microscopic polyarteritis. p-ANCA occurs in idiopathic glomerulonephritis, Churg–Strauss syndrome, polyarteritis nodosa with visceral involvement and vasculitic overlap syndromes.

If the diagnosis of systemic disease is still being considered after the initial screening, other options are available: muscle, renal, rectal and lung biopsies, and arteriography and chest roentgenogram.

In the lymphocytic form of CNV these laboratory tests are usually normal.

Management

The therapy of vasculitis depends on whether or not there is clinical evidence of systemic disease, and the severity of the cutaneous and/or systemic disease.

When possible, identifying and removing the causative agents (drugs, chemicals, infections, foods) represents the aetiological treatment, followed by rapid clearance of skin lesions; no other treatment is necessary. Patients without an identifiable cause or associated phenomenon who require therapy can be treated with a variety of local and systemic therapies.

Local treatments

Topical therapy (corticosteroid creams, antibiotic creams) may be helpful in some cases.

General treatments

These treatments include:

- corticosteroids
- non-steroidal anti-inflammatory drugs
- antimalarial agents
- dapsone
- potassium iodide
- antihistamines
- fibrinolytic agents
- aminocaproic acid
- immunosuppressive agents
- drugs reducing platelet aggregation
- high-dose intravenous immunoglobulin.

A systemic treatment with corticosteroids (prednisone 60–80 mg/day) is advised in the majority of patients for 7–15 days in the acute phase (especially in Schönlein–Henoch purpura, urticarial vasculitis, Behçet's disease).

Non-steroidal anti-inflammatory drugs such as acetylsalicylic acid and indometacin have been used for vasculitis with more persistent or necrotic lesions. Some cases of urticarial vasculitis have responded to indometacin. Phenylbutazone, oxyphenbutazone and ibuprofen are indicated for thrombophlebitis in nodular vasculitis.

Antimalarials such as oral colchicine, which inhibits neutrophil chemotaxis, in doses of 0.6 mg twice daily, may be helpful in the chronic forms of the disease.

Dapsone (50–200 mg/day) has also been used, usually in patients with skin involvement alone (especially in patients with erythema elevatum diutinum).

Potassium iodide (0.3–1.5 g four times daily) is useful for nodular vasculitis.

H_1-antihistamines alone or in combination with H_2-antihistamines are used to alleviate the pruritus and to block histamine-induced endothelial gap formation with resultant trapping of immune complexes.

Fibrinolytic agents can be used in patients in which there is a reduction of plasma and/or cutaneous fibrinolytic activity. Stanozolol (5 mg twice daily), phenformin hydrochloride (50 mg twice daily) plus ethyloestrenol (2 mg four times daily) can be used for about a year. Other fibrinolytic agents such as heparin (5000 units twice daily), mesoglycans (50–100 mg/day) and defibrotide (700 mg/day i.m.) seem beneficial in various types of hypofibrinolytic vasculitis.

Low molecular weight dextran by means of fibrinolytic effect is also indicated in the hypofibrinolytic phase of disease. This seems to produce beneficial effects both in the livedo reticularis and in the livedoid vasculitis.

Aminocaproic acid (8–16 g/day for many months) can be used in the hyperfibrinolytic states.

Immunosuppressive agents such as cyclophosphamide (2 mg/kg per day), methotrexate (10–25 mg/week), azathioprine (150 mg/day) and ciclosporin A (3–5 mg/kg per day) are effective especially in patients with CNV (with a rapidly progressing course or with systemic involvement) not controlled with corticosteroids.

In the course of vasculitis induced by immune complexes with concomitant arterial disease drugs reducing platelet aggregation (dipyridamole, acetylisalicylic acid, ticlopidine) and plasmapheresis can be used.

High-dose intravenous immunoglobulin therapy was associated with improvement in Schönlein–Henoch purpura.

The correction of local factors such as trauma, cold stasis and lymphoedema may also be important.

The future

These treatments include:

- monoclonal antibodies
- low-dose recombinant tissue plasminogen activator
- prostacyclin and prostaglandin E_1
- interferon-α.

Recently a patient with intractable systemic vasculitis has been treated with two monoclonal antibodies, Campath-1H and rat CD4.

Low-dose recombinant tissue plasminogen activator therapy was reported to be successful in one study. Infusions of prostacyclin and of prostaglandin E_1 have been successful in one patient each.

The administration of interferon-α has been associated with clearing of CNV in patients with hepatitis C virus infection.

Further reading

Braun-Falco O, Plewig G, Wolff HH *et al. Dermatology.* Berlin: Springer-Verlag, 1991: 620–3.

Burge S. The management of cutaneous vasculitis. In: Panconesi E, ed. *Dermatology in Europe.* Oxford: Blackwell Scientific Publications, 1991: 328–30.

Callen JP, Kallenberg CGM. The vasculitides: relationship of cutaneous vasculitis to systemic disease. In: Kater L and Baart de la Faille H, eds. *Multi-Systemic Auto-Immune Diseases: an Integrated Approach.* Elsevier, 1995: 267–97.

Chan LS, Cooper KD, Rasmussen JE. Koebnerization as a cutaneous manifestation of immune complex-mediated vasculitis. *J Am Acad Dermatol* 1990; 22: 775–81.

Comacchi C, Ghersetich I, Lotti T. La vasculite necrotizzante cutanea. *G Ital Dermatol Venereol* 1998; 133: 23–49.

Habif TP. *Clinical Dermatology*, 3rd edn. St Louis: CV Mosby, 1996: 567–96.

Isseroff SW, Whiting DA. Low molecular weight dextran in the treatment of livedo reticularis with ulceration. *Br J Dermatol* 1971; 85: 26–9.

Katz SI. Erythema elevatum diutinum. Skin and systemic manifestations, immunologic studies and successful treatment with Dapsone. *Medicine* 1977; 56: 443–52.

Lotti T. The management of systemic complications of vasculitis. In: Panconesi E, ed. *Dermatology in Europe*. Oxford: Blackwell Scientific Publications, 1991: 330–2.

Lotti T, Celasco G, Tsampau D *et al.* Mesoglycan treatment restores defective fibrinolytic potential in cutaneous necrotizing venulitis. *Int J Dermatol* 1993; 32 (5): 368–71.

Lotti T, Comacchi C, Ghersetich I. Cutaneous necrotizing vasculitis. *Int J Dermatol* 1996; 35: 457–74.

Lotti T, Ghersetich I, Comacchi C, Jorizzo JL. Cutaneous small-vessel vasculitis. *J Am Acad Dermatol* 1998; 39: 667–87.

Lotti T, Ghersetich I, Comacchi C, Panconesi E. Purpuras and related conditions. *J Eur Acad Dermatol Venereol* 1996; 7: 1–25.

Lynch PJ. Vascular reactions. In: Schachner LA *et al.*, eds. *Pediatric Dermatology.* New York: Churchill Livingstone, 1988: 959–1014.

Mathieson PW, Cobbold SP, Hale CG *et al.* Monoclonal-antibody therapy in systemic vasculitis. *N Engl J Med* 1990; 323: 250–4.

Resnick AH, Esterly NB. Vasculitis in children. *Int J Dermatol* 1985; 24: 139.

Ryan TJ. Microvascular injury. *Maj Probl Dermatol* 1976; 7: 373–405.

Ryan TJ. Cutaneous vasculitis. In: Rook A *et al.*, eds. *Textbook of Dermatology.* Oxford: Blackwell Scientific Publications, 1992: 1893–961.

Schifferli JA, Saurat JH, Woodley DT. Cutaneous Vasculitis. In: Ruiz-Maldonado R *et al.*, eds. *Textbook of Pediatric Dermatology.* Philadelphia: Grune & Stratton, 1989: 654–61.

Soter NA. Cutaneous necrotizing venulitis. In: Fitzpatrick TB *et al.*, eds. *Dermatology in General Medicine*, 5th edn. New York: McGraw-Hill, 1999: 2044–53.

Van Vroonhoven TJMV, Van Zijl J, Muller H. Low dose subcutaneous heparin versus oral anticoagulants. *Lancet* 1974; i: 375–84.

Darier's disease

C. Varotti and F. Bardazzi

Synonyms

Darier–White disease, keratosis follicularis.

Definition and epidemiology

Darier's disease is a dominantly inherited condition with variable penetrance that has been considered to be a disorder of keratinization. Darier's disease is characterized by a persistent rash of keratotic papules over the whole skin with particular involvement of seborrhoeic areas and nail dystrophy.

Lesions typically appear between 8 and 15 years and rarely before the age of 5; however, onset in adulthood can occur.

Its estimated prevalence ranges from 1/55 000 to 1/100 000.

Aetiology and pathophysiology

The cause of Darier's disease is not known. The autosomal dominant nature of transmission suggests that a genetic defect is operative and the premature keratinization as well as a loss of desmosomes and detachment of tonofilaments usually observed by electron microscopy seem to be the primary abnormalities. Many cases, however, appear to occur as a new mutation.

The histological changes of Darier's disease, characterized by focal acantholytic dyskeratosis, are distinctive but not entirely pathognomonic; they are:

1 Suprabasal lacunae resulting from suprabasal acantholysis.
2 Villi (irregular upward proliferation of dermal papillae lined with a single layer of basal cells).
3 Corps ronds (small groups of cells around the lacunae separated from their neighbours; enlarged and present a darkly staining nucleus surrounded by clear cytoplasm and a glistening ring; they occur in the upper stratum malpighii, particularly on the granular and horny layers).
4 Grains (dyskeratotic small cells with elongated and often grain-shaped nucleus surrounded by shrunken cytoplasm; they are seen in the horny layer and in the suprabasal lacunae).
5 Hyperkeratosis, acanthosis, papillomatosis.
6 Chronic inflammatory infiltrate in the dermis.

Acantholysis occurs first, dyskeratosis later.

Clinical characteristic and course

The fundamental lesions of Darier's disease are firm, persistent, hyperkeratotic, greasy papules which are skin-coloured, yellow–brown or brown. The lesions may coalesce into large plaques or papillomatous masses. The scalp, face, neck, chest, back and groin are usually affected. When the intertriginous areas are involved, the lesions are foul smelling. On the backs of the hands and feet discrete papules resemble acrokeratosis verruciformis of Hopf. The palms and the soles may show pits or punctate keratosis that can often be found in otherwise unaffected relatives.

Mucous membrane lesions consist of white, centrally depressed papules, most frequently of the mucosae of the cheeks, the hard and soft palate and gums; salivary glands obstruction may be associated.

The nails are usually abnormal presenting longitudinal red and/or white lines extending from the base of the nail across the lunula to the free margin of the nail, as well as nail fragility, V-shaped nick at the free edge of the nail, longitudinal ridging of the nail, painful splitting of the nail plate and subungual hyperkeratotic fragments.

General health remains unaffected.

There is no difference in the incidence of the disease in men and women.

Darier's disease is chronic and unremitting for almost all patients, it is exacerbated during summer and after exposure to ultraviolet light or excessive sweating.

Clinical variants are hypertrophic, vesiculobullous and systematized disease.

Diagnosis

Skin biopsy showing focal acantholytic dyskeratosis is mandatory for diagnosis.

Direct and indirect immunofluorescent studies are negative.

Differential diagnosis

This includes chronic benign familial pemphigus (later occurrence lesions starting in different areas—never on hands and feet); acanthosis nigricans (pigmented, flexural lesions); and papillomatosis—reticulated and confluent (flat lesions limited to the upper trunk).

Other dermatological conditions in which the focal acantholytic dyskeratosis histological pattern can be detected (transient acantholytic dermatitis of Grover, linear epidermal naevus with acantholytic dyskeratosis, warty dyskeratomas, focal acantholytic dyskeratoma) are easily ruled out by clinical data.

Treatment

General therapeutic guidelines

At present no entirely effective treatment is available and only one-third of patients

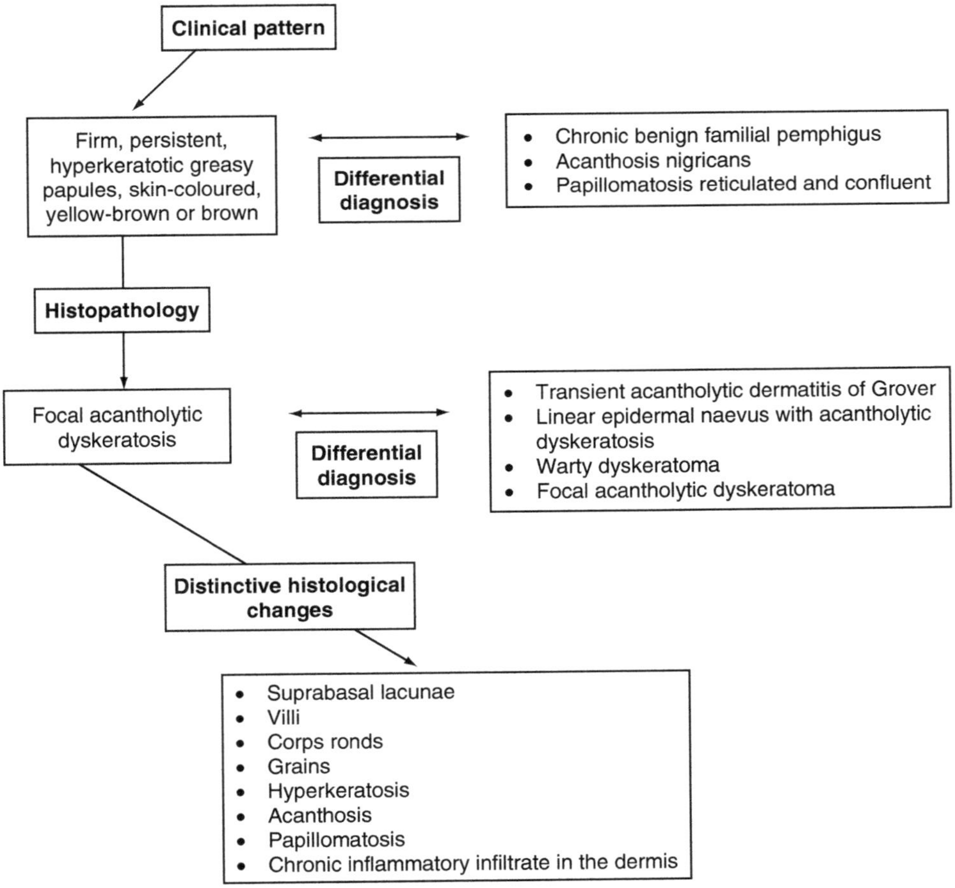

Figure 1 Darier's disease

noted improvement with age. A good doctor/patient relationship to satisfy patients' emotional needs as well as medical requirements is necessary; hot environments should be avoided; cool atmosphere and cotton clothing next to the skin should be suggested.

Recommended therapies

A simple emollient can be used in mild forms.

Oral aromatic retinoids are the most effective management of the severe forms: 0.5–1 mg/kg per day of etretinate, 1–2 mg/kg per day of isotretinoin, or 0.5 mg/kg per day of acitretin. Retinoids are effective in 75% of patients, since they work by temporarily correcting the altered pattern of keratinization; when the treatment is stopped however, the disease more or less promptly recurs.

Retinoids sometimes induce exfoliation giving wet and exudative lesions. Avoidance of the sun is highly recommended; broad-spectrum sunscreen should be applied especially, by sun-sensitive patients.

In the exudative forms, short cycles of topical or systemic corticosteroids can be used.

Surgical treatment such as dermoabrasion or carbon dioxide laser vaporization, have been advocated for recalcitrant, hypertrophic Darier's disease.

Vitamin A acid cream has been effective in some patients particularly when used with occlusion, even though erythema, burning and irritation are constant consequences.

Recently, topical calcipotriol as well as 5–fluorouracil, has been used succesfully in some patients. However further studies are necessary to establish the extent of the efficacy of such treatment in Darier's disease.

Further reading

Burge SM. Darier's disease and other dyskeratoses: response to retinoids. *Pharmacol Ther* 1989; 40: 75–90.

Burge SM, Buxton PK. Topical isotretinoin in Darier's disease. *Br J Dermatol* 1995; 133 (6): 924–8.

Dicken CH, Bauer EA, Hazen PG *et al.* Isoretinoin treatment of Darier's disease. *J Am Acad Dermatol* 1982; 6 (Suppl.): 721–6.

Knulst AC, De La Faille HB, Van Vloten WA. Topical 5–fluorouracil in the treatment of Darier's disease. *Br J Dermatol* 1995; 133 (3): 463–6.

Kragballe K, Steijlen PM, Ibsen HH *et al.* Efficacy, tolerability, and safety of calcipotriol ointment in disorders of keratinization. Result of a randomized, double-blind, vehicle-controlled, right/left comparative study. *Arch Dermatol* 1995; 131 (5): 556–60.

Launaranta J, Kanerva L, Turjanmaa K *et al.* Clinical and ultrastructural effects of acitretin in Darier's disease. *Acta Derm Venereol* 1988; 68: 492–8.

McElroy JA, Meheregan DA, Roenigk RK. Carbon dioxide laser vaporization of recalcitrant symptomatic plaques of Hailey-Hailey disease and Darier's disease. *J Am Acad Dermatol* 1990; 23: 893–7.

Wheeland RG, Gilmore WA. The surgical treatment of hypertrophic Darier's disease. *J Dermatol Surg Oncol* 1985; 63: 420–3.

Dermatitis herpetiformis

C. Gooptu and F. Wojnarowska

Synonym

Dühring's disease.

Definition and epidemiology

Dermatitis herpetiformis (DH) is a rare disease characterized by a chronic, papulovesicular eruption; it is intensely pruritic and associated with immunoglobulin A (IgA) deposition in the papillary dermis. It is accompanied by an underlying gluten-sensitive enteropathy.

In general, men are more commonly affected than women (ratio 2 : 1), though this pattern is reversed in children and young adults. The age of onset varies with geographical location, being in childhood in Italy and Hungary, in middle life in much of northern Europe, and later in southern Sweden. Dermatitis herpetiformis is rare in Malaysia, China and Japan, and in Korea it is seen more commonly in Caucasians than Koreans. The incidence is highest in Ireland, at 1 in 1700, and in Sweden, where it is 39 per 100 000. There is clustering of both DH and coeliac disease in families, with 10.5% of DH patients having affected relatives. There is an immunogenetic association with HLA DR3 DQW2, which is very much more common in Caucasians than Orientals and may be important in the different incidences of DH in different ethnic populations.

Aetiology and pathophysiology

A genetic susceptibility to gluten has been proposed as an aetiological mechanism, since gluten must be present in the diet for DH to be manifested. Differences in daily gluten intake (7–8 g a day in Korea, 15–20 g a day in Scandinavia) may explain why this disease is much less common in Asia than it is in the West, but the exact mechanism by which gluten causes DH has yet to be elucidated. Recently tissue transglutaminase has been shown to be a major autoantigen for IgA antibodies in coeliac disease and dermatitis herpetiformis. This enzyme and its IgA autoantibodies may be involved in the pathogenesis of dermatitis herpetiformis. In some patients, raised titres of antibodies to adenovirus 12 have also been found, suggesting a possible infectious trigger. In addition, iodine may exacerbate dermatitis herpetiformis and has been invoked for its high prevalence in Scandinavia. DH may also be associated with autoimmune disease, particularly thyroid disease.

Clinical characteristics and course

DH is characterized by an intensely pruritic, symmetrical eruption, which can affect the extensor surfaces of the elbows and knees, the buttocks, natal cleft, axillary, folds, trunk, face and scalp. Individual lesions may be erythematous, eczematous, urticarial, papular, vesicular or bullous. Mucosal lesions may also occur but are rare. Pruritus alone may precede lesions.

All patients have an associated gluten-sensitive enteropathy, though this may be asymptomatic. Alternatively, it may lead to bouts of abdominal pain, steatorrhoea, constipation and malnutrition. Removal of gluten from the diet results not only in clearance of the rash but also an increased feeling of well-being. DH tends to run a chronic course punctuated by exacerbations and remissions. Acute infections, emotional stress or reintroduction of gluten can all produce a disease flare.

There is also an association with carcinomas and lymphoma. The life expectancy of patients with DH is nonetheless greater than that of the control population, possibly due to a significant decreased risk of ischaemic heart disease.

Diagnosis (laboratory examinations)

Histology of lesional skin shows microabscesses consisting of neutrophils and eosinophils within the dermal papillae. Subepidermal vesicles and bullae are produced within the lamina lucida as a result of collagen degradation.

Direct immunofluorescence of normal skin shows granular deposits of IgA in the papillary dermis, which gradually clear once gluten has been withdrawn from the diet.

Often these deposits are associated with microfibrils, but the exact target antigen is still unknown. IgG and C3 may also be detected.

Indirect immunofluorescence is negative for basement membrane zone or dermal autoantibodies unless monkey oesophagus is used when IgA endomysial antibodies may be detected. Tissue transglutaminase antibodies may be detected by an enzyme-linked immunosorbent assay (ELISA) technique, but this test is not yet routinely available.

Antithyroid, antireticulin, antigluten and antigliaden antibodies may be detected.

Full blood count and film may show iron or folate deficiency anaemia with Howell–Joly bodies due to splenic atrophy.

Jejunal biopsy reveals signs of gluten-sensitive enteropathy, which are reversed by exclusion of dietary gluten.

Differential diagnosis

This includes scabies (absence of burrows); eczema (histology and lack of IgA deposition); prurigo (histology and lack of IgA deposition); and papular urticaria (histology and lack of IgA deposition).

Treatment

General therapeutic guidelines

1. Treatment with dapsone initially suppresses the eruption, but the long-term treatment of choice is a gluten-free diet, as this not only reverses the gut changes and leads to remission of the rash but also abolishes the risk of lymphoma.
2. All patients should be referred to a dietitian.
3. Contact with a patient support group, such as the Coeliac Society, can also be helpful.
4. Skin cleansers containing iodine should be avoided, as they may produce a disease flare.
5. Topical steroids may be useful.

Recommended therapies

Dapsone

Dapsone is the drug most commonly used to treat DH and, if effective, will improve the irritation within a few days if an adequate dosage is being used, although it does not affect the enteropathy. Treatment is usually commenced at 50 mg/day, increasing by 50 mg every 2 weeks until control is achieved. Most adults are controlled by 100–200 mg daily, although occasionally doses of 400–700 mg are required. Too rapid an increase in dose may result in haemolytic anaemia (which reaches a maximum at 1 month). Glucose-6-phosphate dehydrogenase deficiency (seen particularly in some Afro-Caribbean, Asian and Mediterranean populations) will result in acute haemolysis and must therefore be excluded prior to starting treatment. Methaemoglobinaemia is common, resulting in cyanosis, angina and breathlessness, and these effects limit the usefulness of dapsone in the elderly. Less commonly hepatitis (sometimes accompanied by lymphadenopathy—'the dapsone syndrome') or agranulocytosis may occur, but these are usually early complications. A reversible motor neuropathy may also occur, and treatment may be complicated by headache, lethargy, insomnia and depression. Since side-effects are dose-dependent it is important to find the minimum dose necessary by reducing the dose every 2 months after stable control has been achieved, by 50 mg on alternate days, for example or by 50 mg once a week if the former is not tolerated. Some patients appear to be exquisitely sensitive to the dose of dapsone, with variations of 50 mg/week making a difference to the effect or toxicity. The addition of cimetidine (400 mg three times a day) can reduce the degree if methaemoglobinaemia and increase the plasma dapsone level without increasing haemolysis. Investigations, including full blood count, reticulocyte count and liver function tests, should be monitored at regular intervals—initially fortnightly for up to 3 months after any dose increase and then 3-monthly, with methaemoglobin levels included if clinically indicated.

Dapsone should be avoided in late pregnancy and during lactation, as it may induce haemolytic disease of the newborn. Patients taking dapsone who are trying to conceive are advised to take folic acid supplements.

Other sulphonamides

Sulphapyridine (at doses of 1.5–4 g/day) or sulphamethoxypyridazine (0.5–1.5 g/day) may be used if dapsone is not tolerated. Side-effects include skin rashes, nausea, lethargy, depression, haemolytic anaemia and bone marrow suppression but sulphamethoxypyridazine is often well tolerated at low doses, particularly by the elderly, in whom it is preferable to dapsone. Alternatively, a combination of two or even three of the above drugs may be combined at low doses to achieve therapeutic efficacy with fewer side-effects.

Gluten-free diet

A gluten-free diet is the treatment of choice in the long term, but it must be strictly adhered to for the best results. Gluten occurs in wheat, barley and rye, which must therefore be avoided, but rice, maize and pure oats can be eaten. Unfortunately, many proprietary oat preparations are contaminated with other grain and are therefore unsuitable. A gluten-free diet not only improves the skin lesions but also reverses the enteropathy (leading to an increased feeling of well-being and subsequent weight gain), and often enables the dapsone or sulphonamides to be discontinued. However, in order to follow a strict diet, patients must be intelligent and highly motivated, as it may take many months (on average 2 years) before the drugs can be discontinued. In addition, a gluten-free diet has been shown to reduce the incidence of lymphoma after 10 years. Reintroduction of gluten may lead to a relapse of DH.

Further reading

Dietrich W, Laag E, Bruckner-Tuderman L *et al.* Antibodies to tissue transglutaminase as serologic markers in patients with dermatitis herpetiformis. *J Invest Dermatol* 1999; 113 (1): 133–6.

Fry L. Dermatitis herpetiformis. In: Wojnarowska F, Briggaman R, eds. *Management of Blistering Disease*. London: Chapman & Hall Medical, 1990: 139–62.

Hardman CM, Garioch JJ, Leonard JN *et al.* Absence of toxicity of oats in patients with dermatitis herpetiformis. *N Engl J Med* 1997; 337 (26): 1884–7.

Lewis H, Reunala T, Garioch J *et al.* Protective effect of gluten-free diet against development of lymphoma in dermatitis herpetiformis. *Br J Dermatol* 1996; 135: 363–7.

McFadden J, Leonard J, Powles A *et al.* Sulphamethoxypyridazine for dermatitis, herpetiformis, linear IgA disease and cicatrical pemphigoid. *Br J Dermatol* 1989; 121: 759–62.

Rhodes L, Tingle M, Park B *et al.* Cimetidine improves the therapeutic/toxic ratio of dapsone in patients on chronic dapsone therapy. *Br J Dermatol* 1959; 132: 257–62.

Dermatomyositis

S. Jablonska and M. Blaszczyk

Definition and epidemiology

Dermatomyositis (DM) is a rare chronic idiopathic inflammatory myopathy (IIM), characterized by symmetrical proximal muscle involvement and typical cutaneous lesions. The incidence is approximately 5/1000 000 population. DM occurs in all races, twice more often in females. It is also not rare in childhood (juvenile DM or JDM). In about 10% of patients the cutaneous changes characteristic of DM are not associated with muscle disease (amyopathic DM). DM of adults is associated in about 30% of patients with internal malignancies.

Aetiology and pathophysiology

DM is an autoimmune connective tissue disease (CTD) of unknown aetiology. Both cellular and humoral immune response appear to be involved. Myositis-specific antibody (MSA) Mi2 was found associated with about 15–20% of classical DM of adults and children, and in a small number of patients the immunological marker is tRNA synthetase antibody, mostly anti-histidyl tRNA synthetase antibody (Jo1). The immunogenetics of DM is not homogenous. In about 40% of DM cases the antibodies are of unidentified specificity, and in a proportion of patients they are not detectable. A more benign form of DM associated with Mi2 antibodies was found to have immunogenetic markers DR7, DRw53 and DQ2, whereas polymyositis associated with other myositis-specific antibodies was found to have a significantly increased frequency of HLA-DRB1*0301 and DQA1*0501 alleles.

The membrane attack complex of complement (MAC) deposits in the intramuscular vasculature and persistent expression of interleukin-1 (IL-1), intercellular adhesion molecule-1 (ICAM-1), vascular cell adhesion molecule-1 (VCAM-1) in endothelial cells of capillaries could explain vessel injury, which is especially pronounced in JDM. However cellular immune mechanisms appear also to play an important role, substantiated by the presence of activated T lymphocytes in the inflammatory infiltrates. The role of various viruses (coxsackie B, adenovirus, human immunodeficiency virus (HIV), etc.) is conceivable in the initiation of the autoimmune response (specifically coxsackie virus reacting with human enzyme tRNA synthetase may trigger development of Jo1 antibody). However cell-mediated immune mechanisms might be responsible for perpetuation of the skin and muscle injury.

The significant association with cancers in patients over 50 years of age is well established and these patients should be studied for presence of malignancy.

Clinical characteristics and course

Characteristic cutaneous signs are:

- heliotrope periorbital erythema and oedema
- Gottron's sign: symmetrical erythema overlying the knuckles, elbows, knees, interphalangeal and metacarpophalangeal joints, and Gottron's papules in the latter location
- V-sign: violaceous erythema on the anterior neck and thorax
- erythema on the extensor aspects of the arms and hands, sometimes also present on the posterior trunk (shawl sign)
- characteristic telangiectasia and erythema of the proximal nail fold
- poikilodermatous changes (mostly in chronic cases)

- characteristic for DM and PM (polymyositis) 'mechanic's hand'—keratotic plaques on the palms and the ventral and lateral sides of the fingers, with erythematous changes on the dorsal aspects
- light hypersensitivity
- lipoatrophy (in chronic cases).

Very rare is panniculitis over involved proximal muscles.

The most severe skin changes—necrotic ulcerations, mostly over the elbows, knees and malleoli, and vesiculobullous eruptions—may precede visceral malignancy (paraneoplastic sign). Malignancy can be detected before, simultaneously or within 2 years after the onset of DM.

Muscle disease

Characteristic of the disease is involvement of proximal muscles, with weakness and possible tenderness, leading in chronic disease to muscle wasting.

JDM

JDM is characterized by more severe vascular changes and inflammatory responses, as well as by more pronounced photosensitivity. Calcinosis and visceral involvement are more frequent than in adults. Otherwise the clinical and muscle changes are identical as in adults, and in some cases skin lesions either precede or are not associated with myositis (amyopathic DM). However the course of the disease is often more severe in children.

Amyopathic DM (DM without myositis)

Muscle involvement is not detected in about 10% of patients. The cutaneous changes are similar to those in typical DM but are not associated with muscle weakness and laboratory signs of myositis. Muscle disease may develop within months or years, but there are cases followed up for many years in which cutaneous changes are stable, with no myositis.

The course of DM

The course shows considerable variations. In cases associated with Mi2 antibody it is usually more chronic with milder skin and muscle disease. In rare cases associated with anti-tRNA synthetase antibodies, it is in general more severe, with fever and frequent pulmonary changes (interstitial lung disease—ILD). Thus association with specific antibodies has important therapeutic implications.

In chronic cases, subcutaneous lipoatrophy, atrophy of muscles and calcinosis are not infrequent findings after the regression of cutaneous and inflammatory muscle changes.

Diagnosis

Diagnosis is based on clinical characteristics and should be confirmed by histopathology of the muscle. The cutaneous lesions have no characteristic pattern, and the skin biopsy is usually not contributory. However muscle biopsy is of diagnostic significance. Characteristic of DM are: muscle fibre necrosis and regeneration, microinfarcts, perifascicular atrophy, inflammatory infiltrates of T cells, predominantly of CD4 type, and inflammatory vascular changes or capillary depletion.

Muscles are assessed by manual testing, functional performance, electromyography (preferably quantitative EMG) and muscle enzyme levels (creatine phosphokinase, aldolase). Respiratory function tests should be performed in more severe cases, especially those associated with Jo1 antibody characterized by pulmonary fibrosis (ILD), pronounced Raynaud's phenomenon, arthralgia, not infrequently scleroderma-like cutaneous changes.

In all cases is indicated nail-fold capillaroscopy (which shows characteristic 'bushy', highly enlarged capillaries of the subpapillary flexus and extravasations) and oesophageal radiography or scintigraphy. In adults over 40–50 years of age evaluation of internal malignancy is indicated (in females mammography and pelvic ultrasonography, and serological examination for the ovarian tumour with marker CA-125), and in all patients lung and digestive tract studies. Non-invasive new methods for assessment of muscle in DM: magnetic resonance imaging (MRI) and P-31 magnetic resonance spectroscopy, providing quantitative data, are of special importance for follow-up of treated patients since they are more sensitive than histological evaluation and muscle enzyme levels.

Biological markers of disease activity are serum levels of IL-1ra (IL-1 receptor antagonist), sTNFαr (soluble tumour necrosis α receptor) and—as in all inflammatory CTD—sIL-2r (soluble IL-2 receptor).

Differential diagnosis

The clinical features of DM are in most cases so typical that the diagnosis does not pose any problems.

Cases with very pronounced photosensitivity should be differentiated from systemic lupus erythematosus (SLE) associated with myositis (differs by visceral and cutaneous involvement and by serological markers). JDM cases, displaying pronounced vasculitis and photosensitivity may have somewhat similar cutaneous involvement but serological markers of SLE have diagnostic significance. Scleromyositis (scleroderma/DM overlap syndrome) differs by scleroderma-like cutaneous changes and characteristic immunological marker PM-Scl antibody. The differentiation is of practical importance since patients with scleromyositis do not need such an aggressive therapy as for DM.

Cases of amyopathic DM should be differentiated, besides systemic lupus erythematosus (SLE) and discoid lupus erythematosus (DLE), from polymorphous light eruption, lichen planus, seborrhoeic dermatitis (not infrequent scaling scalp lesions in DM), erythema elevatum and diutinum.

Treatment

General therapeutic outline

Due to the variable course and significant prognostic differences, the therapy must be adjusted to the clinical variety and course of the disease. In DM associated with Mi2 antibody corticosteroids are in general sufficient to control the symptoms (first-line therapy), in cases associated with anti-tRNA synthetase antibodies this therapy must be combined with immunosuppression (second-line therapy). For most severe and treatment-resistant cases the alternative therapy is ciclosporin and intravenous immunoglobulin G (IVIG). In general the better outcome depends on early (not more than 1 year after the onset) start and more aggressive therapy.

Recommended therapies

Corticosteroids

Corticosteroids in a dose of 1 mg/kg body weight produce clinical improvement within 1–6 weeks. After that, the drug is progressively tapered to minimal maintenance dosages which should be applied within at least 1 year to prevent relapses. Such therapy might be sufficient in mild cases, e.g. associated with Mi2, however in our experience only in about 25% of cases could complete control be achieved with corticosteroids alone.

To avoid steroidal side-effects and to improve the response, especially in severe cases, intravenous pulses with methylprednisolone 500–1000 mg/day are indicated on 3 consecutive days, or once every 2 weeks, or once monthly. This therapy proved to be very effective also in JDM with the use of high doses (10–30 mg/kg body weight), 3 pulses monthly. It is not clear whether this regimen could prevent calcinosis, as believed previously. It should be stressed that this therapy must be applied concurrently and followed by oral application of corticosteroids in small doses. However, not all patients respond to pulse therapy, and this indicates the need for combined therapy with immunosuppressive drugs and oral prednisone.

Immunosuppressive agents

The choice of second-line agent is mostly empirical since there are few comparative data and controlled clinical trials, and no reliable predictors of response to particular drug.

- Methotrexate is presently the preferred immunosuppressive agent for DM. It is given in a single weekly oral dose of 7.5–15 mg (max. 25 mg/week). Higher doses (25 mg) are administered weekly by the intramuscular route. Side-effects are stomatitis, mouth ulcers, hepatotoxicity and gastrointestinal symptoms.
- Azathioprine 2–3 mg/kg per day was used most widely, although in controlled clinical trials there was no more benefit when prednisone was used with azathioprine or alone.
- Cyclophosphamide. Oral doses 2.0–2.5 mg/kg per day, or intravenous pulses 500–1000 mg every 1–4 weeks. Side-effects include thrombocytopenia, anaemia, alopecia and gastrointestinal symptoms. Long-lasting application gives an increased risk of malignancy. Cyclophosphamide is more effective in cases associated with vasculitis, mainly in JDM.
- Chlorambucil. This alkylating agent is not widely used in DM, however beneficial effects were reported in some recalcitrant cases. Daily dose 4 mg/day, duration of the therapy 1–2 years. Blood morphology should be monitored during treatment (leukaemia is a possible side-effect).
- Ciclosporin A. This strong immunosuppressive agent should be tried only in patients who are not controlled with corticosteroids. The daily dose is 3 mg/kg per day, adjusted according to the clinical response. Side-effects include nephrotoxicity, rise in blood pressure, headache, hirsutism and thrombocytopenia.

Intravenous immunoglobulins (IVIG)

This therapy was found to have quite excellent effects in patients with drug-resistant DM. The dose of 0.3–0.4 g/kg per day is given over a 5-day period (total 2.0 g/kg), after which 3-day courses are repeated monthly for 3–6 months. An alternative programme is 1 g/kg body weight on two consecutive days every 4 weeks for 10–12 courses. Usually the previous therapy with prednisone or methotrexate is continued.

This treatment is safe (possible headache, fever, itching, exceptionally renal failure) and successful, but expensive. The presumed mode of action is prevention of immune-mediated deposition of activated complement components or binding of anti-idiotypic antibodies produced against circulating autoantibodies.

Plasmapheresis

In our and others experience this is ineffective, and is presently replaced by intravenous immunoglobulin.

Recommended therapy for amyopathic DM

- Hydroxychloroquine is a first-line drug. Daily dose 2–5 mg/kg, preferably with small doses of corticosteroids.
- Use of sunscreens.
- There is no consensus whether corticosteroids should be applied in cases with no frank muscle weakness. However some studies showed that corticosteroids alone or jointly with chloroquine can prevent or delay muscle disease and development of calcinosis.
- For prevention of calcinosis—diphosphonate and colchicin (both are not very effective).

- Recommended therapy for DM associated with malignancy.

After surgery, the same therapy as in other forms. Especially favourable effects have been reported with the use of intravenous immunoglobulin infusions.

Conclusion

New diagnostic procedures, especially highly specific Mi2 antibodies (although present only in about 20% of patients), antisynthetase antibodies and other myositis-specific antibodies allow for early diagnosis and may be useful for the choice of therapeutic regimen. Generally the outcome is excellent if more aggressive therapy is introduced at early stages of illness. However, in our experience, one-third of patients must continue corticosteroids and/or immunosuppressive drugs for several years, both in small doses.

Further reading

Blockmans D, Beyens G, Verhaeghe R. Predictive value of nailfold capillary studies in the diagnosis of connective tissue diseases. *Clin Rheumatol* 1996; 15: 148–53.

Dalakas MC *et al.* A controlled trial of high-dose intravenous immune globulin influsions as treatment for dermatomyositis. *N Engl J Med* 1993; 329: 1993–2000.

Ghate J, Katsambas A, Augerinou G, Jorizzo JL. A therapeutic update on dermatomyositis/polymyositis. *Int J Dermatol* 2000; 39: 81–7.

Huber AM, Lag B, Le Blanc CMA *et al.* Medium- and long-term functional outcomes in a multicenter cohort of children with juvenile dermatomyositis. *Arthritis Rheum* 2000; 43: 541–9.

Jablonska S, Chorzelski TP, Blaszczyk M, Jarzabek-Chorzelska M, Kumar V, Beutner EH. Scleroderma/polymyositis overlap syndromes and their immunologic markers. *Clin Dermatol* 1993; 10: 457–72.

Joffe MM, Love LA, Leff RI *et al.* Drug therapy of the idiopathic inflammatory myopathies: predictors of response to prednisolane, azathioprine and methotrexate and a comparison of their efficacy. *Am J Med* 1993; 94: 379–87.

Kastler JS, Callen JP. Low-dose methotrexate administered weekly is an effective corticosteroid-sparing agent for the treatment of the cutaneous manifestations of dermatomyositis. *J Am Acad Dermatol* 1997; 36: 67–71.

Mattheou-Vakeli G, Ioannides D, Lazaridou E, Kalabalikis D, Batsios P, Minas A. Dermatomyositis sine myositis in five cases. *J Eur Acad Dermatol Venereol* 1997; 8: 208–11.

Pachman LM. Polymyositis and dermatomyositis in children. In: Maddison PJ, Isenberg D, Woo P, Glass DN, eds. *Oxford Textbook of Rheumatology*, 2nd edn. Oxford: Oxford University Press, 1998: 1287–300.

Park JH *et al.* Muscle abnormalities in juvenile dermatomyositis patients. *Arthritis Rheum* 2000; 43: 2359–67.

Sinoway PA, Callen JP. Chlorambucil: an effective corticosteroid sparing agent for patients with recalcitrant dermatomyositis. *Arthritis Rheum* 1993; 36: 319–24.

Zeller V, Cohen P, Prieur AM, Guillevin L. Cyclosporine therapy in refractory juvenile dermatomyositis. Experience and long term follow-up of 6 cases. *J Rheumatol* 1996; 23: 1424–7.

Dermatophyte infections

A. Tosti and B.M. Piraccini

Tinea corporis

Definition and aetiology

Tinea corporis is an infective skin disease resulting from invasion and proliferation by the causal fungi in the stratum corneum. The fungi most commonly involved are *Microsporum canis, Tricophyton rubrum* and *Tricophyton mentagrophytes*. It most commonly involves exposed parts of the body, but can affect any site. Typical lesions are annular in shape, with a raised scaling erythematous edge. The presence of perifollicular granulomatous papules (Majocchi's granuloma) is a definite indication for systemic treatment.

Treatment

Topical treatment

In localized lesions of tinea corporis topical treatment with imidazole derivatives, allylamines, tolnaftate or cyclopiroxolamine is adequate. Treatment period varies between 2 and 4 weeks, except for terbinafine and naftifine that are effective after 1–2 weeks of therapy.

Systemic treatment

Systemic treatment is required in widespread tinea corporis or when follicular lesions (Majocchi's granuloma) are present. Itraconazole (200 mg daily for 1 week) or terbinafine (250 mg daily for 2 weeks), are currently preferred because time of treatment is shorter and they are better tolerated than griseofulvin.

Tinea cruris

Definition and aetiology

This infection mainly occurs in adult men and is usually caused by *Trichophyton rubrum* and *Epidermophyton floccosum*. Tinea cruris presents with an itchy scaling of the groins and inside of the thighs. The margin of the affected area typically presents a raised erythematous border.

Treatment

Topical treatment

In localized lesions topical treatment, as for tinea corporis, may be sufficient.

Systemic treatment

This is mandatory in longstanding lesions or when follicular granulomas are present. Itraconazole (200 mg daily for 1 week), or terbinafine (250 mg daily for 2 weeks) are very effective.

Tinea pedis

Definition and aetiology

Tinea pedis is the most common dermatophyte infection, and is caused in most cases by *Trichophyton rubrum* and *Trichophyton interdigitale*. *Trichophyton rubrum* usually produces non-inflammatory lesions with different degrees of severity ranging from mild scaling to diffuse 'mocassin type' scaly rash. *Trichophyton interdigitale* usually causes interdigital or plantar inflammatory lesions that are often vesicular and pruritic.

Treatment

Topical treatment

Topical antifungals are usually prescribed in association with systemic treatment. They are also commonly utilized to prevent reinfections.

Systemic treatment

Both itraconazole and terbinafine are effective in the treatment of tinea pedis. Terbinafine is administered at a dose of 250 mg/day for 2 weeks and itraconazole at 400 mg/day for 1 week.

Prevention of recurrences

1 Reduction of maceration and humidity can be obtained by regular use of talcum powders.
2 The demonstration that dermatophytes occur in shoes (up to 17% in one study), flooring, carpets (Muslim community) indicates that any treatment directed solely at the feet is inadequate to control the disease. Effective control measures must also include simultaneous eradication of the organisms (such as disinfection of shoes with 1% 8-hydroxycholine sulphate, formaldehyde) and/or the environment to prevent reinfection. However, there is limited data which shows a correlation of such measures and the prevention of athletes' foot. In such circumstances, evaluating the preventing efficacy of these measures against athletes' foot remains guesswork.

Tinea capitis

Definition and aetiology

In Europe tinea capitis is predominantly caused by *Microsporum canis* and *Trichophyton tonsurans*, with *Microsporum canis* being the most common agent of tinea capitis in Italy. Other dermatophytes responsible for tinea capitis include *T. soudanense*, *T. violaceum*, *M. gypseum*, *T. mentagrophytes* and *T. shoenleinii*. The clinical manifestations of tinea capitis range from mild scalp scaling to severe inflammatory reactions. Cervical lymph nodes are often enlarged.

Treatment

Although tinea capitis always requires a systemic treatment, the use of adjunctive topical therapy is important. Periodic hair shaving prevents diffusion of the infection. An antifungal shampoo (ketoconazole 2% shampoo) should be given to the patient and family members in order to reduce transmission of infection. Family members and primary contacts should be screened for asymptomatic disease. Family pets of patients with *Microsporum canis* infection should be treated. Fomites, including toys, phones, clothing, furniture and hair care items, may contribute to spread of the infection and can be sterilized using high temperature or microwaves.

Systemic treatment

In tinea capitis due to *Microsporum canis* griseofulvin remains the treatment of choice. The drug should be administered at 20–30 mg/kg per day for 3–4 months. The azole antifungals itraconazole and fluconazole are effective in the treatment of *Microsporum canis* infection of the hair, with fluconazole being the only one approved in children and available in a pleasant tasting liquid formulation (10–40 mg/mL). Terbinafine is scarcely effective in tinea capitis due to *M. canis*. Suggested regimens are itraconazole 5–10 mg/kg per day, fluconazole 6–8 mg/kg once a week for 8 weeks. In tinea capitis due to *Trichophyton tonsurans* or *T. violaceum* terbinafine can also be utilized. Dosages are 3–5 mg/kg per day for itraconazole, 3–6 mg/kg once a week for fluconazole, 3–6 mg/kg per day for terbinafine. Duration of treatment ranges from 4 to 8 weeks. Pulse therapy with itraconazole is promising, but still under investigation. Oral or topical steroids can be given in association with systemic antifungals to reduce pain, swelling and inflammation.

Onychomycosis

Dermatophytes account for more than 90% of onychomycosis, with *T. rubrum* being the most common pathogen. They may produce four different clinical types of onychomycosis, depending on the modality of nail invasion by the fungus.

Distal subungual onychomycosis

In distal subungual onychomycosis, dermatophytes reach the nail bed horny layer through the hyponychium. The affected nails show subungual hyperkeratosis, onycholysis and yellow discoloration. Distal subungual onychomycosis affects toenails more frequently than fingernails. Since the skin of the palms and soles is the primary site of infection, distal subungual onychomycosis is usually associated with tinea manum or tinea pedis.

Proximal subungual onychomycosis

Proximal subungual onychomycosis is characterized by a primitive invasion of the nail matrix keratogenous zone through the proximal nail fold horny layer. Fungal elements are typically located in the ventral nail plate with minimal inflammatory reaction. The affected nail shows proximal leukonychia that progresses distally with nail growth.

White superficial onychomycosis

In white superficial onychomycosis dermatophytes colonize the most superficial layers of the nail plate without penetrating it. The affected nail presents multiple friable white opaque spots that can be easily scraped away.

Endonyx onychomycosis

Endonyx onychomycosis is characterized by massive nail plate parasitation in the absence of nail bed inflammatory changes. The affected nail is milky-white in colour. The nail plate is firmly attached to the nail bed and there is no nail bed hyperkeratosis or onycholysis.

Treatment

The treatment choice depends on the clinical type of the onychomycosis, the number of affected nails and the severity of nail involvement.

Topical treatment

Penetration of a topical antifungal through the nail plate requires a vehicle that is specifically formulated for transungual delivery. Two transungual delivery systems are currently available in most European countries: amorolfine 5% nail lacquer and cyclopirox 8% nail lacquer. Amorolfine nail lacquer is applied once a week, whereas cyclopirox nail lacquer is applied daily.

Nail lacquers are effective as monotherapy in the treatment of white superficial onychomycosis and of distal subungual onychomycosis limited to the distal nail of a few digits. Treatment should be prolonged for 6–12 months. Nail lacquers are also utilized in severe onychomycosis in combination with systemic antifungals to reduce duration of treatment and increase cure rate.

Weekly application of a nail lacquer may also prevent relapses of onychomycosis after successful treatment.

Systemic treatment

Distal subungual onychomycosis extending to the proximal nail, endonyx onychomycosis and proximal subungual onychomycosis always require a systemic treatment. Systemic treatment with terbinafine or itraconazole produces mycological cure in more than 90% of fingernail infections and in about 80% of toenail infections. These success rates can be increased by associating a topical treatment with a nail lacquer to the systemic treatment. Terbinafine is administered at the dosage of 250 mg daily or as 'pulse therapy' at the dosage of 500 mg daily for 1 week a month. Itraconazole is administered as pulse therapy at the dosage of 400 mg daily for 1 week a month. Treatment duration is 2 months for fingernails and 3–4 months for toenails.

Data about efficacy of fluconazole in the treatment of onychomycosis are recent and require additional studies to establish optimal dosages and treatment duration definitely. The approved dosage of fluconazole is 150 mg once a week, but higher dosages (300 mg once a week) are probably more effective. Treatment should be prolonged for at least 6 months.

Chemical or surgical nail avulsion can be used in association with oral antifungals in order to remove localized fungal masses in total onychomycosis and dermatophytoma. Sequential treatment with itraconazole and terbinafine has been utilized to increase cure rates: the suggested regimen is 2 pulses of itraconazole 400 mg/day for 1 week a month followed by 1 or 2 pulses of terbinafine 500 mg/day for 1 week a month. Mycological cure can be evaluated at the end of treatment. Evaluation of clinical response, on the other hand, requires several months due to the slow growth rate of the nail. Recurrences and reinfection are not uncommon (up to 20% of cured patients). They may be prevented by the regular application of nail lacquers on the previously affected nails and topical antifungals on soles and toe webs.

Further reading

Baran R, Feuilhade M, Datry A *et al.* A randomized trial of amorolfine 5% solution nail lacquer combined with oral terbinafine compared with terbinafine alone in the treatment of dermatophyte toenail onychomycosis affecting the matrix region. *Br J Dermatol* 2001; 142: 1177–83.

Bennet ML, Fleischer AB, Loveless JW *et al.* Oral griseofulvin remains the treatment of choice for tinea capitis in children. *Pediatric Dermatol* 2000; 17: 304–9.

Bräutigam M, Nolting S, Schpf RE *et al.* Randomized double blind comparison terbinafine itraconazole for treatment of toenail tinea infection. *Br Med J* 1995; 311: 919–22.

Ceschin-Roques CG, Hänel H, Pruja-Bougaret SM *et al.* Ciclopirox nail lacquer 8%: in vivo penetration into and through nails and in vitro effect on pig skin. *Skin Pharmacol* 1991; 4: 89–94.

De Doncker P, Decroix J, Piérard GE *et al.* Antifungals pulse therapy for onychomycosis. *Arch Dermatol* 1996; 132: 34–41.

Elewski BE. Tina capitis: a current perspective. *J Am Acad Dermatol* 2000; 42: 1–20.

Gupta AK, Lynde CW, Konnikow N. Single-blind, randomized, prospective study of sequential itraconazole and terbinafine pulse compared with terbinafine pulse for the treatment of toenail onychomycosis. *J Am Acad Dermatol* 2001; 44: 485–891.

Gupta AK, Shear NH. A risk-benefit assessment of the newer oral antifungal agents used to treat onychomycosis. *Drug Safety* 2000; 22: 33–52.

Katsambas A, Antoniou C, Frangouli E *et al.* Itraconazole in the treatment of tinea corporis and tinea curtis. *Clin Exp Dermatol* 1993; 18: 322–5.

Montero JF. Fuconazole in the treatment of tinea capitis. *Int J Dermatol* 1998; 37: 870–3.

Savin RS. Treatment of chronic tinea pedis (athlete's foot type) with topical terbinafine. *J Am Acad Dermatol* 1990; 23: 786–9.

Svejgaard EL. Recalcitrant dermatophyte infection. *Dermatol Ther* 1997; 3: 79–83.

Tosti A, Piraccini BM. Treatment of onychomycosis: a European Experience. *Dermatol Ther* 1997; 3: 79–83.

Tosti A, Piraccini BM, Stinchi C *et al.* Relapses of onychomycosis after successful treatment with systemic antifungals: a three year follow-up. *Dermatology* 1998; 197: 162–6.

Tosti A, Piraccini BM, Stinchi C *et al.* Treatment of dermatophyte nail infections: an open randomized study comparing intermittent terbinafine therapy with continuous terbinafine treatment and intermittent itraconazole therapy. *J Am Acad Dermatol* 1996; 34: 595–600.

Zaias N. Onychomycosis. *Arch Dermatol* 1972; 105: 263–74.

Drug eruption

J. Revuz

The spectrum of adverse cutaneous drug reaction (ACDR) to systemically administered drugs is very large, including benign and severe, life-threatening reactions. An important concern in the patient with common ACDR is to know if the actual eruption may evolve into a more severe, potentially lethal form.

Epidemiology and pathophysiology

There is no comprehensive data on the incidence of ACDR in the general population. In hospital patients one study recorded a 2.2% incidence. Data are lacking about the exact rate for most types of cutaneous reactions. The incidence of toxic epidermal necrolysis (TEN) in European countries is 1.5 per million per year in the general population.

Antibiotics are responsible for more than 70% of ACDR, especially penicillin and, above all, type A penicillins, i.e. amoxicillin and ampicillin; non-steroidal anti-inflammatory drugs, anticonvulsants and sulphonamides are frequently implicated in common and severe ACDR. The observed frequency is the result of the number of prescriptions and of the rate of adverse reactions for a particular drug. The most frequently encountered reactions are: exanthema (maculopapular rash), urticaria and angioedema, fixed eruption, blistering diseases and pustular eruption. The most severe reactions are: the 'drug hypersensitivity syndrome' (preferentially called 'drug rash with eosinophilia and systemic symptoms' or DRESS); Stevens–Johnson syndrome (SJS) and TEN; angioedema, serum sickness and anaphylactic shock; and to a lesser degree acute exanthematic pustulosis and exfoliative dermatitis.

Women, elderly patients and slow acetylators are more prone to develop ACDR. Viral diseases are also precipitating factors: Epstein–Barr virus infection and amoxicillin rash is a well-known association; the risk of developing exanthematous reaction and TEN is approximately 1000 times higher in patients with human immunodeficiency virus (HIV) than in the general population.

The main mechanisms of ACDR are metabolic and immunological. Metabolic susceptibility has been recorded in patients recovering from TEN and from DRESS. The immune mechanism—responsible for most acute ACDR—is exemplified by the chronology of the eruption, occurring 7–21 days after the onset during the first administration of a drug and in less than 48 h in the case of accidental reintroduction after a first ACDR. Cell-mediated immunity and cytokines, especially tumour necrosis factor-α (TNF-α), are involved in exanthematous reactions and TEN. A specific immune mechanism or specific cytokine profile has still to be described for each individual type of drug reaction.

Diagnosis and differential diagnosis

Most drug eruptions, especially exanthematous rashes, have to be differentiated from common viral eruption. Some ACDR have a specific clinical picture, e.g. fixed eruption, TEN that are drug-induced diseases. On the contrary for most drug eruptions, every cutaneous sign, every apparently well-known disease, may be mimicked or be aggravated by drugs (acne, psoriasis, bullous diseases). Specific and/or sensitive biological tests are not yet available. A biopsy should be taken in every case of severe reaction for medico-legal purpose and to strengthen the diagnostic profile. The identification of the responsible drug is mainly based on clinical feature and case history: the time relationship of drug administration and drug reaction on one hand, and the literature search on the other hand, are the two main elements. Dechallenge usually brings little if any information; rechallenge, although not invariably positive with the offending drug, would in most cases give a definite proof, but the risks limit its use to the benign reactions but even in this case the possibility exists of a switch to a more severe reaction.

Treatment—general principles

Drug eruptions are self-limited diseases once the offending drug is stopped. The therapeutic strategy rests on two main principles. Firstly, stop the drug, when it is possible (almost always). Secondly, keep the patient alive and wait for spontaneous healing. Some severe reactions, however, require emergency treatment.

Stopping the offending drug is urgently needed as it has been demonstrated that the earlier its discontinuation, the better the prognosis. It is an easy decision except in two circumstances

1. When the drug is life saving, e.g. sulphonamides in opportunistic infections of the acquired immune deficiency syndrome (AIDS)—the balance of risks and benefits of either case can be difficult to weigh. The prevailing attitude is to stop the drug is if it is a potentially lethal reaction, i.e. TEN or SJS, or if there are severity markers like mucous membrane erosions, high fever, lymphadenopathy or signs of visceral involvement which may announce a severe reaction; conversely, in the case of an exanthematous eruption without any such sign, 'treating through' is the most frequent attitude. It may result in a transient aggravation, but usually the rash vanishes in spite of the continuation of the drug. These results shed a new light on the so-called desensitization procedures which have been claimed to be successful on an uncontrolled basis and do not give better results than 'treating through'.
2. When the patient is receiving several drugs at the same time; in this case, the identification of the responsible drug may be very difficult. Recently introduced drugs (7–30 days) and drugs known to have a high rate of ACDR are considered as the initial suspects.

As patients who have already experienced a drug reaction are more prone to suffer from another, using drugs sparingly in the future is wise.

Severe bullous reactions: SJS and TEN

Management of patients with toxic epidermal necrolysis must be undertaken as soon as possible in an intensive care unit (ICU) or in a burns unit. Medical transport requires soft handling of the patient. Fluid replacement must be started immediately.

The main principles of symptomatic therapy are the same as for major burns: during the first few days, fluids must be replaced intravenously. When possible, it is preferable to use peripheral veins at a distance from affected areas rather than central lines because central lines carry a very high risk of systemic infection by the germs present on the skin. The predicted volume of replacement is proportional to the area of skin lesions, but fluid requirements are only between two-thirds and three-quarters of the amount required for burns patients.

Nutritional support is begun as soon as possible by nasogastric route with a silicone tube to minimize the protein losses and to promote the healing of cutaneous lesions. Because of impaired glycoregulation, intravenous insulin is frequently required.

Infection can arise at any time during the course of TEN. Sterile handling of patients is recommended to decrease the risk of nosocomial infection, and several authors have advocated reverse-isolation nursing techniques. Painting and bathing with topical liquid antiseptics such as 0.5% silver nitrate and 0.05% chlorhexidine is routinely performed. Silver sulfadiazine, very popular in burns units, is avoided, as sulphonamides are frequently implicated in the aetiology. Large operative debridement of non-viable epidermis followed by immediate wound cover with biological dressings has been used in burns units but a more conservative approach, leaving in place the epidermis which has not yet peeled off and using biological dressings on the naked dermis, seems reasonable. Prophylactic antibiotics are not recommended as they carry the risk of secondary sepsis with highly resistant bacteria. The diagnosis of sepsis is difficult and the decision to administer systemic antibiotics must be carefully deliberated. Some indications for antibiotic treatment include: increase in the number of bacteria cultured from the skin with selection of a single strain, sudden drop of fever, drop in diuresis, increase in gastric residue and deterioration in the patient's overall condition. There is no ideal antibiotic and the choice will be directed against the predominant bacterial strains on the skin, i.e. *Staphylococcus aureus* during the first few days and Gram-negative rods later. The administration of unusually high doses of antibiotics may be required to obtain serum levels within the therapeutic range. Frequent determination of serum levels may be useful. Environmental temperature should be raised to 30–32°C. Heat loss can also be limited by raising the temperature of antiseptic baths (to 35–38°C), and using heat shields, infrared lamps and an air-fluidized bed. Thrombosis and pulmonary embolism are causes of morbidity and death and should be prevented by heparin. Antacids reduce the incidence of gastric bleeding. Ocular lesions require daily examination, antiseptic and/or antibiotic eye drops instilled every hour. Developing synechiae are disrupted by a blunt instrument. Oral and nasal debris is to be removed. Pulmonary care includes aerosols and bronchial aspiration; in case of necrolysis of the bronchial epithelium the patient has to be treated in a lung ICU; prognosis is then very poor. Pain, often distressful, must be controlled; emotional and psychiatric support, and tranquillizers are helpful.

Experimental treatments

To date there is no specific treatment. Some authors believe that systemic steroids are helpful if given early, shortly and in high dosage. In fact many cases have occurred during treatment with high doses of corticosteroids; furthermore, systemic corticosteroids have been identified as TEN inducers in an epidemiological study. Three studies found that TEN patients treated with corticosteroids had a worse prognosis with more frequent infections. Beneficial effects of plasmapheresis, ciclosporin and cyclophosphamide have been claimed without consistent evidence. Intravenous immunoglobulins directed against the Fas–Fas ligand conflict, responsible, at least partly, for the necrolysis, have been claimed to be effective but conflicting results have been reported and a definite treatment of TEN is still lacking.

DRESS (drug hypersensitivity syndrome)

The severity is linked to visceral involvement: hepatic and/or renal failure—sometimes lethal—is not improved by any treatment. When eosinophilic infiltration of lung or heart is severe, high doses of systemic steroids given in emergency is life saving. Tapering may be difficult with relapses occurring over several months. Systemic steroids rapidly relieve skin signs, lymph node enlargement and constitutional symptoms, but long-term usefulness may be hampered by relapses on tapering. Systemic steroids are still experimental in DRESS. Topical steroids are useful for the cutaneous manifestations.

Anaphylactic and anaphylactoid reactions

Anaphylactic reactions are observed within the minutes following drug absorption, frequently after a penicillin injection. Early reactions are the most severe and lethal evolutions take place within 1 h. The necessary drugs—mainly epinephrine (adrenaline)—and resuscitation equipment must be present in every place where injections are performed and the risk of anaphylactic shock exists. Anaphylactoid reactions—non-immunologically mediated but mimicking anaphylaxis—are treated in the same way. They are mainly observed with radiocontrast products. This kind of reaction may be at least partially be prevented by prior administration of steroids and antihistamines. The emergency treatment of these reactions includes:

- a tourniquet to stop the diffusion of the drug
- epinephrine 0.2–1 mL of 1/1000 solution subcutaneously; to be repeated every 20 min or given intravenously if blood pressure makes it necessary. Anaphylaxis is particularly dangerous in patients receiving β-blockers as epinephrine may be ineffective
- aerosolized epinephrine in case of laryngeal oedema; mechanical maintenance of airway permeability
- venous access: steroids, fluid and macromolecules, antihistamines
- emergency specialized transport to an ICU.

Further reading

Bocquet H, Bagot M, Roujeau J-C. Drug-induced pseudolymphoma and drug hypersensitivity syndrome (drug rash with eosinophilia and systemic symptoms: DRESS). *Sem Cutan Med Surg* 1996; 15: 250–7.

Breathnach SM, Hinter H. *Adverse drug reactions and the skin*. Oxford: Blackwell Scientific, 1992.

Revuz J, Roujeau J-C. Advances in toxic epidermal necrolysis. *Sem Cutan Med Surg* 1996; 15: 258–66.

Drug-induced pemphigus

S. Albert and M.M. Black

Definition and epidemiology

Drug-induced pemphigus (DIP) is a rare but well-established variety of pemphigus. Several cases have been described worldwide since it was first reported in 1951 in Italy. Two patterns of association have been observed in DIP. In the first group the drug acts as the major aetiological factor, resulting in pemphigus which is usually mild and responds favourably on stopping the drug. In the other group, the drug only acts as a triggering factor in an immunologically and genetically predisposed individual, leading to the development of idiopathic pemphigus, the course of the disease not being influenced thereafter by the removal of the drug.

Aetiology and pathophysiology

The commonest cause of DIP are the thiol compounds, drugs having a sulph-hydryl (–SH) group in their molecule, penicillamine (dimethylcysteine) being the prototype. Others include captopril, bucillamine, thiopronine, piroxicam, pyritinol and gold sodium thiomalate. About 7% of patients who have been on penicillamine for at least 6 months will develop pemphigus. Thiols can cause acantholysis *in vitro* in the absence of antibodies, possibly by influencing plasminogen levels or by competitively incorporating into the keratin molecule because of its chemical similarity to cysteine, but often a combination of biochemical and immunological mechanisms are involved in DIP. Penicillin, ampicillin, amoxicillin (amoxycillin), cephalosporins, rifampicin, phenylbutazone, dipyrone, enalapril and phenobarbital are some of the non-thiol drugs reported to cause DIP. The mechanism is postulated to be either though an active amide group, or by metabolizing sulphur in the molecule to a thiol group, hence termed 'masked' thiols. Antibodies directed against desmoglein 1 and desmoglein 3 antigens of the intercellular substance of the epidermis, similar to idiopathic pemphigus, have been demonstrated.

Clinical characteristics and course

DIP can present as pemphigus foliaceous, pemphigus erythematosus or as pemphigus vulgaris. Patients may develop a non-specific erythematous or papulovesicular eruption before the onset of overt blistering. When fully evolved, clinical features do not differ significantly from that of idiopathic disease. 65–70% of –SH-induced cases develop pemphigus foliaceus with moist erythematous crusted scaling plaques and superficial friable blisters over the seborrhoeic areas of the body. The latent period between drug intake and onset of DIP is longer with –SH drugs. Thiol-induced pemphigus has a high remission rate and excellent prognosis if the drug is stopped. The non-thiol drugs usually precipitate pemphigus vulgaris, with generalized blistering and oral involvement. The course and prognosis is similar to that for idiopathic disease.

Diagnosis

Meticulous history taking is important for eliciting a possible drug aetiology. A skin biopsy may show features of either pemphigus foliaceous, with an acantholytic split in the subcorneal or granular layer of the upper epidermis or that of pemphigus vulgaris, with suprabasal clefting. Other findings such as epidermal spongiosis with eosinophils, keratinocyte necrosis and focal acantholysis resulting in multiple levels of splitting have been reported as characteristic. A recent study did not find any of these histological features to be specific in DIP when compared to spontaneous pemphigus. Direct immunofluorescence (IF) detects intercellular immunoglobulin G (IgG) and C3 deposits in the skin in about 90% while indirect IF demonstrates these antibodies in serum in about 70% of patients. IF tests may be negative in a small group of patients, especially when thiol-induced. Enzyme-linked immunosorbent assay (ELISA) tests to detect antidesmoglein 1 and 3 antibodies are extremely sensitive in detecting low titres of antibodies and useful when routine IF studies are negative. Patch testing and *in vitro* tests like macrophage migration inhibition factor (MIF) and mast cell degranulation (MCD) tests can be useful in providing evidence of drug hypersensitivity.

Differential diagnosis

- Seborrhoeic dermatitis: negative direct and indirect IF studies.
- Steven–Johnson syndrome: history, histology, IF studies.
- Lupus erythematosus: histology, ARA criteria, lupus band on direct IF.

Treatment

In thiol-associated DIP, spontaneous recovery was reported in over 50% of patients while in the non-thiol group this was seen in only 15% of the patients. Hence stopping the offending or suspected drug is important as this may help in reducing disease severity if not a quick remission. Management guidelines are similar to those for pemphigus foliaceous or pemphigus vulgaris. Systemic steroids 40–60 mg/day or 1 mg/kg form the first line of therapy, immunosuppressants such as azathioprine (1.5–2.5 mg/kg) or cyclophosphamide (1–3 mg/kg) are added as steroid-sparing agents with the view to tapering off the steroids. A recent report found low-dose intravenous immunoglobulin, 40 mg/kg per day for 5 days administered at weekly intervals, to be useful in a recalcitrant case of penicillamine-induced pemphigus.

Further reading

Brenner S, Bialy-Golan A, Anhalt GJ. Recognition of pemphigus antigens in drug-induced pemphigus vulgaris and pemphigus foliaceus. *J Am Acad Dermatol* 1997; 36: 919–23.

Brenner S, Bialy-Golan A, Ruocco V. Drug-induced pemphigus. *Clin Dermatol* 1998; 16 (3): 393–7.

Landau M, Brenner S. Histopathologic findings in drug-induced pemphigus. *Am J Dermatopathol* 1997; 19 (4): 411–14.

Mutasim DF, Pelc NJ, Anhalt GJ. Drug-induced pemphigus. *Dermatol Clin* 1993; 11 (3): 463–71.

Ogata K, Nakajima H, Ikeda M *et al.* Drug-induced pemphigus foliaceus with features of pemphigus vulgaris. *Br J Dermatol* 2001; 144 (2): 421–2.

Ruocco V, De Angelis E, Lombardi ML. Drug-induced pemphigus. II. Pathomechanisms and experimental investigations. *Clin Dermatol* 1993; 11 (4): 507–13.

Toth GG, Jonkman MF. Successful treatment of recalcitrant penicillamine-induced pemphigus foliaceus by low-dose intravenous immunoglobulins. *Br J Dermatol* 1999; 141 (3): 583–5.

Drug photosensitivity

P. Santoianni and E.M. Procaccini

Definition

Drug photosensitivity reactions are adverse cutaneous responses to the interactions in the skin of a chemical agent (drug) and a non-ionizing electromagnetic radiation (light). The drug photosensitizer can reach the skin after topical application or systemic ingestion. The term drug refers not only to chemicals employed for therapeutic purposes, but also to cosmetics, food preservatives and agricultural and industrial compounds.

Aetiology and pathophysiology

Drug photosensitivity reactions are divided into two broad types: photoallergic reactions and phototoxic reactions.

Drug-induced photoallergy involves an immunological response. The cutaneous reaction is induced by light, but its pathogenesis is similar to that of an allergic contact dermatitis. The drug in the skin absorbs photons and is then converted to a stable or unstable photoproduct, which interacts with a protein to form a complete antigen.

A phototoxic reaction is similar to an irritative reaction. Phototoxic reactions are likely to occur in 100% of the population if sufficient doses of drugs are administered and appropriate wavelengths of light are present. Since any drug can be activated by specific wavelengths of absorption spectrum, a photosensitivity reaction is characterized by a specific action spectrum. The action spectrum of the photosensitivity reaction is most frequently in the ultraviolet A (UVA) range.

Clinical characteristics and course

Photoallergic drug reactions

These are much less common than phototoxic reactions. Photoallergy occurs only in previously sensitized individuals. The skin eruption generally appears 48 h after the interaction between chemicals and light. Usually photoallergic drug reactions are clinically characterized by an eczematous response that resembles an ordinary allergic contact dermatitis. The primary lesions are vesicles and bullae, which can be followed by crusts and desquamation. Lichenified plaques predominate in the chronic reactions. Skin eruptions are usually localized in the light-exposed body areas and occasionally also involve nearer non-exposed areas. The clinical course depends on how long the photosensitizer lasts in the skin, and on possible cross-reactions with other photosensitizers. Usually the cutaneous involvement lasts for a week after the drug is discontinued. Sometimes, however, the cutaneous reaction can persist and become chronic (persistent light reaction).

Phototoxic drug reactions

The clinical features are confined exclusively to areas of the skin that are exposed to light (face, ears, the 'V' of the neck, hands, extensor surfaces of the forearms). The reaction can appear just after the UVA exposure and is characterized by a burning, painful sensation, erythema, oedema or vesiculation (as occurs with some dyes); delayed reactions can occasionally appear 8–24 h after the light exposure.

Reactions to some phototoxic drugs (e.g. psoralens or bergamot oil) are characterized by marked hyperpigmentation.

Diagnosis

For a clear assessment of the aetiological role of sunlight an exhaustive description of the eruptions and of their relation with the exposure should be obtained. A diagnosis, together with the action spectrum, can be formulated only from the recorded history in some cases.

The anamnesis is useful to assess (a) the latent period between the exposure to light and the cutaneous reaction; (b) the systemic use or topical application of a potential photosensitizer drug; and (c) the existence of family members with a photosensitivity disease.

Phototests can be useful to determine the subject's photosensitivity and to demonstrate the action spectrum of the dermatosis. Photopatch tests are useful to detect the drug involved, in particular for photoallergic drug reactions. Recently, because of numerous false-negative results performed by photopatch testing, photoscratch testing has been proposed, but it does not increase the photopatch testing sensitivity.

Some drugs can induce a photoallergic and/or a phototoxic reaction and most systemic drugs causing photoallergy seem also to cause phototoxicity (these different reactions cannot always be distinguished clinically). Probably the mechanism involved depends on drug and UV doses as well as on topical applications or systemic ingestion of the drug (e.g. systemic photoallergic reactions are much less frequent than topical ones). Furthermore, under the same photosensitizing potential a drug much frequently prescribed will be often more photosensitizing than one less prescribed. In Tables 1 and 2 the main drugs inducing topical and systemic photosensitivity reactions are shown. Table 3 shows some drugs that sometimes increase a subject's photosensitivity to non-ionizing electromagnetic radiation by an unknown mechanism that probably does not involve either a phototoxic or a photoallergic reaction.

Table 1 Topical photosensitizers

Frequently involved in drug photosensitivity reactions
Psoralens: 8-MOP, 5-MOP, bergapten
Phenothiazines: promethazine
Fragrances: musk ambrette, 6-methylcoumarin, oak moss absolute
Dyes: eosin, fluorescein dye, methylene blue, rose bengal
PABA
Sulphonamide (derivatives): blankophor
Tetracyclines
Acridine
Rarely involved in drug photosensitivity reactions
NSAIDS: tiaprofenic acid, suprofen, ketoprofen
Sunscreen ingredients: benzophenones, cinnamates, dibenzoylmethanes
Oil: lavender,vanilla, sandal
Metals: nickel, chromium, cobalt, cadmium
Diphenhydramine
p-Phenylendiamine
5-fluorouracil
Porphyrins
6-ALA
Thiazides
Quinine
Halogenated salicylanilides
Oxytetracicline
Tricloroethilene
Hydrocortisone
Local anaesthetics
Formaldehyde

Differential diagnosis

This includes airborne dermatitis (no relation with sun exposure); atopic dermatitis (anamnesis can assess the existence of a cutaneous involvement during infancy and in non-sun-exposed areas); polymorphous light eruption (isomorphous lesions developing after phototest/photopatch test negative); and solar urticaria (urticarial lesions that disappear some hours after light exposure has stopped).

Treatment

General management

The first essential step for managing a drug-photosensitive patient is to discontinue exposure to the photosensitizer or light or both. Because light is more difficult to control the chemical usually has to be removed. Photosensitizing drugs are numerous including: antibiotics, non-steroidal anti-inflammatory drugs, diuretics, antimitotic drugs, psychiatric drugs,

Table 2 Systemic photosensitizers

Frequently involved in drug photosensitivity reactions
NSAIDS: piroxicam, carprofen, diclofenac
Fluoroquinolones: lomefloxacin, pefloxacin, ciprofloxacin
Nalidixic acid
Phenothiazines: promethazine
Sulphonamide derivatives: sulphonamides, sulfonylureas, thiazides
Tetracyclines: doxycicline, demeclocycline
Amiodarone
Heamatoporphyrin
Rarely involved in drug photosensitivity reactions
Fluoroquinolones: enoxicin, norfloxicin, ofloxacin, rosoxacin, sprafloxacin
Trimethoprim
Phenothiazines: thioridazine, mequitazine, dioxopromethazine
Benzodiazepines
NSAIDS: benoxaprofen, ibuprofen, ketoprofen, nabumetone, naproxen, tiaprofenic acid, meclofenamic acid, sulindac, tenoxicam
Diltiazem
Diuretics: furosemide
Ketoconazole
Tetracyclines: minocycline, methacycline, tetracycline
Griseofulvin
Penicillins: ampicillin
Antituberculous: isoniazid, pyrazinamide
Antineoplastic agents: 5-fluorouracil, dacarbazine, methotrexate, vinblastine, bleomycin, mitomycin
Fibric acid derivatives: bezafibrate, clofibrate
Methyldopa
Chloroquine
Tricyclic antidepressants: imipramine, protriptyline
Quinine
Quinidine
D-Penicillamine
β-blockers: propanolol

amiodarone and fibric acid derivatives; every year new photosensitizing drugs are discovered. Therefore, knowledge of potentially photosensitive drugs is fundamental in general practice.

1 Many patients are just reassured and encouraged; otherwise, topical treatments similar to the ones used for other acute inflammatory dermatosis, such as wet dressings, soothing lotions and topical corticosteroids, may be necessary.
2 Some cases need high doses of systemically administered corticosteroids or hospitalization.
3 However, even after removal, exogenous agents may persist in the skin for several weeks. Patients with chronic photodermatitis often complain more of pruritus and loss of sleep than of pain. These patients usually benefit from sedatives.

Recommended therapies

Topical photoprotection

The aim of photoprotection is to minimize the penetration of photoactive radiation into the skin. Photoprotection must be effective in the action spectra of drug photosensitivity photodermatosis: many photosensitivity eruptions are provoked by UVA. In the choice of a sunscreen different factors must be considered: the wavelengths against which protection is sought, the absorption spectrum and the sunscreen protection factor. Many sunscreens now have high efficacy in the UVB and UVA range.

Table 3 Other photosensitizers (neither photoallergic nor phototoxic)

Acetazolamide
Amantadine
Amiloride
Aminosalicylate sodium (PAS)
Amitriptyline
Betaxolol
Captopril
Carbamazepine
Chlordiazepoxide
Clorazepate
Dapsone
Ethambutol
Flutamide
Fluvastatin
Gold compounds
Heroin (diacetyl-morphine)
Isotretinoin
Loratadine
Methotrexate
Pimozide
Pyrimethamine
Retinoids
Simvastatin
Spironolactone
Triamterene

In general, sunscreens protect by absorbing (chemical sunscreens) or reflecting (physical sunscreens) radiation. For photosensitivity eruptions physical sunscreens with a high protection factor and with high efficacy in the UVA must be chosen. Physical sunscreens are to be selected to obtain absolute photoprotection. However, some sunscreens are sometimes opaque and are not easily accepted by patients. Patients should be advised about the frequency and modality of sunscreen application.

Further reading

Gould JW, Mercurio MG, Elmets CA. Cutaneous photosensitivity diseases induced by exogenous agents. *J Am Acad Dermatol* 1995; 23: 551–73.

Epstein JH. Phototoxicity and photoallergy in man. In: Daynes RA, Krueger G, eds. *Experimental and Clinical Photoimmunology*, Vol. 2. Boca Raton: CRC Press, 1983: 107–14.

Allen JE. Drug-induced photosensitivity. *Clin Pharmacol* 1993; 12: 580–7.

Conilleau V, Dompmartin A, Michel M. Photoscratch testing in systemic drug-induced photosensitivity. *Photoderm Photoimmunol Photomed* 2000; 16: 62–6.

Toback AC, Anders JE. Phototoxicity from systemic agents. *Dermatol Clin* 1986; 4: 223–30.

Marguery MC. Drug-induced photosensitivity. *Rev Pract* 2000; 50: 1315–19.

Eccrine miliaria

H.R. Bruckbauer and H.-J. Vogt

Definition and epidemiology

This is a disease of the eccrine sweat excretion ducts with retention of sweat within the skin. Dependent on the histopathological and clinical findings miliaria crystallina, miliaria rubra and miliaria profunda can be distinguished. Miliaria is a common disorder of children and infants although it can be seen at any age. Miliaria usually occurs during spring and summer, in hot and humid climates, often after extended exposure to the sun.

Aetiology and pathophysiology

The aetiology and pathophysiology of miliaria are controversial. There is agreement that it is a disorder of the sweat ducts of the eccrine glands at various levels but it is not yet clear if miliaria is caused by occlusion or disruption of sweat ducts. Sweat ducts may be occluded by keratinous material, by metabolites of microorganisms or exogenous substances. Increased pH causes hydration of the stratum corneum and may result in miliaria. The primary pathogenic factor seems to be excessive sweating and overhydration of the stratum corneum. High humidity, increased sodium chloride concentrations and occlusion increase hyperhydration. This overhydration can cause transient occlusion of the acrosyringium. These local factors favour bacterial colonization.

According to the level of ductal blockage, miliaria profunda (dermis), miliaria rubra (epidermis) or miliaria crystallina (stratum corneum) can be observed. As a consequence regulation of body temperature is impaired, and life-threatening anhidrotic heat exhaustion may occur. Secondary bacterial infections may complicate the clinical course.

Clinical characteristics and course

Miliaria crystallina (sudamina)

On previously sun-exposed body sites, especially on the trunk, asymptomatic, pinhead sized, clear, subcorneal non-inflammatory vesicles can be seen. Vesicles easily rupture as a result of minimal mechanical stress. After hours to days the disease clears with pityriasiform desquamation. Sweat ducts are affected at the level of the stratum corneum. Histology shows subcorneal vesicles with neutrophils and little perivascular inflammation.

Miliaria rubra (prickly heat)

Sweat is retained in the subcorneal layers of the epidermis and the acrosyringium, and papulovesiculous pruritic and inflammatory eruptions occur. After initial sweating anhidrosis occurs, which in severe cases can lead to hyperpyrexia. If the eruptions become pustular this variant is called miliaria pustulosa. Histology shows spongiosis, vesicle inflammation in the vicinity of eccrine ductal systems within the epidermis.

Miliaria profunda

This affects the sweat ducts at the level of the dermis resulting in non-inflammatory and non-pruritic 'gooseflesh-like' papules. The papules enlarge after sweat stimulation. Miliaria profunda often occurs after recurrent episodes of miliaria rubra. Miliaria profunda tends to be limited to the trunk and limbs. Often a compensatory axillary and facial hyperhidrosis can be observed. Widespread lesions may result in hyperpyrexia. The disease can last a few weeks. Histology shows local oedema in the dermis. Plugging of the intradermal portion of the eccrine ducts with homogenous, eosinophilic material and periductal lymphocytic infiltration may be seen as well as hyperkeratosis of the acrosyringium.

Diagnosis

Diagnosis is from the typical clinical picture. Histological examination of a skin biopsy can be helpful.

Differential diagnosis

Bockhart's superficial folliculitis commonly involves the skin of the face, scalp and limbs. The 2–5-mm sized pustules are found in association with hairs. Coagulase-positive staphylococci can be isolated from the pustules.

Hot tube folliculitis usually occurs at areas covered by bathing suits. It is caused by *Pseudomonas aeruginosa* and is characterized by itchy follicular erythematous papules, macules and pustules.

Erythema neonatorum toxicum is found in about 30% of newborns. Eruptions of erythematous macules, red, white or yellow papules, or vesiculopustules are associated with pilosebaceous glands. The pustules are located subcorneally and are filled with eosinophils.

Acne neonatorum and acne infantum are found in newborns and infants. Hormone-induced acneiform lesions and pustules are located on the cheeks and nose.

Treatment

General therapeutic guidelines

The disease improves within days after changing climatic factors. Air conditioning and light clothes are recommended. Regular showers with synthetic detergents remove salt and bacteria. A gradual increase in exposure to ultraviolet (UV) light and the use of sunscreens prevent UV-induced damage of sweat ducts and help prevent miliaria crystallina.

Recommended therapies

Zinc oxide lotions and cool moist dressings provide cooling and symptomatic relief. Topical anhydrous lanolin is thought to be beneficial. Topical antimicrobial preparations help to prevent bacterial superinfection, if necessary. Irritant and keratolytic agents should be avoided. Symptomatic relief has been described after taking vitamin C (1 g daily).

In severe therapy-resistant cases isotretinoin (0.5 mg/kg) to reduce keratinous plugging in miliaria profunda has been applied successfully.

With anhidrosis due to ductal blockage, it takes about 2 weeks until complete recovery where repair of the affected sweat ducts is achieved.

Further reading

Braun-Falco O, Plewig G, Wolf HH. *Dermatologie und Venerologie*, 4th edn. Berlin: Springer, 1996.

Feng E, Janniger CK. Miliaria. *Cutis* 1995; 55: 213–16.

Henning DR, Griffin TB, Maibach HI. Studies on changes in skin surface bacteria induced miliaria and associated hypohidrosis. *Acta Dermatovener (Stockh)* 1972; 52: 371–5.

Hölzle E, Kligman AG. The pathogenesis of miliaria rubra. *Br J Dermatol* 1978; 99: 117.

Kirk JF, Wilson BB, Chun W, Cooper P. Miliaria profunda. *J Am Acad Dermatol* 1996; 35: 854–6.

Mayser P, Gründer K, Nilles M, Schill W-B. Morbus Fox-Fordyce (Apokrine Miliaria). *Hautarzt* 1993; 44: 309–11.

Mowald CM, McGinley KJ, Foglia A, Leyden JJ. The role of extracellular polysaccharide substance produced by *Staphylococcus epidermidis* in miliaria. *J Am Acad Dermatol* 1995; 33: 729–33.

Orfanos CE, Garbe C. *Therapie der Hautkrankheiten*. Berlin: Springer, 1995.

Shelley WB, Levy EJ. Apocrine sweat retention in man. II. Fox-Fordyce disease (apocrine miliaria). *Arch Dermatol* 1956; 73: 38–49.

Shuster S. Duct disruption, a new explanation of Miliaria. *Acta Derm Venereol (Stockh)* 1997; 77: 1–3.

Stashower LM, Krivda MS, Turiansky LG. Fox-Fordyce disease: diagnosis with transverse histologic sections. *J Am Acad Dermatol* 2000; 42: 89–91.

Epidermolysis bullosa

G. Menchini, B. Bianchi and T.M. Lotti

Definition

Epidermolysis bullosa (EB) is a group of rare dermatoses, mainly inherited, characterized by blistering and erosions of the skin and mucous membranes caused by minor mechanical trauma (mechanobullous disorders). Only acquired EB is not inherited.

Aetiology and pathophysiology

The group of inherited EB are congenital disorders due to a defective composition of one or more components that mediate the adherence of the epidermis to the underlying dermis (Fig. 1). The molecular basis of several major forms of EB are definite. Generalized dominantly inherited forms of simple EB are known to result from mutation in the keratin 5 and 14 genes that are expressed in the cells at the bottom of the epidermis. The Herlitz form of junctional EB results from mutations in three chains of laminin 5, and finally all forms of inherited dystrophic EB result from mutations in the type VII collagen gene.

The classification is based on genetic and clinical features. The level of cleavage is different for each group of syndromes and depends on the site of the defect (Fig. 2). In the simple forms the cleavage is in the basal and suprabasal layers of the epidermis, in junctional types in the lamina lucida and in dystrophic types is beneath the lamina densa. All defects are determined by autosomal dominant (ADI) or recessive (ARI) inheritance. Acquired EB is an autoimmune disorder due to immunoglobulin G (IgG) self-antibody targeting the non-collagenous (NC1) domain of type VII collagen, the major component of anchoring fibrils that connect the basement membrane with the dermal structures.

Clinical characteristics and course

Inherited EB

Simple EB

Generalized simple EB (Köbner) (ADI)

This form appears within the first year of life and sometimes is present at birth. Traumatic bullae are tense, serous and heal without scarring or milia. The entire body is involved in blistering but hands and feet are more affected then other areas. Some patients improve after puberty, but usually blistering continues for the entire lifetime.

Ogna (Gedde–Dahl) (ADI)

The blistering is traumatic and seasonal, largely confined to the hands and feet. There is also a generalized bruising tendency.

Simple EB of hands and feet (Weber–Cockayne) (ADI)

Clinically, there is traumatic blistering of hands and feet, and occasionally elsewhere. Usually the syndrome begins in childhood, sometimes in early adult life. The general state of health is normal.

Herpetiform simple EB (Dowling–Meara) (ADI)

The onset of this occurs normally in infancy, with severe and extensive blistering that involves mucous membranes and nails. Spontaneous herpetiform blistering on the trunk may help with differential diagnosis with junctional and dystrophic forms. The bullae may leave milia and mild hyperpigmentation. This syndrome may improve during fever, with age or warm saline soaks.

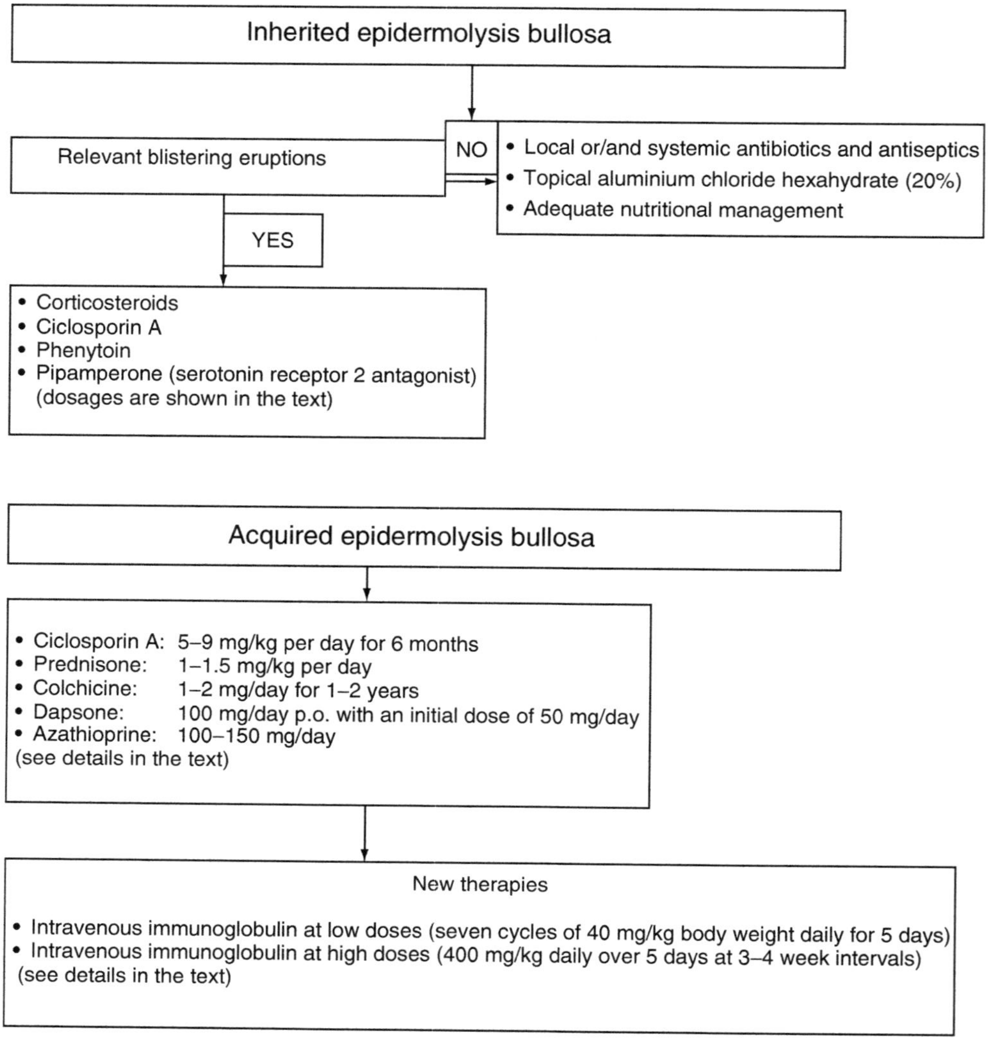

Inherited epidermolysis bullosa
Relevant blistering eruptions
NO
• Local or/and systemic antibiotics and antiseptics
• Topical aluminium chloride hexahydrate (20%)
• Adequate nutritional management
YES
• Corticosteroids
• Ciclosporin A
• Phenytoin
• Pipamperone (serotonin receptor 2 antagonist)
(dosages are shown in the text)
Acquired epidermolysis bullosa
• Ciclosporin A: 5–9 mg/kg per day for 6 months
• Prednisone: 1–1.5 mg/kg per day
• Colchicine: 1–2 mg/day for 1–2 years
• Dapsone: 100 mg/day p.o. with an initial dose of 50 mg/day
• Azathioprine: 100–150 mg/day
(see details in the text)
New therapies
• Intravenous immunoglobulin at low doses (seven cycles of 40 mg/kg body weight daily for 5 days)
• Intravenous immunoglobulin at high doses (400 mg/kg daily over 5 days at 3–4 week intervals)
(see details in the text)

Figure 1 Treatment

Simple EB with mottled pigmentation (ADI)

Except for mottled hyper-and hypopigmentation this syndrome is very similar to Köbner simple EB.

Superficial simple EB (ADI)

This variant involves conjunctive and oral mucous membrane involvement and residual atrophic scarring.

Lethal simple EB (ARI)

This severe variant starts at birth with generalized blistering that involves skin and oral mucosae; patients die from infectious complications and dehydration.

Generalized EB (ARI)

This form is correlated with myasthenia gravis and other muscular dystrophies. Clinically the blisters are widespread

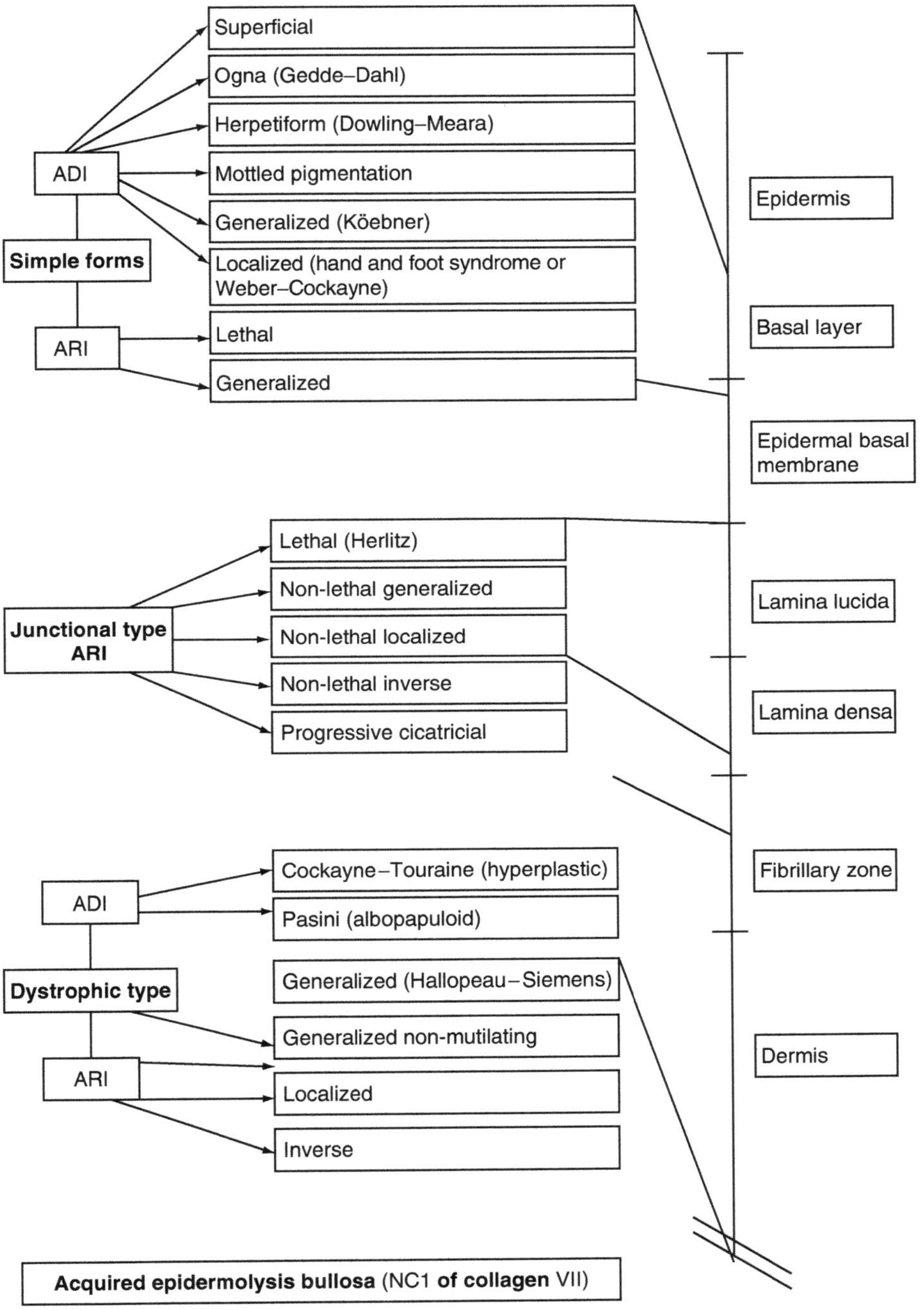

Figure 2 Epidermolysis bullosa inherited and acquired classification and bullae level of cleavage

with residual atrophic scarring, nail dystrophy, milia and scarring alopecia.

Junctional EB

Lethal junctional EB (Herlitz) (ARI)
Blistering and erosions are present at birth and become generalized in a few days. Often there is associated involvement of oral, laryngeal, tracheal, bronchiole and biliary duct mucosae. These lesions heal with difficulty and leave an area of atrophy. Infants die from infectious complications or severe refractory anaemia.

Non-lethal generalized junctional EB (ARI)
Clinically this variant is identical to the lethal form, but there is a gradual lessening in the severity of the blistering with age. Milia and scarring are not present and teeth and nails show few defects.

Non-lethal localized junctional EB (ARI)
Blistering is confined to the lower legs and feet; there are alterations in nail and teeth enamel.

Non-lethal inverse junctional EB (ARI)
Onset of blistering occurs a few months after birth with development of pyoderma-like lesions in the groin, perineum and axillae. Healing of the lesions is difficult and results in small atrophic white streaks.

Progressive junctional EB (ARI)
The onset is late and progressive with blistering on the hands, feet, knees and elbows, and nail distrophy. Healing of the blisters is difficult and results in diffuse atrophic changes in the skin.

Cicatricial junctional EB (ARI)
The blisters heal with scarring and result in the loss of nails, pseudosyndactyly, alopecia and contractures. The mucosae are also involved with stenosis of the anterior nares.

Dystrophic EB

Generalized dystrophic EB (Hallopeau–Siemens) (ARI)
Onset is in early infancy. The bullae are large, flaccid and often haemorrhagic. All the skin and mucosal surfaces are involved. These lesions result in scars, and often pseudosyndactyly is present. Nails are dystrophic and teeth are malformed. Serious problems may arise with eating (oral mucosal, tongue and oesophageal lesions), talking (laryngeal lesions) and vision (corneal erosions). One of the most important complications is dysphagic pneumonitis. Squamous cell carcinomas may involve any chronically scarred area and often are aggressive.

Generalized non-mutilating dystrophic EB (ARI)
This is a milder form of generalized dystrophic EB with milder and more localized involvement.

Inverse dystrophic EB (ARI)
This variant affects the axillae, groin and neck but the skin of hands, feet, knees and elbows is spared. Often there are corneal erosions, nail dystrophy, mucous membrane involvement and malformed teeth.

Cockayne–Touraine dystrophic EB (ADI)
Onset is in infancy or later, the bullae are more numerous on the limbs, but are present on all skin surfaces. The bullae heal with hypertrophic scarring, milia and may result in mutilating effects on the hands. Often the skin is affected by other diseases such as ichthyosis, keratosis pilaris and hypertrichosis. No mucous membranes are involved.

EB pasini (ADI)
This form is very similar to Cockayne–Touraine EB. The peculiar characteristic of Pasini's disease is the development of firm, ivory-white perifollicular papules

which may enlarge to a diameter of 15 mm and last indefinitely, especially on the lumbosacral area; these papules contain degraded chondroitin sulphate.

Acquired EB

The acquired form of EB may mimic a number of bullous dermatoses. The bullae are serous or haemorrhagic, trauma-induced and leave scars. Often blisters heal with milia and hyperpigmentation. The involvement of mucous membranes and scarring alopecia are not very common. Acquired EB is a chronic inflammatory disease, with periods of partial remission and exacerbation. Death as a direct result of the disease is uncommon. However, acquired EB is relatively unresponsive to treatment and can cause significant morbidity. The onset of acquired EB could be at any age and onset of acquired EB in a 3-month-old child has been reported. However, it appears that acquired EB affects the elderly more frequently. The majority of patients with acquired EB experience slow onset and chronic disease affecting the trauma-prone extensor skin surfaces. The scarring nature of the disease usually leads to skin fragility and restricted mobility of the extensor skin surfaces. Acquired EB may present any of various skin and mucous membrane manifestations.

Non-inflammatory or mildly inflammatory acquired EB

This is the most common form of acquired EB, presenting tense blisters and erosions primarily on the extensor surfaces of hands, knuckles, elbows, knees and ankles. Healing leaves significant scar and milia formation; nail dystrophy and scarring alopecia have been observed in some patients. This type of acquired EB resembles the dominantly inherited form of dystrophic epidermolysis bullosa in children.

Generalized inflammatory acquired EB

These subjects have widespread tense blisters in both trauma and non-trauma-prone areas, with some haemorrhagic blisters. Other skin manifestations, such as generalized erythema, urticarial plaques and generalized pruritus, have been observed. This form of acquired EB clinically resembles bullous pemphigoid or linear IgA bullous disease, and usually heals with a minor degree of scarring and milia formation compared to other forms.

Predominant mucous membrane acquired EB

Predominant mucous membrane disease. This form of acquired EB can affect mucous membranes of oral, conjunctival, nasal and oesophageal mucosae. This form of acquired EB clinically resembles cicatricial pemphigoid.

Diagnosis

The family history is very important but may be non-contributory. The clinical aspect in infancy may help in differentiation from other bullous diseases: for example: X-linked incontinentia pigmenti results in swirly patterns of pigmentation especially over the trunk, dominant bullous ichthyosiform erythroderma presents erythroderma and hyperkeratosis and staphylococcal scaled skin syndrome presents necrotic peeling epidermis and generalized erythema. When it is clear that the patient has a mechanobullous eruption, it is important to assess clinical, genetic and histological characteristics for the correct diagnosis. Moreover, immunofluorescence or electron microscopy can help to establish the level of cleavage and detect ultrastructural abnormalities.

- Electron microscopy. This analysis has become the gold standard for the diagnosis and classification of EB because it visualizes the cleavage plane of the blisters and the ultrastructural abnormalities of the junctional structures.

Cytolysis of basal layer cells and the presence of keratinocyte fragments is diagnostic for simple EB; retraction and clumping of tonofilaments of the basal cells is characteristic of the herpetiform type. In junctional EB a reduced number of abnormal structures of hemidesmosomes have been observed; dystrophic EB is characterized by alteration of anchoring fibrils that appear defective and diminished or absent.

- Immunofluorescence. Immunofluorescent mapping of the dermal–epidermal junction represents an additional advance in the diagnosis of EB. In this technique mono-and polyclonal antibodies directed against structural proteins (i.e. type IV collagen, laminin and bullous pemphigoid antigen) are used to identify the various forms of EB. In simple EB all three antigens are localized in the floor of the blister; in junctional EB type IV collagen and laminin are present in the floor of the blister, whereas the bullous pemphigoid antigen is in the roof of the blister; finally in dystrophic EB all three proteins are situated in the roof of the blister. Moreover, the defective expression of monoclonal antibodies against structural proteins may be a diagnostic standard to identify certain subtypes of EB. For example since expression of antigen GB3 is reduced or absent in the Herlitz form, the presence of this protein excludes this junctional EB variant; in dystrophic EB the expression of monoclonal antibodies KF-1 and LH7:2, that recognize two different epitopes of collagen VII, has permitted differentiation of the dominant and the recessive forms.
- Molecular biology. The molecular biology technique has allowed cloning and subsequent mapping of genes corresponding to the components of the basement membrane zone. These technologies are sensitive enough to identify distinct mutations in the various EB forms and have several implications in terms of improved prognostication regarding severity and progress of the disease. Identification of specific mutations in fetal DNA is important in prenatal diagnosis in families at risk for Herlitz junctional EB or Hallopeau syndrome; this test can be performed from chorionic villus samples at the 10th week of gestation or from amniocentesis specimens at the 12th week.
- Preimplantation genetic diagnosis (PGD) is a novel, emerging technology for the prevention of inheritable diseases such as EB. *In vitro* fertilized embryos are examined at the eight-cell stage by removal of one of the eight blastomeres. The DNA contained in the single cell allows the detection of specific mutations, in the event of diagnosis of a normal or carrier genotype, the original pre-embryo is transferred into the uterus.

Diagnosis of acquired EB

The diagnosis of acquired EB is based on the following tests:

- Histological examination of blistered skin shows a subepidermal blister formation and mixed inflammatory cell infiltration.
- Direct immunofluorescent examination of perilesional skin reveals the immune-mediated disease process, a thick band of IgG, and to a lesser extent C3, deposited linearly at the periblistered skin basement membrane zone.
- Indirect immunofluorescent examination of the subject serum on salt-split normal skin substrate usually detects IgG circulating autoantibodies in the patient serum that bind to the dermal floor (lower part) of the salt-split normal skin substrate.

Treatment

General guidelines

Treatment is primarily symptomatic because there is currently no completely effective treatment for EB.

- Local and/or systemic antibiotics and antiseptics to prevent secondary infection with application of Vaseline gauze or saline compresses to protect the blisters are the general therapies for these patients.
- Topical aluminium chloride hexahydrate (20%) is efficacious in reducing blistering because of its antiperspirant property; in fact, especially in summer, sweating increases the friction of the skin causing trauma. Also a topical application of 10% glutaraldeyde is used, but its efficacy is variable and contact sensitization may occur. These drugs are employed mostly in localized simple EB.
- Adequate nutritional management (vitamins, iron, proteins) may improve the course of disease when the oral and gastrointestinal mucosae are involved and provide many benefits, including improved growth, accelerated healing and decreased susceptibility to infection. Moreover in EB, chronic constipation, painful defaecation and faecal impaction frequently contribute to malnutrition and growth failure; especially in chronically constipated children with dystrophic EB, administration of a fibre-containing liquid formula (Enrich) (250–750 mL/day) is recommended.
- Appropriate counselling is important to inform patients and their families about adequate lifestyle to prevent trauma (e.g. the use of soft, well-ventilated clothes and shoes is suggested; sports are not advised).

Therapy for inherited EB

Pharmacological treatments

1 Steroids: high-potency topical steroids (betamethasone dipropionate cream, clobetasol propionate cream, 1% hydrocortisone lotion) are applied continuously for 2–12 months. Alternative dosage consists in weekend topical pulse therapy with clobetasol propionate cream twice daily for 9 months. This treatment is effective in Pasini's variant which is not responsive to other therapies.

In the more severe forms of EB, such as Herlitz JEB and recessive DEB, high systemic dosages of corticosteroids (initially 60–120 mg prednisone, later a minimal maintenance dose) may be used in life-threatening situations.

2 Phenytoin: this anticonvulsant and antiarrhythmic drug is used as a wound-healing agent in DEB although there are contradictory reports about its efficacy. The clinical benefit of phenytoin may be due to its ability to decrease collagenase and collagen peptidase activity. Patients are treated systemically with 3 mg/kg body weight daily, divided into two doses for 10–14 days; the maintenance dose must to be at least 8 fg/mL blood level. Efficacy of systemic phenytoin in the treatment of GABEB has been described, and topical phenytoin has also been used in EBS; the cream (2 or 5% in a hydrophilic base) is applied twice daily at the sites of bulla formation for 6–36 months.

3 Serotonin (5-hydroxytryptamine) receptor 2 antagonists: therapy with pipamperone, a neuroleptic drug, is demonstrated to be useful in the treatment of herpetiform EBS (Dowling–

Meara); a complete clearing of the lesions is obtained at doses of 20 mg/day for children and 120 mg/day for adults. Contraindications for this therapy include drowsiness, torpidity and laziness with slow neuropsychomotor development in children. A progressive reappearance of the bullous lesions is evident 2 months after the therapy is suspended. Another 5–HT2 antagonist, cyproheptadine hydrochloride, seems to be effective in the treatment of this bullous disease with less severe secondary effects than pipamperone and a longer period of latency is observed.

4 Vitamin E: sometimes oral therapy (600–1800 mg/day) is administered to patients with EB, particularly in the Cockayne–Touraine form, with satisfactory clinical reduction of blister formation.

5 Retinoids have been tried in the therapy of the Hallopeau–Siemens syndrome since they inhibit collagenase production by fibroblasts but without convincing results.

6 Ciclosporin: there are reports of good results with ciclosporin in patients with Cockayne–Touraine EB at a dose of 1 mg/kg per day. In recessive dystrophic EB, this drug results in a remarkable decrease in blister formation only at toxic doses. Further studies will be necessary to confirm these data and establish optimum dosages.

Surgical treatments

Serious complications of EB that influence prognosis can be treated with surgical techniques. Generalized enamel hypoplasia and dental caries appear in junctional EB and in generalized recessive dystrophic EB, respectively. Dental therapy, consisting in preventive restorative and surgical procedures with extractions and stainless steel crowns, is the most common treatment modality to maintain a functional dentition. Use of small suction tips, flat tissue retractors and extensive lubrication of all tissues may reduce mucosal blistering. Digital contractures and pseudosyndactyly, common manifestations in recessive dystrophic EB, cause significant functional impairment. The deformities progress with time, although surgery may help with dynamic splinting and coverage of wounds with allogenic keratinocyte sheets. Oesophageal dilatation, reconstruction to alleviate stricture or gastrostomy are employed to control chronic malnutrition. Recently, a new method for oesophageal dilatation, using a microinvasive rigiflex balloon catheter has been described: the catheter is advanced to the stenotic area under radiography and then expanded by injecting contrast medium into the balloon. Feeding gastrostomy consists in a button device (inserted primarily) that supplements oral intake. Laryngeal involvement is rare and associated with junctional EB. Tracheostomy may be suggested to protect the airway in the acute setting and to prevent any further laryngeal injury due to endotracheal intubation.

Nutritional aspect

Extensive cutaneous injury is associated with marked alterations in both haemodynamic and metabolic responses, requiring increased caloric and protein intake for recovery. The burns patient has been studied extensively from both of these perspectives. Studies confirm that the development of nutritional deficiencies inhibits successful wound healing and the body's return to a normal haemodynamic and metabolic profile. Impediments to intake and absorption are oropharyngeal and gastrointestinal lesions which greatly threaten the nutritional well-being of patients with EB. Complications include oral blistering, abnormal oesophageal motility, strictures, dysphagia, diarrhoea, malabsorption and dental problems. Nutritional assessment taking these factors into account is essential for replenishing the malnourished patient.

Complications

1 Dystrophic EB is frequently associated with aggressive secondary squamous cell carcinoma arising on affected skin or mucosae. Surgery and chemotherapy are suggested but the best results have been achieved with radiation (at 4500 cGy dose) with 54% tumour response.
2 Frequently wounds are infected: ointments and creams with an antimicrobial effect are used. These are preferably effective against at least staphylococci and streptococci because these are the main causes of skin infections. Furthermore, the ointment and cream should cause as little sensitization as possible. Examples of ointments and creams with an antimicrobial effect include: tetracycline cream/ointment, chlorhexidine cream 1%, mupirocin calcium cream 2% and fusidic acid.
3 EB patients are often troubled by itching, especially on the sites of wounds that are healing. Here, the skin is dry and quick to scale. It is important to prevent itch as much as possible. Itching is not only annoying but it is also often a reason for the patient to start scratching. This must be prevented as much as possible; because scratching damages the skin again. Ointments or creams that are used to prevent or control itching are usually also the ointments and creams that counteract dry skin; zinc oxide ointment 10% or Eucerin cum aqua. In the case of intractable itching, ointments with corticosteroids are used by EB patients as well. These are applied topically. In the use of corticosteroids prudence is in order. Application of corticosteroids causes a decrease in the local response to chemical, microbial or immunogenic stimuli. This means caution should be exercised when there are conditions in which infections can play a role, that cannot be treated effectively simultaneously. Preferably, a class 1 corticosteroid is applied. A class 1 corticosteroid has a mild potency. An example of a class 1 ointment or cream with corticosteroids is hydrocortisone cream/ointment 1%.

Alternative and experimental treatments

Gene therapies

This technique may be a potential approach for the treatment of inherited EB. For the ADI form it is necessary to suppress *in vitro* the mutant gene product of affected epidermis using either homologeous recombination, antisense or ribozyme strategy. Corrected keratinocyte production employs epithelium for grafting. In the recessive disorders insertion of the normal allele recreates a normal phenotype; normal allele may be inserted using an *in vivo* strategy such as the gene gun or cultured patient keratinocytes which are used then as an autograft. In some studies, for example, keratinocytes from junctional EB patients (containing a β3 gene defect of laminin 5) are immortalized and then transfected with retroviral vectors introducing a wild-type version of the β3 gene; this reversion results in correct laminin 5 heterotrimer production and often in a normal phenotype.

Acquired EB therapies

The acquired EB therapies are based on immunosuppressive, immunomodulatory and anti-inflammatory drugs, such as:

1 Ciclosporin A in dose of 5–9 mg/kg per day for a mean of 6 months has demonstrated great efficacy in reducing blistering and, in some cases, remission even after the discontinuation of therapy.

2 Prednisone is used at 1–1.5 mg/kg body weight/day orally. Special precautions must be taken in patients with high blood pressure and diabetes. This treatment can be associated to ciclosporin administration to increase their efficacy.
3 Colchicine: the mechanism of action of this drugs in EB is probably due to the binding of microtubular proteins, interfering with polymorphonuclear leucocyte mitosis and chemotaxis. Colchicine is administered in a dose of 1–2 mg/day for 1–2 years. No significant side-effects have been noted.
4 Dapsone is used in conjunction with other anti-inflammatory and immunosuppressive drugs to treat acquired EB. The suggested dose is 100 mg/day orally with an initial dose of 50 mg/day. Special precautions are necessary in patients with glucose-6-phosphate dehydrogenase deficiency.
5 Azathioprine is used in conjunction with other anti-inflammatory drugs, for treating acquired EB. The suggested dose is 100–150 mg/day orally. Azathioprine is not safe for pregnant women and children, and bone marrow suppression should be closely monitored in all cases.
6 Photophoresis is a therapeutic method that utilizes ultraviolet (UV)-sensitizing medication and UV irradiation in the A spectrum to expose patient blood cells.

New therapies for this refractory condition are: extracorporeal photochemotherapy, intravenous immunoglobulin at low doses (seven cycles of 40 mg/kg body weight daily for 5 days) and intravenous immunoglobulin at high doses (400 mg/kg daily over 5 days at 3–4-week intervals).

Further reading

Bastin KT, Steeves RA, Richards MJ. Radiation therapy for squamous cell carcinoma in dystrophic epidermolysis bullosa. a case report and literature review. *Am J Clin Oncol* 1997; 20 (1): 55–8.

Campiglio GL, Pajardi G, Rafanelli G. A new protocol for the treatment of hand deformities in recessive dystrophic epidermolysis bullosa. *Ann Chir Main Memb Super* 1997; 16 (2): 91–100.

Cunningham BB, Kirchmann TT, Woodley D. Colchicine for epidermolysis bullosa acquisita. *J Am Acad Dermatol* 1996; 34: 781–4.

Engineer L, Ahmed AR. Emerging treatment for epidermolysis bullosa acquisita. *J Am Acad Dermatol* 2001; 44 (5): 818–28.

Gordon KB, Chan LS, Woodley DT. Treatment of refractory epidermolysis bullosa acquisita with extracorporeal photochemotherapy. *Br J Dermatol* 1997; 136 (3): 415–20.

Harman KE, Black MM. High dose intravenous immune globulin for the treatment of autoimmune blistering diseases: an evaluation of its use in 14 cases. *Br J Dermatol* 1999; 140: 865–74.

Haynes L, Atherthon D, Clayden G. Constipation in epidermolysis bullosa: successful treatment with a liquid containing-fiber formula. *Pediatr Dermatol* 1997; 14: 393–6.

Khavari PA. Gene therapy for genetic skin disease. *J Invest Dermatol* 1998; 110: 462–7.

Kofler H, Wambacher-Gasser B, Topar G *et al.* Intravenous immunoglobulin treatment in therapy resistant epidermolysis bullosa acquisita. *J Am Acad Dermatol* 1997; 36 (part 2): 331–5.

Ladd AL, Kibele A, Gibbons S. Surgical treatment and postoperative splinting of recessive dystrophic epidermolysis bullosa. *J Hand Surg* 1996; 21 (5): 888–97.

Layton AM, Cunliffe WJ. Clearing of epidermolysis bullosa acquisita with cyclosporin A. *Dermatologica* 1990; 181: 44–7.

Megahed M, Scharffetter-Kochanek K. Epidermolysis bullosa acquisita: successful treatment with colchicine. *Arch Dermatol Res* 1994; 286: 35–40.

Shenefelt PD, Castellano LM, Frenske NA. Successful treatment of albopapuloid epidermolysis bullosa (Pasini's variant) with pulse topical corticosteroid therapy. *J Am Acad Dermatol* 1993; 29 (1): 785–6.

Yamasaki H, Tada J, Yioshioka T, Arata J. Epidermolysis bullosa pruriginosa (McGrath) successfully controlled by oral cyclosporin. *Br J Dermatol* 1997; 137: 309–11.

Erysipelas

M. Balabanova

Erysipelas, also known as Saint Anthony's fire, is a distinctive type of superficial cellulites of the skin with prominent lymphatic involvement.

It is almost always due to β-haemolytic streptococci group A (uncommonly, *Streptococcus dysgalactiae* group G or *S. dysgalactiae* group C). Group B streptococci have produced erysipelas in newborns.

Clinical characteristics and course

Erysipelas is more common in infants, young children and older adults. Formerly, the face was most commonly involved, and an antecedent streptococcal respiratory tract infection preceded cutaneous involvement in about one-third of patients even though streptococci might not be found on culture at the time that the skin lesions become evident. Now, the distribution of erysipelas has changed: 70–80% of the lesions are on the lower extremities and 5–20% are on the face.

- The portal of entry commonly includes skin ulcers, local trauma or abrasions, psoriatic or eczematous lesions, or fungal infections; in the neonate, erysipelas may develop from an infection of the umbilical stump.
- Predisposing factors include venous stasis, paraparesis, diabetes mellitus and alcohol abuse. Location, and hepatic and renal disease, are the most important risk factors, while diabetes is probably of less significance than previously suggested. Patients with the nephrotic syndrome are particularly susceptible. Erysipelas tends to occur in areas of pre-existing lymphatic obstruction or oedema (e.g. after a radical mastectomy). Also, because erysipelas itself produces lymphatic obstruction, it tends to recur in an area of earlier infection. Over a 3-year period, the recurrence rate is about 30%, predominantly in individuals with venous insufficiency or lymphoedema.

Streptococcal bacteraemia occurs in about 5% of patients with erysipelas; group A, C or G streptococci can be isolated on throat culture from about 20% of cases.

Erysipelas is a painful lesion with a bright red, oedematous, indurated ('peau d'orange') appearance and an advancing, raised border that is sharply demarcated from the adjacent normal skin. Fever is a feature. A common form of erysipelas involves the bridge of the nose and the cheeks. Local clinical signs, without fever and inflammation, characterize the recurrent forms. Uncomplicated erysipelas remains confined primarily to the lymphatics and the dermis. Occasionally, the infection extends more deeply and produces cellulites, subcutaneous abscess and necrotizing fasciitis.

Diagnosis

The diagnosis is based on the:

- general symptoms: sudden appearance, temperature of 39–40x, fever, nausea
- local symptoms: well-demarcated, indurated, dusky red lesions with advancing, palpable borders
- biopsy
  Gram or Giemsa stain
  direct immunofluorescence
  throat swabs
  culture technique
  swabs from the local portal of entry
  serological tests.

Differential diagnosis

- Early herpes zoster involving the second division of the fifth cranial nerve.
- Contact dermatitis.
- Giant urticaria.

- Diffuse inflammatory carcinoma of the breast.
- Erythema chronicum migrans.
- An erysipelas-like skin lesion in patients with hypogammaglobulinaemia.
- *Campylobacter jejuni* bacteraemia.

Treatment

Mild early cases of erysipelas in an adult

- Intramuscularly procaine penicillin (600 000 units once or twice daily) or oral penicillin V (250–500 mg every 6 h).
- Erythromycin (250–500 mg every 6 h).

More extensive erysipelas

- Hospitalization and parenteral aqueous penicillin G (600 000–2000 000 units every 6 h for 5–10 days).
- Clindamycin should be added in case of septic shock.
- Extensive cellulitis or necrotizing fasciitis requires surgical debridement of the necrotic tissue and intensive care for the shock syndrome.

Alternative treatment

The other macrolides—roxithromycin, clarithromycin, azithromycin—appear to be as effective as parenteral penicillin G. Quinolones are not indicated in the treatment of erysipelas.

Although typical erysipelas can be readily distinguished from cellulitis (which can be of staphylococcal as well as streptococcal aetiology), differentiation may not be clear-cut in occasional circumstances. Under such conditions, particularly in an acutely ill patient, intravenous administration of a penicillinase-resistant penicillin (nafcillin or oxacillin) or a first-generation cephalosporin is warranted.

Prophylactic treatment

- Benzylpenicillin-benzatin (Tardocillin) 2.4 million units every 3 weeks for 1 or 2 years
- Erythromycin 250 or 500 mg twice a day.

Of importance for prophylaxis is the rigorous disinfection of minor injuries that may provide a portal for bacteria, usually streptococci, and the physical oedema therapy described by comprising manual lymph drainage and compression.

Although a possible risk for the development of deep venous thrombosis in the course of erysipelas exists, an anticoagulant treatment should be considered.

Opinions differ about the duration of antibiotic prophylaxis. It has been established that recurrences are reduced, but the effect is not dramatic. Continuous antibiotic prophylaxis is indicated only in patients with a high recurrence rate. Treatment of the local point of entry does not guarantee that there will be no recurrences. The dominant opinion is long-term (lifetime) antibiotic treatment for certain predisposed patients, long-term antibiotic treatment if local point of entry persists, and vigorous treatment of local factors.

Further reading

Dupuy A, Benchikhi H, Roujeau JC *et al.* Risk factors for erysipelas of the leg (cellulitis): case–control study. *Br Med J* 1999; 318: 1591–4.

Herpertz U. Erysipelas and Lymphodema. *Fortschr Med* 1998; 116 (12): 36–40.

Highet AS, Hay RJ, Roberas SOB. Cellulitis and erysipelas. In: Champion RH, Burton JL, Eblings FJG, eds. *Rook–Wilkinson–Ebling: Textbook of Dermatology*, 5th edn. Oxford: Blackwell Scientific, 1992: 968–73.

Mahé E, Toussaint P, Boutchnei S, Guiguen Y. Erysipeles dans la population jeune d'un hôpital militaire. *Ann Dermatol Venerol* 1999; 126: 593–9.

Erythema multiforme

F.M. Brandao

Synonyms

Erythema exudativum multiforme.

Definition and epidemiology

Erythema multiforme (EM) is a distinctive self-limited exanthematic cutaneous reaction to different stimuli, characterized by typical target lesions, with an acral distribution, sometimes with mucosal lesions, but rarely with systemic involvement.

Patients of all ages, predominantly adolescents and young adults, with no sex predominance, may be affected. An association with HLA Bw62 (15), B35 and DR53 has been reported in recurrent cases.

Two variants of EM are usually described: EM minor, without mucosal lesions or systemic symptoms, and EM major, in which cutaneous lesions are more widespread, mucosal (mainly oral) and some general malaise are present. EM major and Stevens–Johnson syndrome (SJS) have been considered for a long time to be the same condition; more recently, there is a tendency to consider EM minor and major as a part of the same spectrum (usually due to viral infections) and SJS and toxic epidermal necrolysis (TEN) a separate entity, more related to drug hypersensitivity.

Aetiology and pathophysiology

Viral infections, namely herpes simplex virus (HSV), account for most cases of EM. Even in the 30–50% of cases, in which no apparent cause can be found, most of them are probably due to subclinical herpes simplex infections. Other viruses (like hepatitis B virus (HBV), HCV, Epstein–Barr virus (EBV), adenovirus, infectious mononucleosis), *Mycoplasma pneumonia*, bacterial and fungal agents, contactants (*Primula obconica*, dinitrochlorobenzene (DNCB), poison ivy, tropical woods) as well as systemic diseases (such as autoimmune progesterone dermatitis, sarcoidosis, polyarteritis nodosa, Wegener's granulomatosis, lymphoma, carcinoma and leukaemia) have been associated with EM.

Drugs, the principal causative agents in SJS/TEN, are of much less importance in this side of the spectrum.

The pathophysiology is not yet completely understood, although it is generally accepted that EM is a hypersensitivity syndrome. Both circulating immune complexes and deposits of immunoglobulin M (IgM) and C3 have been documented, but their role in the pathogenesis of EM has not been demonstrated. A delayed-type hypersensitivity seems to be more plausible. The finding of HSV antigens and DNA in cutaneous lesions of some patients, even in idiopathic cases, supports the hypothesis that a cell-mediated immune reaction, aimed at the destruction of keratinocytes expressing HSV antigens, may be the pathogenetic mechanism.

Clinical characteristics and course

The target or iris lesion is the characteristic lesion in EM. It is defined as being less than 3 cm in diameter, with a well-demarcated border and at least three different zones: a central disk of dusky erythema or purpura that may become necrotic or transform into a tense vesicle, a ring of palpable pale oedema and an outer ring of erythema. Atypical targets may have only two zones and/or a poorly defined border. The eruption is usually pruritic, appears in an abrupt form and is acrally located: hands (dorsum and palms), wrists, elbows, feet and knees; more rarely the face, neck and trunk may be involved.

In EM major the central area may be bullous and haemorrhagic, and there is a more extensive cutaneous involvement (but less than 10%). Mucosal erosions in the oral cavity, with crusting on the lips, are commonly seen. Other mucosae (conjunctival and genital) are affected more rarely. General malaise and cervical lymphadenopathies, accompanying oral lesions, may occur.

Lesions develop in successive crops for a few days, with individual lesions lasting for 1–2 weeks and the whole eruption resolving in 2–3 weeks, usually healing with no scarring or sequelae.

Recurrence is seen mainly in herpes-associated EM and develops 7–10 days after HSV infection, although sometimes only subclinical infection occurs. In some patients EM have an almost continuous and chronic course.

Diagnosis

The diagnosis of EM is clinical and should not be confused with any other skin condition. Laboratory abnormalities are not frequent—elevated erythrocyte sedimentation rate (ESR), and moderate leucocytosis may be seen in EM major.

Histopathology may be helpful in atypical cases. Papillary oedema, vasodilatation and a perivascular lymphohistiocytic infiltrate are the earliest changes, with later extravasation of erythrocytes. A variable degree of necrosis of the lower layers of the epidermis may be found, running from vacuolar degeneration and focal necrosis of keratinocytes, to confluent epidermal necrosis.

Differential diagnosis

- Urticaria vasculitis: no target lesions that last for 24–48 h.
- Drug eruptions: no target lesions, generalized distribution.
- Annular erythemas: larger individual lesions with different localization, protracted course; no mucosal lesions.
- Secondary syphilis: may have annular lesions in palms and soles, but not in other localizations; it is not an acute eruption.
- SJS: individual atypical lesions, with predominance of epidermal necrosis and detachment, severe mucosal involvement.
- Kawasaki's disease: may resemble EM, but red lips, strawberry tongue, swollen palms and soles, lymphadenopathies are characteristic.
- Gingivostomatitis herpetica: no cutaneous lesions or herpes simplex labialis.
- Other diseases with mucosal involvement (erosive lichen planus, pemphigus): chronic diseases with different cutaneous lesions.

Treatment

General therapeutic guidelines

- Most cases, especially of EM minor, have a mild and self-limited course and do not need any specific therapy, but only symptomatic measures to relieve pruritus and malaise.
- In EM major attention should be directed mainly at mucosal lesions, to prevent infection and scarring.
- The use of systemic corticosteroids is controversial, but seems indicated to abort severe reactions.
- In recurrent cases long-term antiviral therapy may be helpful.

Recommended therapies

General symptomatic therapy

In most cases of EM minor simple therapeutic attitudes are enough—oral antihistamines to relieve pruritus (hydroxizine 25 mg b.i.d.), medium potency topical corticosteroids in cutaneous lesions, and saline or Burow's solution dressings in folds. When symptoms are more severe, acetoaminophen and non-steroidal anti-inflammatory drugs (NSAIDs) may be administered. If there is proven secondary infection or if EM is associated with *Mycoplasma pneumoniae* oral antibiotics (erythromycin 0.5–1 g t.i.d.) are indicated.

Systemic corticosteroids are beneficial in EM major—prednisone (or equivalent) should be administered in doses of 0.5–1.0 mg/kg per day, with gradual tapering in 2–4 weeks.

Treatment of mucosal lesions

Good nursing is of the utmost importance in patients with mucosal lesions. Careful oral hygiene with antiseptic solutions—hydrogen peroxide 3%, povidone iodine, chlorhexidine—a soft bland diet, topical anaesthetics (e.g. viscous lidocaine (lignocaine)), liquid antacids and topical corticosteroids (clobetasol propionate, fluocinonide or triamcinolone in orabase) can all be important in alleviating patient discomfort.

In the rare cases with ocular involvement the prevention of scarring and secondary infections are the priorities—saline dressings for removal of crusting, local antibiotics (chloramphenicol), associated or not with corticosteroids and, more important than anything else, atraumatic and frequent debridement of tarsal and bulbar conjunctival adherences. In other mucosae the objectives and therapeutic approaches are the same.

Treatment of recurrent erythema multiforme (REM)

This is a challenge. Long-term oral aciclovir is beneficial in recurrent herpes-associated EM and in some 'idiopathic' cases, which are probably due to subclinical herpes simplex infections: 400 mg twice daily is indicated in these patients. However administration of aciclovir during or immediately after herpes simplex episode may not prevent EM. In cases of aciclovir failure, valaciclovir proves useful.

Thalidomide has been successfully used in chronic EM, in patients resistant to other therapies (prednisone, aciclovir). One hundred milligrams per day reduced the duration of the episodes and remission was maintained with lower-dose treatment.

Patients with non-HSV associated REM may respond to dapsone, hydroxychloroquine or azathioprine.

In refractory cases long-term therapy with low doses of prednisone may be justified, but corticosteroidal side-effects may limit the use of this approach.

Alternative and experimental treatments

Experimental treatments have been used mainly in chronic EM and REM, where other therapies have failed—levamisole (whether or not in association with prednisone), cimetidine and ciclosporin A have all been used with variable degrees of success. In the absence of controlled studies they must be regarded with caution.

A patient with palmoplantar chronic EM was successfully treated with oral PUVA. Another patient with REM and chronic HCV infection resolved with interferon-α.

Further reading

Assier H, Bastuji-Garin S, Revuz J, Roujeau J-C. Erythema multiforme with mucous membrane involvement and Stevens–Johnson syndrome are clinically different disorders with distinct causes. *Arch Dermatol* 1995; 131: 539–43.

Brice SL, Leahy MA, Ong L *et al.* Examination of non-involved skin, previously involved skin and peripheral blood for herpes simplex virus DNA in patients with recurrent herpes-associated erythema multiforme. *J Cutan Pathol* 1994; 21: 408–12.

Cherouati K, Claudy A, Souteyrand P *et al.* Traitement par thalidomide de l'erythème polymorfe chronique formes récidivantes et subintrantes. Étude rétrospective de 26 malades. *Ann Dermatol Venereol* 1996; 123: 375–7.

Dowd PH, Champion RH. Erythema multiforme. In: Champion RH, Burton JL, Burns DA, Breathnach SM, eds. *Rook/Wilkinson/Ebling Textbook of Dermatology*, 6th edn. Oxford: Blackwell Science, 1998: 2081–5.

Dumas V, Thieulent N, Souillet AL *et al.* Recurrent erythema multiforme and chronic hepatitis C: efficacy of interferon alpha. *Br J Dermatol* 2000; 142: 1248–9.

Fritsch PO, Ruiz-Maldonado R. Erythema multiforme. In: Freedberg IM, Eisen AZ, Wolff K *et al.*

eds. *Fitzpatrick's Dermatology in General Medicine*, 5th edn. New York: McGraw-Hill, 1999: 636–44.

Kerob D, Assier-Bonnet H, Esnault-Gelly P *et al.* Recurrent erythema multiforme unresponsive to acyclovir prophylaxis and responsive to valacyclovir continuous therapy. *Arch Dermatol* 1998; 134: 876–7.

Morison WL, Anhalt GJ. Therapy with oral psoralen plus UV-A for erythema multiforme. *Arch Dermatol* 1997; 133: 1465–6.

Tatnall FM, Schofield JK, Leigh IM. A double blind, placebo controlled trial of continuous acyclovir therapy in recurrent erythema multiforme. *Br J Dermatol* 1995; 132: 267–70.

Erythema nodosum

A. Claudy

Definition and epidemiology

Erythema nodosum (EN) is an acquired acute or subacute/chronic disease characterized by deep erythematous, tender nodules, typically over the pretibial areas of the legs. A chronic variant of EN, termed subacute nodular migratory panniculitis (Villanova's disease), has also been described. EN occurs in all races and both sexes and has no genetic inheritance.

Aetiology and pathophysiology

EN is an idiopathic disorder. The evidence for EN as a cutaneous manifestation of an immune response is still circumstantial. EN may be regarded as a reaction pattern that has a number of possible causes. It is thought to be mediated by immune mechanisms that develop in response to a variety of antigenic stimuli such as a viral, bacterial (streptococci), mycobacterial, deep fungal infections (coccidioidomycosis and blastomycosis), sarcoidosis, lymphomas, intestinal inflammatory diseases and drugs (especially oral contraceptives, and possibly halogens). *Yersinia* infection is a common underlying condition. A common pathogenic mechanism may be suggested as a result of the immune host response to circulating immune reagents. This may possibly cause immune complexes that precipitate EN. In inflammatory bowel diseases, EN may be caused as a result of increased intestinal permeability to endogenous or exogenous antigens. EN may also be the result of alterations in cellular immune functions. Recent studies have shown differences in the usage of the T-cell receptor (TCR) Vβ subsets in EN associated with inflammatory bowel diseases, suggesting a potential role of superantigens. EN may also be induced by radiotherapy. Breakdown products of cancer cells destroyed by radiation might activate circulating antibodies and complement to form immune complexes thereby triggering the reaction. Radiotherapy is also known to activate several reactive dermatoses.

Clinical characteristics and course

EN is a septal granulomatous panniculitis. The acute form becomes manifest as red, tender nodules of the anterior surface of the lower leg, which involute within a few weeks. It may be accompanied by fever and arthralgias. Angina, diarrhoea, intermittent abdominal pain, hepatitis or a past history of tuberculosis may be indicative of a causative agent.

In the chronic form, the subcutaneous non-tender nodules coalesce into plaques with central clearing and last for some months.

Diagnosis

The clinical features are generally enough to establish the diagnosis of EN. Skin biopsy shows septal panniculitis, which is mostly useful to rule out lobular panniculitis, nodular vasculitis and periarteritis nodosa. The biopsy should be obtained from the central portion of the lesion and should be deep enough to incorporate subcutaneous fat.

Differential diagnosis

Erythema induratum (Bazin's disease) is a clinical entity that differs from EN in being characterized by recurrent crops of violaceous nodules over the posterior part of the legs, often with tuberculin hypersensitivity and response to antituberculous drugs. Superficial migratory thrombophlebitis may be misdiagnosed as EN. In EN with severe histological vascular involvement, the possibility of cutaneous periarteritis nodosa must be excluded.

Table 1 Treatment of acute and chronic EN

Acute EN	
Without systemic symptoms ('idiopathic type')	
	bed rest
	analgesic drugs (paracetamol, acetyl salicylic acid) *or* potassium iodide
With systemic symptoms	
	bed rest
	potassium iodide *or* NSAIDs (ketoprofen, indomethacin, naproxen)
According to aetiological factors	
	serological test for *Yersinia* + erythromycin or tetracycline
	ASLO titres elevated: penicillin
	Mantoux test + and chest film + antituberculous drugs
	sarcoidosis: no treatment
Chronic EN	
Bed rest	
NSAIDs *or* colchicine *or* hydroxychloroquine	

Treatment (Table 1)

General therapeutic guidelines

Bed rest should be recommended for EN, which may resolve spontaneously in a relatively short period. Since EN is self-limited, the most significant concern remains the identification and treatment of the underlying provocative cause.

Recommended therapies

Treatment of acute EN

Potassium iodide is the treatment of choice. Potassium iodide is a compound made of 76% of the halogen iodide and 23% of the alkali metal potassium by weight. After ingestion, potassium iodide is readily absorbed in the intestinal tract and rapidly distributed through the extracellular space. Iodide concentrates in the thyroid gland but also in other tissues such as salivary glands, gastric mucosa and mammary gland.

Potassium iodide may take effect so promptly that the efficacy of the medication can be easily evaluated. The oral dose is 300 mg 3 times daily. Complete remission of lesions occurs within 10–14 days after administration, especially if the medication is administered shortly after the initial onset of EN. The best response is noted in patients with EN associated with systemic symptoms such as fever and joint pains, and a positive C-reactive protein. Nausea and vomiting occasionally occur, but there is usually no need to discontinue the medication. Adverse cutaneous reactions may include erythematous, purpuric, urticarial, acneiform, nodular, pustular and vegetative lesions. Apart from these rather minor side-effects, major adverse reactions may occur in pregnant patients and those with a history of kidney or thyroid disease. The development of profound hypothyroidism secondary to exogenous intake of iodide has been reported. The inhibition of organic binding of iodide in the thyroid gland by excess iodide, resulting in the cessation of thyroid hormone synthesis, is known as the Wolff–Chaikoff effect.

The mechanism by which potassium iodide exerts its therapeutic effects in EN has not been elucidated. One hypothesis is that potassium iodide may cause heparin to be released from mast cells and heparin, in turn, suppresses cellular immunity. The drug may also modulate the function of neutrophils by suppressing the generation of hydrogen peroxide and hydroxyl radicals. These oxygen intermediates are so strongly reactive that the tissue could be damaged. Potassium iodide, by interfering with the production of oxygen intermediates, confers protection from auto-oxidative tissue injury.

- Bed rest and potassium iodide should be recommended in acute EN whatever the aetiology.
- Treatment with colchicine at a dose of 1 mg/day for 1 month has been proposed in acute EN with fever and arthralgias.
- EN may involve sarcoidosis. In 80% of patients affected, the sarcoidosis resolves spontaneously, and therapy is

seldom indicated. The treatment of EN is then similar to that of acute non-symptomatic EN, as described above.

- EN symptomatic of intestinal infections must be treated with erythromycin, 250 mg four times daily, or tetracycline, 1.5 g daily, for 4–6 weeks.
- EN caused by a fungal infection, especially kerion of the scalp, responds to griseofulvin administered for a 6-week period.
- EN indirectly associated with oral contraceptives often regresses when they are discontinued.
- Acute hepatitis B and C are sometimes associated with EN. The nodules usually resolve slowly after the acute phase. A close temporal association between hepatitis B vaccination and the onset of EN has been reported, with spontaneous disappearance of the lesions.

Treatment of chronic EN

Although EN is a chronic debilitating illness for which many treatment modalities have been suggested, none is universally effective. Although patients readily respond to corticosteroids, the hazards of chronic administration encourage the search for an alternative approach. Chronic cases of EN are often unresponsive to large doses of aspirin, whereas they may respond dramatically to the anti-inflammatory effects of indomethacin in doses of 100–150 mg/day. The suppression of EN by indomethacin could be related to the inhibition of prostaglandin synthetase activity in the subcutaneous fatty tissue, and this may affect both cellular and humoral immune responses. Chronic EN may also be successfully treated with naproxen. However, indomethacin proved superior to systemic corticosteroids and may possibly offer advantages over other, less potent, non-steroidal anti-inflammatory drugs.

Hydroxychloroquine can provide an effective and safe alternative therapy for some patients with chronic EN at a dose of 200 mg twice daily, reduced to 200 mg once daily for 4 months.

In conclusion, EN is a relatively common disorder and most often benign. Generally, the diagnosis is clinical. Treatment is essentially symptomatic, consisting in bed rest and non-steroidal anti-inflammatory drugs or potassium iodide. Since EN is self-limited, the most significant concern remains the identification and treatment of the underlying cause.

Treatment of EN leprosum

Thalidomide is currently the recommended first-line therapy for the treatment of EN leprosum (ENL). Sheskin surveyed data from 4522 cases around the world and found a 99% response rate, although thalidomide has no direct effect against *Mycobacterium leprae*. Resolution of ENL occurs 24–48 h after the start of thalidomide therapy. A beneficial effect on reactional polyneuritis in ENL has also been reported.

ENL is associated with elevated levels of tumour necrosis factor-α (TNF-α and interferon-γ (IFN-γ). After thalidomide therapy, patients show decreased serum TNF-α and a decreased number of helper T cells. Thalidomide is a drug known for its inhibitory effect on TNF-α. The optimal dose to obtain a quick effect in ENL is 400 mg/day, with subsequent maintenance therapy at 100 mg/day. The duration of treatment varies from a few weeks to many years.

Plasma exchanges have also been reported to be efficient in ENL without recurrences after failure of conventional treatments.

Further reading

Alloway JA, Franks LK. Hydroxychloroquine in the treatment of chronic erythema nodosum. *Br J Dermatol* 1995; 132: 661–2.

Barnhill RL, McDougall AC. Thalidomide use and possible mode of action in reactional lepromatous leprosy and in various other conditions. *J Am Acad Dermatol* 1982; 7: 317–23.

Barton Sterling J, Heymann WR. Potassium iodide in dermatology. A 19th century drug for the 21st century. Uses, pharmacology, adverse effects, and contraindications. *J Am Acad Dermatol* 2000; 43: 691–7.

Fearfield LA, Bunker CB. Radiotherapy and erythema nodosum. *Br J Dermatol* 2000; 142: 189.

Heymann WR. Potassium iodide and the Wolff-Chaikoff effect: relevance for the dermatologist. *J Am Acad Dermatol* 2000; 42: 490–2.

Honma K, Saga K, Onodera H, Takahashi M. Potassium iodide inhibits neutrophil chemotaxis. *Acta Dermatol Venereol* 1990; 70: 247–9.

Klausner JD, Freedman VH, Kaplan G. Thalidomide as an anti-TNFα inhibitor: implications for clinical use. *Clin Immunol Immunopathol* 1996; 81: 219–23.

Lehman CW. Control of chronic erythema nodosum with naproxen. *Cutis* 1980; 26: 66–7.

Ochonisky S, Revuz J. Thalidomide use in dermatology. *Eur J Dermatol* 1994; 4: 9–15.

Sheskin J. The treatment of lepra reaction in lepromatous leprosy. Fifteen years experience with thalidomide. *Int J Dermatol* 1980; 19: 318–22.

Takagawa S, Nakamura S, Yokozeki H, Nishioka K. Radiation-induced erythema nodosum. *Br J Dermatol* 1999; 140: 372–3.

Tseng S, Pak G, Washenik K, Pomeranz MK, Shupack JL. Rediscovering thalidomide. a review of its mechanism of action, side effects and potential uses. *J Am Acad Dermatol* 1996; 35: 969–79.

Ubozy Z, Persellin RH. Suppression of erythema nodosum by indomethacin. *Acta Dermatol Venereol* 1982; 62: 265–6.

Erythrasma

E. Koumantaki-Mathioudaki

Definition and epidemiology

Erythrasma is usually described as a mild bacterial infection. It is located in intertriginous areas of the body and is due to disorders of the normal flora of the skin. The incidence increases with age and is higher in middle-aged persons. Both sexes are affected, although the disease is more common in men.

In most cases the diagnosis is based on clinical considerations; as a result the non-identification, with laboratory tests, of the responsible organism precludes accurate statistics on the incidence of erythrasma. In any case, it is usually reported in the literature that the incidence could be over 20% in the general population. A warm and humid climate, diabetes, hyperhidrosis, obesity and inadequate hygiene are predisposing factors. The disease is rarely contagious, if ever.

Aetiology and pathophysiology

Corynebacterium minutissimum is held to be responsible for erythrasma, although, very rarely, other species of *Corynebacterium* can be isolated, individually or in coexistence. This organism is a microaerophilic, pseudodiphtheroid, Gram-positive bacterium, and is to be found among the normal flora of the skin; it produces porphyrins and could cause erythrasma whenever there is a disorder of the local defence mechanism. The composition and classification of these porphyrins have not been defined with certainty.

Clinical characteristics and course

Erythrasma is usually located in the scrotum and the intertriginous groin areas. Less often, lesions may appear in the axillae, the intergluteal and submammary flexures, the skin of the hypogastrium in obese persons, and the toe clefts. Very rarely, in girls and women erythrasma may appear in the vulva.

Morphologically, there is an initial appearance of reddish or brownish macular patches, which gradually spread and can reach the size of a palm. These lesions attain distinct margins; smaller satellite lesions occasionally occur in neighbouring areas. The surface of the skin is usually soft and may wrinkle slightly, while fine scaling is possible. The disease is usually asymptomatic. Occasionally, itching, or burning sensation, may start because of sweating. Without treatment, lesions can persist for months or for years, with exacerbations during the summer.

Diagnosis (laboratory examinations)

1. Direct microscopic examination of scales with Gram stain, or Giemsa or KOH, shows rod-like bacteria and filaments.
2. The use of a Wood's lamp shows red-coral fluorescence. May be negative if patient has bathed recently.
3. Culture under certain microaerophilic conditions in enriched nutritive medium for 5–7 days, yields colonies, which also fluoresce.
4. Histological examination is not much help for confirmation of the diagnosis, because the filamentous bacteria are found at the top of the stratum corneum. However, when Wood's lamp test is negative it might be worth insisting on finding bacterial structures in the histological section.

Differential diagnosis

- Tinea cruris: lesions have a raised erythematous border with central clearing.

- Inverse psoriasis: lesions are usually more inflammatory.
- Seborrhoeic dermatitis.
- Tinea versicolor: smaller lesions that appear in similar locations as those of erythrasma, but elsewhere on the trunk as well.
- Tinea pedis: when erythrasma is located in the toe clefts; difficult.
- *Candida* infection: when erythrasma is located in the vulva; difficult, since in some cases Wood's lamp test is negative.

In all the above cases laboratory confirmation should be obtained.

Treatment

General therapeutic guidelines

Regular washing with an antiseptic is helpful during the treatment; it can also prevent relapses. Acid soaps may impede the action of topical antimycotics, however, the use of strong antiseptics is questionable, since there is a serious probability of producing disorders of the local protective mechanism of the skin's normal flora. Given the fact that there is a pronounced tendency to recurrence, the intertriginous areas should be kept dry with the use of suitable powders, while clothes and/or shoes should be appropriate.

Recommended therapies

Topical

Creams or lotions of imidazoles or broad-spectrum antibiotics twice daily for 15 days are recommended for successful treatment. The broad-spectrum antibiotics for this case include fucidic acid, clindamycin and erythromycin.

Systemic

Erythromycin 250 mg orally every 6 h for 14 days, or 500 mg every 8 h for 7 days, or the same dose every 6 h for 3 days will produce clearing of the lesions within a few weeks. Clarithromycin 1 g orally in a single dose is a safe, cost-effective and well-tolerated alternative treatment.

There is no sure way of knowing which of the above therapies, topical or systemic, should be preferred. It appears, however, that in extensive and/or recurrent lesions the systemic treatment is more effective. The disappearance of the red-coral fluorescence confirms the efficacy of treatment; however, the brownish hyperpigmentation can persist for a while.

Further reading

Allen S, Christmas TI, Mckinney W, Parr O, Oliver GF. The Auckland skin clinic tinea pedis and erythrasma study. *N Z Med J* 1990; 103: 391–3.

Braun-Falco O, Plewing C, Wolff HH, Winkelmann RK. *Dermatology*. Berlin: Springer, 1991: 181–2.

Golledge CL, Phillips G. *Corynebacterium minutissumum* infection. *J Infect* 1991; 23: 73–6.

Haman K, Thorn P. Systemic or local treatment of erythrasma? A comparison between erythromycin tablets and fucidin cream in general practice. *Scand J Prim Health Care* 1991; 9: 35–9.

Marinella MA. Erythrasma and seborrheic dermatitis of the groin (letter). *Am Fam Phys* 1995; 52: 2012.

Mattox TF, Rutgers J, Yoshimori RN, Bhatia NN. Nonfluorescent erythrasma of the vulva. *Obstet Gynecol* 1993; 81: 862–4.

Puissant A. Mycoses cutaneomuqueuses et erythrasma. In: Monsalier JF, Carli A, Dhainaut JG, eds. *Precis de Therapeutique*. Paris: Maloine, 1990: 845–7.

Wharton RJ, Wilson LP, Kincannon MJ. Erythrasma treated with single dose clartithromycin. *Arch Dermatol* 1998; 134: 671–2.

Erythroplasia of Queyrat

B.-R. Balda

Synonym

Epithéliome papillaire nu of Darier.

Definition and epidemiology

Erythroplasia of Queyrat is a carcinoma *in situ* of the mucosa and the transitional epithelia. It resembles Bowen's disease and therefore the terms are frequently equated.

Predominantly uncircumcised men between the age of 40 and 50 are affected. The lesions are localized on the glans penis and the prepuce. Erythroplasia of Queyrat may also be found in the anal region, in the vulva and the oral mucosa.

Aetiology and pathophysiology

Erythroplasia of Queyrat is an intraepidermal carcinoma. For the most part, its histological picture is identical with that of Bowen's disease. Mitoses and numerous dysplastic cells are found, although there is less single cell keratinization than in Bowen's disease. Occasionally type 16 human papillomaviruses (HPV) have been demonstrated.

Clinical characteristics and course

This carcinoma is usually found as singular infiltrated-looking erythemas that are chiefly irregular, but with very sharply defined margins. They are crimson in colour, the exudative surface shiny or erosive. Slightly raised areas usually indicate an invasive carcinoma. When making a prognosis, caution is advised since the onset of primary lymphogenic metastasis can occur at a very early stage.

Diagnosis

When there is a clinically justified suspicion of erythroplasia of Queyrat, a biopsy followed by histological validation of the diagnosis is mandatory. If appropriate, several biopsies should be taken to rule out with certainty an invasive carcinoma. This particularly applies to greater, multilocular and partially raised lesions. Sonographic examination of the regional lymph nodes is also essential.

Differential diagnosis

The pathological spectrum is broad and comprises:

- erosive balanitis
- benign chronic circumscribed plasmocytic balanoposthitis
- genital psoriasis
- fixed toxic drug eruption
- bowenoid genital papulosis (detection of HPV 16)
- lichen planus.

Treatment

General therapeutic guidelines

Treatment should be initiated without delay. The procedure depends on the results of the histological examinations. If there is already evidence of the transition to an invasive carcinoma, surgical excision of the entire lesion followed by grafting is imperative. The tumour should be excised with a safety margin of 3 mm and combined with a sentinel lymphodectomy (for details, see Malignant melanoma chapter).

Other therapeutic options

In the case of purely intraepidermal changes, the following therapeutic options are available in addition to excision:

1. CO_2 laser ablation. This easily controllable procedure of coagulation that is gentle to the surrounding tissue must be followed by local antiseptic treatment.
2. Cryotherapy using the contact method (for smaller lesions) or the spray method (for larger lesions) usually requires three consecutive treatment

cycles. Attention should be paid to the marked oedema that commonly occurs and is the reason that a bladder catheter should be put in place for several days. The healing phase usually takes 3 weeks.

These two methods are conducted under local infiltrative or nerve-blocking anaesthesia. The target sites must be prepared according to standard surgical procedure.

3 Low kilovoltage X-ray technique (40–60 Gy, given in fractions of single doses of 3–5 Gy, 20 kV) is only considered an option in exceptional cases.

Alternative and experimental treatments

Recently, reports on photodynamic therapy modalities using both systemic as well as local (20% aminolaevulinic acid in ointment base) administration of a light sensitizer have been published. However, sufficient evidence on these methods is still outstanding.

Today, electrocoagulation and cauterization (e.g. with 50% zinc chloride solution) are no longer regarded as appropriate techniques. Similarly the external use of 5% 5-fluorouracil ointment, which can result in the transition from Queyrat's erythroplasia to an invasive carcinoma being overlooked is no longer recommended.

Check-up examinations

Patients must be advised to return for regular clinical check-ups over several years. These should include sonographical control of the regional lymph nodes.

Further reading

Beier C, Gregel C, Kaufmann R. Topische photodynamische Therapie mit 5-Aminolaevulinsäure bei M. Bowen. In: Garbe C, Rassner G, eds. *Dermatologie. Leitlinien und Qualitätssicherung für Diagnostik und Therapie.* Heidelberg: Springer, 1998: 341–2.

Factitial dermatitis

N. Tsankov and L. Stransky

Definition and epidemiology

Factitial dermatitis is a disease, partially or totally dependent on friction. It affects all ages and sexes and can coexist with various skin disorders. This coexistence is usually accidental but there are cases when the friction is a triggering factor for eliciting the onset.

The dermatological entities in which friction plays a role can be classified into the following groups:

1 Dermatoses totally dependent on friction
   - hyperkeratotic palmar dermatitis
   - pigment contact dermatitis.

2 Dermatoses in which friction plays an important role
   - juvenile plantar dermatosis
   - frictional dermatitis in children.

3 Dermatoses in which friction plays a limited role
   - atopic dermatitis
   - contact dermatitis.

Aetiology and pathophysiology

Mechanical friction is a widely accepted factor in the induction of dermatitis. Sometimes it is difficult to determine the 'chicken or the egg' since dermatitis induces friction due to pruritus, and friction induces dermatitis. Most cases have been termed 'neurodermatitis', narrowing its nosological position with the development of dermatological research estimating the causative factors. In the induction of contact dermatitis friction has an important role, enhancing the penetration of the allergen, as well as the irritant and thus triggering either the chain of the delayed sensitivity cascade or direct toxic damage causing dermatitis.

Clinical characteristics and course

As the condition consists of a number of entities the clinical chracteristics are variable. The clinical picture includes dermatitis with erythema, desquamation and changes, characteristic for chronic dermatitis and eczema. Lichenification with or without hyperpigmentation is present in atopic dermatitis in children and neurodermatitis in adults, and also in chronic contact dermatitis. In juvenile plantar dermatosis the affected skin has glossy, sometimes hyperkeratotic and fissured appearance on the contact areas of the anterior plantar aspects of the feet. In one communicated case of factitial dermatitis in children, small pinhead papules and warty lesions were noted on the knees, elbows and back of hands. Hyperkeratotic palmar dermatitis is usually connected with trauma and chronic psoriasis.

Diagnosis and differential diagnosis

To specify the eliciting disease careful patch testing should be performed. Once the contact dermatitis is excluded if the clinical picture is obscure a biopsy is a method of choice. Acanthosis, hyperkeratosis, spongiosis and lymphohistiocytic infiltrate in the upper dermis are characteristics.

Histological incontinentia pigmenti is present in cases with pigmented dermatitis. It is connected with friction and in most cases there are no clinical eczematous changes.

Treatment

General therapeutic guidelines

The main trend of treatment is to eliminate friction directly and indirectly by influencing pruritus.

Recommended therapies

Systemic tranquillizers are administered for at least a month and the effect is expected no earlier than the second week. Lichenification and hyperpigmentation can be treated with local steroid ointment once a day for 2 or 3 months. It is recommended that the local treatment be continued at least a week after the disappearance of clinical signs.

Tar preparations remain effective classic reductive therapy. Local retinoids and azelaic acid can be used with some success on hyperpigmented areas.

Alternative treatments

Local baths with radioactive mineral water have been prescribed additionally in some cases with focal lichenification.

High altitude climatotherapy is a nonspecific method with very good results, especially with regard to pruritus.

Further reading

Antony SJ, Mannion SM. Dermatitis artefacta revisited. *Cutis* 1995; 55 (6): 362–4.

Cronin E. *Friction Enhances Cutaneous Penetration of Allergens in Cement*. Edinburgh: Churchill Livingstone, 1980: 277.

Domingez-Soto L, Hojyo-Tomoka T, Vega-Memije E, Arenas R, Cores-Franco R. Pigmentary problems in the tropics. *Dermatol Clin* 1994; 12 (4): 777–84.

Kaplan B, Schewach-Millet M, Yorav S. Factitial dermatitis induced by application of garlic. *Int J Dermatol* 1990; 29 (1): 75–6.

Katsambas A. Quality of life in dermatology and the European Academy of Dermatology. *J Eur Acad Dermatoven* 1994; 3: 211–14.

Lachapelle JM, Bataille AC, Tennstedt D, Marot L. Pseudofactitial dermatitis: a useful clinical and/or histopathological concept. *Dermatology* 1994; 189 (Suppl. 2): 62–4.

Lotti T, Biandu B, Teofoli P. Dermatological Psychoneuroendocrine immunology, Nederlands Tigdschrift voor. *Dermatol Venerol* 1998; 8: 350–2.

Menne T, Hjorth N. Frictional contact dermatitis. *Am J Industr Med* 1985; 8: 401–2.

Nakayama H. Pigmented contact dermatitis and chemical depigmentation. In: Rycroft R, ed. *Contact Dermatitis*. Edinburgh: Churchill Livingstone, 1994: 648–51.

Patrizzi A, De Lernia V, Ricci G. Atopic background of a recurrent popular eruption in children (frictional lichenoid eruption). *Paediatr Dermatol* 1990; 7: 111–15.

Strumia R, Varroti E, Manzato E, Gualandi M. Skin signs in anorexia nervosa. *Dermatology* 2001; 203 (4): 314–17.

Tan HH, Tsu-Li Chan M, Goh Ci. Occupational skin disease in workers from electronic industry, Singapore. *Am J Contact Derm* 1997; 4: 210–14.

Tsankov N, Kamarashev J. Spa therapy, Bulgaria. *Clin Dermatol* 1996; 14: 675–87.

Furuncles and carbuncles

D. Ioannides

Definition, aetiology and pathophysiology

A furuncle (boil) is a deep, necrotizing form of folliculitis with involvement of the subcutaneous tissue. Several furuncles may coalesce to form a carbuncle. *Staphylococcus aureus* is the causative agent.

The initial pathophysiological event involves *S. aureus* colonization of the skin surface and proliferation with spread within the follicles. The organism may spread through follicular walls to the dermis or can be inoculated through cuts and scratches into the dermis leading to the formation of a furuncle. The attraction of polymorphonuclear leukocytes by the *S. aureus* chemotactic factors and the elaboration of several enzymes by the microorganism result in clinical inflammation. These enzymes include enterotoxins, proteases, haemolysins and leukocidins.

Clinical characteristics and course

A furuncle is manifested by a tender, round, subcutaneous nodule, which is usually capped with a small pustule. The follicular abscess enlarges, becomes fluctuant and then softens and ruptures spontaneously to discharge a core of necrotic tissue and pus and may result in scarring. The preferred sites of the furuncle are the hairy parts of areas exposed to friction and maceration, especially the face, scalp, buttocks and axillae. A carbuncle with multiple draining sites is found commonly on the neck, back and thighs. Predisposing factors are obesity, diabetes, prolonged sitting, tight irritating pants or immunodeficiencies.

Systemic symptoms, such as fever and malaise, are more frequently present with carbuncle. When infection occurs in the nasolabial area, extension via the vein draining into the cavernous sinus may lead to thrombosis. Perinephric abscess and osteomyelitis are other complications.

Recurrent furunculosis develops in some patients, in whom there is no evidence of harbouring specific staphylococcal strains or having any deficiency in their host defence mechanism. Such patients, who suffer from repeated infections, are usually nasal carriers of the infecting strain. The anterior nares can serve as a reservoir for spread into the skin and subsequent reinfection. Less common reservoirs for the pathogenic staphylococci may be found in the axillae or perineum.

Differential diagnosis

Furuncles must be differentiated from other bacterial infections, such as anthrax and tularaemia or from some other infections of the follicles, such as conglobate acne and hidradenitis suppurativa. In the latter, the location and multiplicity of lesions usually lead to the correct diagnosis.

Treatment

General therapeutic guidelines

Furuncles or carbuncles associated with fever or located on the face are better to be treated with a systemic antibiotic. Isolated lesions on other areas of the body can only be treated with local care and sometimes surgical drainage of pus.

Eradication of recurrent lesions is often difficult. Prolonged antibiotic therapy, along with adjuvant measures, is often necessary.

Recommended therapies

Systemic antibiotics

Antibiotics can be given systemically in furuncles or carbuncles associated with surrounding cellulites or with fever or located on the forehead, nose, cheeks or upper lid. Patients with recurrent furunculosis and immunocompromised patients are also treated with systemic antibiotics.

Knowledge of antibiotic sensitivity of the organism is desirable for the selection of treatment. If this is unknown, it is reasonable to begin with a semisynthetic penicillinase-resistant penicillin by mouth, such as cloxacillin at a dose of 250 mg every 4–6 h or dicloxacillin at a dose of 500 mg every 6 h for 10 days. For penicillin-sensitive patients, erythromycin (500 mg every 6 h for 10–15 days) or clindamycin (300 mg every 6 h for 10–15 days) are suggested. I prefer to start with azithromycin, one of the relatively newer macrolides, at a dose of 500 mg on day 1, followed by 250 mg on days 2–5. Patient compliance is better with this dose schedule. If the organism is resistant to macrolides, oral therapy with a cephalosporin such as cefaclor or one of the newer quinolones, such as ciprofloxacin, is recommended.

In recurrent furunculosis, which represents a difficult therapeutic problem, the organism's antibiotic sensitivity should be assessed. The appropriate drug, most often a semisynthetic penicillin, is usually given for 1–3 months, but it can be administered for longer periods (6–12 months), if necessary. Rifampin (600 mg daily) or rifabutin (300 mg daily), because of the potential for rifampin of less drug interactions and greater tissue penetration, can be given for 7–10 days, along with a semisynthetic penicillin. In especially stubborn cases, their administration for longer periods, alone or in combination with other antibiotics, can be considered.

Local treatment

Topical therapy consists of the application of warm normal saline compresses (1 teaspoon of table salt in 2 cups of tap water) followed by the application of an antibiotic ointment. A daily bath with antimicrobial soap is advisable. Incision and drainage are particularly helpful to relieve the pressure and pain associated with furunculosis.

Local anaesthetics are usually not required before small furuncles are incised. Spray anaesthesia is in most cases adequate to provide enough local analgesia. The use of a number 11 blade with its sharp tapered end is preferable and, initially, a small (2–4 mm) rather than lengthy incision is better to prevent unsightly scarring. If the furuncle has been present a long time or is large, a longer incision may be required. Pressure is then gently applied to the abscess because sudden rupture of intrafollicular loculi may shoot purulent material from the wound. Sometimes, it is necessary to probe into the abscessed cavity with a curved mosquito forceps or curette to break these loculi, but only after injecting a small amount of 2% lidocaine (lignocaine) into the skin overlying the abscess.

In recurrent furunculosis, topical antibiotic ointment should be applied to the potential reservoir areas, e.g. the nostrils, axillae and perineum. Special measures for maintaining topical hygiene have also been proposed in repeated infections. It is not clear whether these measures add anything of benefit to the care of such patients. According to these instructions, patient and family should bathe and shampoo 1–2 times daily, nails should be clipped short to avoid scratching, precautions should be taken during shaving to soak the beard with hot water and discard or boil the blade, and clothing, including underwear, should be changed daily and laundered thoroughly.

Alternative and experimental treatments

Interferon-gamma, iron supplements, zinc sulphate, levamisole, pentoxyfilline and vitamin C have been used in the treatment of furunculosis in clinical and experimental settings.

Long-standing improvement of recurrent furunculosis was noted in patients with human immunodeficiency virus (HIV), following the administration of interferon-α. It was given at a dose of 50 μg on days 1, 2 and 3 of the first week, with a new cycle every 4 weeks.

Treatment with iron supplements for a period of 4 weeks was very beneficial in patients with furunculosis and hypoferraemia without anaemia. Recurrences of furunculosis were prevented after treatment with oral zinc sulphate, in cases with low serum zinc levels.

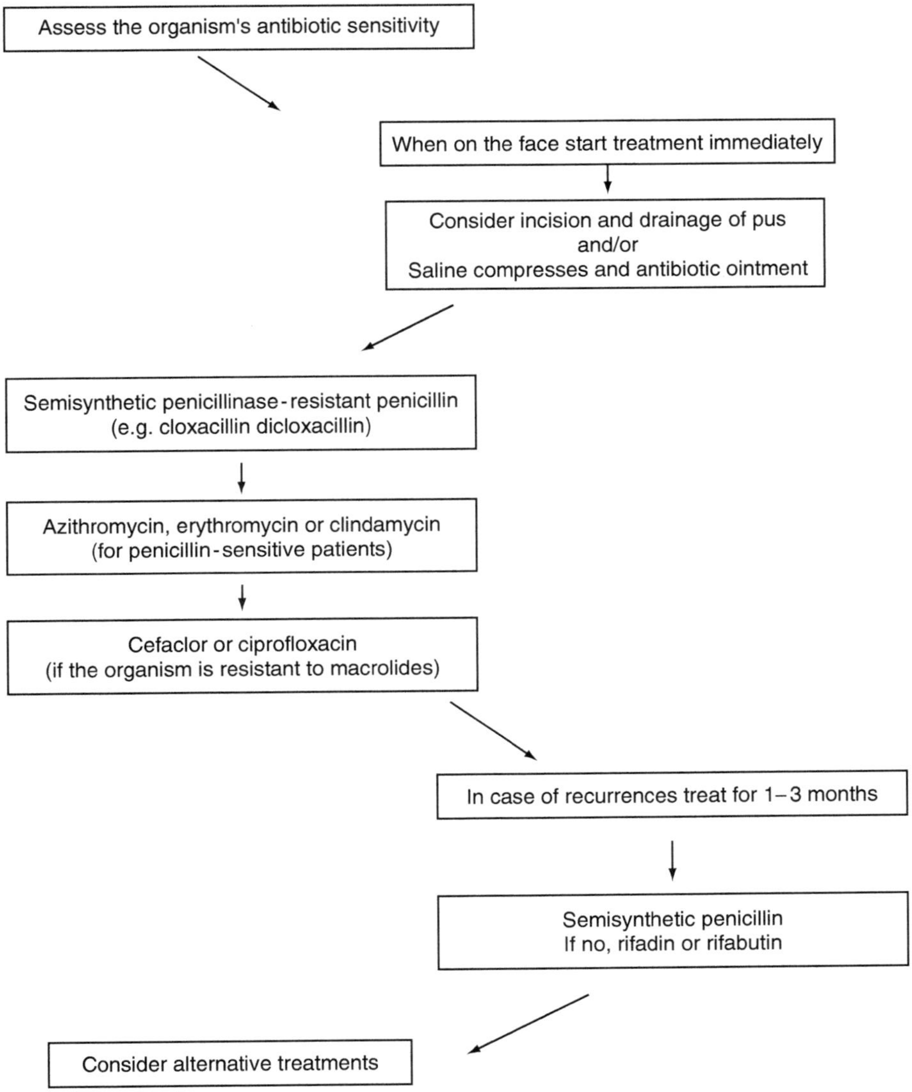

Pentoxifylline 400 mg t.i.d. for 2 months was successful in reducing recurrences in patients with chronic furunculosis.

Vitamin C has been found to be effective in the treatment of recurrent furunculosis in patients with impaired neutrophil function. It was administered alone at a dose of 500–1000 mg/day for at least 30 days, or in combination with levamisole at a dose of 2.5 mg/kg for 3 days per week.

Further reading

Brody I. Treatment of recurrent furunculosis with oral zinc. *Lancet* 1977; 2(8052–3): 1358.

Dahl M. Furuncles and carbuncles. In: Roenigk R, Roenigk H, eds. *Dermatologic Surgery*. New York: Marcel Dekker, 1989: 745–8.

Gentry LO. Therapy with newer oral beta-lactam and quinolone agents for infections of the skin and skin structures: A review. *Clin Infect Dis* 1992; 14: 285–97.

Hass DM, Feder HM Jr. Addition of rifampin to conventional therapy for recurrent furunculosis. *Arch Dermatol* 1995; 131: 647–8.

Katsambas A. Quality of life in dermatology and the EADV. *J Eur Acad Dermatovener* 1994; 3: 211–14.

Levy R, Shriker O, Porath A, Riesenberg K, Schlaeferr F. Vitamin C for the treatment of recurrent furunculosis in patients with impaired neutrophil functions. *J Infect Dis* 1996; 173: 1502–5.

Mallory S. Azithromycin compared with cefalexin in the treatment of skin and skin structure infections. *Am J Med* 1992; 91(suppl.): 36–9.

Rebora A, Dallegri F, Patrone F. Neutrophil dysfunction and repeated infection: influence of levamisole and ascorbic acid. *Br J Dermatol* 1980; 102: 49–56.

Shegren JN. Staphylococcal infections of the skin and skin structures. *Cutis* 1985; 36: 2–6.

Thoma-Greber E, Froschl M, Stoltz W, Landthaler M, Plewig G. Interferon-gamma. Therapy of recurrent furunculosis in HIV infections. *Hautartz* 1993; 44: 587–9.

Wadha-Yahar AV. Intractable chronic furunculosis: prevention of recurrences with pentoxifylline. *Acta Dermatol Venereol* 1992; 72: 461–2.

Weimer MC, Neering H, Welten C. Preliminary report: furunculosis and hypoferraemia. *Lancet* 1990; 336(8713): 464–6.

Granuloma annulare

C. Ligeron, L. Meunier and J. Meynadier

Definition and epidemiology

Granuloma annulare (GA) is a benign inflammatory acquired dermatosis of unknown aetiology, characterized by flesh-coloured or violaceous papules often arranged in rings.

GA occurs most frequently in children and young adults, although it can start at any age. There is a predilection for females (sex ratio 2.5 : 1). Rare familial cases and occurrence in identical twins have been reported, which is suggestive of a hereditary predisposition, but most cases of GA are sporadic.

Aetiology and physiopathology

Sometimes viral infections—human immunodeficiency virus (HIV), hepatitis C virus (HCV), Epstein–Barr virus (EBV), herpes simplex virus (HSV) and varicella-zoster virus (VZV)—can act as precipitating factors. GA associated with immunodeficiency (HIV, liver transplant) is more often generalized. It can present at all stage of HIV infection but it is slightly more common in patients with acquired immune deficiency syndrome (AIDS).

GA following insects bites, local trauma, intradermal reaction, HBV immunization, sunlight exposure or psoralen and ultraviolet A (PUVA) therapy, vitamin D_3 treatment or stressful events have also been described.

The generalized type of GA is most often associated with diabetes mellitus and requires a carbohydrate metabolism investigation.

The question of associated internal diseases like sarcoidosis, thyroiditis and malignant lymphoproliferative diseases remains a subject of debate.

Viruses could induce an atypical delayed hypersensitivity reaction. The presence of VZV DNA in early lesions of GA (demonstrated by the polymerase chain reaction) without histological viral cytopathic changes at sites of resolved VZV reactivation infection provides an argument for this hypothesis. It is likely that this delayed-type hypersensitivity mechanism (Th1) occurs in GA lesions, whatever the aetiology.

Activated helper T lymphocytes (following unknown antigenic stimuli) in cooperation with Langerhans' cells produce lymphokine, which recruit and activate histiocytes and macrophages. New studies suggest that interferon-γ is the most important Th1–associated cytokine and demonstrated that cytokine-like tumour necrosis factor-α and matrix metalloproteinases produced by macrophages elicit matrix degradation. In parallel, activation-induced apoptosis in lymphocytes and macrophages may serve to restrict the destructive potential of inflammatory cells.

Clinical characteristics and course

There are several forms of GA.

Localized GA

This is the most common form, predominantly affecting children and young adults.

Lesions are flat, firm, well limited, flesh coloured or red papules of variable size; they are usually asymptomatic. The epidermal surface is mostly undisturbed. The arrangement of papules is often annular and arciform. They are electively distributed on the back of hands and feet, on the fingers, and less frequently over the joints (ankles, wrists, elbows), the face (especially periorbital areas) and the scalp are rarely affected.

Generalized GA

About 15% of all patients with GA have more than 10 lesions. It occurs in patients younger than 10 or older than 40 years. It is a widespread papular eruption often involving the trunk, neck and extremities. Macules, nodules and papules may be present. Lesions do not always have annular configuration. Symmetry is a common feature. It shows a more chronic, relapsing course, only rarely resolves spontaneously and has a poorer response to therapy than the localized form.

Subcutaneous GA

This is a painless soft-tissue nodule of the extremities (especially pretibial location) or scalp and occurs almost exclusively in healthy children.One case of subcutaneous granuloma associated with immunoglobulin A (IgA) and IgG_2 deficiency has been reported. Nevertheless, because nodules are benign and may recur with or without surgical biopsy; reassurance is the best managment.

Perforating GA

This is a very rare disease, affecting both children and adults, characterized by multiple umbilicated and/or crusted papules on the dorsum of the hands and by pustular lesions and scars.

Most GA lesions resolve spontaneously over a period of several months to years without scars. But scars have been described after the perforating or the generalized forms sometimes with secondary anetoderma.

Diagnosis

Clinical investigation is the cornerstone of the diagnosis. Skin biopsy confirms in doubtful cases, such as when generalized or subcutaneous types are suspected.

Histology reveals focal degeneration of collagen in the upper and middle dermis surrounded by a palisading granuloma of histiocytes under a normal epidermis. In older lesions, numerous T lymphocytes and fibroblasts may appear. Tuberculoid reaction with many giant cells is unusual. Sometimes elastic fibre degeneration can be observed in sun-exposed lesions of GA.

Laboratory tests are usually not necessary except in the disseminated type in which glycosylated haemoglobin, HIV, HBV and HCV serodiagnostic should be investigated.

It may be advantageous to consider checking the thyroid-stimulating hormone and antithyroid antibodies before administrating medications that could affect thyroid function in patients with GA.

Magnetic resonance imaging can be helpful for the diagnosis of disseminated GA but must be confirmed by histology.

Differential diagnosis

Other annular dermatoses such as tinea corporis, lichen planus annularis, annular sarcoidosis, erythema migrans of Lyme disease, insect bites, late secondary or tertiary syphilis and erythema annulare centrifugatum should be distinguished from GA.

The subcutaneous type may occasionally simulate rheumatoid nodules, both clinically and histologically. However, children are healthy and there is no connective tissue disorder.

Clinical and histological differentiation between the plaque type of GA and necrobiosis lipoidica may sometimes be difficult. However, later sclerosis, atrophy and telangiectasia are more usual.

Perforating GA must be distinguished from other perforating dermatoses, such as elastosis perforans serpiginosa, reactive perforating collagenosis, calcinosis cutis. Histology confirms the diagnosis.

Nosological boundaries between GA and actinic granuloma are not yet clearly defined but most authors consider actinic granuloma as a specific entity. It is characterized by annular lesions on actinically damaged skin areas in patients older than those who have a classical GA. Histological examination shows, in addition to the lymphohistiocytic and giant-cell granuloma of the superficial dermis, an elastosic degeneration of elastic fibres.

Treatment

General therapeutic guidelines

GA is a benign asymptomatic dermatosis with a capricious and unpredictable course. Numerous therapies have been proposed, but at present no entirely effective treatment has an influence on outcome.

Most reports are of uncontrolled studies or individual cases, so that it is difficult to carry out a good evaluation of treatments. Treatment should be chosen after consideration of the age of the patient, clinical form, the extent of disease and the cosmetic and functional disability. Spontaneous healing and recurrences are frequent, so that treatment is not always indicated; it depends on the patient's wishes.

Several therapeutic measures have been proposed for localized GA, with varying degrees of success. Sometimes, lesions heal after biopsy, but some authors find this inefficient because of the frequent recurrences.

Internal treatment is virtually never indicated, except for the disseminated forms, which have a more chronic course.

Recommended therapies

Localized GA

Cryosurgery proved effective and safe in a prospective trial of 31 patients. Excellent cosmetic results may be achieved. The authors used nitrous oxide as a refrigerant, with a single freeze–thaw cycle of 20 s, covering the entire surface of small lesions and the active rim of larger lesions (> 4 cm diameter). Pain, bulla formation and local oedema are the major temporary adverse effects; lesional hypopigmentation and peripheral hyperpigmentation are the most commonly occurring long-term complications.

Intralesional injection of triamcinolone can also be used with the risk of secondary atrophy.

Topical corticosteroids (i.e. clobetasol propionate) under occlusion may be employed, but care should be taken to avoid side-effects such as atrophy of the near skin.

Some cases of localized GA have been treated with PUVA therapy but with a worse response than for generalized GA.

Subcutaneous GA

Excision of the lesions can be proposed when there is severe functional discomfort.

Generalized GA

This is often resistant to treatment. Modalities that are effective in localized GA, such as cryotherapy or intralesional injections of glucocorticosteroids, are inadequate for generalized GA, in which large areas of the body need to be treated.

In the first place, sulphones (dapsone 100 mg/day for 6–8 weeks) can be proposed. The major side-effects of sulphone therapy are haemolytic anaemia and methaemoglobinaemia, so that regular haematological monitoring is necessary.

PUVA therapy may improve the eruption and apparently even cure it but prolonged maintenance therapy is needed to preserve a disease-free state. It is not recommended for children under 12 years of age. The initial dose of UVA is determined by the patient's skin type (range 2–4 J/cm^2) and is increased by 0.5–1 J/cm^2 at each treatment, provided no significant erythema is present. Treatments are given two to three times a week during the clearance phase. Maintenance PUVA therapy is administered at weekly or biweekly intervals once patients are completely free of lesion.

The mechanism of action of PUVA therapy in GA is unclear; one possibility is selective elimination of the cells that are responsible for initiating the disease.

An alternative approach, psoralen bath and UVA therapy (PUVA bath therapy), avoids the adverse effects associated with oral PUVA therapy and is increasingly being used, with good responses in patients with generalized GA. High cumulative UVA (92 J/cm^2) doses were required and improvement was usually first noticed after 15–20 treatment sessions.

UVA1 is known to suppress delayed-hypersensitivity responses in the skin and patients with chronic generalized GA may benefit from this phototherapy. High dose should be given once daily 5 times per week for 3 weeks. This therapy seems to be well tolerated with improvement or clearance of lesions.

Retinoids, such as etretinate (0.8 mg/kg per day) and isotretinoin (0.5 mg/kg per day) may sometimes be effective. They must be used for at least 3 months. These drugs have an immunomodulatory action and inhibit delayed hypersensitivity responses. They also reduced fibroblast proliferation and collagen synthesis of human cultured fibroblasts, with a decreased production of collagenase.

Some authors have proposed a three-stage regimen of therapy. They initiate monotherapy with etretinate (up to 0.8 mg/kg per day) and switch to a low-dose treatment over a longer period of response; if there is no response, they switch to the second stage, i.e Re-PUVA therapy. The third stage is then low-dose etretinate to prevent relapses.

Antimalarials (chloroquine or hydroxychloroquine at the initial dose of 3 mg/kg per day and 6 mg/kg per day, respectively, for 3 weeks and then at half dose for 3 weeks) proved effective and safe in the control of disseminated GA in children. The first signs of regression of the skin lesions were noted after 10 days and complete remission was achieved within 4–6 weeks. Blood smears, serum creatinine levels and creatinine clearance and liver enzyme determinations were monitored every 2 weeks. The eyes were examined before and 2 weeks after therapy. No side-effects were observed. No relapses occurred during a mean follow-up period of 2.5 years.

Alternative and experimental treatments

Localized GA

- Topical vitamin E has been used twice daily, once under occlusion. After 2 weeks, the lesions were almost completely cleared. A possible explanation for the efficiency of this therapy could be its potential as an antioxidant and as a scavenger of oxygen free radicals.
- Vitamin PP.
- Laser CO_2 destruction.
- Intralesional fibroblast interferon.

Generalized GA

Little information is available on any of these treatments.

Three cases of GA that did not exhibit a self-limited course were treated with tranilast at a dose of 300 mg daily. The treatment resulted in the resolution of skin lesions within 3 months of administration.

Pentoxifylline has been used in one case of chronic GA. A dramatic clearing of the majority of papules was observed after 4 weeks of treament, without side-effects.

Potassium iodide has been used in few cases (initial dose of 450 mg/day, progressively increased to 1500 mg/day for 3–6 months) with little success. But it had no significant advantage over placebo and there is a risk of hypothyroidism.

Ciclosporin (6 mg/day for 1 month, then 3 mg/day for 3 months) was effective in one patient. Ciclosporin levels and serum creatinine levels were monitored twice monthly throughout treatment. After 4 months, complete clearing was obtained and there was no recurrence during the following year.

Therapy with low doses of alkylating agents, such as chlorambucil 2 mg twice daily for 4–12 weeks may be effective but should be used with care and in only the most severe cases because of severe side-effects such as induction of leukaemia and bone marrow depression.

One case of generalized GA associated with HCV totally regressed during α-interferon treatment prescribed for the chronic hepatitis.

Further reading

Burg G. Disseminated granuloma annulare: therapy with vitamin E topically. *Dermatology* 1992; 184: 308–9.

Derancourt C, Senser M, Atallah L, Becker MC, Laurent R. Granuloma annulare of the photo-exposed areas in two liver transplants. *Ann Dermatol Venereol* 2000; 127 (8–9): 723–7.

Filotico R, Vena GA, Coviello C *et al.* Cyclosporine in the treatment of generalized granuloma annulare. *J Am Acad Dermatol* 1994; 30: 487–8.

Grogg KL, Nascimento AG. Subcutaneous granuloma annulare in childhood: clinicopathologic features in 34 cases. *Pediatrics* 2001; 107 (3): E42.

Kerker BJ, Huang CP, Morison WL. Photochemotherapy of generalized granuloma annulare. *Arch Dermatol* 1990; 126: 359–61.

Muchenberger S, Schopf E, Simon JC. Phototherapy UVA1 for generalized granuloma annulare. *Arch Dermatol* 1997; 133: 1605.

Oberlin P, Revuz J. Granulome annulaire: quelles thérapeutiques? *Ann Dermatol Vénéréol* 1989; 116: 519–21.

Ohata C, Shirabe H, Takagi K, Kawatsu T. Granuloma annulare in herpes zoster scars. *J Dermatol* 2000; 27 (3): 166–9.

Rubel DM, Wood G, Rosen R *et al.* Generalized granuloma annulare successfully treated with pentoxyfilline. *Australas J Dermatol* 1993; 34: 103–8.

Schleicher SM, Milstein HJ, Lim SJM *et al.* Resolution of granuloma annulare with isotretinoin. *Int J Dermatol* 1992; 31: 371–2 (letter).

Schmutz JL. PUVA therapy of granuloma annulare. *Clin Exp Dermatol* 2000; 25 (5): 451.

Simon JC, Pfieger D, Schopf E. Recent advances in phototherapy. *Eur J Dermatol* 2000; 10 (8): 642–5.

Simon M, Von den Driesch P. Antimalarials for control of disseminated granuloma annulare in children. *J Am Acad Dermatol* 1994; 31: 1064–5.

Smith JB, Hansen CD, Zone JJ. Potassium iodide in the treatment of disseminated granuloma annulare. *J Am Acad Dermatol* 1994; 30: 791–2.

Toro JR, Chu P, Yen TS, Leboit PE. Granuloma anulare and human immunodeficiency virus infection. *Arch Dermatol* 1999; 135 (11): 1341–6.

Volden G. Successful treatment of chronic skin diseases with clobetasol propionate and hydrocolloid occlusive dressing. *Acta Derm Venereol* 1992; 72: 69–71.

Wolf F, Grezard P, Berard F, Clavel G, Perrot H. Generalized granuloma annulare and hepatitis B vaccination. *Eur J Dermatol* 1998; 8 (6): 435–6.

Wong WR, Yang LJ, Kuo T, Chan HL. Generalized granuloma annulare associated with granulomatous mycosis fungoides. *Dermatology* 2000; 200 (1): 54–6.

Yamada H, Ide A, Sugiura M *et al.* Treatment of granuloma annulare with tranilast. *J Dermatol* 1995; 22: 354–6.

Hand dermatitis

K. Thestrup-Pedersen

Definition and epidemiology

Hand dermatitis is a pruritic skin disease of the hands with intraepidermal vesicles (known to the patient as water blisters) followed by scaling and painful fissuring. Three main clinical pictures exist: contact dermatitis, pompholyx and keratotic hand dermatitis, and each will be described below.

Hand dermatitis is a disease both of children, and of adults early in their professional career. It is quite common. In Scandinavia, hand dermatitis has a cumulative 1-year prevalence of 10%. One important contributing factor is the high prevalence of atopic dermatitis. The risk of developing hand eczema in a person with previous atopic dermatitis is 35–50%.

Aetiology and pathophysiology

Hand dermatitis occurs mostly in predisposed persons except in cases of allergic contact eczema arising after exposure to potent allergens.

There are two anatomical types of skin on the hands: dorsal 'thin skin' and palmar 'thick skin' which includes the palmar aspects of the fingers and periungual skin (Fig. 1). The treatment principles differ for each category of hand dermatitis.

Contact dermatitis is primarily elicited by contact with triggers in the environment the most important of which are irritants and sometimes also allergens. Approximately 90% of cases with hand eczema are caused by contact dermatitis. It is located in thin skin and on the hands, including the volar aspects of the lower arms. Two-thirds of the patients are women.

Pompholyx or recurrent vesicular hand eczema is mostly located in palmar skin, though it can also appear in plantar skin. This type of eczema is sometimes called dyshidrotic eczema. The disease takes a cyclic course and seems mostly to depend on endogenous factors, although secondary contact allergies are common.

Keratotic dermatitis of the hands is a hyperkeratotic disorder of palmar and/or plantar skin. A prominent feature is painful fissuring. The disease is provoked by multiple repetitive trauma of palmar skin.

Activated T lymphocytes together with the antigen-presenting cells in the skin are important elements of eczema. The expression of adhesion molecules and secretion of chemokines and inflammatory cytokines are also involved. How the pathophysiology of toxic-irritant contact dermatitis differs from allergen-induced dermatitis is not quite certain. Also, the pathophysiology behind the different forms of hand eczema is not known.

Clinical characteristics and course

Contact dermatitis is primarily located to the thin dorsal skin of the fingers and finger webs, and the volar aspects of the wrists. Severity of the symptoms varies from patient to patient and over time. This type of hand eczema often occurs early in the patient's professional life and can be of an occupational nature. In the acute phase oedema and vesicle formation are the most prominent symptoms. It is closely related to exposure to irritants or allergens (Table 1). The acute phase is followed by a chronic phase in which scaling, infiltration and painful fissures are prominent features and pruritus is limited. Almost three-quarters of patients do not have contact allergies.

Pompholyx, or recurrent vesicular hand eczema, affects palmar and/or plantar skin either partly or completely. The disease starts with a sudden eruption of very severely itching vesicles which can last up to a week and is followed by scaling and

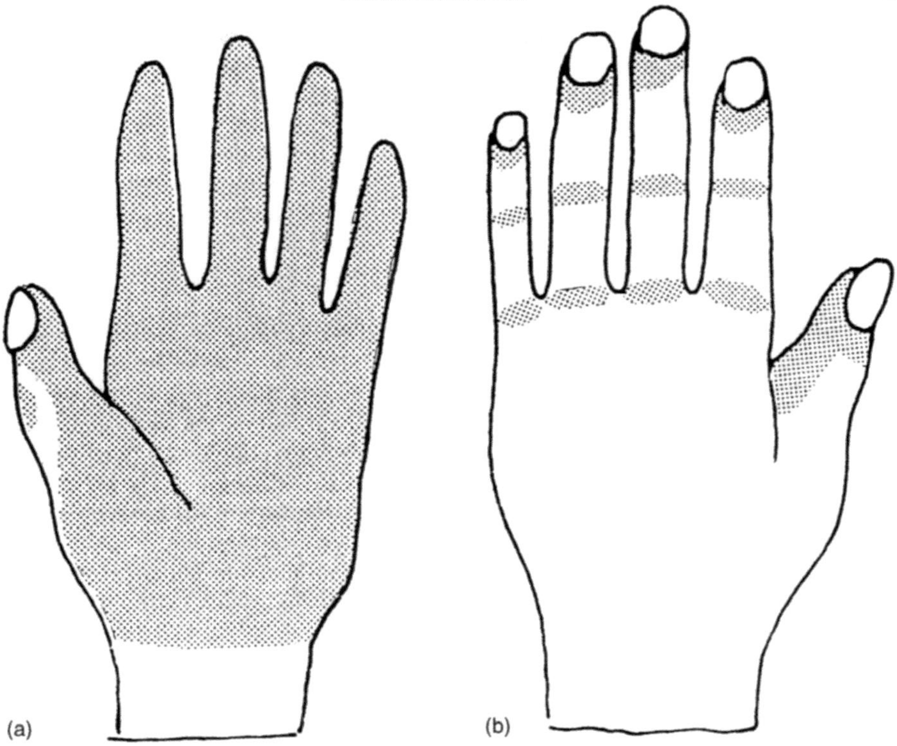

Figure 1 Palmar skin ('thick skin') is shown by the *grey shading*. Note that the border between (a) palmar and (b) dorsal skin goes round the sides of the fingers and that palmar skin extends around the nails up to the distal phalangeal joints. Palmar skin stops at the wrists

painful fissuring. Within a few weeks new vesicular eruptions occur. Patients with pompholyx are older than those with contact dermatitis and there seems to be an equal distribution between men and women. The course of the disease is not predictable. It may last for a few years and then dissappear. Relapse can occur. An Italian study has found that three-quarters are smokers, half have had previous atopic disease and one-fifth have nickel allergy. Other contact allergies, e.g. allergy to Compositae, are common, but although allergens and irritants may be eliciting factors they do not seem to be of primary importance for the course of the disease. At its worst pompholyx can incapacitate the patient, leading to a change of job or even permanent job loss and early retirement.

Table 1 The most common irritants and allergens found among 16 688 patients with hand dermatitis notified to the Danish Board of Occupational Health

Detergents and cleaning agents
Water and waste water
Metals
Food items
Rubber

Keratotic dermatitis of the hands is most common among 30–60-year-old men and is less frequent than pompholyx. The symptoms consist of abnormal hyperkeratosis in the palmar skin. There are no vesicles and pruritus is non-existent or limited to periods of aggravation. It is the painful fissuring of the hyperkeratotic skin that is most troublesome. The eczema often runs a chronic, constant course for years.

The overlap cases are those of hand dermatitis that do not strictly follow the regional anatomical differences in the hands. Very severe dermatitis can include all the skin on the hands. Potent allergens such as acrylates, epoxy resins and plant allergens can cause allergic contact dermatitis at every site of contact, irrespective of the thickness of the skin.

Diagnosis

Diagnosis and classification are based on the patient history and on clinical examination. Diagnostic patch testing with the standard series, supplemented with relevant allergens according to the patient's exposure, is very important. This author considers that patch testing and the interpretation of the results combined with guidance of the patient must be performed by an experienced dermatologist.

A clinically relevant, positive patch test(s) will identify the hand eczema as allergic contact hand dermatitis. If no contact allergy is found and the patient has had relevant exposure to irritants, the dermatitis is classified as irritant contact dermatitis. However, allergic contact dermatitis often involves a significant contribution from irritant factors.

Patients with pompholyx do almost always have contact allergies which are probably mostly acquired following the outbreak of the disease. The most common allergens are nickel and chromium followed by allergy to perfumes, rubber additives, colophony, preservatives and plants such as sesquiterpene lactones from Compositae plants. However, it is important to know about these allergies in order to reduce contact allergy as an aggravating factor in pompholyx. Allergen avoidance may improve the eczema considerably, but it rarely leads to a complete cure, underlining the multifactorial causes of eczema.

Keratotic dermatitis of the hands is rarely accompanied by contact allergies.

Differential diagnosis

Hand dermatitis is mostly due to the disease described above. Secondary infection of hand dermatitis with *Staphylococcus aures* is quite common.

Table 2 lists diseases which should be considered as differential diagnoses.

Treatment

General therapeutic guidelines

Although there are differences in the therapeutic principles for the three groups of hand eczema, all patients with hand dermatitis should adhere to measures designed to reduce the impact of both allergens and irritants on their skin. Table 3 lists measures that should be considered.

Table 2 Differential diagnoses

Reasonably common hand dermatosis
Physiological hyperkeratosis
Trichophyton rubrum infection of hands
Psoriasis
Pustulosis palmo-plantaris
Acrodermatitis continua Hallopeau (localized pustular psoriasis which involves fingers and nails)
Pompholyx-like reactions in palms seen in patients with athlete's foot (fungal infection)
Rare hand dermatosis
Lichen planus
Lupus erythematosus
Hyperkeratosis due to internal malignancies
Pityriasis rubra pilaris
Inherited palmar/plantar hyperkeratosis (Papillon–LeFevre syndrome, Mal de Meleda, Jadasohn–Lewandowsy's syndrome and others)

Table 3 Factors to be considered by persons with hand dermatitis

1	Reduce the amount of manual work in the family and discuss the various parts where the partner could—and should—help, e.g. cleaning, dish-washing, helping the children with their baths, changing of nappies, etc.
2	Short-term prophylatic measure of using gloves; however, do not use gloves for a long time as this will induce sweating of the hands. Use cotton gloves and loosely fitting neoprene gloves
3	Short-term use of disposable gloves when shampooing
4	Short-term use of disposable gloves to avoid contact with irritants: washing powder, dish-washing liquid, cleaning liquid such as toilet cleaner, etc.
5	Wash hands with mild, non-perfumed soap to reduce amount of skin bacteria
6	Avoid contact with certain food items: tomatoes, peeling of oranges, citrus fruits and such like. Avoid juice from fish, meat and certain vegetables. The patient's own experience will show what must be avoided
7	Buy dish-washing machine
8	Avoid hair-dying and potent allergens (e.g. certain plants, acrylic compounds, epoxy, etc.)

Allergen avoidance may also be beneficial, but not all contact allergies are clinically relevant.

Recommended therapies for hand dermatitis

Contact dermatitis

- Use moderate to strong topical steroid cream once or twice daily until all clinical signs of eczema are gone. Do not exceed 25 g/week on the hands. Then use the steroid twice or thrice weekly—irrespective of clinical signs of eczema. Do not exceed 10 g/week.
- Concomittantly, use emollients.
- Ensure compliance.
- Instruct patient about prophylactic measures (see Table 2).
- Grenz X-ray may be given as 10 kV 2 Gy weekly for a maximum of 6 weeks.
- Local PUVA can be given for up to 20–30 treatments (three times per week) and continued at a maintenance dosage once or twice weekly. A maximum of 200 therapies is recommended for a lifetime.

Pompholyx

- Potent topical steroids during the vesicular phase of the eczema.
- Emollients in the chronic phase.
- Desinfection using chlorhexidine bath 0.005%—or potassium permanganate 3% in a volume of 1 : 100.
- Systemic and local PUVA in severe cases.
- Methotrexate 15 mg weekly in severe cases.
- Ciclosporin 3–4 mg/kg per day in severe cases.

Keratotic hand dermatitis

- Keratolytic compounds such as an emollient with salicylic acid 5% or 10% preferably in an ointment base.
- Potent topical steroids.
- Tar containing ointment.
- Etretinate 25 or 50 mg daily.

Additional therapeutic comments

Contact dermatitis is often secondarily infected. It must be explained to the patient that if oozing becomes prominent the eczema is probably infected with *Staphylococcus aureus*. Daily use of mild soap diminishes this risk, but if the eczema is infected use either steroids combined with antibacterial compounds and/ or baths of hands containing an antiseptic. Systemic antibiotics efficacious against penicillinase producing *Staphyloccocus aureus* may be necessary.

Systemic use of steroids is not recommended in contact dermatitis, but may be used in severe cases.

Pompholyx is not easily treated. Systemic treatment with corticosteroids, methotrexate or ciclosporin has been found useful in selected patients with incapacitating pompholyx.

Patients with keratotic hand eczema benefit from keratolytic compounds, i.e. ointments containing salicylic acid. Tar therapy can also be quite effective whereas topical steroids are not sufficiently efficaceous unless a keratolytic agent is added. In severe cases systemic retinoids are effective.

Compliance is very important. The physician should stress to the patient that because of the recurring nature of hand dermatitis counselling and compliance are particulary important issues.

Further reading

Aberer W, Anderen KE, White IR. Should patch testing be restricted to dermatologists only? *Contact Dermatitis* 1993; 28: 1–2.

Halkier-Sorensen L. Occupational skin diseases. *Contact Dermatitis* 1996; 1 (Suppl.): 1–120.

Halkier-Sorensen L, Thestrup-Pedersen K. Effects of long-term application of a moisturizer: electrical capacitance, transepidermal water loss and skin surface temperature. A field study. *Contact Dermatitis* 1993; 29: 1–9.

Hersle K, Mobacken H. Hyperkeratotic dermatitis of the palms. *Br J Dermatol* 1982; 107; 195–202.

Larsen FS, Hanifin JM. Secular change in the occurence of atopic dermatitis. *Acta Dermato-Venerol* 1992; 176 (Suppl.): 7–12.

Lodi A, Betti R, Chiarelli G, Urbani CE, Crosti C. Epidemiological, clinical and allergological observations on pompholyx. *Contact Dermatitis* 1992; 26: 17–21.

Meding, B, Järvholm B. Hand eczema in Swedish adults—changes in prevalence between 1983 and 1996. *J Invest Dermatol* 2002; 118: 719–23.

Olesen AB, Ellingsen AR, Olesen H, Juul S, Thestrup-Pedersen K. Atopic dermatitis and birth factors. *Br Med J* 1997; 314: 1003–8.

Panconesi E, Lotti T. Steroids versus nonsteroids in the treatment of contaneus inflammation. Therapeutic modalities for office use. *Arch Dermatol Res* 1992; 284: 537–41.

Paulsen E, Andersen KE. Compositae dermatitis in a Danish dermatology department in 1 year (II). Clinical features in patients with Compositae contact allergy. *Contact Dermatitis* 1993; 29: 195–201.

Reitamo S, Granlund H. Cyclosporin A in the treatment of chronic dermatitis of the hands. *Br J Dermatol* 1994; 130: 75–8.

Sheehan-Dare RA, Goodfield MJ, Rowell NR. Topical psoralen photochemo-therapy (PUVA) and superficial radiotherapy in the treatment of chronic hand eczema. *Br J Dermatol* 1989; 121: 65–9.

Thestrup-Pedersen K, Andersen KE, Menne T, Veien NK. Treatment of hyperkeratotic dermatitis of the palms (eczema keratoticum) with oral acitretin. A single-blind placebo-controlled study. *Acta Dermato-Venerol (Stockh)* 2001; 81: 353–5.

Veien NK, Larsen P, Thestrup-Pedersen K. Efficacy and safety of longterm intermittent treatment of hand eczema with mometasone furoate fatty cream. *Br J Dermatol* 1999; 140: 882–6.

Herpes genitalis

S. Kroon

Definition and epidemiology

Genital herpes is a sexually transmitted infection with herpes simplex virus type 1 or 2 (HSV-1 or HSV-2), causing ulceration in the genital area.

Types of infection include:

- First episode primary infection in a person without prior HSV-1 or HSV-2 antibodies.
- First episode non-primary infection in a person with prior antibodies to the alternative virus.
- First recognized recurrence, which is HSV-1 or -2 in a person with prior HSV-1 or -2 antibodies.
- Recurrent genital herpes, which is caused by reactivation of latent HSV infection.
- Subclinical genital herpes, which is caused by reactivation of latent HSV infection in a person without clinically recognized symptoms.

Seroprevalence studies show genital herpes infections to be among the most common sexually transmitted diseases. In the USA 22% of adults have HSV-2 antibodies, in Scandinavia 17–30% of the pregnant population are infected and for the rest of Europe figures vary according to risk factors and age, between 7% to over 20%. More first episode diseases are caused by HSV-1, specifically in women, but the majority of recurrences are caused by HSV-2 because of the significantly higher reactivation rate. Seropositivity for HSV-2 is associated with viral shedding in the genital tract, and the rate of subclinical shedding is similar between persons with clinical symptoms and persons without a reported history of genital herpes.

Aetiology and pathophysiology

HSV-1 and HSV-2 are transmitted through direct contact with infected skin lesions, mucus membranes and secretions. HSV can be transmitted from mother to child during delivery or by nosocomial spread after delivery.

The herpes viruses are cytotoxic causing necroses of the infected epithelial cells and infiltration of inflammatory cells, mainly mononuclear, into the underlying connective tissue.

During natural infection with HSV a variety of humoral, cytokine and cell-mediated immune responses terminate virus replication and limits the infection.

The success of HSV as a pathogen and its key to survival depends on its ability to establish latent infection in the sensory sacral ganglia for the lifetime of the host. Viral fusion and entry into the nerve cell body occur rapidly after axonal contact and nucleocapsids travel to the neuronal nucleus through retrograde axonal flow. Available evidence suggests that HSV replication during the maintenance stage of latency is blocked at the level of viral early gene expression.

Clinical characteristics and course

First episode disease

In a prospective study 40% of newly acquired HSV-2 infections and 60% of HSV-1 infections were symptomatic. Men were more likely than women to acquire asymptomatic HSV-2 infection.

Clinical severity may vary depending on antibody status. In primary disease most patients are ill with a combination of systemic and local symptoms. Fever, headache, malaise and myalgia are experienced by 39% of men and 68% of women, HSV viral pharyngitis in 19% of patients. Pain, itching, dysuria, vaginal or urethral discharge, and tender bilateral inguinal adenopathy are the predominant local symptoms. Patients develop bilateral lesions in the genital area with erythema, oedema and multiple vesicles, followed by painful ulcerations. New vesicles may continue to evolve during the second week of the disease. Healing is the result of crusting (on skin) or re-epithelialization (on mucus membranes). HSV cervicitis or urethritis may occur as the only manifestation in 8% of women and 5% of men, respectively.

Transient systemic complications are common as aseptic meningitis and autonomic nervous dysfunctions in homosexual men with HSV proctitis: urinary retention, decreased sphincter tone or impotency. Autoinoculation may occur in up to 26% of women and 10% of men, predominantly in the second week, located on the buttocks, thighs, fingers or the eyes. Local complications as bacterial and fungal superinfections may occur in both men and women.

Patients with non-primary disease have a reduction in symptoms and complications are more rare. Less than half of the patients have bilateral lesions and the rate of extragenital autoinoculation is diminished.

Patients with first recognized recurrence have clinical symptoms corresponding to a recurrent episode of genital herpes. They have contracted the disease from months to years back in time either asymptomatic or without recognizable symptoms.

Recurrent episodes

The majority of patients with HSV-2 infection experience a recurrence during the first year after acquisition compared to around 60% of those with HSV-1 infection.

More than half the patients experience prodromal symptoms such as numbness, local tingling, neuralgia and itching as warning signs of an attack evolving. Prodromal pain may mimic sciatica. The prodromal phase may last from less than an hour up to several days. Not all prodromal symptoms are followed by a recurrence. Itching, erythema and oedema, but no vesicles, ulcers or crusts define abortive lesions.

Local and systemic symptoms are significantly less prominent. Lesions involve a smaller area that tends to be unilateral. New formation of vesicles, duration of viral shedding (mean 2–3 days) and time to complete healing, are shorter lasting 7–10 days. Women experience pain more often than men (88% vs. 67%), and the pain is of longer duration. Men seem to have more recurrences than women.

Known triggers of reactivation are:

- febrile illnesses
- stressful life events (controversial)
- premenstrual tension
- local traumatization
- sexual activity
- ultraviolet radiation (UVR) exposure (extra genital herpes).

Diagnoses

Viral culture is the gold standard test, allowing viral amplification and subtyping. In addition, drug resistance can be identified. Other specific tests are antigen detection, producing results within a few hours. In late healing lesions, in atypical disease or defining subclinical shedding, HSV polymerase chain reaction (PCR) may be more sensitive. HSV-PCR is now available for routine laboratory testing in some European countries and offers high detection rates in any HSV lesion. Serological testing (total antibodies) can help to diagnose primary infection and identify HSV-seronegative individuals. Detection of type-specific antibodies (Western blot or laboratory or office-based tests for detection of type-specific glycoproteins G1 and G2) can in some instances help identify discordant couples. Positive serology for HSV-1 cannot differentiate between oral and genital infection.

Differential diagnoses

- Apthae: viral culture, clinical examination.
- Recurrent erythema multiforme: viral culture, clinical examination.
- Adamantiades–Behçet's disease: viral culture, clinical examination.
- Primary syphilis: darkfield microsopy.
- Chancroid: microsopy.
- Epstein–Barr virus (EBV) ulcerations: viral culture.
- Fungal infections: culture.

Treatment

General therapeutic guidelines

- Aims for treatment are to reduce the morbidity of first episode disease, to reduce the risk for recurrent disease after a first episode and to prevent further transmission.
- Patients need advice to help them deal with the impact of psychosocial morbidity.
- Pregnant women with an established diagnosis of genital herpes before pregnancy have a very low risk for transmitting the virus to the neonate, even if they have a recurrence at term.
- Pregnant women who contract genital herpes in late pregnancy have a high risk for transmitting the virus to the neonate, and should deliver by caesarean section.
- Systemic treatment is more effective than topical antiviral treatment and is recommended by international guidelines.
- The use of a condom is encouraged to decrease the risk for contracting other sexually transmitted diseases and human immunodeficiency virus (HIV): HSV-2 infection may increase the risk for HIV acquisition and transmission.
- Patients need help to recognize minor symptoms. Most people contract the virus without symptoms but can still learn to recognize the disease when educated.

Recommended therapies

Antiviral therapy (Table 1)

First episode

Several randomized placebo-controlled trials have shown oral antiviral treatment to decrease the duration of antiviral shedding (2 vs. 10 days), time to healing of lesions (8 vs. 14 days) and prevent formation of new lesions. Neurological complications as aseptic meningitis and urinary

Table 1 Antiviral treatment of genital herpes

First episode	Oral aciclovir 200 mg five times a day for 7–10 days Oral valaciclovir 1.000 mg twice a day for 7–10 days Oral famciclovir 250 mg three times a day for 7–10 days
Recurrent episode	
Episodic	Oral aciclovir 200 mg five times a day for 5 days 400 mg three times a day for 5 days 800 mg twice a day for 5 days Oral valaciclovir 500 mg twice a day for 5 days Oral famciclovir 125 mg twice a day for 5 days
Suppressive	Oral aciclovir 400 mg twice a day Oral famciclovir 250 mg twice a day Oral valaciclovir 250 mg twice a day 500 mg once a day* 1.000 mg once a day

*Valaciclovir 500 mg appears less effective in patients with more than 10 recurrences per year

retention were also reduced. No significant differences have been found between oral aciclovir, valaciclovir and famciclovir. Adverse effects such as headache and nausea were rare and occurred with similar frequency in the placebo groups. In the studies aciclovir 200 mg five times a day for 7–10 days were compared with valaciclovir 1000 mg twice daily or famciclovir 125, 250 or 500 mg three times a day. The new antiviral drugs offer a more convenient dosing compared to aciclovir.

Episodic treatment of recurrent genital herpes

Mainly patients with a well-defined prodromal phase will benefit. Treatment must be patient-initiated by the first prodromal sign and patients should have their medication at home. One study comparing valaciclovir to placebo has found an effect on aborted recurrences. A number of randomized studies have shown oral antiviral treatment to be effective on duration of lesions, symptoms and viral shedding. The benefits of episodic treatment are however, minor compared to daily suppressive treatment.

In randomized controlled studies famciclovir 125–500 mg twice daily for 5 days vs. placebo decreased episode duration from 5 to 4 days and viral shedding from 3 to 2 days; valaciclovir 500 or 1000 mg twice daily for 5 days vs. placebo decreased the episode duration from 6 to 4 days and viral shedding from 4 to 2 days. Two studies that compared valaciclovir to aciclovir found no significant difference between the two drugs. In studies comparing aciclovir to placebo, 200 mg five times a day or 800 mg twice daily for 5 days, active treatment decreased duration of lesions from 6 to 5 days and decreased viral shedding from 2 to 1 days.

Suppressive or prophylactic oral treatment

Suppressive oral aciclovir treatment in immunocompetent patients has been evaluated in a number of placebo-controlled trials and has been proven to be highly efficacious for patients with frequently recurring genital herpes. The long-term safety and efficacy have been evaluated after suppressive treatment with aciclovir 400 mg twice daily for 5 years. Side-effects were few and drug-related toxicity was not registered. The study did not evaluate viral resistance prospectively, but treatment failures caused by viral resistance was not proven. Aciclovir treatment was associated with a reduction in the recurrence rate by 74–93% and in the duration of recurrences from 5 to 3.5 days. In patients treated with valaciclovir 500 mg or 1000 mg twice daily, 250 mg twice daily or aciclovir 400 mg twice daily for 1 year 40–50% had no recurrences compared to 5% who received placebo. In another trial patients were treated with famciclovir 250 mg twice daily for 1 year, the median time to first recurrence was 11 months compared to 1.5 months with placebo. Daily suppressive antiviral treatment with any of the three drugs reduced antiviral shedding up to 94–95% on days with and without lesions compared to 6 days on placebo.

The patients eligible for this kind of treatment are patients with:

- frequent recurrent episodes
- severe and prolonged episodes
- severe psychological disturbance
- patient withdrawn, and unable to function
- sex-life severely affected by recurrences.

Counselling and psychosocial support

The diagnosis of genital herpes elicits a shock reaction in most patients with feelings such as guilt, anger, denial and depression. Common concerns relate to the stigma of a sexually transmitted disease, the risk of transmission and the fear of telling potential sexual partners who may reject them. Frequently recurring genital herpes can be associated with psychological morbidity and restrictions on sexual ability. Suppressive antiviral treatment has been shown to reduce the stress and to improve psychosocial morbidity on a genital herpes quality-of-life scale.

Use of condoms

In a prospective study of 528 couples discordant for HSV-2 infection, use of condoms was associated with a lower risk of HSV-2 acquisition. But only 7.6% used them consistently. Condoms may offer some protection from lesions in men and women, but published data on subclinical shedding have proven reactivation of the virus to be in multiple locations both in men and women, a fact that may limit the protection rate significantly. Condoms are generally recommended as protection for not contracting other sexually transmitted diseases and HIV. This is important as HSV-2 infected persons have an increased risk for transmission and acquisition of HIV.

Specific patient populations

Pregnancy

The safety of systemic aciclovir therapy in pregnant women has not been established. A registry on aciclovir use in pregnancy has not found an increased risk for major birth defects after aciclovir treatment but the accumulated case histories represent an insufficient sample for definitive conclusions. First clinical episode of genital herpes in pregnancy may be treated with oral aciclovir (or intravenous aciclovir in disseminated maternal infections).

Routine administration of aciclovir to pregnant women who have a history of recurrent genital herpes is not recommended. Prenatal exposure to valaciclovir and famciclovir is too limited to provide useful information and the drugs are not recommended in pregnancy.

HIV infection

The dosage of antiviral drugs in HIV-infected patients is controversial. A randomized, double-blind multicentre trial has provided limited evidence for the clinical equivalence of valaciclovir and aciclovir for the suppression of genital herpes in HIV patients with CD4+ cell counts over 100 cells/γL. Valaciclovir 500 mg twice a day and aciclovir 400 mg twice daily were equally effective. Famciclovir 500 mg twice a day has been effective in decreasing the rate of recurrences and subclinical shedding in HIV-infected patients. Regimens such as aciclovir 400 mg three to five times a day until clinical resolution is attained have been useful for other immunocompromised patients. If lesions persist, resistance of the HSV strain should be suspected. All aciclovir-resistant strains are resistant to valaciclovir, and most are resistant to famciclovir. Foscarnet i.v. or topical cidofovir gel 1% may be alternative regimens.

Alternative and experimental treatments

Vaccines

Large-scale randomized controlled trials with prophylactic and therapeutic vaccines based on recombinant HSV-2 glycoproteins have now been completed. Unfortunately, the results from the trials have been generally disappointing. One of the trials did show effect on disease prevention, but the effect was only demonstrated in women who had no pre-existing antibody to HSV-1 or HSV-2. New vaccines based on a live-attenuated single-gene modified virus (DISC) are now in trial and results are awaited with interest.

Immunomodulators

A new class of drugs, imiquimod and its related derivate, resiquimod, act as topically active immune response modifiers that selectively induce cytokines, including interferon-α and interleukin-12. In a smaller randomized study, resiquimod delayed the recurrence of genital herpes significantly compared to placebo-treated patients (169 days vs. 57 days). Further studies are in progress.

Further reading

Goldberg L, Kaufman R, Kurtz T *et al.* Continuous five-year treatment of patients with frequently recurring genital herpes simplex virus infection with aciclovir. *J Med Virol Supplement* 1993; 1: 45–50.

Kroon S. Genital herpes. clinical disease, antiviral therapy and vaccines. In: *Bailliere's Clinical Infectious Diseases*, Vol 3, no 3. November 1996: 391–414.

Kroon S. Optimizing the management of genital herpes—psychological perspective. In: *Optimizing the Management of Genital Herpes*. Royal Society of Medicine Press, Round Table Series, no. 69: 2000: 47–52.

Langenberg GMA, Corey C, Ashley RL *et al.* A prospective study of new infections with herpes simplex virus type 1 and type 2. *N Engl J Med* 1999; 341: 1432–8.

Stone K, Whittington W. Treatment of genital herpes. *Rev Infect Dis* 1990; 12 (Suppl. 6): 610–19.

Wald A. New therapies and prevention strategies for genital herpes. *Clin Infect Dis* 1999; 28: 4–13.

Wald A. Genital herpes. Treating a first episode of genital herpes; treating recurrent genital herpes; preventing transmission. *Clin Evidence* 2000; 3: 756–63.

Wald A, Zeh J, Barnum G, Davis LG, Corey L. Suppression of subclinical shedding of herpes simpex virus type 2 with aciclovir. *Ann Intern Med* 1996; 124: 8–15.

Wald A, Zeh J, Selki S *et al.* Reactivation of genital herpes simplex virus type 2 infections in asymptomatic seropositive persons. *N Engl J Med* 2000; 342: 844–50.

Herpes simplex virus infection (orofacial)

S. Kroon

Epidemiology

The prevalence of herpes simplex virus type 1 (HSV-1) infections is high in all areas of the world. In the 1950s more than 90% of the general population over 30 years of age had serological evidence of infection with HSV-1. In recent years there has been a slight decline in some Western countries to around 60–80%. This decline has been attributed to improved hygiene.

The infection tends to have two peaks, the first occurring between 6 months and 3 years of age; the second after sexual maturity as a result of oral-to-oral and oral-to-genital transmission.

Aetiology and pathophysiology

In most cases orofacial HSV infections are caused by HSV-1, but HSV type 2 (HSV-2) infections have been reported in some cases of sexually active persons and in HIV-positive patients. HSV-1 and HSV-2 are transmitted from person to person through direct contact with infected skin lesions, mucous membranes and secretions.

The herpes viruses are cytotoxic causing necroses of the infected epithelial cells and infiltration of inflammatory cells, mainly mononuclear, into the underlying connective tissue.

Distinctive microscopic features are oedematous ballooning of epithelial cells, formation of giant cells, and presence of inclusion bodies in cell nuclei.

The success of HSV as a pathogen and its key to survival depends on its ability to establish a latent infection in the sensory ganglia (the trigeminal for orofacial HSV) for the lifetime of the host. Viral fusion and entry into the nerve cell body occur rapidly after axonal contact and nucleocapsids travel to the neuronal nucleus through retrograde axonal flow. Following HSV infection of cells, the virus encodes 80 or more different genes, most of which are expressed during viral replication resulting in the production of infectious virus and the death of the cell. In general, replication involves expression of three classes of genes, immediate early (α), early (β) and late (γ). Available evidence suggests that HSV replication during the maintenance stage of latency is blocked at the level of viral early gene expression. The interaction between the virus and the immune system of the host is complex and involves a balance of transcription factors, prostaglandins, humoral and cell-mediated immunity.

Clinical characteristics and course

Primary infection

In most instances, primary infections are asymptomatic and clinical lesions occur in a minority of infected persons. The most common clinical manifestation of primary HSV-1 infection is gingivostomatitis in children and young adults. Fever is common, lasting 2–7 days, as is malaise, myalgia, inability to eat, irritability, and cervical adenopathy. An exudative or ulcerative pharyngitis may be present. Multiple ulcers may appear on the anterior parts of the mouth and oral lesions may persist for 2–3 weeks. Dehydration in children secondary to refusal to take oral liquids is the most commonly associated complication and may require hospitalization.

In sexually active individuals, HSV-2 may cause primary infection with oral lesions and pharyngitis associated with moderate to severe pain and systemic symptoms mimicking bacterial tonsillitis.

Common complications to primary infections are:

- eczema herpeticum in atopic individuals
- keratoconjunctivitis
- autoinoculation
- disseminated HSV infection in other skin conditions such as Darier's disease, mycosis fungoides, ichthyosis vulgaris and congenital ichthyosiform erythroderma.

Recurrent infection

Based on the natural history of HSV-1, the infection should be redefined as a persistent, chronic infection of the sensory ganglia with varying degrees of epithelial expression. Up to 40% of the HSV-1 infected population have at some stage a recurrent clinical outbreak. Asymptomatic shedding of HSV-1 in saliva has been reported in 1–10% of adult cases.

Known triggers of reactivation are:

- UVR exposure
- febrile illnesses
- stress
- premenstrual tension
- surgical procedures
- dental surgery
- dermabrasion including laser therapy
- neural surgery.

The majority of those who develop a recurrent infection have a prodromal phase with tingling, itching, numbness and/or pain. This phase occurs within 6–12 h followed by clinical symptoms. Grouped vesicles appear on an erythematous or papule base at the mucocutaneous junction of the lips, and on intraoral keratinized sites such as the hard palate and gingiva. The ulcerative phase is very short-lived lasting a median of 30 h, and is followed by a longer lasting crusting phase, with a median duration of 133 h. The total healing time is 7–10 days.

Immunocompromised patients with HSV-1 infection have an increased activation rate of up to 70–80%. They develop ulcerations mainly periorally and intraorally, both on the keratinized and non-keratinized sites. Herpetic geometric glossitis was first described in 1993 as a distinctive pattern of lingual HSV infection in organ-transplanted and HIV-infected patients.

Complications of recurrent orofacial HSV infection are:

- eczema herpeticum
- recurrent erythema multiforme
- nosocomial spread including neonatal herpes
- herpetic whitlow in dentists and other health-care workers.

Diagnoses

Viral culture is the gold standard test, allowing viral amplification and subtyping. In addition, drug resistance can be identified. Other specific tests are antigen detection, producing results within hours. In late healing lesions, in atypical disease or defining subclinical shedding, HSV-PCR may be more sensitive. In the near future, HSV-PCR will be available in routine laboratory testing, offering high detection rates in all HSV lesions. In the absence of lesions, serological testing is the best way to identify infected persons.

Differential diagnoses

Other causes of oral ulcerations must be excluded like recurrent aphthae, traumatic ulcerations and chemotherapy-associated ulcers. Bacterial and fungal infections may alter the clinical picture and cause diagnostic problems.

Recurrent aphthae. Ulcers are located on non-keratinized sites. HSV culture negative.

Impetigo. Inflammation more intense. Spreading in a different pattern. In atopic dermatitis the two conditions often coexist. Bacterial and viral culture important.

Treatment

General therapeutic guidelines

- The majority of those infected do not develop clinical disease requiring treatment.

- Primary infection with clinical symptoms in seronegative children and adults can be treated with oral or intravenous antivirals.
- Around 20% of those infected develop recurrent clinical disease and can be treated with topical antivirals.
- Education to avoid oral-to-oral and oral-to-genital spread is important. The rate of genital herpes caused by HSV-1 is increasing in Europe.
- Sunscreens can prevent attacks in those patients who develop UVR-related recurrences.
- Patients with very frequent or severe recurrences can be treated with suppressive oral antivirals.
- Immunocompromised and atopic patients should receive systemic treatment. The dose may need to be higher and the treatment period longer.
- HSV-associated recurrent erythema multiforme can be reduced with oral suppressive antiviral treatment.

Recommended therapies

Antiviral therapy (Table 1)

Primary infection

Two randomized placebo-controlled trials in children have both found a beneficial effect with oral aciclovir treatment. The larger of the studies included 72 children aged 1–6 years with gingivostomatitis of less than 3 days duration, and compared oral aciclovir 15 mg/kg five times a day for 7 days versus placebo. Time to healing was reduced from 10 to 4 days. Additional symptomatic and supportive treatment is important, with pain relief, antiseptic mouthwash to prevent secondary infection, and fluid intake.

No studies in adults are available, and no randomized data from topical antiviral treatment have been published. Primary infection in atopic patients and any serious infections with risk of dissemination should be treated with oral or intravenous aciclovir. Oral administration of one of the new antiviral drugs, valaciclovir or famciclovir, may offer increased oral availability.

Table 1 Treatment of orofacial herpes simplex infections

Primary infection
Oral aciclovir 15 mg/kg five times a day for 7 days (children)
Oral aciclovir 400 mg five times a day for 7 days (adolescent/adult)
Recurrent infection
Topical episodic
Aciclovir crème five times daily for 5 days
Penciclovir crème every 2 hours for 5 days
Systemic episodic
Oral aciclovir 400 mg five times daily for 5 days
Suppressive
Oral aciclovir 400 mg twice daily

Episodic treatment of recurrent disease

Only patients with a well-defined prodromal phase will benefit. Treatment must be patient-initiated by the first prodromal sign. Aborted lesions, not evolving beyond the erythematous/papular stage, are not influenced.

Topical treatment

In four randomized placebo-controlled clinical trials of topical aciclovir 5% cream, applied five times daily for 5 days, no significant impact on lesion pain was observed and results for lesion healing time were inconsistent. Topical penciclovir 1% cream applied every 2 h for 4 days, while the patients were awake, decreased healing time of classical lesions by 0.7 days, and the duration of pain by 0.6 days.

In two randomized, double blind, placebo-controlled studies, *n*-Doconasol 10% cream increased healing time by 18 hours compared to placebo.

Small, short duration trials have studied the effect of several drugs/alternative medications. None had sufficient power to draw conclusions.

Systemic treatment of individual episodes

Two randomized controlled trials have been published. In one trial oral aciclovir, 400 mg five times daily for 5 days, reduced the mean duration of pain by 1.4–2 days and the mean healing time to loss of crusts by 2.1 days. The second trial showed a reduced healing time by 0.98 days and duration of pain by 0.04 days.

Data from a preliminary multicentre, randomized, double blind study comparing valaciclovir 1000 mg twice daily for one day with valaciclovir 500 mg twice daily for a 3 day treatment period showed aborted lesions (primary endpoint) in 42.2 versus 46.7% of patients in the two regimens respectively. Most patients initiated treatment in prodrome or macule phase of the disease.

Suppressive or prophylactic oral treatment

Oral aciclovir, 400 mg twice a day, can reduce the frequency of recurrences during treatment by 50–78%. Oral famciclovir, 500 mg three times a day for 5 days, beginning 48 h after exposure to artificial light, reduced the mean time to healing by 2 days.

The patients eligible for this kind of treatment are:

1 Patients with
   - frequent recurrent episodes (>6 episodes/year)
   - severe and prolonged episodes (including atopic patients)
   - severe UVR-associated episodes
   - herpes simplex associated recurrent erythema multiforme.

2 Patients undergoing
   - chemical or abrasive facial procedures for cosmetic reasons
   - surgical procedures on the trigeminal ganglion.

3 Selected health-care professionals to lower the potential for virus transmission.

Sunscreen

Two randomized double-blind crossover trials found that sunscreen significantly reduced the rate of recurrence.

Further reading

Amir J, Harel L, Smetana Z, Varsano I. Treatment of herpes simplex gingivostomatitis with aciclovir in children: a randomised double blind placebo controlled trial. *BMJ* 1997; 314: 1800–3.

Doucoulombier H, Cousin J, DeWilde A. La stomato-gingivite herpetique de l'enfant: essai a controlle aciclovir versus placebo. *Ann Pediatr* 1988; 35: 212–16.

Duteil L, Quelle-Roussel C, Loesche C, Verschoore M. Assessment of the effect of a sunblock stick in the prevention of solar-simulating ultraviolet light-induced herpes labialis. *J Dermatol Treat* 1998; 9: 11–14.

Laiskonis A, Thune T, Neldam S *et al.* Valaciclovir in the treatment of facial herpes simplex virus infection. *J Infect Dis* 2002; 186 (Suppl 1): S66–70.

Rooney JF, Bryson Y, Mannix ML *et al.* Prevention of ultraviolet-light-induced herpes labialis by sunscreen. *Lancet* 1991; 338: 1419–21.

Rooney JF, Strauss SE, Mannix ML *et al.* Oral aciclovir to suppress frequently recurrent herpes labialis: a double-blind, placebo controlled trial. *Ann Intern Med* 1993; 118: 268–72.

Sacks SL, Thisted RA, Jones TM *et al.* Clinical efficacy of topical docosanol 10% cream for herpes simplex labialis: A multicenter placebo-controlled trial. *J Am Acad Dermatol* 2001; 45: 220–30.

Spruance SL. Prophylactic chemotherapy with aciclovir for recurrent herpes simplex labialis (review). *J Med Virol* 1993; 41(suppl. 1): 27–32.

Spruance SL, Rea TL, Thoming C, Tucker R, Saltzman R, Boon R. Penciclovir cream for the treatment of herpes simplex labialis. *JAMA* 1997; 277: 1374–9.

Spruance SL, Stewart JCB, Rowe NH *et al.* Treatment of recurrent herpes simplex labialis with oral aciclovir. *J Infect Dis* 1990; 161: 185–90.

Worral G. Update on herpes labialis: Effects of treating a first attack of herpes labialis, of treating a recurrent attack and of prophylaxis. *Clin Evidence* 2000; 3: 826–30.

Herpes zoster

S. Georgala

Synonyms

Shingles, zoster.

Definition and epidemiology

Herpes zoster (HZ) is an acute localized infection of a sensory nerve and ganglion characterized by pain and vesicular eruption in a dermatomal distribution, resulting from the reactivation of a lifelong latent infection with the varicella-zoster virus (VZV) acquired during an earlier attack of varicella (chickenpox).

HZ may occur at any stage in a person's life, with the incidence increasing with advancing age. More than two-thirds of the patients are over the age of 50 years. The incidence rate is estimated to be 1.3–5.0/1000 population per year, while the cumulative lifetime incidence is 10–20%. There is no seasonal prevalence for HZ. Both sexes are equally affected.

HZ development is determined by the interaction between VZV and host immunity. Thus, immunocompromised patients due to congenital or acquired disease, malignancy, especially lymphoproliferative disorders, radiotherapy or immunosuppressive chemotherapy, including organ and bone transplant recipients, are at high risk for severe HZ. HZ develops in up to 25% of human immunodeficiency virus (HIV)-infected individuals and it is sometimes the first manifestation of HIV infection. It occurs in 13–15% of Hodgkin's disease patients and in 7–9% of renal or cardiac transplant recipients.

Zoster patients are infectious for up to 7 days from the onset of the rash. Susceptible contacts may develop varicella.

Aetiology and pathophysiology

HZ is caused by herpes virus varicellae or VZV, an icosahedral, enveloped, DNA-containing α-herpes virus. Primary infection results in varicella. During the course of varicella, VZV travels along the sensory nerve from the skin lesions to the respective sensory ganglion, where it establishes a latent infection. Immunity (both cellular and humoral) to VZV suppresses viral replication. Impairment of the immune status, particularly of the cell-mediated immunity, is due to:

- age
- physical or emotional stress
- local irradiation or trauma
- immunosuppressive or corticosteroid therapy
- underlying acquired or congenital immunodeficiency.

It permits reactivation of the virus, which travels antidromically to produce dermatomal pain and skin lesions. In patients with defective immunity, anamnestic immune mechanisms often fail to terminate direct or haematogenous spread, leading to extensive skin and visceral dissemination of the VZV.

VZV tends to be reactivated only once in a lifetime, with the incidence of second attacks being <5% and recurrent HZ occurring in <1%. It is noteworthy that the virus in the live-attenuated varicella vaccine has the potential to become reactivated. However, reactivation occurs much less often after immunization than after natural infection.

Clinical characteristics and course

Pain, often severe, itching, tingling, burning, paraesthesia or hyperaesthesia, confined to areas of one or more dermatomes, usually precede the appearance of the eruption. Few patients complain of constitutional flu-like symptoms, such as headache, fever or malaise.

After 1–14 days from the onset of the prodrome stage, the characteristic vesicular eruption develops in a continuous or interrupted band. Lesions present as erythematous macules, papules or plaques (24 h). Oval or round, umbilicated, clear or haemorrhagic vesicles or bullae arise in clusters on the plaques, giving the classical picture of closely grouped vesicles on an erythematous base (48 h). Successive crops may appear for up to 1 week. Vesicles evolve to pustules (96 h) and, finally, dry to crusts that fall off in 2–4 weeks. Mucous membranes within the affected dermatome are also involved (vesicles and erosions). Regional tender lymphadenopathy is commonly present.

Distribution is highly distinctive of HZ. Lesions are localized to the dermatome corresponding to the involved sensory ganglion, with some overflowing into the adjacent dermatomes. Two or more contiguous dermatomes may be involved. The rash is almost invariably unilateral. Although HZ can involve any area of the body, it affects more often the cranial nerves (20%), especially the ophthalmic division of the trigeminal nerve, or the spinal nerves, particularly T3 to L2. More than half of the reported cases involve the thoracic region (55%). Haematogenous dissemination to other skin sites occurs in up to 10% of healthy individuals.

In some cases, pain due to nerve involvement is not followed by eruption (zoster sine eruptione).

Clinical presentation in the immunocompromised host includes HZ with cutaneous and/or visceral dissemination, HZ with persistent dermatomal infection (hyperkeratotic or verrucous papules and nodules) and chronic cutaneous VZV infection after haematogenous dissemination.

Ophthalmic zoster (HZ ophthalmicus), i.e. involvement of any branch of the ophthalmic nerve, is not uncommon (10–15% of cases). When the nasociliary branch is involved, as evidenced by the presence of vesicles on the tip and the sides of the nose (Hutchinson sign), ocular infection may occur. It may present as conjunctivitis, keratitis, scleritis or anterior uveitis. Complications are not unusual, including cicatricial lid retraction, paralytic ptosis, extraocular muscle palsies, secondary glaucoma, chorioretinitis and optic neuritis. Corneal anaesthesia may lead to neurotrophic keratitis with ulceration that may result in scarring and loss of vision. Ophthalmic zoster merits referral to an ophthalmologist.

Ramsay–Hunt syndrome is a combination of facial palsy and auditory symptoms (tinnitus, vertigo, deafness, nystagmus) associated with HZ of the external ear or tympanic membrane (HZ oticus). It results from the involvement of the facial and auditory nerves (herpetic inflammation of the geniculate ganglion). The course is not uncommonly unfavourable. More than 75% of patients have consequences of paralysis (paresis, hemispasm, synkinaesia, etc.). It may be also associated with sensorineural hearing disorder, vertigo and paralysis of other cranial nerves. Many patients are left with functional and cosmetic deficits.

In otherwise healthy individuals, HZ runs a self-limited course with extremely low direct mortality. Fatal cases are seen almost exclusively among immunocompromised patients. In these patients, HZ often has a more severe and prolonged course and it may be associated with serious complications.

Postherpetic neuralgia (PHN) is an exhausting intractable chronic neuropathic pain that persists or recurs after healing of cutaneous lesions. Its definition is controversial, ranging from pain persisting after the rash heals to pain persisting 30 days or 6 months after the onset of HZ. Some experts consider all pain during and after HZ as a continuum. It is the most common complication occurring in 10–20% of all zoster patients. Although very unusual in patients under 40 years of age, it affects more than one third of patients aged over 60 years. It may last for months to years, but usually resolves spontaneously in 1–6 months (95%). PHN is very common (30%) following ophthalmic zoster. The incidence increases with age, as well as in patients with severe pain or severe rash during the acute episode or in patients with prodrome dermatomal pain. In contrast, PHN in immunocompromised individuals is as common as in the general population. PHN is associated with scarring of the dorsal root ganglion and atrophy of the dorsal horn on the affected side, which follows the extensive inflammation that occurs during HZ.

Bacterial superinfection of cutaneous lesions is frequent and may lead to scarring. Other local complications include haemorrhage and gangrene.

Presence of vesicles remote from the involved dermatome is not unusual. However, generalized HZ manifested by a varicelliform eruption, occurs in 2–10% of the patients 6–10 days after the onset of localized lesions, most commonly in debilitated or immunosuppressed individuals.

Motor paralysis occurs in 5% of cases. It is more prominent when cranial nerves are affected or when the extremities are involved. Spontaneous recovery is the rule.

Central nervous system (CNS) or visceral complications result from uncontrolled viral spread and replication. These are mainly seen among individuals with defective immune mechanisms. Visceral complications include pneumonitis, hepatitis, pericarditis/myocarditis, arthritis, gastritis, enterocolitis and cystitis. Of these patients, 10–25% die. CNS complications are manifested by headache, fever, altered sensorium, meningismus and palsies. Zoster encephalomyelitis is often fatal. VZV polymerase chain reaction (PCR) in the cerebrospinal fluid (CSF) may allow rapid diagnosis and early specific antiviral treatment. HZ is uncommonly followed by cerebrovascular accident. The pathophysiological mechanism remains uncertain, although granulomatous angiitis of the cerebral arteries has been suspected.

Diagnosis

Diagnosis is mostly clinical. In atypical cases, the following diagnostic procedures may establish diagnosis:

- Tzanck smear, prepared with material scraped from the base of a vesicle, shows multinucleated giant cells and acidophil intranuclear bodies containing epithelial cells, as in herpes simplex and varicella.
- Rapid (30 min) identification of herpes virus particles in vesicle fluid or biopsy material by electron microscopy.
- Direct immunofluorescence antibody staining of infected cells from the vesicle fluid.
- Identification of complement-fixing antigens in vesicle fluid.
- VZV can be grown in cell cultures. Cytopathogenicity of VZV may be evident after several days. Isolated VZV can be tested for antiviral sensitivity. This may be necessary in immunocompromised patients.
- Identification of VZV DNA by PCR.
- Titration of complement-fixing antibody in acute and convalescent sera. Most immunocompetent patients show an anamnestic increase (fourfold or more) in antibody titre. Presence of VZV-specific immunoglobulin M (IgM) is indicative of recent active infection.
- Histopathology. In the nuclei of the vesicle epithelium, acidophilic inclusion bodies can be seen. There is marked intracellular and intercellular oedema (ballooning) in the vicinity of the vesicle. In the papillary dermis, there is vascular dilatation with perivascular inflammatory infiltrate. Inflammatory and degenerative changes are also noted in the corresponding sensory nerve and ganglion.

The diagnosis of neurological disorders produced by VZV should be assessed by viral culture, PCR analysis and antibody testing of CSF.

Differential diagnosis

Pre-eruptive pain may be easily mistaken for pleurisy, myocardial infarction, intervertebral disk prolapse, abdominal disease, migraine headache, and so on. An electrocardiogram and chest X-rays may be warranted.

Zoster eruption should be differentiated from the following:

- Zosteriform herpes simplex. Often impossible to distinguish. History of multiple recurrences is indicative of HSV infection. Reliable diagnosis can be based on virus isolation or identification of VZV antigens or nucleic acid.
- Contact dermatitis, mostly phytoallergic, e.g. poison ivy, poison oak.
- Burns (history)
- Vaccinia autoinoculation (history).
- Localized bacterial skin infection, e.g. erysipelas, bullous impetigo, necrotizing fasciitis (bacterial culture).

Disseminated HZ may be confused with varicella. Concentration of lesions at the site of the primarily involved dermatome is indicative of HZ.

Treatment

General therapeutic guidelines

Treatment strategies for HZ have three major objectives:

1 To control signs and symptoms and to accelerate local healing.
2 To reduce the severity and the duration of the disease and to prevent cutaneous and visceral dissemination by inhibiting viral replication and spread.
3 To prevent or relieve PHN and to prevent other complications.

Recommended therapies

Symptomatic treatment

Symptomatic therapy aims to alleviate acute pain and itching and to promote healing.

For vesicular skin lesions, the following topical preparations may have a soothing and drying effect:

- cool compresses with cool tap water, normal saline solution or Burow's solution, several times a day
- flexible collodion tincture or tincture with equal parts of benzoin and flexible collodion
- lotion containing alcohol, menthol and/or phenol, or solution of ethyl ether and ethyl alcohol in equal parts, calamine lotion, cornstarch or baking soda.

For crusted lesions, bland ointment or olive oil dressings may help to separate adherent crusts.

For secondarily infected skin lesions, warm soaks and topical antibiotics should be applied.

Analgesics are often necessary to relieve pain, e.g. oxycodone with acetaminophen, 1 tablet p.o. every 4–6 h. Opiates may be needed in more severe cases. Subcutaneous (under the lesion) injection of corticosteroids (triamcinolone acetonide) or anaesthetics (lidocaine (lignocaine) 0.5%, 4–5 mL) or in combination, has succeded to eliminate pain. Therapy with levodopa and benzerazide (peripheral decarboxylase inhibitor), emetine or dehydroemetine have been reported to ameliorate acute pain of zoster. Systemic corticosteroids during acute zoster have shown efficacy in alleviating pain. Sympathetic blocks with 0.25% bupivacaine terminates acute pain and prevent PHN in more than 80% of the treated patients.

Bed rest is helpful.

Antiviral treatment

Antiviral therapy involves several chemotherapeutic agents, mostly nucleoside or nucleotide analogues, which act as virostatics. Their mechanism of action is based on the interaction of their active intercellular metabolite with the viral DNA polymerase, resulting in termination of the viral DNA chain synthesis.

Aciclovir (ACV)

ACV, a purine nucleoside analogue, has emerged as an important and reliable antiviral agent over the past 15 years. ACV is selectively phosphorylated by the viral thymidine kinase to its active metabolite, ACV triphosphate, that in turn halts viral DNA synthesis. ACV is a more potent inhibitor of viral DNA polymerases than of cellular DNA polymerases, ensuring efficacy with a remarkable safety profile. Randomized double-blind placebo-controlled studies have concluded that early treatment with ACV significantly reduces time to healing, viral shedding and acute pain. In addition, it prevents or aborts visceral or cutaneous dissemination in both immunocompetent and immunocompromised zoster patients. However, it has no significant effect on PHN occurrence. To be most effective, ACV should be administered within 48 h from the appearance of the rash and may be given orally (800 mg five times a day for 5–10 days) or in more severe cases intravenously (500 mg/m^2 or 10 mg/kg every 8 h for 7 days or until there is no evidence of continuing VZV replication). Side-effects are rare, including transient recurrence of pain on discontinuation of therapy and nephrotoxicity. ACV dosage must be reduced in patients with renal insufficiency.

VZV resistance to ACV is a rare event among immunocompetent zoster patients. In contrast, it is increasingly detected among patients with acquired immune deficiency syndrome (AIDS) or transplant recipients, especially those who have received repeated ACV treatment. Foscarnet, a direct inhibitor of the viral DNA polymerase not requiring activation by the viral thymidine kinase, is considered the drug of choice for ACV-resistant VZV infections. The drug, 40 mg/kg i.v. every 8 h, should be initiated within 7–10 days and should be continued for 10 days or until all lesions are completely healed. Foscarnet-resistant strains are sensitive to cidofovir, an acyclic nucleoside phosphonate, which depends only on cellular enzymes for its activation.

New oral antivirals

Recently, new oral antivirals have been approved for the treatment of HZ in adults. These agents are characterized by enhanced *in vivo* and *in vitro* activity against VZV and enhanced oral bioavailability that permits more convenient dosing and improved compliance, compared to ACV.

Valaciclovir is the L-valyl ester of ACV that produces increased plasma levels of ACV following oral administration. The recommended dosage is 1 g three times a day for 7 days. In a large comparative study valaciclovir was at least as effective as ACV in controlling acute HZ. However, valaciclovir alleviated zoster-associated pain and PHN significantly faster than ACV.

Famciclovir is a synthetic acyclic guanine derivative. After oral administration, it is rapidly metabolized to penciclovir, a highly bioavailable antiviral compound that is efficiently phosphorylated to its active metabolite (penciclovir triphosphate). It is administered at a dosage of 500 mg three times a day for 7 days (dose reduction is necessary in patients with diminished renal function).

Ideally, antivirals should be administered as soon as possible or within 72 h from the onset of the rash. However, in a recent observational study, starting treatment with valaciclovir later than 72 h did not significantly reduce the beneficial effect. In a large double-blind, randomized, controlled, multicentre clinical trial of otherwise healthy immunocompetent outpatients, aged 50 years and older, both valaciclovir and famciclovir have been shown to attenuate significantly the acute signs and symptoms and, more importantly, to decrease the duration and incidence of PHN. Side-effects are minor (nausea, headache).

Alternative and experimental treatments

Vidarabine

Vidarabine (10 mg/kg over 12 h each day for 7 days) represents as alternative antiviral treatment for HZ. It has proved effective in limiting the severity and duration of acute zoster and in reducing the incidence of complications. Comparative studies have shown that vidarabine is less effective than ACV, while it is far more toxic. Current recommendations favour intravenous ACV vs. intravenous vidarabine.

Human interferon-α

Human interferon-α (1.7 or 5.1×10^5 units/kg per day i.m. for 7 days) has been shown to reduce the severity of HZ, as well as the incidence of PHN and to prevent dissemination of VZV. However, its use is associated with increased toxicity (flu-like syndrome, bone marrow suppression).

Soriduvine

Sorivudine is a new nucleoside analogue with excellent oral bioavailability and increased efficacy against VZV. It is administered once daily in a dose that is one-hundredth that of ACV. It appears to be superior to ACV for the treatment of localized HZ in patients with HIV.

Several other antiviral compounds are under clinical development, including lobucavir, brivudine, cyclocreatine, 882C87 and cidofovir (HPMPC). The latter, confers prolonged antiviral action allowing infrequent dosing (every week or every 2 weeks).

In conclusion:

1 All patients may benefit from symptomatic therapy.
2 In immunocompetent individuals under 50 years of age, only symptomatic measures are necessary.
3 In elderly otherwise healthy individuals, oral antivirals may be administered.
4 In ophthalmic HZ, antiviral therapy should be considered due to the increased risk for ocular or CNS complications.
5 In Ramsay–Hunt syndrome, oral antivirals are recommended. There is weak evidence to suggest benefit of oral steroids, but their use can be supported in immunocompetent individuals. Facial nerve decompression surgery may benefit patients at high risk for persistent deficits.
6 Immunocompetent patients of any age with significant cutaneous dissemination or with evidence of visceral or CNS involvement, should receive antiviral therapy with intravenous ACV.
7 Immunocompromised patients of any age at high risk for dissemination and visceral complications should receive, with no delay, ACV intravenously.

Management of PHN

Prevention of PHN is of great importance, especially in the elderly. Although ACV has no significant effect on the incidence of PHN, new antivirals such as famciclovir and valaciclovir may reduce the duration of PHN. The hypothesis that PHN should be attributed to inflammation, necrosis and subsequent scarring of neural structures, has led to the use of systemic corticosteroids during the acute phase of HZ. The results are conflicting and the indication is still a subject of controversy. Small or uncontrolled trials have shown a favourable effect on PHN occurrence. On the contrary, a more recent large double-blind controlled trial found no significant effect of corticosteroids on PHN prevention. It is noteworthy that systemic corticosteroids neither affect adversely the course of the disease nor increase the risk of dissemination. Moreover, they reduce local pain and oedema during the acute phase. The starting dose is usually 40–60 mg prednisolone continued over 3–4 weeks in a tapering fashion. A convenient regime is 40 mg prednisolone for 5 days, lowered to 20 mg for 5 more days and finally to 10 mg for 5 days. In another study, epidural administration of local anaesthetic and methylprednisolone is significantly more effective in preventing PHN at 12 months compared to intravenous ACV combined with prednisolone.

Once instituted, PHN is refractory to treatment. Evaluation and management of patients is better left to pain clinics. Emotional support, preferably by specialists, is of crucial importance.

Pharmacological approaches can be classified into three groups: (a) drugs that act topically in the affected skin area; (b) drugs that act on nerve excitability and conduction in sensory axons; and (c) drugs that act on neural damage related synaptic changes.

Various therapeutic modalities are currently available:

- Conventional analgesics should be tried, but most often fail. Semisynthetic narcotic analgesics, e.g. oxylodone, may be useful. Narcotics, even when at an optimal dose, may prove ineffective for the long-term control of pain from PHN and are associated with unacceptable side-effects in the elderly, such as lethargy, confusion, unsteadiness, constipation and headache.
- Tricyclic antidepressants, e.g. amitriptyline 50–100 mg daily per os, have resulted in pain relief in two-thirds of patients with PHN. It has recently been demonstrated that nortriptyline provides equivalent analgesic benefit when compared with amitriptyline, but is better tolerated. Based on these results, nortriptyline can now be considered the preferred antidepressant for the treatment of PHN. Desipramine may be used if the patient experiences unacceptable sedation from nortriptyline.
- Tranquillizers, such as aloperidin, levopromazine, clonazepam, have been reported to provide relief.
- Carbamazepine, an antiepileptic drug, is particularly effective for lancinating pain. Gabapentin (300 mg t.i.d.), a new anticonvulsant, can be considered a first-line oral medication for PHN based on the efficacy and safety results of a recently completed double-blind trial. In addition to positive effects on PHN, sleep, mood and overall quality of life were significantly improved.
- Chloroprothixene can be given 25–50 mg p.o. every 6 h for 4–10 days. For severe pain an initial 50–100 mg i.m. injection is recommended.
- Intralesional corticosteroids, e.g. triamcinolone acetonide 10 mg/mL. Up to 60 mg can be administered per session. Multiple injections over several months are necessary.
- Epidural injection of local anaesthetics or corticosteroids.
- Topical anaesthetics: EMLA cream applied for a 24-h period; topical lidocaine gel, with or without occlusion; double-blind, vehicle-controlled studies have demonstrated that patients with PHN obtain pain relief from a topical lidocaine patch.
- Capsaicin cream 3–5 times daily for many weeks. Capsaicin depletes peripheral nerve endings of their substance P content and prevents its

resynthesis. Substance P is a neuropeptide that acts as mediator for centripetal nociceptive stimuli.

- Combination of a tricyclic antidepressant and a substituted phenothiazine administered over several months.
- Combination of carbamazepine (600–800 mg daily) or phenytoin sodium (300–400 mg daily) with nortriptyline (50–100 mg) or clomipramine (75 mg daily).
- A novel but still controversial approach includes the administration (in a hospital setting where cardiovascular resuscitation is available) of intrathecal methylprednisolone and lidocaine (3 mL of 3% lidocaine with 60 mg of methylprednisolone acetate) to treat persisting inflammation. However, it is associated with increased neurotoxicity, and haemodynamic and respiratory adverse effects (due to lidocaine).
- Transcutaneous electrical nerve stimulation (TENS) which supplies electrical current to the affected dermatome.
- Frequent rubbing with a dry towel for several weeks.
- Repeated cryotherapy to limited areas to reduce sensation of trigger points.
- Gamma knife radiosurgery as a noninvasive, relatively successful and safe method for patients even in poor condition.
- Neurosurgical intervention (rhizotomy or surgical separation of pain fibres) should be considered in patients with intolerable pain.

Prevention

Reactivation of latent endogenous VZV in populations with declining VZV-specific immunity, may be prevented by stimulating immunity to VZV. The live-attenuated varicella vaccine (Oka strain) has safely increased the VZV-specific T lymphocytes following vaccination. In this way, it may prevent or modify HZ in high-risk patients, including the immunocompromised or the elderly. Long-term suppression therapy with ACV in bone marrow transplant recipients and patients with HIV has been tried. The results were poor and there was an increased risk of selection of resistant strains of VZV. However, short-term chemoprophylaxis (400 mg p.o. b.i.d. for 4–6 weeks) may prove useful during the peritransplant period, or in individuals at high risk for reactivation of VZV infection.

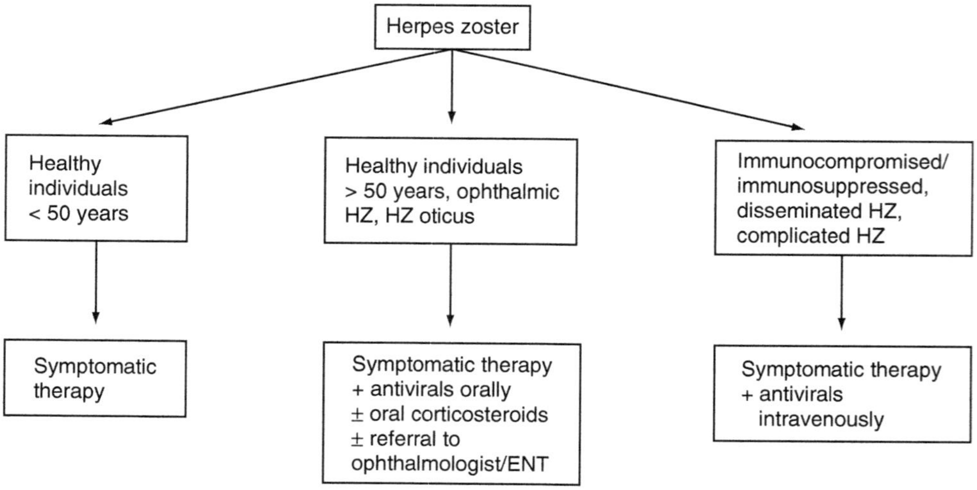

Further reading

Alrabiah FA, Sacks SL. New antiherpesvirus agents. Their targets and therapeutic potential. *Drugs* 1996; 52 (1): 17–32.

Cerelli R, Herne K, McCrary M *et al.* Famciclovir: review of clinical efficacy and safety. *Antiviral Res* 1996; 29: 141–51.

Cunningham AL, Dworkin RH. The management of post-herpetic neuralgia. *BMJ* 2000; 321: 778–9.

Harding SP. Management of ophthalmic zoster. *J Med Virol* 1993; 1: 97–101.

Kanazi GE, Johnson RW, Dworkin RH. Treatment of postherpetic neuralgia: an update. *Drugs* 2000; 59: 1113–26.

Naoum C, Perissios A, Varnavas V, Lagos D. Treatment of herpes zoster with interferon alpha-2A. *Int J Dermatol* 1996; 35 (10): 749–50.

Ormrod D, Goa K. Valacyclovir: a review of its use in the management of herpes zoster. *Drugs* 2000; 59: 1317–40.

Reusser P. Herpesvirus resistance to antiviral drugs: a review of the mechanisms, clinical importance and therapeutic options. *J Hosp Infect* 1996; 33 (4): 235–48.

Tyring SK, Beutner KR, Tucker BA, Anderson WC, Crooks RJ. Antiviral therapy for herpes zoster: randomized, controlled clinical trial of valacyclovir and famciclovir therapy in immunocompetent patients 50 years and older. *Arch Fam Med* 2000; 9: 863–9.

Wagstaff AJ, Faulds D, Goa KL. Acyclovir: a reappraisal of its antiviral activity, pharmakokinetic properties and therapeutic efficacy. *Drugs* 1994; 47 (1): 153–205.

Whitley RJ. Sorivudine: a promising drug for the treatment of varicella-zoster virus infection. *Neurology* 1995; 45 (12) (Suppl. 8): S73–5.

Whitley RJ. Therapeutic approaches to varicella-zoster virus infections. *J Infect Dis* 1992; 166 (Suppl. 1): S51–7.

Wood MJ, Johnson RW *et al.* A randomized trial of acyclovir for 7 days or 21 days with and without prednisolone for treatment of acute hepres zoster. *N Engl J Med* 1994; 330: 896–900.

Hirsutism

D. Rigopoulos

Definition and epidemiology

Hirsutism is a term used to describe the condition in women, in whom the pattern of terminal hair growth follows a similar mode to that which develops in men after puberty, in other words, in androgen-dependent sites. So, hirsutism by definition, refers only to females. The androgen-dependent sites include cheeks, the upper lip, chin, chest, lower abdomen inner aspect of the thighs, back and legs. In females, only vellus hair is normally found at these sites.

There are serious differences among subjects in defining hirsutism, according to racial, cultural and social factors. So, what is pathological for North European women is normal to Mediterraneans.

Hair, facial and body, is rarer in black people, mongoloids and American Indians.

Aetiology and pathophysiology

Hirsutism may be the result of increased androgen production, enhanced sensitivity of the hair follicle in sexual areas to normal levels of circulating androgens, increased concentration of free testosterone, or increased 5α-reductase activity. Circulating androgen levels in females depend upon direct secretion by the ovaries and adrenal glands, peripheral conversion of androgen precursors and metabolic clearance rate, which is related to androgen production.

All these conditions lead to the conversion of vellus to terminal hair, in sex hormone-responsive follicles. Causes of hirsutism are listed in Table 1.

Table 1 Causes of hirsutism

Idiopathic
Ovarian
polycystic ovary syndrome
ovarian tumours
Adrenal
congenital adrenal hyperplasia
adrenal tumours
Prolactinoma
Iatrogenic
Pregnancy
Postmenopausal

Idiopathic

Probably the most common cause. It results from hypersensitivity of hair follicles to androgens, decreased sex hormone-binding globulin (SHBG) or increased activity of 5α-reductase. This kind of hirsutism is usually noted at puberty and, in most cases, there is a positive family history.

Ovarian

- Polycystic ovary syndrome (PCO): these patients present (usually just before or at the time of puberty) with hirsutism, acne, dysfunctional uterine bleeding or amenorrhoea, infertility and obesity. In some cases, PCO may exist in the absence of gross pathology and can be the result of abdominal ultrasound investigation.
- Ovarian tumours: functional ovarian tumours, present less than 1% of all ovarian tumours. In these cases, hirsutism usually has a sudden onset between the ages of 20 and 40 years, with a rapid progression.

Adrenal

- Congenital adrenal hyperplasia (CAH): Three types of CAH exist: (a) the severe form, with masculinization of the female at the time of birth; (b) the less severe form, with masculinization at childhood with girls being very tall at an early age but with comparatively diminished height later; and (c) the late-onset type, with onset

at puberty or after pregnancy. In CAH, the most common deficiency in 95% of all cases, is that of 21-hydroxylase.
- Adrenal tumours: these are rare causes of hirsutism. They can appear at any age but usually occur before puberty or after menopause. Symptoms arise suddenly and have a rapid progression.

Prolactinoma
This can result from pituitary adenoma, hypothalamic disease or hypothyroidism. It is reported that prolactin might have a direct effect on androgen production from the adrenals.

Iatrogenic
This can result as a side-effect of systemic administration of various compounds, such as testosterone, danazole, oral contraceptives (in less than 5% of all cases), adrenocorticotropic hormone (ACTH), phenothiazines, minoxidil, metyrapone, ciclosporin and synthetic glucocorticosteroids.

Pregnancy
This is a rare cause of hirsutism and results in the development of PCO or virilizing tumours during the first or the third trimester.

Postmenopausal hirsutism
This is poorly understood. Ovarian or adrenal tumours and hyperthecosis or hypertrophy of the ovarian stroma are possible causative diseases.

Treatment

General therapeutic guidelines
History and physical examination is extremely critical and important, in order to differentiate idiopathic hirsutism from other forms of the disease. Laboratory investigations and echogram is added whenever it is needed.

Recommended therapies

Physical and chemical measures
These are used in those cases where little can be done or can be expected by the patients, such as cases of mild familial or idiopathic hirsutism. Physical measures include the following.
- Hair bleaching. It is an excellent, easy, safe and cheap technique, used only by fair-skinned women.
- Shaving. The most widely used method for removing unwanted hair from the legs and bikini area. Rarely it is used also for removing hair from the face.
- Depilation with tweezers. An easy, cheap and safe technique, to remove isolated hair especially from eyebrows, chin and periareolar areas.
- Depilation with wax. Widely used for legs and upper lip. It is repeated every 2–6 weeks.
- Depilation with chemicals. Calcium thioglycolate 5% is the main substance used for chemical depilation. This method is not recommended for fair-skinned or allergic women, since it can result in allergic contact dermatitis. Other common side-effects are recurrent folliculitis and hyperpigmentation.

Systemic treatment
This includes androgenic receptor antagonists, 5α-reductase inhibitors, drugs that can cause ovarian suppression and corticosteroids.

Cyproterone acetate (CPA)
This acts by inhibiting the binding of testosterone and dihydrotestosterone to the androgen receptors and increases the metabolic clearance rate of testosterone, by inducing hepatic enzymes and decreasing SHBG levels. CPA is a potent progestogen, but it has to be prescribed with a cyclical oestrogen to become a reliable

ovulation inhibitor. Therefore it can be given either with 0.050 mg ethinyl oestradiol from days 5 to 26 of the cycle, or with 0.035 mg ethinyl oestradiol, from days 1 to 21 for the first cycle and from days 5 to 26, for the rest of the cycles. It should be prescribed for at least 2–3 years. Side-effects include decreased libido, mastodynia, nausea, headache, depression, emotional alterations, increase of height and elevation of blood pressure.

Spironolactone

This is a steroidal androgen receptor which can also inhibit 5α-reductase activity and, at high doses, decrease cytochrome P450 activity. It is given at a dose of 50–20 mg/day, for at least 6 months. After 12 months of administration, a reduction of 83% of facial hair was noticed. Side-effects, which are usually mild, include menstrual disturbances, decreased libido, increased breast tension, headache, vertigo, nausea, vomiting, anorexia, diarrhoea, hypercalcaemia and increased serum creatinine. It can also cause cutaneous side-effects.

Flutamide

This is a pure non-steroidal antiandrogen, with no glucocorticoid, progestational, androgenic, oestrogenic or antigonadotropic activity, both *in vivo* and *in vitro*. Its active metabolite, hydroxyflutamide acts by inhibition on the androgen receptor of the target organ of the follicle. It is usually used in a dosage of 250–375 mg/day, for a period of 6–24 months. Improvement is noticed after 3 months of administration.

Toxic hepatitis and digestive side-effects, are usually seen with doses as high as 500 mg/day.

Finasteride

This is a potent inhibitor of 5α-reductase type 2. It has been used in females with facial hirsutism in a dosage of 2.5 mg/day with oral contraceptives used for a period of 2 years. Results were considered good and equal to those achieved with CPA.

Finasteride can cause feminization of the male fetus and in association with oral contraceptives, it can cause increased cholesterol levels.

Oral contraceptives

These act as suppressors of the ovaries. Usually they are a combination of an oestrogen (ethinyl oestradiol) and a progestogen (ethinodiol diacetate, linestranol, norethindrone acetate, norgestrel, desogestrel, norefinodrel or levonorgestrel). The action of oestrogens is based mainly on the fact that they stimulate the production of SHBG, which leads to a decrease of free testosterone levels. They can also modify the binding of dihydrotestosterone (DHT) to its receptor and after a prolonged period of administration, they reduce the activity of 5α-reductase.

Oral contraceptives are contraindicated in women suffering from thromboembolic disease, carcinoma of the breast or uterus and hypertension.

Antagonists of gonadotrophic-releasing hormone

Nafarelin and lenprolide, synthetic analogues of gonadotrophin-releasing hormone (GnRH), have been used successfully to treat hirsutism. They act by reducing the production of luteinizing hormone (LH) and follicle-stimulating hormone (FSH) by the pituitary gland.

A newer antagonist of GnRH is triptorelin which has been recently introduced in the treatment of hirsutism.

Corticosteroids

This is the treatment of choice for CAH. They lower androgen levels in plasma. Prednisone is used at a dose of 7.5 mg/day, for 2 months reducing to 5 mg/day for 2 more months and finally, 2.5 mg/day for the next 2 months.

Electrolysis

This is a widely used technique for removing unwanted hair. It is perfomed by isolated insulated and non-insulated epilating needles, which are inserted into the hair follicle. Hyperpigmentation and scars are the most common, although rare, side-effects.

Photodynamic therapy

This method, using topical aminolaevulinic acid (ALA), is mainly used for treating cutaneous malignancies. Since ALA is absorbed by hair follicles, the exposure to red light may cause selective cell damage and the destruction of unwanted hair.

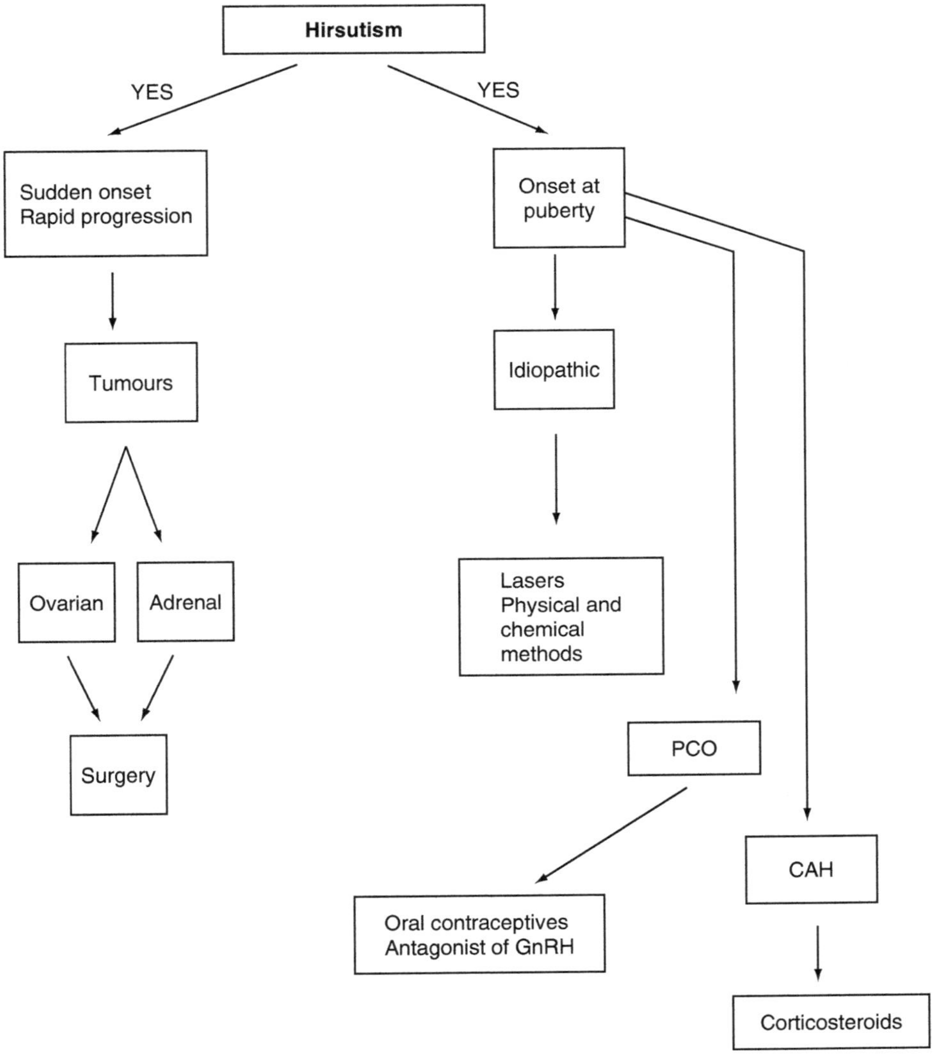

Table 2 Laser used for hair removal

Laser	Wavelength (μm)	Pulse width (ms)
Ruby		
Epilaser	694	3
Epitouch Silk	694	1.2
Chromos	694	0.5–1.2
Alexandite		
Photogenica	755	5, 10, 20
Apongee	755	5, 10, 20
Epitouch 5100	755	2
Gentle Lase	755	.
Diode		
Light Sheer	800	5–30
Nd : YAG		
Softlight	1064	tons

This method is still in the early stage of development.

Lasers

The use of lasers for treating excess unwanted hair is based on the principle of selective photothermolysis. This does not provide a permanent solution for hirsutism, since in the first 3–6 months, there is hair regrowth. The main target of laser hair removal is to increase the temperature of the hair follicle to 200°C in order to destroy it. It is mainly used in cases of idiopathic hirsutism. All lasers used for hair removal are listed in Table 2.

Alternative and experimental treatments

Recently a new medication has been used in some cases of hirsutism. Eflornithine hydrochloride acts as an irreversible inhibitor of ornithine decarboxylase, an enzyme which is required for dihydrotestosterone production of polyamines, which are necessary for hair matrix proliferation. Hair growth rate is affected, but this agent unfortunately provides only temporary hair removal.

Further reading

Camacho FM. Drug treatment of hirsutism. In: Camacho FM, Randall V, Price VH, eds. *Hair and its Disorders. Biology, Pathology and Management*. UK: Martin Dunitz, 2000: 368–81.

Crossman M, Winberly J, Owyer P *et al*. PDT for hirsutism. *Laser Surg Med* 1995; 7: 44–6.

Falsetti L, Fusco D, Elefteriou G *et al*. Treatment of hirsutism by finasteride and flutamide in women with PCO syndrome. *Gynecol Endocrinol* 1997; 11: 251–7.

Olsen EA. Methods of hair removal. *J Am Acad Dermatol* 1999; 40: 143–55.

Shaw JC. Antiandrogen therapy in dermatology. *Int J Dermatol* 1996; 35: 770–8.

Yucelten D, Erenus M, Gurbuz O *et al*. Recurrence rate of hirsutism after three different antiandrogen, therapies. *J Am Acad Dermatol* 1999; 41: 64–8.

HIV infection and AIDS: present status of antiretroviral therapy

R. Husak and C.E. Orfanos

Definition and epidemiology

The epidemic of human immunodeficiency virus (HIV) infection and acquired immunodeficiency syndrome (AIDS) emerged in the last two decades of the 20th century and has now affected over 190 countries. At the end of 2000 approximately more than 35 million human beings were infected with HIV worldwide, 95% of them in countries of the developing world.

In Western Europe, approximately 520 000 individuals were infected with HIV at the end of 1999 and with a present incidence of 40 000 new infections per year. Recently, a dramatic increase of new HIV infections in eastern European countries has been observed where the HIV epidemic started in the early 1990s. The regional statistics of the UNAIDS/WHO counts 420 000 adults and children living with HIV/AIDS in eastern Europe and central Asia at the end of 1999. Among the European countries Spain, Switzerland, France and Italy had the highest cumulative AIDS incidences, as related to their population. Interestingly, there is an obvious North–South gradient in the distribution of the main risk groups of HIV infection in Europe: in northern countries homo- and bisexual men are predominantly affected, whereas i.v. drug use (IDU) represents the main transmission route in southern European countries.

Aetiology

HIV infection can be caused by HIV-1 and HIV-2. The spread of HIV-2 is mainly restricted to West Africa, with foci in Angola and Mozambique. However, some cases have also been reported in Europe, namely from Portugal, Spain and France, all countries with former ties to Western or Central Africa. Compared with HIV-1, the spread of HIV-2 is slower, it appears less transmissible through sexual intercourse, and its clinical course is generally less progressive, especially in terminal stages of the infection. Throughout this chapter, the abbreviation of HIV refers to HIV-1.

Treatment

General therapeutic guidelines

With the expanding arsenal of new antiretroviral agents in recent years more progress in the treatment of HIV infection has been achieved than in 16 years before. The availability of new sensitive laboratory techniques together with a better understanding of the complex pathogenesis of HIV infection, particularly the viral dynamics and the immune response, were an important precondition for this development. It has now become clear that HIV burdens are substantial at all stages of the infection. The daily turnover of HIV has been estimated to be at least 10^{10} viral particles, with a similar rate for the CD4 cell turnover. Even during the early, clinically asymptomatic phase of HIV infection, replication of the virus in lymphoid tissues is extensive. The high virus turnover drives the pathogenic process and the development of genetic variations resulting in the emergence of resistance mutations under the pressure of drug therapies.

As a rule, the homeostasis between HIV replication and CD4+ cell production collapses after several years, followed by permanent decline of the CD4+ cell counts, which ultimately result in the clinical symptomatology of AIDS. Today, the rate of viral replication can be easily estimated from the viral levels in plasma based on measurements of HIV RNA. Assays employing either reverse transcriptase polymerase chain reaction (RT-PCR) or branched-chain DNA (bDNA) technology are commercially available and are routinely used for that purpose.

The HIV viral load is the strongest predictor for disease progression in HIV infection to AIDS or death. It is important to realize that this marker is a better predictor of the general outcome than the numbers of CD4+ cells in the peripheral blood. In addition, changes of plasma viral load indicate rapidly the success or failure of antiretroviral therapy, and may thus serve for management control.

The goals of highly active antiretroviral treatment (HAART) are maximal and sustainable suppression of HIV viral load to restore and preserve immunological function. This is usually associated with improvement of life quality due to reduction of HIV-related morbidity and mortality.

Recommended therapies

Antiretroviral agents

A number of new antiretroviral agents for the therapy of HIV infection have been introduced over the last 5 years. In particular, the introduction of HIV protease inhibitors (PI) and non-nucleoside reverse transcriptase inhibitors (NNRTI) have substantially enriched the treatment modalities and allowed effective anti-HIV combination therapies. At present six nucleoside analogues, three non-NRTI and six PI are available for treatment (Table 1).

NRTI

The first drug to be approved for use in HIV-infected individuals was zidovudine (AZT, ZDV), a potent inhibitor of reverse transcriptase. Since then five other drugs of this class have been approved for treatment of HIV infection: zalcitabine (ddC), didanosine (ddI), stavudine (d4T) lamivudine (3TC) and abacavir (ABC). ABC is the most recent NRTI with *in vitro* synergistic effects to other NRTI. Drug formulations including AZT and 3TC (Combivir) and AZT, 3TC together with ABC (Trizivir) are now available and allow a triple antiretroviral therapy with only two tablets daily.

The major adverse effects of this group of antiretroviral agents include bone marrow toxicity, peripheral neuropathy and pancreatitis (Table 1). In addition, ABC shows as a major side-effect a potentially fatal hypersensitivity syndrome with fever, rash, nausea, malaise, fatigue and respiratory symptoms. This syndrome occurs in up to 5% of the treated patients usually between the first and fourth week of treatment. Patients who develop signs or symptoms of hypersensitivity syndrome should discontinue ABC as soon as the syndrome is suspected. In these cases ABC should not be restarted. For the other NRTI counts when toxicity occurs, doses should be reduced or discontinued until symptoms become tolerable or resolve. A rare but potentially life-threatening toxicity with the use of all NRTI is lactic acidosis with hepatic steatosis.

Most NRTI, particularly AZT and d4T, penetrate into the central nervous system (CNS), with cerebrospinal fluid concentrations ranging from 10% to 100% of simultaneous plasma levels. In general, the group of NRTI are relatively well-tolerated drugs and are 'the backbone' in nearly any antiretroviral combination therapy.

Non-NRTI (NNRTI)

Reverse transcriptase can be inhibited by agents that are not nucleoside analogues. Nevirapine, delavirdine and efavirenz belong to this class of antiretroviral agents. Combination of nevirapine and NRTI improves surrogate markers of HIV infection and has been recommended for clinical use. A major adverse reaction associated with the use of NNRTI are rashes (Table 1), which occur in around 20–40% of patients, mostly during the first 4 weeks after initiation of treatment. In some

Table 1 Antiretroviral agents

Nucleoside reverse transcriptase inhibitors (NRTI)						
Generic name	Zidovudine (AZT/ ZDV)	Zalcitabine (ddC)	Didanosine (ddI)	Lamivudine (3TC)	Stavudine (d4T)	Abacavir (ABC)
Trade name	Retrovir	Hivid	Videx	Epivir	Zerit	Ziagen
Dosing recommendations	250 mg b.i.d., or 300 mg b.i.d. with 3TC as Combivir 1 b.i.d., or with 3TC and abacavir as Trizivir 1 b.i.d.	0.75 mg t.i.d.	< 60 kg: 125 mg b.i.d.; > 60 kg: 200 mg b.i.d., 400 mg q.d.	150 mg b.i.d., or with ZDV as Combivir 1 b.i.d., or with ZDV and abacavir as Trizivir 1 b.i.d.	< 60 kg: 30 mg b.i.d.; > 60 kg: 40 mg b.i.d.	300 mg b.i.d., or with ZDV and 3TC as Trizivir 1 b.i.d.
Food effect	None	Take 30 min before or 2 h after meal	Take 30 min before or 2 h after meal	None	None	None
Major side-effects	Bone marrow suppression: anaemia and/or neutropenia, GI intolerance, headache	PNP (20–30%), stomatitis, headache	PNP (20%), pancreatitis (6%), GI intolerance, headache	Minimal toxicity: bone marrow suppression, GI intolerance, headache	PNP (20%), pancreatitis, GI intolerance, headache, insomnia	Hypersensitivity reaction (5%, can be fatal), GI intolerance, headache
Non-Nucleoside Reverse Transcriptase Inhibitors (NNRTI)						
Generic name	Nevirapine (NVP)	Delavirdine (DLV)	Efavirenz (EFV)			
Trade name	Viramune	Rescriptor	Sustiva			
Dosing recommendations	200 mg q.d. × 14 days, then 200 mg b.i.d.	400 mg t.i.d.	600 mg q.h.s.			
Food effect	None	None	Avoid taking after high-fat meals			
Major side-effects	Rash (up to 40%), increased transaminase levels	Rash (up to 50%), GI intolerance, headache, increased transaminase levels	CNS, GI intolerance, rash, increased transaminase levels, hyperlipidaemia			

(Continued)

Table 1 (*Continued*)

Protease Inhibitors (PI)

Generic name	Saquinavir hard gel capsule (SQV-hgc)	Saquinavir soft gel capsule (SQV-sgc)	Indinavir (IDV)	Ritonavir (RTV)	Nelfinavir (NFV)	Amprenavir (APV)	Lopinavir/Ritonavir
Trade name	Invirase	Fortovase	Crixivan	Norvir	Viracept	Agenerase	Kaletra
Dosing recommendations	400 mg b.i.d. with ritonavir; otherwise not recommended	1200 mg t.i.d.	800 mg t.i.d.	600 mg b.i.d.; dose escalation: Day 1–2: 300 mg b.i.d.; day 3–5: 400 mg b.i.d.; day 6–13: 500 mg b.i.d.; day 14: 600 mg b.i.d.	750 mg t.i.d. or 1250 mg b.i.d.	1200 mg b.i.d.	400 mg lopinavir + 100 mg ritonavir b.i.d.
Food effect	No food effect when taken with ritonavir	Take with meal	Take 1 h before or 2 h after meals; may take with skimmed milk or low-fat meal, daily drinking: 2–3 L	Take with meal; this may improve tolerability	Take with meal	None	Take with meal
Storage	Room temperature	Refrigerator	Room temperature	Refrigerator, oral solution should not be refrigerated	Room temperature	Room temperature	Up to 7 days at room temperature, refrigerator: stable for 2 months
Major side-effects	GI intolerance, headache, LDS, rare: haemolytic anaemia	GI intolerance, headache, LDS, rare: haemolytic anaemia	Nephrolithiasis, GI intolerance, CNS, rash, hyperbilirubinaemia, LDS, rare: haemolytic anaemia	GI intolerance, paraesthesias-circumoral, taste perversion, asthenia, LDS, rare: haemolytic anaemia	GI intolerance, rash, LDS, headache, rare: haemolytic anaemia	GI intolerance, headache, rash, LDS, oral paraesthesias, rare: haemolytic anaemia	GI intolerance, asthenia, LDS, rare: haemolytic anaemia

CNS, central nervous system symptoms (dizziness, somnolence, insomnia, abnormal dreams, dysphoria etc.);
GI intolerance, gastrointestinal side-effects (nausea, vomiting, diarrhoea, etc.);
LDS, lipodystrophy syndrome;
PNP, peripheral neuropathy.

patients serious reactions of intolerance, including the development of Steven–Johnson syndrome, may appear if medication is not discontinued. In addition, major side-effects of efavirenz are CNS symptoms including dizziness, somnolence, abnormal dreams, impaired concentration and others. These symptoms usually subside spontaneously over 2–4 weeks.

Bioavailability of nevirapine is good (93%) and cerebrospinal fluid concentrations reached 45%. Development of resistance is still an emerging problem with the use of NNRTI and cross-resistances occur among all NNRTI. Again, interactions to other drugs must be carefully studied by health-care providers. In summary, the NNRTI represent a class of antiretroviral agents which have their position in the initial combination of antiretroviral drugs as an alternative to PI with comparable antiviral potency.

PI

Inhibition of virally produced protease ('HIV protease') provides another possibility for therapeutic action and several appropriate agents have been shown to be effective for treatment of HIV infection. Saquinavir was the first inhibitor of HIV protease approved for treatment, shortly followed by ritonavir and indinavir. Three other PIs including nelfinavir, amprenavir and lopinavir + ritonavir have enriched the arsenal of PIs and offer more treatment choices. The use of lopinavir in a fix formulation with ritonavir in one drug (Kaletra) is a new concept which reflects the widespread practice of using ritonavir for increasing the plasma concentration of other PIs ('booster effect'). In addition, these dual PI combinations often lead to more convenient regimens in terms of pill burden, scheduling and elimination of food restrictions.

Indinavir has been associated with nephrolithiasis which may result in renal atrophy in some patients. Ritonavir may cause gastrointestinal intolerance as well as peripheral neuropathy, particularly perioral paraesthesia, as major adverse effects, leading to poor compliance in some patients. Saquinavir alone has a poor bioavailability that may limit its efficacy therefore it is mainly used in combination with ritonavir. Shortly after introduction of PI-containing regimens observations about the induction of diabetes mellitus and hyperglycaemia as well as fat maldistributions and hyperlipidaemia were made which are now better known as 'lipodystrophy syndrome' (Table 2). The lipodystrophy syndrome is strongly associated with the use of PI and will be discussed separately.

Development of drug resistance, including cross-resistance to other PI, have been reported and may limit the use of these agents. PI therefore should be only used in combination with other groups of antiretroviral agents. In addition, the list of interactions between PI and other drugs is long; ritonavir particularly interacts with more than 200 different drugs. All other drugs taken by the patient therefore

Table 2 Symptoms of the lipodystrophy syndrome

Clinical signs	Laboratory findings
Peripheral fat wasting	Hypertriglyceridaemia
Visceral fat accumulation	Hypercholesterolaemia
Dorsocervical fat accumulation ('buffalo hump')	(e.g. LDL and VLDL)
Breast enlargement	Hyperuricaemia
Facial thinning	Hyperinsulinismus
Lipomas	Peripheral insulin resistance
Extremity wasting with venous prominence	Hyperglycaemia

must be checked carefully by the physician when PIs are prescribed. PI are very powerful in durable HIV viral load suppression but their use brings long-term side-effects which may have fatal implications.

Lipodystrophy syndrome

Changes in body fat distribution with or without laboratory findings (Table 2) have been observed in up to 80% of patients receiving PI-containing antiretroviral regimens, usually during the first months of therapy. These clinical and laboratory changes have been called lipodystrophy syndrome; however, no uniform definition of this syndrome exists. It is still unclear whether the clinical manifestations represent distinct entities with different aetiologies, or whether they occur as a result of a single pathological process. Lipodystrophy has been primarily associated with the use of PI, but may occur also with the use of NRTI (especially d4T including combinations) or, even in the absence of therapy. Although the long-term consequences of this syndrome are unknown, substantial increases of serum lipids are of concern because of the possible association with cardiovascular diseases and pancreatitis. Only a few case reports exist describing premature coronary artery disease, cerebrovascular disease, pancreatitis and cholelithiasis in HIV-infected patients receiving PI including antiretroviral therapy. Altogether, therapeutic interventions reversing or halting the progression of lipodystrophy are limited. Switching to other classes of antiretroviral agents together with exercise training, dietary changes and smoking cessation may be of help. The effectiveness of lipid-lowering drugs is not clear and must be undertaken with caution due to potential drug interactions.

Guidelines for treatment with antiretroviral agents

Initial treatment

The optimal time to initiate multidrug antiretroviral therapy is still unknown. It is becoming clear that HAART is a field of complex and sometimes difficult treatment with major side-effects. For many patients difficulties with adherence, and serious potential consequences from the development of viral resistance due to non-adherence to the drug regimen, are common experiences. Therefore for each individual patient, HAART requires a careful balance of risks and benefits, and especially in the asymptomatic patient.

Potential benefits of early therapy in asymptomatic patients include (a) earlier suppression of viral replication; (b) preservation of immune function; (c) prolongation of disease-free survival; and (d) decreased risk of viral transmission. Potential risks include (a) the adverse effects of the drugs with sometimes serious toxicities; (b) the inconvenience of most of the suppressive regimens currently available; (c) development of drug resistance over time because of early initiation of therapy; (d) limitation of future treatment options; and (e) the risk of transmission of drug-resistant virus strains. However, therapy should be strongly considered in patients with plasma HIV RNA concentrations $> 30\,000$ (bDNA) to $55\,000$ (RT-PCR) copies/mL, regardless of the CD4+ cell counts. On the other hand, CD4+ counts of $< 350/\mu L$, particularly $< 200/\mu L$, and clinically severe symptoms including AIDS-defining diseases, should result in ini-

Table 3 When to initiate antiretroviral treatment. Every point of this list is a marker for starting therapy

1	HIV viral load: $> 30\,000$–$55\,000$ copies/mL
2	CD4+ count: $< 350/\mu L$
3	Clinically symptomatic HIV infection (AIDS, severe symptoms)

tiation of antiretroviral treatment (Table 3). In patients with < 30 000 HIV RNA copies/mL, > 350/μL CD4+ cells and no clinical symptoms of HIV disease a more 'wait-and-see' attitude appears justifiable, especially if the patient is not committed to antiretroviral therapy and shows poor compliance. These patients should be carefully re-evaluated every 3–6 months, reconsidering antiretroviral management, or if they are committed to therapy treatment should be offered participation in clinical trials. In addition, HAART in patients with acute HIV infection should be restricted to clinical trials because of the very preliminary data regarding benefits and risks of such an early intervention.

When making decisions regarding the initiation of therapy, the CD4+ cells and HIV viral load should be performed on two occasions to ensure accuracy and consistency of measurement because intercurrent infections, resolution of symptomatic illnesses or immunization may interfere especially with the HIV viral load. It is important to know that there is some variability among viral load assays and plasma HIV RNA values may vary. In addition, there are differences regarding variable levels of detection and their capacity to determine HIV RNA of non-B HIV subtypes. For that reason, control measurements of HIV RNA levels should be obtained using the same assay and, if possible, the same laboratory in every single patient.

Combinations of antiretroviral agents

In general, monotherapy with a single antiretroviral agent is rather obsolete. The aim of every initial combination is to reduce the plasma viral load as low and as long as possible, to increase the CD4+ cell counts and to improve the overall clinical status of the patient.

Today, antiretroviral administration including two NRTI and one or two PI (Table 4) is most likely to reduce and maintain the HIV viral load levels below the detection limit, to achieve partial immunological restoration, and decreased incidence of AIDS and death. These drug combinations are especially recommended for patients with initial high viral load levels, low numbers of CD4+ cell counts and clinical symptoms of advanced HIV infection or AIDS.

Alternatively, a regimen including two NRTI plus an NNRTI or a three NRTI regimen can be considered (Table 4). The advantage of a class-sparing regimen is to preserve one or two classes of drugs for later use. Moreover, this strategy makes it possible selectively to delay the risk of certain side-effects uniquely associated with a single class of drugs. A recent drug trial has established a major principle for the use of nevirapine: showing the highest antiretroviral activity when combined with other drugs to which the patient is naive. This observation suggests that the best chance to use nevirapine is to include this drug into initial multidrug combinations. Viral load suppression and CD4+ T-cell responses that are similar to those observed with PI-containing regimens have been achieved with selected PI-sparing regimens, such as efavirenz + two NRTI or ABC + two NRTI; however, it is not yet known whether such PI-sparing regimens

Table 4 Initial antiretroviral treatment combinations

Groups of agents	Examples
NRTI-1+NRTI-2+PI	AZT+3TC+IDV; d4T+3TC+NFV
NRTI-1+NRTI-2+PI-1+PI-2	AZT+3TC+SQV+RTV; d4T+3TC+IDV+RTV
NRTI-1+NRTI-2+NNRTI	AZT+3TC+EFV; d4T+ddI+NVP
NRTI+NNRTI+PI	d4T+NVP+NFV; AZT+EFV+IDV
NRTI-1+NRTI-2+NRTI-3	AZT+3TC+ABC; d4T+ddI+3TC

will provide comparable efficacy in patients with advanced HIV infection or AIDS. Although antiretroviral drug regimens including PI are very potent, they may not be practical for every patient. This applies particularly in asymptomatic cases during the early phases of the disease, in IDUs or in patients who are intellectually limited due to cerebral HIV manifestations. In these individuals such a regimen may be a major challenge. In our experience, some HIV-infected patients who are symptomless and otherwise in a good healthy condition start to feel sick as soon as they are confronted with a daily drug regimen including 20 or more pills and combinations of three NRTI or two NRTI plus an NNRTI may be more appropriate for initial management in this group. In addition, patients with a history of non-compliance to other medication, or others who signal only limited overall compliance should be first treated with a combination including a triple NRTI regimen or NNRTI-based regimen which are generally easier to use and adhere than PI-containing regimens. Less than excellent adherence may result in viral breakthrough and the emergence of drug-resistant strains. Even short-term non-compliance to aggressive combinations may be followed by rapid virus reproduction in lymph nodes and the potential cross-resistance among the available PI can diminish future treatment options.

For initial treatment AZT or d4T should be part of the combination because of their potency to penetrate the blood–brain barrier. Some combinations (e.g. d4T and ddC) should be avoided due to overlapping toxicity profiles whilst d4T and AZT may be antagonistic.

Under all circumstances, it is of utmost importance to inform the patient on the aim of any therapeutic measures, possible complications and side-effects before initiating effective antiretroviral drug combinations. Information on the correct use of particular drugs and a detailed time schedule for their use are necessary preconditions in order to integrate the therapy into the patient's daily life and to ensure his commitment to what will be a costly and potentially toxic medication (Fig. 1).

The issue of poor adherence

Several studies have shown that poor adherence increases with drug therapies in the asymptomatic stages of disease and

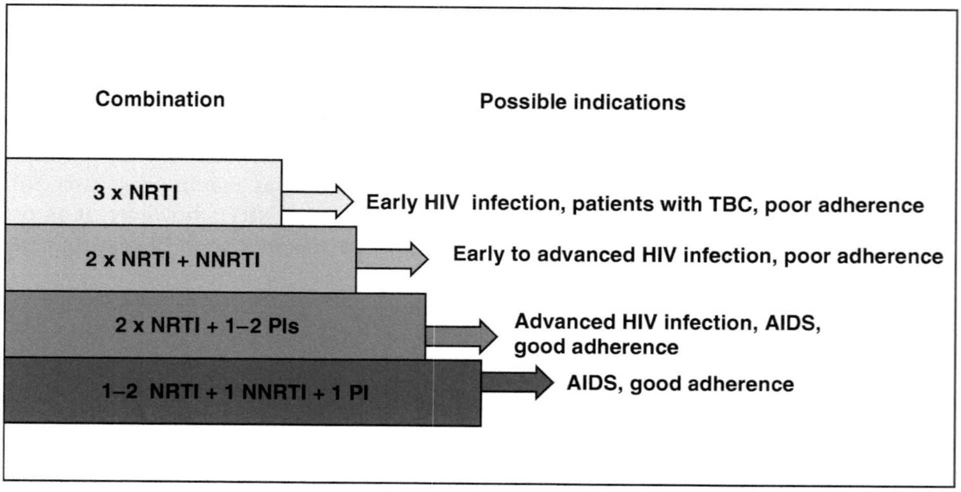

Figure 1 Possible indications for initial treatment combinations

with the number of toxic adverse effects. In addition, it is well known that poor adherence is highest among young patients and that the rate of compliance does not correlate with the severity of the disease. The ability of the HIV-infected patient to adhere to the regimen is essential for successful treatment. Excellent adherence has been shown to increase the likelihood of sustained virus suppression. Conversely, poor adherence has been shown to increase the likelihood of virological failure and has been associated with increased morbidity and mortality. In addition, poor adherence leads to the development of drug resistance, limiting the effectiveness of therapy. Surveys have shown that one-third of patients missed doses within 3 days of the survey. It is therefore not surprising that the issue of adherence in HIV-infected individuals under antiretroviral multidrug therapy is a major concern and must be carefully considered when the physician decides to introduce the appropiate management in each particular patient.

Indications for changing antiretroviral medication

HIV viral load levels and CD4+ cell counts should be evaluated at least every 3 months in patients under antiretroviral therapy. Together with the clinical examination of the patient these surrogate markers will best indicate a possible treatment failure after introduction of antiretroviral multidrug therapy. The nadir of HIV RNA levels usually occurs between 8 and 16 weeks after initiation of therapy. However, in patients with high pretreatment plasma HIV RNA levels, maximal suppression may not be seen until 16–24 weeks, even after an aggressive multidrug regimen.

In treating naive patients reduction of the viral load below the detection limit (< 50 copies/mL) is most likely associated with slow or non-progression of HIV infection and therefore should be the therapeutic goal. If this goal cannot be achieved consideration should be given to changing the drug regimen administered. Less than a 0.5–0.75 $\log_{10}$ reduction in plasma HIV RNA by 4 weeks, or less than a 1 $\log_{10}$ reduction by 8–12 weeks, or failure to suppress plasma HIV RNA to undetectable levels within 4–6 months after starting therapy requires modification of the regimen (Table 5).

In patients who have already achieved a viral load below the detection limit under treatment a new rise of HIV RNA levels (e.g. >5000–50 000 copies/mL) suggests the development of drug resistance and is an indication to change the medication (Table 5). However, in patients whose plasma HIV RNA increases from undetectable to low-level detectability (e.g. 50–5000 copies/mL) the physician may consider short-term further observation and patients should be followed very closely. Not only viral resistance but also other factors such as recent vaccination, intercurrent infections or lack of compliance will influence the HIV viral load measurements. For this reason every increase of HIV viral load, defined as threefold or greater from the nadir not attributable to intercurrent infections or vaccination should be confirmed twice

Table 5 When to change antiretroviral therapy

1	Viral load reduction < 1 $\log_{10}$ by 8–12 weeks or less than the detection limit after 4–6 months after initiating therapy
2	New rise of HIV RNA levels, defined as threefold or greater from the nadir of viral load
3	Progressive declining CD4+ cell counts
4	Clinical symptoms indicating progression of HIV infection
5	Unacceptable side-effects or non-adherence to the initial treatment regimen
6	Current use of suboptimal treatment combinations (e.g. overlapping toxicity, monotherapy)

and exploration of patient adherence should be done before the decision to modify therapy is taken. When changing because of possible non-compliance the individual reasons (e.g. low-grade side-effects, number of pills, psychosocial factors) should be carefully analysed and simpler regimes with less toxicity may appear more appropriate and, in the long term, be more successful.

There may be some lack of correlation between HIV RNA levels in plasma and the CD4+ cell counts measured. As a rule, an increase of the CD4+ cell count is seen with a time shift to the decrease of viral load, however, falling CD4+ cell counts may be measured in some patients with sustained decrease of viral load levels below detectable limits. This phenomenon has been reported in patients treated with multidrug regimen including PI. Similarly, a discordance may also occur when the plasma viral load returns to pretreatment levels while the CD4+ cell counts remain substantially above their pretreatment values. At present, the reasons for such observations are not clearly understood. In agreement with other authors we recommend switching antiretroviral regimen if the CD4+ cell counts are falling rapidly and progressively, even if the viral load indicates effective antiretroviral activity. Possibly, the immune deficiency may be markedly disturbed due to HIV infection and opportunistic infections may occur even in the presence of low viral load levels and rising CD4+ cell counts. Therefore, the appearance of a new HIV-associated disease is not necessarily a sign indicating treatment failure.

In cases of intolerable adverse effects, dose reduction should be avoided if possible. If the reason for the toxic side-effect is not clear, brief and complete interruption of the full therapeutic regimen is rather recommended. Clinical experience with the use of antiretroviral agents together with the options of available alternative drugs are necessary to decide whether to replace a single drug of the prior regimen or to introduce an entirely new multidrug combination. In patients with antiretroviral monotherapy or with combinations of two NRTI the entire medication should be changed.

How to switch antiretroviral therapy

As stated above, there is a number of factors to consider once the decision has been made to change the drug regimen. Careful evaluation of the possible reasons for treatment failure in every single patient should be done before switching therapy. The guiding principle should be to change all agents of the initial regimen, if possible, or at least two of three drugs of a prior insufficiently suppressive multidrug combination. Examples of alternative therapeutic settings to a prior regimen are listed in Table 6. Today, the practice of adding or replacing only a single new agent is not recommended because of the rapid development of resistant strains in this setting. If susceptibility testing indicates resistance to only one agent in a combination regimen, it may be possible to replace only that drug.

Table 6 Examples for switching an initial regimen

Initial regimen	Alternative combinations
NRTI-1+NRTI-2+PI-1	NRTI-3+NRTI-4+PI-2; NRTI-3+NRTI-4+PI-2+PI-3; NRTI-3+NRTI-4+PI-2+NNRTI
NRTI-1+NRTI-2+NNRTI	NRTI-3+NRTI-4+PI-1; NRTI-3+NRTI-4+PI-1+PI-2
NRTI-1+NRTI-2+PI-1+PI-2	NRTI-3+NRTI-4+PI-3+NNRTI; NRTI-3+NRTI-4+PI-3+PI-4+NNRTI
NRTI+NNRTI+PI-1	NRTI-2+NRTI-3+PI-2+PI-3
NRTI-1+NRTI-2+NRTI-3	PI-1+PI-2+NNRTI; PI-1+PI-2+NRTI-4; PI-1+PI-2+NNRTI+NRTI-4

Change of a successful medication due to side-effects should be managed by replacing the responsible drug with another of similar potency and mode of action, but with non-overlapping toxicity profile (e.g. substitution of AZT with d4T in the case of haematological toxicity). This will avoid loss of therapeutic benefit.

For patients in late-stage disease with no rational options who have virological failure with return of viral load to pretreatment levels and declining CD4+ cell counts, discontinuation of any antiretroviral therapy should be considered. There is limited information about the value of restarting a drug that the patient has previously received. Susceptibility testing (phenotypic or genotypic resistance) may be useful in this situation if clinical evidence suggestive of the emergence of resistance is observed. Changing from ritonavir to indinavir or vice versa for drug failure should be avoided, since high level cross-resistance is likely. The decision to change therapy and the choice of a new regimen has a tremendous impact on the life of the patient and requires a clinician with considerable expertise in the care of HIV-infected individuals.

Outlook

So far we know eradication of HIV infection cannot be achieved with currently available antiretroviral regimens, possibly due to the establishment of a pool of latently infected CD4+ cells during the very earliest stages of acute HIV infection. This pool of cells persists with an extremely long half-life, even with durable suppression of plasma viraemia to the detection limit.

With the newly developed agents and the introduction of multidrug combinations, the treatment of HIV infection seems to be in a more optimistic stage. Nevertheless, the long-term outcome and toxicity of recently introduced multidrug combinations is still unknown. We can overlook the side-effects of the currently used agents only when patients are treated over a longer period of time. The complexity of existing combination therapies should spur efforts to develop equivalent agents with easier dosing regimens. This is extremely important because poor adherence to complex drug regimens—resulting in multidrug resistance—is becoming an increasing problem.

There is a series of new antiviral agents for HIV infection under development. Drugs which inhibit the viral integrase will open new therapeutic approaches in antiretroviral therapy. In addition, chemokines from lymphocytes (e.g. interleukin-16), have been isolated, which may interfere with a recently described coreceptor involved in HIV infection and have possible therapeutic potential. Hydroxyurea is a promising candidate as an adjunct in the treatment of HIV infection; however, only few data are currently available from controlled clinical trials providing support for the clinical utility of this drug.

The ongoing progress of multidrug treatment for HIV infection challenges each physician involved in the management of HIV-infected patients. Since treatment options are now considerably more complicated and complex, physician experience, training and permanent updating become even more important in the management of this disease.

Further reading

Cameron DW, Japour AJ, Xu Y *et al.* Ritonavir and saquinavir combination therapy for the treatment of HIV infection. *AIDS* 1999; 13: 213–24.

Carpenter CCJ, Fischl MA, Hammer SM *et al.* Antiretroviral therapy for HIV Infection in 1998: Updated recommendations of the International AIDS Society–USA Panel. *JAMA* 1998; 280: 78–86.

Carr A, Samaras K, Chisholm DJ, Cooper DA. Pathogenesis of HIV-1-protease inhibitor-associated peripheral lipodystrophy, hyperlipidaemia, and insulin resistance. *Lancet* 1998; 351: 1881–3.

Carr A, Samaras K, Thorisdottir A *et al.* Diagnosis, prediction, and natural course of HIV-1 protease-inhibitor associated lipodystrophy, hyperlipidaemia, and diabetes mellitus: a cohort study. *Lancet* 1999; 353: 2093–9.

Cohen OJ, Fauci AS. Transmission of multidrug-resistant human immunodeficiency virus–the wake-up call. *N Engl J Med*, 1998; 339: 341–3.

Deeks SG, Smith M, Holodniy M, Kahn JO. HIV-1 protease inhibitors: a review for clinicians. *JAMA* 1997; 277: 145–53.

Detels R, Munoz A, McFarlane G *et al.* Effectiveness of potent antiretroviral therapy on time to AIDS and death in men with known HIV infection duration. *JAMA* 1998; 280: 1497–503.

Dietrich U, Ruppach H, Gehring S *et al.* Large proportion of non-B HIV-1 subtypes and presence of zidovudine resistance mutations among German seroconvertors. *AIDS* 1997; 11: 1532–3.

Dietrich U, Wolf E, Jäger H *et al.* Increasing prevalence of protease-resistance mutations in therapy-naive HIV-1 positive Germans. *AIDS* 1999; 13: 2304–5.

Flexner C. HIV-protease inhibitors. *N Engl J Med* 1998; 338: 1281–92.

German-Austrian Guidelines for Antiretroviral Therapy in HIV Infection. *Eur J Med Res* 2000; 5: 129–38.

Hartmann M, Petzoldt D. Lipodystrophiesyndrom bei der HIV-Infektion. *Hautarzt* 2000; 51: 159–63.

Henry K, Melroe H, Huebsch J *et al.* Severe premature coronary artery disease with protease inhibitors. *Lancet* 1998; 351: 1328.

Herry I, Bernard L, de Truchis P, Perronne C. Hypertrophy of the breasts in a patient treated with indinavir. *Clin Infect Dis* 1997; 25: 937–8.

Husoli R, Orfanos CE. HIV-Infektion und Kaposi-Sarkom. In: Orfanos CE, Garbe C, eds. *Therapie der Hautkrankheiten*. 2. Auflage. Berlin: Springer-Verlag: 1015–74.

Ickovics JR, Meisler AW. Adherence in AIDS clinical trials. A framework for clinical research and clinical care. *J Clin Epidemiol* 1997; 50: 385–91.

Levy JA. Caution: should we be treating HIV infection early? *Lancet* 1998; 352: 982–3.

Lo JC, Mulligan K, Tai VW *et al.* 'Buffalo hump' in men with HIV-1 infection. *Lancet* 1998; 351: 867–70.

Lonergan JT, Behling C, Pfander H *et al.* Hyperlactatemia and hepatic abnormalities in 10 human immunodeficiency virus-infected patients receiving nucleoside analogue combination regimens. *Clin Infect Dis* 2000; 31: 162–6.

Max B, Sherer R. Management of the adverse effects of antiretroviral therapy and medication adherence. *Clin Infect Dis* 2000; 30 (Suppl. 2): 96–116.

Mellors J, Munoz A, Giorgi J *et al.* Plasma viral load and CD4+ lymphocytes as prognostic markers of HIV-1 infection. *Ann Intern Med* 1997; 26: 946–54.

Miller KD, Jones E, Yanovski JA *et al.* Visceral abdominal-fat accumulation associated with use of indinavir. *Lancet* 1998; 351: 871–5.

Palella FJJR, Delaney KM, Moorman AC *et al.* Declining morbidity and mortality among patients with advanced human immunodeficiency virus infection. HIV Outpatient Study. *N Engl J Med* 1998; 338: 853–60.

Pezzotti P, Napoli PA, Acciai S *et al.* Increasing survival time after AIDS in Italy: The role of new combination therapies. *AIDS* 1999; 13: 249–55.

Racoosin JA, Kessler CM. Bleeding episodes in HIV-positive patients taking HIV protease inhibitors: a case series. *Haemophilia* 1999; 5: 266–9.

Treudler R, Husak R, Raisova M *et al.* Efavirenz-induced photoallergic dermatitis in HIV. *AIDS* 2001; 15: 1085–6.

Ungvarski IPJ. Improving patient compliance with HIV treatment regimens. *JAMA* 1998; 280: 1745–6.

Visnegarwala F, Krause K, Musher D. Severe diabetes associated with protease inhibitor therapy. *Ann Intern Med* 1997; 127: 947.

Von Bargen J, Moorman A, Holmberg S. How many pills do patients with HIV infection take? *JAMA* 1998; 280: 29.

Wali RK, Drachenberg CI, Papadimitriou JC *et al.* HIV-1-associated nephropathy and response to highly-active antiretroviral therapy. *Lancet* 1998; 352: 783–4.

Walli R, Herfort O, Michl GM *et al.* Treatment with protease inhibitors associated with peripheral insulin resistance and impaired oral glucose tolerance in HIV-1-infected patients. *AIDS* 1998; 12: 167–73.

Walsh JC, Dalton M, Gazzard BG. Adherence to combination antiretroviral therapy assessed by anonymous patient self-report. *AIDS* 1998; 12: 2361–3.

Hyperhidrosis

B. Brazzini, G. Campanile, G. Hautmann and T.M. Lotti

Definition

Physiological sweating from cutaneous eccrine glands maintains normothermia and skin hydration. Hyperhidrosis is unphysiological and, although not life-threatening, it can have a substantial effect on the quality of life, causing considerable social, psychological and occupational problems.

Primary hyperhidrosis is a disorder of excessive sweating caused by a dysfunction of the neuroexocrine interplay between the nervous system and eccrine glands. It is independent from thermoregulation phenomena. It most commonly involves the axillae, palms, soles and armpits, where the eccrine sweat glands are mostly concentrated, but in a small number of cases it occurs over the whole body surface. The diagnosis is based on the patient's history and visible signs of excessive sweating.

Primary hyperhidrosis is increased by stress and emotion, and results from the stimulation of postganglionic cholinergic fibres. It cannot be confined within the limits of a general illness like pathological hyperhidrosis, which accompanies fever, certain neurological diseases (e.g. syringomyelia, Parkinson's disease and Riley–Day syndrome), endocrinopathy (e.g. diabetes mellitus, hypoglycaemia, thyrotoxicosis, hyperpituitarism), trauma (e.g. medullary accidents, Frey's syndrome) or other various disorders (e.g. dumping syndrome, carcinoid, alcohol or drug withdrawal, Hodgkin's disease, menopausal state, anxiety, congestive heart failure and obesity).

Treatment (Fig. 1)

Topical treatments

Perfumes, deodorants and antimicrobials

Perfumes have been used for centuries to hide unpleasant body odours. However, the successors of perfumes, deodorant soaps and cosmetic deodorants, are not strong enough to hide bad odour for a long period of time. Antimicrobial fragrances have been used to suppress the microorganism responsible for bromhidrosis. However, effective products, such as antiseptic benzalkonium chlorides and quaternary ammonium compounds, are inactivated very rapidly and therefore are not useful. Other antiseptics like triclosan and triclocarban, are effective for long periods but very irritating.

Antiperspirants

Satisfying results have been obtained with topical antiperspirant salts. The best results are obtained with topical applications of aluminium salts, in particular hexahydrated aluminium chloride in 20–25% solution in absolute ethanol. The effect is optimal and lasts for several days in patients with moderate hyperhidrosis, but in severe cases it is ineffective. These very effective products, used for axillary hyperhidrosis are less efficient on palmoplantar sites. Shelley and Hurley have achieved good results by applying 20% aluminium chloride in absolute ethanol at night, when the axilla is dry, with or without polythene occlusion, at first daily and then every 2–4 weeks. The mechanism of action is still not clear. The occurrence of anhidrosis could be a transient functional disturbance of the duct or secretory coil of the sweat glands. In addition, the application of aluminium salts can cause irritation and soreness.

Aqueous solutions of gluteraldehyde (gluteraldehyde 10% in a buffered

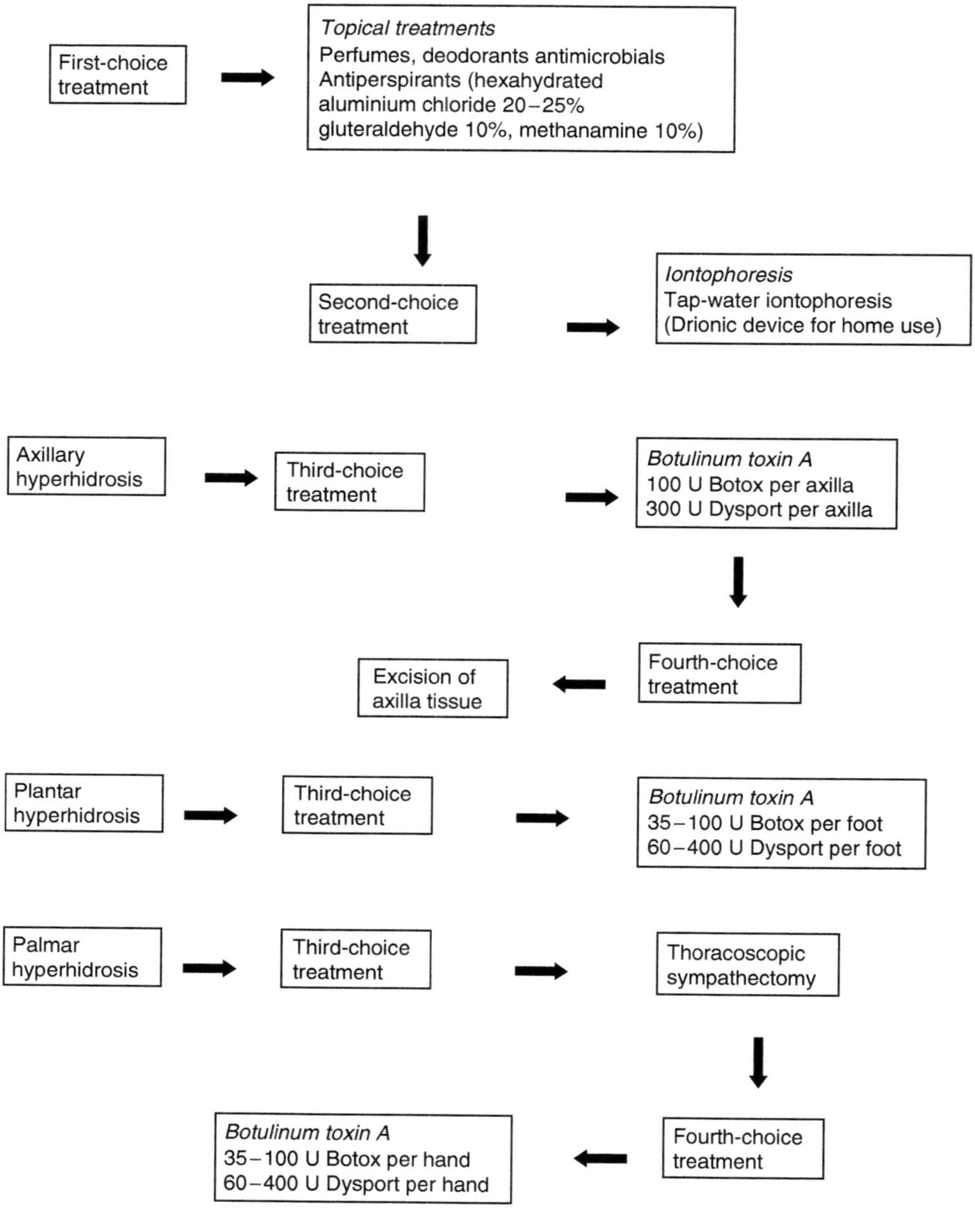

Figure 1

solution pH 7.5) applied to palms and soles can control hyperhidrosis. At the beginning it must be applied on alternate days until control is achieved. Thereafter it can be decreased to a once-weekly application or used only when needed. However, a yellow coloration of the skin and clothes is frequent, and also irritation and allergic reactions occur commonly.

A 10% methenamine, which is hydrolysed to ammonia and formaldehyde when applied to the skin, is effective in mild hyperhidrosis and rarely produces allergic reactions.

Anticholinergic topical drugs

Topical anticholinergic drugs are absorbed sufficiently to produce a beneficial local effect without producing systemic side-effects but none of those available at present can be relied upon.

Iontophoresis

Iontophoresis is a simple and effective solution to mild and moderate palmar and plantar hyperhidrosis. In 1952 the principle of tap-water iontophoresis was introduced by physiotherapists. Since then it has been adopted for the treatment of hyperhidrosis and its efficacy has been proved by several studies. In particular, two recent studies have demonstrated that iontophoresis is effective in about 90% of patients, free of hazardous side-effects and well accepted by almost all patients.

The procedure consists in the exposure of the patient's hands and feet to a 15–20 mA electrical current, which may be conducted through a diluted solution of an anticholinergic drug or tap water (the mechanism of action of tap-water iontophoresis remains unknown). The duration of each session varies between 10 and 40 min, with an accepted average of 20 min. Usually a euhydrotic state can be achieved with an attack treatment (2–6 sessions a week until euhydrosis) and maintained with treatments repeated every 3–6 weeks. The interval between two sessions should be constant because there is no structural alteration in the sweat glands. In theory the treatment should be carried on indefinitely, although the pathology generally decreases with age.

Once the major problem of electrical security is solved, tolerance is excellent. Shortcomings of iontophoresis using direct current include: (a) discomfort, with burning and tingling; (b) skin irritation, erythema and vesicles; and (c) deep burning in cases of defective devices and badly protected electrodes. No adverse effects of long-term maintenance therapy have been observed.

Contraindications to treatment include pregnancy, cardiac pacemaker and metal orthopaedic implants.

To minimize side-effects and to increase technical and safety standards without loss of efficacy, a new method using alternating current and direct current can be used.

Treatments need quite expensive equipment. Multiple patient visits are required and treatment is time-consuming for patients and clinical staff. Moreover, iontophoresis offers only symptomatic relief and therapy has to be continued on a maintenance schedule over many years. This overloads clinical or office facilities and alters patient lifestyle. A battery-operated apparatus, the Drionic device, has been designed for home use.

Systemic treatments

Anticholinergic drugs

Anticholinergic drugs are used to block the effect of acetylcholine on sweat glands. These drugs are certainly useful and reduce hyperhidrosis. However, their benefit/risk ratio is still very controversial. Some authors consider their side-effects (e.g. dry mouth, vision disturbance, glaucoma, hyperthermia, impaired micturition, reduced bronchial secretion, constipation, confusion, nausea and vomiting) extremely troublesome, while according to others such side-effects do not occur in all patients and are frequently moderate and acceptable. According to Klaber and Catteral very good results can be obtained using glycopyrronium bromide 2 mg up to three times a day, for as much as 25 years.

Ganglion-blocking drugs

These drugs can inhibit sweating, but side-effects from hypotension are usually too troublesome.

Others

Diltiazem has been useful in some cases. In cases with a pronounced emotional factor, sedative or tranquillizing drugs are helpful associated with a psychiatric treatment.

Surgical treatments

The nerves innervating the sweat glands are the sympathetic postganglionic fibres, which consist of unmyelinated C fibres. The sympathetic nerves to the arm arise from spinal cord segments T2–T6 and leave the spinal canal in the corresponding ventral rami to synapse or pass through the 2nd to 6th thoracic sympathetic ganglia. All postganglionic sympathetic fibres to the hand, forearm and arm except the axilla run with the somatic nerves of the brachial plexus. Consequently, division of the sympathetic trunk between the first and second thoracic ganglia will interrupt all the sympathetic innervation to the arm, comprising preganglionic and postganglionic fibres.

To achieve axillary euhidrosis it is necessary to perform a thoracoscopic excision or destruction of the T2 and T3 sympathetic ganglia, which is very difficult. But, unless both ganglia are ablated, sweat glands are still innervated by sympathetic fibres in the 2nd and 3rd intercostal nerves. However, a successful improvement of axillary hyperhidrosis can be achieved by the removal of subcutaneous axillary tissue through three parallel transverse incisions. The complications of this technique are quite rare and are represented by: infections, skin necrosis, abscesses, scarring, cutaneous anaesthesia and limitation of shoulder abduction.

For plantar hyperhidrosis, sympathectomy of L2 and those nerves of the lower lumbar extremities relieves symptoms efficaciously. However, lumbar sympathectomy has no place in the treatment of pedal hyperhidrosis since ejaculatory impotence and anorgasmia are almost certain consequences.

There are three main approaches for upper thoracic sympathectomy: the classical posterior approach with rib resection, the supraclavicular approach, and the axillary approach. However, all of these surgical procedures carry risks of intra- and postoperative complications: Horner's syndrome, pleural tear, vascular damage, injury to the phrenic nerve or brachial plexus, postsympathetic neuralgia, persistent postoperative pain, cosmetically unattractive scars and infections.

Thoracic endoscopic sympathectomy has been advocated as a closed percutaneous procedure, which is less invasive and cosmetically acceptable. However, it requires specialized equipment and an experienced anaesthetist; moreover, this approach is limited by pleural adhesions.

In conclusion, thorascopic sympathetic truncotomy and gangliotomy can be considered one of the first-choice treatments for palmar hyperhidrosis, with low risk of operative complications. The symptoms usually remit for 12 months to even 3 years, because of nerve regeneration and/or individual anatomical variations of alternative pathways by which sympathetic outflow reaches the brachial plexus. Compensatory sweating is uncommon after unilateral sympathectomy but frequent after bilateral T2, T3 ganglionectomy, if the two sides are treated at the same time.

Sympathetic ganglion blockade with a neurolytic solution is a closed percutanoeus technique, which has been widely used in pain centres. This technique offers some advantages over surgery because it can be done on an outpatient basis, allowing patients a rapid return to their home environment. This reduces postoperative morbidity and decreases the duration and cost of hospitalization. In addition, when the effects of the blockade vanish, the procedure can be repeated. Side-effects are also rare.

Botulinum A toxin subcutaneous injection

Botulinum toxin A is one of seven neurotoxins produced by *Clostridium botulinum*, that binds to presynaptic nerve membranes and then inhibits release of acetylcholine by disrupting the Ca^{2+}-dependent K^{+}-evoked release mechanism.

Botulinum toxin is approved in many countries to treat spasticity, including blepharospasm, focal dystonia, achalasia and chronic anal fissures.

Botulinum toxin A is available in Europe as Botox or Dysport (manufactured by Ipsen Biopharm, Wrexham, UK) and in the USA as Botox (manufactured by Allergan, Irvine, California, USA). In terms of clinical efficacy in humans, 1 U of Botox is estimated to be equal to 3–4 U of Dysport.

Recently botulinum toxin A has been efficaciously employed to treat primary hyperhidrosis. Many studies have been performed to analyse the dose necessary to achieve euhidrosis, and the number of treatments necessary, but there is no agreement among the different authors. However, in the various studies the doses employed vary between 100 and 500 U Dysport/36–300 U Botox per axilla, and 60–400 U Botox (Dysport 35–100 U) for palmar and plantar hyperhidrosis. Relief from symptoms lasts from 4 to 11 months according to the different studies, and additional injections can be repeated several times, but antibody formation can reduce long-term therapeutic potency.

Intradermal injection of botulinum toxin A is a safe, effective and well-tolerated treatment for axillary hyperhidrosis, and should be considered as a second-choice treatment in patients that do not have a response to topical treatments.

The treatment of palmar hyperhidrosis with botulinum toxin A is complicated by severe pain and paresis of the intrinsic muscles of the hand.

Pedal hyperhidrosis is tedious and uncomfortable to treat because of the large surface area and sensitivity of the feet. However, local toxin diffusion in the axilla or foot is unlikely to produce symptomatic muscle weakness.

Recently, some authors have reported different procedures to relief pain during palmar injection of botulinum toxin A. Vollert B *et al.* proposed an intravenous regional anaesthesia, while De Almeida *et al.* suggest a wrist block.

Further reading

Ashton AC, Dolly JO. Characterization of the inhibitory action of botulinum neurotoxin type A on the release of several transmitters from rat cerebrocortical synaptosomes. *J Neurochem* 1988; 50: 1808–16.

Beach NM. Axillary hyperhidrosis: surgical cure with aesthetic scars. *Ann R Coll Surg Eng* 1979; 61: 295–7.

Bonerandi JJ, Lota I. La ionophorèse. *Derm Prat* 1990; 48: 2–3.

Braune C, Erbguth F, Birkliein F. Dose thresholds and duration of the local anhidrotic effect of botulinum injections: measured by sudometry. *Br J Dermatol* 2001; 144: 111–17.

Collin J. Treating hyperhidrosis. Author's reply. *BMJ* 2000; 321(16): 702–3.

Collin J, Whatling P. Treating hyperhidrosis: surgery and botolinum toxin are treatments of choice in severe cases. *BMJ* 2000; 320(6): 1221–2.

De Almeida AR, Kadunc BV, De Oliveira EM. Improving botulinum toxin therapy for palmar hyperhidrosis: wrist block and technical considerations. *Dermatol Surg* 2001; 27(1): 34–6.

Desnos P, Henriet JP, Vigneron JL *et al.* Traitement de l'hyperhidrose par ionophorèse: principe, matériel, méthodologie, résultats. A propos de 93 cas. *Nouv Dermatol* 1988; 7: 551–4.

Haxton HA. The sympathetic nerve supply of the upper limb in relation to sypathectomy. *Ann R Coll Surg Eng* 1954; 14: 247–66.

Heckmann M, Ceballos-Baumann AO, Plewig G *et al.* Botulinum toxin A for axillary hyperhidrosis (excessive sweating). *N Engl J Med* 2001; 344(7): 488–93.

Holze E, Ruzicka T. Treatment of hyperhidrosis by a battery-operated iontophoretic device. *Dermatologica* 1986; 172: 41–7.

James WD, Schoomaker EB, Rodmann OG. Emotional eccrine sweating. 1987; 123: 925–9.

Karamfilov T, Konrad H, Karte K *et al.* Lower relapse rate of botulinum toxin A therapy for axillary hyperhidrosis by dose increase. *Arch Dermatol* 2000; 136: 487–90.

Klaber M, Catteral M. Treating hyperhidrosis: anticholinergic drugs were not mentioned. *BMJ* 2000; 321(16): 703.

Lin TS *et al.* Video-assisted thorascopic T2 sympathectomy block by clipping for palmar hyperhidrosis: analysis of 52 cases. *J Laparoendosc Adv Surg Tech A* 2001; 11(2): 59–62.

McWilliam SA, Montgomery I, Jenkinson DM *et al.* Effects of topically applied antiperspirant on sweat gland function. *Br J Dermatol* 1987; 120: 907–8.

Murphy R, Harrington CI. Treating hyperhidrosis: iontophoresis should be tried before other treatments. *BMJ* 2000; 321(16): 702–3.

Nicolas C *et al.* Endoscopic sympathectomy for palmar and plantar hyperhidrosis: results in 107 patients. *Ann Dermatol Venereol* 2000; 127(12): 1053–4.

Odia S, Vocks E, Rakoski J *et al.* Successful treatment of dyshidrotic hand eczema using tap water iontophoresis with pulsed direct current. *Acta Derm Venereol* 1996; 76: 472–4.

Reinauer S, Neusser A, Schauf G *et al.* Pulsed direct current iontophoresis as a possible new treatment for hyperhidrosis. *Hautartz* 1995; 46: 543–7.

Shelley WB, Hurley HJ. Studies on topical antiperspirant control of axillary hyperhidrosis. *Acta Derm Venereol* 1975; 95: 241–60.

Vollert B, Blaheta HJ, Moehrle E *et al.* Intravenous regional anaesthesia for the treatment of palmar hyperhidrosis with botulinum toxin A. *Br J Dermatol* 2001; 144: 632–3.

Weight CS *et al.* Thorascopic sympathectomy: a one-port technique. *Aust N Z J Surg* 2000; 70(11): 800.

Ichthyosis

M. Paradisi and A. Giannetti

Definition and epidemiology

The ichthyoses represent a large group of disorders of keratinization (cornification), clinically characterized by the presence of visible scales on much or all of the body surface.

This can be acquired or genetic. The first scales appear in adulthood following neoplasms, and nutritional, metabolic or drug disorders.

The inherited forms of ichthyoses can be classified into (a) autosomal dominant ichthyosis vulgaris (ADI); (b) recessive X-linked ichthyosis (X-LI); (c) epidermolytic hyperkeratosis (EH); (d) congenital lamellar ichthyoses (LI); and (e) complex syndromic ichthyoses (Table 1).

Aetiology

The typical thickening of the stratum corneum in ichthyoses, can occur either as a result of an increase in the proliferative activity of the basal cells or from intercellular adhesion disorders due to proteic and/or lipidic anomalies of the epidermis cells (Table 1).

Clinical characteristics and course

Recessive X-LI affects males and the clinical picture is characterized by large dark brown scales, fold involvement, corneal opacity, hypogonadism and placental sulphatase deficiency syndrome in carrying mothers.

In EH and related syndromes (Siemens ichthyosis and Curth–Macklin ichthyosis) there are erythroderma, verrucose scales prevalent on the folds, bullae and superficial erosions, cutaneous macerations with a consequent unpleasant smell and itching. In complex syndromic ichthyoses there is a variable association with serious neurological, ocular and skeletal damage. ADI, the most common of the genetic ichthyoses, is characterized by small grey–white scales, mainly found on the extensor surfaces without fold involvement. There is a strong association with atopia (50% of cases) and with keratosis pilaris and hyperlinear palms. ADI improves with age, unlike the other types of ichthyosis which remain substantially stable or become worse. The congenital lamellar ichthyoses that first manifest

Table 1 Classification of the ichthyoses

Ichthyoses	Heredity	Incidence	Disorder	Clinical form
Ichthyosis vulgaris	AD	1 : 300	Defect in profilaggrin/ filaggrin expression	
Recessive X-linked ichthyosis	AR	1 : 6000	Deficiency of steroid sulphatase	
Lamellar ichthyoses	AR AD	1 : 300 000	Deficiency of transglutaminase	Lamellar ichthyoses with erythroderma (ELI) and non-erythroderma (NELI), harlequin fetus, ADLI
Epidermolytic hyperkeratosis (bullous ichthyosiform erythroderma)	AD	1 : 200 000	Cytokeratin alterations K1, K10, K2e	Generalized bullous ichthiosiform erythroderma, Siemens ichthyosis, Curth–Macklin ichthyosis
Complex syndromic ichthyoses	AD AR		Variable lipidic metabolic disorder, enzymopathy unknown	For example: Sjögren–Larsson syndrome, Rud's or Refsum's syndrome

themselves as colloidon baby, successively evolve into a form with (ELI) or without (NELI) persistent erythroderma, fat, thick scales, a variable degree of ectropion and a possible electrolytic imbalance. In some cases of harlequin fetus, which is usually lethal, etretinate enables them to survive as ELI. Acquired ichthyosis is different from ichthyosis vulgaris as it has a sudden onset in adulthood, and is often associated with an underlying systemic disease such as Hodgkinson's disease, leprosy, lymphoma, renal failure and hypothyroidism. X-LI is recessive, affecting males only (1 : 6000). The scales are larger and darker than those of ichthyosis vulgaris, and the flexures are not spared. Palms and soles are normal, there is no keratosis pilaris, and associated findings include corneal opacities. Histologically, the granular layer is normal. It is thought that this form of ichthyosis is caused by a deficiency of a specific enzyme (steroid sulphate) which affects cholesterol metabolism in the epidermis.

Diagnosis

A diagnosis of ichthyosis is easy in ichthyosis vulgaris. In the majority of cases, however, a comparison between clinical, histological, ultrastructural and biochemical data is required. Histology shows orthokeratotic laminar hyperkeratosis with a reduction of the granular layer in ichthyosis vulgaris, while this last appears normal or slightly thickened in X-LI. There is a lipoprotein electrophoresis anomaly in X-LI. The diagnostic test is the enzymatic dosage of the steroid sulphatase in the cultured fibroblasts. Some authors classify the lamellar ichthyoses into four forms on the basis of ultrastructural data.

Treatment

General therapeutic guidelines

The type of treatment depends on the type of ichthyoses and the severity of the clinical picture. In fact while in the less severe forms of ichthyosis vulgaris or recessive X-LI a localized treatment is sufficient in the severe ichthyoses such as lamellar, complex syndromic ichthyoses or EH an associated systemic therapy is necessary.

The treatment must be clearly linked to the patient's age, the involved areas and to the extent of the disease. As the total dosage of the drug absorbed through the skin depends on the relationship between the cutaneous layer and the weight of the patient (this relationship is higher in newborn babies than in adults), it is better to avoid, particularly in childhood, the use of potentially toxic drugs. For example, the use of salicylic acid as a keratolytic at concentrations between 5% and 10% as previously recommended, has recently been excluded because of the risk of toxicity both in adults and children. In children acute toxicity—resulting in tinnitus, hyperthermia, convulsions, respiratory depressions—can be lethal. Particular attention must always be paid to internal problems linked to the serious forms of congenital ichthyoses as well as to the risk of hydroelectrolytic imbalances, sunstroke and alterations in thermoregulation especially in the erythrodermic forms. Treatment has the aim of improving hydration, obtaining keratolysis and modulating keratinization.

Recommended therapies

Therapies that normalize keratinization

Systemic retinoids

Systemic retinoids like etretinate and its active metabolite acitretin produce good results in the treatment of the ichthyoses because they can operate selectively on the keratinization disorders. Etretinate was the retinoid first used for serious cases of ichthyosis with the dosage of 1 mg/kg per day at the initial stage, for 1–3 months, with a successive reduction to 0.5 mg/kg per day. Acitretin is more manageable and better tolerated. The therapeutic index of the retinoids restricts their use to the most serious forms of ichthyosis. Above all they are found most useful in the treatment of LI and EL, while only moderately so in EH. In fact in EH, given that aromatic retinoids can increase the cutaneous fragility acting on the interkeratinocyte adhesion, an increase of the bullous component of the disease can be observed. It is therefore advisable to begin with lower dosages (0.3–0.5 mg/kg per day) and always in association with topical treatment. Even in the treatment of Netherton's syndrome they have shown very little evidence of success.

The collateral effects are dose-dependent. Those of the skin appearing almost constantly include: cheilitis, xeroderma and cutaneous desquamation, reduced tolerance to light, long-term cutaneous fragility and sometimes paronychia. Other possible collateral effects include migraine, reversible alopecia, a temporary increase in transaminases, bilirubin and triglycerides, modification of night vision, epistaxis, arthromyalgia and occasionally intracranial hypertension and skeletal anomalies. Some studies have shown that the collateral effects (e.g. hyperostosis, osseous condensation, extraskeletal calcification of the soft tissues and ligaments) are always present after 4–6 years of therapy, whereas the total bone growth and development is normal even if early closure of the epiphysis has been registered.

The potential for bone damage caused by retinoids has, however, been reviewed in the last few years. To diminish the incidence of such risks, it is advisable, when possible, to alternate cycles of therapy with periods of abstension from treatment, especially during the summer when there is greater cutaneous sensitivity caused by the retinoids to the accentuated light of the sun. Radiographic monitoring of children does not seem to offer significant advantages in comparison to clinical observation. Radiographic checks for bone lesions are advisable only in symptomatic cases. However, before beginning treatment with systemic retinoids, laboratory analyses should be undertaken to ensure that patients with dyslipidaemia, hepatoses and presumed and verified pregnancy are excluded from this therapy. A measure of lipid balance and hepatic function should be repeated monthly in the initial phase of treatment and then at greater intervals.

The main collateral effect of systemic retinoids is teratogenicity. This is important in women of fertile age both during the treatment and for 2 years after the end of therapy. To avoid collateral systemic effects, in some cases topical application of retinoic acids is preferable. Some recent studies show the effectiveness of retinoic acid 13-*cis* (isotretinoin) cream 0.1% in the treatment of ichthyoses because of its capacity to reduce desquamation and to improve cutaneous smoothness. Although the use of the *trans*-retinoic acid (tretinoin) can produce less irritation its use is not recommended in the erythrodermic form and in the presence of atopia.

Vitamin D_3 analogues

Topical calcipotriol, tacalcitol or the biologically active form of vitamin D_3 (1.25-dihydroxy vitamin D_3), is effective above all in the treatment of the lamellar and epidermolytic ichthyoses, because of its capacity to stimulate the terminal differentiation of the epidermic keratinocytes and to inhibit their proliferation. Topical application of vitamin D_3 analogues twice a day for at least 12 weeks is found to be moderately effective and well tolerated. It is also possible to treat 15–20% of the cutaneous surface, though not exceeding the weekly dose of 120 g because of the risk of hypercalcaemic crisis.

Keratolytic substances

Urea cream or ointment

As a 10–20% cream or ointment this is effective in the treatment of ichthyoses and psoriasis. The mechanism of action is only partially known, but it seems linked to proteolytic activity (for concentrations of 6–30%), to keratolytic activity that reduces the stratum corneum through the elimination of scales and also to the increased links between water and the stratum corneum. Therefore urea cream helps in the hydration of the stratum corneum, induces epidermic differentiation, reduces epidermic hyperproliferation and does not result in any undesired side-effects though it can cause burning on atopic, irritated skin.

The α-hydroxy acids (AHA)

These simple organic hydroscopic acids are so called because they present an oxydrile in their chemical structure that links to the carbon atom in the α position. Among the numerous AHA, e.g. lactic, pyruvic, malic and glycolic acids, the first is the most effective in ichthyosis therapy. These are different from the normal keratolytics because they act by reducing the cohesion of the newly formed corneocytes at the deep stratum corneum level without exercising any effect on the more superficial cells. They stimulate the turnover of the epidermis and also favour the penetration of other associated substances. Creams with lactic acid (8%) are effective in reducing the hyperkeratosis associated with ichthyoses and in increasing the hydration of the stratum corneum.

The following is a simple effective formula with lactic acid base:

- lactic acid 5 g
- water 40 ml
- ethanol 35 ml
- propylenic glycol 20 g.

This preparation should be applied four times a day for 1–3 weeks. Afterwards the medication is reduced to once or twice a day, depending on the clinical situation.

The mechanism of action explains the greater effectiveness of the lactic acid in the treatment of recessive X-LI. This is characterized by increased cellular cohesion in the lamellar ichthyoses and by altered cell kinetics.

Propylene

Propylene is an effective keratolytic and is used to remove the scales in ichthyoses at a concentration of 40–70% in water with occlusive medication at bedtime, covering the treated parts with a layer of impermeable film. It is important to avoid use on extensive areas of the skin surface, particularly in children.

Propylene glycol can be used in lower concentrations together with other substances. It also possesses a moistening action which increases the content of water in the stratum corneum. This can, however, cause cutaneous irritation and contact dermatitis even at low concentrations.

Alternative therapies

PUVA

This therapy seems useful in the treatment of Netherton's syndrome. Some studies have reported an association between etretinate and PUVA which has resulted in patients responding positively to this combination but only poorly to etretinate when given alone.

Liarozole

This is a new hymidazolic derivative recently used in the treatment of various forms of ichthyoses. It acts by inhibiting hydroxylation at position 4 of retinoic acid which depends on cytochrome P450 for its physiological degradation. Oral administration is also convenient (150 mg twice a day for 12 weeks), with undesired subjective effects similar to those of retinoids.

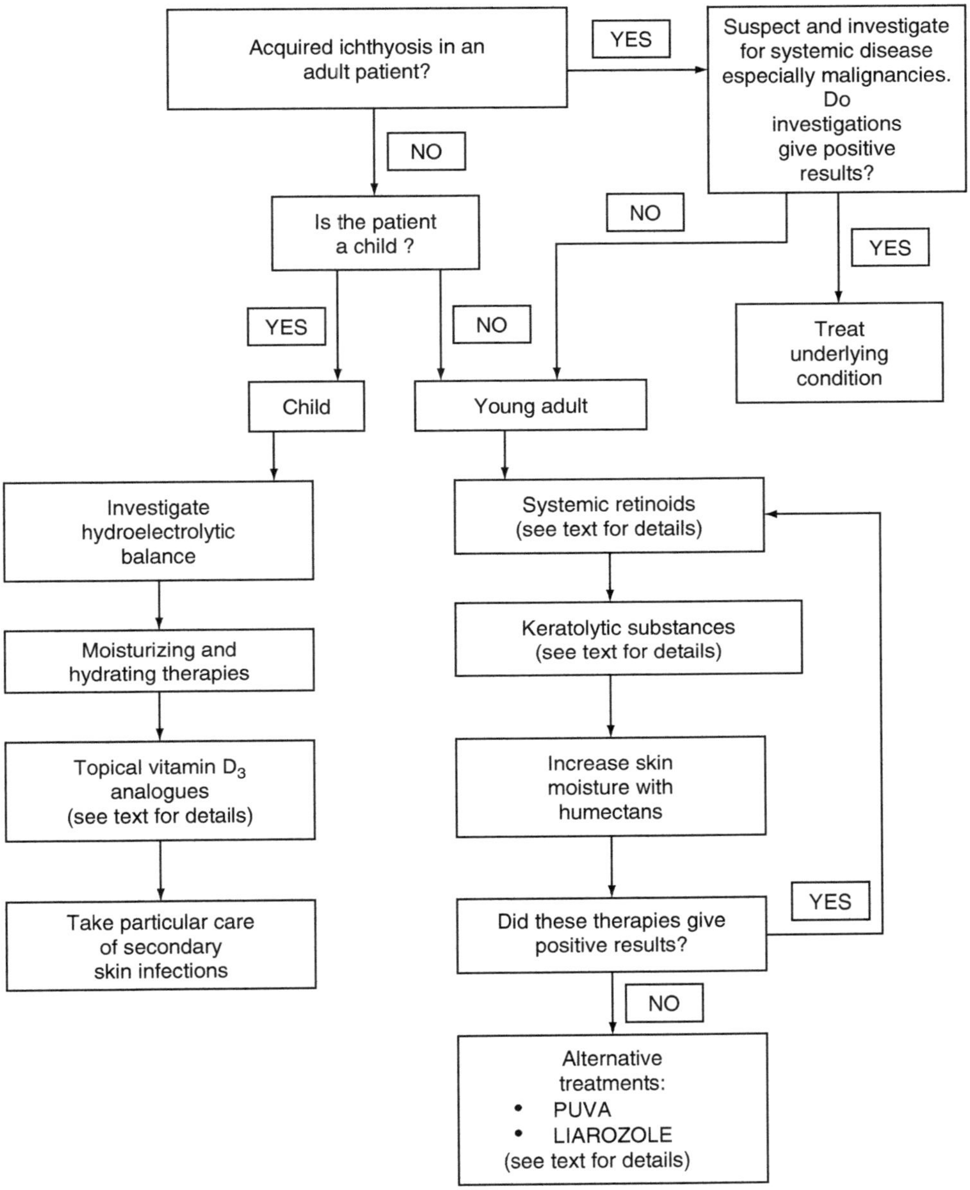

Figure 1 Treatments for ichthyosis

Further reading

Burton JL. *Essentials of Dermatology*. Edinburgh: Churchill Livingstone, 1990.

Delfino M, Fabbroncini G, Sammarco E, Procaccini EM, Santoianni P. Efficacy of calcipotriol versus lactic acid cream in the treatment of lamellar and X-linked ichthyoses. *J Dermatol Treat* 1994; 5: 151–2.

Effendy I, Kwangsukstith C, Lee JY, Maibach HI. Functional changes in human stratum corneum induced by topical glycolic acid: comparison with all-trans retinoic acid. *Acta Derm Venereol* 1995; 75 (455): 458.

Fitzpatrick E, Wolff Freedberg Austen. *Dermatology in General Medicine*, 4th edn. New York: McGraw-Hill, 1993.

Hagemann I, Proksch E. Topical treatment by urea reduces epidermal hyperproliferation and induces differentiation in psoriasis. *Acta Derm Venereol* 1995; 76: 353–6.

Kragballe K, Steijlen PM, Ibsen HH *et al.* Efficacy, tolerability, and safety of calcipotriol ointment in disorders of keratinization. *Arch Dermatol* 1996; 131 (556): 560.

Lacour M, Mehta Nkhar B, Atherton DJ, Harper JI. An appraisal of acitretin therapy in children with inherited disorders of keratinization. *Br J Dermatol* 1996; 134: 1023–9.

Lucker GP, Heremans AM, Boegheim PJ, van der Kerkhof PC, Steijlen PM. Oral treatment of ichthyosis by the cytochrome P-450 inhibitor liarozole. *Br J Dermatol* 1997; 1: 71–5.

Steijlen PM, Refenschweiler DOH, Ramaekers FCS *et al.* Topical treatment of ichthyoses and Darier's disease with 13–cis retinoic acid. *Arch Dermatol Res* 1993; 285: 221–6.

Steijlen PM, Van Dooren-Greebe RJ, Van De Kerkhof PCM. Acitretin in the treatment of lamellar ichthyosis. *Br J Dermatol* 1994; 130: 214.

Traupe H. *The Ichthyoses. A Guide to Clinical Diagnosis, Genetic Counselling and Therapy.* Berlin: Springer, 1989.

Vallat VP, Gileaudeau P, Battat L *et al.* PUVA bath therapy strongly suppresses immunological and epidermal activation in psoriasis: a possible basis for remittent therapy. *J Exp Med* 1994; 180: 283–96.

Impetigo

S. Veraldi and R. Caputo

Definition and epidemiology

Impetigo is a superficial infection of the skin caused by staphylococci and/or streptococci. It is the most frequent bacterial dermatitis in infancy. It occurs mainly in preschool-aged children, particularly during the summer.

The disease is very contagious especially among neonates and breast-fed babies. In fact, it is not rare to observe minor epidemics in kindergarten schools.

The transmission is prevalently by direct person-to-person contact and is favoured by:

1 Environmental factors:
- high temperatures
- high humidity
- overcrowding
- poor hygiene.

2 Personal factors:
- malnutrition
- poor hygiene
- abnormalities in humoral or cellular immunity
- presence of debilitating diseases
- previous or concomitant systemic therapies with antibiotics, corticosteroids, immunosuppressives or antitumorals.

Impetigo often develops on a pre-existing skin disease (mainly atopic dermatitis, as well as other eczemas, traumatic or vascular ulcers, burns, chickenpox, pediculosis, scabies, stings or bites of arthropods). In these cases it is more appropriately referred to as secondary impetigo or impetiginization.

Aetiology and pathophysiology

The term 'impetigo' consists of two distinct entities from the aetiopathogenetic and clinical point of view: impetigo contagiosa (or non-bullous or vulgaris) and bullous impetigo. The first may be caused by staphylococci or streptococci or both. In the past, streptococcal aetiology was most common. Now, staphylococcal infections are more frequent, although marked geographical differences exist; staphylococcal forms are followed by mixed forms and then by streptococcal ones. Group A β-haemolytic streptococci (*Streptococcus pyogenes*) are isolated with greater frequency. Very rare are the infections caused by groups B, C and G.

Bullous impetigo is always caused by *Staphylococcus aureus* (phagic II group in about 80% of cases); furthermore, about 60% of staphylococci are of type 71.

The pathogenesis of impetigo is known particularly in regard to staphylococcal bullous infections. Staphylococci belonging to the phagic II group synthesize some exotoxins with exfoliative properties both *in vivo* and *in vitro* (in media enriched with 10% CO_2). These toxins induce a real acantholysis of keratinocytes of the upper layers of the epidermis, with consequent development of vesicles and bullae.

Clinical characteristics and course

Impetigo contagiosa is initially characterized by the appearance of one or more round vesicles, small in size, containing a clear fluid, and surrounded by an erythematous halo. Because of the superficial localization, these vesicles can rupture, resulting in erosions, or they may remain intact; however, the fluid becomes purulent, with development of a pustule. Subsequently, both erosions and pustules dry up, transforming into crusts: these are rather thick, poorly adherent, present a characteristic yellowish colour similar to honey and are surrounded by an erythematous halo. Their removal shows an underlying surface which is erythemato-erosive, moist and bright red in colour.

Uncovered areas are characteristically affected, particularly the nose, cheeks, lips and chin; subsequently, covered areas can be involved by self-inoculation.

Bullous impetigo presents as isolated vesicles and/or bullae which are widespread on the trunk and skin folds. These lesions are round, often very large (several centimetres in diameter), flaccid, containing initially a clear fluid which becomes frankly purulent, surrounded by very slight or no erythema. The removal of the roof reveals moist erosions which eventually become yellow–brown crusts.

Both varieties of impetigo may be accompanied by mild pruritus.

General health is fairly good: only in diffuse infections may fever sometimes be observed. Even regional lymphadenitis (often painful) is rare.

Both varieties of impetigo can resolve spontaneously within some weeks; with adequate therapy, the duration is 5–10 days.

The disease heals without leaving scars; transitory hyper- or hypopigmentation may persist for some weeks.

Complications (lymphangitis, suppurative lymphadenitis, erysipelas, septicaemia) are extremely rare. Acute glomerulonephritis, although rare today compared to the past, is frightening all the same. Glomerulonephritis is caused by strains of 'nephritogenic' streptococci, mainly M49 and less frequently 55 and 57. Glomerulonephritis generally occurs 3–4 weeks (up to 7 weeks) after the appearance of the skin lesions and is initially characterized by proteinuria and microhaematuria.

Recurrences of impetigo are possible if bacterial foci are not adequately eradicated in the patient, in his/her family and in the community.

Diagnosis

Bacteriological examination of the fluid or the pus removed from a vesicle, bulla or pustule and then Gram-stained enables the observation of both extracellular and intracellular (particularly in the cytoplasm of neutrophils) Gram-positive cocci, which are arranged in bunches or chains.

The same modality of collection may be followed for bacterial culture and antibiogram.

Antistreptolysin and antistaphylolysin titres increase in an inconsistent and delayed fashion. Slightly more specific are anti-DNAse B antibodies. A mild leukocytosis with neutrophilia may be present. Sometimes, an increase in inflammatory tests (erythrocyte sedimentation rate, C-reactive protein, α_1–acid glycoprotein, fibrinogen) may be observed.

Three to four weeks after cure, it is necessary to test the urine to exclude a poststreptococcal glomerulonephritis.

Differential diagnosis

- Herpes simplex: small grouped vesicles, which always recur at the same sites.
- Allergic contact dermatitis: tiny vesicles accompanied by intense pruritus.
- Herpetiform dermatitis: also papular lesions at characteristic sites (shoulders, elbows, lumbosacral region, back, knees) accompanied by intense pruritus.
- Tinea corporis: scaling is almost always present—microbiology.

Treatment

General therapeutic guidelines

A quick diagnosis and an adequate therapy limit the extension of the infection and its diffusion within the family and the community.

Therapy must be preceded or accompanied by a careful search in the patient, in his/her family and in his/her contacts for any possible infective reservoir:

1 For staphylococci:
   - nares and external auditory canal
   - major skin folds (axillae, inguinal, intergluteal and perineal folds).

2 For streptococci:
- pharynx
- tonsils and external auditory canal
- major skin folds.

The patient should be isolated until cure is achieved. During the course of the disease, the patient must use personal bed sheets and underwear.

Recommended therapies

Topical treatment

It is necessary to open vesicles, bullae and pustules with the tip of a scalpel or needle, and then clean and disinfect erosive lesions. This can be achieved with potassium permanganate—250 mg in 3 L of water (dilution 1 : 10 000, approximately) with 2–3 soaks or spongings/day or one bath/day for 7–10 days. Since potassium permanganate is toxic, maximum caution must be taken and its use on the face must be avoided.

In early and localized impetigo, treatment with a topical antibiotic can be sufficient. Topical antibiotics should not be used for more than 14 days, with the aim of minimizing the possibility of the development of resistant strains (particularly staphylococci).

Mupirocin

This is active *in vitro* and *in vivo* even against methicillin-resistant staphylococcal strains. The development of resistant strains and sensitization are so far rare events. Furthermore, due to its chemical structure, mupirocin does not cross-react with other antibiotics. The drug is used as 2% ointment or cream both on cutaneous lesions and in the nares, external auditory canal and skin folds. The dosage is 2–3 applications/day for 7–10 days.

Fusidic acid

Fusidic acid 2% cream is also effective to treat staphylococcal and/or streptococcal impetigo.

Gentamicin sulphate

As 0.1% cream, this is active against staphylococci, but much less active against streptococci; therefore, gentamicin sulphate is more indicated in bullous impetigo and staphylococcal impetigo contagiosa. In the case of topical use, gentamicin must not also be used by the systemic route. The dosage is 2–3 applications/day for 7–10 days on both skin lesions and external auditory canal and skin folds.

Other antibiotics

The use of other topical antibiotics (amikacin sulphate, bacitracin, chlortetracycline hydrochloride, clindamycin phosphate, erythromycin, meclocycline sulphosalicilate, neomycin and polymixin B) should be banished because of the frequency with which bacterial resistance and/or allergic contact dermatitis develop.

Five per cent benzoylperoxide can be successfully used as a cleansing agent for the prevention of recurrences (2–3 washings or baths/week).

Systemic therapy

Streptococcal impetigo

In babies and young children:
- erythromycin ethylsuccinate: 30–50 mg/kg per day orally in 4 administrations for 10 days, or
- clarithromycin: 15 mg/kg per day orally in 2 administrations for 10 days.

In the adult:
- erythromycin ethylsuccinate: 2–3 g/day orally in 4 administrations for 7–10 days, or
- clarithromycin: 500–1000 mg/day orally in 2 administrations for 7–10 days.

In our experience, 7-day therapy in adults is sufficient, as is a daily clarithromycin dosage of 500 mg.

Staphylococcal impetigo

In babies and young children:

- amoxicillin combined with clavulanic acid: 50 mg/kg per day orally in 2 administrations for 10 days.

In the adult:

- amoxicillin combined with clavulanic acid: 2 g/day orally in 2 administrations for 7–10 days.

Also in this case, a 7-day therapy in adult patients is sufficient.

Staphylococcal impetigo caused by methicillin-resistant strains

- Minocycline hydrochloride: 200 mg/day orally in 2 administrations for 10–14 days, or
- Ciprofloxacine hydrochloride: 1 g/day orally in 2 administrations for 7 days.

Further reading

Dagan R, Bar-David Y. Comparison of amoxicillin and clavulanic acid (Augmentin) for the treatment of nonbullous impetigo. *Am J Dis Child* 1989; 143: 916–18.

Feder HM Jr, Abrahamian LM, Grant-Kels JM. Is penicillin still the drug of choice for nonbullous impetigo? *Lancet* 1991; 338: 803–5.

Hebert A, Still JG, Reuman PD. Comparative safety and efficacy of clarithromycin and cefadroxil suspensions in the treatment of mild to moderate skin and skin structure infections in children. *Pediatr Infect Dis* 1993; 12: 112S–117S.

Mertz PM, Marshall DA, Eaglstein WH, Piovanetti Y, Montalvo J. Topical mupirocin treatment of impetigo is equal to oral erythromycin therapy. *Arch Dermatol* 1989; 125: 1069–73.

Pappa KA.The clinical development of mupirocin. *J Am Acad Dermatol* 1990; 22: 873–9.

Spelman D. Fusidic acid in skin and soft tissue infections. *Int J Antimicrob Agents* 1999; 12 (Suppl. 2): S59–S66.

Wilkinson JD. Fusidic acid in dermatology. *Br J Dermatol* 1998; 139: 37–40.

Kaposi's sarcoma

J.D. Stratigos, A.C. Katoulis and A.J. Stratigos

Synonyms

Multiple idiopathic haemorrhagic sarcoma.

Definition and epidemiology

Kaposi's sarcoma (KS) is a systemic multifocal angiomatous tumour of undefined aetiopathogenesis and histogenesis. It was originally described by Moriz Kaposi in 1872.

Clinicoepidemiologically, KS is classified into four distinct forms.

- Classic or sporadic KS (CKS) predominantly affects elderly males of Jewish, Eastern European or Mediterranean descent. It most often arises on the legs, but it may spread to lymph nodes and viscera. The course is most often chronic and indolent.
- African or endemic KS affects children and adults in tropical Africa. Four clinical patterns have been described: nodular, florid, infiltrative and lymphadenopathic.
- Iatrogenic KS occurs in organ transplant recipients and cancer patients undergoing immunosuppressive chemotherapy.
- Epidemic or acquired immune deficiency syndrome (AIDS)-related KS (AIDS-KS) mainly affects homosexual/bisexual human immunodeficiency virus (HIV)-positive males under 50 years of age. It is an AIDS-defining illness and represents the most common opportunistic neoplasm associated with HIV infection. It runs a rapidly progressive and aggressive course, characterized by extensive skin and systemic involvement. However, highly active antiretroviral therapy has substantially decreased the incidence and severity of AIDS-KS in the Western world.

Classic KS

Epidemiology of CKS varies greatly by geographical area, age and gender. In the USA, the annual incidence of CKS was found to be 0.34 and 0.08 per 100 000 population for males and females, respectively. The respective figures for New South Wales in Australia were 0.065 and 0.29. In countries of the Mediterranean basin, CKS is much more common, with an estimated annual incidence rate per 100 000 population of 0.62 for males and 0.32 for females (mean age-standardized incidence of 0.47 per 100 000 total population per year) in Greece, or 1.02 and 0.31, respectively, in Italy.

Foci of CKS have been described in Sardinia, Italy and the Peloponnese, Greece.

In Northern European countries lower annual incidence rates have been reported, e.g. 0.40 and 0.14 per 100 000 per year for males and females, respectively, in Sweden, or 0.014 for both genders in England and Wales.

The highest incidence of the disease is observed in the sixth to eighth decade of life. Mean age at diagnosis is more often 63–65 years.

Males predominate in all forms of KS.

Aetiology and pathogenesis

The aetiopathogenesis of KS remains an unsolved mystery. Even its nature is still controversial. It has not been clarified whether KS is a true neoplasm, an opportunistic malignancy likely to develop in the setting of immunodeficiency, or a reactive hyperplasia in response to angiogenic substances. KS is rather multifocal than metastatic.

KS is an angioproliferative disease. At least in the early stage, KS behaves as a benign reactive and reversible polyclonal hyperplasia. However, in time it can become monoclonal, evolving into a true sarcoma. The development of KS lesions seems to result from the interaction of exogenous and endogenous agents, including angiogenic growth factors, oncogenes and cytokines. Angiogenesis appears to be an important feature and recent experimental studies have demonstrated the role of vascular endothelial growth factor (VEGF) and its receptors in the pathogenesis of KS.

A multifactorial aetiology has been suggested. Immunodeficiency is an inducing factor for KS development. Geographical and racial distribution of CKS indicates that genetic and/or environmental factors may be implicated. It has been speculated that the predisposition to the disease could be linked with HLA-DR5 antigen, while resistance could be linked with HLA-DR3. However, more recent studies are not in agreement with this hypothesis. Male predominance suggests that hormonal factors may play a role.

Infectious agents have long been incriminated in KS aetiology. Epidemiological data regarding AIDS-KS suggest that a second infectious, sexually transmitted agent may play a causal role. Cytomegalovirus involvement has been studied, but without convincing evidence. Retrovirus-like particles have been detected in CKS lesions, supporting a retroviral aetiology.

Kaposi's sarcoma-associated herpes virus (KSHV), or human herpes virus type 8 (HHV-8), is a novel α-herpes virus that has been identified in all clinical types of KS through both DNA and serological studies. It still remains controversial whether HHV-8 is the long suspected infectious aetiological factor of KS, a cofactor, or represents an opportunistic infection.

Clinical manifestations and course

CKS is manifested by single or, more frequently, multiple red to purple or violaceous macules or papules, slowly evolving to nodules or plaques. Lesions may coalesce, may become eroded or ulcerated, or may form nodular or fungiform tumours. Most commonly, lesions first appear in the distal part of the extremities (feet, legs, hands). Involvement of the trunk or the face is rare in CKS. Almost all lesions are palpable. Although unilateral at the onset, lesions develop bilaterally and later spread in a more disseminated multifocal pattern. Every part of the skin can be involved, as well as mucous membranes, especially those of the oral cavity. Mucocutaneous lesions are usually asymptomatic, but are associated with significant cosmetic stigma. Lesions of the feet, especially those ulcerated or associated with oedema, may be particularly painful. Oral lesions may cause pain or dysphagia.

Non-pitting oedema of the surrounding tissues often accompanies skin lesions of KS. It is most commonly located on the lower extremities and causes considerable discomfort. It is probably due to infiltration and pressure of the lymph nodes by KS lesions. Occasionally, lymphoedema due to lymphadenopathy follows the appearance of cutaneous lesions. Long-standing oedema can evolve to fibrosis, contracture and atrophy, resulting in dysfunction of the affected limb.

Viscera, lymph nodes and underlying bones can also be involved. The gastrointestinal (GI) tract is the most common extracutaneous site of involvement. Although usually asymptomatic, GI involvement may cause haemorrhage or obstruction. Detailed examination has revealed gastrointestinal KS in up to 90% of patients. Other visceral organs may be affected, including lung, liver, spleen, heart and adrenals. Pulmonary KS may cause intractable coughing, dyspnoea or progressive respiratory failure. It has a high short-term mortality rate.

Occurrence of systemic KS in the absence of cutaneous manifestations is extremely rare.

CKS has been associated with other primary malignancies that may precede, coincide with or follow the occurrence of KS, with a reported incidence varying between 15% and 37%. Second primaries most often originate from the reticuloendothelial system, such as Hodgkin or non-Hodgkin lymphoma, chronic lymphocytic leukaemia, multiple myeloma, and so on.

CKS usually runs a protracted, indolent course with a survival similar to that of age-matched controls. Most patients die of unrelated causes that befall the elderly, as well as of second primary malignancy. However, it appears that subsets of CKS exist, including a fulminant disseminated type with early visceral involvement that has a poor prognosis.

Diagnosis

The diagnosis is suspected by the distinctive colour and typical distribution on the extremities, leading to clinical diagnosis in almost 80% of cases. Histological confirmation is necessary in all patients.

Histological features of KS are pathognomonic. The disease process takes place mainly in the middle and lower dermis.

Testing for HIV antibodies should be performed to exclude AIDS-KS.

Staging of the disease, as well as investigation for coexisting malignancy warrants detailed clinical and laboratory investigation including:

- haematological and chemistry analysis
- chest, bone and GI tract radiography
- GI tract endoscopy and bronchoscopy
- computed tomography of the abdomen and of the thorax
- bone or liver scintiscan (when indicated)
- lymph node or bone marrow biopsy (when indicated)
- HLA typing
- Venereal Disease Research Laboratory (VDRL) testing.

Staging of KS is difficult. There is no widely accepted staging system available.

Differential diagnosis

The following conditions should be considered in the differential diagnosis, especially when evaluating a single pigmented lesion:

- haemangioma
- dermatofibroma
- angiokeratoma
- echymosis
- purpura
- pyogenic granuloma
- melanocytic naevus
- lymphangioma, lymphangiosarcoma
- glomus tumour
- mycosis fungoides
- sarcoidosis, tuberculosis, leprosy
- lichen planus
- bacillary angiomatosis
- stasis dermatitis
- filariasis, Madura foot (in endemic countries)
- insect bite reactions.

Treatment

General therapeutic guidelines

There is no definitive treatment for KS. Management of KS aims to relieve symptoms, to improve cosmetic appearance, to alleviate psychological stress and to control widespread, progressive or visceral disease. Unfortunately, all treatments are only temporarily effective. Consequently, the primary goal is to ameliorate the patient's quality of life and to prolong survival. Furthermore, many authorities recommend a policy of observation in asymptomatic elderly immunocompetent patients.

Treatment can be divided into local and systemic. The choice of treatment depends on:

- type (morphology and histology) of lesions
- localization of lesions
- extent of the disease

- extracutaneous involvement
- coexistence with other disease
- patient's general condition, especially regarding immune status.

The lack of unanimity in staging and response criteria makes it difficult to design rational treatment strategies.

Recommended therapies

Topical therapies

Topical therapeutic modalities are first-line therapies because they are:

- safe
- easy to perform
- cost-effective
- available on an outpatient basis
- able to offer considerable palliation.

The mechanism of action is based on induction of an inflammatory response that will resolve KS lesions. However, they cannot favourably modify the course of the disease.

Local therapy is indicated for:

- patients with a limited number of lesions
- localized disease of the hands, feet, face, oral cavity or genitals
- large or disfiguring lesions
- lesions that cause symptoms (bleeding, pain), oedema or functional disturbances.

Topical therapies can be applied alone or in combination with systemic therapy.

Radiotherapy

This is a traditional therapeutic tool for CKS. Lesions are particularly radiosensitive with a response rate greater than 80%.

Various techniques have been employed including local field treatment for solitary lesions, and extended field or half-limb irradiation for large tumours or multiple lesions of the extremities accompanied by lymphoedema.

Radiotherapy can effectively control local disease that is too extensive to be treated with intralesional chemotherapy but not extensive enough to warrant systemic therapy. It is indicated for:

- early vascular macules and nodules
- bulky, bleeding or ulcerated lesions
- oral lesions
- conjunctival lesions with periorbital oedema
- localized lymphadenopathy
- oedema.

It has been successfully used for visceral KS, including KS of the lung or the bowel, as well as for mediastinal or intra-abdominal lymphadenopathy.

In conclusion, radiotherapy provides significant palliation and satisfactory cosmetic result. However, recurrence is the rule. Side-effects depend on technique, dosing and irradiation volume. Most commonly, adverse effects are minor, including actinic dermatitis, residual hypopigmentation or hyperpigmentation, and telangiectases. In a few patients, an idiosyncratic painful mucositis, following irradiation of mucosal surfaces, has been reported.

Liquid nitrogen cryotherapy

This is an easily applied method that is particularly useful for treating cosmetically undesirable lesions. It is ideal for small (< 1 cm) macular or papular lesions, especially of the extremities or the face. A clinical response of more than 70% has been achieved. However, cosmetic improvement often results from superficial scarring, while the disease is not eradicated from the deep reticular dermis.

Patients receive an average of three treatments per lesion every 3 weeks. A hand-held spray or cryoprobes are usually used. Each treatment consists of two freeze–thaw cycles, with thaw time ranging from 10 to 60 s (10–30 s for macular lesions and 30–60 s for papular lesions). Cryotherapy is well tolerated. Side-effects are minor (pain, topical erythema and oedema, blistering). It often results in hypopigmentation and scarring.

Intralesional cytotoxic chemotherapy

Especially with vinca alkaloids, this treatment is indicated for isolated papulonodular lesions (> 1 cm), or symptomatic oral lesions. It is a fast and inexpensive modality. The dose of vinblastine is 0.1–0.2 mg/cm^2 for cutaneous lesions and 0.2 mg/cm^2 for oral lesions. Maximal total dose is 2 mg. After a healing interval of 3 weeks, one or two additional injections may be required. Vinblastine has a response rate in the range of 70%. The most frequent side-effects are: pain, skin irritation, ulceration and postinflammatory hyperpigmentation.

Intralesional bleomycin (median dose 1.5 mg per cutaneous lesion) is also effective, particularly for macular lesions. It has no side-effects, except for local pain and hypopigmentation.

Sclerosing agents

Injection of sclerosing agents (3% sodium tetradecyl sulphate) is a fast, convenient (one treatment is enough), inexpensive and effective therapeutic modality that induces long remission by producing ischaemic necrosis. Pain, scarring and ulceration are the most frequent side-effects.

Intralesional interferon (recombinant IFN-α_{2b})

This has been shown to be efficacious for single cutaneous or oral lesions, or infiltrated plaques. However, in some studies it has failed to show superiority over placebo. It is administered at a dose of 3–9 mega units (MU), two to three times weekly for 4–8 weeks. The high cost and the more frequent treatments required, compared to cryotherapy or intralesional vinblastine, are major disadvantages. The most common side-effect is local pain. In general, it has fewer side-effects than systemic IFN. Addition of interleukin-2 has been associated with a more rapid involution of KS lesions.

Intralesional recombinant GM-CSF

Intralesional recombinant granulocyte–macrophage colony-stimulating factor (GM-CSF) is an effective but expensive modality. Its action is probably based on induction of inflammation with subsequent local necrosis.

Surgery

Shave excision has been used for pedunculated lesions. Surgical excision may prove beneficial in selected cases.

Lasers

Argon laser can improve KS lesions, but this method is time-consuming. The carbon dioxide laser is faster, but the presence of infectious viral particles in its vapours has limited its use. Macular lesions have been treated with pulsed-dye laser, but recurrences within 3 months are frequent after the initial response. Long-term therapy is required to maintain cosmetic improvement. Adverse reactions include local pain and blistering.

Systemic therapy

Systemic therapy is indicated for widespread cutaneous disease, locally aggressive or rapidly progressive disease, as well as for KS with visceral or extracutaneous involvement. Concurrently, patients may benefit from local therapy. Systemic treatment may be applied either as immunotherapy using biomodulators, such as IFN, or as cytotoxic chemotherapy using single or multiple agent regimes.

Interferon

IFN-α_{2b} is the most widely used. Interferons β and γ are ineffective for KS.

Experience with IFN-α_{2b} in CKS is limited. Although the response rate is dose-dependent, satisfactory results have been reported with low doses of rIFN-α_{2b} (1–5 MU subcutaneously three times per week for 6–12 months) for cutaneous as well as for visceral CKS. The discrepancy between efficacy of IFN in CKS and AIDS-KS is related to differences in the immunological status between patients of these two forms. Although unable to cure definitively, IFN can induce long-term regression even when other treatments have failed. No maintenance therapy is necessary. Relapse is usually delayed and limited, and can be responsive to treatment with IFN. Occasionally, CKS can become refractory to IFN. Unfortunately, IFN therapy is associated with significant toxicity, which can be divided into constitutional (most notably flu-like symptoms), neuropsychiatric, haematological or hepatic effects, and GI distrurbances. In some patients, these events may have a major impact on the quality of life, leading to discontinuation of treatment.

Chemotherapy

This is the treatment of choice for rapidly progressing disease or extracutaneous KS. Various agents have been employed as single-agent regimens. Vinca alkaloids have been shown to have satisfactory effect on KS. The recommended total weekly dose is 0.1 mg/kg i.v. for vinblastine and 2 mg i.v. for vincristine.

An alternating regimen of vinblastine and vincristine has produced a better response and reduced toxicity compared to those of either drug when used as a single agent.

Bleomycin represents an alternative monotherapy. It is given at a dose of 5–10 mg/m^2 per week. Toxicity includes skin eruption, alopecia, Raynaud's phenomenon and mild myelosuppression.

Oral etoposide (VP-16) is considered by some authors as the most potent single agent studied to date, ensuring a higher response, longer duration of remission and better compliance. It is given at 100 mg daily for 3–14 days every 3–4 weeks for 10–12 times.

Dactinomycin, doxorubicin, epirubicin and other cytotoxic drugs have also been tested with good results.

Liposomally encapsulated anthracyclines doxorubicin (20 mg/m^2 i.v. every 2 weeks) or daunorubicin (40 mg/m^2 i.v. every 2 weeks), enables targeted drug delivery. Intravenous administration has been associated with improved efficacy and reduced toxicity. A high response rate in patients previously resistant to other cytotoxic treatments has been found. Myelosuppression is the commonest adverse event.

Polychemotherapy

This is reserved for advanced KS in an attempt to halt the progression of the disease. Several regimens employing combinations of actinomycin D, adriamycin, bleomycin, dacarbazine, doxorubicin, vinblastine and vincristine have been used. Polychemotherapy is reasonably safe and more effective for palliative management of KS. Myelotoxicity and immunosuppression represent its major disadvantages. Neutropenia caused by cytotoxic chemotherapy may be reduced by administration of GM-CSF or G-CSF.

Alternative and experimental treatments

Several alternative and experimental therapies are currently being evaluated.

Topical agents and retinoids

Docosanol inhibits a broad spectrum of lipid-enveloped viruses *in vitro*. In a pilot clinical study with docosanol 10% cream as a topical treatment for AIDS-KS (five times daily for 4 weeks), a 20% average decrease in lesion area for all target lesions was found.

Preliminary data support the use of retinoids (tretinoin and isotretinoin) in both AIDS-KS and non-AIDS-KS. Retinoids show *in vitro* evidence of inhibition of proliferation of KS cells and regulation of apoptosis. In randomized, controlled clinical trials of topical alitretinoin gel 0.1% (2–4 times daily), the results showed that alitretinoin (9-*cis*-retinoic acid) is safe, effective and generally well tolerated in the treatment of cutaneous AIDS-related KS lesions. Alitretinoin gel may be a useful alternative or adjunct to other treatments for the management of cutaneous KS lesions. Oral 9-*cis* retinoic acid has been associated with tumour regression.

New cytotoxic chemotherapeutic agents

Paclitaxel (100 mg/m^2 given every 2–3 weeks) has yielded response rates as high as 75% with acceptable toxicity (alopecia, myalgia/arthralgia, bone marrow suppression) in patients with advanced AIDS-KS, whose disease progressed on the first-line chemotherapy. The median duration of response is among the longest observed. Paclitaxel has recently been shown to be effective in recalcitrant CKS as well. Paclitaxel appears to be active against KS as a single agent. Paclitaxel stabilizes microtubules, interfering with KS possibly by downregulating Bcl-2 antiapoptotic effect.

Gemcitabine (1.2 g/week i.v. for 2 weeks, followed by a 1-week interval, until maximal response is reached), an analogue of deoxycytidine with cytotoxic activity in the treatment of solid tumours, has been shown to be useful in the treatment of recurrent aggressive CKS, resistant to conventional chemotherapy.

Vinorelbine (30 mg/m^2 every 2 weeks by intravenous bolus), a semisynthetic vinca alcaloid, is safe and effective in the treatment of patients with advanced KS who have been previously treated with one or more chemotherapy regimens. Toxicity, including neurologic toxicity, is mild and reversible. Neutropenia is the most frequent dose-limiting toxicity.

Systemic physical therapy

A single 1-h session of systemic hyperthermia at 42°C has given encouraging results. Intravenous immunoglobulin is being evaluated in KS, as well in several viral infections.

Antiangiogenesis agents

Many investigators have high hopes for the inhibitors of angiogenesis. Two agents, TNP-470 (a fumagillin analogue) and thalidomide, have been determined to induce some responses in KS, and others are currently being tested, such as pentosan polysulphate sodium, sulphate polysaccharide–peptidoglycan compound, recombinant platelet factor, antioestrogens, somatostatin, metalloproteinase inhibitors (e.g. COL-3), inhibitors of protein kinase C, IM862 (a naturally occurring peptide given as intranasal drops), and sulphated polysaccharide dextrin 2- or 6-sulphate.

More than three decades after its withdrawal due to its teratogenic effects, thalidomide is attracting growing interest. It is now known that these teratogenic effects are due to potent antiangiogenic and immunomodulatory actions. Current evidence indicates that thalidomide reduces the activity of the inflammatory cytokine tumour necrosis factor (TNF)-α by accelerating the degradation of its messenger RNA. These properties have lead to the testing of thalidomide in a number of infective, inflammatory and malignant conditions. Oral thalidomide is tolerated at doses up to 1000 mg/day for as long as 12 months and was found to induce clinically meaningful anti-KS responses in a sizeable subset of the patients.

Therapeutic agents that target the VEGF pathway may be an effective strategy in KS. Phase I study results with SU5416, a synthetic low molecular weight inhibitor of the VEGF-Flk-1/KDR receptor tyrosine kinase, demonstrate that this agent is well tolerated and clearly has biological activity (it flattens, shrinks or dissolves lesions, and reduces or resolves oedema) or stabilizes the disease.

A gene therapy approach for constant and local delivery of type I IFNs can effectively inhibit tumour angiogenesis and growth of vascular tumours.

Other therapies

Other experimental therapies include immune modulators such as interleukin-12; recombinant apolipoprotein E-3; phosphorothioate antisense oligonucleotide; TNF; and bacterial cell wall complex.

Inhibitors of cytokines, including tretinoin, interleukin-4, platelet factor 4, and pentoxifylline, may prove effective for KS.

Hormonal treatment with chorionic gonadotrophin has been tried with encouraging results. Preliminary studies suggest that a urinary protein (antineoplastic urinary protein) found in preparations of human chorionic gonadotrophin also has activity.

Future therapies will probably be targeted on inhibition of angiogenesis, suppression or eradication of HHV-8, cytokine overexpression and/or virus-induced tumorigenesis and the process of cellular differentiation. Evidence of viral aetiology for KS suggests that antiviral

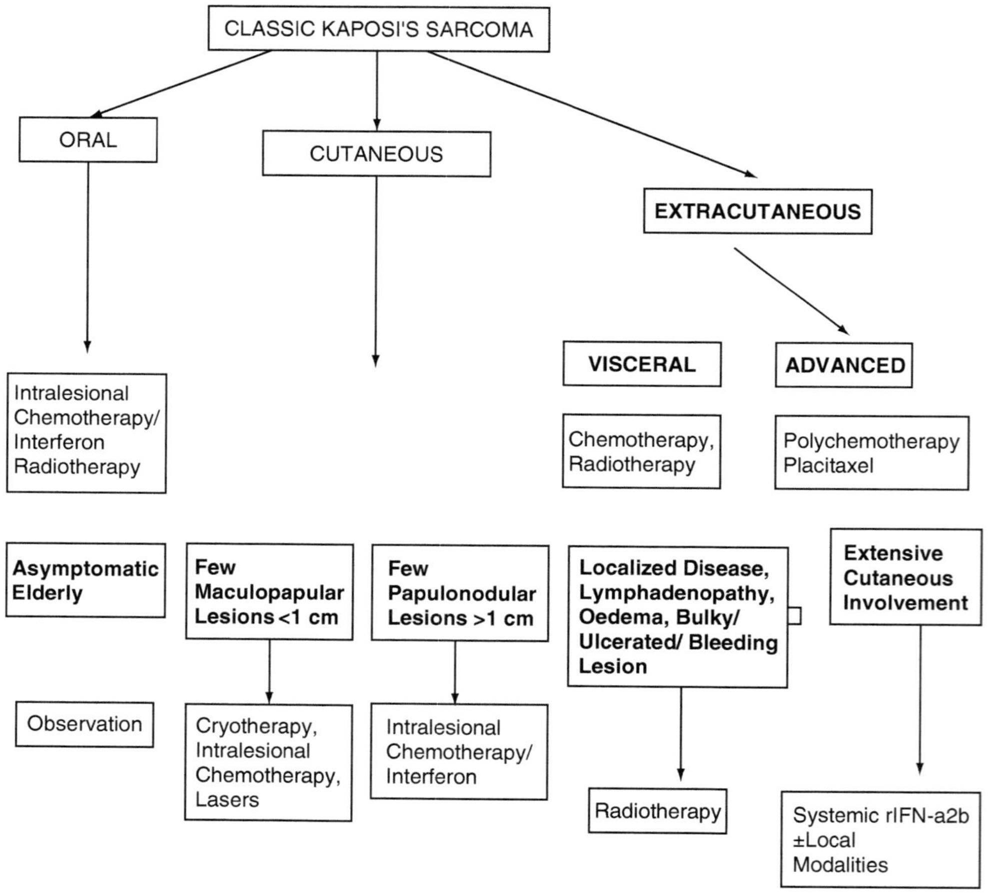

therapy could play a pivotal role in the treatment for KS. In AIDS-KS highly active antiretroviral therapy alone has achieved regression of KS. In addition, good results have been reported with foscarnet. Gene therapy also represents a promising option for the future.

In conclusion, several therapeutic modalities are currently in use for KS and several others are under development. Our long experience with CKS patients has shown that rational treatment choice and, most importantly, individualization of treatment offers satisfactory results with minor adverse effects. New experimental therapies targeting the pathogenic mechanisms of KS allow us to envision the future treatment of KS with optimism.

Further reading

Blauvelt A. The role of human herpesvirus 8 in the pathogenesis of Kaposi's sarcoma. *Adv Dermatol* 1999; 14: 167–206.

Branbilla L, Labianca R, Boneschi V *et al.* Mediterranean Kaposi's sarcoma in the elderly: a randomized study of oral etoposide versus vinblastine. *Cancer* 1994; 74: 2873–8.

Chao SC, Lee JY, Tsao CJ. Treatment of classical type Kaposi's sarcoma with Paclitaxel. *Anticancer Res* 2001; 21: 571–3.

Costa de Cunha CS, Lebbe C, Rybojad M *et al.* Long-term follow-up of non-HIV Kaposi's sarcoma treated with low dose recombinant interferon alfa-2b. *Arch Dermatol* 1996; 132: 285–90.

Duvic M, Friedman-Kien AE, Looney DJ *et al.* Topical treatment of cutaneous lesions of acquired immunodeficiency syndrome-related Kaposi sarcoma using alitretinoin gel: results of phase 1 and 2 trials. *Arch Dermatol* 2000; 136: 1461–9.

Finesmith TH, Shrum JP. Kaposi's sarcoma. *Int J Dermatol* 1994; 33: 755–62.

Gascon P, Schwartz RA. Kaposi's sarcoma. New treatment modalities. *Dermatol Clin* 2000; 18: 169–75.

Kuflic E. Cryosurgery updated. *J Am Acad Dermatol* 1994; 31: 925–45.

Mitsuyasu RT. Update on the pathogenesis and treatment of Kaposi sarcoma. *Curr Opin Oncol* 2000; 12: 174–80.

Stavrianeas NG, Polydorou D, Paparizos V *et al.* Treatment of AIDS-associated Kaposi's sarcoma. The experience of Athens University Hospital for Skin and Venereal Diseases. *Skin Cancer* 1996; 11: 95–101.

Stratigos JD, Katoulis AC, Stavrianeas NG. An overview of classic Kaposi's sarcoma in Greece. *Adv Exp Med Biol* 1999; 455: 503–6.

Stratigos JD, Potouridou I, Katoulis AC *et al.* Classic Kaposi's sarcoma in Greece: a clinico-epidemiological profile. *Int J Dermatol* 1997; 36: 735–40.

Tombolini V, Osti MF, Bonanni A *et al.* Radiotherapy in classic Kaposi's sarcoma (CKS): experience of the Institute of Radiology of University 'La Sapienza' of Rome. *Anticancer Res* 1999; 19: 4539–44.

Trattner A, Reizis Z, David M *et al.* The therapeutic effect of intralesional interferon in classical Kaposi's sarcoma. *Br J Dermatol* 1993; 129: 590–3.

Keloids and hypertrophic scars

G. Hautmann, A. Mastrolorenzo, G. Menchini and T.M. Lotti

Definition and epidemiology

Hypertrophic scars and keloids are benign cutaneous lesions produced by an overgrowth of dense fibrous tissue for uncontrolled synthesis and deposition of dermal collagen. The former remain confined to the site of the primary lesion, the latter invade the surrounding skin extending for variable distances beyond the site of injury.

Occasionally a keloid will form after acne (or during isotretinoin treatment), while the patient's rapid growth phase in the teenage years occurs. They are more common in young patients and are rare in infancy and old age. Women are more often affected than men.

Dark-skinned individuals, Hispanic and Asian people are more susceptible to keloid formation than whites. As a rule, not all people are capable of developing keloids, and keloids do not arise on all anatomical sites.

Aetiology and pathophysiology

The factors that trigger this fibrous tissue proliferation are unknown. Keloids may develop spontaneously, but most commonly they form at the site of dermal trauma, following surgical incision (even if uncomplicated), laser therapy or thermal burns. Furthermore, burn wounds or scalds often lead to keloids in patients who otherwise would not have them.

Keloids most frequently develop on the upper back and chest, neck, shoulders, jaw, ear lobes and legs. These areas all share the quality of high tension on healing wounds. Keloids rarely appear on the eyelids, genitals, palms and soles.

Hypertrophic scars may occur in patients of all ages, everywhere but usually in the same sites as keloids. They are the result of surgical wounds poorly or not at all approximated, wounds closed under tension or with improper surgical incision or hygiene. The presence of foreign material either exogenous (e.g. suture material, foreign bodies) or endogenous (e.g. embedded keratin from hair) is liable to induce scar hypertrophy.

Keloids and hypertrophic scars commonly develop in areas where the muscle's pull across the wound is strong, such as on the deltoid area or the upper arm in muscular young men.

Many individuals have a hereditary predilection (autosomal dominant and recessive factors) for hypertrophic scars or keloids.

Many endocrine factors influence the growth of keloids but the mode of action is unknown. They often occur after thyroidectomy and form readily in acromegalies or enlarge during pregnancy.

Clinical characteristics and course

A keloid in the early stages is soft and pink and looks like an overgrown scar. Then, after 2 or 3 months, it becomes firm and white, protuberant and more extensive than the original trauma, with irregular border and claw-like extensions. Its surface become smoother and rounder.

A hypertrophic scars usually appear 3–4 weeks following a penetrating injury as an elevated, smooth-surfaced lesion, firm, pink or red linear plaque as a reflection of the course of the blade of a scalpel that most commonly was the cause of it. The variability in the size of hypertrophic scars is related to the nature of the original injury.

The usual course of a keloid is that of gradual enlargement to a steady-state size.

Keloids are much less likely to regress than hypertrophic scars, but in any case, the time course for regression, if it occurs at all, is measured in years.

Diagnosis and differential diagnosis

The clinical picture of hypertrophic scars and keloids is typical. Nevertheless, in some cases the macroscopic differentiation of keloids from hypertrophic scars sometimes may be difficult, as these are confined to the site of trauma, e.g. to the surgical scars. However, hypertrophic scars tend to regress within a few months and their excision is not followed by recurrence.

Treatment

General therapeutic guidelines

Hypertrophic scars and keloids are both examples of fibrosing inflammations that tend to regress, to a greater or lesser degree over time, yet rarely may disappear completely, with none transforming into neoplasms.

Successful treatment can be predicted by differentiating a true hypertrophic scar from a keloid. Hypertrophic scars respond fairly well to treatment whereas keloids almost always have a questionably poor prognosis, related to selection of proper treatment and long-term follow-up. Generally, older keloids are less responsive to therapy.

Each treatment modality provides different mechanisms of action on suppression of the growth of the scars. So far, there has been no universally accepted treatment modality resulting in permanent hypertrophic or keloid scar eradication. The current management or prevention of scars is based on three different therapeutic approaches: manipulation of the mechanical properties of wound repair, correction of abnormal balance of collagen synthesis and degradation, and alteration of immune/inflammatory response.

Recommended therapies

Surgery, as an isolated treatment modality, has been almost abandoned due to the high recidivation rates, which are near 100% and generally occur within the first postoperative year. The surgical excision—together with postoperative corticoid injections, radiotherapy or compression—presents better results and each combination is discussed below.

Surgical techniques

Appropriate surgical techniques include simple elliptical excision with wide undermining and careful reapproximation of the wound edges, proximal flaps (rotation, transposition flaps), or island-pedicle flaps depending on technical reasons such as shape, size and site of the lesion, Z-plasty scar revisions, or 'shelling out' of the fibrous keloid with the use of the resulting redundant free skin for closure. The keloid is usually excised by removing a lozenge of skin including the keloid, so that a flat and linear scar is obtained. The deep layers are sutured with reabsorbable material while the superficial layers are sutured by separated stitches with silk or other material. For sites where there is no superficial tension the stitches are removed in the first few days (third day). From the central areas of the wound where tension is greatest the stitches are also removed, at the latest by the seventh day. Unfortunately, the risk of a second keloid forming is 50% or more and sometimes that second keloid is larger than the one originally excised.

Larger keloids may be excised and grafted with a full-thickness skin graft. A full-thickness excision of the keloid is carried out with retention of a rim to which the skin graft is attached. This rim serves as a splint to decrease the transmission of tensile forces to the central area of the graft. This method however has not been widely accepted.

Extremely wide keloids can be shaved off with a scalpel or razor blade and not closed primarily. Excisions which have been shaved must be treated immediately and for prolonged periods with intralesional corticosteroids. Linear keloids or spheroidal keloidal masses (such as found in the ear lobes) can be excised and the scar revised simultaneously to reduce tension across the defect, thereby discouraging new keloid formation.

Intralesional injections

For intralesional injections, we use triamcinolone acetonide diluted with plain lidocaine (lignocaine) or physiological saline to concentrations between 5 and 40 mg/mL. The injection should be given every 3–6 weeks for as long as necessary to obtain flattening of the keloid. Some physicians like to use triamcinolone hexacetonide. However, the crystals of this medication remain in the skin for many months, which makes reinjection with this or other triamcinolones a calculated guess. The width and length of the keloidal scar will not be altered by the intralesional injections alone.

A 30-gauge needle on a disposable Luer-Lok syringe is our favourite instrument for injecting keloids. A three-ring dental syringe is also comfortable for the physician's hand. There are disposable three-ring syringes or adapters available. The needle should be passed back and forth through the scar tissue to fill the entire keloid so that the surface blanches.

A Dermojet is sometimes helpful for the initial softening of the outer portion of the keloid. These needleless injectors have different thrust strengths. It is important to know the way they are calibrated and the setting of the particular instrument. Usually for general dermatological work, the penetration strength will allow only superficial penetration into firm keloids. However, if the keloid is already softened, a Dermojet may be adequate for penetrating the entire lesion. If there are no medical counterindications and the keloid is extremely firm, triamcinolone acetonide, 40 mg i.m., will soften the keloid. This will permit easier intralesional injections 2–3 weeks later.

Twenty-four hours prior to intralesional injection, liquid nitrogen cryotherapy helps the penetration of the steroid into the keloid. This probably is due to the interstitial oedema of the freezing injury.

Some patients experience severe pain during and after injection. For these patients, a field block using lidocaine 1% will prevent or alleviate the discomfort. As the keloid softens with repeated injection, pain lessens and the block may not be necessary.

Begin the injections with triamcinolone acetonide at low concentrations (5 mg/mL) and increase the concentration slowly until softening or atrophy of the keloid occurs. If the low concentrations do not produce a therapeutic response, gradually increase the concentration up to the full 40 mg/mL, remembering that triamcinolone crystals sometimes remain in the tissue longer than 4 weeks.

Increasing the dose and injecting repeatedly without adequate time between injections leads to a build-up of triamcinolone crystals, possibly leading to overtreatment and prolonged atrophy around the lesion. Some patients are extremely sensitive and atrophy develops quickly even at low concentrations. Repeated injections beneath the skin or even in nearby normal skin will also cause atrophy and worsen the appearance of the keloid. Unintentional injection or diffusion of the steroid into the surrounding skin and subcutaneous fat make long-acting triamcinolone hexacetonide less acceptable.

When injecting the area where a keloid was excised, infiltrate the triamcinolone acetonide around the suture line. The first injection may be given immediately after the wound is closed or 1 week postoperatively. Some physicians prefer to inject a few days prior to excision. Continue these injections throughout the healing phase, at 3-week intervals, until the wound shows no sign of keloid development. The wound should be watched carefully for up to 2 years. Sometimes it will do well and then at 6 months or so start to develop another keloid.

Cryotherapy

Cryotherapy is popular with some physicians for the treatment of keloids, but we believe that it has the best results on hypertrophic scars, particularly those located on the chest, shoulders, and back. Several moderate-to-hard freezes 4–6 weeks apart on these postacne scars will flatten them, although the outline of the scar remains, as will its abnormal colour and texture. Cryosurgical media such as liquid nitrogen, affect the microvasculature and causes cell damage via intracellular crystals leading to tissue anoxia. Generally, one to three freeze–thaw cycles lasting 10–30 s are used for the desired effect. The cryotherapy as an isolated form of treatment presents a positive response in 55–70% of the patients and, at the majority of the cases, two sessions, with a 20-day interval, are required. Treatment may need to be repeated every 20–30 days. Cryotherapy in combination with intralesional corticosteroids yielded 'excellent results' after 1.5 years. This is generally well tolerated with only local pain during freezing and/or shortly after treatment and hypo/hyperpigmentation being the most frequent side-effect.

Radiation therapy

This can be combined with excision for single keloids and may reduce the incidence of recurrence. An evaluation of the previous lack of response to any other treatments, of the large size of the lesion and its functional importance should be taken into account. Using 1.7 mm of aluminium half-value layer, a one-time-only dose of 300–500 R or three alternate-day doses of 300–500 R are adequate. Radiation should be started on the day of or the day following surgery. A time interval of 6 days between surgical excision and the beginning of radiotherapy seems to avoid complications at the suture sites. Appropriate shielding is necessary and radiation therapy should not be used on keloids on the neck. The dose is dependent on the anatomical site as well as on the size of the keloid—the dorsal (scapular and paralumbar) and parasternal sites exhibit the least favourable cosmetic outcomes. Some surgeons highlight the good results obtained from a postoperative interstitial radiotherapy right after the total excision, leaving the 'Curie therapy needles' in site for 24–48 h. The success rate of surgery followed by radiation in the prevention of keloid recurrence is 85%.

Application of constant pressure

Another successful treatment for keloids and hypertrophic scars is the application of constant pressure. Firm wrapping with a woven elastic bandage, surgically designed straps and corsets, and sometimes even plastic clamps are used. A continuous pressure clamp on both sides of an ear lobe will help reduce the size of the keloid and help prevent recurrence. This treatment is limited to those areas where pressure can be safely applied for a prolonged period. The most effective results are when the pressure is at least 24 mmHg (to exceed the capillary pressure) and has been in place 12 h/day for several months, sometimes even up to a year. Silicone elastomer pads have been used underneath pressure garments for a mean duration of 10 months. Good results are reported in most cases (see section on silicone plates below). This method is effective only in areas where pressure can be maintained, particularly on extremities. A reduction in fibroblast content, total chondroitin-4 sulfate content, probably mediated by local tissue hypoxia induced by pressure-treated scars are additional mechanisms by which this modality reduces excessive scarring.

Retinoids

It has been recently reported that the effect of retinoic acid cream on keloids is most readily observed in recent injuries. Initially it is used in concentrations of 0.01% once a day, and then increased to twice a day. Once the skin is accustomed to the drug, the concentration can be increased to 0.025% and then to 0.05%. It should be used for no less than 8–12 months. The clinical changes observed are a lightening colour on the surface, softening of the keloid, and, in some cases, its total remission. Sometimes it is difficult to assess the results of various treatments obtained by others from reading the literature. Often, the differential diagnosis between a keloid and a hypertrophic scar is not made carefully. More important, the necessary long-term follow-up sometimes is lacking. It is essential to follow each treatment for several years before any kind of cure rate is assessed.

Interferons

The use of interferons has been recently studied and presented consistent results. They act by decreasing type I, II, III and possibly IV collagen production. Its use is intralesional, with weekly applications of up to 0.05 mg. The studies presented decreases of up to 50% at the linear dimensions, with the flattening of elevated lesions. Headaches are the most frequently reported adverse effect. According to Grandstein *et al.* changes at the dermis and epidermis can occur. The epidermis presents slender suprapapillar plates and the corneal extract presents focal hyperkeratosis with the vacuolization of the basal layer. The authors have demonstrated a meaningful decrease of the collagen bundle number and an increase of the mucin quantity at the dermis and epidermis. The use of pharmaceuticals is prevented due to the necessity of preliminary results confirmation.

UV-A1

Recently, UV-A1 has been shown to be effective in the treatment of morphoea and scleroderma. When given in localized scleroderma in high doses, UV-A1 produced better results than low-dose therapy, with maximal therapeutic effect reached after an average of 25 treatments. The mechanism of action seems to be related to apparently dose-dependent induction of collagenase enzyme. The advantages of UV-A1 include deep penetration into the skin allowing treatment of deeper tissues, and less DNA absorption than occurs with shorter, more erythemogenic UV radiation, thus offering a theoretical decrease in the risk of burns and cancer formation. Asawanonda *et al.* report a treatment with UV-A1, generated by a light box (model SOL5; UVATEC Inc, Sherman Oaks, California, USA) fitted with a UV-A1 filter allowing only wavelengths between 340 and 450 nm. Treatment was administered to only two thirds of the keloid 4 times weekly for 6 weeks, with two treatments missed, for a total of 22 treatments, while the untreated third of the keloid served as a control. The post-treatment section shows the reappearance of normal-looking collagen and elastic fibres in this keloid. Results of routine histological tests supported these findings. At present, there are no definitive long-term data regarding the carcinogenic risks of UV-A1. The only reported short-term adverse effect is transient hyperpigmentation.

Silicone plates

According to Sawada and Sone, this method's beneficial effects are not due to the pressure, temperature or capillary occlusion, but to the corneal extract occlusion and hydration, which would be the major related factors. Several authors reported this modality's efficiency in hypertrophic scars and keloids. Gold assessed the method's efficiency applying a silicone plate covering only half of the area to be treated. After 4 weeks, approximately 20% of patients did not show evidence of improvement in their lesions, but in the authors' assessment, approximately 95% of patients presented some kind of positive response. The plates can be used singly or as a prophylactic postoperative treatment. The patient should apply them for at least 12 h/day. It is a painless and easy to apply method, except for the scars at irregular surface zones due to problems with plate adhesion. According to Palmieri *et al.*, the results can be higher if vitamin E is added. To date, the obtained response is not enough to justify its use as a monotherapy, but some studies support its use as an assistant to surgical treatment. The lower price of silastic plate treatment has not been proved and there are no studies comparing the two plates.

Laser

The response to carbon dioxide laser varies from 39 to 92%. Similar controversial rates were identified for the argon

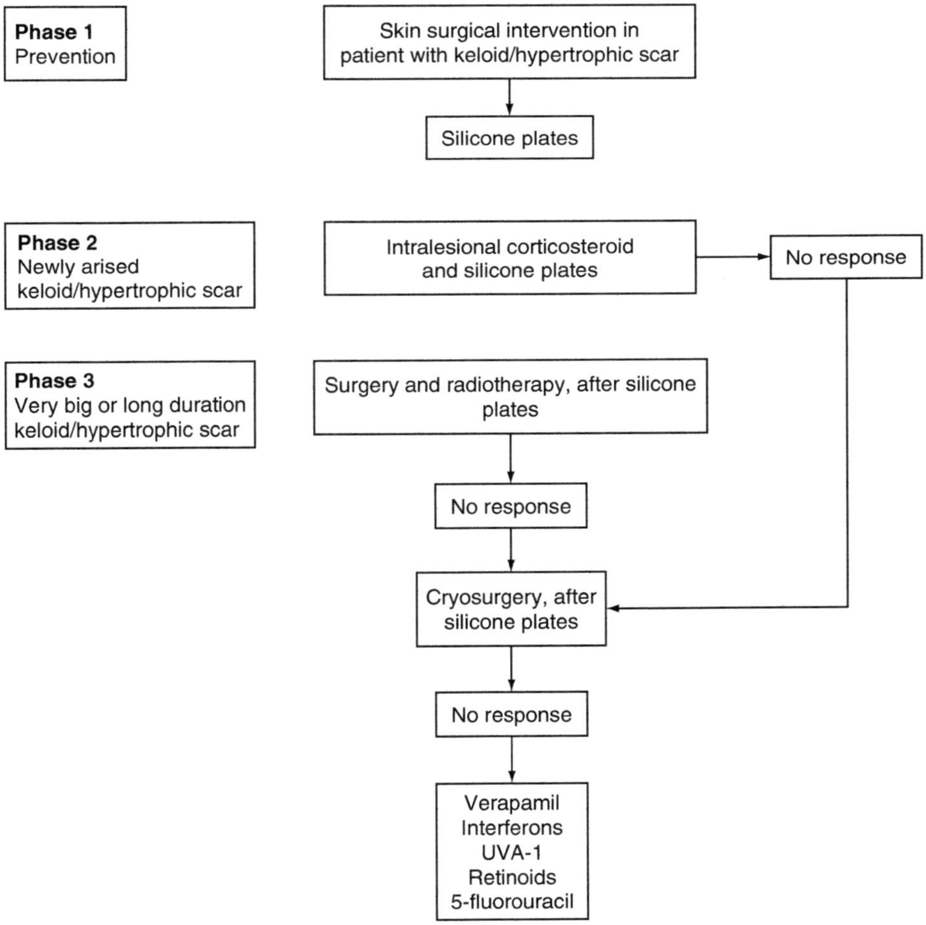

Figure 1

laser, between 45 and 93%. In experimental trials, laser surgical excision has shown a high capacity for delay in collagen synthesis. Unfortunately, according to Henderson, this effect is only temporary and the advantages demonstrated *in vitro* have not been confirmed in clinical trials. Norris has demonstrated the laser's ineffectiveness. Initial responses were followed by recidivation in those treated with corticoids, therefore the use of lasers in keloid treatment has not been defined.

5-fluorouracil (5-FU)

5-FU has been shown to inhibit fibroblast proliferation *in vitro* and *in vivo*, and is believed to reduce postoperative scarring by decreasing fibroblast proliferation. Fitzpatrick observed that the composite solution of 0.1 mL of 10 mg/mL triamcinolone acetonide mixed with 0.9 mL of 50 mg/mL of 5-FU in the same syringe offered the best efficacy with less pain. Corticosteroids (triamcinolone acetonide) is believed to provide an adjunctive inhibition effect on scar proliferation. Xylocaine mixtures were found to be ineffective in alleviating pain, as pain is caused by the injection procedure itself and the medication as well.

Calcium channel blockers

Lee reported that calcium channel blockers produced a 50% reduction in the incorporation of the proline tritiated to the extracellular matrix. They probably induce meaningful changes in fibroblast configuration and formation and therefore increase extracellular matrix degradation. The same reported hypertrophic scar control with intralesional verapamil. These pharmaceuticals should have new studies in order to achieve better assessment of their efficacy.

References

Asawanonda P, Khoo LS, Fitzpatrick TB, Taylor CR. *Arch Dermatol* 1999; 135: 348–9.

Berman B, Bieley H. Keloids. *J Am Acad Dermatol* 1995; 33: 117–23.

Blumenkranz MS, Ophir A, Claflin AJ, Hajek A. Fluorouracil for the treatment of massive periretinal proliferation. *Am J Ophthalmol* 1982; 94: 458–67.

Brent B. The role of pressure therapy in management of car lobe keloids: preliminary report of a controlled study. *Ann Plast Surg* 1978; 1: 579–81.

Campanile G, Hautmann G, Lotti T. A topical pharmacological approach to wound healing. *Current* 1994; 1: 33–8.

Ceillev RI, Babin RW. The combined use of cryosurgery and intralesional injections of suspensions of fluorinated adrenocorticosteroids for reducing keloids and hypertrophic scar. *J Dermatol Surg Oncol* 1979; 5: 54–6.

Cordero A Jr. Non-conventional uses of retinoic acid. In: Burgdorf WHC, Katz SI, eds. *Dermatology: Progress and Perspectives*. Proccedings of the 18th World Congress of Dermatology. New York: Parthenon Publishing, 1993: 542–43.

Cosman B, Crikelair CF, Ju DMC *et al.* The surgical treatment of keloids. *Plast Reconstr Surg* 1961; 27: 335–58.

Datubo-Brown DD. Keloids: a review of the literature. *Br J Plast Surg* 1990; 43(1): 70–7.

Fitzpatrick RE. Treatment of inflamed hypertrophic scars using intralesional 5-FU. *Dermatol Surg* 1999; 25: 224–32.

Gold M. A controlled clinical trial of topical silicone gel sheeting in the treatment of hypertrophic scars and keloids. *J Am Acad Dermatol* 1994; 30(3): 506–7.

Grandstein RD, Rook A, Flotte TJ. A controlled trial of intralesional recombinant interferon γ in the treatment of keloid scarring. *Arch Dermatol* 1990; 126: 1285–302.

Griffith BH, Monroe CW, McKinney P. A follow-up study on the treatment of keloids with triamcinolone acetonide. *Plast Reconstr Surg* 1970; 46: 145–50.

Gruss C, Stucker M, von Kobyletzki G *et al.* Low dose UVA-1 phototherapy in disabling pansclerotic morphoea of childhood (letter). *Br J Dermatol* 1997; 136: 293–4.

Henderson D. The effect of carbon dioxide laser surgery on the recurrence of keloids: discussion. *Plast Reconstr Surg* 1991; 87(1): 53–6.

Kerscher M, Volkenandt M, Gruss C *et al.* Low-dose UVA1 phototherapy for treatment of localized scleroderma. *J Am Acad Dermatol* 1998; 38: 21–6.

Kiil JC. Keloids treated with topical injections of triamcinolone acetonide (Kenalog): immediate and long term results. *Scand J Plast Reconstr Surg* 1977; 11: 169–72.

Kischer CW, Shetiar MR, Shetlar CL. Alteration of hypertrophic scars induced by mechanical pressure. *Arch Dermatol* 1975; 111: 60–4.

Lee R. The response of burns scars to intralesional verapamil. *Arch Surg* 1994; 129: 107–11.

Lee R, Ping A. Calcium antagonist retard extracellular matrix production in connective tissue equivalent. *J Surg Res* 1990; 49: 463–6.

Levy DS, Salter MM, Roth RE. Postoperative irradiation in the prevention of keloids. *Am J Roentgenol* 1976; 127: 509–10.

Malaker K, Ellis E, Paine CH. Keloid scars: a new method of treatment combining surgery with interstitial radiotherapy. *Clin Radiol* 1976; 27: 179–83.

Mallick KS, Hajek AS, Parrish RK. 5-Fluorouracil (5-FU) and cytarabine (ara-C) inhibition of corneal epithelial cell and conjunctival fibroblast proliferation. *Arch Ophthalmol* 1985; 103: 1398–402.

Murray JC, Pollack SV, Pinnel SR. Keloids: a review. *J Am Acad Dermatol* 1981; 14: 461–70.

Norris J. The effect of carbon dioxide laser surgery on the recurrence of keloids. *Plast Reconstr Surg* 1991; 87(1): 50–3.

Petersen MJ, Hansen C, Craig S. Ultraviolet A radiation stimulates collagenase production in cultured human fibroblasts. *J Invest Dermatol* 1992; 99: 440–4.

Sawada Y, Sone J. Hydration and occlusion treatment for hypertrophic scars and keloids. *Br J Plast Surg* 1992; 45(8): 599–603.

Scharfetter K, Wlaschek M, Hogg A *et al.* UVA irradiation induces collagenase in human dermal fibroblasts in vitro and in vivo. *Arch Dermatol Res* 1991; 283: 506–11.

Sproat JE, Dalcin A, Weitauer N *et al.* Hypertrophic sternal scars: silicone gel sheet versus kenalog injection treatment. *Plast Reconstr Surg* 1992; 90(5): 988–92.

Stege H, Berneburg M, Humke S *et al.* High-dose UVA1 radiation therapy for localized scleroderma. *J Am Acad Dermatol* 1997; 36: 938–44.

Vallis CP. Intralesional injection of keloids and hypertrophic scars with the Dermojet. *Plast Reconstr Surg* 1967; 40: 255–62.

Keratoacanthoma

I. Danopoulou

Synonyms

Molluscum sebaceum.

Definition and epidemiology

Keratoacanthoma is a benign, relatively common and rapidly growing tumour, arising from the pilosebaceous follicles. If left to run its natural course, it regresses spontaneously, leaving behind an unsightly scar. Fair-complexioned persons living under conditions of sun exposure or in industrial zones are most likely candidates, whereas African black people and Japanese are not prone to this disorder. It is commoner in the middle-age and the elderly; males are afflicted 2–3 times more than females. The ratio of squamous cell carcinoma to keratoacanthoma ranges, according to the literature, from 2 : 1 to 4.8 : 1. In Greek patients, however, it was found to be 10 : 1. These differences may reflect the frequency variance of squamous cell cancer in different parts of the world, and also the difficulty sometimes in distinguishing keratoacanthoma histologically from the early stages of squamous cell carcinoma.

Aetiology and pathophysiology

The location of the tumour on exposed parts of the body suggests that it may be related to solar irradiation. It has also been established with experimental data that chemical carcinogens, such as tar and mineral oils, can provoke keratoacanthomas in animals, which is consistent with the occurrence of this tumour in smoky areas. Keratoacanthoma has also been found to be more common in smokers than in non-smokers. Genetic factors may predispose to it, since members of the same family have been reported to develop such tumours. Mutations in the *p53* gene and detectable oncoprotein in biopsy specimens of keratoacanthomas have also been reported. Mechanical trauma is considered to be a triggering factor in some cases. There are reports referring to keratoacanthomas arising secondarily from other skin lesions such as eczema and psoriasis, and also after skin resurfacing with carbon dioxide (CO_2) laser. Although virus-like particles have been found by electron microscopy in keratoacanthomas, the viral nature of these particles is disputed by other investigators. There have been reports of several human papillomaviruses (HPVs) detected by the polymerase chain reaction in tissues of keratoacanthomas, but the significance of these findings are again challenged by other researchers. The viral origin of at least some keratoacanthomas, such as multiple keratoacanthomas in immunosuppressed patients after transplants, seems reasonable, but the subject has to be further elucidated.

The rapid growth of keratoacanthoma, followed by a resting phase and spontaneous involution and healing, is believed to reflect the cyclic phases of the hair follicles and has been supported with experimental data. On the contrary, most researchers dispute the involvement of immune mechanisms.

Clinical characteristics and course

Keratoacanthoma occurs in exposed areas favouring the middle parts of the face and the dorsal areas of the hands. It may, however, appear on any part of the body. Sometimes keratoacanthomas may be located subungually, causing pain of the underlying tissues. In rare cases they may occur on mucous membranes, such as the oral mucosa and the conjunctiva, probably developing from ectopic sebaceous glands. Keratoacanthoma starts as a small hemispheric molluscum contangiosum-like nodule, flesh or reddish coloured, and grows rapidly within 4–6 weeks attaining a diameter of 1–2.5 cm, followed by a resting phase and thereafter by a more slow, spontaneous involution within 4–6 months. As the tumour grows, it presents a bud or dome-shaped appearance with a characteristic central keratinous crater sometimes covered by a skin layer. As time goes by, the central keratinous mass detaches, leaving behind a puckered or pitted and hypopigmented scar. In some cases the keratinous mass may build up to a horn.

A variant of solitary keratoacanthoma is the so-called giant keratoacanthoma, which may be larger than 5 cm in diameter; it can also grow deep, disturbing the underlying structures. Another rare variant is the keratoacanthoma centrifugum marginatum type, which exhibits peripheral growth with concomitant central healing and atrophy. Sometimes spontaneous resolution may occur, but it may also grow for years. It occurs on the face, trunk or extremities and may reach 20 cm and even larger diameters.

Multiple keratoacanthomas are rare. The Grzybowski type, also known as eruptive multiple keratoacanthoma, consists of hundreds or even thousands of small, 2–3 mm pruritic follicular lesions; it occurs in adults and is quite persistent and treatment-resistant. Another variant is the Ferguson–Smith type, inherited as an autosomal dominant trait and consisting of hundreds of follicular, flesh-coloured papules, growing rapidly to the size of an ordinary keratoacanthoma that regresses spontaneously and leaves a scar behind. The rare Witten–Zak variant is a combination of the lesions seen in the two above-mentioned types. Multiple keratoacanthomas may also be part of the Muir–Torre syndrome, inherited probably by the autosomal dominant trait, in which multiple keratoacanthomas are combined with sebaceous adenomas and internal malignancies, usually of gastrointestinal or urological origin.

Malignant transformation of keratoacanthoma to squamous cell carcinoma cannot be excluded, although it is difficult to prove, because one cannot be sure that the lesion had not been malignant from the beginning.

Recurrences may occur after spontaneous healing, as well as after treatment.

Diagnosis

The characteristic regular, round shape with the central keratinous crater, the undamaged surrounding skin and the typical growth pattern, are usually sufficient for diagnosis in most cases.

Despite their typical morphology, some tumours, such as ulcerating keratoacanthomas, may at some stages mimic squamous cell carcinomas. Biopsy and histological examination solve the diagnostic problem in most cases. The biopsy specimen should include the centre of the lesion. In the early stages of squamous cell carcinoma it may be sometimes difficult to distinguish between the two tumours. Surgical excision is a must in such cases.

Differential diagnosis

- Squamous cell carcinoma: less rapid development, absence of keratinous central crater, cells more undifferentiated with less tendency to keratinize.
- Viral warts: papillomatous surface, absence of central keratinization.
- Granulomas: absence of keratinous crater, presence of epithelioid and giant cells.
- Molluscum contangiosum: umbilicated centre with crud-like substance; no tendency to keratinize, characteristic intracytoplasmic inclusion bodies.
- Hypertrophic actinic keratosis: irregular shape and borders, no rapid growth, irregular hyperplasia of stratum Malpighii, atypical nuclei.

Treatment

General therapeutic guidelines

Taking into consideration the benign nature of keratoacanthoma and its spontaneous regression and self-healing capacity, the first question that arises is to treat or not to treat?

Most dermatologists agree that one should treat keratoacanthomas for several reasons—above all, to rule out the possibility of squamous cell carcinoma. The second reason is the unsightly scar left behind and the much better cosmetic results achieved in treated than untreated tumours, considering also that most keratoacanthomas are located over the face and may cause anxiety to patients.

The treatment of choice, especially in cases where squamous cell carcinoma is suspected, is surgical excision, allowing histological examination of the whole specimen.

Other factors that have to be taken into account when treating these tumours are size and location, as well as the age and general condition of the patient. Multiple lesions and very large or aggressive cases may require systemic therapy; however, one should always treat benign lesions in the less harmful way, and use systemic treatment, especially with cytostatics, only if absolutely indicated and/or when all other methods have failed.

Recommended therapies

The following treatments are indicated in solid keratoacanthomas.

Surgical excision

This is the treatment of choice for most cases of solitary keratoacanthomas, giving much better cosmetic results than spontaneous healing and allowing histological examination of the full specimen.

Radiotherapy

Keratoacanthoma is radiosensitive and responds well to relatively small doses of X-rays (600–1000 rad). Electron beam therapy may also be used. Radiotherapy should be applied in recurrent tumours and in extensive lesions where the patient's age and general condition do not allow major surgical procedures.

Mohs chemosurgical technique

This involves minimal loss of tissue and histological examination of the full specimen. It may be useful in extensive and/or recurrent tumours.

Curettage electrodesiccation

This simple technique can be applied in small lesions with quick and acceptable cosmetic results.

Cryotherapy

Cryosurgery using liquid nitrogen has been reported to be of value in the early stages of keratoacanthomas.

Argon laser therapy

The concentrated non-specific thermal effect of argon laser has been reported to have good and acceptable cosmetic results and is recommended for keratoacanthomas not exceeding 1 cm in special locations, such as the auricles and the upper lid where major surgical procedures can be avoided.

Corticosteroids

Intralesional triamcinolone has been used with very good results in 10 out of 17 patients, with solid keratoacanthomas up to 2 cm without residual scar formation. The number of injections ranged between 2 and 4, applied at 1- or 2-week intervals, after local anaesthesia or in a 1:2 or 1:3 part dilution with procaine or lidocaine (lignocaine). This simple treatment may be a useful alternative in case of recurrences and in tumours situated in difficult and cosmetically important locations.

Podophyllin

Podophyllin has been mentioned to be effective as a 30–50% preparation alone, either in combination with curettage or radiotherapy. However, local application has also been reported to provoke keratoacanthomas and therefore it is questionable whether it should be used to treat this specific tumour.

The following methods of treatment are indicated mainly for multiple and/or very extensive lesions involving aggressive tumours.

Systemic retinoids

Retinoids are the treatment of choice in syndromes with multiple keratoacanthomas such as the Grzybowski type, the Ferguson–Smith type and the Witten–Zak variety. Effectiveness in keratoacanthomas has been attributed to their antikeratinizing effect, but immunomodulating action has also been reported.

Both etretinate and isotretinoin (1 mg/kg per day and 1.5 mg/kg per day, respectively) have been used successfully in such cases; some patients, however, are treatment-resistant and may need more aggressive treatment. A maintenance dose may be necessary in order to avoid recurrence. Isotretinoin has also been reported to be effective in giant keratoacanthoma and in keratoacanthoma centrifugum marginatum. A large starting dose may be indicated.

Cytostatics

5-Fluorouracil (5-FU)

5-FU is applied locally with good results either as a cream, 2–5 times daily, or intralesionally (1–3 mL of a 50-mg/mL solution) once a week; because of local pain, local anaesthesia with 1% lidocaine should precede the injections. Treatment may take up to 8 weeks. 5-FU is recommended for large tumours situated in critical locations, where surgical excision is difficult or contraindicated. It has been stressed that this treatment is effective only at the growing phase of the tumour, because of 5-FU's selective action for tissues with high mitotic rate. If there is not more than 70% reduction after 3–4 injections, treatment should be discontinued.

Bleomycin

Bleomycin is applied intralesionally once weekly for 3–4 weeks (1 mg/mL) and may be combined with an equal amount of 0.5% lidocaine. It is a rather effective and safe treatment that has been reported to have very good results in the classic solitary keratoacanthoma but also in large lesions, such as keratoacanthoma centrifugum marginatum.

Methotrexate

Methotrexate can be applied either intralesionally or systemically, with good results in extensive keratoacanthomas and multiple lesions. Intralesional therapy is applied weekly and the doses range from 5 to 37.5 mg weekly according to different studies. Some authors maintain that it is less painful and results are achieved quicker than with intralesional 5–FU. If there is no complete regression after the second injection, treatment should be stopped. Methotrexate has also been applied intramuscularly (25 mg weekly) in multiple keratoacanthomas.

Cyclophosphamide

Cyclophosphamide has been reported to be very effective in a case with generalized eruptive keratoacanthomas, which was treatment-resistant to retinoids and methotrexate. It was administered in a dosage of 100 mg daily for over 8 months, but the lesions reappeared after cessation of treatment and, after repeating, treatment had to be stopped because of side-effects. If applied at all, cyclophosphamide should be restricted to very severe cases and a limited time.

Interferon-a

There are some reports, in restricted numbers of patients, claiming very good results achieved by injections of interferon, applied intra- and perilesionally in a dosage of 3 million IU weekly for 6–15 weeks. It is recommended for large keratoacanthomas occurring in sites difficult to treat surgically.

Photodynamic therapy

Local photodynamic therapy with δ-aminolevulinic acid (ALA)-induced endogenous porphyrins has been recently reported to have good results in a small number of patients, with complete regression in some cases of large keratoacanthomas, and in patients where surgery was not feasible. In some of them, however, spontaneous regression could not be excluded. As a result, this treatment will have to be applied in larger series of patients for its benefit to be fully established.

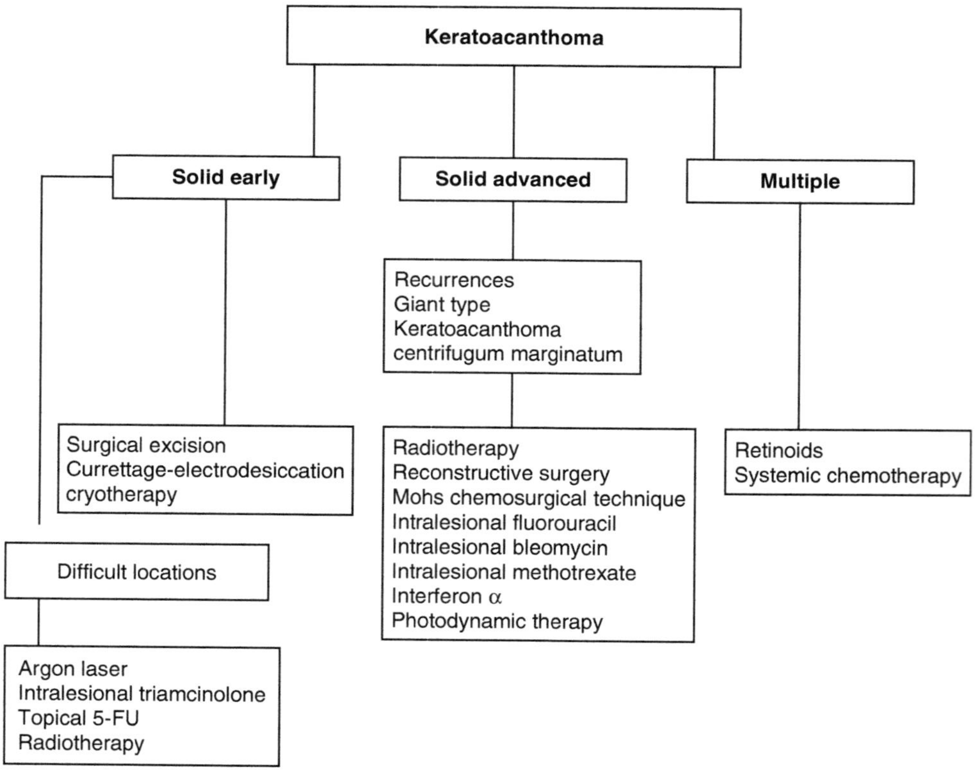

Figure 1

Further reading

Danopoulou I, Laskaris G, Nikolis G, Stratigos J. Clinical and histopathological study in 112 cases of keratoacanthoma. *Proceedings of the 3rd Hellenic Congress of Dermatology,* Thessaloniki, 1978: 193–202 *(Engl. Abstract).*

De la Torre C, Losada A, Cruces J. Keratoacanthoma centrifugum marginatum. Treatment with intralesional bleomycin. *J Am Acad Dermatol* 1997; 37: 11010–11.

Ghadially R, Ghadially FN. Keratoacanthoma. In: Freedberg IM, Eisen AZ, Wilff K, Austen F, eds. *Dermatology in General Medicine,* 5th edn. New York: McGraw-Hill, 1998: 578–89.

Grine RC, Hendris JD, Greer KE. Generalized eruptive keratoacanthoma of Grzybowski: response to cyclophosphamide. *J Am Acad Dermatol* 1997; 36: 786–7.

McNairy D. Intradermal triamcinolone therapy of keratoacanthomas. *Arch Dermatol* 1978; 89: 136–40.

Radakovic-Fisan S, Hoenigsman H, Tanew A. Efficacy of topical photodynamic therapy of a giant keratoacanthoma demonstrated by partial irradiation. *Br J Dermatol* 1999; 141: 936–8.

Schwartz RA. Keratoacanthoma. *J Am Acad Dermatol* 1994; 30: 1–19.

Somlai B, Hollo P. Use of interferon-alpha (IFN-alpha) in the treatment of keratoacanthoma. *Hautarzt* 2000; 51: 173–5.

Spieth K, Gille J. Intralesional methotrexate as effective treatment in solitary giant keratoacanthoma of the lower lip. *Dermatology* 2000; 200: 317–19.

Street ML, White JW, Gibson LE. Multiple keratoacanthomas treated with oral retinoids. *J Am Acad Dermatol* 1990; 23: 862–6.

Leg ulcers

A.A. Ramelet

Definition and epidemiology

A chronic leg ulcer may be defined as any wound located above the foot and under the knee that does not heal within a 6-week period.

Most leg ulcers (70–90%) are of venous aetiology (varicose or postphlebitic), many of them (10–20%) having an additional arterial component. Both the frequency and significance of pure arterial ulcer and ulceration of other origin (Table 1) should not be underestimated.

The overall prevalence of venous ulcers (open or healed) is about 1% in adults and up to 8.5% in elderly people (over 70), with a predominance in females.

Leg ulcers are a major public health concern, representing about 2% of the UK health-care budget or yearly costs over 1.5 billion DM in Germany.

Aetiology and pathophysiology

Venous leg ulcers result from ambulatory venous hyperpressure induced by superficial and/or deep venous reflux. Both are mainly consecutive to valvular and/or perforator impairment (destruction as in postphlebitic syndrome or incompetence following venous dilatation), and dysfunction of muscular and articular pump (which no longer ensures the progression of the blood column from the foot to the heart).

Superficial vein insufficiency is a major cause of leg ulcers, up to 60% as demonstrated by Duplex investigations in most recent series. This frequency should not be underestimated, as minimal surgery assures definitive healing of the ulcer.

Either deep or superficial, venous hyperpressure induces major microcirculatory disorders including the following.

1 Dilatation, lengthening and microthrombosis of capillaries.
2 Distension of venular endothelial pores, allowing large plasmatic molecules to escape into the interstitial fluid and thereby inducing pericapillary deposits of fibrin. Increased onco-

Table 1 Main aetiologies of leg ulcers

Venous insufficiency	Primary, secondary, atrophie blanche
Arterial disorders	Hypertensive ulcers, occlusive arterial diseases, arterial embolisms, arteriovenous fistulas
Vasculitis	Primary and secondary
Haematological disorders	Fibrinolytic disorders, hypercoagulability states, thrombocythaemia, polycythaemia, drepanocytosis, chronic haemolytic anaemia
Neurological disorders	Paraplegia, poliomyelitis, peripheral neural traumas
Traumatisms	Animal and insects bites, physical, thermal or chemical traumas, self-inflicted wounds
Infections	Ecthyma, *Pasteurella multocida*, tularaemia, cat-scratch disease, osteomyelitis, mycobacterioses (tuberculosis, lepra, Buruli's ulcer), tropical ulcer, syphilis and other treponematoses, deep mycoses, parasitoses (leishmaniasis, filariasis)
Cutaneous disorders	Pyoderma gangrenosum, necrobiosis lipoidica, scleroderma, radiodermatitis, chillblain, halogenides, sarcoidosis, bullous diseases, amyloidosis
Tumours	Carcinomas (basal cell, squamous cell, verrucous), melanoma, Kaposi's sarcoma, other sarcomas, lymphomas, metastases
Drug-induced	Hydroxyurea
Various	Chromosomal abnormalities (Klinefelter, Werner), prolidase deficiency, chronic renal insufficiency, hyperparathyroidism, calcinosis

tic pressure then favours the subsequent development of oedema, lymphatic overload and lymphangiopathy.

3 Accumulation and 'trapping' of white blood cells in the distal medial part of the dependent legs of chronic venous insufficiency (CVI) patients, plugging of capillaries, and releasing of cytokines as well as toxic metabolites.
4 Fibrosis and thickening of the fascia superficialis of the leg, histologically well demonstrated, altering calf muscle pump function.

Taken together, these alterations disturb oxygen diffusion and metabolic exchanges, inducing hypoxia, anoxia and leg ulcers.

Clinical characteristics and course

A venous ulcer is typically located at or above the medial malleolus, but lateral and/or other localization may occur, in particular in the case of lesser saphenous vein insufficiency. Its size is highly variable. Pain is inconstant, but may be considerable. The ulceration may be covered with fibrin. Its borders are well delimited and thickening of the edges is associated with a chronic evolution. Surrounding tissues may present associated alterations such as:

- purpura
- dermite ocre
- gravitational and contact dermatitis
- papillomatosis
- dermatofibrosclerosis
- atrophie blanche.

Complications include infection (lymphangitis, cellulitis), haemorrhages and malignant transformation.

Without treatment, evolution is long lasting, with exceptional remissions and frequent relapses.

Recurrences occur if venous hyperpressure is not definitely corrected.

Diagnosis

Aetiological diagnosis is mandatory and should include the following, as described in Fig. 1.

1 A medical history: familial and personal history of varicose veins, deep venous thrombosis (DVT), accidents and operations, drug intake, concomitant disorders, date and modalities of leg ulcer onset.
2 Inspection: varicose veins, oedema, trophic skin changes, aspect and odour of the ulcer.
3 Physical examination: skin temperature, peripheral arterial pulsation, varicose veins or incompetent perforators (Schwartz and Trendelenburg's tests), signs of peripheral neuropathy.
4 Duplex (or at least Doppler) investigation, determining the competence of superficial (greater and lesser saphenous), deep (femoral, popliteal, tibialis posterior) veins and perforators.
5 Ankle arterial pressure measurement to control arterial supply.
6 In selected cases: plethysmography, varicography, phlebography, arteriography, bone or soft-tissue radiograph and other specialized investigations.

Differential diagnosis

A large number of systemic and skin diseases may induce skin ulceration (Table 1). Every atypical or treatment-resistant ulcer should be referred to an experienced dermatologist and laboratory investigations, including histology, bacteriology, and/or blood examination, performed. Main differential diagnosis include the following.

1 Arterial ulcers: these are preferentially located on the foot or toe. Deep ulcerations are often covered with a black eschar, with possible exposition of the

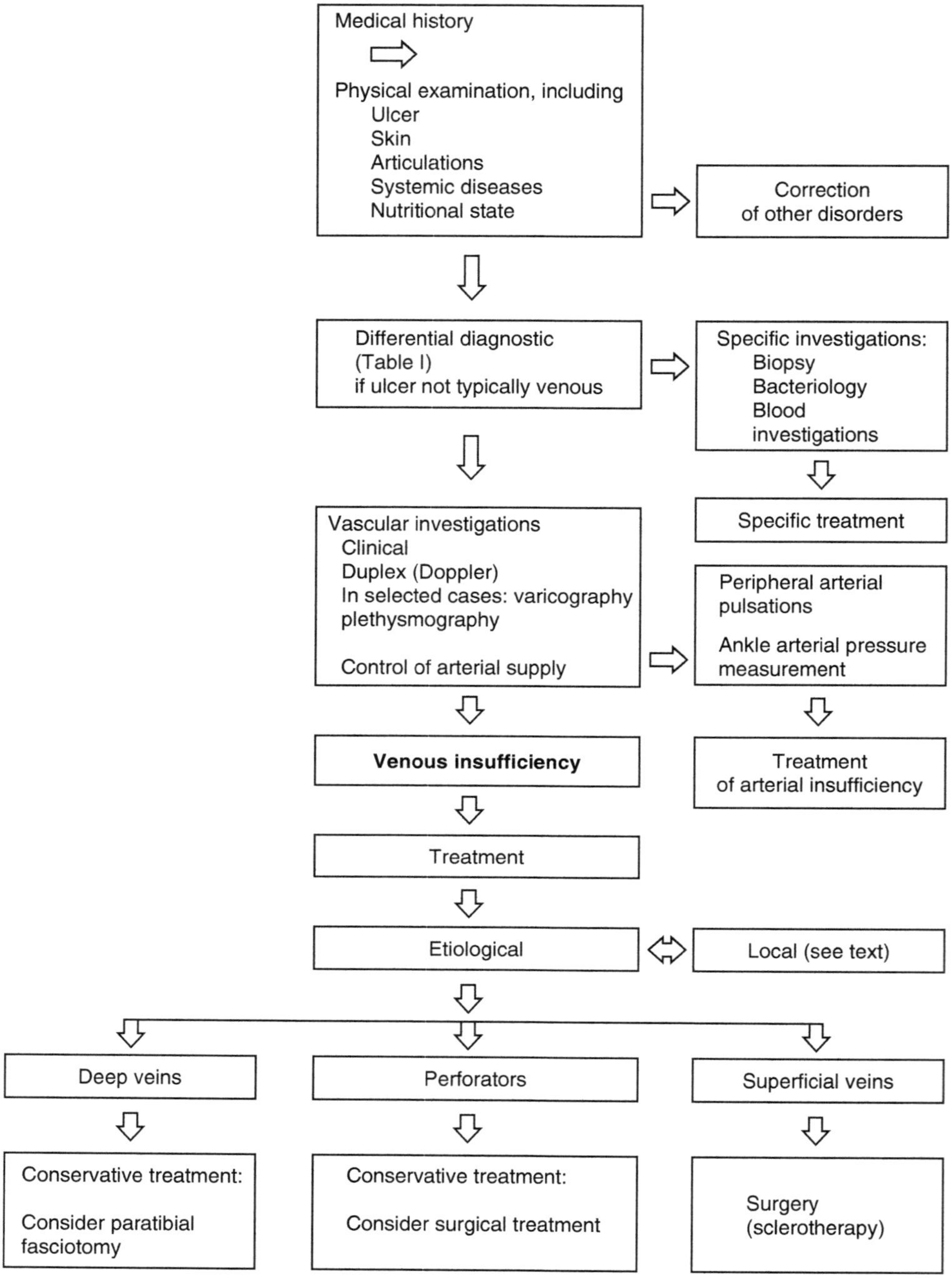

Figure 1 Algorithm: leg ulcer evaluation

underlying tendon. Pain is inconstant. Thorough arterial investigations are mandatory, as best treatments are angioplasty and arterial reconstruction.

2 Ulcerated atrophie blanche is very painful and refractory to treatment. It is associated in a majority of cases with CVI, although it occurs in other conditions. Smooth ivory, atrophic, sclerotic patches, speckled with telangiectasias are located on the dorsum of the foot or on the ankles. Paratibial fasciotomy is the treatment of choice (see below).
3 Martorell's hypertensive ulcer (necrotic angiodermatitis) is very painful. Ulcerations are typically located on the lateral part of the leg, corresponding to a skin infarction. Evolution is long lasting, before slow healing. Acute phases may respond to systemic steroids. Grafts achieve rapid relief of pain, but have usually to be repeated several times before healing. Recurrences are frequent.
4 Tumours (primary or cancerization of a chronic ulceration): biopsies and histology should always be discussed in case of atypical and therapy-resistant ulcers.
5 Vasculitis, infections, pyoderma gangrenosum and other causes.

Treatment

General therapeutic guidelines

Local treatment of venous and arterial ulcers does not fundamentally differ. General treatment is rarely indicated. An ulcer should be objectively and regularly examined for aspect, and size (measurement).

Concomitant diseases should be listed and treated:

- hypertension
- cardiac insufficiency
- diabetes
- arthropathies
- oedema: correction of peripheral oedema is particularly important.

Aetiological treatment

This should always be considered first. Up to 60% of venous ulcers result from greater and/or lesser saphenous insufficiency, which should absolutely be corrected, to ensure healing and prevent relapses.

Compression therapy

Compression therapy is more effective than any sophisticated treatments of venous ulcer. Compression therapy is the cornerstone of phlebology, and:

- reduces distension of superficial veins
- may correct valvular dysfunction
- enhances blood velocity in both superficial and deep venous compartments
- improves the efficacy of the calf muscle pump
- corrects microcirculatory alterations
- reduces oedema.

Compression is only counterindicated when arterial ankle pressure is under 80 mmHg (however, prudent application of passive compression with short stretch bandage is possible).

Compression treatment may be achieved with long stretch (exerting compression when standing and lying) or short stretch bandages (no-resting pressure, efficacy when walking = working pressure). Applying a bolster to the ulceration may selectively enhance compression. Excellent results are achieved with new techniques, such as four-layer bandages.

Compression stockings (sometimes difficult to apply in elderly patients) are mainly indicated at treatment's end and for preventing relapses. New stockings concepts and gliders have been developed, which are easier to wear and secure a higher compression in the gaiter area, e.g. Tubulcus, CircAid, UlcerCare or Venotrain Ulcertec.

Bed rest
This may be important, as the postural vasoconstrictive effect is diminished or abolished in CVI patients. However, regular exercise, such as walking, with compression bandage or stockings, is imperative. Stimulation of ankle mobility and of the calf muscle pump is essential to promote ulcer healing.

Risks of infection
Bacteria and yeast, saprophytes or pathogens, colonize most ulcers. Only 15% of ulcers are sterile. Bacterial colonization is, however, well tolerated and does not prohibit healing. Systemic or local antibiotics are exceptionally required. Local disinfectants and topical antibiotics are cytotoxic, irritant and potentially sensitizing.

As tetanus may complicate leg ulcers, vaccination should be controlled and repeated if necessary.

Follow-up after healing
This is too frequently overlooked: surgical correction (if possible) of venous hyperpressure or long-term compression therapy is essential to prevent relapses.

Recommended therapies
Some general rules apply to all leg ulcers.

Compression
Correction of venous reflux and microcirculatory dysfunction by compression which is essential during and after the whole treatment. This may be achieved with short or long stretch bandages and compression stockings, as described above.

Local treatment

Wound debridement
This is achieved either chemically (autolytic debridement with hydrocolloid dressings, long-lasting application of fibrinolytic enzymes) or surgically (by use of scissors, tweezers, curettage or CO2 laser, under surface anaesthesia).

Vacuum-assisted closure (VAC)
This new technique is intended to remove chronic oedema and fluid from exudative wounds, stimulate granulation, increase local blood flow, impede nosocomial infection of the wound and isolate infected ulcers. A foam dressing under occlusion is hermetically applied on the ulcer, and connected with an aspirating device assuring a controlled continuous or intermittent subatmospheric pressure (between 55 and 200 mmHg below ambient pressure). This technique may induce granulation in refractory venous ulcers, decubitus, infected wounds or even in arterial ulceration.

Calcifications
Either clinically visible or detected by X-rays, these must be surgically removed.

Regular cleaning of the wound
Using ample amounts of warm tap water (e.g. hand shower) ensures elimination of secretions and debris, and limits bacterial proliferation. Sterile saline is not necessary, except in freshly applied grafts, neither is disinfection of the wound. Infected ulcers (β-haemolytic streptococci type A; in case of lymphangitis) may require antibiotherapy (although this is exceptional). Silver sulphadiazine or polyvidone-iodine may be applied locally to control bacterial proliferation, although it will not suppress it.

Dressing change
Dressings have to be changed quite regularly in exudative ulcers. Later, it is preferable to avoid frequent changes of dressing, as this interferes with healing and may compromise newly formed tissue, disturb the patient's life and enhance the costs of treatment. In a prospective medicoeconomic French study, care concerned 48% of costs and drugs 33%.

Surrounding tissues

These must be carefully handled to prevent inflammation, infection, dermatitis and/or ulcer enlargement. Applying zinc paste may protect perilesional skin. Usually, gentle cleaning whilst changing the bandage may be sufficient. Local corticosteroids are indicated in gravitational or contact dermatitis. It is important to consider the high risk of sensitization in leg ulcer patients. Conservatives, emulsifiers, antiseptics, Peru balsam, antibiotics and corticosteroids are all potential sensitizers.

Dressing

This has to be adapted to a wound's aspect. The tendency of leg ulcers to heal is highly variable. Recent ulcers may heal quickly, even with inappropriate dressing. Long-lasting leg ulcers are regularly quite resistant to treatment. Therefore it is mandatory to treat leg ulcers and their cause immediately and carefully, as they tend to 'autonomize' and then have a tendency to heal poorly, due to their progressively fibrotic and badly vascularized base.

Local treatment may be divided into several steps, depending on the aspect and evolution of the wound.

1 Excessive exudation. This may be controlled by applying wet dressings, dextranomer, cadexomer-iodine, and new dressings, as alginates and hydrofibres. These all have a good bacterial adsorbing effect too.
2 Ulcers with a tendency to heal poorly. These may do so consecutively due to insufficient blood supply. Angiological evaluation is required. The wound may be stimulated, either with scarification or with topical autohaemotherapy, a simple, economical and highly effective treatment. This requires application of heparinized venous blood (1 mL mixed with 0.1 mL of heparin 25 000 UI for 4 cm^2) to the ulcer, covered with occlusive hydrocolloid dressing and repeated every second day. Topical haemotherapy probably works by supplying essential growth factors and cytokines to the wound. Application of growth factors or new skin equivalents is an expensive but effective alternative.
3 Granulation phase. Hydrocolloid dressings are quite effective and well tolerated. Occlusion secures maintenance of moisture of the wound, mediates local fibrinolysis, stimulates capillary proliferation, enhances the concentration of growth factors within the wound fluid and increases the rate of re-epithelialization. Hydrocolloid dressings are also effective in relieving pain. They are relatively expensive, but treatment is simplified, as they only have to be changed every 2–7 days. The dressing must be gently removed to avoid damaging surrounding skin and freshly developed epithelialization. The malodorous exudate underlying the dressing must be washed out with tap water, the wound dried and a new hydrocolloid plaque simply applied. Vaseline gauze dressings are a cheaper alternative. They do not adhere to the ulcer bed and achieve some hydration. The efficacy of 'healing ointments' and topical antibiotics has not been confirmed in reliable controlled trials. Sensitization to one or more of their constituents is a common occurrence. These preparations are of little interest and should not be used.

Surgery

Skin grafting

Skin grafting dramatically shortens the time to complete healing. The wound has to be well prepared, with a good granulation tissue. Pinch and punch grafting may be performed in the outpatient department. Thick-split and meshed graft can be considered in poorly healing ulcers, usually after large excision of fibrotic ulcer bed and ligation of underlying insufficient perforators. Pinch-grafts can be effectively applied to hypertensive ulcers, even on an insufficiently prepared wound, so as to promote healing and abolish pain.

Cultured keratinocytes and tissue-engineered skin equivalent

These strongly stimulate wound granulation and may secure ulcer cicatrization. Autologous keratinocyte cultures (derived from the hair shaft, or more recently from fetal cells, among others) are very effective and promising alternatives. These techniques are however, quite expensive. Recurrences are not prevented as long as an aetiological treatment, as surgical, has not been undertaken. As many dermatologists have poor knowledge in angiology, there is presently a high risk of choosing sophisticated and expensive substitutive skin rather than an effective and simple aetiological treatment.

Surgical indications

These are largely underestimated by dermatologists and surgeons alike. Besides debridement and grafting, one should envisage surgery for each patient with an active or healed ulcer to correct venous hyperpressure and prevent relapses. Long-term results are excellent. Operations may be performed under rachianaesthesia. They are well tolerated, even in the elderly. The following techniques may be indicated.

1 Phlebectomy, sclerotherapy or echo-guided sclerotherapy of a feeding vein in the neighbourhood of the ulceration are simple, ambulatory and cost-effective treatments. They induce healing and may be completed later, if necessary by a more definitive operation, with reduced infectious risks.
2 Flush ligation and stripping of insufficient greater and/or lesser saphenous veins suppresses reflux and venous hyperpressure. Photoplethysmography is useful to determine the impact of venous reflux and can predict the improvement to be achieved with surgical removal of the incompetent vein(s). Up to 60% of leg ulcers are consecutive to isolated superficial venous insufficiency, which is quite easy and economical to correct.
3 Endoscopic perforator dissection is easily performed through a single 4-cm incision, medially under the knee, in healthy skin. The incompetent perforators, visualized with an endoscope and video camera, are ligated or coagulated.
4 Paratibial fasciotomy, as described by Hach, yields excellent results in post-thrombotic syndromes or in painful atrophie blanche ulcers. It now usually completes perforator dissection and is performed through the same incision. The fascia is split down to the malleolus with long scissors or with a fasciotome. Its mode of action is not clearly understood, but it certainly compensates a chronic compartment syndrome, by re-equilibrating sub- and epifascial venous pressure. Fibrotic alteration of the fascia induces a fatty degeneration of the muscles and impedes its effect on the venous return. These changes are partially reversible after fasciotomy. Postoperative improvement of the microcirculation is immediate, as demonstrated by transcutaneous pO_2 measures.
5 Large excision of the ulcer and surrounding tissues, including the fascia, associated if necessary to endoscopic dissection of perforators, stripping and fasciotomy may be the single solution to heal refractory long-lasting ulcers, which become 'autonomous', definitively. Long-term results are excellent.
6 Shave excision and grafting are indicated in circular superficial ulcers on dermatofibrosclerosis.

Refractory ulcers must be carefully re-examined, to exclude arterial disorders, neglected venous reflux or incorrect diagnosis, as in, for example, an overlooked infection or tumour.

Alternative and experimental treatments

Many treatments have been proposed in ulcer healing. Few controlled studies have been undertaken. Most of them are anecdotal, limited to exceptional cases or are presently research tools, which might lead to future improvements in everyday practice.

Systemic treatments

These are controversial. Oedema-protective agents (such as diosmine, rutosides or dobesilate) have some effect in promoting healing, as demonstrated in several clinical studies. Oral anticoagulants, heparin, aspirin, pentoxyphilline and prostaglandins have been suggested to improve microcirculation; stanozolol to reduce dermatofibrosclerosis. Excessive intake of drugs should, however, be avoided, as many other crucial treatments are often necessary in elderly patients. Oral diuretics have no place in the treatment of CVI oedema, but may be usefully prescribed for cardiac insufficiency.

Manual lymphatic drainage

This improves lymphatic microcirculation, which may be considerably altered in severe CVI. It is indicated only in the long-term therapy of refractory leg ulcers.

Biosurgery

Maggot therapy appears to be quite effective for debridement and stimulation of granulation, although it appears unpopular with both nurses and patients.

Experimental treatments

These include application of various growth factors or granulocyte–macrophage colony-stimulating factors, laser or ultrasound stimulation of the ulcer, hyperbaric oxygen and others. Controlled studies and serious evaluation of the costs of these alternatives have yet to be established.

Future perspectives

These rely on a better evaluation and correction of macro-and microcirculatory abnormalities (including a more frequent surgical approach). Hydrocolloid dressings containing fibrinolytic enzymes or growth factors, fetal cells or extracts, and new commercial allografts are in development. Limiting factors for their introduction in therapy will be essentially financial, although CVI and leg ulcers are a major problem in health care.

Present treatment modalities are quite effective. Most patients suffering from leg ulcers may be effectively and definitively healed if correctly treated.

Further reading

Bello M, Scriven M, Hartshorne T, Bell PRF, Naylor AR, London NJM. Role of superficial ulceration in the treatment of venous ulceration. *Br J Surg* 1999; 86: 755–9.

Gardon-Mollard C, Ramelet AA. *Compression Therapy.* Paris: Masson, 1999.

Grabs AJ, Wakely MC, Nyamekye I, Ghauri ASK, Poskitt KR. Colour duplex ultrasonography in the rational management of chronic venous leg ulcers. *Br J Surg* 1996; 83: 1380–2.

Hafner J, Botonakis I, Burg G. A comparison of multilayer bandage systems during rest, exercise, and over 2 days of wear time. *Arch Dermatol* 2000; 136: 857–63.

Hafner J, Ramelet AA, Schmeller W, Brunner U, eds. Management of leg ulcers. In: *Current Problems in Dermatology,* Vol. 27. Basel: Karger 1999.

Hafner J, Schaad I, Schneider E, Burkhardt S, Burg G, Cassina PC. Leg ulcers in peripheral arterial disease (arterial leg ulcers). Impaired wound healing above the threshold of chronic critical limb ischemia. *J Am Acad Dermatol* 2000; 43: 1001–8.

Joseph E, Hamori CA, Bergamn S, Roaf E, Swann NF, Anastasi GW. A prospective randomized trial of vacuum-assisted closure versus standard therapy of chronic nonhealing wounds. *Wounds* 2000; 12: 60–7.

Lévy E, Lévy P. Les attitudes thérapeutiques des médecins français face à l'ulcère veineux de jambe: diversité et coûts induits. *J Mal Vasc* 2001; 26: 39–44.

Marklund B, Sülau T, Lindholm C. Prevalence of non healed and healed chronic leg ulcers in an elderly rural population. *Scand J Prim Health Care* 2000; 18: 58–60.

Mumcuoglu KY, Ingber A, Gilead L *et al.* Maggot therapy for the treatment of intractable wounds. *Int J Dermatol* 1999; 38: 623–7.

Ramelet AA. Ulcère veineux, approche dermato-chirurgicale et chirurgicale. *Ann Dermatol Venereol* 1996; 123: 361–6.

Ramelet AA. Ulcère de jambe—Bactériologie. *Phlébologie* 1999; 52: 393–7.

Ramelet AA. Clinical benefits of Daflon 500 mg in the most severe stages of chronic venous insufficiency. *Angiology* 2001; 52 (Suppl. 1): S49–S56.

Ramelet AA, Monti M. *Phlebology, the Guide*. Paris: Elsevier, 1999.

Schmeller W, Schwahn-Schreiber C, Hiss U, Gaber Y, Kirschner P. Vergleich zwischen Shave-Therapie und kruraler Fasziektomie bei der Behandlung therapieresistenter venöser Ulzera. *Phlebology* 1999; 28: 53–60.

Triquet B, Ruffieux P, Mainetti C, Salomon D, Saurat JH. Topical haemotherapy for leg ulcers. *Dermatology* 1994; 189: 418–20.

Leishmaniasis

M. Onder and M. Ali Gurer

Synonyms

Aleppo boil, Oriental sore, Delhi boil, Baghdad sore, Rose of Jericho, Chiclero's ulcer, uta, espundia (mucous form), forest yaws, dumdum fever (visceral form), kala-azar and black fever.

Definition and epidemiology

Leishmaniasis is a protozoan disease with different clinical manifestations depending on both the infecting species of *Leishmania* and on the immune response of the host. Its transmission occurs through the bite of a sandfly infected with *Leishmania* parasites.

It occurs in two forms, visceral and cutaneous leishmaniasis. Visceral leishmaniasis, also known as kala-azar, is a systemic disease and it is usually diagnosed by demonstrating the organisms in spleen, lymph gland or bone marrow aspirates. Cutaneous leishmaniasis usually occurs in the form of an ulcer or nodule on the skin.

It is seen in all races and both sexes. It is a common disease especially in the southeast of Anatolia in Asia. Aproximately 400 000 new cases occur each year and 400 million people are at risk of the disease.

Aetiology and pathophysiology

Leishmaniasis is caused by parasites of the genus *Leishmania*. Sandflies from the genus *Phlebotomus* transmit the disease. Only the female sandflies are blood sucking and they prefer to feed at night. The *Leishmania* parasite exists in two forms, the promastigote or leptomonal form and the amastigote or leishmanial form. The first is seen in the gut of the sandfly. It is flagellated and extracellular. The amastigote form occurs in the human host where the organism exists intracellularly and non-flagellated. Transmission occurs when the exposed area of skin is bitten by an infected sandfly; at that time, the organisms are engulfed by dermal macrophages. The sandfly becomes a vector by either biting the lesions of infected humans or feeding on animals which harbour the organism.

Clinical characteristics and course

Leishmaniasis usually affects the face, neck, arms and legs which are easily bitten by a vector. The bite commonly presents as a solitary red papule which enlarges to a plaque or nodule. The lesion often develops into an ulcer, which is well demarcated. Itching and pain are very mild. After approximately 6–12 months, the ulcer spontaneously regresses. It leaves a depressed scar with hypo- or hyperpigmentation. The wound may become superinfected, leading to misdiagnosis. A generalized papular eruption may also develop representing a hypersensitivity reaction.

In patients with acquired immune deficiency syndrome (AIDS), atypical manifestations of cutaneous leishmaniasis occur as an opportunistic infection. One to three per cent of patients with AIDS in endemic areas suffer from visceral leishmaniasis.

Diagnosis

Leishmaniasis is diagnosed by demonstrating the organisms in a superficial smear or biopsy of the ulcer. The smears stained with Giemsa or Wright's stain are often not satisfactory, because the lesion usually contains secondary infection. Moreover the parasites are found much deeper in the tissue.

Skin biopsy reveals epidermal or dermal changes depending on the type and stage of the disease. Epidermal changes are hyperkeratosis, parakeratosis and follicular plugging. Epidermal atrophy and acanthosis may be seen. The basal layer may be degenerated. In the dermis, there is predominantly a mononuclear infiltrate consisting primarily of lymphocytes and histiocytes. The histiocytes may be filled with leishmaniasis bodies.

In suspected cases, both biopsy and touch preparation (imprint) from a biopsy specimen improve the sensitivity of diagnosis.

The intradermal *Leishmania* test (Montenegro reaction) and other serological tests are of little value in regions where the disease is endemic because of previous exposure to the parasite. Immunofluorescence studies should be interpreted with caution and only if antibody levels are very high. Cultures of aspirated material from the lesions on NNN (Nicolle–Novy–MacNeal) blood agar were found to be moderately sensitive monoclonal antibodies to parasite surface antigens and have been used to identify *Leishmania* species. Polymerase chain reaction (PCR) can be used to distinguish between the different species of *Leishmania*.

Differential diagnosis

The natural history of cutaneous leishmaniasis is characteristic. It should be suspected in any patient with chronic inflammatory skin lesions who has visited or resided in the areas where leishmaniasis is endemic. The disease is on the rise due to travel, immigration and military activity. The differential diagnosis may differ depending on the location of skin manifestations. Lip leishmaniais is fairly common. It resembles herpes labialis, syphilitic chancre, squamous cell carcinoma and fixed drug eruption.

Table 1 Differential diagnosis of leishmaniasis

Acute infections	
Fungal	
Sporotrichosis	Microbiology, culture
Blastomycosis	Microbiology, culture
Bacterial	
Mycobacteriosis	
leprosy	Microbiology, culture
lupus vulgaris	Diascopia, histopathology
tuberculosis verrucosa	Violeceous border,
Trepenomatoses	
yaws	
pinta	
syphilitic gumma	
Staphylococcal/streptococcal pyodermas	
impetigo	
ecthyma	
furunculosis	
insect bite	
Viral	
Orf	
Chronic infections	
Inflammatory	
Sarcoidosis	
Discoid lupus erythematosus	Histopathology
Foreign body granuloma	
Keloids	
Neoplastic	
Cutaneous T-cell lymphoma	Histopathology
Jessner's lymphocytic infiltrate	Histopathology
Basal cell carcinoma	Histopathology
Keratoacanthoma	Histopathology

The differential diagnosis is outlined in Table 1.

Treatment

General therapeutic guidelines

- Leishmaniasis is a worldwide health problem and to date there is no ideal therapy. Treatment depends on the clinical form of the disease.
- The important measures to control leishmaniasis in areas where it is endemic are health education, elimination or control of reservoir, hosts and vectors and early treatment of patients.
- Patients with lesions on the face or another cosmetically important area should be treated to reduce the size of the resultant scar.
- The most successful therapy is intralesional therapy. Systemic chemotherapy is recommended for very extensive lesions. Uncomplicated lesions do not need be treated aggressively. Simple excision, cryosurgery and topical therapy are usually sufficient.

Recommended therapies

Systemic chemotherapy

Antimonials have been used to treat most forms of leishmaniasis. They inhibit the amostigote's glycolytic activity and fatty acid oxidation. Two available preparations of pentavalent antimony are sodium stibogluconate (Pestostam) and meglumine antimonate (Glucantime). The recommended dosage is 20 mg/kg per day for 20 days intravenously or intramuscularly. The parenteral route of administration is expensive and impractical in rural areas in which leishmaniasis is so prevalent. Moreover the side-effects, such as arthralgias, reversible elevations of hepatocellular enzymes, leukopenia, thrombocytopenia and electrocardiogram changes make systemic antimonials an unattractive choice for treatment. All side-effects resolve spontaneously after treatment.

Several oral agents have been tried instead of the parenteral antimonials. Amphotericin-B, dapsone and allopurinol have shown effective activity against *Leishmania* organisms. Rifampicin 1200 mg/day in two divided doses is well tolerated. It is simple to administer, cheap, more effective and less toxic than other available oral drugs.

Pentamidine at a dose of 3–4 mg/kg once weekly for at least 4 months may help in diffuse cutaneous leishmaniasis.

A 600-mg dose of ketaconazole has been shown to be effective. Itraconazole 7 mg/kg per day for 4–8 weeks has been encouraging, but it cannot be used as the single agent.

Intralesional therapy

Intralesional antimonial regimen involves the application of 0.2–0.4 mL sodium stibogluconate intradermally 3 times a week for a total of 15 injections. The recurrence rate with this regimen is only 4%. It is advocated, because of its efficacy, absence of toxicity and low cost.

Topical therapy

Today topically applied drugs are being used to minimize systemic toxicity and concentrate medication to specific sites on the skin. Recently paromomycin sulphate 20% was found to be a promising topical medication. It is an aminoglucoside and has an antibiotic spectrum. It is applied twice daily for 10–20 days. Some redness and irritation can be seen.

Local measures

Cryotherapy, local excision, CO_2 lasers and localized heat have all been tried with variable results. Freezing the lesions for 30–60 s until 2-mm margins are obtained has proved lethal to *Leishmania* organisms. Liquid nitrogen is a relatively simple and safe alternative with few or no systemic adverse effects.

Alternative and experimental treatments

Interferon (IFN)

More recently subcutaneous injection of IFN-γ has proved effective for regression of lesions by stimulating the macrophages of the Th line.

Vaccination

This has been performed on animal models and human beings with virulent promastigotes. Reduced rates of subsequent infection have been noted in the vaccinated populations. The development of an effective, non-infectious vaccine is problematic.

Immunotherapy

The mixture of heat-killed cultured *Leishmania* promastigotes plus live lyophilized bacille Calmette-Guérin (BCG) can be combined for chemotherapy. It is recommended as a single intradermal injection and applied every 6 weeks.

WR 6026

This is a primaquine analogue that has shown effectiveness in animal models.

Liposomal amphotericin

This has proved effective but is still undergoing clinical trials.

Oral zinc sulphate

Zinc sulphate 5 mg/kg orally can be recommended in the prophylaxis of cutaneous leishmaniasis.

Further reading

Boletis JN, Pefani SA, Stathakis C *et al.* Visceral leishmaniasis in renal transplant recipients; successful treatment with liposomal amphotericin B (AmBisome). *Clin Infect Dis* 1999; 28: 1308–9.

Convit J, Castellanos PL, Ultich M, Castes M *et al.* Immunotherapy of localized, intermediate and diffuse forms of American cutaneous leishmaniasis. *J Infect Dis* 1989; 160: 104–15.

Davidson RN. AIDS leishmaniasis. *Genitourin Med* 1997; 10: 298–319.

Grevelink SA, Lerner EA. Leishmaniasis. *J Am Acad Dermatol* 1996; 34: 257–72.

Herwaldt B. Leishmaniasis. *Lancet* 1999; 354: 1191–9.

Herwaldt BI, Berman JD. Recommendations for treating leishmaniasis with sodium stibo-gluconate (Pentostam) and review of pertinent clinical studies. *Am J Trop Med Hyg* 1992; 46: 296–306.

Higashi GI. Vaccines for parasitic diseases. *Ann Rev Public Health* 1988; 10: 560–86.

Katsambas A. Quality of life and the European Academy of Dermatology. *JEADV* 1994; 3: 211–14.

Kochar DK, Aseri S, Sharma BV *et al.* The role of rifampicin in the management of cutaneous leishmaniasis. *QJM* 2000; 93: 733–7.

Kolde G, Luger T, Sorg C *et al.* Successful treatment of cutaneous leishmaniasis using systemic interferon gamma. *Dermatology* 1996; 192: 56–60.

Memisoglu HR, Kotogyan A, Acar MA *et al.* Cryotherapy in cases with leishmaniasis cutis. *J Eur Acad Dermatol Venereol* 1995; 4: 9–13.

Moskowitz PF, Kurban KA. Treatment of cutaneous leishmaniasis; Retrospectives and advances for the 21st century. *Clin Dermatol* 1999; 17: 305–15.

Mujtaba G, Khalid M. Weekly vs fortnightly intralesional meglumine antimoniate in cutaneous leishmaniasis. *Int J Dermatol* 1999; 38: 607–9.

Oliveria M, Armondo A, Mathots M *et al.* Intralesional therapy of American cutaneous leishmaniasis with pentavalent antimony in Rio de Janeiro, Brazil an area of leishmania transmission. *Int J Dermatol* 1997; 36: 463–8.

Samady JA, Schwartz RA. Old World cutaneous leishmaniasis. *Int J Dermatol* 1997; 36: 161–6.

Sharquie VE, Najim RA, Farjou IB, Al Timimi DJ. Oral zinc sulphate in the treatment of acute cutaneous leishmaniasis. *Clin Exp Dermatol* 2001; 26: 21–6.

Stanimirovic A, Stipic T, Skerlev M, Basta A. Treatment of cutaneous leishmaniasis with 20% paromomycin ointment. *J Eur Acad Dermatol Venereol* 1999; 13: 214–17.

Uzun S, Uslular C, Yücel A, Acar M, Özpoyraz M, Memisoglu HR. Cutaneous leishmaniasis. evaluation of 3074 cases in the Çukurova region of Turkey. *Br J Dermatol* 1999; 140: 347–50.

Vardy D, Barenholes Y, Cohen R *et al.* Topical amphotericin B for cutaneous leishmaniasis. *Arch Dermatol* 1999; 135: 856–7.

Xaidara A, Kakourou T, Klontza D *et al.* Cutaneous leishmaniasis response to cryotherapy treatment. *Eur J Pediatr* 1999; 158: 530.

Zakai HA, Zimmo SK. Effects of itraconazole and terbinafine on leishmania major lesions in BALC/C mice. *Ann Trop Med Parasitol* 2000; 94: 787–91.

Lentigo maligna

R. Dawber

Synonyms

Hutchinson's melanotic freckle.

Definition and epidemiology

Lentigo maligna (LM) is characteristically a single, impalpable, irregularly pigmented, brownish-black lesion occurring on the exposed parts, mainly the face of elderly individuals.

Hutchinson first described the entity as lentigo melanosis in 1894; it is sometimes called Hutchinson's melanotic freckle. Since that time it has been recognized as a specific type of melanoma *in situ*, arising from epidermal melanocytes.

Published figures show LM in individuals over 40 years, with a mean age of 65 years; the increasing age-related frequency peaks in the seventh and eight decades.

Aetiology and pathophysiology

Descriptive epidemiology of LM suggests that it is due to chronic cumulative sun exposure. It occurs on sun-exposed areas of mainly white-skinned individuals and microscopically shows solar elastosis and epidermal atrophy.

Clinical characteristics

LM typically presents as a single, hyperpigmented macular lesion on the most prominently sun-exposed sites such as the cheeks, nose, forehead or ear. The brownish-black colour is variegating with a clearly defined, irregular edge. Patchy pale areas may be seen within the hyperpigmentation areas, a clinical sign of regression. LM slowly increases in size over many years; since it is often asymptomatic, the diameter at initial diagnosis may be from one to several centimetres. If it has nodules within it or is palpably thickened it is not LM and may be malignant—lentigo maligna melanoma (LMM) or superficial spreading melanoma.

Diagnosis (laboratory examinations)

The diagnosis is based on clinical and histological correlates. The latter is crucial in all cases in which the diagnosis is suspected in view of its preinvasive melanoma (LMM) status and the difficulty of accurate clinical diagnosis. Some authorities dispute the use of incisional or punch biopsy in staging LM vs. LMM: but in practice dermatologists do biopsy, which enables the differential diagnosis to be resolved. One study supported this, showing that clinical acumen plus a single punch biopsy was good enough to judge diagnosis and premelanoma status accurately —all these lesions were subsequently fully excised.

LM histology is characterized by proliferation of atypical dendritic, often spindle-shaped, melanocytes containing cytoplasmic vacuolation and irregular hyperchromatic, often angular nuclei. These cells may palisade and involve adnexial epithelium. Pigmentation may involve the whole thickness of the epidermis including the stratum corneum. The upper dermis shows prominent solar elastosis and there is epidermal atrophy. Assessing excision margins for residual and atypical melanocytes is difficult; recently HMB-45 immunolabelling has proved to be a valuable adjunct.

Treatment

General therapeutic guidelines

In the century since Hutchinson described LM, there have been many treatments proposed. It would appear from the literature that micrographic Mohs' surgery (MMS) has the lowest recurrence rates, although there is only a limited number of studies and small series of patients.

The other modalities which appear to have relatively equivalent recurrence rates in the order of 7–10% include conventional surgery, cryosurgery and radiotherapy. Despite the drawbacks for cryosurgery and radiotherapy there does not appear to be any significant difference in recurrence rate when these modalities are compared. Therefore, all three could equally be recommended as a primary treatment of LM if the physician is adequately trained in the appropriate technique. Close follow-up of the patient is extremely important in the destructive therapies because a full histological assessment has not been possible. The use of destructive therapies may be especially helpful in the very elderly or the infirm patient where surgery may be declined or inappropriate.

No treatment should ever be carried out without prior histological confirmation since the differential diagnosis includes benign lesions—seborrhoeic keratosis, solar lentigo, pigmented solar keratosis; and malignant changes of LMM or superficial spreading melanoma.

Recommended therapies

Surgical methods

Surgery

Surgical excision is generally taken to be the most reliable method of adequately removing LM. It has been said by most surgeons and some dermatologists, that the treatment of choice for LM is wide excision on the basis that 'destructive' techniques are done 'blind' with no specimen for full diagnosis or histological guide to adequacy of treatment. To support this, cure rates of 91% and above have long been quoted. It has been shown that from 85 pigmented lesions diagnosed as LM prior to treatment, 45 had foci of LMM. These studies have been used to show the necessity of surgery and the provision of a full specimen for histological diagnosis. However, other studies showed that a single punch biopsy was appropriate as a representative sample, if non-excisional methods are to be used.

This surgical management regimen has been followed for many years. For the continued acceptance of wide excision margins as the primary treatment of LM, a much larger series of patients is required for a controlled prospective study with long-term follow up.

Micrographic mohs surgery

The advantage of MMS over conventional surgery and the destructive methods include almost 100% evaluation of the tumour margin, detection of disease extending beyond the clinical margin and preservation of maximal amount of tissue. The latter is especially important as most LM cases involve the head and neck region. The major disadvantage is the difficulty in distinguishing normal from abnormal melanocytes on frozen sections. To overcome this, the use of rush permanent sections and HMB-45 monoclonal antibody has been advocated. The major problem with HMB-45 is its lack of sensitivity in melanoma cell detection.

From reports reviewed, it would appear that MMS seems to be the logical surgical treatment of both LM and LMM. The most likely source of progression to metastases would be the presence of satellite foci of abnormal melanocytes away from the microscopic margin of the lesion. A larger series of patients looking at both treatments of primary and recurrent lesions needs to be undertaken. Also the technical and financial constraints, as well as the general health of the patient, may preclude one using this treatment. Such longer follow-up studies would also answer the question (if many recurrences develop) of whether LM/LMM is a pathological field defect. If so, this would be an indication for the use of non-surgical methods.

Non-surgical methods

Cryosurgery

Cryosurgery has long been used as an alternative to surgical excision for LM and, in some cases, for early LMM. In standard dermatology textbooks it is recommended for use in elderly and infirm patients in whom surgery is not appropriate.

It is known that melanocytes can be killed by temperatures of −4°C to −70°C. This is not as low as the temperatures required to kill squamous epithelial cells.

The technique for cryosurgery does vary from centre to centre. However, it has been suggested that aggressive treatment is required where double freeze–thaw cycles must be used with a 1-cm margin and temperatures of −40 to −50°C at the base of the lesion.

There have been many reports on the success or otherwise of cryosurgery for LM; the recurrence rates range from 0 to 50%.

Taking the total number of patients from all the reported studies on the use of cryosurgery for LM over the past 15 years, there are 169 patients and 16 recurrences at a recurrence rate of 9.5%. It has been noted that recurrences, if they do occur, will happen in the first 3 years after treatment. The most common side-effects include hypopigmentation, atrophy, hypertrophic scarring and postinflammatory transient halo hyperpigmentation. Reactive lentiginous hyperpigmentation can occur and, if present, needs to be biopsied to exclude recurrences, if the pigment remains for more that 2–3 months after treatment.

A review of the cryosurgical literature shows that the problem with assessing the value of cryosurgery is often the lack of standardization of treatment both within individual groups ('freeze time was dependent on the size of the lesion') and between centres. These studies have a similar problem to those assessing conventional surgery in that they lack significant patient numbers.

The main argument levelled against cryosurgery is the lack of histological confirmation of cure. However, the follow-up studies recorded are not inferior to the surgical recurrence rates (excluding MMS).

It is important to state that 'cold' is a powerful stimulus of lymphocyte-mediated immunity. It may therefore be possible that cryosurgery will lessen systematization of the tumour as compared with other treatment methods, if LMM occurs.

Radiotherapy

The use of radiotherapy has been especially proposed for the elderly and for lesions where surgical repair would be difficult. In Europe, Miescher's technique, or a variant thereof, is frequently employed for the treatment of LM. It involves:

- the use of an X-ray tube with beryllium window producing 12 kV: 15 mA
- a target skin distance at 20 cm
- a 50% depth dose occurs at 1–1.3 mm of skin
- a dose of 20 Grays per treatment with five treatments given 3–4 days apart
- a 5-mm margin of normal skin is included in the treatment field.

The major drawbacks with this technique is rapid radiation fall-off and a limited depth of penetration of X-ray beams.

We feel that radiotherapy is a totally acceptable treatment for LM if used by experienced clinicians. The follow-up of postradiotherapy wounds and the expected hyperpigmentation will also require experience in distinguishing this from recurrences.

Alternative and experimental treatments

Azelaic acid

Azelaic acid is a competitive concentration-dependent inhibitor of different oxidoreductive enzyme systems. It has been shown to be effective in the treatment of melasma and postinflammatory melanoderma. Its effect on hyperfunctioning and abnormally proliferating melanocytes is achieved by reversible inhibition of tyrosinase and inhibition of mitochondrial enzymes.

On this basis, 20% azelaic acid in a cream or 15–35% in ointment has been used for a period of months to over a year by a number of investigators in the treatment of LM. The results, however, have varied between studies.

The large availability in the results is mainly due to the use of different formulations and concentrations of azelaic acid, variability in the length of treatment and selection of lesions to treat, that is previously treated with other modalities, or foci of LMM not diagnosed on pretreatment biopsy. In conclusion, we have found 81 patients in the literature who have been treated with azelaic acid; 58 of whom had complete clearance, 17 who had no improvement, three who had partial improvement, two who had progressed to LMM and one who had been lost to follow-up.

Further modification of the molecular structure of azelaic acid may enable their results to be enhanced. The initial recurrence and the relatively long time to total clearance would require very close follow-up to ensure no progression to LMM. We feel that the recurrence rate of 22% is too high and that the time to response period is too long for this treatment modality to be regarded as a main choice of treatment for LM.

5-Fluorouracil (5-FU)

The topical use of 5-FU in the treatment of LM was reported in 1975. There is no clear evidence that 5-FU is of significant benefit in the treatment of LM and it is not recommended as a therapeutic option for its treatment.

Laser methods

The argon laser, a blue–green light laser with 80% output at 488 and 514.4 nm, is preferentially absorbed by haemoglobin and melanin with very poor absorption by non-chromophore containing tissue. With only three patients reported in the literature, it is not possible to make an adequate judgement on the efficacy of this treatment regimen. There are currently no long-term follow-up reports on laser-treated LM and LMM; therefore comparison with other modalities is not possible.

The carbon dioxide laser emits infrared light at a wavelength of 10 600 nm. This light energy is absorbed by water and converted into heat. Kopera has used this laser on four patients with LM and followed them up for an average of 15 months with no recurrences. As with the argon laser, although these results are encouraging, the study had only four patients with a short follow-up.

Topical tretinoin

It has been shown that retinoids inhibit proliferation and induce differentiation of cultured murine melanoma cells. Topical retinoids have been tried on invasive melanoma, dysplastic naevi and LM. This method cannot be recommended for routine clinical practice.

Figure 1 is constructed using the data collected on UK current practice regarding the management of LM and the literature data on recurrence rates. It is however, acknowledged that there is a relative

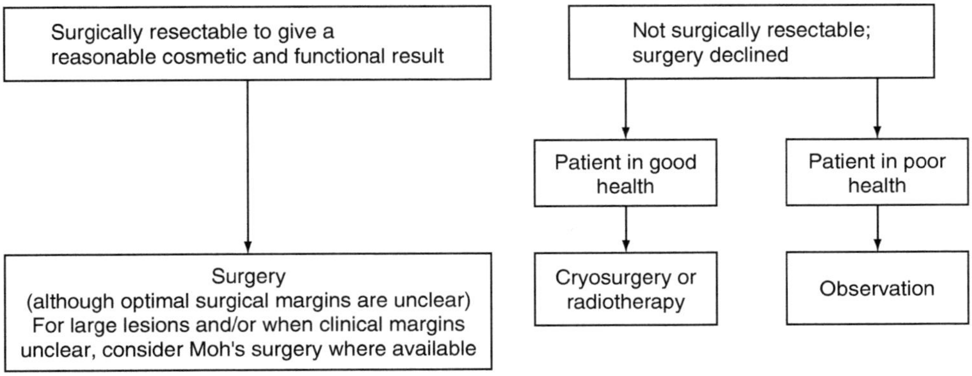

Figure 1

paucity of data on natural history and outcome in terms of treatment morbidity.

Further reading

Cohen LM, McCall MW, Zax RH. Mohs' micrographic surgery for lentigo maligna and lentigo maligna melanoma: a follow-up study. *Dermatol Surg* 1998; 24: 673–7.

Ellwood JM, Gallagher RP, Worth AJ. Etiological differences between subtypes of cutaneous malignant melanoma: W. Canada Melanoma study. *J Natl Cancer Inst* 1987; 78: 37–44.

Fersht N, Spittle MF. Some aspects of radiotherapy for melanoma. *Br J Dermatol* 2001; 144: 1–3.

Holman CDJ, Armstrong BK. Cutaneous malignant melanoma and indicators of total accumulated exposure to the sun: an analysis separating histogenic types. *J Natl Cancer Inst* 1984; 73: 75–82.

Hutchinson J. Lentigo melanosis. *Arch Surg* 1894; 5: 252.

Kuflik EG, Gage AA. Cryosurgery for lentigo maligna. *J Am Acad Dermatol* 1994; 31: 75–8.

Little JH, Holt J, David N. Changing epidemiology of malignant melanoma in Queensland. *Med J Austr* 1980; I: 66–9.

Litwin MS, Kremetz ET, Mansell PW, Reed RJ. Topical chemotherapy of lentigo maligna with 5-fluorouracil. *Cancer* 1975; 3: 721–33.

Mahendran R, Newton-Bishop JA. Survery of UK current practice in the treatment of lentigo maligna. *Br J Dermatol* 2001; 144: 71–6.

McKee PH. *Pathology of the Skin with Clinical Correlations*, 2nd edn. London: Mosby-Wolfe, 1996: 14.39.

Nazzaro-Porro M, Passi S, Zina G. 10 years' experience of treating lentigo maligna with topical azeleic acid. *Acta Derm Venereol* 1989; 143 (Suppl.): 49–57.

Orten SS, Waner M, Dinehart SM. Q-switched neodymium. yttrium-aluminium-garnet laser treatment of lentigo maligna. *Otolaryngol Head Neck Surg* 1999; 120: 296–302.

Robinson JK. Margin control for lentigo maligna. *J Am Acad Dermatol* 1994; 31: 79–85.

Schmid-Wendtner M, Brunner B, Konz B. fractionated therapy of lentigo maligna and lentigo maligna melanoma in 64 patients. *J Am Acad Dermatol* 2000; 43: 477–82.

Stevens G, Cockerell CJ. Avoiding sampling errors in the biopsy of pigmented lesions. *Arch Dermatol* 1996; 132: 1380–1.

Yell JA, Baigrie C, Dawber RPR, Millard PR, Goodacre T. Cryotherapy for lentigo maligna—is clinical acumen combined with a single punch biopsy good enough for staging? *J Eur Acad Derm Ven* 1996; 7: 39–43.

Leprosy or Hansen's disease

B. Flageul and I. Dubertret

Definition and epidemiology

Leprosy is a chronic infectious disease due to *Mycobacterium leprae* (*M. leprae*) or Hansen's bacillus that mainly affects the skin and the peripheral nerves. It is a very unevenly distributed disease between and within countries. In 1999, the World Health Organization (WHO) reported a global prevalence rate of about 1.4 per 10 000 population. Thirteen endemic countries contributed to 90% of the global burden with a combined prevalence of 4.4 per 10 000. The prevalence by WHO Regions was of 4.3 in South-East Asia, 1.1 in the Americas, 1.2 in Africa, 0.2 in the Eastern Mediterranean and 0.1 in Western Pacific. In Europe, small endemic areas persist in Portugal, Spain, Greece and Sicily. However, most patients seen in Europe come from countries where it is endemic.

Aetiology and pathophysiology

M. leprae, discovered in 1873 by Hansen in Norway, is an obligate intracellular acid-fast bacillus (AFB) multiplying mainly in macrophages of the skin (histiocytes) and the peripheral nerves (Schwann cells). It still cannot be cultivated *in vitro*.

Infected humans, especially untreated multibacillary cases, are considered as the only source of infection. In these patients, nasal discharges are the most contagious while the intact skin is not: only ulcerated or abraded skin may be an occasional portal of exit for bacilli. The most likely mode of entry of bacilli in contact patients is by inhalation of bacilli-laden droplets and penetration through the nasal mucosa. Inoculation through abraded or damaged skin has been reported in exceptional cases.

However, some animals have been discovered as naturally infected (armadillo, Mangabey monkeys) or as experimentally sensible to the bacillus (normal or nude mouse). These animals are used as a source of bacilli or to test the resistance of *M. leprae* strains to antibiotics.

The occurrence or non-occurrence of a clinical disease is directly linked to the ability of the exposed patient to develop a specific cellular immune response to *M. leprae*. Most individuals living in a closed vicinity with multibacillary patients eliminate the bacilli without clinical infection. The remaining patients develop the disease in a clinical form depending of the level of their immunity: an indeterminate form that may heal spontaneously or evolute in one of the following forms, a tuberculoid-paucibacillary (PB) form (fair host's resistance) or a lepromatous-multibacillary (MB) form (poor or non-host resistance).

The period of incubation is long, about 3–5 years in tuberculoid and 5–7 years in lepromatous leprosy. Shorter (6 months) and longer (20 years) periods have been reported.

Clinical characteristics and course

According to the individual's specific response, leprosy presents a broad spectrum of clinical lesions. For this reason in 1966, Ridley and Jopling have proposed a five-group classification of leprosy that includes clinical, histological, bacteriological and immunological criteria (see Table 1).

Cutaneous involvement

In tuberculoid (TT, BT) leprosy, skin lesions are few (1–10), large, over 5 cm in diameter, asymmetrically distributed, maculous or infiltrated, hypopigmented or erythematous, often slightly squamous, well demarcated from the normal

Table 1 Ridley and Jopling classification

	Polar tuberculoid (TT)	Borderline tuberculoid (BT)	Borderline borderline (BB)	Borderline lepromatous (BL)	Polar lepromatous (LL)
Skin lesions	1 or 2 well-demarcated lesions, anaesthetic	Few lesions (< 10), well-demarcated, hypo- or anaesthetic, asymmetrical	Exclusively annular lesions with large borders, normo- or faintly hypoaesthetic, symmetrical	Numerous (> 10), both annular and papulonodular lesions, symmetrical, normoaesthetic	Very numerous lesions (up to 100 or more); papulonodular (leproma), normoaesthetic, symmetrical or diffuse infiltration
Nerves involvement	1 or 2 nerves, severe	Few nerves, severe, asymmetrical	More or less severe, and symmetrical	More or less severe, symmetrical	Initially slight, symmetrical
Bacteriological index (BI)	0	1–2+	3–4+	4–5+	5–6+
Histology	Epithelioid infiltrate with numerous lymphocytes, epithelioid and giant (Langerhans) cells. Nerve destruction	Epithelioid infiltrate with less lymphocytes than TT. Granuloma-free subepidermal zone. Nerve destruction	Epithelioid infiltrate with rare lymphocytes. Granuloma-free subepidermal zone. Nerves slightly infiltrated	Virchowian infiltrate: vacuolated 'spumous histiocytes' with few lymphocytes. Granuloma-free subepidermal zone. Nerves slightly infiltrated	Virchowian infiltrate: vacuolated 'spumous histiocytes' with rare lymphocytes. Granuloma-free subepidermal zone. Nerves enlarged slightly infiltrated
Lepromin test	+++	++/+	–	–	–
Antibodies	+/–	+	++	+++	++++
Type 1 reaction	0	+	++	+	0
Type 2 reaction	0	0	0	+	++

surrounding skin, sometimes annular and always hypo- or anaesthetic.

In lepromatous (BB, BL, LL) leprosy, the lesions are multiple (10 up to 100 or more) and symmetrically distributed over the whole body. In LL form, they are small, less than 2 cm in diameter, macular, ill defined and hypopigmented or papulonodular and erythematous (leproma), with a shiny surface and normo- or slightly hypoaesthetic. In advanced cases, the lesions coalesce giving the 'facies leonina' look, a lion-like appearance with loss of eyebrows and eyelashes. In BB and BL forms, more or less annular with large edges and normoaesthetic or faintly hypoaesthetic lesions are associated with LL lesions.

Close to these five forms exists an indeterminate form, rarely observed, as it more often heals spontaneously, with one or two blurred hypopigmented macules, normoaesthetic or faintly hypoaesthetic.

Histoid leprosy is a rare clinical and histological variant of lepromatous leprosy with firm erythematous nodules and plaques sometimes ulcerated and subcutaneous nodular lesions. Lucio–Latapi leprosy is another unusual form of lepromatous leprosy that appears as a diffuse shiny infiltration of all the skin of the body.

Neurological involvement

Leprosy affects the peripheral nerves especially:

- the ulnar nerve at the elbow
- the median nerve at the wrist
- the lateral popliteal nerve at the knee
- the posterior tibial nerve near the medial malleolus
- the facial nerve.

The main sign of involvement is the enlargement of these nerves. Damage may result in local pain and in sensitive (hypo- or anaesthesia), or motor loss (weakness or paralysis) in the corresponding innervated areas. All these features are responsible for:

1 Contractures.
2 Deformities.
   - claw-hand
   - wrist-drop
   - foot-drop
   - claw-toes
   - mask-face
   - lagophthalmos.
3 Tissue necrosis.
4 Plantar ulceration.
5 Cellulitis.
6 Osteomyelitis.
7 At least progressive loss of digits of the hands and feet.

In tuberculoid leprosy, nerves involvement is often rapid, serious and asymmetrical, affecting one to three nerves while in lepromatous leprosy it is more often slow and symmetrical.

Other organ involvement

In lepromatous leprosy, the following organs may be involved, especially in the evoluted form:

1 Ocular (keratitis, iritis, uveitis).
2 Upper respiratory tract
   - nose (deformation, destruction)
   - mouth
   - larynx
   - pharynx.
3 Bone (osteitis)
   - digits, hands, feet.
4 Kidney.
5 Testis.

Leprosy reactions

The course of leprosy may be marked by the occurrence of acute immunological complications named 'reactions'.

Type 1 reactions

These include ugrading or reversal reaction (RR) and downgrading reaction. The former, the most frequent, is due to a sudden increase in cell-mediated immunity (CMI) and occurs in borderline BT, BB or BL patients usually during the first months of treatment. Suddenly, in a few hours or days, without general symptoms, pre-existing skin lesions become more erythematous, swollen and shiny, and may ulcerate. One or more nerves commonly become painful and tender. A rapid occurrence or increase of a sensitive and/or motor deficit is frequent and may be irreversible in the absence of adequate treatment. Enhancement of the CMI results in a positive lepromin test result and the occurrence of more histological tuberculoid features.

The downgrading reaction occurs in untreated borderline patients. Skin lesions become more numerous and progress towards the lepromatous pole.

Type 2 reactions

Erythema nodosum leprosum (ENL), an immune-complex disease (Arthus phenomenon), occurs in BL and LL lepromatous patients mostly during the first 2 years of treatment. Clinical features include fever, malaise and sudden appearance, in crops, of transient painful, tender and erythematous nodules which disappear within a few days while pre-existing lepromatous lesions do not change. Neuritis affecting several nerves is frequent with painful and tender nerves, and more or less complete loss of sensitivity or motor function. Iritis, iridocyclitis, arthralgia, arthritis, orchitis and glomerulonephritis may occur. ENL is often recurrent and may even become chronic.

Lucio's phenomenon is a peculiar and severe form of type 2 reaction that occurs in cases of diffuse Lucio–Latapi leprosy.

Diagnosis

Bacteriological examination

Research for bacilli must be made in all suspected leprosy patients. Smears are taken by the slit and scrape method from ear lobes and at least from a skin lesion and nasal smear by nose-blow in the morning. Slides are stained using the Zielh–Neelsen or the Fite–Faraco methods.

The bacteriological index (BI) is defined as the number of AFB seen in the microscopic field and is expressed according to the Ridley's logarithmic scale:

- 0 = no BH found in any of the 100 fields
- 1+ =1–10 BH in 100 fields
- 2+ =1–10 BH in 10 fields
- 3+ =1–10 BH in each field
- 4+ =10–100 BH in each field
- 5+ =100–1000 BH in each field
- 6+ =more than 1000 BH in each field.

The morphological index (MI) is the percentage of uniformly stained BH (presumably living bacilli) in relation to the total number of bacilli seen in the smears.

BI is negative or lower than 3+ and MI is negative in tuberculoid patients while in lepromatous cases, BI is higher than 2+ to 6+ and MI more or less positive.

Histological evaluation

Histology is essential to make the diagnosis and the classification. Detailed features are given Table 1. Briefly, tuberculoid leprosy exhibits a perinervous and periadnexial lymphoepithelioid granuloma with none or rarely any bacilli and lepromatous leprosy is characterized by a spumous histiocytic ('Virchow cells') infiltrate containing numerous bacilli.

Immunological evaluation

The lepromin test (Mitsuda reaction) is a guide to evaluate the CMI of the patient against *M. leprae* but it is not of diagnostic help in leprosy. Read between 3 and 4 weeks after intradermal injection of standardized lepromin, it is positive in tuberculoid patients (and in a significant number of normal subjects not exposed to *M. leprae*) and always negative in lepromatous patients.

Infection by *M. leprae* induces an humoral immune response with production of antibodies in a level correlated with the bacillary load. Despite great advances made during the last two decades in serological techniques (ELISA) and in the determination of *M. leprae* specific antigens (phenolic glycolipid I) no reliable serological test is yet available.

Differential diagnosis of skin lesions

Macular lesions

- Pityriasis alba.
- Seborrhoeic dermatitis.
- Hypochromic sarcoidosis.
- Hypopigmented mycosis fungoides.
- Naevus anaemicus.
- Vitiligo.
- Tinea versicolor.
- Occupational leucoderma.
- Postinflammatory hypopigmentation.
- Nutritional dyschromia.
- Post-kala-azar dermal leishmaniasis.
- Onchocerciasis.

Infiltrated papulous or nodular lesions

- Granuloma annulare.
- Tinea corporis.
- Sarcoidosis.
- Granuloma multiforme (Leiker).
- Lupus erythematosus.
- Psoriasis.
- Lichen planus.
- Tuberculosis (lupus vulgaris, tuberculosis verrucosa cutis).
- Syphilis (syphylides).
- Leishmaniasis (dermal or post-kala-azar dermal leishmaniasis).
- Onchocerciasis.
- Kaposi sarcoma.
- Leukaemia cutis.

Treatment

Recommended therapies

Current antibacillary drugs

Dapsone (Disulone)

Dapsone or 4,4′-diaminodiphenylsulphone (DDS) was the first effective antileprosy drug, first used in 1946. It is mainly bacteriostatic against *M. leprae*. Daily dosage in adult patients is of 100 mg (2 mg/kg in a child). At this dosage, it is well tolerated. Side-effects are rare and mainly consist in haematological disturbances: methaemoglobinaemia, acute haemolytic anaemia in case of glucose-6-phosphate dehydrogenase (G6PD) deficiency, macrocytic anaemia and leucopenia–agranulocytosis.

The 'DDS syndrome', an allergic manifestation, associates fever, exfoliative dermatitis, generalized lymphadenopathy, eosinophilia, monocytosis, hepatitis and nephritis and sometimes may be lethal. A motor polyneuropathy has been reported in other dermatological diseases in long-term and high-dosage treated patients. Its occurrence in leprosy is hardly detectable.

Dapsone is not teratogenic and currently it is not contraindicated during pregnancy.

Rifampicin (RMP)

RMP was the first bactericidal antileprosy drug and has been used since 1970. Its daily dosage in adult is 600 mg (10 mg/kg in a child). Its side-effects are rare. The most common is a red coloration of urine, sweat, tears, faeces and sputum. Anorexia, nausea, vomiting and gastrointestinal pains may be seen at the onset of treatment. The 'flu syndrome', of allergic origin, occurs every day, a few hours after intake of the drug and is manifest by malaise, fever, chills, headaches, muscle and bone pain. Toxic hepatitis is rare except in the presence of other hepatotoxic factors such as other hepatotoxic drugs. Some cases of allergic anaemia, thrombocytopenia and hepatitis, porphyria cutanea tarda, pemphigus, Stevens–Johnson syndrome and psychosis have been reported. RMP acts on the metabolism of other drugs such as steroids and oral contraceptives and reduces their effectiveness.

It has been shown to be neuroteratogenic in animals but not in humans. However, it seems preferable to avoid its use at least during the first 3 months of pregnancy.

Clofazimine (CLO; Lamprene)

CLO, a rimino-phenazine dye, was developed initially as an antituberculosis drug. Of little value in this disease, it appears effective (bacteriostatic) in leprosy and has been used since 1962. In addition, CLO has an anti-inflammatory effect, which is clinically valuable in leprosy reactions.

The daily dosage in adults is of 100 mg (10–20 mg/kg in a child). It induces few side-effects. The most common, and often not tolerated by patients, is the red to purple–brownish coloration and the dryness of the skin. This pigmentation, due to the deposition of the drug, disappears within 6 to 12 months after cessation of the drug. It may also affect the cornea, the conjunctiva and the macula.

Transient gastrointestinal symptoms such as mild abdominal or epigastric pain and mild diarrhoea may occur at the onset of the treatment. However, more severe symptoms mimicking Cröhn's disease may appear including:

- severe abdominal or pseudo-occlusive abdominal pain
- severe diarrhoea
- nausea or vomiting
- weight loss.

This 'CLO-induced enteropathy' is seen after several months of treatment and more often in patients receiving a dosage higher than 100 mg daily. This is due to deposition of crystals of CLO in the small bowel mucosa that induces effacement of the mucosal villosities and partial or complete obstruction. Symptoms rapidly decrease after discontinuation of the drug. Fatal outcome has been reported.

CLO is neither embryotoxic nor teratogenic nor mutagenic and may be prescribed during pregnancy. The only known effect in the child is a congenital transient discoloration.

New drugs

Other antibiotics have been more recently found which exhibit an antibacillary bactericidal effect. These drugs are promising in the treatment of leprosy. However they are all still being evaluated in human trials. Thus the WHO recommends, that they are not to be used except in two conditions: the 'single lesion paucibacillary leprosy' (see Table 2) and when the usual antileprosy drugs are contraindicated in a particular patient.

Quinolones

Among fluoroquinolones, ofloxacin (200 mg twice a day) has the most potent antibacillary activity. Gastrointestinal symptoms, headaches and dizziness are common side-effects. However it has other, sometimes severe, side-effects including photosensitivity, tendinitis and tendon rupture.

Table 2 WHO leprosy classifications

Bacteriological classification	Paucibacillary leprosy: negative BI Multibacillary leprosy: positive BI (>1+)
Clinical classification*	*Single lesion paucibacillary leprosy* 1 hypopigmented or reddish anaesthetic skin lesion without nerve involvement *Paucibacillary leprosy* 2–5 hypopigmented or erythematous, asymmetrically distributed anaesthetic skin lesions and only one nerve affected *Multibacillary leprosy* More than five skin lesions, symmetrically distributed with loss of sensation and many nerves involved

*Any patient showing a positive skin smear, irrespective of the clinical classification, should be considered as multibacillary leprosy and treated with the MDT regimen for multibacillary leprosy.

It is contraindicated in infants and children and during pregnancy because of osteocartilaginous involvement.

Cyclines

Minocycline (100 mg/day) is the only cycline that exhibits an antibacillary effect. Common side-effects include gastrointestinal symptoms. More severe side-effects have been reported: pigmentation of the skin and mucous membrane, photosensitivity, autoimmune hepatitis, lupus erythematosus and hypersensitivity syndrome that may sometimes be lethal.

It is contraindicated in infants, children and pregnant women.

Macrolides

Clarithromycin (500 mg/day) has a significant bactericidal effect. It is usually well tolerated. Its side-effects include nausea, vomiting and diarrhoea. It may be given in children and during pregnancy.

Recommended multidrug regimens

The treatment of leprosy consists in a combined multidrug therapy (MDT) including RMP and one or two of the usual drugs, CLO and DDS.

MDT is the only way to prevent the occurrence of secondary and primary drug resistances as seen after dapsone or RMP monotherapy.

WHO-recommended MDT

Taking into account the medical and socioeconomic conditions in developing countries, the WHO initially recommended in 1982 a simplified bacteriological classification of leprosy patients into two groups. However, in practice, bacteriological examination was difficult and so, in 1995 and 1999, another clinical classification into three groups was proposed (Table 2). Each classification may be used.

The relationship between the WHO and the Ridley and Jopling classifications is as follows: SL includes only polar tuberculoid TT; PB includes indeterminate and most borderline tuberculoid (BT) leprosy; and MB includes some borderline tuberculoid (BT), borderline borderline (BB), borderline lepromatous (BL) and polar lepromatous (LL) leprosy.

According to the form of leprosy, the following regimens are allowed:

- Single lesion paucibacillary leprosy: one single dose of RMP (600 mg) + OFLO (400 mg) + MINO (100 mg)
- Paucibacillary leprosy: RMP (600 mg once a month, given under supervision) + DDS (100 mg daily, taken at home) for 6 months.

- Multibacillary leprosy: RMP (600 mg once a month given under supervision) + CLO (300 mg once a month given under supervision and 50 mg daily, taken at home) + DDS (100 mg daily, taken at home) for at least 12 months, preferably 24 months.

Daily MDT

In most developed countries, MDT is given daily with the drug regimen dependent on the classification of Ridley and Jopling:

- Tuberculoid TT and BT forms: RMP (600 mg) + CLO (100 mg) (likely in case of neuritis and RR) or DDS (100 mg) until clinical cure (6–18 months).
- Lepromatous BB, BL and LL forms: RMP (600 mg) + CLO (100 mg) + DDS (100 mg) until bacteriological negativity (2–5 years).

Treatment of leprosy reactions

If these reactions occur while MDT is given, it must be maintained and additional therapy given to counteract the acute immunological complications.

Type 1 reactions

Reversal reaction

Corticosteroids are the treatment of choice in RR. It has to be prescribed as soon as possible after the onset of RR. Prednisolone or prednisone should be started at 1 mg/kg per day, maintained until clinical (neuritis) improvement and then slowly decreased (over 4–6 months). In the absence of a rapid (1–2 weeks) motor and/or sensitive loss recovery, neurolysis of the affected nerve(s) has to be performed.

In moderate RR, acetylsalicylic acid (2–3 g/day) may be sufficient.

Although controversial, the use of CLO (100 mg/day) may prevent or attenuate the RR.

Downgrading reaction

This implies the onset of MDT.

Type 2 reactions

ENL

Thalidomide is the best treatment of the acute phase of ENL, effective on all the symptoms (cutaneous lesions, neuritis, iritis, and so on). The initial dose, 300–400 mg/day, is maintained until cessation of symptoms (about 2 days to 1 week) and then gradually decreased by 100 mg, every week until 100 mg/day and further by 50 mg every week thereafter.

Because of its high neuroteratogenicity, thalidomide use has to be severely limited in fertile women; however, if it must be prescribed many precautions must be taken (e.g. very effective contraception, as RMP given in MDT diminishes the effectiveness of oestroprogestatives).

In dermatological diseases other than leprosy, it has been shown that thalidomide may induce peripheral sensitive neuropathy sometimes irreversible. This side-effect has not been obvious in leprosy patients; however, it implies that the maintenance of high dosages for long periods should be limited as far as possible.

In the case of moderate ENL or contraindication for thalidomide, the following drugs may be useful:

- Corticosteroids: prednisolone or prednisone at an initial dose of 1–1.5 mg/kg per day is effective against ENL but less rapid than thalidomide. A slow decrease of the dose is necessary, as recurrent attacks are frequent if the dosage is diminished too quickly.
- Pentoxifylline: at a dose of 1200–2400 mg/day pentoxifylline is effective in the treatment of acute ENL. The delay in response is longer than that observed with thalidomide but it is the same as that reported for corticosteroids.

- Acetylsalicylic acid: 2–3 g/day.
- Antimalarials: chloroquine at an initial dose of 300–400 mg/day.
- Colchicine: 100–200 mg/day.
- In severe ENL, ciclosporin and plasmapheresis have been used successfully in few cases.
- In the case of recurrent or chronic ENL, CLO must be prescribed systematically because of its antireactional effect. The usual dosage is 100 mg/day. Higher doses can cause gastrointestinal side-effects. If this proves insufficient, prevention of attacks may be obtained with additional low doses of thalidomide such as 50 mg every other day or twice a week, for 6 or more months.
- Lucio's phenomenonL relatively high doses of corticosteroids (2 mg/kg per day) are needed in the management of this severe type 2 reaction. Addition of thalidomide and CLO may be useful although their efficacy has never been proved. Plasmapheresis has given excellent results in some cases.

Surgical treatment in leprosy

Surgery is often needed in addition to MDT in two conditions: acute neuritis and deformities.

Acute neuritis

This is defined as acute pain and tenderness of a nerve with more or less complete loss of sensitive and/or motor functions; more often this occurs during leprosy reactions. It may respond to medical treatment but sometimes requires additional surgical decompression including neurolysis and disentrapment of nerves in anatomical osteotendinous channels. The sooner it is performed after the onset of neuritis, the better the results.

Surgery

- Correction of primary involvement: facies leonina; eyebrow and eyelash loss; nasal deformities; claw-hand (ulnar and/or median nerve); wrist-drop (radial nerve); foot-drop (lateral popliteal nerve); and claw-toes (posterior tibial nerve).
- Correction of secondary deformities: palmar and plantar ulcers; osteitis; fracture and disintegration.

Chemoprophylaxis

Dapsone or RMP chemoprophylaxis are not recommended, the former in view of the widespread dapsone-resistant strains of *M. leprae* (up to 40% in some countries), the second because of the risk of RMP-resistant *M. leprae* occurrence.

Vaccination

Starting in the 1980s, numerous trials of vaccination by BCG, heat-killed *M. leprae* or other mycobacteria have been carried out. Recent evaluation shows that all afforded some protective effect but at a level insufficient to justify a mass vaccination programme.

Further reading

Arbiser JL, Moschella S. Clofazimine. A review of its medical uses and mechanism of action. *J Am Acad Dermatol* 1985; 32: 241–7.

De Carsalade GY, Wallach D, Spindler E, Pennec J, Cottenot F, Flageul B. Daily multidrug therapy for leprosy: a fourteen years experience. *Int J Lepr* 1997; 65: 37–44.

Jolliffe DS. The reactional states in leprosy and their treatment. *Br J Dermatol* 1977; 97: 345–52.

Joppling WH. Side effects of antileprosy drugs in common use. *Lepr Rev* 1983; 54: 261–70.

Joppling WH. References to 'Side effects of antileprosy drugs in common use'. *Lepr Rev* 1985; 56: 61–70.

Lafitte E, Revuz J. Thalidomide. *Ann Dermatol Venereol* 2000; 127: 603–13.

Moreira AL, Kaplan G. Comparison of pentoxyfilline, thalidomide and prednisone in the treatment of ENL. *Int J Lepr* 1998; 66: 61–5.

Waldinger TP, Siegle R, Weber W. Dapsone-induced peripheral neuropathy. *Arch Dermatol* 1984; 120: 356–9.

WHO. *Rapport d'une Réunion Spéciale du Groupe Consultatif sur L'élimination de la Lèpre.* WHO/LEP/99.1. Geneva: WHO.

WHO Expert Committee on Leprosy. *Technical Report Series 874.* Geneva: WHO, 1998.

Lichen planus

A. Rebora

Definition and epidemiology

Lichen planus (LP) is an acquired chronic disease characterized by small cutaneous papules and mucosal striae erosions. It affects 0.3–0.8% of the population occurring in all races and both sexes. Children are rarely affected.

Aetiology and pathogenesis

LP is a specific pattern of cell-mediated cutaneous reactivity to a variety of antigens. The latter vary from viruses (hepatitis C and hepatitis B virus in the Mediterranean countries and USA), drugs and contact antigens, e.g. expressed on keratinocytes, which are the target of lymphocytotoxicity. LP may associate with visceral disease, in particular chronic active hepatitis, primary biliary cirrhosis and ulcerative colitis, and with other autoimmune cutaneous disorders, such as alopecia areata.

Clinical characteristics and course

Lesions are small violet, polygonal papules, which coalesce into larger papules or plaques. On the surface of plaques, a whitish reticulum can be observed. On the skin, a typical site is the volar aspect of the wrist, but widespread lesions are not uncommon. Mucosae are often involved usually by the whitish reticulum, more rarely by erosions. Nail plates may be dystrophic. Clinical features vary according to the body region. On the shins, LP is verrucous, while on the scalp it presents as a scarring alopecia plaque. Unusual varieties include:

- annular LP of the scrotum
- ulcerative form of the sole
- lichen planopilaris
- vesicobullous lichen
- pigmentary forms (lichen actinicus, lichen pigmentosus).

The course is chronic, accompanied by pruritis of varying severity. Mucosal erosions may result in cancer.

Diagnosis

Diagnosis is mainly clinical. Histopathology may help in doubtful cases, revealing a typical mononucleate infiltrate, which impinges the basal line of the keratinocytes. Immunofluorescence is not contributory.

Differential diagnosis

- Lichenoid drug eruptions: parakeratosis and eosinophils.
- Lupus erythematosus: lupus band in direct immunofluorescence, but there may be overlapping cases.
- Secondary syphilis: lymph nodes, serology.
- Psoriasis: parakeratotic scales, typical histopathology.
- Leucoplakia: involving the anterior part of the mouth, rough surface, typical histopathology.
- Candidiasis: easily removed whitish patches, severe immunodeficiency.
- Erythema multiforme: target-like lesions on the skin, typical histopathology.
- Bullous diseases: typical histopathology and immunofluorescence.

Treatment

General therapeutic guidelines

Usually, LP is a chronic, but benign and often symptomless disease, which does not require systemic treatment. As an immune disease, LP responds to all immunosuppressants. Those should be used only if a severe visceral involvement is documented or whenever the mucosal erosions prevent efficient eating and speaking.

Recommended therapies

Local treatment

Topical corticosteroids

These are in most cases the treatment of choice. Class I and II corticosteroids should be used. Occlusive dressings with class I drugs are recommended on verrucous plaques. Intralesional preparations have been advocated, but they should be used only in very resistant verrucous plaques. They have been tried in pitted nails, but discomfort discourages the patient. In any case, injectable triamcinolone is preferable. On lichen planopilaris of the scalp, corticosteroids may be useful if they are spread around the plaque rather than in its centre. A foamy preparation of betamethasone is very useful in this particular location.

A particular problem is oral lesions, especially when they are eroded or ulcerated. Oral pastes or gels containing triamcinolone have been claimed to improve 65% of such patients in 2 weeks. Fluocinolone 0.025% in 4% hydroxycellulose gel associated with clorexidine and miconazole gel as antimicotics improved 50% of patients to avoid oral candidiasis.

It may be helpful as well to rinse the mouth for 5 min, with one tablet of an effervescent preparation of betamethasone originally meant for systemic use. It should be stressed, however, that this swishing technique is useful only on lesions which are erosive *de novo* and not in those which have become eroded from mechanical trauma.

Fluocinonide 0.025% applied 6 times daily for over 2 months proved active in comparison with placebo without side-effects. Betamethasone valerate in aerosol has also been tried for 2 months obtaining good results in eight out of 11 patients. Clobetasol propionate 0.05% was recently found more effective than fluocinonide 0.05%.

Intralesional corticosteroid have been used in oral lichen planus as well. Triamcinolone acetonide is the preferred preparation and is given 5–10 mg/mL weekly or twice weekly over 3–4 weeks.

Retinoids

These have been used topically in oral LP. Fenretinide, for example, in twice daily applications has been claimed to give excellent responses and no local or distant side-effects. Retinoic acid 0.1%, tretinoin 0.025% and isotretinoin gel 0.1% were all found to be effective, but less than topical triamcinolone or fluocinonide, however.

In conclusion, several local treatments have been tried, but conclusive findings from adequately controlled trials are lacking. Results originate from anecdotal reports of from small series. A recent review provided only weak evidence for the superiority of the assessed interventions over placebo. Finally, there are only few data concerning the long-term effects of the medical treatments upon the course of the disease and it is unknown whether therapy influences malignant evolution.

Systemic treatments

Cyclosporin A (CyA)

Being specifically aimed at cell-mediated hypersensitivity reactions, CyA could be the drug of choice. Usually 5 mg/kg per day is the dose to start with. It should be tapered to 2 mg/kg per day as soon as possible: regimens longer than 6 months should be avoided. Blood pressure should be monitored weekly and kidney function monthly. The best indication for systemic CyA is severe erosive LP.

Corticosteroids

Systemic corticosteroids may also be used to replace CyA. Prednisone 1 mg/kg per day (or lower dosage) may be used and tapered over 1 month. Rebound phenomena may occur at withdrawal. The usual adverse effects of corticosteroids are commonly observed.

Azathioprine

Azathioprine (50–100 mg/day) may be used in erosive LP with chronic active hepatitis. Usually, transaminase level improves with oral lesions. If the patient is hepatitis C virus antibody positive, however, all immunosuppressive treatments should be avoided as immunosuppressives may help hepatocarcinoma to develop.

Other drugs that have been claimed to be of some benefit are thalidomide, hydroxychloroquine, retinoids and levamisole.

Thalidomide

This has obtained a dramatic response in one patient.

Hydroxychloroquine

This has been used at 200–400 mg/day for several months in patients with oral lesions. Retinal adverse effects should be considered in the risk/benefit ratio and thoroughly monitored.

Retinoids

Etretinate (0.3–0.6 mg/kg per day), acitretin (0.25–0.75 mg/kg per day) and isotretinoin (0.25–0.50 mg/kg per day) have also been used with success. Such drugs cannot be used in fertile women for their well-known teratogenicity.

Levamisole

This has been used successfully (150 mg/day) in China in order to limit the use of steroids, but the study was not controlled.

PUVA

PUVA therapy may be useful for severe forms of erosive oral lichen planus that do not respond to conventional treatment.

A dose of 0.6 mg/kg 8-methoxypsoralen is administered orally 2 h before long-wave ultraviolet light irradiation is done. In one study, irradiation was given 12 times at intervals of 2–3 days, at a total dosage of 16.5 J/cm^2. In another study, 20 sessions were held, three weekly, at a total cumulative dose of 35.9 J/cm^2. After the treatment was concluded, clinical symptoms and erosive lesions disappeared. Side-effects were similar to those seen after whole-body irradiation PUVA treatment.

Alternative and experimental treatments

Topical CyA and tacrolimus

CyA 10% in olive oil (for 5 min, 3 times a day for 8 weeks) or as a syrup preparation may be of benefit in erosive LP, sometimes greater than 0.1% triamcinolone, even though its effect has been denied. In my experience, benefit is minimal.

Tacrolimus has been found to be of benefit. Three patients with severe recalcitrant erosive mucosal LP obtained complete resolution with topical application of tacrolimus ointment after 4 weeks of treatment while the other three patients experienced a substantial improvement. Prolonged treatment resulted either in further improvement or in complete healing. All patients reported rapid relief from pain and burning. No severe side-effects were observed.

Basiliximab

Basiliximab is an interleukin-2 receptor monoclonal antibody used in the prevention of rejection of solid organ transplantation and in the treatment of acute graft-vs-host reaction. My experience is limited to one case of severe bipolar erosive LP in which basiliximab replaced CyA successfully. Basiliximab has been given intravenously at a dose of 20 mg 4 days apart.

No short-term side-effects have been noted. Medications for the treatment of severe hypersensitivity reactions, including anaphylaxis, must be available for immediate use. Such reactions may occur within 24 h following initial exposure and/or following re-exposure to the drug.

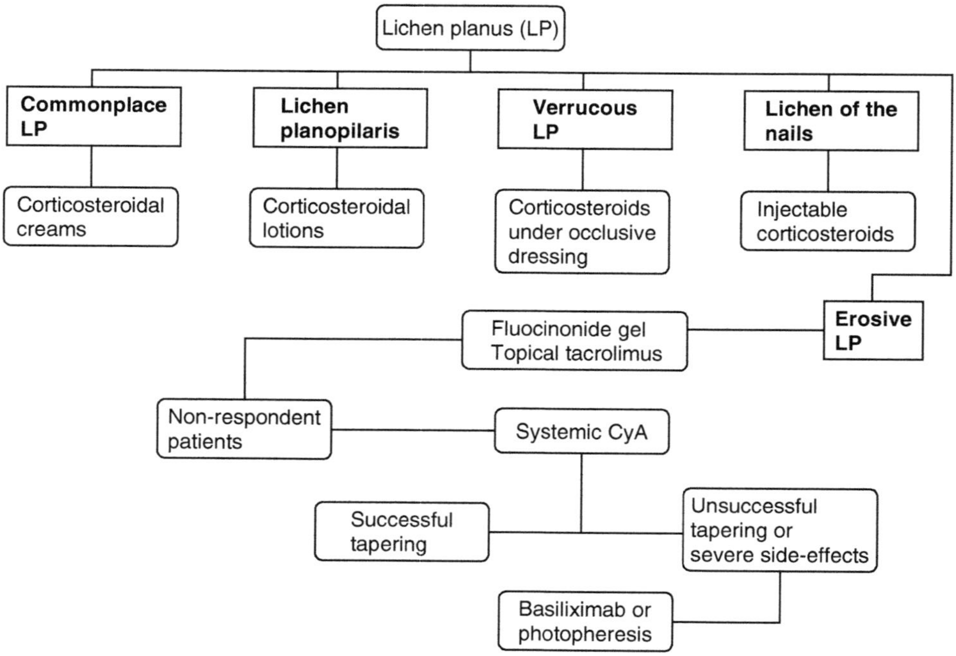

Figure 1 Treatment of lichen planus

Extracorporeal photochemotherapy

Extracorporeal photochemotherapy has been found to improve generalized LP and its oral lesions. The procedure has been applied twice a week for 3 weeks and then tapered according to the patients' needs. All seven patients treated had complete remission. Improvement began after an average of 1.5 months and remission was reached after a total of 24 sessions (19–27). The longest follow-up was 24 months. The treatment was well tolerated.

Further reading

Becherel PA, Bussel A, Chosidow O *et al.* Extracorporeal photochemotherapy for chronic erosive lichen planus. *Lancet* 1998; 351: 805.

Bratel J, Hakeberg M, Jontell M. Effect of replacement of dental amalgam on oral lichenoid reactions. *J Dent* 1996; 24: 41–5.

Buajeeb W, Kraivaphan P, Pobrurska C. Efficacy of topical retinoic acid compared with topical fluocinole acetonide in the treatment of oral lichen planus. *Oral Surg Oral Med Pathol Oral Radial Endo* 1997; 93: 21–25.

Carbone M, Carrozzo M, Broccoletti R, Mattea A, Gandolfo S. The topical treatment of atrophic-erosive oral lichen planus with fluocinonide in a dioadhesive gel, chlorhexidine and miconazole gel. A totally open trial. *Minerva Stomatol* 1996; 45: 61–8.

Dereure O, Basset-Seguin N, Guilhou JJ. Erosive lichen planus: dramatic response to thalidomide. *Arch Dermatol* 1996; 132: 1392–3.

Gorsky M, Raviv M, Moskona D, Laufer M, Bodner L. Clinical characteristics and treatment of patients with oral lichen planus in Israel. *Oral Surg Med Oral Pathol Radiol Endo* 1996; 82: 644–9.

Lu SY, Chen WJ, Eng HL. Dramatic response to levasimole and low-dose prednisolone in 23 patients with oral lichen planus: a 6-year prospective follow-up study. *Oral Surg Oral Med Pathol Oral Radiol Endo* 1995; 80: 705–9.

Panconesi E, Lotti T. Steroids versus nonsteroids in the treatment of cutaneous inflammation. Therapeutic modalities for office use. *Arch Dermatol Res* 1992; 284: 537–41.

Salim A, Emerson RM, Dalziel KL. Successful treatment of severe generalized pustular psoriasis with basiliximab (interleukin-2 receptor blocker). *Br J Dermatol* 2000; 143: 1121–2.

Setterfield JF, Black MM, Challacombe SJ. The management of oral lichen planus. *Clin Exp Dermatol* 2000; 25: 176–82.

Tradati N, Chiesa F, Rossi N *et al.* Successful topical treatment of oral lichen planus and leukoplakias with fenretinide (4-HPR). *Cancer Lett* 1994; 76: 109–11.

Lichen simplex chronicus

M.L. Gantcheva

Synonyms

Lichen simplex chronicus, neurodermitis circumscripta, lichen Vidal, circumscribed neurodermatitis.

Definition and epidemiology

Lichen simplex chronicus (LSC) is an acquired severely itching chronic dermatosis with circumscribed lichenified lesions, which are due to rubbing and scratching of the skin previously apparently normal, the so-called primary lichenification. There is no known predisposing skin disorder and underlying cause of the development of the lichenification but it could develop as a secondary process due to a chronic eczematous process. Variants in clinical morphology, size and location have led to several clinical variants, which affect the population worldwide. LSC is particularly common in Orientals and is comparatively rare in black people. Women are predominantly affected with the peak incidence between 30 and 50 years.

Aetiology and pathophysiology

Pruritus seems to be the cause and not just a symptom of LSC. It is the main factor for the development of the lichenification and probably results from mediator release or proteolytic enzyme activity. Nervous stress and psychovegetative disorders unlock an unconscious habit of rubbing and repeated scratching, which lead to thickening of the skin with accentuation of the skin markings.

Lichenification may occur secondary to many pruritic dermatoses and some authors suggest that LSC is a minimal variant of atopic eczema in adults with a personal or family history of atopic disorders. Others suppose that the occurrence of the disease is related to internal disorders such as gastrointestinal or liver cholecystopathies, diabetes mellitus or constipation. Lichenification also develops in the course of other irritant dermatoses or complicates persistent skin lesions of many types, such as chronic contact dermatitis, asteatotic and nummular eczema, seborrhoeic and stasis dermatitis, lichen planus, pruritus ani et vulvae and rarely psoriasis.

The distinction between lichenification and some forms of prurigo is not so clear in nomenclature and in practice. In some subjects chronic rubbing and scratching produce nodules—nodular prurigo or nodular lichenification. The increase in neuropeptides, calcitonin gene-related peptide and substance P-immunoreactive nerve fibres can be related to the intense pruritus. Other patients (e.g. black people) develop papular and follicular lichenification. Presumably there is a native predisposition to the development of lichenification and its persistence.

Clinical characteristics and course

Pruritus is severe and paroxysmal and usually occurs at night. It is often out of proportion to the extent of the objective changes. The original lesion is usually isolated and a three-zone structure could be distinguished:

- central: infiltration and the primary flat lichenification
- middle: closely set lichenoid papules
- peripheral: slight thickening and pigmentation.

There are different forms of lichenification with their own characteristics depending on the localization and the duration. In early lesions the two external zones may be absent. In some cases leucoderma can be seen accompanied by vitiligo-like macules and depigmented area of infiltrated plaques. Rarely LSC is presented with isolated lichenoid papules without central lichenification.

Almost every skin area may be affected, but the most common locations are those that are conveniently reached: the nape of the neck, scalp, extensor aspect of forearm, sacrum, inner thighs, lower legs and ankles, vulva, pubis and scrotum.

Lichen nuche occurs on the back of the neck, particularly in women under emotional stress or in patients with atopic dermatitis. This area is easily reached and patients will scratch it. In both cases the disease is characterized by scaly and psoriasiform plaque and frequent episodes of secondary infection.

Nodular neurodermatitis of the scalp presents with pruritic and excoriated papules. The epidermal thickening on the scalp in this situation is enough to form nodules.

Giant lichenification of Pautrier, consisting of warty, cribriform plaques, develops in the genitocrural region when the pruritus is persistent for many years. Sharply demarcated patches of verrucoid hyperplasia can be elevated above the surrounding surface and tumour-like plaques may be formed.

The clinical evidence of 'pebbly' lichenification are plaques of coalescing smooth papules or discrete small nodules resembling lichen planus. They could also be seen in patients with atopic dermatitis, photodermatitis and seborrhoeic dermatitis.

The course of LSC is chronic and the lesions persist indefinitely depending on individual variation.

Diagnosis (laboratory examinations)

LSC requires elimination of primary causes of lichenification. A skin biopsy specimen shows some variations with site and duration. Hyperkeratosis and acanthosis are constant. The rete ridges are lengthened. Sometimes spongiosis is present and small areas of parakeratosis are seen. Hyperplasia is everywhere.

Differential diagnosis

- Atopic eczema: present at childhood; presence of atopic stigmata; symmetrical lichenified lesions of predilection; positive radioallergosorbent test (RAST) or skin prick tests; elevated immunoglobulin E (IgE).
- Nummular eczema: absence of lichenified plaques.
- Psoriasis: presence of psoriatic lesions elsewhere; thick adherent white scars and the underlined deep red colour; biopsy specimen; usually without itch.
- Lichenified chronic eczema: presence of more inflammatory changes, biopsy specimen.
- Hypertrophic lichen planus: involvement of the mucosa in about 50% of patients; Wickham's striation.
- Lichen amyloidosus: biopsy; infiltrated itchy papules with typical ripple appearance are not usually localized in plaques, symmetrical distribution.
- Prurigo nodularis Hyde: single nodules on normal skin.
- Tinea (dermatophyte infection): microbiology, Wood's lamp.
- Dermatitis contacta: anamnesis; patch testing; usually symmetrical involvement.
- Drug reactions (gold, trimethoprim–sulphamethoxazole duflunisal, bupivacaine, quanidine, quinacrine): discontinuing the medication leads to improvement.
- Cutaneous T-cell lymphoma: biopsy.
- Stasis dermatitis: skin lesions on the lower leg in the presence of venous insufficiency.

Treatment

General therapeutic guidelines

- The treatment of LSC must be tailored for every patient depending on different inducing factors and on the localization and duration of the given lesions.

- Patients should be given treatment for any underlying stresses. The lesions worsen during periods of fatigue and emotional tension, and improve with rest and relaxation.
- In most cases the rubbing and scratching exist as a reflexive and unconscious habit. Explanation to the patient of the itch–scratch mechanism and its relationship to the disease could be helpful to suppress this habit.
- Some patients need a psychiatric consultation and psychotherapy is recommended, if necessary. These are usually individuals who feel themselves emotionally disturbed or have functional complaints.
- It is imperative to search for underlying disease, which could be related to the lichenification development.
- During active treatment, the patient must avoid washing the involved areas with soaps and detergents and having their nails cut.

Recommended therapies

Systemic

Pruritus is the leading symptom of the disease and the treatment must be directed to stop it.

- Antihistamines are widely accepted and are most useful as oral and parenteral administration in the course of treatment. Hydroxyzine hydro chloride, diphenhydramine hydrochloride, chlorpheniramine and promethazine are well-known classic antihistamines, blocking H1-receptors, and recommended against itching. Cetirizine, loratadine and mizolastine are second-generation antihistamines, which are preferred to prevent the pruritus in socially active patients, as they have no sedative effect. Cyproheptadine hydrochloride may be another useful medicine for control of the pruritus.
- Antidepressant and anxyolitics. In many cases the antipruritic effect of antihistamines is not enough and it could be replaced by some psychotrophic agents. Tranquillizers inhibit the wish to scratch and diminish nervous tension. Tricyclic antidepressant medications might be another alternative for the control of pruritus because of strong H1 binding. Amitriptyline could be prescribed in patients with neurosis and depression in view of the tendency to scratch and rub.
- Antibiotics. Appropriate administration is required in cases complicated with secondary infection. *Staphylococcus aureus* is often the major pathogen in these patients.

Topical

Glucocorticoids

External therapy without steroid treatment is not conceivable, although there are side-effects connected with them. High-potency glucocorticoids tend to relieve the itching and infiltration of the lesions. Very potent topical steroids as a local application and under occlusive dressing are recommended for a short time in both cases. If the lesion is located in the genital area it is preferable to use mild potent steroid.

Intralesional applications of triamcinolone acetonide (crystalline suspension) 10 mg/mL, 1 : 4 dilution in 1% local anaesthetic should be tried in small lesions. Care must be taken to avoid the risks of atrophy and depigmentation. Injection should not be made into excoriated or infected lesions.

Tar

The anti-inflammatory property of tar and tar products are well known. Liquor carbonis detergents or pure coal tar could be prescribed for a few days. It is better prescribed together with emollients because tar dries the skin. Photosensitization, contact dermatitis and folliculitis may also occur as side-effects. Combined therapy is well tolerated, including steroids and tar with or without salicylic acid.

Urea

Urea preparations have been applied with great success in therapy, follow-up and prophylaxis of neurodermatitis. Efficacy is based on its properties to elevate the water-binding capacity of the corneal layer, on its keratoplastic abilities, antipruriginous effect and proliferation-suppressing action. The combination of hydrocortisone and urea may prove useful in the treatment of LSC.

Doxepin

Topical application of 5% doxepin cream has significant antipruritic activity in patients suffering from LSC. Doxepin cream provides pruritus relief with transient and mild adverse effects, which include stinging at the site of application and drowsiness.

Other therapy

- Topical treatment with antibiotic alone or in combination with glucocorticoids gives good results if secondary infection is present.
- If substance P or calcitonin gene-related peptide is considered as a possible mediator of severe pruritus, the use of capsaicin cream might be helpful. It is also used in the treatment of prurigo nodularis.
- Cryotherapy with liquid nitrogen or CO_2 may be justified for infiltrated lesion. It has an anti-itching effect.
- Dripping with trichloracetic acid (10–33%) or podophyllin (2–10%), used several times depending on the duration of the lesion, reduces the infiltrate and relieves the itch.
- Soft X-rays or Grenz rays may be successfully used especially in tumour-like lichenification.
- Local application of tretinoin 0.05% or aromatic retinoid might be successful in some cases of LSC.

Alternative and experimental treatments

- Alternative local PUVA therapy three times weekly (3–5 J/cm^2) is recommended for about 20 procedures.
- Bulgarian dermatologists have been pioneers in the successful treatment of LSC using high-mountain climatotherapy. Itching is reduced by a cooling off in the atmosphere at 2000 m above sea level. Pathologically changed reactivity of the organism modifies itself to a state of hyposensibilization. The beneficial effects of high-mountain climatotherapy are based on the relative cleanliness of the air, the abundance of ultraviolet radiation and the low partial pressure of O_2, stimulating the hormonal activity of adrenal glands.
- Acupuncture is also helpful in the relief of pruritus and could be recommended as follow-up care.
- Cool to tepid baths are another commonly used method of reducing itching.

Further reading

Drake L, Millikan L. The antipruritic effect of 5% doxepin cream in patients with eczematous dermatitis. Doxepin Study Group. *Arch Dermatol* 1995; 131 (12): 1403–8.

Kantor G, Resnik K. Treatment of LCS with topical capsaicin cream (letter). *Acta Derm Venereol* 1996; 76 (2): 161.

Katsambas A. In: Milikan L, ed. *Antihistamines. Drug Therapy in Dermatology.* New York: Marcel Dekker, 2000: 243–51.

Lotti T, Hautmann G, Panconesi I. Neuropeptides. *Skin* 1995; 33: 482–96.

Peters M, Löwenberg H. Prognose und Behandlungserfold bei stationärer psychotherapentisch—dermatologischer Behandlung von Neurodermitis patienten. *Hautarzt* 1993; 44: 210–14.

Voalasti A, Suomalainen H. Calcitonin gene-related peptide immunoreactivity in prurigo nodularis: a comparative study with neurodermatitis circumscripta. *Br J Dermatol* 1989; 120: 619–23.

Lupus erythematosus

B. Crickx and S. Belaich

Definition and epidemiology

The term lupus erythematosus (LE) refers to a disease group that may involve one or many organ systems. Skin involvement is a major feature of LE in 100% of patients with cutaneous LE and in 70–85% of patients with systemic LE. The spectrum of LE is usually divided into two opposite poles (the cutaneous and systemic poles) with intermediate subsets. But cutaneous and systemic forms are variants of the same disease as follows.

1 Some clinical or biological immunological features are found in both conditions.
2 Patients with cutaneous LE occasionally develop evidence of overt systemic LE (SLE).
3 In both conditions the disease takes the form either of a latent morbidity occasionally interrupted by acute intermittent flares or very slowly evolving lesions.
4 Both conditions are observed in all races and modulate by genetic, immunological and environmental factors as sunlight.

But the genetic predisposition is probably not the same as the age and sex distribution, and natural history may be quite different. SLE occurs primarily in women during their childbearing years with a prevalence of 12.5/100 000 women (North Europe) to 24/100 000 in Afro-Caribbean or Chinese women. In cutaneous LE, the peak age of onset is in the fourth decade and the female prevalence is less marked.

Aetiology and pathophysiology

LE is a multifactorial disease: genetic, immunological, infectious, hormonal and other environmental factors may modulate disease expression and clinical course in a particular individual. It is an autoimmune disease characterized by the development of autoantibodies directed against a variety of nucleoprotein antigens. The precise aetiology, however, remains unknown.

Clinical characteristics and course

Subsets of LE were identified by grouping patients with similar clinical and/or laboratory features, thus defining more homogeneous groups of patients.

Clinical forms of histologically LE-specific skin lesions

Chronic cutaneous LE (15–20%)

- Localized or generalized.
- Predominant in photoexposed areas.
- Scarring (discoid) or congestive (tumidus).
- Usually no extracutaneous disease (5% will develop SLE).
- Antinuclear antibodies occasionally present in low titre.

Subacute cutaneous LE (10–15%)

- Papulosquamous or annular-polycyclic lesions with photosensitive distribution and exacerbation.
- Usually associated with extracutaneous disease but severe visceral involvement is uncommon.
- Antinuclear antibodies frequently present (60%) with anti RO-SSA specificity (50%).

Lupus panniculitis (lupus profundus): (5–10%)

- Subcutaneous nodules with evolution to cupuliform atrophy (face, upper portions of the arms, thighs and buttocks).

- May be associated with typical discoid lesions.
- Fifty per cent have mild systemic involvement.
- Antinuclear antibodies are usually present.

Systemic acute LE (30–50%)

- Localized, indurated erythematous lesions (butterfly rash) or widespread indurated erythema (face, upper chest, back of hands).
- Multisystem disease.
- Antinuclear antibodies usually present and anti-double-stranded (ds) DNA positive in 60–80%.

Clinical forms of LE: non-specific skin lesions

- Vascular lesions: dermal vasculitis thrombotic manifestations of antiphospholipid syndrome (ulcers, livedo reticularis, etc.).
- Bullous lesions: in photo-exposed areas (anticollagen VII antibodies).
- Amicrobial pustulous lesions: in skin folds, hair and genital area.

Diagnosis

During recent years, establishing the diagnostic criteria has played a major role in standardizing classification of patients with SLE. A person is classified as having SLE if any four or more of the 11 ARA (American Rheumatism Association) criteria (revision 1982) are present either simultaneously or serially:

1 = malar rash
2 = discoid rash
3 = photosensitivity
4 = oral ulcers
5 = arthritis
6 = serositis
7 = renal disorder
8 = seizures or psychosis
9 = haematological disorders such as haemolytic anaemia, leukopenia, thrombopenia
10 = anti-dsDNA, anti-Sm antibodies
11 = antinuclear antibodies (Hep-2 cells) without drug inducing.

They are frequently and wrongly used as a diagnostic tool. The main problem in the application of the set is that many patients do not fulfil four criteria (cutaneous LE and mild SLE). It should be emphasized here that the definition of cutaneous LE has never required features other than erythematous lesions that occur in a photo-exposed distribution and have an LE-specific histopathology:

- hydropic degeneration of the epidermal basal cell layer with focal epidermal atrophy
- heavy mononuclear cell infiltrate in upper dermis, periappendageal and perivascular regions extending to the deep dermis
- subepidermal immunoglobulin deposits commonly found in lesions (lupus band test).

Differential diagnosis

- Polymorphous light eruption (cutaneous LE, SLE). The link with exposure to the sun is constant with immediate rash (anamnesis). Absence of scarring atrophy, and negative lupus band test. Immunofluorescence (IF)
- Lymphocytic infiltration of the skin (cutaneous LE). Usually no link with sun exposure. Negative lupus band test. IF
- Tinea facia: microbiology
- Rosacea: facial erythrosis, flush, pustules.
- Dermatomyositis (SLE). Oedema, periorbital involvement. Myositis (muscular enzymes, electromyogram, muscular biopsy). Non-specific histopathology: cutaneous biopsy (histology, IF).

Treatment

General therapeutic guidelines

The current concepts concerning the pathogenesis of LE imply that management strategies which suppress inflammation and/or immune function should prove beneficial in treatment of the disease. A detailed understanding of the exact mechanisms of action of many of the disease-modifying therapies is lacking. It is a suspensive treatment. As such, the therapies are based largely on successful clinical experiences, in some instances confirmed by randomized controlled trials.

Therapy of cutaneous LE is both an art and a science. The interplay of cosmetic and environmental or systemic factors must be understood by the physician who must discuss prognosis and lifestyle modification with the patient. Finally, therapeutics are administered and frequently modified to control the disease.

Evaluation

On the first visit, the patient is completely evaluated in order to classify the patient into a subset, and to discuss prognosis. Some patients with chronic cutaneous LE are concerned about the possibility of developing SLE. This possibility must be evaluated by appropriate tests (complete blood cell count, urinalysis, sedimentation rate, antinuclear antibodies, anti-dsDNA, total haemolytic complement and C3). Testing for RO (SSA) antibodies or antiphospholipid antibodies is utilized in some particular subsets.

Education

There should be an extensive discussion with the patient concerning prognosis and therapy.

In chronic cutaneous LE, too often the patient believes the disease is far more serious than it really is: the patient with completely negative laboratory test results should be informed that the problem is primarily cosmetic and that the possibility of developing SLE is minimal; he must understand that he has a chronic, usually slowly progressive disease over many years. Effective forms of camouflage by cosmetic cover up are available and help morale.

In SLE, the course is very variable but acute fulminating cases are much less common than the subacute cases. Survival is related to systemic involvement and to frequency of flares. Prolonged survival is associated with an increased risk of atherosclerosis and secondary infection. The overall prognosis is not as bad as popular opinion might suggest. The physician will aim to use immunosuppressive therapy sparsely or the minimal effective dosage to control the disease.

Progressive flares can, at least to some degree, be prevented by taking a number of simple precautions.

- Minimize exposure to ultraviolet rays. It is not certain if this precaution is really necessary for all LE patients. Nevertheless, it is necessary to follow-up patients with a previous history of photosensitivity; they should be advised to wear a broad-brimmed hat and avoid short-sleeved shirts and shorts. A sunscreen should be prescribed (protection factor > 15).
- A second preventive measure (in SLE patients only) is to avoid medications containing oestrogens. The advisability of pregnancy must be discussed extensively with each patient, since there is the possibility of a flare during pregnancy or during the immediate postpartum period. Women with discoid LE and mild SLE have an optimistic outlook if pregnancy occurred during remission. If RO-SSA or antiphospholipids are positive, the obstetrician and paediatrician should be informed. Pregnancy is contraindicated in SLE with active visceral involvement. The risks, adverse effects of medications and effect on the fetus of LE, must be discussed.
- In SLE, it is also important to guard against the use of particular drugs

(including isoniazide, hydralazine, phenothiazines)
- Patients should be warned against overtiredness and excessive daily activities.

Treatment

Treatment approaches to acute lupus flares is different in chronic cutaneous LE and SLE. Referral to appropriate specialists (i.e. nephrologist) must be made. The mode of administration must be appropriate for dosage and until remission is obtained. Once the patient's condition has completely stabilized, which may require a period of several weeks, medications should be tapered gradually over weeks or months. In some patients, even in SLE, complete termination is possible.

Regular follow-up is necessary to ensure the correct treatment is being given, to assess whether repeat non-medical therapy and/or preventive treatment for lupus flares are needed and to identify any side-effects resulting from the prescribed treatment.

Recommended therapies

Topical therapy

These form the basis of therapy for cutaneous LE, and are particularly beneficial for early lesions and erythematous plaques. Medium- or high-potency (class II or I) topical corticosteroids are usual but should be used with caution if needed for long periods on the lips and face (risk of telangiectasia or atrophy). Intralesional corticosteroids are less useful since the availability of class I topical corticosteroid (clobetasol cream).

Systemic therapy

Antimalarials

Efficacy and usage

Best responses are achieved in patients with mild systemic disease and those with prominent skin involvement (excellent or good response in 70–80%). A Canadian study concluded that antimalarials have a preventive effect on lupus flares and improve constitutional symptoms and arthritis/arthralgias. Improvement is first evident after 1–6 weeks of treatment. If the efficacy is incomplete, combination antimalarial therapy (i.e. quinacrine + hydroxychloroquine or chloroquine), or the substitution of one antimalarial for another, is often effective. Once complete healing of skin lesions has occurred, the dose should be slowly decreased to the lowest effective maintenance dose (Table 1).

Side-effects include mild gastrointestinal disturbance or cutaneous eruptions.

Haematological side-effects (leukopenia, anaemia, thrombocytopenia) can be seen as myopathy or neurological signs. But the main side-effect is retinal toxicity which occurs when a dose higher than the safe daily dose is used. Ophthalmological examinations should be performed before and during therapy. The frequency is determined by a specialist. A simple clinical examination is sufficient in most cases but controversy still exists over the use of complex and costly electrophysiological instrumentation. Pregnancy is not an absolute contraindication.

Table 1 Antimalarials dosage guidelines

Drug	Usual daily dose (mg)	Safe daily dose (mg/kg per day)
Hydroxychloroquine	400	6.0–6.5
Chloroquine	200–250	3.5–4.0
Quinacrine	100	2.0

Systemic corticosteroids and non-steroidal anti-inflammatory drugs (NSAIDs)

In SLE disease, manifestations can be grouped into three broad categories: (a) those treated primarily with NSAIDs; (b) those treated primarily with corticosteroids; and (c) those treated with symptomatic agents (tranquillizers, antihypertensive drugs) (see Table 2).

NSAIDs

Many different NSAIDs are available. Selection of the most effective agent for any given patient remains an empirical clinical exercise. In general, and in the absence of adverse reactions, an NSAID should be continued for at least 2 weeks at maximum dose before switching to a second agent due to lack of efficacy. Lupus nephritis is a risk factor for NSAID-induced acute renal failure, but not for rare idiosyncratic toxic renal reactions to NSAIDs. In refractory nephrotic syndrome, NSAIDs have been used successfully. Cutaneous and allergic reactions to NSAIDs are increased in SLE patients as well as hepatotoxic effects, particularly with high-dose aspirin. Whereas a variety of central nervous system side-effects of NSAIDs are probably no more common in SLE patients than others, aseptic meningitis has been reported more frequently.

In summary, treatment of SLE with NSAIDs requires awareness for the increased frequency of some side-effects and close monitoring of toxicity.

Systemic corticosteroids

If NSAIDs do not control the disease or some disease manifestations require their use, high-dose corticosteroids are used approximately equivalent to 1 mg/kg per day in two divided doses. As disease activity is controlled (6–8 weeks) tapering of the daily dosage proceeds, usually with a single daily dosage. The clinician must rely on experience and judgement over stopping corticosteroids or keeping them to a minimal dosage (5–15 mg/kg per day). Side-effects of corticosteroids are proportional to the dosage given: follow-up requires determination of blood pressure, weight, blood cell count and chemical profile. Intravenous methyl prednisolone pulse therapy had been used for severe SLE but a higher responsiveness than oral corticosteroids cannot always be predicted and side-effects are not less with this therapy as compared with oral corticosteroids.

Alternative and experimental treatments

Cutaneous lupus erythematosus

Thalidomide

Thalidomide gives 70–90% of complete remission for cutaneous LE, refractory to conventional therapy.

Table 2 Treatment of SLE: corticosteroids and anti-inflammatory drugs

Disease manifestation	Therapeutic approach
Fever Arthralgia/arthritis Serositis	Aspirin → other NSAIDs → antimalarials or steroids (low dose)
Pulmonary Haematological signs Nephritis CNS	Steroids → immunosuppressives
Hypertension Raynaud's Rash	Antihypertensives Ca^{++} channel blockers Topical steroids/antimalarials

Initial treatment is started at 100 mg daily. If the cutaneous lesions vanished, the dose is lowered to 50–25 mg daily as a maintenance therapy for at least 6 months. Despite thalidomide's potential for producing clinical improvement, serious side-effects, e.g. teratogenicity and permanent sensory neuropathy (15–25% of patients), preclude its use routinely. Nevertheless, in a recent American study with low-dose thalidomide therapy for severe cutaneous LE, peripheral neuropathy is not as common as suggested by other studies.

Retinoids

Isotretinoin (80 mg/day) or acitretin (50 mg/day) have been used for hyperkeratotic discoid lupus. However, a multicentre double-blind trial comparing the efficacy of acitretin with hydroxychloroquine showed better tolerance with antimalarials.

Dapsone

This drug is useful at 25–100 mg/day in vasculitis lesions of LE and especially in bullous clinical forms.

Cefuroxime axetil

This oral cephalosporin was used with success, without side-effects, in three patients with subacute cutaneous LE lesions.

Laser therapy

Argon laser or pulsed dye laser may be powerful alternative approaches in the treatment of vascular lesions of cutaneous LE.

Systemic lupus erythematosus

Immunosuppressives

Where there is an inability to control severe disease or side-effects, immunosuppressives are a good alternative.

Methotrexate (7.5–15 mg/week), especially in patients with active arthritis and skin lesions are frequently used.

Azathioprine (2–4 mg/kg per day) or oral cyclophosphamide (2–3 mg/kg per day) are other possible therapies.

Intermittent intravenous pulse cyclophosphamide is the standard of treatment for diffuse proliferative lupus nephritis and also an indication in most other forms of serious lupus affecting major organ systems, in particular lupus vasculitis and acute central nervous system manifestations.

Cyclosporin A (CSA) can be of use in proteinuric nephritis although the incidence of hypertension with this drug is high. CSA could be used as a steroid sparer in the earliest stages of active disease.

Mycophenolate mofetil (1500–2000 mg/day) during 8–16 months seems a promising option in immunosuppressive treatment of patients with moderate and severe SLE who did not show a satisfactory response to other immunosuppressives.

Plasmapheresis

Results of plasmapheresis have not been convincing in the literature. Nevertheless, plasmapheresis in association with CSA gave a good improvement in a prospective trial of about 28 patients with SLE.

Intravenous immunoglobulins (IVIg)

This therapy has a high response rate among SLE patients. A combination of clinical manifestations, autoantibodies and complement levels may aid in the future in predicting who among SLE patients will benefit most from IVIg treatment.

Stem cell transplantation

Stem cell transplantation, in association with high-dose chemotherapy has been used in highly resistant cases or those with a poor prognosis.

Others

Other recently developed molecules including anti-CD40L monoclonal antibodies are still under investigation.

Further reading

Bambauer R, Schware U, Schiel R. Cyclosporin A and therapeutic plasma exchange in the treatment of severe systemic lupus erythematosus. *Artif Organs* 2000; 24: 852–6.

Dammacco F, Della Casa Alberighi O, Ferraccioli G, Racanelli V, Casatta L, Bartoli E. Cyclosporine-A plus steroids versus steroids alone in the 12-month treatment of systemic lupus erythematosus. *Int J Clin Lab Res* 2000; 30: 67–73.

Duong DJ, Spigel GT, Moxley RT III, Gaspari AA. American experience with low-dose thalidomide therapy for severe cutaneous lupus erythematosus. *Arch Dermatol* 1999; 135: 1079–87.

Gaubitz M, Schorat A, Schotte H, Kern P, Domschke W. Mycophenolate mofetil for the treatment of systemic lupus erythematosus: an open pilot trial. *Lupus* 1999; 8: 731–6.

Kimberly RP. Systemic lupus erythematosus. Treatment, corticosteroids and anti inflammatory drugs. *Rheum Dis Clin North Am* 1988; 14: 203–21.

Kuhn A, Becker-Wegerich PM, Ruzicka T, Lehmann P. Successful treatment of discoïd lupus erythematosus with argon laser. *Dermatology* 2000; 201: 175–7.

Levy Y, Sherer Y, Ahmed A *et al.* A study of 20 SLE patients with intravenous immunoglobulin—clinical and serologic response. *Lupus* 1999; 8: 705–12.

Ortmann RA, Klippel JH. Update on cyclophosphamide for systemic lupus erythematosus. *Rheum Dis Clin North Am* 2000; 26: 363–75.

Ostensen M, Villiger PM. Nonsteroidal anti-inflammatory drugs in systemic lupus erythematosus. *Lupus* 2000; 9: 566–72.

Raulin C, Schmidt C, Hellwig S. Cutaneous lupus erythematosus—treatment with pulsed dye laser. *Br J Dermatol* 1999; 141: 1046–50.

Rudnicka L, Szymanska E, Walecka I, Slowinska M. Long-term cefuroxime axetil in subacute cutaneous lupus erythematosus. A report of three cases. *Dermatology* 2000; 200: 129–31.

Ruzicka T, Sommer GC, Goerz G, Kind P, Mensing H. Treatment of cutaneous lupus erythematosus with acitretin and hydroxychloroquine. *Br J Dermatol* 1992; 127: 513–18.

Samsoen M, Grosshans E, Basset A. La thalidomide dans le traitement du lupus érythémateux chronique. *Ann Dermatol Venereol* 1980; 107: 505–23.

Toubi E, Rosner I, Rozenbaum M, Kessel A, Golan TD. The benefit of combining hydroxychloroquine with quinacrine in the treatment of SLE patients. *Lupus* 2000: 9–92–5.

Traynor AE, Schroeder J, Rosa RM *et al.* Treatment of severe systemic lupus erythematosus with high-dose chemotherapy and haemopoietic stem-cell transplantation: a phase I study. *Lancet* 2000; 356: 701–7.

Lyme borreliosis

J. Hercogova

Synonyms

Lyme disease, cutaneous borreliosis, borreliosis. Cutaneous manifestations of Lyme borreliosis had different names—erythema migrans was called erythema chronicum migrans and borrelial lymphocytoma was named lymphadenosis cutis benigna.

Definition and epidemiology

Lyme borreliosis is an inflammatory disease caused by the spirochaete *Borrelia burgdorferi* which is transmitted by ticks (mainly of the genus *Ixodes*). It is anthropozoonosis which manifests itself as a multisystem disorder in the skin and in other organs (joints, nerves, heart, eye, etc.).

Lyme borreliosis is the most common vector-borne disease in Europe and the USA. Ticks of the genus *Ixodes* are the vectors that transmit the infection to mammals in endemic areas—in the North American and Eurasian continents. In Europe Austria, Slovenia, Sweden and the Czech Republic belong to the most endemic areas (incidence could raise to 100 cases per 100 000 inhabitants). *B. burgdorferi* has not been isolated yet from patients suffering from symptoms similar to those of Lyme borreliosis in Australia, Africa and South America. Cutaneous involvement is the most frequent manifestation of the disease: it represents 60–80% of all reported cases. Concerning cutaneous symptoms, erythema migrans is the most prevalent (approximately 85%), followed by acrodermatitis chronica atrophicans (10%) and borrelial lymphocytoma (5%). Concrete cutaneous manifestations affect different age groups—erythema migrans is mainly present in middle-aged adults (30–50 years), borrelial lymphocytoma is typical for children, and acrodermatitis is a disease of the elderly.

Aetiology and pathophysiology

The aetiological agent, *B. burgdorferi sensu lato*, has been subdivided into three genospecies causing the human disease: *B. burgdorferi sensu stricto*, *B. afzelii* and *B. garinii*. Strains of all three species have been isolated from patients in Europe, whereas only the first species is involved in the USA. Some studies show that *B. afzelii* represents a dominant human skin isolate in Europe. Antigenic differences of three genospecies may explain the variability of clinical manifestations in patients with Lyme borreliosis. Genetic analysis of *B. garinii* OspA serotype 4 strains are correlated with the development of neuroborreliosis. *B. afzelii* OspA serotype 2 closely correlates with the development of acrodermatitis chronica atrophicans.

After the tick-bite, borreliae spread in the dermis causing cutaneous symptoms of the early localized stage (erythema migrans and borrelial lymphocytoma). Antibody immune response could be demonstrated in 3–4 weeks (IgM class), resp. in 4–6 weeks (IgG class). Haematogenic spread of borreliae follows weeks to months after the tick-bite and can manifest itself as the early disseminated stage of the disease. The development of the chronic stage is a subject of ongoing studies. The question is whether borreliae are still present or whether the symptoms are a result of the host immune response against organism or even against tissue autoantigens. T-cell mediated immunity might be responsible for inducing and exacerbating cardiac and joint symptoms. T-cell mediated immunopathology may result from the antigenic specificity of T cells, the activation of a specific T-cell subset, or ability of persisting antibodies to induce hypersensitive autoreactive T cells in the joint and heart. Autoreactive B lymphocytes as well as significantly raised concentrations of IgA rheumatoid factor were proven in the serum of patients with the chronic stage of Lyme borreliosis; production of these antibodies may be a result of B-cell autoreactivity.

Clinical characteristics and course

Cutaneous manifestations of Lyme borreliosis include erythema migrans, borrelial lymphocytoma, and acrodermatitis chronica atrophicans; morphoea and its initial stage, lichen sclerosus et atrophicus, are considered to be polyaetiological entities in which borreliae (*B. afzelii* and *B. garinii*) were isolated from morphoea lesions. Extracutaneous manifestations are variable (Table 1).

Erythema migrans is defined as a red patch, bigger than 4 cm in diameter at the site of the tick-bite which spreads centrifugally and can reach several decimeters in diameter. Three main clinical types are known: (a) homogenous (a red, sharply demarcated patch without a central clearing); (b) annular (a red, sharply demarcated patch with a central clearing); and (c) iris-like (concentric annular patches). A central reddish macule, representing the site of the tick-bite, may be apparent in any of these three clinical types. Erythema migrans can be present anywhere on the body surface, but lower extremities are the most frequent sites. In children, head and neck are also usually affected.

Table 1 Clinical manifestations of Lyme borreliosis

Early stage
Localized infection
Erythema migrans
Borrelial lymphocytoma
Disseminated infection
Multiple erythemata migrantia
'Flu-like' symptoms
Meningitis, meningoradiculoneuritis
Endocarditis, myocarditis, pericarditis
Arthritis, tendosynovitis
Hepatitis, keratitis, conjunctivitis
Chronic stage
Acrodermatitis chronica atrophicans
Morphoea, lichen sclerosus et atrophicus
Chronic encephalitis, encephalomyelitis, polyneuritis
Chronic arthritis

Borrelial lymphocytoma is a bluish-red papule, nodule or plaque, 1–3 cm in diameter, localized on the ear lobe. The areola mammae, scrotum and nose are other typical sites.

Acrodermatitis chronica atrophicans starts as an inflammatory stage which evolves into an atrophic stage. Firstly, bluish-red, not sharply demarcated patch(es) or plaque(s) appear on the dorsal aspect of the foot or hand. Predilection sites include above the bony prominences (on the lower extremities, the ankle, lateral aspects of the foot, fingers and knee, and on the upper extremities, fingers and elbow). Lesions usually spread from distal to proximal sites, including the trunk and face. Four clinical types of lesions can be differentiated: (a) erythematous lesions (bluish-red patches, plaques in cases of swelling); (b) teleangiectatic lesions (teleangiectasias predominately red patches); (c) fibrous lesions (firm, bluish-red or skin-coloured nodules or funiculus, mainly above the elbow, ulna or small joints of the hand); and (d) atrophic lesions (thin skin with wrinkles, prominent vessels).

Diagnosis

The diagnosis of Lyme borreliosis is based on the history of tick exposure, the characteristic clinical picture and confirmation of *B. burgdorferi* infection (with the exception of early typical cutaneous manifestations of the disease, e.g. annular erythema migrans or borrelial lymphocytoma which is localized on the ear lobe and is present in children). Histopathological examination should be performed in acrodermatitis chronica atrophicans patients and in those where the diagnosis is not clear from a clinical point of view.

Direct proof of borrelial infection includes isolation (allowing the demonstration of live *B. burgdorferi*, e.g. in the skin, synovial fluid, myocardium), histopathological detection of the microorganisms in the tissue by a modified Dieterle's stain or a modified Steiner method, electron microscopy, DNA hybridization and polymerase chain reaction (PCR).

Indirect methods include indirect immunofluorescence and enzyme-linked immunosorbent assay. Two-step serological testing is recommended in which a serum specimen with a positive test result is further tested with immunoblotting. In Europe immunoblotting is regarded as an additional test with an increased emphasis on specificity which supports the clinical diagnosis rather than confirms it. True standardization of an immunoblotting method for the diagnosis of Lyme borreliosis would require agreement on the strains used for antigen preparation. This approach would not be possible in Europe due to different local prevalences of genospecies of *B. burgdorferi sensu lato* and also to heterogenity within those strains. To date, none of the serological tests should be termed as a 'screening' test.

Histopathological examination of the erythema migrans lesion shows superficial perivascular dermatitis, composed of lymphocytic infiltrate with plasma cells and eosinophils. Borrelial lymphocytoma is a pseudolymphoma, lymphocytes are top-heavy, without nuclear atypia, and plasma cells can be present. Acrodermatitis chronica atrophicans shows superficial perivascular or lichenoid dermatitis, lymphocytic infiltrate with plasma cells, epidermal atrophy, dilated vessels in the upper part of the dermis and orthohyperkeratosis. Later on, degeneration of elastic and collagen fibres, as well as gland adnexae, could follow.

Differential diagnosis

Erythema migrans should be differentiated from erysipelas, superficial tinea, fixed drug eruption, lupus erythematoses, granuloma anulare, morphoea and contact dermatitis.

Borrelial lymphocytoma could be similar to histiocytoma, keloid, angioma, Kaposi's sarcoma, granuloma faciale, granuloma annulare, sarcoidosis and lupus erythematoses. In all cases, histopathological examination is helpful. Malignant lymphoma can be distinguished by immunohistochemical examination.

Acrodermatitis chronica atrophicans can mimic circulatory insufficiency, perniones, morphoea and dermatomyositis; fibrotic papules and nodules are considered to be rheumatic nodules or gouty tophi.

Treatment

General therapeutic guidelines

Antibiotic therapy should be started as soon as possible after the diagnosis has been made. Some studies demonstrate that even an appropriate antibiotic regimen may not always eradicate the spirochaete. On the one hand, the treatment of disseminated Lyme borreliosis for 3 months may not be sufficient: the spirochaetes can remain in serum, skin and other tissues, and clinical relapses can occur. However, it remains unresolved whether the prognosis of patients with disseminated Lyme borreliosis could be improved by longer initial treatment. On the other hand, the outcomes of most persons diagnosed as having Lyme borreliosis who are treated with antimicrobial agents are excellent. Extracutaneous manifestations of Lyme borreliosis are described after any antibiotic regimen in up to 10% patients. No significant differences were found in the outcome of erythema migrans after 1 year in patients whose immune system was impaired compared to previously healthy individuals.

The immunological response after antibiotic therapy appears to be abrogated, so levels of antiborrelial antibodies cannot be used as proof of successful therapy. Cutaneous manifestations disappear after the therapy, but immediate disappearance of borrelial lymphocytoma and acrodermatitis chronica atrophicans during antibiotic therapy is exceptional. These lesions begin to fade and loose the swelling, but resolution can take up to 6 months. The degenerative changes in acrodermatitis are not reversible.

Recommended therapies

Borreliae are sensitive to four groups of antibiotics—penicillins, cephalosporins (third generation and cefuroxim axetil), tetracyclines and macrolides. The drugs of choice for oral treatment of Lyme borreliosis are doxycycline and amoxicillin, for parenteral treatment ceftriaxone, cefotaxime and penicillin G. Ceftriaxone is primarily used as a treatment for patients with extracutaneous (joint, neurological, cardiac), and multiple cutaneous manifestations. If the coinfection with ehrlichiosis is suspected, doxycycline is the drug of choice. Doxycycline is also preferred in cases of penicillin–cephalosporin allergy since erythromycin has inferior efficacy. Children with solitary erythema migrans could be treated with phenoxymethyl penicillin and cefuroxime axetil, however, drug-related side-effects were more frequently observed with cefuroxim axetil. Minocycline causes teeth discoloration even in young adults, discoloration of the skin, nails, sclerae and conjunctivae. Vertigo, ataxia and dizziness have been described during minocycline therapy. These symptoms are a major disadvantage, in particular for patients with neurological symptoms, as in Lyme disease.

Recommended therapies for uncomplicated erythema migrans include oral doxycycline 200 mg daily (divided into two doses every 12 h) or amoxycillin 3 g daily (divided into three doses every 8 h) for 15 days. If any general signs or symptoms (subfebrilia, malaise, fatigue, arthralgias, myalgias, meningism, conjunctivitis, etc.) are present even if for 1 day, the duration of antibiotic therapy is 20 days. In case of penicillin or tetracycline allergy, azithromycin is prescribed (500 mg daily p.o. for 10 days, resp. for 15 days in the presence of general signs or symptoms).

Borrelial lymphocytoma is treated with the same antibiotic regimen, only the duration of therapy is at minimum 20 days, resp. 25 days. Acrodermatitis chronica atrophicans patients are given the same oral antibiotics for 25–30 days, but in the presence of any extracutaneous manifestations, parenteral therapy is needed—ceftriaxone 2 g i.v. daily in one dose or penicillin G i.v. 20 million units daily (divided into four doses of 5 million units every 6 h) for 15 days followed by oral antibiotic (as in the early stage) for the next 15 days.

Special attention should be given to pregnant women with Lyme borreliosis. Penicillins, macrolides and/or ceftriaxone are used, but antibiotic administration depends on the time of tick-bite; if the tick-bite is suspected during the first trimester, parenteral antibiotics are used. On the other hand, if the tick-bite occurs later in pregnancy, and the patient has no extracutaneous symptoms or signs, oral antibiotics are sufficient for therapy.

Prevention

Prevention of Lyme borreliosis include avoiding exposure to tick-bites by limiting outdoor activities in endemic areas, using tick repellents, tucking in clothing and frequent skin inspection for early detection and correct removal of ticks. Antibiotic prophylaxis has not been shown to be effective in reducing the risk of acquiring Lyme borreliosis. Some authors recommend local antibiotics after the tick-bite.

Vaccination trials showed that a single recombinant outer surface protein A (OspA) appears to be safe and immunogenic in man. A single antigen OspA vaccine is not effective in Eurasia, where more heterogenous species of *Borrelia* and more variable OspA are present. In Eurasia, compared to the USA, a vaccine must be effective against all subgroups of the *Borrelia* spirochaete. Some protective immunity against *Borrelia* infection in laboratory animals were demonstrated by some other *B. burgdorferi* proteins, e.g. OspB and OspC.

Further reading

Aberer E, Kehldorfer M, Binder B, Schauperl H. The outcome of Lyme borreliosis in children. *Wien Klin Wochenschr* 1999; 111 (22–23): 941–4.

Arnez M, Radsel-Medvescek A, Pleterski-Rigler D *et al.* Comparison of cefuroxime axetil and phenoxymethyl penicillin for the treatment of children with solitary erythema migrans. *Wien Klin Wochenschr* 1999; 111 (22–23): 916–22.

Cunha BA. Minocycline versus doxycycline in the treatment of Lyme neuroborreliosis. *Clin Infect Dis* 2000; 30 (1): 237–8.

Dotevall L, Hagberg L. Adverse effects of minocycline versus doxycycline in the treatment of Lyme neuroborreliosis. *Clin Infect Dis* 2000; 30 (2): 410–11.

Gilmore RD Jr, Mbow ML. Conformational nature of the *Borrelia burgdorferi* B31 outer surface protein C protective epitope. *Infect Immun* 1999; 67 (10): 5463–9.

Hayney MS, Grunske MM, Boh LE. Lyme disease prevention and vaccine prophylaxis. *Ann Pharmacother* 1999; 33: 723–9.

Hercogova J, Brzonova I. Lyme disease in central Europe. *Curr Opin Infect Dis* 2001; 14: 133–7.

Maraspin V, Lotric-Furlan S, Cimperman J *et al.* Erythema migrans in the immunocompromised host. *Wien Klin Wochenschr* 1999; 111 (22–23): 923–32.

Oksi J, Marjamaki M, Nikoskelainen J, Viljanen MK. *Borrelia burgdorferi* detected by culture and PCR in clinical relapse of disseminated Lyme borreliosis. *Ann Med* 1999; 31 (3): 225–32.

Seltzer EG, Gerber MA, Cartter ML *et al.* Long-term outcomes of persons with Lyme disease. *JAMA*, 2000; 283 (5): 609–16.

Shadick NA, Phillips CB, Sangha O *et al.* Musculoskeletal and neurologic outcomes in patients with previously treated Lyme disease. *Ann Intern Med* 1999; 131 (12): 919–26.

Stanek G, Breier F, Menzinger G *et al.* Erythema migrans and serodiagnosis by enzyme immunoassay and immunoblot with three *Borrelia* species. *Wien Klin Wochenschr* 1999; 111 (22–23): 951–6.

Wahlberg P. Vaccination against Lyme borreliosis. *Ann Med* 1999; 31: 233–5.

Warshafsky S, Nowakowski J, Nadelman RB *et al.* Efficacy of antibiotic prophylaxis for prevention of Lyme disease. *J Gen Intern Med* 1996; 11: 329–33.

Lymphomas (primary cutaneous)

W.A. van Vloten

Definition and classification

Primary cutaneous T- and B-cell lymphomas (CTCL and CBCL) are a heterogeneous group of lymphomas with a wide range of clinical manifestations, histology and prognosis. They belong to the group of non-Hodgkin's lymphomas. The non-Hodgkin's lymphomas are clonal proliferations of lymphoid cells with morphological and membrane properties of different maturation stages of T and B lymphocytes. They were classified according to histological classification schemes such as the classification of Rappaport in 1966, Lukes and Collins in 1970, the (updated) Kiel classification in 1988 and the working Formulation of the World Health Organization (WHO) in 1982, and recently in 1994 the Revised European–American Lymphoma (REAL) classification.

Primary cutaneous lymphomas are defined as lymphomas of the skin without concurrent extracutaneous disease at the time of diagnosis. Recent studies demonstrated that primary cutaneous lymphomas have highly characteristic clinical and histological features and a clinical course and prognosis different from primary nodal lymphomas. Moreover molecular biological differences such as expression of oncogenes, specific translocations and adhesion receptors suggest that primary cutaneous lymphomas should be considered as a distinctive group. The well-defined entities of primary cutaneous lymphomas cannot be categorized adequately in the above-mentioned classification schemes of nodal lymphomas. These findings resulted in a proposal from the Cutaneous Lymphoma Study Group of the European Organization for Research and Treatment of Cancer (EORTC) for a classification of primary cutaneous lymphomas.

This classification should give the clinician all the necessary information for management and treatment (Table 1). It is based on a combination of clinical, histological, immunohistochemical and genetic criteria. It includes distinct disease entities with well-defined clinical and histological features, including a predictable course, response to treatment and prognosis.

When discussing the treatment of cutaneous lymphoma in this chapter, all the different entities will be dealt with separately.

Diagnosis and staging of cutaneous lymphomas

A careful history should be taken from the patient and the skin lesions photographed. Skin biopsies should be taken from representative skin lesions for routine haematoxylin and eosin histopathology (H & E) and frozen skin specimens for immunophenotyping. In selected cases electron microscopy may be helpful in the diagnosis.

Complete blood cell count with cytomorphology should be performed in addition to routine blood biochemistry. In patients with erythroderma, immunophenotyping of peripheral leucocytes should be carried out. Studies for T-cell rearrangement has to be performed in selected cases.

Bone marrow examination is necessary in B-cell lymphomas and in patients with cutaneous T-cell lymphomas with abnormal blood smears.

Histopathological examination of lymph nodes is mandatory in cases with palpable enlarged lymph nodes. Histology is superior to lymph node needle cytology.

Table 1 EORTC classification for primary cutaneous lymphomas

Primary CTCL	
Indolent	
Mycosis fungoides	
Mycosis fungoides and follicular mucinosis	
Pagetoid reticulosis	
Large cell CTCL, CD30+	
anaplastic	
immunoblastic	
pleomorphic	
Lymphomatoid papulosis	
Aggressive	
Sézary syndrome	
Large cell CTCL, CD30–	
immunoblastic	
pleomorphic	
Provisional	
Granulomatous slack skin	
CTCL, pleomorphic small/medium sized	
Subcutaneous panniculitis-like T-cell lymphoma	
Primary CBCL	
Indolent	
Follicle centre cell lymphoma	
Immunocytoma (marginal zone B-cell lymphoma)	
Intermediate	
Large B-cell lymphoma of the leg	
Provisional	
Intravascular large B-cell lymphoma	
Plasmacytoma	

From Willemze *et al.* (1997) *Blood* 90, 354–71.

Chest radiography and computed tomography of the chest and/or abdomen and pelvis should be carried out to evaluate mediastinal, retroperitoneal and pelvic nodes especially in T3 and T4 disease.

The TNM staging classification, as also recommended for other tumours, enables us to make a detailed recording of characteristics that describe each patient (Table 2).

Clinical end-points in evaluating response to treatment

The most important indicator of the effect of any treatment is the complete response rate.

No patient with cancer has ever been cured without first attaining a complete remission (CR). For every study, definition of remission has to be made.

CR is complete resolution of all measurable disease. The quality of a complete response is the relapse-free survival from the time all treatment is discontinued.

Partial remission (PR) is at least 50% reduction of measurable disease and absence of new lesions.

Stable disease (SD) is less than 50% reduction of measurable disease.

Progressive disease (PD) is increase of disease or development of new lesions.

Table 2 TNM classification of cutaneous lymphomas

Skin	
T0	Clinically or histopathologically suspicious lesions
T1	Patch or plaque/lesions <10% of skin surface
T2	Patch and/or plaque/lesions >10% of skin surface
T3	Tumours
T4	Generalized erythroderma
Lymph nodes	
N0	No clinical abnormal lymph nodes
N1	Clinical enlarged nodes, histology negative
N2	Clinical no enlarged nodes, histology positive
N3	Clinical enlarged nodes, histology positive
Visceral organs	
M0	No visceral involvement
M1	Visceral involvement confirmed

Treatment

General therapeutic guidelines

The treatment of primary cutaneous lymphomas is quite different from nodal lymphomas. The disease presents first in the skin and subsequently involves the lymph nodes and visceral organs. Hence early stage disease localized only in the skin has a great chance of cure with therapy directed to the skin. When involvement of other systems occurs one of the systemic treatment modalities should be chosen.

All skin-directed therapies are capable of destroying malignant lymphocytes directly, probably by triggering lymphocyte apoptosis and interference with the local production of cytokines.

In the approach of cutaneous lymphomas different combination therapies are often used.

Combination chemotherapy provides maximal cell kill within the range of toxicity tolerated by the patient for each drug. It covers a broader range of resistant cell lines in the heterogeneous tumour population. It prevents the development of new resistant lines.

Treatment of CTCL

Mycosis fungoides (MF)

MF is the most well-known type of CTCL. Described in 1806 for the first time by Alibert, three stages can be recognized, the eczematous, plaque and tumour stage. The disease starts mostly in the fourth decade of life with eczematous lesions. In the course of several years, plaques and tumours may develop. In the last stage, lymph nodes and other internal organs may become involved in the disease process. There is still a debate over whether MF is a lymphoproliferative disorder from the outset or a reactive process initially evolving into true malignancy.

The diagnosis may be very difficult especially in the eczematous stage. Histopathologically MF is characterized by an epidermotropic band-like infiltrate in the upper dermis. The infiltrate is composed out of small, medium and occasionally large mononuclear cells with hyperchromatic, indented (cerebriform) nuclei and a variable number of inflammatory cells. The infiltrate can invade the epidermis forming the highly characteristic Pautrier's microabscesses.

In the tumour stage of MF, these cerebriform mononuclear cells transform into blast cells of T-cell origin, losing several of their membrane markers and is often associated with an aggressive clinical course.

Treatment of MF depends on the stage of the disease, i.e. whether there is lymph node or visceral involvement (Table 3).

MF stage I and II

Topical corticosteroids class III or IV

These can induce clinical remission in the very early limited patch stage. It can be given also as additional therapy in one of the other topical modalities.

Ultraviolet B (UVB) phototherapy

This is reported to give CR in 25/35 (71%) of patients with early patch MF with a median duration of remission of 22 months. Using a two to three times weekly regime of irradiation the median time to remission was 6 months. UVB should start with 50% of the minimal erythema dose, with subsequent increase of the dose determined by the individual skin reaction.

Table 3 Treatment by stage in mycosis fungoides (MF)

Stage Ia: MF confined to the skin (T1, N0) (< 10% surface area involved)
- Topical corticosteroids
- Phototherapy with UVB

Stage Ib: MF confined to the skin (T2, N0) (> 10% surface area involved)
- Phototherapy with UVB
- Photochemotherapy (PUVA)
- Photochemotherapy with retinoids (RePUVA)
- Photochemotherapy with IFN-α
- Topical mechlorethamine (nitrogen mustard)
- Topical carmustine (BCNU)
- Total skin electron beam irradiation
- Local radiotherapy of solitary tumours

Stage II: MF with dermatopathic lymphadenopathy (T1–3, N0–1)
- As in stage Ib

Stage III: MF with lymph node involvement (T1–4, N2)
- Systemic (poly) chemotherapy
- Local radiotherapy of tumours

Stage IV: MF with visceral involvement (T1–4, N2, M1)
- As in stage III

Ultraviolet A (UVA) phototherapy

Psoralen in combination with UVA (PUVA) was reported for the first time in 1976 for the treatment of MF and in many other studies subsequently. It is an effective and relatively safe treatment modality in early patch/plaque stage MF. Psoralen (8-methoxypsoralen) is activated by UVA. The activated psoralen binds to DNA forming mono- and bifunctional adducts to pyrimidine bases. The overall effect may be caused by preferential mitotic inhibition or killing of the neoplastic T-lymphoid cells in the skin or in the cutaneous capillaries. Moreover PUVA interferes with antigen presentation and cytokine production in the skin.

PUVA therapy requires the ingestion of 0.6 mg/kg of 8-methoxypsoralen 2 h prior to the irradiation of the whole skin with UVA. Treatment should start with a regime of two to three times weekly with a 50% of the minimal phototoxic UVA dosage, increasing every time depending on the presence of erythema. This schedule should be maintained for 3–6 months, until CR is achieved. For maintenance therapy irradiation can be given once a week or once in 2 weeks for several months. However, not all investigators agree that maintenance treatment is necessary.

In most patients PUVA therapy is well tolerated. Side-effects such as erythema, nausea and pruritus may occur in 10–20% of patients. Long-term side-effects including the increased risk of squamous cell carcinoma, development of pigmented macules, nail pigmentation and cataract formation have been described. So all patients should be monitored accordingly.

PUVA therapy in MF will result in a 80–90% CR.

The combination of PUVA with retinoids (RePUVA) results in an equal complete response rate compared to PUVA alone. However the addition of retinoids reduces the number of PUVA treatments. Isotretinoin is given in a dosage of 0.5 mg/kg.

Combination of PUVA with interferon-α_{2a} (INF-α_{2a}) enhances the effect of PUVA. However in most of the patients side-effects include fever, chills, fatigue and muscular aches. IFN is given intermuscularly (3 million IU three times a week). In his study, Kuzel (1995) had the IFN dose escalated in increments of 3 million IU over a 6–8-week period to the final dose of 12 million IU. The dosage has to be reduced in many patients because of the side-effects.

UVA-1 (340–400 nm) is an effective and well-tolerated treatment for patients with MF in stage I and II. Eleven out of 13 patients showed CR.

Topical chemotherapy with mechlorethamine (nitrogen mustard, NH_2)

This may give CR up to 60% depending on the extent of the skin involvement. The technique is simple and can be carried out by the patient at home whether or not assisted by a helper.

Dissolve 10 mg HN_2 in 50 mL tap water and apply the fresh prepared solution to the whole skin surface daily (except eyelids and lips). Duration and frequency of the treatment may differ among institutions. In the Netherlands we start with daily application for 5 days a week for at least 3 months. If the lesions disappear we give a maintenance treatment once or twice a week for several months or even years. Delayed-type hypersensitivity or a toxic reaction may occur. In those cases, open patch tests with several concentrations are valuable, since this enables continuation with the concentration which gives the least erythema. For reasons of sensitization the helper is advised to use protective double plastic (PVC) gloves as well as a mouth and nose cap while applying the solution. Ointment based HN_2 is less likely to induce allergic reactions. The formulation is 10 mg mechlorethamine in 100 g eucerine anhydricum. Side-effects of topical HN_2 are erythema, itching, telangiectasia, hyperpigmentation and long-term effects such as secondary squamous cell carcinoma of the skin. No bone marrow or lung abnormalities have been observed. Topical HN_2 therapy seems to be a relatively safe therapy for patients with early MF.

Topical chemotherapy with carmustine (BCNU)
This is an alternative therapy for patients with MF. It is not immunologically cross-reactive with HN_2 and for that reason it is used in those patients who developed contact allergy to HN_2. BCNU is formulated as a 0.5% ointment and is stable at room temperature. With BCNU bone marrow suppression may occur if the total dose exceeds 600 mg, therefore haematological monitoring is necessary.

Total skin electron beam (TSEB) therapy
This is an excellent treatment for patients with widespread involvement of the skin with plaques and small tumours. The six-field technique gives the best homogeneity of the dose delivered to the total skin surface of the patient. Most of the dose (80%) is delivered within the first centimetre of skin thus sparing the deep dermis. In the Netherlands we use 4 MeV with a total dose of 30–35 Gy. The scalp, perineum and soles are treated supplementary. Side-effects are dry skin, pigmentation, telangiectasia and sometimes permanent loss of scalp hair. Secondary skin cancer especially in those patients receiving follow-up treatment with topical HN_2 or PUVA may occur. About 50% of patients will relapse in 1–2 years. They can then be treated with a booster dose of irradiation or topical HN_2 or PUVA.

Local radiotherapy
This should be considered for solitary tumours or recalcitrant plaques in patients with MF. MF lesions are extremely responsive to radiotherapy, so even low-dose radiotherapy will give a complete response rate of 90%.

MF stage III and IV

Systemic chemotherapy with the regimen CHOP
CHOP is the first treatment of choice for MF in stage III and IV. It is wise to obtain experience with one or two systemic therapy modalities instead of changing every time to a new treatment modality.

Combination with TSEB or total nodal irradiation is possible, but the efficacy is controversial and the cumulative side-effects have to be considered.

The CHOP regime can give a 45% response rate. In Utrecht we have obtained a 5-year survival in 35% of the patients treated with CHOP.

The CHOP regime consists of six to eight cycles every 4 weeks depending on blood monitoring. Each cycle consists of: cyclophosphamide 750 mg/m^2 i.v. on day 1; adriamycin 50 mg/m^2 i.v. on day 1; vincristine (Oncovin) 1.4 mg/m^2 i.v. on day 1; and prednisone 40 mg/m^2 orally on days 1–5. This regimen is well tolerated regarding all side-effects. Vincristine may give paraesthesia of the fingers in which case it should be withdrawn from the regimen.

The dosages may be adapted due to bone marrow reserve. In older patients this may be a problem. Additional drugs against nausea may be given. Patients should be warned that hair loss may occur.

More aggressive regimes and experimental regimes should be considered for second-line polychemotherapy and should be given in collaboration with a haematologist.

Variants of MF

Several variants of MF exist, however, most of them such as the hypo-, and hyperpigmented and bullous variants have the same clinical course as classical MF. In contrast to classical MF, there is an association with follicular mucinosis, pagetoid reticulosis and granulomatous slack skin which show a distinct clinical course.

MF associated with follicular mucinosis is difficult to treat since the malignant cells are located deeper in the dermis and therefore not suitable for PUVA or topical treatment. Radiotherapy is the treatment of choice.

Pagetoid reticulosis characterized by a solitary plaque is best treated by radiotherapy or even surgery.

Granulomatous slack skin can be treated by radiotherapy or strong topical corticosteroids.

Large cell CD30+ cutaneous lymphoma

Large cell CD30+ lymphoma presents in the skin with solitary nodules or tumours. This type of cutaneous lymphoma has been designated formerly as 'mycosis fungoides d'emblee'. Histologically they show a diffuse non-epidermotrophic infiltrate with sheets of CD30+ lymphoid tumour cells showing round, oval or irregularly shaped nuclei with prominant nucleoli. CD30 antigen must be expressed by >50% of malignant cells. Rearrangement of T-cell receptor (TCR) genes can be demonstrated in most cases. The prognosis is good with a 5-year survival of 90%.

Treatment

Radiotherapy is chosen in cases of a solitary or very localized lesion. In patients with widespread disease or extracutaneous involvement, polychemotherapy should be given. The first choice is the CHOP regime.

Lymphomatoid papulosis (LyP)

LyP is defined as a chronic recurrent self-healing eruption of papules and nodules with histological features of cutaneous lymphoma. In a small percentage of patients LyP is associated with MF, CD30+ lymphoma or Hodgkin's disease. Three different histological types can be recognized.

1 LyP type A with a wedge-shaped infiltrate with clusters of large atypical CD30+ Reed–Sternberg-like cells.
2 LyP type B shows a perivascular epidermotropic infiltrate with atypical cerebriform lymphoid cells similar to MF.
3 LyP type C has a monotonous infiltrate with large clusters of CD30+ cells.

The prognosis of LyP is very good with a 5-year survival of 100%.

Treatment

This consists of PUVA, topical chemotherapy or low-dose methotrexate. Patients should be kept under medical scrutiny in case of transformation into a more aggressive form.

Large cell CD30– cutaneous lymphoma

Large cell CD30– lymphoma presents with solitary or generalized plaques, nodules or tumours. Development of rapid-growing tumours is more common than in CD30+ lymphoma. Patients show an aggressive clinical course with a 5-year survival of 15%. The large malignant cells should represent > 30% of the tumour population. CD30 staining is negative.

Treatment

Treatment should consist of polychemotherapy as the CHOP regime.

Sézary syndrome

Sézary syndrome is characterized by generalized erythroderma, generalized lymphadenopathy, alopecia, onychodystrophy, palmoplantar hyperkeratosis and the presence of atypical lymphoid cells, the so-called 'Sézary cells', in the skin, lymph nodes and peripheral blood. The criterion of 1000 Sézary cells/mm^3 in peripheral blood for the diagnosis of Sézary syndrome is not generally agreed upon.

Additional criteria are the presence of an expanded CD4+ T-cell population

Table 4 Diagnosis in 102 patients with erythroderma

Origin of erythroderma	Incidence (%)
Pre-existing dermatosis such as eczema and psoriasis	53
Drug reactions	5
CTCL (MF and Sézary syndrome)	13
Paraneoplastic conditions	2
Miscellaneous	1
Idiopathic erythroderma	26

resulting in an increased CD4/CD8 ratio (> 10). Sézary syndrome has to be differentiated from other forms of erythroderma as shown in Table 4.

Treatment

Systemic chemotherapy

The combination of chlorambucil 4 mg/day and prednisone 15 mg/day is an established modality with a remission of 94% in 34 Sézary syndrome patients.

Low-dose methotrexate with 25 mg given as a single weekly oral dose or up to 125 mg s.c. resulted in 41% CR and 17% PR. The median survival time was 8.4 years.

Extracorporal photopheresis

This a successful treatment modality for erythrodermic patients with CTCL. A 73% response rate was obtained with 21% CR lasting 3–13 months in 33 patients. However other studies resulted in a 50% overall response rate and did not achieve this high remission rate. Side-efffects are nausea, erythema, transient fever, hypovolaemia and hypervolaemia.

Treatment of CBCL

Follicle centre cell lymphoma

Follicle centre cell lymphoma presents with non-scaling plaques and/or tumours, surrounded by erythema. The skin lesions are mostly confined to a regional area of the head and neck or trunk. The lesions show a slow progression. Dissemination to internal organs is rare.

Histopathologically, the lesions show a nodal pattern of a mixture of centrocytes and centroblasts depending on the stage of the disease. The B cells express B-cell associated antigens and show monotypic staining for surface immunoglobulin. The cells show a clonal immunoglobulin rearrangement.

The 5-year survival is 97%.

Treatment

Radiotherapy is the first choice of treatment if no visceral involvement has been detected. Chemotherapy should be considered when the skin lesions are widespread or extracutaneous localizations are present. In those cases, the polychemotherapy regimen CHOP is given.

Primary cutaneous immunocytoma

Mostly solitary tumours are present on the extremities and they have a good prognosis. Histopathologically they are characterized by a nodular or diffuse proliferation of small lymphocytes, lymphoplasmacytoid cells and plasma cells showing monotypic surface immunoglobulin.

The 5-year survival is 100%.

Treatment

Radiotherapy is the treatment of choice.

Large B-cell lymphoma of the leg

Large B-cell lymphoma of the leg is a specific entity in elderly persons. Red/purple nodules and tumours are present on the legs mostly the lower part. The prognosis is less favourable than with follicle centre cell lymphoma on the trunk. Histopathologically they are characterized by a diffuse infiltrate of centrocytes and centroblasts and immunoblasts. They express monotypic surface immunoglobulin.

Treatment

Radiotherapy is given only in patients with a solitary lesion. In all other cases polychemotherapy is given (CHOP regimen).

Intravascular large B-cell lymphoma

Intravascular large B-cell lymphoma is a rare disease presenting with purple indurated plaques on the legs or trunk. Histopathology shows dilated blood vessels extended by a proliferation of large atypical lymphoid cells. Clonal rearrangement of Ig genes can be demonstrated.

Treatment

This consists of polychemotherapy.

Alternative and experimental therapies in CTCL

Besides the above-mentioned treatment modalities several additional and/or more experimental therapies are available for CTCL. Some of these can be considered as alternative, second-or third-line treatment in cases of PD.

Etoposide (VP16-213)

This a derivative of epipodophyllotoxin and is used as single agent treatment in non-Hodgkin's lymphoma. Oral etoposide has been reported to induce CR in cutaneous large cell lymphoma. Etoposide can be given in a dosage of 50 mg/m^2 daily for 2–3 weeks. Further courses can be given. Even low doses with 50 mg daily for 2 weeks and 2 weeks of rest as maintenance treatment with oral etoposide may be considered.

2′-Deoxycoformycin (pentostatin, Nipent)

This is a purine analogue and potent inhibitor of adenosine deaminase which is a key enzyme in purine metabolism. Adenosine deaminase regulates intracellular adenosine levels through irreversible deamination of adenosine and deoxyadenosine. Pentostatin is a good drug for low-grade T-cell lymphomas. It is administered in patients with advanced stage CTCL. Pentostatin is given in a dose regime of 4–5 mg/m^2 intravenously every 2 weeks. Several studies showed good results in a total of 63 patients with CTCL with a response rate of 41%. However the response duration varied from 1 to 16 months. The drug is well tolerated with few side-effects. Side-effects observed were nausea, dizziness, cough, loss of weight, exanthema, thrombocytopenia and abnormal liver function tests. All side-effects were reversible.

The combination of deoxycoformycin and high doses of intermittently given IFN-α_{2a} can be an active regimen in patients with very advanced stage disease.

2-Chlorodeoxyadenosine (2-CdA, cladribine)

As a purine analogue this has been used in 27 patients with CTCL as second-line therapy. The overall response rate was 33–47% after 1–6 courses each of 0.1 mg/kg per day cladribine given for 7 days with monthly interval between courses. Five patients achieved CR and six patients a partial response. The median response duration was 5–6 months.

Methotrexate

This was given in a moderately high dose parenterally followed by leucovorin rescue in 11 patients with MF resulted in 80% clearance in nine patients with prolonged survival and minimal side-effects. Methotrexate in a dose of 60–240 mg/m^2 was infused over a 24-h period, followed by leucovorin 25 mg 8 h later. This procedure was repeated four times at intervals of 5 days.

A recent study showed even better results with methotrexate infusion followed by fluorouracil and leucovorin rescue. After hydration methotrexate 60 mg/m^2 is administered intravenously over 24 h. After completion of the methotrexate infusion, fluorouracil 20 mg/kg per 24 h is given over a 36–48-h period. Leucovorin 10 mg/m^2 is given intravenously 6 h after cessation of the methotrexate infusion and then orally every 6 h for five additional doses. Patients receive several courses at varying time intervals as required for control of their disease. Methotrexate and fluorouracil show a synergistic effect. Following methotrexate and fluorouracil therapy, leucovorin potentiated the effect of fluorouracil. Leucovorin prolonges the stability of the thymidylate synthetase-*N*-methylene tetrahydrofolate–fluorouridine monophosphate complex which prolonged the inhibition of DNA synthesis in the S phase of the cell cycle.

Leucopheresis

The application of leucopheresis in the treatment of Sézary syndrome was reported some time ago. A recent study in 22 patients with this syndrome showed CR in 10 (45.5%) patients, PR in four (18%) patients and failure in eight (36.5%) patients. Each patient was treated on average with 33 sessions of leucopheresis, 1–3 times a month. The mean survival was 90 months.

IFN-α

This acts upon the proliferation of keratinocytes and has an immunomodulatory effect. It is possible that INF-α restores the imbalance of the T-helper 1 and 2 cells in CTCL. A literature summary of 207 patients treated with IFN-α showed an overall response rate for INF-α of 52%, with 17% CRs. The median duration of response is 4–28 months. The response can be predicted by the stage of the disease, with lower response rates in advanced stages. The dose suggested by many investigators is 3 million units administered 3 times a week.

IFN-α in combination with retinoids

Treatment with this combination in 102 patients resulted in an overall response of 60%, with complete response of 11%.

IFN-α in combination with PUVA

In 26 patients this combination resulted in an overall response of 96%, with complete response of 65%. Combination therapy can enhance the therapeutic effect and diminish the side-effects of the single therapy modalities.

IFN-α in combination with extracorporeal photopheresis

This resulted in a total response rate of 56% in 14 male patients with MF stage II. The treatment was well tolerated.

Retinoids

As single agents these have been used in CTCL in a small number of patients. They inhibit proliferation and arrest dedifferentiation of the lymphoma. All retinoids together showed an overall response rate of 58%, with a complete response of 19%. The median duration of response ranged from 3 to 13 months. Etretinate alone showed an overall response of 67% with complete response of 21%, with a median duration of 3 months.

Ciclosporin A

This has been reported in several studies for patients with advanced stage disease. PR was achieved in only a few patients for some weeks. Some patients became worse after initial improvement and died. The natural course of the disease can be accelerated. Moreover it may cause serious side-effects. Ciclosporin A is not indicated in cutaneous lymphomas.

Interleukin-2 (IL-2)

This acts by stimulating the immune system with enhancement of both CD8+ cells and natural killer cytotoxic activities.

Recombinant IL-2 in high doses was given to seven patients with advanced stage CTCL. The dose given was 20 × 10 million IU/m^2 per day for 3–5 days administered by continuous infusion. Three initial cycles every 14 days were followed by 5 monthly cycles of 2 days. Three complete and two partial responses were obtained. The complete responses were ongoing at 6, 28 and 33 months after completion of the therapy. Side-effects were chills, nausea, hypotension, anaemia and elevated creatinine levels.

IL-2 fusion toxin

A new strategy for treatment is the use of recombinant cytokine molecules to direct toxins to tumour cells via specific receptors. A number of tumours including CTCLs express the high-affinity IL-2 receptor on the malignant cells. This receptor is not displayed on normal lymphocytes and only transiently expressed on activated T lymphocytes, B lymphocytes and macrophages. The IL-2 fusion toxin is a hybrid of IL-2 and diphtheria toxin. The first generation of this fusion toxin (DAB486IL-2) gave a favourable effect on IL-2R expressing tumours. The generation of DAB389IL-2 has a smaller molecular weight and better antitumour characteristics. In a recent study 35 patients with cutaneous lymphoma in whom prior therapy had failed and whose malignant cells were expressing IL-2 receptors, were treated with DAB389IL-2. Thirteen patients (37%) obtained an objective response, including five patients with complete response. The median duration of the CR was 15.3 months (range 10.1–22.7). The median duration for PR was 3.3 months. The side-effects such as chills, fever, hypotension, nausea and elevation of liver transaminases were reversible.

Autologous bone marrow transplantation

This is an experimental treatment for CTCL. When used in patients with advanced stage CTCL a prolonged remission can be achieved. In two studies a total of 13 patients were treated with high-dose combination chemotherapy with or without total body irradiation followed by autologous bone marrow transplantation. Seven out of 13 patients achieved CR with a duration of 3–46 months. Prolonged remission is seen in patients given total body irradiation. It is debatable whether autologous bone marrow transplantation should be given earlier in the course of the disease to obtain even better results.

Aciclovir

This has been used in only nine patients with a response rate of 22%, without complete response. It is not advised as treatment in cutaneous lymphoma.

Monoclonal antibodies

These have been used in cutaneous lymphomas since the antigens expressed on the malignant helper T cells are potential targets for immunotherapy with monoclonal antibodies. Anti-CD5 (T101) was given in 43 patients which resulted in an overall response rate of only 11% without any complete responses.

Conclusion

It is important to establish the correct diagnosis with all the possible techniques available. A uniform classification should be used. Treatment should be given according to the stage of the disease. Collaboration between dermatologist, pathologist, haemato-oncologist and radiotherapist is essential for the management of cutaneous lymphoma. All patients should be followed for at least 5 years, preferably by the dermatologist.

Further reading

Bekkenk MW, Geels FAMJ, van Voorst Vader P *et al.* Primary and secondary cutaneous CD30+ lymphoproliferative disorders; a report from the Dutch Cutaneous Lymphoma Group in the long-term follow-up data of 219 patients and guidelines for diagnosis and treatment. *Blood* 2000; 95: 3653–61.

Beljaards RC, Kaudewitz P, Berti E *et al.* Primary cutaneous CD30-positive large cell lymphoma. definition of a new type of cutaneous lymphoma with a favourable prognosis. *Cancer* 1993; 71: 2097–103.

Beljaards R, Meijer CJLM, van der Putte SCJ *et al.* Primary cutaneous T-cell lymphomas. clinicopathological features and prognostic parameters of 35 cases other than mycosis fungoides and CD30–positive large cell lymphoma. *J Pathol* 1994; 172: 53–60.

Benchikhi H, Zeitoun Ch, Bagot M *et al.* Syndrome de Sézary traité par cytaphérèses. *Ann Dermatol Venereol* 1996; 123: 247–50.

Bigler RD, Crilley P, Micaily B *et al.* Autologous bone marrow transplantation for advanced stage mycosis fungoides. *Bone Marrow Transplant* 1991; 7: 133–7.

Bunn PA, Hoffman SJ, Norris D, Goltitz LE. Systemic therapy of cutaneous T-cell lymphomas (mycosis fungoides and the Sézary syndrome). *Ann Intern Med* 1994; 12: 592–602.

Bunn PA, Lamberg SI. Report of the committee on staging and classification of cutaneous T-cell lymphomas. *Cancer Treatm Rep* 1979; 63: 725–8.

Cooper DL, Braverman IM, Sarris AH *et al.* Ciclosporin treatment of refractory T-cell lymphomas. *Cancer* 1993; 71: 2335–41.

DeVita VT, Hellmann S, Rosenberg SA. *Cancer Principles and Practice of Oncology*, 5th edn. Philadelphia: Lippincott, 1997: 334–6.

Doorn van R, van Haselen CW, van Voorst Vader P *et al.* Mycosis fungoides; disease evaluation and prognosis of 309 Dutch patients. *Arch Dermatol* 2000; 136: 504–10.

Duvic M, Hester JP, Lemak NA. Photopheresis therapy for cutaneous T-cell lymphoma. *J Am Acad Dermatol* 1996; 35: 573–9.

Edelson RL, Berger C, Gasparro F, Jegosothy B, Heald P, Wintrob B. Treatment of cutaneous T-cell lymphoma by extracorporal photochemotherapy. *N Engl J Med* 1987; 316: 297–303.

Foss FM, Ihde DC, Breneman DL *et al.* Phase II study of pentostatine and intermittent high dose recombinant interferon alfa-2a in advanced mycosis fungoides mycosis/Sézary syndrome. *J Clin Oncol* 1992; 10: 1907–13.

Gather RC, Scherschun L, Malick F *et al.* Narrow band UVB phototherapy for early-stage mycosis fungoides. *J Am Acad Dermatol* 2002; 47: 191–7.

Grange F, Bekkenk MW, Wechsler J *et al.* Prognostic factors in primary cutaneous large B-cell lymphomas: a European multicenter study. *J Clin Oncol* 2001; 19: 3602–10.

Greiner D, Olsen EA, Petroni G. Pentostatin (2′-deoxycoformycin) in the treatment of cutaneus T-cell lymphoma. *J Am Acad Dermatol* 1997; 36: 950–5.

Harris NL, Jaffe ES, Stein H *et al.* A revised European-American classification of lymphoid neoplasms: a proposal from the the International Lymphoma Study Group. *Blood* 1994; 84: 1361–92.

Herrmann JJ, Roenigh HH, Hurria A *et al.* Treatment of mycosis fungoides with photochemotherapy (PUVA); long term follow-up. *J Am Acad Dermatol* 1995; 33: 234–42.

Hoppe RT, Fuks Z, Bagshaw MA. Radiation therapy in the management of cutaneous T-cell lymphomas. *Cancer Treatm Rep* 1979; 63: 625–32.

Jones GW, Kacinsky BM, Wilson LD *et al.* Total skin electron radiation in the management of mycosis fungoides: consensus of the European Organization for Treatment of Cancer (EORTC) cutaneous lymphoma project group. *J Am Acad Dermatol* 2002; 47: 364–70.

Kuzel TM, Roegnik HH, Samuelson E *et al.* Effectiveness of interferon alfa-2 combined with phototherapy for mycosis fungoides and the Sézary syndrome. *J Clin Oncol* 1995; 13: 257–63.

Lambert WC, Giannotti B, van Vloten WA eds. *Basic Mechanisms of Physiological and Aberrant Lymphoproliferation in the Skin.* New York: Plenum Press, 1994.

Marolleau JP, Baccard M, Flageul B *et al.* High-dose recombinant interleukin-2 in advanced cutaneous T-cell lymphoma. *Arch Dermatol* 1995; 131: 574–9.

Ramsey DL, Lish KM, Yalowitz CB, Soter NA. Ultraviolet-B phototherapy for early stage cutanepous T cell lymphoma. *Arch Dermatol* 1992; 128: 931–3.

Rijlaarsdam JU, Huygens PL, Beljaards RL, Bakels V, Willemze R. Oral etoposide in the treatment of cutaneous large cell lymphoma. *Br J Dermatol* 1992; 127: 524–8.

Rijlaarddam JU, Toonstra J, Meijer CJLM, Noordijk EM, Willemze R. Treatment of primary cutaneous B-cell lymphomas of follicular center cell origin. A clinical follow-up study of 55 patients treated with radiotherapy or polychemotherapy. *J Clin Oncol* 1996; 14: 549–55.

Rijlaarsdam JU, van der Putte SCJ, Berti E *et al.* Cutaneous immunocytomas. a clinicopathological study of 26 cases. *Histopathology* 1993; 23: 117–25.

Saleh MN, LeMaistre CF, Kuzel TM *et al.* Antitumor activity of DAB389 IL-2 fusion toxin in cutaneous T-cell lymphoma. *J Am Acad Dermatol* 1998; 39: 63–73.

Savin A, Piro LD. The newer purine analogs. Significant therapeutic advances in the management of lymphoid malignancies. *Cancer* 1993; 72: 3470–83.

Schappell DL, Alper JC, McDonald CJ. Treatment of advanced mycosis fungoides and Sézary syndrome with continuous infusions of methotrexate followed by fluorouracil and leucovorin rescue. *Arch Dermatol* 1995; 131: 307–13.

Sigurdsson V, Toonstra J, Hezemans-Boer M, van Vloten WA. Erythroderma. a clinical and follow up study of 102 patients, with emphasis on survival. *J Am Acad Dermatol* 1996; 35: 53–7.

Suchin KR, Cucchiari AJ, Gottleib SL, *et al.* Treatment of cutaneous T-cell lymphoma with combined immunomodulatory therapy: a 14 year experience at a single institution. *Arch Dermatol* 2002; 138: 1054–60.

Taylor A, Gasparro P. Extracorporeal photochemotherapy for cutaneous T-cell lymphoma and other diseases. *Sem Hematol* 1992; 29: 132–41.

Vermeer MH, Geelen FAMJ, van Haselen CW *et al.* Primary cutaneous large B-cell lymphomas of the legs. *Arch Dermatol* 1996; 132: 1304–8.

Vloten WA, Cooijmans ACM, Poel J, Meulenbelt J. Concentrations of nitrogen mustard in the air during topical treatment of patients with mycosis fungoides. *Br J Dermatol* 1993; 128: 404–6.

Vloten WA, de Vroome H, Noordijk E. Total skin electron beam irradiation for cutaneous T-cell lymphoma (mycosis fungoides). *Br J Dermatol* 1985; 112: 697–702.

Vonderheid EC, Bernengo MG, Burg G *et al.* Update on erythrodermic cutaneous T-cell lymphoma: report of the International Society for cutaneous lymphomas. *J Am Acad Dermatol* 2002; 46: 95–106.

Vonderheid EC, Saijadian A, Kadin ME. Methotrexate is effective therapy for lymphomatoid papulosis and other primary cutaneous CD30 positive lympho-proliferative disorders. *J Am Acad Dermatol* 1996; 34: 470–6.

Vonderheid EC, Tan E, Kantor AF, Shrager L, Micaly B, van Scott EJ. Long term efficacy, curative potential and carcinogenicity of topical mechlorethamine chemotherapy in cutaneous lymphoma. *J Am Acad Dermatol* 1989; 20: 416–28.

Willemze R, Kerl H, Sterry W *et al.* EORTC classification for primary cutaneous lymphomas. A proposal from the cutaneous lymphoma study group of the European Organization for Research and Treatment of Cancer. *Blood* 1997; 90: 354–71.

Winkelmann RK, Diaz-Perez JL, Buechner SA. The treatment of Sézary syndrome. *J Am Acad Dermatol* 1984; 10: 1000–3.

Wollina U, Looks A, Meyer J *et al.* Treatment of stage II cutaneous T-cell lymphoma with interferon-alfa-2a and extracorporal photochemotherapy; a prospective controlled trial. *J Am Acad Dermatol* 2001; 44: 253–60.

Zackheim HS, Epstein H Jr, Crain W. Topical carmustine (BCNU) for cutaneous T-cell lymphoma: a 15 year experience in 143 patients. *J Am Acad Dermatol* 1990; 22: 802–5.

Zackheim HS, Kashani-Sabet M, Hwang ST. Low-dose methotrexate to treat erythrodermic cutaneous T-cell lymphoma: results in 29 patients. *J Am Acad Dermatol* 1996; 34: 626–31.

Zane C, Leali C, Airo P, DePanfilis G, Pinton PC. 'High dose' UVA 1 therapy of widespread plaque-type, nodular, and erythrodermic mycosis fungoides. *J Am Acad Dermatol* 2001; 44: 629–33.

Zeitoun C, Baccard M, Marolleau JP *et al.* Autogreffe de moelle osseuse dans le traitement des lymphomes cutanés. *Ann Dermatol Venereol* 1996; 123: 79–84.

Zic J, Arzubiaga C, Salhany KE *et al.* Extracorporeal photopheresis for the treatment of cutaneous T-cell lymphoma. *J Am Acad Dermatol* 1992; 27: 729–36.

Malignant melanoma

B.-R. Balda and H. Starz

Synonym

Black skin cancer.

Definition and epidemiology

Malignant melanoma is a malignant tumour originating from the transformation of melanocytes or naevus cells. These cells, arising from the neural crest are not only encountered in the skin and the adjacent mucous membranes, but also in the uvea, retina and central nervous system. Nonetheless, between 85% and 90% of melanomas arise on the outer skin.

Since it is not rare (up to 22%) that associations have been observed between naevus cell clusters and malignant melanoma by histology, it can be assumed that at least some melanomas evolve from common naevi. In any event, the risk of developing a melanoma increases markedly with the number of naevi present. In Central Europe, up to 50 naevi per person is considered to be normal.

Special attention is required for dysplastic (atypical) naevi. Their features are characterized both clinically (ill-defined as well as irregular borders and colour shifts from light brown to reddish to black, macular and papular elements) and histologically (cellular and nuclear atypia, concentrical connective tissue septa, inflammatory cells) and occur both sporadically as well as hereditarily (*f*amilial, *a*typical *m*ole and *m*elanoma (FAMM) syndrome, B-K mole syndrome). One subtype of the latter variant implies an individual risk of up to 100% to develop at least one melanoma within the course of a lifetime. Congenital naevus cell naevi, especially when presenting as giant cell naevi should be regarded as melanoma precursors. Their earliest possible surgical removal in specialized and experienced centres is therefore recommended. However, benign nodules (pseudomelanoma), frequently develop from these lesions. Their differentiation from true melanomas may be very difficult.

Naevus cell naevi, and atypical naevi in particular, prove to change colour and can grow during pregnancy. It has not yet been proven with certainty whether this is associated with a higher risk of melanoma.

Malignant melanoma occurs with a frequency of approximately 2–5% among all malignancies. In Central Europe, the morbidity is about 15–20 per 100 000 per year. In the past decades, it has been doubling around every 6–10 years. This fact is very worrisome since, as in the USA, projections indicate that if the tendency stays the same, around one in every 90–100 persons will develop a malignant melanoma over the course of a lifetime by now.

The major, if not the only cause, is assumed to be increased exposure to ultraviolet light (solar radiation), especially in childhood. Although cytological and molecular genetic tests have shown that melanomas of varying degrees of severity can be associated with changes in chromosomes 1, 6–11, 19 and 20 and others corresponding to oncogenes, tumour-suppressor genes or apoptosis genes, respectively, that have meanwhile been identified, it has not yet been possible to derive a general pattern that has any diagnostic or prognostic validity, except for some restrictions regarding the acral lentiginous melanoma (discussed below). It seems rather that the genetic instability increases with disease progression.

Clinical characteristics and course

Based on clinical and histological criteria, four major types of malignant melanoma can be differentiated:

- superficial spreading melanoma
- nodular melanoma

- lentigo maligna melanoma
- acral lentiginous melanoma.

More than two-thirds of the tumours are classified as superficially spreading melanoma with a history of 2–5, sometimes even many more, years. The epidermis shows pagetoid proliferation of tumour cells which causes a discrete and flat elevation of the involved vs. the surrounding skin. Characteristically, coloration ranges from red to blackish-brown, with scar-like whitish areas, called regression zones. These facilitate diagnosis. Around 20% of melanoma exhibit primarily nodular growth and have a rather short history. Almost all lentigo maligna melanomas are encountered in areas exposed to sunlight, preferentially the face. The intraepidermal growth phase, lasting many years (precancereous circumscribed melanosis Dubreuilh, Hutchinson's freckle, lentigo maligna) is only clinically remarkable as a macula with different shades of brown that gradually becomes larger and shows elevation. Visible and palpable tissue changes, accompanied by shifts in colour similar to a superficially spreading melanoma, do not occur until the onset of the vertical growth phase. This group constitutes about 5–10% of all melanomas. Acral lentiginous melanoma occurs with an even rarer frequency, characteristically localized on the palms, soles or beneath the nail beds. This melanoma type is also encountered in the oral mucosa and anogenital region. Recently described specific molecular genetic features support its distinct position in the classification of melanoma subtypes. Similarly characteristic genetic profiles are still lacking for the other mentioned categories.

Unclassifiable melanoma and melanoma variants like desmoplastic melanoma are very rare and should therefore not be discussed in detail in the context of this chapter.

Nodular and acral lentiginous melanomas have been considered to have a less favourable prognosis than the superficial spreading type. Multivariate analyses, however, have shown that the crucial prognostic factor in all melanomas, including lentigo maligna melanoma, is the depth of invasion of tumour cells. Ulceration and bleeding as well as area dimension and sex can also play a role. The tumour thickness is measured in mm according to Breslow rather than in relation to anatomical structures (level of invasion) according to Clark because it is much more reproducible and indeed the dominant prognostic predictor. Melanomas with a thickness of up to 0.75 mm have a low risk of metastasis, up to 1.5 mm a relatively low risk, from 1.5 to 4.0 mm a moderate risk, and over 4.0 mm a high risk of metastasis.

Clinical staging is mainly determined by the presence versus absence of lymphatic and/or haematogenous metastases. If metastases are not detectable, an additional distinction is made between stage I and stage II based on the thickness of the primary melanoma. The internationally accepted breakpoint used to be 1.5 mm. It has recently been changed to 2 mm according to the updated staging system of the American Joint Committee on Cancer (AJCC) (Table 1).

Stage I and stage II melanoma patients have 10-year survival rates of 85% and 55% respectively, if micrometastases detected by SLNE are not taken into consideration. Clinically or sonographically apparent nodal or cutaneous metastases, equivalent to the previous definition of stage III, reduce the 10-year survival rate to about 30%, distant metastases (= stage IV) to 15%. Such macrometastases, however, are rare at the time when the primary melanoma is diagnosed.

A further leading criterion for staging appears to be the micrometastatic involvement or the lack of tumour cells in regional lymph nodes. This must be demonstrated by histological testing of the first node draining the primary tumour

Table 1 TNM classification (AJCC 2000/2002)

T classification		
T1	≤ 1.0 mm	a: without ulceration
T1		b: with ulceration or Clark-level IV or V
T2	1.01–2.0 mm	a: without ulceration
T2		b: with ulceration
T3	2.01–4.0 mm	a: without ulceration
T3		b: with ulceration
T4	> 4.0 mm	a: without ulceration
T4		b: with ulceration
N classification		
N1	One lymph node	a: micrometastasis (diagnosed after sentinel lymphadenectomy) b: macrometastasis
N2	2–3 lymph nodes	a: micrometastasis (diagnosed after sentinel lymphadenectomy) b: macrometastasis c: in-transit met(s)/satellite(s) without metastatic lymph nodes
N3	4 or > metastatic lymph nodes, matted lymph nodes, or combinations of in-transit met(s)/ satellite(s) and metastatic lymph node(s)	
M classification		
M1a	Distant skin or lymph node metastases	Normal LDH
M1b	Lung metastases	Normal LDH
M1c	All other visceral or	Normal LDH
	any distant metastases	Elevated LDH

site, i.e. the sentinel lymph node, which is an indicator for the entire region. Sentinel lymphonodectomy provides both the opportunity and the need for a new staging system characterized by a more accurate prognostic relevance. This new staging tool combines a minimally invasive operative intervention with adequate histological and immunohistochemical techniques using labelling with anti S-100 and HMB45 antibodies to investigate the sentinel lymph nodes as described in The Augsburg Consensus (see below).

Melanoma-positive sentinel lymph nodes are associated with a 10-year survival rate of about 55%. The mentioned prognostic implications are well reflected by the new pTNM staging system, which has been proposed by the American Joint Committee on Cancer in 2000 and has become valid internationally in 2002 (Tables 1 and 2). Macro- and microscopic ulcerations of the primary tumour as well as lactate dehydrogenase (LDH) blood levels are further determinants in this new classification due to their predictive relevance.

Even more precise prognostic differentiation is achieved by a micromorphometric subclassification of the sentinel

Table 2 Stage groupings for cutaneous melanoma

0	Tis	NO	MO
IA	T1a	NO	MO
IB	T1b	NO	MO
	T2a	NO	MO
IIA	T2b	NO	MO
	T3a	NO	MO
IIB	T3b	NO	MO
	T4a	NO	MO
IIC	T4b	NO	MO
IIIA	T1-4a	N1a	MO
IIIB	T1-4a	N1b	MO
	T1-4a	N2a	MO
IIIC	any T	N2b, N2c	MO
	any T	N3	MO
IV	any T	any N	M1a, M1b, M1c

lymph node micrometastases into three so-called S categories. The depth of invasion of metastatic cells towards the centre of the sentinel lymph node measured in mm from the interior margin of the lymph node capsule is the leading parameter to distinguish between the highest S category S3 (>1 mm) and the lower ones. This principle of measuring is quite analogous to Breslow's method regarding primary melanomas. The same applies for its prognostic relevance.

Diagnosis and differential diagnosis

The diagnosis of a malignant melanoma is based on clinical examination and epiluminescence microscopy. 20 or 50 MHz sonography provides a preoperative estimation of tumour thickness. The need for biopsy should be decided judiciously since it is possible that not enough representative tissue is obtained for correct diagnostic decision-making. In addition to this, metastasis may be promoted by this intervention. As a general rule in cases of doubt, an excision biopsy only is permitted.

Various marker systems have been developed to detect low numbers of circulating melanoma cells in blood or bone marrow. Examples are soluble S-100 beta protein, melanoma inhibitory activity protein (MIA), 5-S-cysteinyldopa, RT-PCR for detecting tyrosinase mRNA and others. While, for example, increasing S-100 blood levels may be an early indicator of recurrent disease during follow-up, there is still no convincing evidence for their predictive value at the initial staging.

The most important differential diagnoses encompass the different variants and manifestations of naevus cell naevi, seborrhoeic keratosis, granuloma pyogenicum, pigmented basal cell carcinoma, histiocytoma, complemented by more than 70 further pigmented and non pigmented lesions.

Treatment

General therapeutic guidelines

In general, surgical removal of the tumour and its metastases (reduction of tumour mass) has priority over all other interventions. This applies to all stages of the disease, in so far as it is technically feasible and reasonable for the patient. This is currently the only curative measure. In the early stages or if the tumour thickness is minor, this method can cure the disease. The procedure has been standardized (described later); any deviations depend on the localization (e.g. head, hands, feet, anogenital region). In the case of extended lentigo maligna melanoma of the face, the central, 'thicker' portion of the tumour can be excised and the peripheral areas irradiated with X-rays.

In melanomas with a high risk for metastasis, adjuvant systemic treatment modalities are sometimes initiated following surgery. All previously published data on this subject have given cause for disappointment regardless of whether chemotherapy, immunotherapy, hormone therapy or corresponding combinations were involved.

According to the published data, single drug cytostatic therapy (DTIC/dacarbazine) has achieved objective remission of the tumour in only about 20% of patients with metastatic melanoma. Originally reported higher percentages had to be corrected downwards with increasing evidence from multiple centres. The same response has been achieved with combinations of cytostatics.

In particular, the outcome of treatment with interferons and interleukin-2 alone or in various combinations has not been convincing. The reason that melanoma appears to be so resistant *per se* is not known, even though a number of resistance mechanisms have recently been detected. For example, this includes the overexpression of drug-transporting molecules and detoxification enzymes as well as the resistance to therapeutically induced apoptosis (cf. remarks on genetic instability).

Recommended therapies

Surgical procedure

The surgical treatment of melanoma decisively depends on the individual stage of the disease. Preoperative staging usually reveals no macrometastases. In this case, melanomas thinner than 0.76 mm are sufficiently treated by excision with a security margin of 1 cm. For *in-situ* melanomas, even 0.5 cm appears to be curative in most patients. If a melanoma thicker than 0.75 mm is suspected due to its clinical, dermatoscopic or sonographic features, or if such a melanoma has been diagnosed by excisional biopsy, then the respective patient should immediately be referred to a dermato-oncology centre with experience in sentinel node technology. The rationale is that lymphoscintigraphy must precede any (further) surgery at the site of the primary tumour, starting from 6–12 intracutaneous injections of 99m-technetium-labelled colloid (either sulphur colloid or colloidal human albumin) within a margin of 0.5 cm around the melanoma or its scar. The relevant lymph drainage can thus be followed by repeated scintigrams in at least two planes over a period of 1–6 hours up to the sentinel lymph nodes. They are defined as those target nodes that receive direct lymph drainage from the primary tumour site, i.e. without passing previous lymph nodes.

On the next day, the suspected tumour including the radioactivity depots is excised with a safety margin of 1 cm and immediately examined histologically using the rapid section technique. If the suspicion of malignancy is confirmed and depending on the tumour thickness, an extended excision with a margin of up to 3 cm and a depth down to the fascia is made and the defect closed by grafting or by primary closure appropriate to the location.

In a second step, the sentinel lymph node is located by placing a collimated gamma probe through a small skin incision at the previously marked site and then selectively removed for histological examination. Special attention should be given to ensure the lymphatic vessels supplying and draining the area are meticulously ligated and that wound closure is performed layer by layer. In exceptional cases, several sentinel lymph nodes may be found that should be treated accordingly.

In our experience, lymphatic mapping using patent blue dye as originally described by Morton *et al.* is clearly inferior to gamma-probe guidance. Therefore, we only use it from time to time in addition to the technetium method. When the technique is applied correctly and a suitable radioactive carrier and optimized probe are used, sentinel lymphonodectomy is an extremely reliable procedure.

The same method can even be employed in patients who have had previous surgery, i.e. who have already undergone tumour excision, although the detection of the sentinel lymph node is subject to greater imprecision.

If tumour cells in this sentinel lymph node are detected, the final step is the radical extirpation of the entire affected lymph node region (radical completion lymphadenectomy). Since involvement of non-sentinel lymph nodes seems to be very rare in cases of S1-classified sentinel lymph nodes, the radical lympadenectomy can be omitted. Nevertheless, this opinion needs critical appraisal by prospective randomized multicentre trials.

While some other authors prefer 1.0 mm instead of 0.75 mm as the break point, we also strongly recommend sentinel lymphonodectomy for all patients with melanoma of 0.76–1.0 mm thickness because about 12% of them present a sentinel lymph node positive for micrometastases.

Chemotherapy

A discussion of the numerous published and ongoing studies on melanoma drug therapy would exceed the scope of this chapter. This fact alone reflects the impossibility of making convincing recommendations for treatment. The most recommended single agents and drug combinations are listed in Tables 3 and 4. The high remission rates reported by some authors did not stand up to critical appraisal.

Table 3 The most recommended drugs used as monotherapy of metastasized melanoma and their published remission rates

Agent	Remission rate (%)
Fotemustine	24.2 (10–47)
Dacarbazine	23.4 (14–33)
Carmustine	17.1
Cisplatin	15.8
Vindesine	14.9
Cyclophosphamide	12.5
Vinblastine	12.1
Lomustine	11.1
Vincristine	11.0
Hydroxyurea	8.1
Bleomycin	2.5
Taxol	15.0
Tamoxifen	7.9

Table 4 The most recommended drug combinations for melanoma treatment and their published remission rates

Agent	Remission rate (%)
Dacarbazine/cisplatin	10.0–42.5
Dacarbazine/fotemustine	27.2
Dacarbazine/vincristine/carmustine	22.7–42.5
Carmustine/hydroxyurea/dacarbazine	12.5–31.05
Cisplatin/vinblastine/bleomycin	47.0
Cisplatin/vindesine/dacarbazine	24.0–44.0
Bleomycin/vincristine/lomustine/ Dacarbazine (BOLD)	4.0–46.0
Bleomycin/vindesine/lomustine/ Dacarbazine (BELD)	41.0–45.0
Dacarbazine/carmustine/cisplatin/ tamoxifen (DBCT)	29.0–55.0

DTIC (dacarbazine (5-(3,3-dimethyltriazeno)-4-imidazolcarboxamide)

This is still the standard drug. The administration of a single infusion of 850 mg/m^2 body surface area and repetition at 4-week intervals (over a total of 10–12 cycles) appears to be the most favourable for practical reasons. Since DTIC/dacarbazine can cause considerable nausea and vomiting, it should be given together with modern antiemetic 5HT$_3$ antagonists. The agent should be protected from light when stored and administered. Despite an enormous amount of publications the efficacy of this drug was not proved to be indisputable.

MTIC/temozolomide (3-methyl-(triazene-1-yl)-4- imidazolcarboxamide)

This successor of DTIC/dacarbazine can be taken orally and passes the blood–brain barrier. However, the therapeutic benefit is doubtful like that of DTIC itself.

Fotemustine

This third-generation nitroso-urea derivative also passes the blood–brain barrier, but it has not been possible to date to validate its efficacy in brain metastases on a broader patient population.

Cytokines

The intravenous administration of high-dose interleukin-2 has been rejected because of its severe side-effects. Neither has subcutaneous low-dose therapy in combination with interferon-α yielded very convincing results. Although some data suggest that immune activation takes place, the progressive course of the disease has not been improved as far as metastasis and survival is concerned.

Interferon-α was and is currently being tested in numerous studies using low and medium doses (1.5–5 million units/m^2 body surface area, 3–5 times weekly over 6–36 months) and given as a single agent or in combination with DTIC/dacarbazine, temozolomide, vindesine or vincristine or other drugs. Unfortunately, the results from a greater number of patients tend to indicate that efficacy is poor or lacking regarding overall survival.

A recently published American trial (ECOG 1684) reports on an adjuvant high-dose interferon-α therapy (20 million units /m^2 body surface area 5 times a week for 4 weeks, then 10 million units/m^2 3 times a week given over 11 months). According to its findings, the patients in the treatment group have shown significant benefits with regard to relapse rate and survival after 5 years compared to the untreated patients, but critical appraisal reveals that the rate of complications was extremely high. Furthermore, a subsequent multicentre trial performed by the same group (ECOG 1690) could not confirm this significant survival benefit induced by high-dose interferon-α in comparison to control patients without adjuvant treatment. Hence, the use of this protocol cannot be recommended as a standard. Similarly, further evidence must be collected on the palliative approach with inhalative interleukin-2 for the treatment of patients with lung metastases (see Table 5 for details).

Hyperthermic limb perfusion

This form of regional, extracorporeal, mechanically driven therapy, performed under hyperthermic conditions, was administered with cytostatics like melphalan and DTIC/dacarbazine and others as well as cytokines like tumour necrosis factor-α and interferon-α. Therapy with melphalan in particular led, at least temporarily, to good responses in locally inoperable tumours, in-transit metastases and local recurrences. The effect of this intervention on overall survival is questionable. Moreover, this method is technically very complicated and therefore reserved to experienced centres.

Radiation therapy

Flat lentigo maligna melanomas that have been partially excised or are not accessible to surgical interventions respond well to treatment with a total dose of 80–100 Gy, given in fractions of four single doses of 10 Gy per week. Otherwise, radiation therapy is reserved for the palliative treatment of brain and painful bone metastases and to other locations of the body that can be exposed to higher doses of irradiation, depending on the individual case. Pre- and postoperative radiation of regional lymph node localizations in conjunction with radical lymphadenectomy is obsolete.

Experimental therapies

Various experimental models including most sophisticated vaccination therapies with hybrid cells or tumour antigen-loaded dendritic cells have been developed, but there does not appear to be

Table 5 Study protocol for inhalative use of interleukin-2

First cycle							
Day 1	Day 2	Day 3	Day 4	Day 5	Day 6	Day 7	Day 8
DTIC (850 mg/m^2)	18 MIU IL-2	21 MIU IL-2	24 MIU IL-2	27 MIU IL-2	30 MIU IL-2	36 MIU IL-2	36 MIU IL-2
From the second cycle							
Day 28, 55, 82, 109		Day 29, etc.	Day 30, etc.	Day 31, etc.			
DTIC (850 mg/m^2)		36 MIU IL-2	36 MIU IL-2	36 MIU IL-2 inhalant			

After the fourth administration of DTIC, inhalation of 36 MIU IL-2 is given alone, up to the end of the 6-month period.
MIU, million international units.

any tendency to a broader clinical use until now.

Currently a randomized prospective multicentre trial for stage II melanoma patients has been initiated by the EORTC melanoma group using GM2 ganglioside in combination with the immune response enhancers keyhole limpet haemocyanin (KLH) and QS-21.

Other vaccines based on irradiated melanoma cell lines with multiple melanocytic antigens (Canvaxin) are being applied in two other randomized prospective international trials initiated by D.L. Morton for stage III and stage IV melanoma patients after R0 resection of their metastases.

Conclusion and follow-up

It should be stated that for advanced melanoma disease there exists no satisfactory therapeutic approach, rather an urgent need for introduction of new pharmaceuticals and therapeutic strategies.

Every treatment regimen should include a comprehensive follow-up programme involving appropriate clinical and laboratory testing conducted at set intervals and covering at least a period of 5, or better 10, years.

In high-risk cases it is necessary to control periodically the brain for metastases by nuclear magnetic resonance (NMR) analyses.

The recently introduced proton emission tomography (PET) is especially helpful for the discrimination between scars and tumour recurrences or metastases, respectively, often also for the detection of clinically still occult organ metastases.

Further reading

Andreassi L, Balda B-R, Landi G. Current trends in the treatment of melanoma. *Skin Cancer* 1993; 8: 103–13.

Bachter D, Balda B-R, Vogt H, Büchels H. Die 'sentinel' Lymphonodektomie mittels Szintillationsdetektor. *Hautarzt* 1996; 47: 754–8.

Bachter D, Balda B-R, Vogt H, Büchels H. Primary therapy of malignant melanomas: Sentinel lymphadenectomy. *Int J Dermatol* 1998; 37: 278–82.

Balch C, Buzaid AC, Atkins MB *et al.* A New American Joint Committee on Cancer Staging System for Cutaneous Melanoma. *Cancer* 2000; 88: 1484–91.

Balch C, Buzaid AC, Soong S-J, *et al.* Final version of the American Joint Committee on Cancer Staging System for Cutaneous Melanoma. *J Clin Oncol* 2001; 19: 3635–48.

Balda B-R, Herrmann R. Neoplasien der Haut. In: Huhn D, Herrmann R, eds. *Medikamentöse Therapie Maligner Erkrankungen*, 3rd edn. Stuttgart: Fischer, 1995: 393–405.

Balda B-R. Die Sentinel-Lymphonodektomie bei malignen Melanomen—mehr als ein Diagnostikum? In: Konz B, Plewig G, eds. *Fortschr Dermatol.* Darmstadt: Steinkopf, 2002: 7–14.

Bastian B, LeBoit P, Hamm H, Bröcker EB, Pinkel D. Chromosomal gains and losses in primary cutaneous melanomas detected by comparative genomic hybridization. *Cancer Res* 1998; 58: 2170–5.

Bastian B, Kashani-Sabet M, Hann H. Gene amplifications characterize acral melanoma and permit detection of occult tumor cells surrounding skin. *Cancer Res* 2000; 60: 1968–73.

Berger W, Ebling L, Micksche M. Chemoresistance of human malignant melanoma. *Cellular Mol Aspects Onkol* 1998; 21: 105–10.

Cochran A, Balda B-R, Starz H, Bachter D, Krag DN, Cruse CW, Pijpers R, Morton DL. The Augsburg Consensus. Techniques, lymphatic mapping, sentinel lymphadenectomy, completion lymphadenectomy, cutaneous malignancies. *Cancer* 2000; 89: 236–41.

Elsässer-Beile U, Schöpf E, Neumann HA, Drews H, Hundhammer K, Balda B-R. Rekombiniertes Leukozyten-A-Interferon beim metastasierten malignen Melanom. *Dtsch med Wschr* 1987; 112: 373–7.

Enk AH, Nashan D, Knop J. Therapie von Lungenmetastasen des malignen Melanoms mit inhalativem IL-2. *Hautarzt* 1997; 48: 894–6.

Falkson CI, Ibrahim J, Kirkwood JM, Coates AS, Atkins MB, Blum RH. Phase III trial of dacarbazine versus dacarbazine with interferon alpha-2b versus dacarbazine with tamoxifen versus dacarbazine with interferon alpha-2b and tamoxifen in patients with metastatic malignant melanoma: an Eastern Cooperative Oncology Group Study. *J Clin Oncol* 1998; 16: 1743–51.

Katsambas A, Nicolaidou E. Cutaneous malignant melanoma and sun exposure. Recent developments in epidemiology. *Arch Dermatol* 1996; 132: 444–50.

Kirkwood JM, Hunt-Straderman M, Ernstorff MS, Smith TJ. Interferon alpha-2b adjuvant therapy of high-risk resected cutaneous melanoma: the Eastern Cooperative Oncology Group Trial EST 1684. *J Clin Oncol* 1996; 14: 7–17.

Krämer K-U, Prang N, Balda B-R. Evaluation of plasma 5-*S*-cysteinyldopa as a tumor marker of malignant melanoma. *Ann Ital Dermatol* 1999; 53: 75–9.

Morton DL, Wen DR, Wong JH, Economou JS, Cagle LA, Storm FK, Foshag LJ, Cochran AJ. Technical details of intraoperative lymphatic mapping for early stage melanoma. *Arch Surg* 1992; 127: 392–9.

Serrone L, Hersey P. The chemoresistance of human malignant melanoma: an update. *Melanoma Res* 1999; 9: 51–8.

Starz H, Balda B-R. Sentinel lymphonodectomy and micromorphometric S-staging, a successful new strategy in the management of cutaneous malignancies. *G Ital Dermatol Venereol* 2000; 135: 161–9.

Starz H, Balda B-R, Büchels H. Sentinel-Lymphonodektomie bei malignen Melanomen. Eine vorläufige Bilanz aus histomorphologischer Sicht. In: Garbe C, Rassner G, eds. *Dermatologie. Leitlinien und Qualitätssicherung für Diagnostik und Therapie.* Heidelberg: Springer, 1998; 274–7.

Starz H, Balda B-R, Kramer KU, Büchels H, Wang JH. A micromorphometry-based concept for routine classification of sentinel lymph node metastases and its clinical relevance for patients with melanoma. *Cancer* 2001; 91: 2110–21.

Starz H, De Donno A, Balda B-R. The Augsburg Experience: Histological Aspects and Patient Outcomes. *Ann Surg Oncol* 2001; 8(9S): 48–51.

Starz H, Cochran AJ, Balda B-R. Die Sentinel-Lymphonodektomie aus histopathologischer Sicht. *Akt Dermatol* 2002; 28: 273–8.

Volkenandt M, Schmidt M, Konz B, Gummer M, Hein R, Plewig G, Hölzel D. Klinisch-epidemiologische Daten von Patienten mit malignen Melanomen aus dem Bereich des Tumorzentrums München von 1977 bis 1997. *Hautarzt* 1999; 50: 470–78.

Mastocytosis

A.P. Oranje and D. Van Gysel

Definition and epidemiology

Mastocytosis covers a wide spectrum of proliferative mast cell disease. Mastocytosis is a primary abnormal proliferative accumulation of mast cells. Mast cell infiltrates may be present anywhere in the body, but appear most commonly in the skin. In particular, as a second organ the bones may be involved. There are six different recognized subtypes of mastocytosis: (a) urticaria pigmentosa; (b) mastocytoma; (c) diffuse cutaneous mastocytosis; (d) telangiectasia macularis eruptiva perstans (TMEP); (e) systemic mastocytosis; and (f) mast cell leukaemia. The most common manifestation of mastocytosis is urticaria pigmentosa. Recent advances in research on mastocytosis lead to a new classification based on *C-kit* mutation. Whereas mastocytosis in adults usually is persistent and progressive, the course in children is often transient and limited.

The exact prevalence of mastocytosis in the general population is unknown. One estimate predicts the incidence at dermatology units to be about 1 in every 5000 patients. Mastocytosis may start at any age, but in about 65% of cases, the onset is in childhood. No sex or racial predominance has been described. No clear-cut genetic factors have been identified, although some familial cases have been reported.

Aetiology and pathophysiology

Mastocytosis represents a hyperplastic response to an abnormal stimulus and can be considered as a proliferative process of the mast cell. Recent studies indicate that the disease in children is different from that in adults with respect to clinical pattern and pathogenesis.

Molecular biology techniques have identified the way in which the growth of mast cells is regulated. We now better understand the variations in the clinical course of mastocytosis. Research in mastocytosis is focused on mutations in proto-oncogen receptor *C-kit*. Analysis of *C-kit* mutations in the skin by polymerase chain reaction (PCR) may differentiate patients likely to have a chronic disease (*C-kit* mutation positive; mostly adults) from those likely to have a transient form of mastocytosis (mostly children).

Clinical characteristics and course

Urticaria pigmentosa (UP) is by far the most common variant of mastocytosis, representing 70% of cases. The lesions commonly appear in the first year of life, or may even be present at birth. The eruption consists of slightly elevated, skin-coloured, brown–red or yellow macules, plaques or nodules. The lesions may occur anywhere on the body and may present in a generalized distribution. The highest density of the lesions is on the trunk, sparing the acral areas. Urticarial flare-ups are frequent. Contact with triggering agents may induce a contact urticarial reaction. Darier's sign is positive (rubbing the lesions) in active lesions, and dermatographism is present in one-third of patients. In the first 2 years vesicles and bullae may occur spontaneously or after rubbing the lesion.

When the lesions of UP first present before the age of 5 years, the disease is almost always limited to the skin. Systemic extension occurs in about 10% of patients with UP, presenting after the age of 5 years. The organs most frequently involved besides the skin, are bones, gastrointestinal tract, liver and spleen. Headaches, bone pain, flushing, diarrhoea, fainting and growth retardation are all signs of systemic involvement.

The second most common cutaneous presentation of childhood-onset mastocytosis is solitary mastocytoma. In adults solitary mastocytoma is rarely observed. Solitary mastocytoma consists of one to several (but less than five) separate lesions. It is encountered in 25% of cases of childhood-onset mastocytosis. An asymptomatic solitary lesion may be overlooked or be mistaken for a mole or juvenile xanthogranuloma. Additionally, although rare, xanthogranuloma and mastocytomas may occur together. Solitary mastocytoma invariably follows a mild course with in almost all cases a complete resolution. Most mastocytomas have disappeared by puberty.

Diffuse cutaneous mastocytosis is a rare manifestation starting early in life, often as a neonatal erythroderma giving the patient an orange thickened skin. TMEP is another rare manifestation occurring more often in adults and only extremely rarely in children. Mastocytosis without any skin abnormalities has been observed, but is extremely rare. Non-cutaneous systemic mastocytosis will not be discussed in this chapter.

Diagnosis

The diagnosis of mastocytosis can often readily be made by the clinical history and the visible cutaneous lesions. Rubbing or trauma of the affected skin results in a wheal with flare (Darier's sign) in more than 90% of patients. A biopsy is indicated to verify the diagnosis in all cases.

Measurement of released mediators (histamine, prostaglandin D2, tryptase) and their metabolites (e.g. *N*-methyl histamine) can be used to support the diagnosis, although none of these tests is 100% specific. Most laboratories now use urinary *N*-methyl histamine (NMH) and serum tryptase measurements. We confirmed that NMH values, adjusted for age, were significantly higher in the group of children with active mastocytosis than in the control group of children. There was a significant difference, but there was also an overlap in NMH values between the groups of children with diffuse cutaneous mastocytosis, active UP and active mastocytomas. There is less overlap in adults. We recommend measurement of urinary NMH level once at the time of diagnosis and repeated measurements during further follow-up only in cases in which the initial values were elevated or when systemic signs have developed.

Further diagnostic evaluation to determine the presence of systemic involvement should be reserved for those children with very extensive cutaneous lesions and high urinary NMH or serum tryptase values, and those children who exhibit evidence of organ involvement (including haematemesis, melaena and severe bone pain, haematological abnormalities such as anaemia, leukopenia or mast cells in peripheral blood). A diagnostic internal investigation should be performed in adults with abnormal function tests or with systemic signs.

Diagnostic work-up (Fig. 1)

Screening for systemic involvement of mastocytosis

A complete blood cell count with peripheral smear and a blood chemistry study should be routinely and repeatedly performed to rule out associated haematological diseases and systemic involvement of mastocytosis. Anaemia, leucopenia, leucocytosis or thrombocytopenia may indicate bone marrow involvement. New studies suggest that measurement of α-protryptase may be an even more sensitive screening test than a bone marrow biopsy for suspected systemic mastocytosis.

Other invasive diagnostic procedures may be limited to patients presenting with specific symptoms that suggest systemic mastocytosis. Abdominal pain may require abdominal ultrasound, contrast

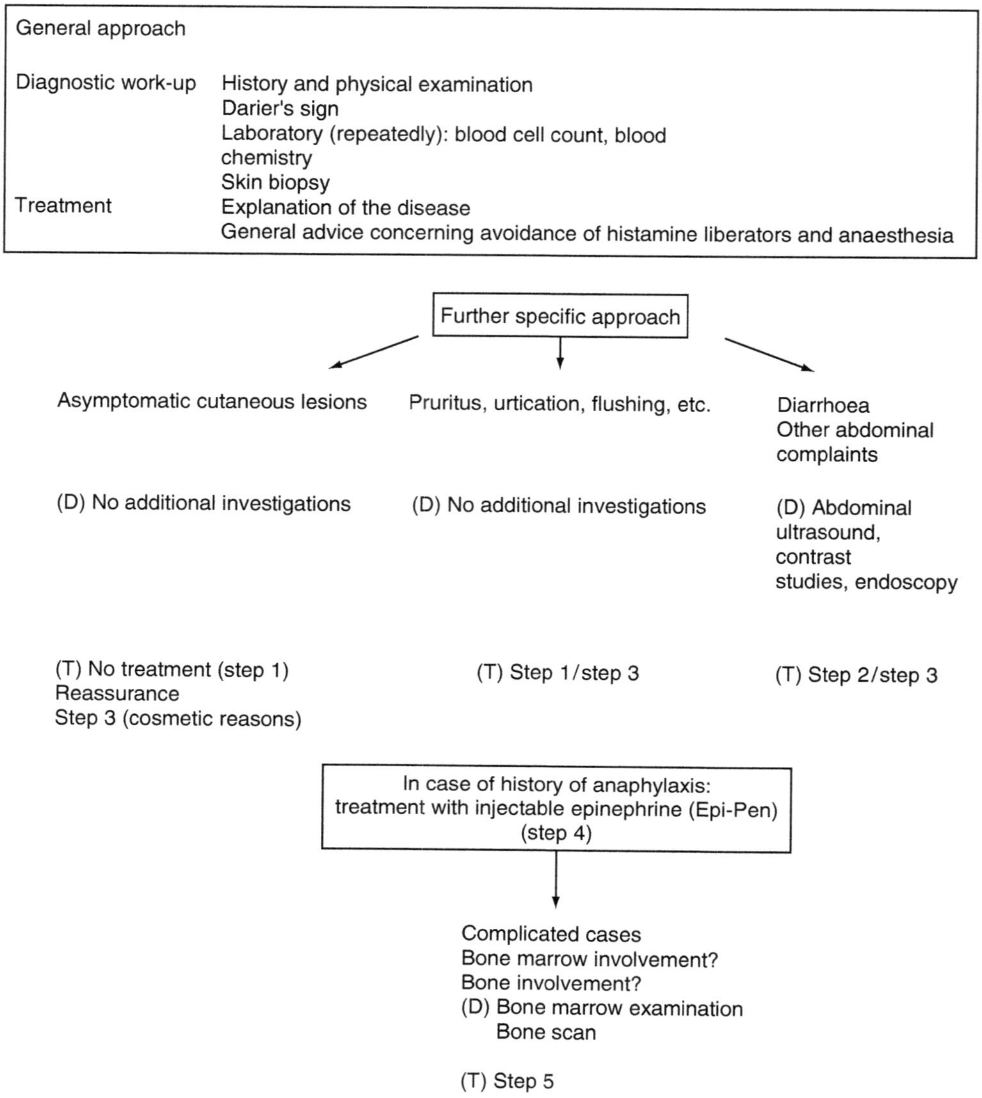

Figure 1 Diagnostic work-up (D) and treatment (T) of mastocytosis (see text for steps 1–5 in the treatment section)

studies and/or endoscopy; bone scans may be necessary if bone involvement is suspected. The usefulness of skeletal surveys should be considered carefully as skeletal lesions may be transient and no correlation between skeletal abnormalities and systemic involvement has been found.

Differential diagnosis

- Lentigines: brown macules, Darier's sign is negative.
- Freckles.
- Histiocytosis: rare, Darier's sign is negative.
- Café-au-lait freckling: in neurofibromatosis.

- Juvenile xanthogranuloma: red–yellow–brown macules, Darier's sign negative, only in children.
- Staphylococcal scalded skin syndrome: neonates, only in bullous forms.
- Incontinentia pigmenti: neonates.
- Rarely: bullous dermatosis of childhood, bullous pemphigoid and epidermolysis bullosa.

Treatment

General therapeutic guidelines

Treatment is indicated only when symptoms are present and is directed towards alleviation of symptoms. A more pathophysiological approach to mast cell hyperplasia is unavailable at present. UP usually follows a benign course. A multidisciplinary approach is advisable. The team will at least include a dermatologist, allergologist, haematologist and dietitian.

Therapy can often be limited to reassurance of the patient and, in children, his or her parents. A basic approach is avoiding factors known to stimulate mast cell degranulation.

Step 1

H_1-receptor antagonists (e.g. hydroxyzine maximum 2 mg/kg daily in 3 doses, cetirizine 10–20 mg daily, children aged 2–6 years 5 mg 2 times daily, older than 6 years as in adults) can control symptoms such as pruritus, urtication and flushing.

Step 2

The addition of a H_2-receptor antagonist (e.g. cimetidine 20 mg/kg daily in 3 doses, ranitidine 4 mg/kg daily in 2 doses) may be warranted in children who exhibit gastrointestinal symptoms of hyperacidity or ulceration. Patients with diarrhoea may benefit from treatment with an H_2-receptor antagonist, with or without disodium cromoglycate (a stabilizer of mast cell membranes) orally 100 mg 4 times daily. Disodium cromoglycate may also have a beneficial effect on flushing, pruritus, cutaneous and central nervous system symptoms.

Another mast cell stabilizer, ketotifen 1 mg/kg 2 times daily, has been demonstrated to reduce whealing and pruritus in patients with UP, although a more recent controlled comparison with hydroxyzine in paediatric cutaneous mastocytosis showed no advantage.

Step 3

Topical corticosteroids (especially those without systemic side-effects) under plastic dressings led to effective responses and even showed regression of the lesions. Patients with significant malabsorption may need oral prednisone treatment at a dose of 1–2 mg/kg daily at start, slowly tapering off (stress dose = 2 mg/kg daily). However, it includes a real danger of accentuating concomitant bone disease caused by the mast cells in the marrow. High doses of aspirin have found favour in the treatment of patients with recurrent episodes of flushing and a marked overproduction of prostaglandin D2.

As aspirin is a potential histamine releaser itself, treatment should be initiated under hospital supervision and should never be started without concomitant administration of a H_1-receptor antagonist.

Ultraviolet B (UVB)/UVA or UVA combined with oral psoralens (PUVA) may be used in adolescents and adults for skin manifestations that are resistant to more standard therapy. Much success has been claimed when using UVA1 light.

Step 4

Patients with mastocytosis and a history of anaphylaxis should be equipped with injectable epinephrine (adrenaline) in the form of either an Epi-Pen or an Ana-Kit and be prepared to self-medicate.

Step 5 (non-dermatological)

To date, treatment for patients with aggressive lymphadenopathic systemic mast cell disease or true mast cell leukaemia has so far been unsatisfactory. Interferon-α therapy has been successful in some adults.

For treatment evaluation one needs a scoring system. Until now a scoring system has been missing. Therefore we developed a scoring system that we called the scoring index of mastocytosis (SCORMA).

Prognosis

Children with mastocytoma or UP generally have a good prognosis. Lesions may continue to increase in number after onset, but then gradually resolve. About half of the children with UP will experience resolution of lesions and symptoms by adolescence, with the remainder experiencing a marked reduction in symptomatic cutaneous lesions and dermatographism. Partial regression is often noted within 3 years after onset. However systemic involvement develops in 10% of children with UP, in whom the first manifestations appeared after the age of 5 years.

Table 1 Clinically relevant mast cell degranulators

Immunological stimuli (IgE)
Complement-derived anaphylotoxins (C3A and C5A)
Physical stimuli (cold, heat, sunlight, friction)
Polymers (Compound 48/80; dextran)
Bacterial toxins
Wasp stings
Snake venoms
Hymenoptera venoms
Biological polypeptides (released by *Ascaris*, jellyfish, crayfish and lobster)
Drugs
Acetylsalicylic acid
Alcohol
Narcotics (e.g. codeine, morphine)
Procaine
Polymyxine B
Amphotericin B
Atropine
Thiamine
D-Tubocurarine
Quinine
Radiographic contrast media containing iodine
Scopolamine
Gallamine
Decamethonium
Reserpine

From Van Gysel & Oranje (2000).

Diffuse cutaneous mastocytosis with an onset before the age of 5 years carries the same good prognosis as mastocytomas and UP. Children who manifest diffuse cutaneous mastocytosis prior to bullous eruptions appear to have a better chance of a gradual improvement in their disease than infants, who manifest bullae as the initial symptom of mastocytosis. Blistering usually disappears by the age of 1–3 years, and 90% of children are free of symptoms by puberty.

Prevention

Factors triggering mast cell degranulation should be avoided by all patients with symptoms. Clinically relevant mast cell degranulators are shown in Table 1. The most important stimuli are stroking, scratching, extremes of temperature, physical exertion, intake of histamine-releasing nutrients and medicines. The preventive management of patients with mastocytosis undergoing anaesthesia is controversial. We adopted the following perioperative measures for the management of children with mastocytosis. Close monitoring of most patients, the avoidance of known histamine-releasing drugs and the continuous availability of resuscitative drugs are sufficient therapy. Patients with an extensive form of mastocytosis and with systemic symptoms are hospitalized 1 day before surgery. Prednisone at a stress dose (2 mg/kg daily) and antihistamines are initiated. Oral diazepam is given, as a sedative premedication, and all histamine-releasing products are avoided perioperatively. Epinephrine is continuously available.

Further reading

Czarnetzki BM. A double-blind cross-over study of the effect of ketotifen in urticaria pigmentosa. *Dermatologica* 1983; 166: 44–7.

Czarnetzki BM, Behrend H. Urticaria pigmentosa. clinical picture and response to oral disodium cromoglycate. *Br J Dermatol* 1981; 105: 563–7.

Fowler JF, Parsley WM, Cotter PG. Familial urticaria pigmentosa. *Arch Dermatol* 1986; 122: 80–1.

Guzzo C, Lavker R, Roberts J *et al.* Urticaria pigmentosa: systemic evaluation and successful treatment with topical steroids. *Arch Dermatol* 1991; 127: 191–6.

Hartmann K, Henz BM. Mastocytosis: recent advances in defining the disease. *Br J Dermatol* 2001; 144: 682–95.

Heide R, Middelkamp Hup MA, Mulder PGH, Oranje AP. Clinical scoring of cutaneous mastocytosis. The Mastocytosis Study Group Rotterdam. *Acta Derm Venereol* 2001.

Kettelhut BV, Berkebile C, Bradley D, Metcalfe DD. A double-blind, placebo-controlled, cross-over trial of ketotifen versus hydroxizine in the treatment of systemic mastocytosis. *J All Clin Immunol* 1989; 83: 866–70.

Kettelhut BV, Metcalfe DD. Pediatric mastocytosis. *J Invest Dermatol* 1991; 96 (Suppl.): 15–18.

Lucaya J, Pérez-Candela V, Celestina A *et al.* Mastocytosis with skeletal and gastrointestinal involvement in infancy. Two case reports and a review of the literature. *Radiology* 1979; 131: 363–6.

Oranje AP, Widowati S, Sukardi A *et al.* Diffuse cutaneous mastocytosis mimicking staphylococcal scalded skin syndrome [report of three cases]. *Pediatr Dermatol* 1991; 8: 147–51.

Parris WCV, Scott HW, Smith BE. Anesthetic management of systemic mastocytosis: experience with 42 cases. *Anesth Analg* 1986; 65: 117S.

Van Gysel D, Oranje AP. Mastocytosis. In: Harper J, Oranje AP, Prose N, eds. *Textbook of Pediatric Dermatology*, 1st edn. Oxford: Blackwell Science, 2000: 600–9.

Van Gysel D, Oranje AP, Vermeijden I, Lijster J, de Raadt Toorenenbergen van A. Evaluation of urinary *N*-methylhistamine measurement in patients with mastocytosis. *J Am Acad Dermatol* 1996; 35: 556–8.

Melasma

A.D. Katsambas, A.J. Stratigos and T.M. Lotti

Synonyms

Chloasma, mask of pregnancy.

Definition and epidemiology

Melasma (a term derived from the Greek word 'melas' meaning black) is an acquired blotchy, irregularly patterned, brown or sometimes grey–brown hypermelanosis of the face and occasionally the neck, of poorly understood aetiology but attributable to sunlight and genetic predisposition.

Epidemiological studies regarding incidence of melasma have not yet been published. A limitation to valid results is also dictated by the fact that many patients prefer to use over-the-counter bleaching products rather than consult the dermatologist. Although women are predominantly affected, men are not excluded from melasma, representing approximately 10% of cases.

Although no race is spared, melasma appears to be far more common in darker-skinned individuals of Hispanic, Oriental and Indo-Chinese origin who live in places with strong solar radiation. People, especially women of these origins, tend to develop melasma at a rather young age. Melasma is quite common in black patients.

Aetiology and pathogenesis

The exact cause of melasma is unknown. However, many factors have been implicated in the aetiopathogenesis of this disease. Natural and synthetic oestrogen and progesterone hormones have been incriminated for its pathogenesis. This is due to the association of the disease with pregnancy, oral contraception and ovarian tumours. Extensive endocrinological measurements in female patients with melasma, revealed increased levels of luteinizing hormone (LH) and lower levels of serum oestradiol, abnormalities suggesting subclinical evidence of mild ovarian dysfunction. Male patients with melasma have also been shown to have an abnormal hormonal profile with increased levels of circulating LH and low serum testosterone levels. Although the mechanism of oestrogen in precipitating melasma is unknown, it has been reported that melanocytes contain oestrogen receptors that stimulate these cells to become hyperactive.

The use of cosmetics with certain components (oxidized linoleic acid, salicylate, citral, preservatives, etc.) and the use of certain drugs (antiseizure, etc.) and photosensitizing agents are often implicated as aetiological factors.

As mentioned above, the two most important causative factors are sunlight and genetic predisposition. The role of solar radiation is of great importance. Exacerbations of melasma are almost inevitably seen after uncontrolled sun exposure and conversely melasma has been seen to fade during periods of sun avoidance. Genetic and racial factors appear to predominate as suggested by familial occurrence and the fact that the disease is far more common in people of Hispanic, Oriental and Chinese origin.

Clinical characteristics and course

The number of hyperpigmented patches may range from one single lesion to multiple patches located usually symmetrically on the forehead, cheeks, dorsum of the nose, upper lip (moustache-like melasma), chin and occasionally on the V-neck area. Melasma does not involve the mucous membranes.

According to the distribution of lesions, the following three clinical patterns of melasma are recognized: the centrofacial, the malar and the mandibular pattern. Histologically, melasma can be classified into three types: epidermal, dermal and mixed. The histological type of melasma can be detected with Wood's light examination.

- The epidermal type is characterized by intensification of the colour contrast between the melasma and the normal skin.
- In the dermal type, the pigmentation of the epidermis is not intensified under Wood's light and the contrast between the lesions and the uninvolved skin becomes less apparent.
- In the mixed type some areas become more apparent while others become less apparent under Wood's light in the same individual.

The prognostic significance of this classification is very important to the beneficial effects of the treatment. Patients with epidermal type respond much better to the use of depigmenting agents. In the case of dermal melanin depositions, elimination of pigment is governed by transport via macrophages and is not accessible to depigmenting agents.

Diagnosis

The diagnosis is clinical. The initial interview with the patient will give all available information (pregnancy, use of oral contraceptives, genetic and racial involvement, response to sun exposure). The use of Wood's lamp will assist in the classification into the three afore-mentioned histological types.

Differential diagnosis

- Postinflammatory hyperpigmentation: distribution of the eruption; history of inflammation.
- Pigmented cosmetic dermatitis: reddish-brown pigmentation, reticulate pattern.
- Hyperthyroidism: thyroid tests.
- Actinic lichen planus: papular lesions—histology.
- Infection with human immunodeficiency virus: serology.
- Hydantoin intake: history.

Treatment

Melasma is a cosmetic problem that sometimes causes great emotional suffering. At present there is no universally effective agent for the treatment of melasma. The majority of the existing treatments may temporarily depigment the melasma, but the condition usually relapses. There are, however, various therapeutic modalities that can offer a significant benefit. Before attempting to treat melasma, it is important to consider the factors that are associated with the abnormality of pigmentation. The objects of melasma therapy should be (a) the retardation of proliferations of melanocytes; (b) the inhibition of melanosome formation; and (c) the enhancement of melanosome degradation.

General therapeutic guidelines

Avoidance of solar exposure. Broad-spectrum sunscreens should be used, as the melanocytes in melasma are easily stimulated not only by ultraviolet B (UVB) but also by UVA and visible radiation. The sunscreen must be applied daily both during treatment and when treatment has stopped, throughout the sunny months of the year for an indefinite period. Sunbathing is absolutely contraindicated as a few minutes of sunbathing can reverse the benefit of months of therapy.

Women, in whom melasma develops during pregnancy, should avoid exposure to sunlight and should use a broad-spectrum sunscreen every day throughout the pregnancy. These patients should have patience because melasma may fade or clear spontaneously within months after pregnancy.

Patients taking contraceptive pills must discontinue them.

Recommended therapies

Bleaching agents

Hydroquinone (HQ)
From the numerous agents that have been employed at different times for the treatment of melasma HQ seems to be the most effective. The mode of action of HQ as depigmenting agent is based on the following properties:

1 HQ retards melanin biosynthesis by inhibiting the conversion of tyrosine to melanin.
2 HQ inhibits the formation or increases the degradation of melanosomes or both.
3 HQ inhibits the DNA and RNA synthesis of melanocytes.

The effectiveness of HQ is related directly to the concentration of the preparation, to the vehicle used and to the chemical stability of the final product. Concentrations of HQ vary from 2% (over the counter) to as high as 10% that are prescribed extemporaneously for resistant cases. These extemporaneous preparations of HQ are often effective in patients who have failed to respond to lower concentrations. With controlled use and monitoring, the side-effects from these preparations are minimal.

The most suitable vehicle for the formulation is an hydroalcoholic solution (equal parts of propylene glycol and absolute ethanol) or an hydrophilic ointment, or a gel containing 10% α-hydroxy acids (AHA).

The chemical stability of the HQ formulations is of great importance. HQ is easily oxidized and loses it potency. Therefore, antioxidants such a 0.1% sodium bisulphate and 0.1% ascorbic acid should be used to preserve the stability of the formulation.

Taking into consideration the desired HQ concentration, the vehicle and the chemical stability, the following formula can be prescribed:

- HQ 3–10%
- in ethanol and propylene glycol 1 : 1 (or in a cream base or an AHA 10% gel).

Ascorbic acid 0.1% (as preservative)
The side-effects of HQ include allergic contact dermatitis, irritant contact dermatitis (more probable with the higher concentrations), postinflammatory hyperpigmentation and nail discoloration. These side-effects are temporary and resolve on HQ discontinuation. A very rare complication of HQ use is ochronosis (a permanent blue–black postinflammatory discoloration) in black individuals.

Combination of HQ and other agents
It has been demonstrated that the skin-lightening effect of HQ can be enhanced by adding various topical agents such as tretinoin and corticosteroids. The following combination has been proposed (the Kligman and Willis formula):

- HQ 5%
- tretinoin 0.1%
- dexamethasone 0.1%
- in ethanol and propylene glycol 1 : 1 or in hydrophilic ointment.

Tretinoin stimulates the cell turnover promoting the rapid loss of pigment via epidermopoieses. Moreover, it acts as a mild irritant and therefore facilitates the epidermal penetration of HQ. Tretinoin acts as an antioxidant preventing the oxidation of HQ. Corticosteroids may inhibit melanin synthesis through a depression of the general metabolic activity of the cell. Moreover, corticosteroids can eliminate the irritation caused by HQ and/or tretinoin. Depigmentation begins within 3 weeks after twice daily application and it is used for a maximum of 5–7 weeks. This formulation is not preserved by antioxidants, and therefore should never be more that 30 days old.

A slight modification of the Kligman and Willis formula is the following:

- HQ 4%
- tretinoin 0.05%
- hydrocortisone acetate 1%
- in ethanol and propylene glycol 1 : 1 or in hydrophilic ointment.

In this formula the concentration of tretinoin is 0.05% and hydrocortisone acetate 1% is used instead of dexamethasone. By lowering the concentration of tretinoin and the use of a non-fluorinated steroid, the aim is to minimize the irritation caused by tretinoin and eliminate local steroid side-effects. These two formulations should be dispensed in a 25-mL volume in a dark-coloured bottle with an airtight screw cap and it should be kept in a refrigerator at 2–4°C. Another treatment suggestion is the use of 0.05% tretinoin, 2% HQ and 1% hydrocortisone acetate cream successively through the day.

Azelaic acid (AZA)

AZA is a naturally occurring, straight-chain saturated dicarboxylic acid. It has been reported that AZA acts as a competitive inhibitor of tyrosinase and interferes directly with melanin biosynthesis. AZA does not affect normal melanocytes. AZA cream has been reported to be of benefit in the treatment of melasma. The cream is applied twice daily and most patients report a mild but transient irritation and dryness of the skin at the beginning of the treatment. Various studies report 'good' to 'excellent' results in 63–80% of the patients with epidermal or mixed-type melasma after 6 months of treatment with 20% AZA cream in conjunction with a broad-spectrum sunscreen. As already mentioned, AZA has practically no effect on normal melanocytes and its long-term use is not associated with ochronosis. Since treatment of melasma with AZA requires several months, a combination of AZA with other drugs deserves consideration as a further therapy option.

Chemical peels

Superficial and medium depth chemical peels can be used for the treatment of melasma in fair-skinned individuals. All types of chemical peels but especially trichloracetic acid and AHA peels of various concentrations have been used alone or in combination with other depigmenting agents. It has to be emphasized that the response of melasma to chemical peels is rather unpredictable—there is a tendency for pigmentation changes and therefore melasma can be aggravated after chemical peel as a result of the postinflammatory hyperpigmentation, especially in dark-skinned individuals.

Alternative and experimental therapies

Lasers

The treatment of melasma with various types of laser has been tried during the last few years, but unfortunately without considerable success. Whereas the treatment of facial and hand lentigines with the Q-switched, pigment-specific lasers resulted in an excellent outcome, the treatment of melasma has failed and often resulted in hyperpigmentation. The use of a Q-switched ruby laser had initially given some encouraging results, especially in patients with a fair complexion and epidermal-type melasma, but a quick recurrence took place when the treatment stopped. Since the laser treatment is not without adverse effects (hyperpigmentation, mild scarring, atrophy, etc.) the role of lasers in the treatment of melasma has yet to be established. Encouraging results have been observed in the treatment of the more refractory dermal-type melasma by using a resurfacing laser (pulsed/scanned CO_2 or erbium : YAG lasers) to ablate the superficial portions of the skin, including the abnormal melanocytes.

Patients with refractory melasma who were treated with an erbium:YAG laser (2940 nm) showed significant pigment lightening 6 months after the procedure, despite the initial development of postinflammatory hyperpigmentation in virtually all patients. Another approach to dermal-type melasma involves the combined use of pulsed CO_2 laser resurfacing followed by Q-switched alexandrite laser treatment to eliminate the dermal melanin selectively.

Kojic acid

This is a fungal metabolic product that inhibits the catecholase activity of tyrosine. It has been used alone in concentration 2–4% and it has also been combined with HQ 2% in an AHA gel base.

N-Acetyl-4,5-cysteaminyl alcohol

This is another phenolic compound that has been considered much more stable and less irritating than HQ. It acts on functioning melanocytes and it has been used in 4% concentration with marked improvement or clearing in 75% of cases with minimal side-effects.

The efficiency of all the above agents warrants further investigation.

Summary

The approach to treatment of melasma can be summarized as follows.

1 Female patients must stop oral contraception.
2 Pregnant women must be patient because melasma often fades without treatment after pregnancy.
3 Sunlight exacerbates melasma. Sun avoidance and daily use of a strong broad-spectrum sunscreen is needed for an indefinite period of time.
4 HQ 2% alone is often ineffective. It is recommended for maintenance therapy.

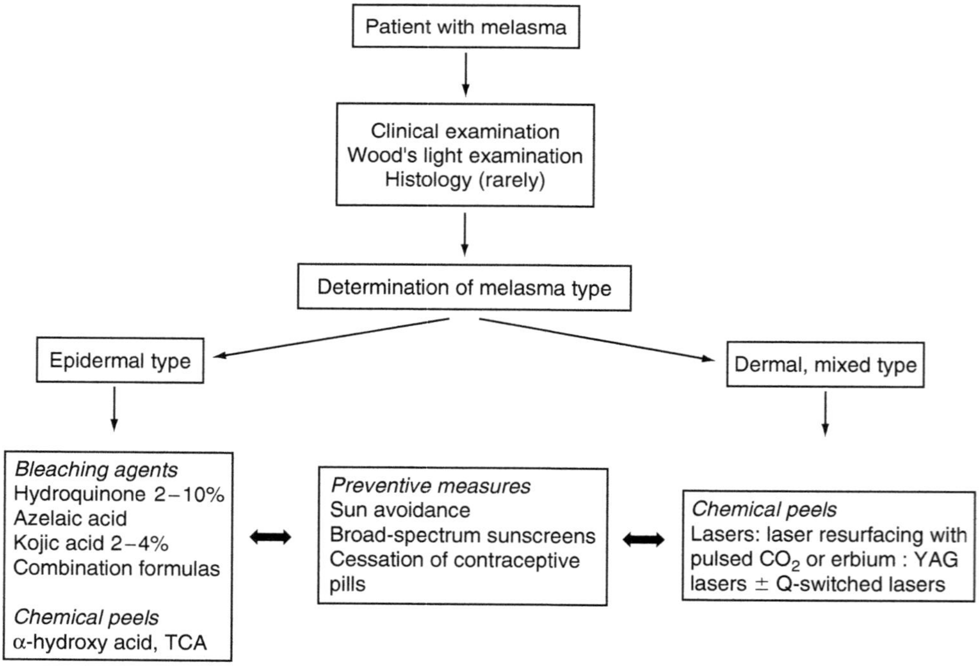

Figure 1

5 Good depigmentation can be achieved with 3–4% HQ alone in a hydroalcoholic solution or in a 10% AHA gel or in a cream base.
6 HQ 5–10% is very effective but it causes irritation.
7 A very effective combination is the use of 3–5% HQ with 0.05% tretinoin with or without corticosteroids in a hydroalcoholic lotion.
8 The prolonged use of fluorinated steroids on the face is not advised because telangiectasia or atrophy, for example, can develop.
9 The use of lasers has not been rewarding to date. However, they may prove effective in the future.
10 Chemical peeling alone or in combination with other depigmenting agents is effective in selected cases.

Further reading

Ballina LM, Graupe K. The treatment of melasma 20% ajelonic acid versus 4% hydroquinone cream. *Int J Dermatol* 1991; 30: 893–5.

Goldberg DJ. Benign pigmented lesions of the skin: Treatment with a switched ruby laser. *J Dermatol Surg Oncol* 1993; 18: 366–79.

Grimes P. Melasma. Etiologic and therapeutic considerations. *Arch Dermatol* 1995; 113: 1453–7.

Katsambas A, Antoniou C. Melasma. Classification and treatment. *J Eur Acad Dermatol Venerol* 1995; 4: 217–23.

Kligman AM, Willis J. A new formula for depigmenting human skin. *Dermatology* 1975; 11: 40–8.

Lim JT. Treatment of melasma using kojic acid in a gel containing hydroquinone and glycolic acid. *Dermatol Surg* 1999; 25: 282–4.

Manaloto RM, Alster T. Erbium : YAG laser resurfacing for refractory melasma. *Dermatol Surg* 1999; 25: 121–3.

Nouri K, Bowes L, Chartier T, Romagosa R, Spencer J. Combination treatment of melasma with pulsed CO_2 laser followed by Q-switched alexandrite laser: a pilot study. *Dermatol Surg* 1999; 25: 494–7.

Sialy R, Hassan I, Kaur I, Dash RJ. Melasma in men: a hormonal profile. *J Dermatol* 2000; 27: 64–5.

Mite bites

G. Leigheb

Definition and epidemiology

Besides the acarus of human scabies (*Sarcoptes scabiei hominis*) (0.3–0.5 mm), many other acari which are parasitic on animals or which infest various plant species, foods, organic waste or soil may occasionally attack man (facultative parasitism vs. obligatory parasitism in the case of scabies). The bites of the mites considered in this chapter are the cause of accidental dermatoses. These represent very frequent events, especially in certain geographical areas, but they often are not diagnosed.

Aetiology and pathogenesis

The most common acariasis are the various type of animal scabies, or pseudoscabies. Frequent forms are dog scabies (due to *S. scabiei canis*), cat scabies (due to *Notoedres cati*), rabbit scabies and other domestic or pet animals. *Cheiletiella* (0.3–0.5 mm), a parasite of dogs (*C. yasguri*), cats (*C. blackei*) and rabbits (*C. parasitivorax*), can also infest man, causing serious itching. Avian gamasid mites that infest domestic poultry or birds nesting in or near human habitation may parasitize man. Acari present in the environment include so-called harvest mites and trombiculid mites. *Neotrombicula autumnalis* (1–2 mm) is the most common in Europe and lives on vegetals feeding on small arthropods. The larvae (0.2–0.3 mm) (called red bugs or chiggers) can attack man. The affliction is known as trombidiasis. Mites of the genera *Tyroglyphus* and *Glyciphagus* (0.4–0.5 mm) can cause lesions in warehouse personnel and grocers. *Pyemotes ventricosus* (0.16–0.22 mm) is also an occasional parasite.

Clinical characteristics and course

Animal pseudoscabies (animal scabies) is characterized by small erythematopomphoid or erythematopapular lesions, sometimes with a small vesicle or pustule. The lesions cause severe itching. They are present on exposed parts of the skin or on the edge of tight-fitting garments. The absence of cuniculi is an essential feature in the differential diagnosis with scabies. Contagion may be direct or indirect, e.g. clothing, seats. The symptoms appear rapidly after contact with the acari. The infection heals promptly once contact with the affected animals is interrupted or when these are suitably treated, but reappear every time the patient comes into contact again with the affected animals. The bite of gamasid mites of the genera *Ornithonyssus* (*O. bacoti* 0.8–1.4 mm) and *Dermanyssus gallinae*, a parasite of poultry, birds and mice, causes intense itching and numerous, often haemorrhagic, papulae in man.

Diagnosis

The history is important including factors such as the presence of animals, the patient's profession and the presence of other affected persons in the same family. The lesions are rather characteristic and very itchy. It is usually difficult to demonstrate the responsible acari in the cutaneous lesions. Infestation by *Tyrogliphus* and *Pyemotes* and other environmental mites is associated with multiple or very numerous lesions, preceded by intense itching.

Differential diagnosis

- Human scabies.
- Papular urticaria.
- Prurigo.
- Lichen planus.
- Dermatitis herpetiformis.
- Toxicodermatitis.

Treatment

General therapeutic guidelines

It is not strictly necessary to treat animal scabies because the dermatosis heals spontaneously when contact with the affected animal ceases.

In the case of mite infestation, repellents such as dimethylphthalate, diethyltoluamide, benzylbenzoate and permethrin can be used also to impregnate clothing. Sprays containing pyrethroids, malathion or Propoxur may be employed.

Recommended therapies

In many cases the use of an acaricide is helpful:

- Polysulphide creams and pastes.
- Benzylbenzoate.
- Gamma hexane (not available in some countries).
- Permethrin.
- Soapy baths are useful in infestation by gamasid acari. Oral antihistamines will mitigate itching. Bedding, arm chairs and chairs, for example, should be disinfested with gamma hexane or malathion powder. The use of DDT is inadvisable. New very active molecules are Cifluthrin and Transfluthrin (Propoxur). Antibiotics are given in the case of superimposed bacterial infections. Topical or systemic corticoids are useful in the case of intense itching or infiltrated and refractory lesions. Polysulphides are effective against the acari.

Further reading

Alexander JO. *Arthropods and Human Skin*. Berlin: Springer Verlag, 1984.

Grob M, Dorn K, Lautenschlager S. Grain mites. A small epidemic caused by *Pyemotes* species. *Hautarzt* 1998; 49: 838–43.

Leigheb G. *Terapia Galenica in Dermatologia*. Rome: Lombardo Edit, 1987.

Lucky AW, Sayers C, Argus JD, Lucky A. Avian mite bites acquired from a new source—pet gerbils. Report of 2 cases and review of the literature. *Arch Dermatol* 2001; 137: 167–70.

Paradis M. Mite dermatitis caused by *Cheyletiella blakei*. *J Am Acad Dermatol* 1998; 38: 1014–15.

Taplin D, Meinkig TL. Pyrethrins and pyrethroids in dermatology. *Arch Dermatol* 1990; 126: 213–21.

Uesugi Y, Aiba S, Suetake T, Tagami H. Multiple infestations with avian mites within a family. *Int J Dermatol* 1994; 33: 566–7.

Molluscum contagiosum

M.V. Milinković and
L.M. Medenica

Definition and epidemiology

Molluscum contagiosum (MC) is a benign, self-limited viral disease of the skin and mucous membranes caused by the MC virus (MCV). The disease mainly affects children, sexually active adults and immunocompromised individuals.

MC is primarily a disorder of children, with peak incidence at 10–12 years of age. In the sexually active population the greatest number of cases occurred among patients 20–29 years old, and affected women are younger than affected men. Published data estimate the incidence of MC to be between 1.2% and 22% of the population worldwide. The prevalence of MC among human immunodeficiency virus (HIV)-infected individuals ranges from 5% to 18%.

Several routes of transmission are recognized for MC. Viral transmission in children occurs by close contact with infected individuals or with fomites, or by autoinoculation. The possibility of sexual abuse should be considered when MC is seen on the genital, perianal and surrounding skin of children, even though the vast majority acquire infection by casual contacts. Infectivity is enhanced in warm, humid, crowded environments. Use of swimming pools also correlates with childhood infection. In adults, MC is most often sexually transmitted. It has also been reported in isolated cases among wrestlers, masseurs and surgeons.

MC is associated with several diseases with impaired cell-mediated immunity including atopic dermatitis, epidermodysplasia verruciformis and HIV infection. Unusually disseminated MC has been reported in patients with sarcoidosis, chronic lymphocytic leukaemia, patients on immunosuppressive therapy and with HIV disease, suggesting that cell-mediated immunity is significant in the control and elimination of the infection.

Aetiology and pathophysiology

MCV is a double-stranded DNA poxvirus which cannot be grown in tissue culture cells nor in an animal model. It is the largest true human virus infecting only human beings. It replicates in the cytoplasm of infected cells and induces hyperplasia.

Three different MCV subtypes have been identified: MCV type I, MCV type II and MCV type III. Lesions produced by either of the subtypes are indistinguishable. Type I is more prevalent than the others, accounting for more than 75% of lesions.

The pathogenesis of the lesions is uncertain, but an epidermal growth-like polypeptide has been postulated to have a role. In the basal layer of lesional skin, the rate of cell division is twice that of normal skin. The number of receptors for epidermal growth factor (EGF) increases in infected cells, which is indirect evidence that MCV synthesizes an EGF-like growth factor. The infected keratinocytes move more quickly through the epidermis than uninfected keratinocytes. Free virus cores have been found in all layers of the epidermis.

Although the role of humoral immunity in these disorders is not clear, dependence on the presence of viral antigen in infected cells, virus-specific antibodies, can be detected in 73% of patients with MC. Most patients infected with MCV produce antibodies predominantly of the immunoglobulin (IgG) class. Anticellular IgM antibodies and fibrillar anticellular IgM antibodies can be found in over 60% of infected patients. Cell-mediated immunity is probably more important in the pathogenesis of the disease.

Clinical characteristics and course

The incubation period is in the range of 7 days to 6 months. The typical lesion is a shiny, pearly white, hemispherical papule with central umbilication and an average diameter of 3–5 mm. Giant lesions may be as large as 3 cm in diameter. The lesions may be flesh-coloured, white, translucent or light yellow in colour. The number of lesions is usually less than 20, although several hundred can be seen. There may be a surrounding eczematous reaction (so-called 'molluscum dermatitis'). Patients with MC are usually asymptomatic, but a few may complain of pruritus or tenderness.

In children, lesions are distributed on the face, trunk and extremities, although the anogenital region may be also involved. In healthy adults, lesions are usually located on the genital region and on the lower abdomen. The disease also appears on the oral mucosa, rarely involving conjuctiva and cornea.

MC is a common viral disorder associated with HIV infection; its clinical features are often atypical, and its course is usually progressive and recalcitrant to treatment. The lesions most often involve the face, neck and trunk.

In immunocompetent patients MC is a benign disorder that resolves spontaneously within 6–8 months, although it may persist as long as 5 years. No individual lesion persists for more than 2 months. Temporary remission of up to 2 months has occurred. Disseminated lesions, as seen in immunocompromised patients, are persistent and recurrent, and they may be a marker of advanced disease.

Diagnosis—laboratory examinations

Diagnosis of MC is usually made relatively easily on the basis of clinical presentation. Rapid freezing with ethyl chloride or liquid nitrogen may accentuate their distinctive umbilication. Direct light microscopic examination of an unstained expressed core, skin biopsy or ultrastructural studies of the lesional skin establishes the diagnosis. Histopathological examination reveals a hyperplastic, cup-shaped invagination of the epidermis composed of multiple lobules. Characteristic intracytoplasmic inclusion bodies, molluscum bodies, are formed.

Differential diagnosis

The differential diagnosis includes: basal cell carcinoma, hystiocytoma, trichoepithelioma, keratoacanthoma, intradermal naevus, syringoma, hidrocystoma, sebaceous adenoma, warts, varicella, pyoderma, papillomas, lichen planus, Darier's disease and dermatitis herpetiformis.

In HIV-infected patients MC must be differentiated from basal cell carcinoma, keratoacanthoma and cutaneous horn. Conversely, in patients with acquired immune deficiency syndrome (AIDS) cryptococcosis and histoplasmosis may mimic MC; for these reasons biopsy of atypical appearing cutaneous lesions is often warranted.

Treatment

There is no specific treatment for MC.

General therapeutic guidelines

- The main question, as with warts, is whether to treat or not. In many cases lesions resolve spontaneously within 8 months without scarring. The decision is crucial and must take into account that MC is a benign, self-limited condition and that treatment is far from being perfect.
- Care should be taken not to traumatize patients unnecessarily with painful treatments, particularly children, who are the largest patient group. Benign neglect may be the most appropriate approach in immunocompetent children with the infection.
- Although MC may be self-limited and asymptomatic in healthy individuals,

therapy is warranted to prevent autoinoculation or transmission of the virus to close contacts, to relieve symptoms (if any) and, often, for cosmetic considerations.

- Treatment method should be chosen after consideration of the age and immunocompetence of the patient, the extent of the disease and the areas involved.
- Patients should be advised to avoid swimming pools, communal baths, contact sports and shared towels, until clear.
- In general, treatment has focused on removing the cutaneous lesions either by surgery or by producing epidermal injury and subsequent desquamation of the molluscum and surrounding uninvolved skin.
- Sexual partners should be examined and treated, to prevent reinoculation.

Recommended therapies (Fig. 1)

Mechanical methods—curettage

Curettage is relatively painless and an easy to perform procedure. It should be performed if the lesions are young and small in number. A sharp curette is used to scrape the lesion. In children, pretreatment with topical anaesthetic, such as the eutectic mixture of local anaesthetics lidocaine (lignocaine) and prilocaine (EMLA cream) may be necessary. One hour before the treatment, a maximum of 10 g of EMLA cream should be applied to the mollusca. One gram of the cream is sufficient to cover a skin area of approximately 2.5×2.5 cm. The cream is covered with an occlusive dressing (Tegaderm) and after 60 min it is wiped off. The curettage usually commences within 5 min after the cream has been wiped off. Local reactions to the cream could include redness, pallor and oedema.

Other simple mechanical methods like expression of the contents of the papule by squeezing it with forceps held parallel to the skin surface, superficial curettage or shaving off the lesion with a sharpened wooden spatula, may suffice, although it is usual to apply a caustic agent, such as silver nitrate stick, phenol, podophyllin or strong iodine solution.

Cryotherapy with liquid nitrogen

Cryosurgery can be completed with specially designed liquid nitrogen spray or with cotton-tipped swabs (dipstick technique). It is less painful and it is not necessary to use local anaesthetics. The lesion and a narrow border of normal surrounding skin should turn white before application is stopped. This usually takes only a few seconds. Destruction of the molluscum body (white, smooth, walled core) will result in resolution of an individual lesion. The treatment should be repeated at weekly intervals if lesions persist. Cryotherapy, though effective at controlling the problem, is also uncomfortable and often requires many weekly treatment sessions.

Electrodesiccation

Electrosurgical destruction by electrodesiccation can be done with little, if any, scarring. Small lesions may be treated without anaesthetic. Subepidermal local anaesthesia is required for big ones. The lesions should be prepared with a non-alcohol-containing skin cleanser. The electrode is brought into contact with the mollusca. Only a low spark should be generated in order to minimize excessive tissue destruction and to avoid scarring. The lesion usually changes in colour and consistency as it is destroyed. It can be easily removed with a curette or simply by rubbing the site with gauze. Punctate bleeding can be controlled with pressure, spot electrocoagulation or topical haemostatic agents such as aluminium chloride.

Chemical agents

Cantharidin

Cantharidin is an extract from the blister beetle. It is a protein phosphatase inhibitor that penetrates the epidermis and induces vesiculation through acantholysis. Cantharidin is available in a collodion-type vehicle. It should be used by precise application of a small amount to each lesion using a pointed stick (a toothpick) with treatment of a maximum of 20 lesions per visit. The patient should be immobilized for 3–5 min until the medication has completely dried to restrict the blistering agent to the lesions. Occlusion should only be used on lesions not responding to uncovered applications. When occlusive tape is used, it is mandatory to ensure complete drying before applying the tape. Patients are

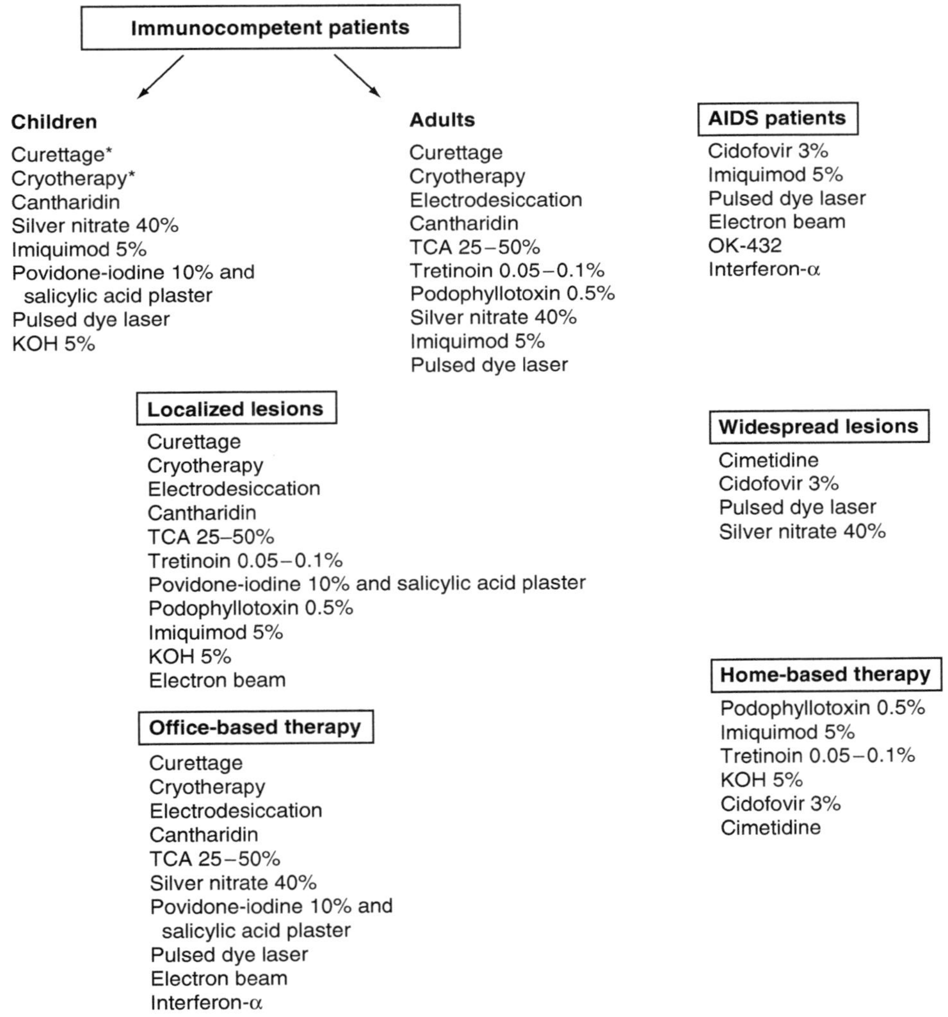

Figure 1 Molluscum contagiosum—therapeutic guidelines. *Pretreatment with topical anaesthetic

instructed to rinse the treated areas with water after 4–6 h. Usually between two and four such treatments, with a 7-day interval, are required to eradicate molluscum lesions.

Application of cantharidin is very effective in children. It has the advantage of being a painless office procedure. However, it may cause significant local irritation with blister formation several hours later, depending on the quantity applied, the duration of application and the individual patient's sensitivity. Testing it on a few lesions at the initial office visit before treating all lesions is recommended. Residual erythema and depigmentation can occur temporarily, but scarring is absent.

Trichloroacetic acid (TCA)

Application of 50% TCA with cotton-tipped swabs often causes sufficient destruction to cure these lesions. The solution should be applied to individual papular lesions for a few seconds until they turn white. This causes a burning sensation that lasts a few minutes. The white treated papules will slowly form crusts and heal within 10 days.

A TCA peel 25–50% is a useful adjuvant therapy in the treatment of extensive MC in immunocompromised patients. MC lesions are typically recalcitrant to therapy in HIV-infected persons. First of all, a test site measuring 2.5×2.5 cm and including the greatest density of lesions on the face, should be chosen to determine the most effective concentration of TCA. Serial peeling of the same test site is performed at 2–3 week intervals to determine the lowest effective concentration of TCA (25, 30, 35, 40 or 50%). After that, full or partial peels should be performed every 2–3 weeks. The concentration of TCA is usually 25–35%. There is no superinfection, delayed healing or scarring.

Topical vitamin A acid (tretinoin)

Successful therapy with topical vitamin A acid has been described in patients with genital lesions. Twice daily application of 0.1% or 0.05% tretinoin cream or nightly in the highest tolerated concentration is proposed. The mechanism of action of vitamin A may relate to its ability to produce marked inflammatory reaction of the skin. Local irritation is common. It is not recommended to be used in children.

Silver nitrate paste

Widespread, small MC lesions, as often seen in atopic children, can be successfully treated with 40% silver nitrate paste. It is as effective as the aqueous solution, but does not run on to normal skin causing irritation. With a blunt toothpick, a small amount of the paste is dabbed on the centre of each lesion which gradually spreads to the entire lesion. Within 1 day, black crusts form. After 2 weeks MCs drop off the skin. Lesions heal without leaving scars. It has a high cure rate, it is painless in most cases and is cost-effective.

Povidone-iodine solution and salicylic acid plaster

Ten per cent povidone-iodine solution and 50% salicylic acid plaster is recommended for (a) children and patients with multiple lesions as it is not painful; (b) diabetic patients as the infection is less frequent; and (c) for use in the dermatology office without equipment for liquid nitrogen therapy, therefore being less expensive.

The combined treatment is much more successful and shorter in duration than 10% iodine solution or 50% salicylic acid plaster alone. The procedure is performed once daily. The 10% iodine solution is applied and left to dry. The 50% salicylic acid plaster is cut into small pieces and patched onto the lesions, covering the area with micropore sticking tape. When the lesion becomes reddened, usually in 3–7 days, it is sufficient to apply only iodine solution until the lesion becomes flat. If necessary, the whole procedure can be repeated. The inflammatory sign (erythema) appears after 3–7 days. However, the more marked the erythema after the application, the more quickly the lesions disappear.

Podophyllotoxin cream

Podophyllotoxin cream as a 0.5% preparation is a safe, home-based first line of therapy for curing MC. It is easily self-administeredtwice daily for 3 consecutive days. If total elimination is not achieved with one trial (6 topical applications), the same treatment can be extended to 3 more weeks (24 topical applications), when 95% of lesions are cured. Tolerable moderate to mild frequent side-effects are erythema and pruritus.

Imiquimod cream

Imiquimod, 1-(2-methylprolyl)-1H-imidazo(4,5-c)quinolin-4-amine, is an immune response modifier capable of inducing high levels of interferon (IFN)-α, a potent antiviral agent, localized to the site of skin application. Patients are instructed to apply imiquimod 5% cream on each lesion with a cotton-tipped applicator before bedtime, 3–5 days per week, for up to 16 weeks, and to wash the areas in the morning. Adverse reactions—erythema, erosions and postinflammatory hyperpigmentation—are limited to application sites and are tolerable. Imiquimod cream is suitable and safe for both children and adults. It appeared to be the most efficacious in patients with HIV-1 disease and in the genital area in immunocompetent adults.

Alternative and experimental treatments

Topical agents

Potassium hydroxide solution (KOH)

Five per cent KOH aqueous solution may be an effective and inexpensive alternative for the management of MC in children. It is based on its property of dissolving epithelial compounds. Parents are instructed to apply a small amount of the solution twice daily with cotton swabs to all lesions for 6 weeks. The stinging sensation is absent or minimal. Even perivaginal and perianal lesions can be treated the same way. A 5% KOH solution proved to be as effective and less irritating when compared to the 10% KOH solution.

Cidofovir

Cidofovir is a potent nucleoside analogue of deoxycytidine monophosphate that has antiviral activity against a broad range of DNA viruses, when applied topically or administrated by intralesional injection. No significant systemic side-effects have been noted, although application site reactions are common and can occasionally be severe. Successful use of topical 3% cidofovir in a combination vehicle (Dermovan), once a day, 5 days a week for 2–8 weeks, in the treatment of recalcitrant MC in children and adults with AIDS, have been reported.

Nitric oxide (NO)

NO has been shown to have antiviral effects in DNA, RNA, enveloped and encapsidated viruses. Topical acidified nitrite cream is an NO-liberating cream. It is shown to be an effective treatment for MC. Five per cent sodium nitrite coapplied with 5% salicylic acid, once a day for 3 months, is recommended. The treatment is time-consuming and can provoke local irritation.

Systemic agents

Griseofulvin

This can be used orally for 4–6 weeks, at dosages of 500 mg daily to patients over 14 years of age, and 250 mg to younger ones. No recurrence was seen in the 6–8-month follow-up period.

Cimetidine
Cimetidine, a histamine (H_2) receptor antagonist with potent immunomodulatory effects, appears to offer a safe alternative form of therapy for multiple, widespread lesions of MC, particularly in atopic patients. It is started at a dosage of 40 mg/kg per day orally in 3–4 divided doses. A 2–3-month course may be safe and cost-effective.

Intralesional agents

Topical injection of OK-432
OK-432 (penicillin-treated and heat-treated lyophilized powder by a substrain of *Streptococcus pyogenes* A) was expected to be effective for immunosuppression. The skin lesions disappeared almost completely within 3 months.

Intralesional IFN-α
This has been used to treat recalcitrant MC. Each lesion was injected with one megaunit of IFN-α weekly for 4 weeks. Molluscum less than 0.5 cm in diameter and those in patients without AIDS are more likely to respond.

Other agents

Pulsed dye laser
Pulsed dye laser treatment may offer another therapeutic modality that is effective, quick and safe in the treatment of widespread and recurrent MC. The lesions are treated by double-pulsing them with a 585-nm pulsed dye laser with a pulse duration of 450 fs at 1 Hz (one pulse per second). Two spot sizes are usually used (to match the diameter of the lesions): 3 mm at fluences of 7.0–8.0 J/cm^2 and 5 mm at fluences of 6.8–7.2 J/cm^2. The lesions could be quickly treated at the rate of one every 2 s. The laser is generally non-scarring and produces a brief snapping sensation on the skin. Because of a possibility of viral particles in the laser plume, a smoke filtration system is utilized.

Electron beam therapy
The use of electron beam radiation is a promising alternative treatment for patients with localized MC lesions. It is administered by using megaelectron voltage (9 or 12 MeV) electron beam energy, five times per week for up to 18 treatments per site. The daily proposed radiation dose is 180 cGy (face and neck) or 200 cGy (body). Response to irradiation is rapid and complete. Mild skin erythema is the only reported side-effect.

Further reading

Barba AR, Kapoor S, Berman B. An open label safety study of topical imiquimod 5% cream in the treatment of molluscum contagiosum in children. *Dermatol Online J* 2001; 7 (1): 20.

Diven DG. An overview of poxviruses. *J Am Acad Dermatol* 2001; 44: 1–14.

Garrett SJ, Robinson JK, Roenigk HH. Trichloroacetic acid peel of molluscum contagiosum in immunocompromised patients. *J Dermatol Surg Oncol* 1992; 18: 855–8.

Hengge UR, Esser S, Schultewolter T *et al.* Self-administered topical 5% imiquimod for the treatment of common warts and molluscum contagiosum. *Br J Dermatol* 2000; 143: 1026–31.

Hughes PSH. Treatment of molluscum contagiosum with the 585-nm pulsed dye laser. *Dermatol Surg* 1998; 24: 229–30.

Inui S, Asada H, Yoshikawa K. Successful treatment of molluscum contagiosum in the immunosuppressed adult with topical injection of streptococcal preparation OK-432. *J Dermatol* 1996; 23: 628–30.

Katsambas A. Quality of life in dermatology and the European Academy of Dermatology. *JEADV* 1994; 3: 211–14.

Lewis EJ, Lam M, Crutchfield CE III. An update on molluscum contagiosum. *Cutis* 1997; 60: 29–34.

Liota E, Smith KJ, Buckley R *et al.* Imiquimod therapy for molluscum contagiosum. *J Cutan Med Surg* 2000; 4: 76–82.

Nelson MR, Chard S, Barton SE. Intralesional interferon for the treatment of recalcitrant molluscum contagiosum in HIV antibody positive individuals—a preliminary report. *Int J STD AIDS* 1995; 6: 351–2.

Niizeki K, Hashimoto K. Treatment of molluscum cotagiosum with silver nitrate paste. *Pediatr Dermatol* 1999; 16: 395–7.

Ohkuma M. Molluscum contagiosum treated with iodine solution and salicylic acid plaster. *Int J Dermatol* 1990; 29: 443–5.

Ordoukhanian E. Warts and molluscum contagiosum. Beware of treatments worse than the disease. *Postgrad Med* 1997; 101: 223–33.

Ormerod AD, White MI, Shah SAA *et al*. Molluscum contagiosum effectively treated with a topical acidified nitrite, nitric oxide liberation cream. *Br J Dermatol* 1999; 141: 1051–3.

Romiti R, Ribeiro AP, Romiti N. Evaluation of the effectiveness of 5% potassium hydroxide for the treatment of molluscum contagiosum. *Pediatr Dermatol* 2000; 17: 495.

Scolaro MJ, Gordon P. Electron-beam therapy for AIDS-related molluscum contagiosum lesions: preliminary experience. *Radiology* 1999; 210: 479–82.

Sharma AK. Cimetidine therapy for multiple molluscum cotagiosum lesions. *Dermatology* 1998; 197: 194–5.

Silverberg NB, Sidbury R, Mancini AJ. Childhood molluscum contagiosum: Experience with cantharidin therapy in 300 patients. *J Am Acad Dermatol* 2000; 43: 503–7.

Singh OP, Kanwar AJ. Griseofulvin therapy in molluscum contagiosum. *Arch Dermatol* 1977; 113: 1615.

Syed TA, Lundin S, Ahmad M. Topical 0.3% and 0.5% podophillotoxin cream for self-treatment of molluscum contagiosum in males. *Dermatology* 1994; 189: 65–8.

Toro JR, Wood LV, Patel NK *et al*. Topical cidofovir. *Arch Dermatol* 2000; 136: 983–5.

Zabawski EJ Jr. A review of topical and intralesional cidofovir. *Dermatol Online J* 2000; 6 (1): 3.

Morphoea: circumscribed scleroderma

U.-F. Haustein

Definition and epidemiology

Morphoea is a disorder of localized sclerosis of the skin. Its cause is unknown. The condition can be subdivided clinically into the following types:

- plaque-like (single/multiple lesions)
- small macules (guttate, lichen sclerosus like, erythematous-atrophic Pasini–Pierini disease)
- linear (band-like at extremities) (disabling)
- frontoparietal (en coup de sabre, hemiatrophia progressiva faciei)
- generalized large plaques
- disabling pansclerotic (deep involvement with nodules and fixation of underlying tissue)
- localized nodular–subcutaneous.

It affects females three times more than males at all ages with the peak being between 20 and 40 years.

Aetiology and pathophysiology

Histology and histochemistry of the skin are similar to systemic sclerosis. Collagen type I is increased on the protein and the mRNA expression level as well due to enhanced synthesis by fibroblasts. Oedematous swelling and discrete perivascular lymphocytic infiltrates precede fibrosis with thickened dense collagen fibres. Associations with *Borrelia* infection are rather accidental than causative. The same is with other infections, trauma, menopause and pregnancy.

Clinical characteristics and course

Round or oval plaques are characterized as indurated areas of faintly purplish colour, later in the course they are waxy and ivory-coloured with a lilac ring at the periphery. Sometimes multiple plaques occur, occasionally with deep involvement. Guttate lesions resemble lichen sclerosis (white spot disease). Linear lesions are usually single and unilateral; the legs are more frequently affected than the arms. This form may rarely involve the subcutaneous fat tissue, fascia, underlying muscle, nerves and bone leading to severe disabling deformities. The generalized type can markedly involve the chest wall leading to constriction of the thorax.

Within months to years, plaques tend to soften leaving hyperpigmentation, which may persist for a long time.

Diagnosis—laboratory examinations

Skin biopsy is the only significant examination, but usually not necessary. Anti-single-stranded (ss) DNA antibodies can be found in children with linear morphoea and in the generalized type. In some geographical areas diagnostics of associated *Borrelia* infection is recommended.

Differential diagnosis

- Vitiligo: depigmented macules.
- Anetoderma: macular atrophy.
- Lichen sclerosus et atrophicus: follicular hyperkeratosis, destruction of elastic fibres.
- Polyarteritis nodosa: minimal induration, reticulate lilac lesions (livedo racemosa).
- Scleroderma adultorum (Buschke's disease): acute onset, postinfectious event.
- Atrophoderma idiopathica et progressiva (Pierini–Pasini disease): benign atrophy without sclerosis, coexistence with morphoea observed.
- Pseudoscleroderma: after injections of vitamin K, bleomycin, pentazocin and other drugs.
- Systemic sclerosis versus generalized morphoea (no Raynaud's phenomenon, rare visceral involvement).

Treatment

General therapeutic guidelines

- The natural course of spontaneous resolution can be awaited.
- Active treatment is indicated in cases of progression, generalization and in linear disabling forms.
- At present, no entirely effective treatment is available.

Recommended therapies

- Topical application of mild or moderate glucocorticosteroid solutions or creams can inhibit the inflammatory process (e.g. hydrocortisone, mometason furoate prednicarbate). Infiltration of triamcinolone acetonide 0.1–0.3 mL (5–10 mg/mL) into the lesion is difficult to perform. If softening occurs injections every 3–4 weeks can be done more easily. Beware atrophy.
- Physiotherapy in the form of massage, ultrasound daily for 15 min.
- In linear forms active and passive stretching exercises of the extremities may increase mobility; in addition, use lymph drainage or underwater massage.
- Infusions with penicillin G, 10 million IU per day within 30 min for 14 days showed beneficial results in our hands. This can be repeated after 3 months. Alternatives are erythromycin (2 × 500 mg/day), cephalosporins (2 × 500 mg/day), doxycycline (2 × 100 mg/day) and tetracycline (2 × 500 mg/day) for 2–3 weeks.
- A moderate dose of systemic glucocorticosteroid (30–40 mg/day) may help control inflammation during the early stages. It should be gradually reduced to zero within 3–6 weeks.
- Psoralen and ultraviolet A (PUVA) bath photochemotherapy enhances collagenase activity of fibroblasts and improves skin sclerosis, in particular in generalized morphoea.
- UVA_1 high-dose therapy not only depletes skin-infiltrating T cells through the induction of apoptosis, but it also upregulates the expression of matrix metalloproteinase-1 (collagenase-1). UVA_1 phototherapy treated skin lesions were markedly softened after 9–29 exposures.

Alternative treatment

- Penicillamine (150–600 mg/day in gradually increasing doses) takes a

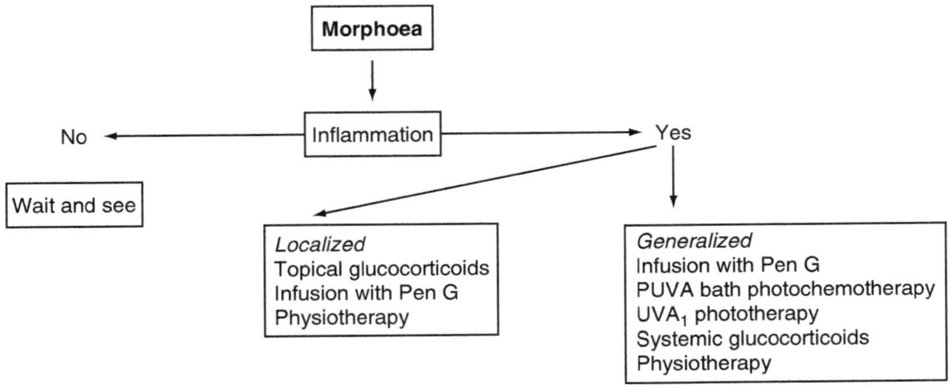

long time and it has a high risk of side-effects. It can no longer be recommended, even in generalized and pansclerotic types, even more so because recently it has been shown that high-dose therapy (750–1000 mg/day) is not superior to low-dose therapy (125 mg every other day) and similar to placebo in systemic sclerosis.

- Controlled studies for phenytoin, sulfasalazine, antimalarials and etretinate do not exist.
- Plastic surgery may be helpful in individual cases with scarring and contractures.

Further reading

Clements PJ, Furst DE, Wong W-K *et al.* High-dose versus low-dose D-penicillamine in early diffuse systemic sclerosis. *Arthritis Rheum* 1999; 42: 1194–203.

Kerscher M, Meurer M, Sander C *et al.* PUVA bath photochemotherapy for localized scleroderma. *Arch Dermatol* 1996; 132: 1280–2.

Stege H, Bernburg M, Humke S *et al.* High-dose UVA_1 radiation therapy for localized scleroderma. *J Am Acad Dermatol* 1997; 36: 939–44.

Ghersetich I, Matucci-Cerinic M, Lotti T. A pathogenetic approach to the management of systemic sclerosis (scleroderma). *Int J Dermatol* 1990; 29 (9): 616–22.

Ghersetich I, Teofoli P, Benci M, Innocenti S, Lotti T. Localized scleroderma. *Clin Dermatol* 1994; 12: 230–92.

Naevi (benign melanocytic)

N.G. Stavrianeas and A.C. Katoulis

Synonyms

Melanocytic naevocellular naevi, pigmented naevi, benign melanocytic tumours or lesions, 'moles'.

Definition and general considerations

Melanocytic naevi (MN) are benign tumours clinically appearing as well-circumscribed pigmented lesions and histologically consisting of naevus cells.

Naevus cells are derived from the neural crest. Through a process of maturation and downward migration type A epidermal naevus cells (epithelioid) evolve into type B (lymphocytoid) and then into type C (neuroid) dermal naevus cells. The following morphological features differentiate naevus cells from melanocytes:

- absence of dendrites
- arrangement in cell nests
- larger size
- more abundant cytoplasm containing coarse granules
- location in the epidermis and/or in the dermis, and rarely in the subcutis.

It has been suggested that naevus cells represent the final stage of evolution of a neural crest precursor cell, the naevoblast. On the other hand, some authorities believe that differences between naevocytes and melanocytes are secondary adjustments and that both these cells originate from the melanoblast.

Acquired MN are believed to have been developed from epidermal melanocytes that have completed their migration from the neural crest to the dermoepidermal junction in fetal life or to arise from dermal melanocytes that have become arrested in the dermis during fetal migration and have never reached their normal site.

MN are classified into:

- common acquired MN
- congenital MN
- halo naevus
- naevus spilus
- Spitz spindle cell naevus
- blue naevus
- dysplastic MN
- dermal MN.

Common acquired MN

Synonyms

Acquired melanocytic naevocellular naevi, moles.

Definition and epidemiology

Common acquired MN (CAMN) are small (< 1 cm), well-circumscribed, pigmented lesions that are composed of naevus cells. Depending on the location of the groups of naevocytes, CAMN are subdivided into junctional (cells at the dermoepidermal junction above the basement membrane), dermal (cells exclusively in the dermis) and compound naevi (cells in both the epidermis and the dermis).

Caucasians, especially those with lighter skin colour, have a greater prevalence of CAMN than black people or Asians, who have more naevi on the palms/soles and nail beds. Both sexes are equally affected. The number of CAMN increases with age, reaching a peak during adolescence and early adulthood. Thereafter, they may undergo involution. Increased number of CAMN has been observed among members of the same family. A strong positive correlation between sun exposure and number of naevi has been documented.

Aetiology and pathogenesis

Naevus cells are thought to derive either from naevoblasts or from melanoblasts, which migrate from the neural crest to the epidermis. Junctional naevi result from the proliferation of naevus cells within the epidermis. Migration and proliferation of naevus cells into the dermis give rise to compound naevi, or to dermal naevi when no residual cells are found in the epidermis. It is believed that the three types of CAMN represent sequential developmental stages of their life history (evolution from junctional naevus to compound, then to dermal, and finally involution with fibrosis).

Genetic and environmental factors (e.g. solar radiation) seem to play a pathogenetic role.

Clinical characteristics and course

CAMN are asymptomatic, well-defined, round to oval lesions, smaller than 1 cm in diameter, with regular or slightly irregular borders and uniformly distributed colour, usually shades of brown and black. They may occur anywhere on the body. Junctional naevi appear as macular hairless lesions, medium to dark brown in colour, most commonly located on the trunk, the upper extremities, or the face (sun-exposed areas). Compound naevi are variably elevated papular lesions with smooth or slightly warty surface and dark brown to black coloration. Bristle-like terminal hair may be present. The face is the most frequent site. Dermal naevi are papular or nodular, dome-shaped or, occasionally, papillomatous or pedunculated lesions. They are skin-coloured to light brown in colour. Telangiectasias are often present. They are usually located on the face, neck or trunk. CAMN of the nail bed present as brown longitudinal bands (melanonychia striata) with regular distinct margins and uniform pigmentation.

CAMN tend to remain unchanged in colour and in shape. Increase in size and in pigmentation may occur at puberty or during pregnancy. Although most of CAMN appear in childhood and adolescence, few may appear later in adult life and most of them disappear spontaneously with progressive age. CAMN have a very low malignant potential. However, the association of CAMN with cutaneous malignant melanoma (CMM) is well established. Histological studies have shown that one-third of CMMs are associated with naevus remnants. In addition, increased numbers of CAMN is a risk factor for CMM.

Diagnosis

Diagnosis is mostly clinical. Evaluation of the patient should include:

- personal and family history for CMM or dysplastic naevi
- total body examination (presence and number of CAMN or dysplastic naevi), which can be assisted by side-lighting or epiluminescence microscopy.

In difficult cases, excisional biopsy and histological examination can document diagnosis (naevus cells arranged in clusters in the epidermis and/or in the dermis).

According to our observations, recently heavily sun-exposed CAMN may develop histological features that simulate a dysplastic naevus or an *in situ* melanoma.

Differential diagnosis

Macular pigmented lesion:

- freckle, solar lentigine
- lentigo simplex
- lentigo maligna
- pigmented actinic keratosis.

Papular pigmented lesion:

- seborrhoeic keratosis
- dermatofibroma
- neurobifroma
- epidermal naevus
- Spitz naevus

- blue naevus
- dysplastic naevus (larger size; asymmetry; not well-defined, irregular border; red, blue, white, grey and black hues)
- trichoepithelioma
- pigmented basal cell carcinoma
- nodular melanoma.

Treatment

General therapeutic guidelines

For CAMN no treatment is necessary. There is no reason to remove CAMN on a routine basis, although it is not contraindicated, should removal be thought necessary. However, it has yet to be clarified if manipulations, such as plucking hair from a mole, or trauma may result in malignant degeneration.

Recommended therapies

Any suspicious pigmented lesion must be removed completely by excisional biopsy down to the subcutaneous tissue and should be histologically evaluated, often with sectional examination. Reference to specialists is also a good practice.

Indications for excision of a CAMN are the following:

- atypical clinical appearance, suspicious for CMM
- changing lesion, e.g. size has increased or the colour has become variegated or the border has become irregular
- symptomatic lesion, i.e. if pain, pruritus or bleeding is present
- evidence of malignancy detected by epiluminescence microscopy
- sites of repeated irritation, or sites associated with increased risk of CMM, or sites that do not permit self-examination, such as palms, soles, penis, scalp, mucous membranes, anogenital region
- cosmetically disfiguring lesion.

Removal of CAMN should be performed by simple complete excision and closure by sutures. An histological examination should always follow, even when there are no clinical indications for atypicality. Destruction of the lesion by electrocautery, cryotherapy or laser surgery is wisely avoided because these modalities do not allow histological evaluation and do not ensure complete excision. However, after an incomplete surgical excision, the residual macular pigmentation at the scar site can be removed using electrodesiccation or cryotherapy, if atypicality or malignancy has been excluded.

Congenital MN

Synonyms

Congenital naevomelanocytic naevi, giant pigmented naevi, giant hairy naevi, naevus pigmentosus et pilosus, garment naevus, bathing trunk naevus.

Definition and epidemiology

Congenital MN (CMN) are benign pigmented neoplasms composed of naevomelanocytes that are usually present at birth. According to their size, they can be distinguished as small ($<$ 1.5 cm in diameter), intermediate (from 1.5 to 9.9 cm), large (from 10 to 19.9 cm) and giant ($\geq$ 20 cm).

Population-based prevalence of CMN was estimated to be 0.6% to 6%. Large and giant CMN occur in 1 in 20 000 and 1 in 500 000 newborns, respectively. There is no race or sex predilection. Familial tendencies have been described.

Aetiology and pathogenesis

Naevomelanocytes are derived from the neural crest as a result of a developmental defect of melanoblasts. CMN probably develop between the tenth and the twenty-fourth week of gestation.

Clinical characteristics and course

CMN are almost invariably present at birth (birthmarks). Only rarely, they may arise during infancy over a period of weeks (congenital naevus tardive).

Small, intermediate and large CMN appear as slightly elevated, round or oval, well-demarcated, hairy or hairless plaques with uniform light to dark brown coloration and regular or irregular contours. The surface is sometimes pebbly, rugose or coarse. CMN may appear at any site. They are usually solitary. Fewer than 5% are multiple.

Giant CMN present as deeply pigmented, irregularly shaped plaques with focal nodules or papules and coarse terminal dark hair. They cover large areas of the head, trunk or the extremities, often having the distribution of a garment, such as a bathing trunk, a cap, a sleeve or a stocking. Multiple smaller satellite lesions may also be present.

With advancing age, CMN increase proportionally to the anatomical area they occupy. Occasionally, they become darker, or assume a verrucous appearance, or develop a halo. The potential for malignant transformation is well documented for all CMN, regardless of size. Lifetime risk for CMM development is 6.3–12% for giant CMN or 1–5% for small CMN. Histological features of CMN have been found in 8.1% of primary melanoma specimens studied. CMN-associated melanoma usually occurs early in childhood and has a poor prognosis. Rarely, malignant soft-tissue tumours may arise on CMN. Additionally, they can be associated with an involvement of the leptomeninges (neurocutaneous melanosis), and may cause considerable cosmetic and psychic problems.

Diagnosis

Clinical diagnosis based on history and physical examination. Histological examination documents diagnosis (naevomelanocytes arranged in theques in the epidermis and the dermis, which often invade the lower reticular dermis or the subcutaneous fat, the walls of blood and lymphatic vessels, the skin appendages, the nerve fascicles and the arrectores pilorum muscles).

Differential diagnosis

- Common acquired melanocytic naevus
- Naevus spilus
- Dysplastic naevus
- Congenital blue naevus
- Becker's naevus
- Malignant melanoma
- Pigmented epidermal naevus
- Pigmented basal cell carcinoma
- Seborrhoeic keratosis
- Paget's disease with pigmentation.

Treatment

General therapeutic guidelines

All CMN should be considered for prophylactic excision due to the cosmetic disfigurement they produce and, most importantly, due to the potential for CMN development.

Lesions should be monitored clinically with photography on a regular basis for life and patients must seek medical advice when a change in the lesion has occurred.

Recommended therapies

Treatment is individualized depending on age, location, size, appearance and risk for CMM. Excision of small CMN can be delayed until late childhood, because the risk for CMM increases in puberty. On the contrary, giant CMN should be removed as soon as possible due to the high risk for early aggressive CMM. However, excision should be performed after the perinatal period when the risks from general anaesthesia are diminished.

Surgical excision is the only acceptable method. Full-thickness skin graft, swing flaps, tissue expanders or patient's skin grown in tissue culture, may be required. Small and medium size naevi (up to 5 cm in diameter) can be removed in a one-stage procedure with suturing of the wound, local plasty or free-tissue skin graft. Blepharal and central facial lesions are best reconstructed with full-tissue skin grafting. Large naevi (over 5 cm in diameter) mandate a staged excision or removal at one stage with prior use of a tissue expander or presuturing. Giant naevi require staged treatment with the use of an intermediate thickness skin graft.

Alternative and experimental therapies

Partial removal of superficial naevus cells by dermabrasion, laser therapy (Q-switched ruby, Q-switched alexandrite), curettage or shave excision is less traumatic than excision surgery and produces an acceptable cosmetic result. Chemical peeling, e.g. with phenol, is an acceptable alternative method of therapy for those lesions that are too large for excision and primary closure or for lesions in which excision would result in unacceptable scars in areas such as the face. However, none of these techniques completely removes the risk of malignant transformation.

Halo naevus

Synonyms

Leukoderma acquisitum centrifugum, Sutton's naevus, perinaevoid vitiligo.

Definition and epidemiology

Halo naevus (HN) is a melanocytic naevus surrounded by a depigmented zone or halo. The melanocytic naevus, which often undergoes spontaneous involution, may be a common acquired (dermal or compound), congenital or atypical melanocytic naevus, a Spitz naevus or a blue naevus. According to a recent concept, HN should not be regarded as a distinct entity, but as a halo phenomenon occurring in a wide variety of naevus types.

It most commonly affects adolescents and young adults with an overall incidence of 1% in individuals under 20 years of age. Family history is not unusual. Of the patients, 18–26% have vitiligo. Furthermore, it may be a heralding manifestation of vitiligo.

Aetiology and pathogenesis

HN results from an immune response (both humoral and cellular) directed against either antigenically altered naevus cells undergoing dysplastic changes or against non-specifically altered naevus cells in response to various influences. Immune mechanisms have been implicated for the involution of the central naevus. Cytokines may act as mediators for the development of the white halo.

Clinical characteristics and course

HN is composed of a central macule or papule with uniform dark brown to pink colour and regular well-defined border, encircled by a symmetrical round or oval, white or hypopigmented, sharply demarcated annulus. It is usually asymptomatic or slightly pruritic. It is most often located on the trunk, especially on the back. Any site may be affected. In 25–50% of patients, multiple lesions are present.

The halo develops around pre-existing melanocytic naevus within months. The course is variable. Only occasionally HN remains unchanged. More often, the central naevus spontaneously regresses completely, followed by repigmentation of the white halo. This process lasts from months to years. In some cases, a depigmented macule remains, or in others the halo repigments while the central naevus remains unchanged.

Malignant transformation may complicate HN. Occasionally, a depigmented halo may develop around a primary malignant melanoma. In older adults, the sudden appearance of multiple halo naevi has been associated with the development of a primary CMM at another site.

Diagnosis

Diagnosis of HN is easy on the basis of a distinctive clinical presentation. However, it is very important to evaluate clinically central naevus for malignancy because a halo can develop around primary CMM. Family history and total skin examination for HN, dysplastic naevi, vitiligo or CMM, is crucial. To exclude malignancy, histological assessment may be necessary.

Differential diagnosis

Common acquired MN with halo must be differentiated from other pigmented naevi with halo:

- Spitz naevus
- blue naevus
- congenital melanocytic naevus
- dysplastic naevus.

An asymmetrical irregular halo surrounding a large lesion with striking irregularity of colour and notched borders, suggests a halo phenomenon occurring on a primary CMM.

Non-melanocytic lesions with halo could be considered to be:

- dermatofibroma
- seborrhoeic keratosis
- flat warts
- molluscum contagiosum
- lichen planus
- psoriasis
- sarcoidosis.

Treatment

HN with benign appearance does not require excision. The patient should be reassured and followed up periodically. HN with atypical clinical features should be excised for histological examination. Individuals over 40 years old, or with a family history of CMM or dysplastic naevi, should be carefully evaluated for CMM.

Naevus spilus

Synonyms

Speckled lentiginous naevus, zosteriform lentiginous naevus.

Definition and epidemiology

Naevus spilus (NS) is a slightly hyperpigmented macular lesion dotted with darker flat or raised spots.

It is usually acquired in childhood. An incidence of 2–3% among Caucasians has been reported.

Aetiology and pathogenesis

These are similar to that of CAMN. Ultraviolet radiation has no pathogenetic role. Segmental or zosteriform distribution suggests localized malformation.

Clinical characteristics and course

Oval or irregularly shaped, light brown, hairless macule (1–20 cm in diameter) containing scattered dark brown to black macules or papules (2–3 mm in diameter). Large lesion may exhibit a lateral, segmental or zosteriform distribution.

NS persists indefinitely. CMM very rarely may arise in NS.

Diagnosis

The diagnosis is clinical. The macular pigmented lesion exhibits histological features of lentigo simplex, while the spots are usually junctional or compound naevi, or rarely dysplastic or Spitz naevi.

Differential diagnosis

- Congential melanocytic naevus
- Becker's naevus.

Treatment

Risk of CMM development warrants periodic follow-up (with baseline photography), especially for congenital or large lesions. Changing clinical picture or atypical features must be assessed histologically. Complete surgical excision and closure with sutures is required.

Spitz naevus

Synonyms

Spindle and epithelioid cell naevus, Spitz tumour, benign juvenile melanoma, epithelioid cell/spindle cell naevomelanocytic naevus.

Definition and epidemiology

Spitz naevus (SN) is a benign nodular melanocytic naevus with distinctive histopathological features that may be confused with CMM. Perhaps SN and CMM exist along one continuum of disease.

Estimated incidence rate of SN in Australia is 1.4 cases per 100 000. It represents 1% of all surgically excised MN. It is usually acquired. One-third of the patients are under 10 years of age, 36% are between 10 and 20 years and only 31% are over 20 years. No familial distribution has been recognized.

Aetiology and pathogenesis

SN derives from cells originating from the neural crest. No pathogenetic associations have been documented.

Clinical characteristics and course

SN presents as an asymptomatic, well-circumscribed, hairless, dome-shaped or flat papule or nodule, 2 mm to 2 cm in diameter, varying in colour from pink to tan or dark brown. The colour is uniformly distributed. The surface is smooth or verrucous. It is most commonly located on the head and neck. There are cases with multiple or clustered SN. Usually there is a history of sudden onset and rapid growth.

The biological behaviour of SN remains obscure. SN may evolve into conventional compound melanocytic naevus. Some undergo fibrosis, eventually resembling dermatofibromas. Very rarely SN may involute spontaneously. CMM may arise within SN, but this event is uncommon.

Malignant SN is an aggressive variant of SN that results in regional lymph node metastases.

Diagnosis

Clinical picture and recent onset suggest diagnosis. Histological confirmation is always necessary (nests of admixed epithelioid and spindle cells extending from a hyperplastic epidermis into the reticular dermis in an inverted-wedge configuration). Atypical SN is characterized by prominent cellularity and increased mitotic activity. The greater the atypia, the more difficult the differentiation from CMM.

Differential diagnosis

Non-pigmented SN must be differentiated from:

- pyogenic granuloma
- haemangioma
- verruca
- molluscum contagiosum
- dermatofibroma
- mastocytoma
- juvenile xanthogranuloma
- dermal melanocytic naevus.

Pigmented SN may be confused with:

- dysplastic naevus
- cutaneous malignant melanoma.

In order to differentiate SN from CMM, which is rare in childhood, excisional biopsy is warranted to establish the diagnosis.

Treatment

Complete surgical excision of the lesion is recommended (with margins of 5 mm to

1 cm for atypical variants) followed by re-excision of positive margins, if present. Incomplete excision often results in recurrence. Periodic follow-up at 6–12-month intervals is advisable.

Blue naevus

Synonyms
Blue naevus of Jadassohn–Tieche, blue neuronaevus, dermal melanocytoma.

Definition and epidemiology
Blue naevus (BN) is a benign, grey to dark blue, papular or nodular lesion of the skin or mucous membranes, representing a localized proliferation of melanin-producing dermal melanocytes.

BN is usually acquired, appearing in childhood and adolescence. Both sexes are equally affected.

Aetiology and pathogenesis
BN results from ectopic accumulation (in the dermis) of melanin-producing melanocytes, which have migrated from the neural crest during fetal life, but have failed to reach the epidermis. The blue colour is due to the Tyndall effect (brown pigment absorbs longer wavelengths of light and scatters blue light).

Clinical characteristics and course
Three types of BN have been identified:

- Common BN: small (0.5–1.0 cm), well-circumscribed dome-shaped papules or nodules, most commonly located on the dorsa of the hands or feet. Although usually solitary, it may be multiple, clustered or may form a plaque. Malignant transformation does not occur in common BN.
- Cellular BN: blue–grey to black nodule, 1–3 cm or larger, with smooth or irregular surface. Sites of predilection include the buttocks, sacrococcygeal region, scalp, face and feet. Malignant transformation can occur rarely.
- Combined BN: nodular blue–brown to blue–black lesions with smooth surfaces. The face is the most common site. It represents an association of BN with overlying melanocytic naevus.

There are occasional reports of BN in the vagina, cervix, prostate, spermatic cord and lymph nodes.

BN usually remains unchanged or, less often, it regresses. Persons with blue naevi are considered at higher risk for CMM development.

Diagnosis
Clinical findings and epiluminescence microscopy suggest the diagnosis. Histopathological examination confirms diagnosis.

Differential diagnosis
The following skin conditions should be considered:

- dermatofibroma
- sclerosing haemangioma
- vascular lesions (angiokeratoma, venous lake)
- glomus tumour
- apocrine hydrocystoma
- pigmented basal cell carcinoma
- pigmented spindle-cell naevus
- dysplastic naevus
- primary or metastatic malignant melanoma.

Treatment
BN smaller than 1 cm without atypical clinical features does not require excision. On the other hand, *de novo* appearance, or a changing lesion, or multinodular or plaque-like lesions warrants excisional biopsy and histological evaluation. Complete prophylactic excision of cellular type BN should be considered due to its malignant potential. Incomplete excision of BN may be followed by recurrence that is difficult to distinguish from malignant BN.

BN have been successfully treated with the Q-switched ruby laser. Dermal injection of riboflavin and exposure to near-ultraviolet/visible radiation (ribophototherapy) has been tried in blue naevi, which are recalcitrant to laser therapy

Dysplastic melanocytic naevus

Synonyms

Atypical naevus, B-K mole, Clark's melanocytic naevus, naevus with architectural disorder and cytological atypia.

Definition and epidemiology

Dysplastic melanocytic naevus (DMN) is an acquired melanocytic lesion with atypical clinical and histological features, compared to CAMN. DMN occupies an intermediate position in the disease spectrum ranging from common acquired naevi to malignant melanoma. It is considered a potential precursor of CMM and a marker of persons at high risk for CMM. The atypical mole and melanoma syndrome is defined as the presence of a large number (> 50) of MN, some of which have atypical features. It is classified into familial and sporadic, depending on the presence or not of family history of CMM.

DMN are found in 5% of the general white population in the USA and in 1.8–18.0% of various populations. DMN are present in almost all patients with familial CMM and in 30–50% of patients with sporadic CMM. White race is predominantly affected. There are no sex differences. Familial distribution has been identified. Most DMN appear during childhood and adolescence, sometimes by crises. Sporadic lesions may appear at any time in life (as late as the sixth decade).

Aetiology and pathogenesis

For familial DMN, an autosomal dominant mode of inheritance with fairly high penetrance, has been recognized. Multiple loci, including 1p36, 9p21, have been incriminated. A polygenic aetiology has been suggested. Sun exposure, especially a pattern of acute and intermittent exposures, is considered as a precipitating factor for DMN development. However, DMN may occur in completely covered areas of the body. Immunosuppression provides a favourable setting for DMN progression to malignancy. Endocrine, dietary and environmental factors may also play a part.

Clinical characteristics and course

Clinically, DMN are characterized by:

- macular lesion with papular components
- asymmetry
- greatest diameter larger than common acquired naevi, usually ranging between 5 and 15 mm
- irregular and ill-defined border
- flat, pebbled or cobblestone surface. Accentuation of skin markings visible by side-lighting
- irregular pigmentation pattern including shades of brown, tan, flesh, pink and brown–black.
- Erythema may be present within or around the lesion (halo)
- round, oval or ellipsoid shape
- solitary or, more often, multiple (up to hundreds) randomly dispersed lesions, especially in familial cases
- distribution: trunk, arms, legs, dorsa of the hands and feet, buttocks and scalp (exposed and covered areas). Mucosae may be involved
- no symptoms are present.

Unusual clinical subtypes include: fried-egg compound DMN, bull's eye or targetoid variant, lentigo-like or seborrhoeic keratosis-like, erythematous and simulant of melanoma variant.

Although most lesions remain stable or evolve into benign dermal MN, DMN is one of the most important precursor lesions of CMM. Patients with familial or sporadic atypical mole syndrome are at increased risk for CMM. Anatomical association with DMN has been observed in 8–36% of patients with sporadic CMM, in about 70% of patients with familial CMM and in >90% of persons with familial atypical mole and melanoma syndrome.

In the USA, lifetime risk of developing primary CMM was estimated to be 0.8% for the general population. In patients with DMN, the risk for CMM is significantly increased reaching 6% or 10–15%, when family history of CMM is present or not, respectively. CMM risk increases with: increasing number of DMN; increasing atypia; and family history of DMN or CMM. CMM in DMN patients may arise either *de novo* (on normal skin) or within pre-existing DMN, more often during the fourth decade of life.

Diagnosis

Clinical diagnosis may be assisted by dermoscopy or epiluminescence microscopy. Wood's lamp examination accentuates the epidermal hyperpigmentation of the lesion. Histological examination confirms diagnosis.

Differential diagnosis

DMN must be differentiated from:

1 Naevomelanocytic lesions:
   - common acquired naevi
   - small congenital MN
   - pigmented spindle cell naevus
   - naevus spilus
   - Spitz naevus
   - melanoma *in situ*, and especially CMM (greater asymmetry, irregular margins with prominent notching, striking variations of colour, including shades of grey, white and blue–black).

2 Keratinocytic lesions:
   - pigmented seborrhoeic or actinic keratosis
   - pigmented basal cell carcinoma.

Treatment

General therapeutic guidelines

Management depends on the number of DMN, history of CMM and family history of DMN or CMM.

Patients with DMN should be followed up periodically for life. Evaluation should include (a) total skin surface examination; (b) clinical photography (baseline 1:1 Polaroid photographs or total body 35-mm slides); and (c) body charts that are periodically updated. Patients should be warned of the potential hazards of sun exposure and should be educated in methods of protecting themselves and their children. Sun avoidance and use of sunscreens should be encouraged. Sunbathing and tanning parlours must be avoided. Blood relatives should also be examined for DMN and CMM and should be followed up regularly as well.

Clinically atypical naevi do not require excision as a routine procedure. Patients with few lesions must be followed up yearly, or every 6 months if there is a family history of CMM. Patients with numerous lesions should be followed up every 6 months, or every 3 months if there is personal or family history of CMM.

Recommended therapies

Lesions that require excision include:

- all lesions suspicious for CMM
- changing lesions, i.e. increasing in size or changing in pigmentation, in shape and/or in border
- lesions that cannot be easily followed by self-examination (scalp, genitalia, upper back) or if the patient is unreliable for follow-up
- lesions at selected sites, such as palms, soles or nail bed.

Complete surgical excision is the treatment of choice. Initial margins of 5 mm are sufficient. If lesion is atypical or present in margins, excision with clear margins is necessary. If severe atypia is present, re-excision with 5–10-mm margins is recommended. Histological examination, preferably by specialists, to document diagnosis and to exclude malignancy, should always follow.

Lasers, electrosurgery, cryotherapy or other modalities resulting in physical destruction of the lesion, should be avoided,

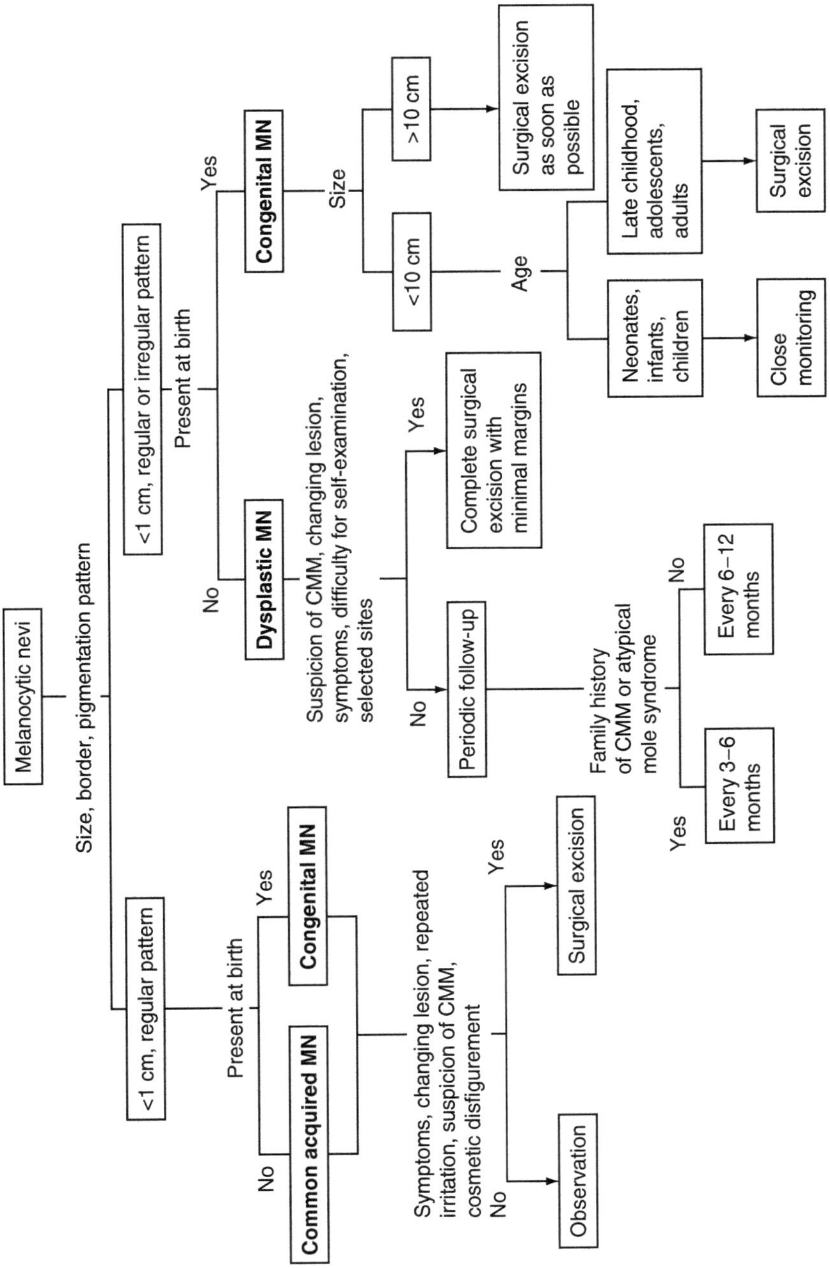
Melanocytic nevi
Size, border, pigmentation pattern
<1 cm, regular pattern
<1 cm, regular or irregular pattern
Present at birth
No
Yes
Common acquired MN
Congenital MN
Symptoms, changing lesion, repeated irritation, suspicion of CMM, cosmetic disfigurement
No
Yes
Observation
Surgical excision
Present at birth
No
Yes
Dysplastic MN
Congenital MN
Suspicion of CMM, changing lesion, symptoms, difficulty for self-examination, selected sites
No
Yes
Periodic follow-up
Complete surgical excision with minimal margins
Family history of CMM or atypical mole syndrome
Yes
No
Every 3–6 months
Every 6–12 months
Size
<10 cm
>10 cm
Surgical excision as soon as possible
Age
Neonates, infants, children
Late childhood, adolescents, adults
Close monitoring
Surgical excision

because they do not permit histopathological examination of the lesion.

Dermal MN

Definition, epidemiology and clinical characteristics

Dermal MN include pigmented lesions consisting of dermal melanocytes, which have never completed their migration from the neural crest to the dermoepidermal junction during fetal life.

Mongolian spot is a congenital, oval or rounded, up to 10 cm in diameter, blue–grey macular lesion, most commonly located on the lumbosacral region. It is found in more than 90% of infants of Asiatic or Amerindian origin, and in about 1% of Caucasoid infants. It almost invariably disappears during early childhood.

Naevus of Ota is a macular lesion consisting of an admixture of diffuse blue pigmentation and patchy reticular or geographical brown pigmentation. It is usually located on the area of distribution of the first and second division of the trigeminal nerve. It is rather common among Asiatics, but it rarely affects also the other races. It most commonly appears in childhood or in puberty and persists for life. Malignant melanoma has been reported to arise in a naevus of Ota.

Naevus of Ito shows a mottled appearance with bluish and brownish macules located on the acromioclavicular region and the upper chest. It differs from the naevus of Ota only in the area of involvement. It almost exclusively affects the Japanese. Malignant change is extremely rare.

Diagnosis and differential diagnosis

Diagnosis of dermal MN is clinical and can be documented by histological examination.

Differential diagnosis includes:

- blue naevus
- melasma
- café-au-lait macule
- naevus spilus
- contusion
- argyria
- ochronosis
- drug eruptions
- lentigo maligna.

Treatment

Camouflage with opaque make-up can diminish cosmetic disfigurement.

Cryotherapy, dermabrasion or electrodesiccation have been used, but they are often associated with hypopigmentation or scarring. For the naevus of Ota, a combination of sequential dry ice, epidermal peeling and argon laser has given satisfactory results. Laser treatment, especially with the Q-switched ruby laser, offers excellent cosmetic outcome. Q-switched alexandrite laser is a very effective and safe tool for treating Ota's naevus.

Long-term follow-up is warranted because of the potential for melanoma development, especially in cases with eye involvement.

Further reading

Barnhill RL, Flotte TJ, Fleischli M, Perez-Atayde A. Cutaneous melanoma and atypical Spitz tumors in childhood. *Cancer* 1995; 76 (10): 1833–45.

Casso EM, Grin-Jorgensen CM, Grant-Kels JM. Spitz naevi. *J Am Acad Dermatol* 1992; 27: 901–13.

Crickx B. Melanocytic naevi. *Rev Pract* 1999; 15: 829–32.

Halpern AC, Guerry D IV, Elder DE *et al*. Dysplastic naevi as risk markers for sporadic (non-familial) melanoma: A case controlled study. *Arch Dermatol* 1991; 127: 995–9.

Helm KF, Schwartz RA, Janniger CK. Juvenile melanoma (Spitz naevus). *Cutis* 1996; 58: 35–9.

Imayama S, Ueda S. Long- and short-term histological observations of congenital naevi treated with the normal-mode ruby laser. *Arch Dermatol* 1999; 135: 1211–18.

Lawrence CM. Treatment options for giant congenital naevi. *Clin Exp Dermatol* 2000; 25: 7–11.

Marchac D, Larregue M. Exerese radicale des naevus geants de l'abdomen chez le nourrisson. A propos de 3 cas. *Ann Dermatol Venereol* 1985; 112: 43–8.

Marghoob AA. The dangers of atypical mole (dysplastic naevus) syndrome. Teaching at risk patients to protect themselves from melanoma. *Postgrad Med* 1999; 105: 147–54.

Milgraum SS, Cohen ME, Auletta MJ. Treatment of blue naevi with the Q-switched ruby laser. *J Am Acad Dermatol* 1995; 32: 307–10.

Rivers JK. Management of precursors and primary lesions of melanoma. *Curr Opin Oncol* 1993; 5: 377–82.

Sau P, Graham JH, Helwig EB. Pigmented spindle cell naevus: a clinicopathologic analysis of ninety-five cases. *J Am Acad Dermatol* 1993; 28: 565–71.

Stavrianeas NG, Katoulis AC, Koumantaki-Mathioudaki E *et al.* Seasonal influences on melanocytic naevi assessment for malignancy. *Skin Cancer* 1997; 2: 289–91.

Necrobiosis lipoidica

E.M. Grosshans

Synonyms

Oppenheim–Urbach disease.

Definition and epidemiology

Necrobiosis lipoidica is a chronic granulomatous disease. Most often it involves the skin of the anterior aspect of the legs in its typical presentation related to diabetes mellitus (necrobiosis lipoidica diabeticorum). The primary event seems to be a degeneration of collagen and elastic fibres with a secondary granuloma continuously spreading around and an extracellular fat storage mainly in diabetics.

Aetiology and pathophysiology

Only a minority of patients with necrobiosis lipoidica have diabetes mellitus. Approximately 10% have diabetes which is already known and treated. In a further 10% a long medical surveillance shows a delayed onset of metabolic disorders of carbohydrates. Necrobiosis lipoidica is a rare complication of diabetes, usually correlated to the severity of the diabetic microangiopathy. It occurs only in 0.3% of diabetic patients; in 2.0% if one considers juvenile diabetics exclusively.

In non-diabetic patients, the aetiology is unknown. Necrobiosis lipoidica unrelated to any metabolic disorders is usually described as granulomatosis disciformis of Miescher. It also occurs most often on the legs, but it may be disseminated in other body areas, especially on the face and scalp in a macular and annular variant.

The triggering factors of focal degeneration of collagen are unknown but may include:

- Focal disturbance of the blood supply and haemostasis due to microangiopathy in diabetics.
- Primary degeneration or defective synthesis of collagen fibres directly related to diabetes or to microtrauma in non-diabetics.
- Secondary degeneration due to the spreading granuloma which may itself be induced by immune complex depositions.

Clinical characteristics and course

Necrobiosis lipoidica usually begins as bilateral nodular lesions of the pretibial areas. These nodules flatten and extend in ovalar plaques for several years and decades. In fully developed forms, it presents as single or multiple scleroatrophic plaques of 5–15 cm. Their borders are polycyclic, raised and red, with numerous telangiectasias and sometimes scales or hyperkeratotic plugs. The centre is depressed, brown or yellowish (in the case of pronounced fat storage), and often adhering to the underlying aponeurosis or periosteum. Chronic and painful ulcerations occur especially in diabetic patients. Rare carcinomas complicate longstanding verrucous or ulcerated lesions.

Lesions may also occur outside the pretibial areas: on the ankles, feet, upper limbs and even on the face and scalp, where they are usually annular and associated with scarring alopecia. The granulomatosis disciformis of Miescher is a polycyclic plaque, more often unilateral, whose surface is smooth, slightly depressed and brownish, spreading over years and involving finally the whole length of the leg without any local complication.

Diagnosis

The diagnosis may be done by biopsy. It is important to be cautious in diabetics with arterial insufficiency because of the risk of persistent ulceration. The histological aspects of non-diabetic necrobiosis are not specifically distinctive: the foci of degenerative collagen are rare or lacking, granulomas of the foreign body type are more extensive, and small blood vessels do not disclose the main characteristic of the diabetic microangiopathy, namely a thickening of the periodic acid-Schiff (PAS) positive basal membranes narrowing the vessel lumina.

Differential diagnosis

In its typical pretibial localization, the clinicopathological aspects are quite specific. In the early stage, pretibial patches of a diabetic dermatopathy ('spotted legs') and common scars should be discussed.

In other localizations with atypical presentation, differential diagnosis must be made with the following.

- Granuloma annulare: disseminated granuloma annulare presenting as large polycyclic lesions with a raised papular border are more frequent in diabetic patients or in patients with a disturbed metabolism of carbohydrates; even with the help of multiple biopsies it may be quite impossible to differentiate both conditions.
- Other non-infectious granulomatous diseases: annular lesions of sarcoidosis can mimick disseminated macular lesions of necrobiosis lipoidica in non-diabetic patients; some cases of Miescher's disciform granulomatosis after a long follow-up time proved to be scarring variants of sarcoidosis; conversely, patients with necrobiosis lipoidica sometimes have an elevated serum angiotensin-converting enzyme level and their lesions are positive in a gallium scan as in sarcoidosis.
- In sun-exposed skin areas of the face and the neck, elastolytic giant cell granulomas (O'Brien's actinic granulomas) must be considered.

Treatment

The incidence of necrobiosis lipoidica diabeticorum has seemingly decreased in the last decades. This is probably related to the preventive effect of better medical care of young and insulin-dependent diabetic patients. On the other hand, necrobiosis lipoidica which is already present is not expected to be influenced by the specific treatment of the diabetes. This is the paradox of this condition which represents a quite specific complication of diabetes mellitus but cannot be controlled through diabetic glycaemic control alone. It must however be stressed that tight diabetic control, even if it does not improve the clinical aspect, provides a better prognosis and reduces the risk of complications.

In non-diabetic patients, spontaneous remission can occur independently of any treatment.

General therapeutic guidelines

No controlled therapeutic studies are available and therefore no general guidelines can be recommended. Topical and systemic medical treatments and physical, especially surgical, approaches have been proposed.

Recommended therapies

Topical therapies

The topics which show some efficacy are corticosteroids. Occlusive dressings or intralesional injections can reduce the inflammatory borders and stop the progression of scleroatrophic plaques. However they do not improve the scarring aspect of the centre and most often the patient does not agree with the practitioner that there has been any improvement. The corticosteroid needs to be potent: clobetasol propionate or betamethasone dipropionate 0.05% in a gel or cream for 3–4 weeks. If the periphery flattens and becomes less inflammatory, maintenance therapy with open applications can be proposed. The results are actually better in the early stages than in fully developed atrophic lesions. In ulcerated lesions, 20% benzoyl peroxide preparations and dressings with hydrocolloid gels or bovine collagen provide some improvement.

Topically applied tretinoin has been tried with some success.

Topical once- or twice-weekly psoralen and ultraviolet A (PUVA) therapy has been shown to be effective in some patients, even with ulcerated lesions, irrespective of the association with diabetes. After topical administration of a 0.15% emulsion of 8-methoxypsoralen the lesions are treated with an initial dose of 0.5 J/cm^2 UVA, with 20% increments at each treatment visit, if tolerated. Complete clearance or a substantial improvement can be expected with a mean cumulative UVA dose of less than 100 J/cm^2 if the lesions are not too atrophic.

Systemic drugs

The list of systemic drugs whose efficacy has been tested in short case reports or in open series is impressive:

- Aspirin 40–300 mg/day
- Clofazimine 200 mg/day
- Ciclosporin A 3–5 mg/kg per day
- Dipyridamole 300 mg/day
- Heparin
- Methylprednisolone
- Mycophenolate mofetil
- Nicotinamide 1.5 g/day
- Pentoxifylline 800–1200 mg/day
- Prostaglandin E1 2 × 4 mg i.v. per day
- Ticlopidine 500 mg/day.

These drugs have been selected among antiplatelet agents, vasodilators, anticoagulants, anti-inflammatory drugs and even immunosuppressors, such as ciclosporin A and mycophenolate mofetil. Patients treated with ciclosporin A (3–4 mg/kg per day for 3–4 months) had a marked improvement of the clinical picture without relapse after withdrawal of the drug.

Only aspirin has been tested in controlled studies but failed to show any benefit, even if associated with dipyridamol, when compared with placebo.

Good benefits are ascribed to systemic steroids under close surveillance of the glycaemia. In a series of six patients treated with methylprednisolone (1 mg/kg per day for 1 week than 40 mg/day for 4 weeks followed by a progressive withdrawal for 2 further weeks), the granulomatous border resolved completely in all patients and only the central atrophic area with its waxy, yellowish appearance persisted. There was no recurrence during a follow-up period of 7 months and the lesions remained stable in size and appearance. Isolated case reports emphasizing similar results have been published.

Surgical procedures

Surgical removal of painful ulcerated necrobiosis followed by split-thickness skin grafting or by tissue-engineered dermal skin grafting can be proposed. The lesion is replaced by a large scar adhering to the underlying muscles and bones. There is a risk of recurrence of the necrobiosis around the scar and the patient should be informed of this. Such surgical treatment must be avoided if the arterial blood supply is insufficient and also if the cosmetic disability is of greater concern to the patient.

If a 6-week regimen of oral systemic corticotherapy (prednisone in decreasing doses starting with 1 mg/kg per day), under tight control of the glycaemia in diabetic patients, proves unsuccessful in the treatment of disabling lesions, a surgical approach can be proposed to the patient. Topical PUVA therapy or a systemic therapy with ciclosporin A should also be proposed in severe ulcerated necrobiosis lipoidica before the surgical treatment.

Other therapeutic procedures

Hyperbaric oxygen therapy has also been tried with apparent success, alone or plus local corticosteroids.

No new therapeutic procedures are in the experimental phase.

Further reading

Beck HI, Bjerring P, Rasmussen I, Zachariae H, Stenbjerg S. Treatment of necrobiosis lipoidica with low dose acetylsalicylic acid: a randomized double-blind trial. *Acta Derm Venereol* 1985; 65: 230–4.

Bouhanick B, Verret JL, Gouello JP, Berrut G, Marre M. Necrobiosis lipoidica: treatment by hyperbaric oxygen and local corticosteroids. *Diabetes Metab* 1998; 24: 156–9.

Cohen O, Yaniv R, Karasik A, Trau H. Necrobiosis lipoidica and diabetic control revisited. *Med Hypotheses* 1996; 46: 348–50.

D'Argento V, Curatoli G, Filatico R, Foti C, Vena GA. Cyclosporin A in the treatment of necrobiosis lipoidica diabeticorum. *J Dermatol Treat* 1997; 8: 123–5.

Darvay A, Acland KM, Russell-Jones R. Persistent ulcerated necrobiosis lipoidica responding to treatment with cyclosporin. *Br J Dermatol* 1999; 141: 725–7.

McKenna DB, Cooper EJ, Tidman MJ. Topical psoralen plus ultraviolet A treatment for necrobiosis lipoidica. *Br J Dermatol* 2000; 143: 1333–5.

O'Toole EA, Kennedy U, Nolan JJ, Young MM, Rogers S, Barnes L. Necrobiosis lipoidica: only a minority of patients have diabetes mellitus. *Br J Dermatol* 1999; 140: 283–6.

Reinhard G, Lohmann F, Uerlich M, Bauer R, Bieber T. Successful treatment of ulcerated necrobiosis lipoidica with mycophenolate mofetil. *Acta Derm Venereol* 2000; 80: 312–13.

Nummular eczema

H.R. Bruckbauer, S. Karl and J. Ring

Synonyms

Nummular dermatitis, microbial eczema, nummular-microbial eczema, dysregulative microbial eczema, discoidal eczema.

Definition

Eczema is defined as non-contagious epidermodermatitis with typical clinical aspects (pruritus, erythema, papule, seropapule, vesicle, desquamation, incrustation, lichenification with synchronous or metachronous polymorphism) and typical histopathological appearance (spongiosis, akanthosis, parakeratosis, lymphocytic infiltration). It often results from various endogenous activators or exogenous noxious substances due to hypersensitivity.

The classification of Hornstein distinguishes between three different groups of eczema (Fig. 1): exogenous eczema, endogenous eczema and dysregulative microbial (e.g. nummular) eczema.

The nummular eczema is a special subtype of chronic eczema with coin-shaped, sharply demarcated erythematous oozing and crusting lesions.

The nummular eczema is more common in males. The manifestation is usually between the ages of 50 and 70 years.

Aetiology

The pathogenesis is unclear; a multifactorial aetiology with functional epidermal dysregulation is probable. Dysregulation may result from chronic dystrophic vascular (e.g. chronic venous insufficiency) or subtoxic cumulative exogenous irritation with reversible impairment of the epidermal physicochemical protection barrier. Conditioning factors are listed in Table 1. Microbial antigens can be a further possible cause of sensitization. Internal disease or infections (sinusitis, chronic tonsillitis, chronic bronchitis, bronchiectases, chronic prostatitis, chronic dental infections) are sometimes relevant bacterial reservoirs and triggers. To date microbial agents have not been implicated as causative factors but contact allergy to microbial allergens may be responsible for the persistent and chronic nature of nummular eczema. Recently, nummular eczema has also been discussed as a skin reactivation to environmental aeroallergens. Often, no triggering factor can be detected.

Clinical characteristics and course

The eruption occurs typically on the distal limbs particularly on the back of hands, feet, forearms and legs. In more extensive cases the shoulders and upper back are involved. The disease starts with small coin-shaped, sharply margined, erythematous, slightly elevated patches of papules and vesicles. After an acute exudative phase the vesicles erode. As a result oozing, crusting and scaling can be noticed. Isolated eczematous lesions are 1–5 cm in diameter but also can show extensive confluence. The disease can be localized, but also spread rapidly with numerous lesions. Differential diagnosis includes psoriasis and tinea corporis. Patients suffer from severe pruritus. It is typical for the response to treatment to be poor and a protracted course to follow with exacerbations and remissions over months to several years. Recurrence rates are high. Mucous membranes are not affected.

Diagnosis

Careful history

A careful history helps in finding any triggering factors like internal diseases, infections or drugs.

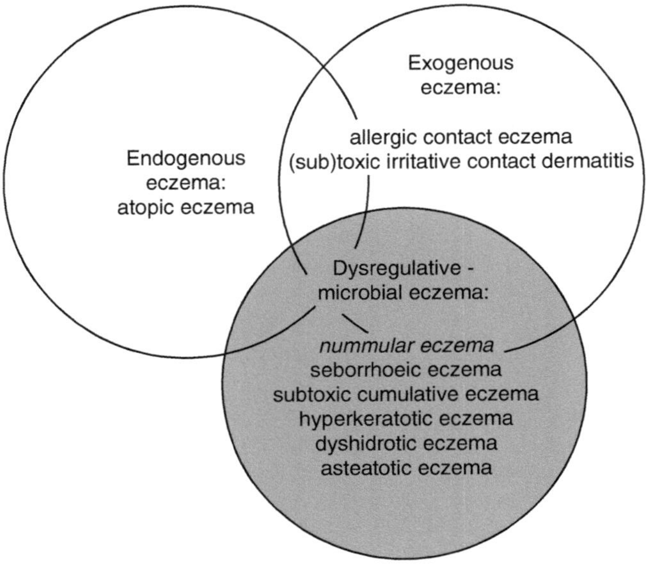

Figure 1 Classification of eczema into three main groups (according to Hornstein).

Blood tests for inflammatory signs

Blood tests—blood cell counts, erythrocyte sedimentation rate (ESR), antistreptolysine —should be performed to find out if there are any signs of underlying infections.

Bacteriological swabs

Bacterial swabs are necessary to detect superinfections.

Skin biopsy

The skin histology shows psoriasiform thickening of the epidermis (acanthosis, hyper- and parakeratosis) with exudative inflammatory exocytosis and spongiotic vesicles. In the upper dermis a perivascular lymphocytic infiltrate is found.

Table 1 Conditioning factors for nummular eczema (according to Hornstein)

Pathogenic factor	Effect
Hyperhidrosis	Vasomotoric dysfunction Swelling of stratum corneum
Dysseborrhoea	Impairment of barrier function
Exsiccation	Impairment of barrier function Reduced elasticity Increased roughness
Physical stress (pressure, rubbing, heat, light, radiation)	Impairment of barrier function Reduced elasticity Increased roughness
Chemical stress	Exsiccation and delipidation of stratum corneum
Microcirculatory disorders	Oedema, circulatory disturbance, acrocyanosis
Nerval irritation or lesion	Vasomotoric dysfunction
Endogenous visceral disorder	Dysproteinaemia, accumulation of metabolites (e.g. renal, hepatic)
Diabetes mellitus	Microcirculatory disturbance
Bacterial foci	Circulating microbial antigens and metabolites

Search for underlying disease

Depending on the history appropriate examinations and laboratory tests should be performed to find provocative factors.

Differential diagnosis

- Tinea: mycological culture.
- Psoriasis: no vesicles; histopathology.
- Nummular atopic eczema: early manifestation; atopy; lichenification.
- Asteatotic eczema: extensor sites; asteatosis.
- Parapsoriasis en plaques (Brocq): not exudative (no crusts, no vesicles); trunk preferred in the lines of cleavage.
- Impetigo contagiosa: localized; massive bacterial (staphylococci, streptococci) superinfection.
- Allergic contact eczema: patch test positive; spreading characteristic.

Diagnostic tests for exclusion of relevant differential diagnoses

- Mycological cultures of scales for exclusion of tinea.
- Patch test for exclusion of allergic contact eczema.
- Total immunoglobulin E, radioallergosorbent test, prick-test (atopy patch test) for exclusion of atopic eczema.

Treatment

General therapeutic guidelines

Eliminate triggering factors and underlying disease. Infections should be treated with antibiotics, suspected provoking factors and drugs should be withdrawn.

Irritating skin contacts should be avoided.

Anti-inflammatory and antieczematous treatment (e.g. glucocorticosteroids, tars, dyes, antiseptic preparations and ultraviolet (UV) irradiation) correlated with the clinical appearance.

In severe and extensive cases, systemic treatment with glucocorticosteroids (0.5–1.0 mg/kg body weight prednisolone) and antibiotics should be considered.

Systemic antihistamine medication is often needed to manage the pruritus.

Recommended therapies (Table 2)

These include:

- topical glucocorticosteroids
- topical antiseptics
- systemic glucocorticosteroids
- systemic antibiotics
- astringents
- tar preparations
- UVB (selective ultraviolet phototherapy, narrow band UVB 311 nm) phototherapy
- topical calcineurin inhibitors (?).

Topical stage-adequate treatment

Acute nummular eczema

To avoid exacerbation of the acute exudative stage preparations should not be greasy. Initially, glucocorticosteroid cream (if necessary a fluorinated steroid) in combination with a wet dressing (clioquinol or $KMnO_4$ solutions) is useful. Astringent dyes will dry moist superinfected eczema and disinfect the lesions. Here Solutio pyoctanini (gentian violet aqueous 1%) and Sol. castellani are appropriate. In severe cases oral glucocorticosteroids (e.g. 40 mg prednisolone daily for 2 weeks with gradual dose reduction) with simultaneous antibiotic protection (e.g. doxycycline or cephalosporin) should be given. Systemic H_1-antihistamines (e.g. dimetindine, hydroxyzine) mitigate pruritus.

Subacute or chronic nummular eczema

If lesions have dried, less potent steroids (prednicarbate, mometasone) on a non-fatty base (lotion, cream, paste), if necessary combined with antiseptic substances like clioquinol, can be chosen. Gradually the steroid content should be reduced and substituted with glucocorticosteroid-free preparations. Tar mixtures (ichthyol

Table 2 Stage-adequate treatment

Clinical stage	Clinical characteristics	Treatment	General measures
Acute nummular eczema	Vesicles, exudation, erosion, crusts	• In *severe and extended cases*: systemic therapy with steroids (0.5–1.0 mg/kg prednisone) for about 1 week in tapering dose	Treatment of underlying disease
		• In *superinfected eczema*: systemic antibiotic therapy (e.g. cephalosporins)	Antipruritic therapy with antihistamines
		• *Topical exsiccating, antiseptic and anti-inflammatory treatment*: dyes (Sol. pyoctanini, Sol. castellani), glucocorticoid cream (O/W) in combination with wet dressings (clioquinol or $KMnO_4$ solutions)	Psychosomatic counselling Avoid triggering factors
Subacute nummular eczema	Erythema, oedema, papules, seropapules, scales	• Mild exsiccation: dyes, glucocorticoid cream (O/W) with wet dressing, zinc oil, soft paste, lotion (powder in water) on non-exudative lesions	
Chronic nummular eczema	Dry scaling, psoriasiform scaling, lichenification, infiltrated papules	• Glucocorticoid cream or ointment occlusive	Ultraviolet B phototherapy Oil bath
		• Soft paste lipophilic ointment	
		• Tars (ichthyol–tumenol liquor carbonis detergens-Pix lithanthracis) 3–5% in soft paste or ointment	
	Hyperkeratotic lesions	• Keratolytic ointments (urea 10% or salicylic acid 5%)	

2–5%, liquor carbonis detergens 3–5%, tumenol 3–10% on a base of lotion, zinc paste or cream) show good antieczematous, antipruritic and antimicrobial effects.

Markedly infiltrated and therapy-resistant lesions can be treated with intralesional injections of glucocorticoids (e.g. triamcinolone).

Oil and oil–tar baths support the therapeutic effect. Exsiccation with soaps, detergents and inappropriate skin care should be avoided.

The subacute stage of the nummular eczema is the proper moment for starting UV therapy. Phototoxic effects of tar preparations should be considered.

UVB whole body irradiation

After determination of individual mean erythematous dosage in order to avoid sunburn reactions, whole body UVB irradiation (UVB 280–320 nm, SUP 305–325 nm, narrow band UVB 311 nm) is performed 3–5 times per week for 3–6 weeks. Starting with an initial dose of about 80% of the MED the dose is increased 15–30% daily for maintaining the erythema reaction. After a moderate erythema reaction is achieved the dose is maintained at this level. The individual initial dose varies between 25 and 70 mJ/cm^2. To shield against UV damage protective glasses should be worn, and the face and genitalia in male patients should be protected. UVB therapy is contraindicated in patients with increased UVB sensitivity.

Alternative and experimental treatments

PUVA photochemotherapy

UVA (320–400 nm) irradiation is performed 2 h after oral administration of the photosensitizing furocumarine 8-methoxysoralen (0.6–0.8 mg/kg). Starting with an initial dose of 0.5–1.0 J^2, with individual dose adjustments depending on the patient's sensitivity. The irradiations are performed 3–4 times per week for about 3–4 weeks. From the point of intake of the psoralen, protective UVA glasses should be worn for 24 h to prevent cataract formation. Male genitalia should be protected by tin foil.

Possible side-effects are sunburn, premature ageing, high risk for basal cell carcinoma and spinocellular carcinoma, nausea, liver function disturbances. Rarely blisters, pain and induction of lupus erythematosus.

According to published results there is no apparent difference between SUP or PUVA. Treatment periods seem to be shorter with PUVA therapy. UV therapy in nummular eczema gives longer periods of remission once the systemic or topical steroid treatment has ceased, and the relapse risk decreases.

Balneophototherapy

In recent times systemic PUVA is replaced by balneophototherapy. No clinical studies about the effect of balneophototherapy on nummular eczema are available.

Calcineurin inhibitors

The immunosuppressive drug ciclosporin A has been applied with reasonable success in different inflammatory dermatological diseases such as atopic eczema and psoriasis. Its use is limited due to systemic side-effects. Topical forms have been tried but were shown to be ineffective. Possibly the new topicals tacrolimus and pimecrolimus, which are able to penetrate the human skin may be an effective alternative for topical application. In some cases low blood concentrations were detected, systemic side-effects have not yet been seen. Since they can suppress skin inflammation in man they may also be useful for treating nummular eczema. Positive effects have been seen in patients with atopic eczema. For nummular eczema specific clinical studies are required.

References

Aoyama H, Tanaka M, Hara M, Tabata N, Tagami H. Nummular eczema: An addition of senile xerosis and unique cutaneous reactivities to environmental aeroallergens. *Dermatology* 1999; 199: 135–9

Braun-Falco O, Plewig G, Wolff HH. *Dermatologie und Venerologie.* Berlin: Springer, 1996.

Breit R, Schmiel G. UV-Therapie des nummulären Ekzems. In: Rüping KW, Stary A, Tronnier H eds. *2. Dermatologisches Forum: Neues in der Therapie.* Neufahrn vor München: Medical Concept, 1987: 223–6.

Hannuksela M. Balneo-Photochemotherapie. In: Braun-Falco O, Ring J, eds. *Fortschritte der Praktischen Dermatologie und Venerologie 12.* Berlin: Springer, 1989: 450–3.

Hornstein OP. Klassifikation der Ekzemkrankheiten. *Z Hautkr* 1986; 61: 1281–96.

Hornstein OP, Nürnberg E. *Externe Therapie von Hautkrankheiten.* Stuttgart: Thieme, 1985.

Lauerma AI, Maibach HI. Topical FK506—clinical potential or laboratory curiosity? *Dermatology* 1994; 188: 173–6.

Michel G, Kemeny L, Homey B, Ruzicka T. FK506 in the treatment of inflammatory skin disease: promises and perspectives. *Immunol Today* 1996; 17: 106–8.

Nakagawa H, Etoh T, Ishibashi Y *et al.* Tacrolimus ointment for atopic dermatitis. *Lancet* 1994; 344: 883.

Ring J. Endogenous and exogenous eczema. *Semin Dermatol* 1990; 9: 195–6.

Ring J. Zum Wandel des Ekzem-Begriffes: Klassisches versus atopisches Ekzem. *Z Hautkr* 1996; 71: 752–6.

Ruzicka T, Bieber T, Schöpf E *et al.* A short-term trial of tacrolimus ointment for atopic dermatitis. *NEJM* 1997; 337: 816–21.

Pediculosis

E. Tsoureli-Nikita, G. Campanile, G. Hautmann and J. Hercogova

Definition and epidemiology

Pediculosis is an ubiquitous, contagious and debilitating skin dermatosis. It is an epizoonose, caused by parasites living on the skin surface. Pediculosis is caused by insects of the order Anoplura and, although only two species (*Phthirius pubis* and *Pediculus humanus*) are host-specific parasites of humans, three clinical forms of infestation exist concerning head, body and pubic area. The incidence of infestation varies from 5% to 30% in certain populations. Children and long-haired people are most likely to become infested. The transmission takes place from person to person and it is favoured by poor personal hygiene and by living in closed communities. Clusters of infestation occur, e.g. affecting patients and staff in hospitals, nursing homes for the elderly, schoolchildren or homeless people, since *P. capitis* may be transmitted by shared hats, caps, brushes, combs and even pillows. Associations with other disorders are common, e.g. pediculosis can be often associated with trench fever or exanthematous typhus.

The head infestation is caused by *Pediculus humanus* var. *capitis* (synonym: *P. capitis*); the body (or clothes) infestation is caused by *Pediculus humanus* var. *corporis* (synonyms: *P. vestimentorum*, *Pediculus humanus humanus*, *Phthirius corporis*); the pubic infestation is determined by *Phthirius pubis* (synonyms: *Pediculus pubis*, *Phthirius pubis*, *Phthirius inguinalis*). No age or economic strata are immune to *P. capitis*.

Unlike *P. capitis*, the body louse has become relatively more rare in many affluent populations. Clothes lice are rarely associated with ordinary social lifestyles. In fact, they occur more frequently among the tramps and vagabonds in the city and countryside, although they may become more common in times of war and deprivation.

Parasites and aetiopathogenesis

Lice have three pairs of strong legs ending in claws. The fertilized female attaches its 150–300 eggs (nits)—which are oval and approximately 0.8 mm long—to the hair of the scalp or to pubic hair (head louse, crab louse) or to the seams of underwear (clothes louse) by means of a water-insoluble cement secreted by a gland appended to the ovary.

The *Pediculus humanus* var. *capitis* is 2–4 mm long with three pairs of legs that are of equal length. The body is dorsoventrally flattened. The entire lifecycle is spent in the scalp hair. Visible eggs or nits are deposited on the hair shaft, singly and close to the scalp.

The large body louse (*Pediculus humanus* var. *corporis*) resembles the head louse in configuration. It lives and reproduces in the lining of clothes and leaves the clothing for feeding only, being rarely found on the skin.

The pubic louse (*Phthirius pubis*), or crabs, is smaller (1.5–2 mm long), shorter than either the head or clothes louse. It has a squat, shield-like shape, is broad-shouldered, and has a narrow head. The miniature crab-like body is dorsoventrally flattened and has three pairs of legs. Unlike the other types of louse, crab lice hardly move and are therefore more difficult to see. Their rate of reproduction is relatively slow.

The louse larvae hatch out after about 1 week. They moult their cuticle three times and reach sexual maturity at 2–3 weeks. Lice suck blood every few hours and cannot survive a fast of more than a few days.

Clinical characteristics and diagnosis

Pediculosis capitis

Infestation of the scalp by *Pediculus humanus* var. *capitis* begins with an itching of the scalp that may vary from moderate to severe. The saliva of the louse produces the marked pruritus. Excoriations are produced, and these soon become secondarily infected, with crusting. The posterior aspect of the scalp commonly shows the greatest degree of involvement. The skin lesions (that may be noticed even after some days) consist of deep-red, urticarial papules which provoke intense itching. A typical louse eczema often develops at the back of the neck and the posterior occipital nodes are enlarged and tender (also due to the secondary infection). The *P. capitis* favours the scalp, and beards and pubic hair are often spared. The adult *P. capitis* is often not observed; fewer than 10 lice are detected in over half of the cases.

P. capitis is frequently diagnosed by barbers and beauticians who readily observe the nits when the hair is wet. Medically, secondary infections of the scalp or neck with chronic pruritus lead the examiner to inspect the hair shafts closely with a hand lens or Wood's lamp for attached nits. In fact, close examination of the hair shaft will show minute white eggs (nits) firmly attached in series, that fluoresce under Wood's light.

These oval structures, which are attached to the hair like buds, are protected by a chitin case. They are initially found close to the scalp, but as the hair grows, they move with it to the tip, by which time they are empty. Unlike dandruff, nits cannot be easily rubbed off but are firmly attached.

Non-specific findings such as occipital lymphadenopathy, cervical adenopathy or mild systemic symptoms make some cases of pediculosis capitis difficult to diagnose.

Pediculosis corporis

Infestation of the body by *Pediculus humanus* var. *corporis* is characterized by pruritus and by parallel linear excoriations that are frequently secondarily infected. The primary lesion, which is seldom found because of the excoriations, is an urticarial wheal with a central haemorrhagic punctum. Small red macules are seen in early cases, with initial lesions often best seen on the back or under the arms. In cases of prolonged infestations, the skin becomes dry, scaly and hyperpigmented with extreme pruritic excoriations, urticarial and pigmentary changes (vagabonds' disease or cutis vagantium). In addition to the scratches, the skin may show many small light scars surrounded by areas of hyperpigmentation or depigmentation.

The adult louse, which measures 1–4 mm in length, feeds on the skin, but lives on the seams of clothing. The nits are attached to the seams in a rosary pattern. Clothes lice may transmit rickettsioses, spotted fever, relapsing fever and trench fever.

When long pruritic excoriations are found on the body, the clothes should be carefully examined for lice.

Pediculosis pubis

Crab lice seem to favour regions with apocrine sweat glands such as pubic hair, the anogenital region and the axillary region, but may be found also in very hairy regions of the chest and abdomen. In severe or long-standing cases, the lice may infect the chest and axillary hair, as well as the eyelashes, the edge of the scalp, the eyebrows, thighs, abdomen, and the axillae. Eyebrows, eyelashes and scalp are most commonly affected in children. Infestation by *Phthirus pubis*, or the crab louse, is primarily manifested by itching. Pruritus tends to be only moderate although it tends to be more severe at night. The urticarial lesions and secondary infections are seldom found with this type of infestation. Pruritus or secondary infection may be the only sign of infestation. Small blue–grey macules occasionally are seen and are useful diagnostic signs. These dusky grey–blue macules (taches bleuâtres or maculae ceruleae), 1–3 cm in diameter, often may be observed on the trunk, thighs and axillae. These are the result of the reaction of the insect's saliva with bilirubin, converting it to biliverdin.

Another clinical feature of the infestation, could be the reddish brown 'dust' apparent on underclothing, which is formed from the excreta of the insects. On close examination, the 1–2-mm long reddish brown louse may be found with its head buried in the hair follicle. The nits are darker than those found in head and body infestations.

The crab louse, *Phthirius pubis*, is generally transmitted by close personal contact, usually by sexual contact but may be transferred by articles of clothing or by infested hairs, also from parents to children.

Careful search with a hand lens for the yellowish adult lice or their ova is the best diagnostic method.

Differential diagnosis

- Scabies: small excoriated lesions in the interdigital webs of the fingers, on the wrists and the penis.
- Flea bites: excoriated papular lesions due to fleas are usually limited to the lower half of the legs.
- Infestation with bedbugs: the papular lesions caused by bedbugs are uniform in size, with central puncta and arranged in rows on exposed areas.
- Tinea capitis: hairless, discrete areas of scalp involvement. Depending on the type of fungus, the lesions may be crusted, swollen and tender, and may appear secondarily infected. The fungus will be found on microscopic examination and culture of the infected hair.

Treatment (Fig. 1)

Recommended therapies

Pediculosis capitis

In pediculosis capitis it is essential to kill not only the lice but also the embryos within the nits. The drug of choice is γ-benzene hexachloride (lindane) as an emulsion or gel (1%). This preparation must be thoroughly rubbed into the hair and left (under a shower cap) for 12–24 h. The hair is then shampooed. The treatment should be repeated after 3–5 days. Treatment may require systemic antibiotics. In addition to topical pediculocidal agents (such as lindane, DDT, malathion, pyrethrins, copper oleatetetrahydronaphthalene, or trimethoprim/sulfamethoxazole (sulphamethoxazole)) systemic antibiotics may be required.

In infants, young children and pregnant women potential neurotoxicity of lindane commonly leads to alternative methods of therapy. This drug has been replaced by other insecticides such as the acetylcholinesterase-inhibitors malathion and carbaryl, following evidence of the development of resistance to organochlorines. Malathion (0.5% liquid) is adsorbed onto keratin, a process which takes approximately 6 h, and has a residual protective effect against reinfection for about 6 weeks. Malathion preparation (0.5% liquid) should remain on the scalp for 12 h before being washed off. Malathion and carbaryl are degraded by heat, and a hot hairdryer should not be used. Treatment should be repeated after 10 days.

Pyrethrins, naturally occurring insecticides extracted from chrysanthemum, are also demonstrated to be effective as pediculocides and ovicides. A synthetic pyrethroid, permethrin (1%) is generally the

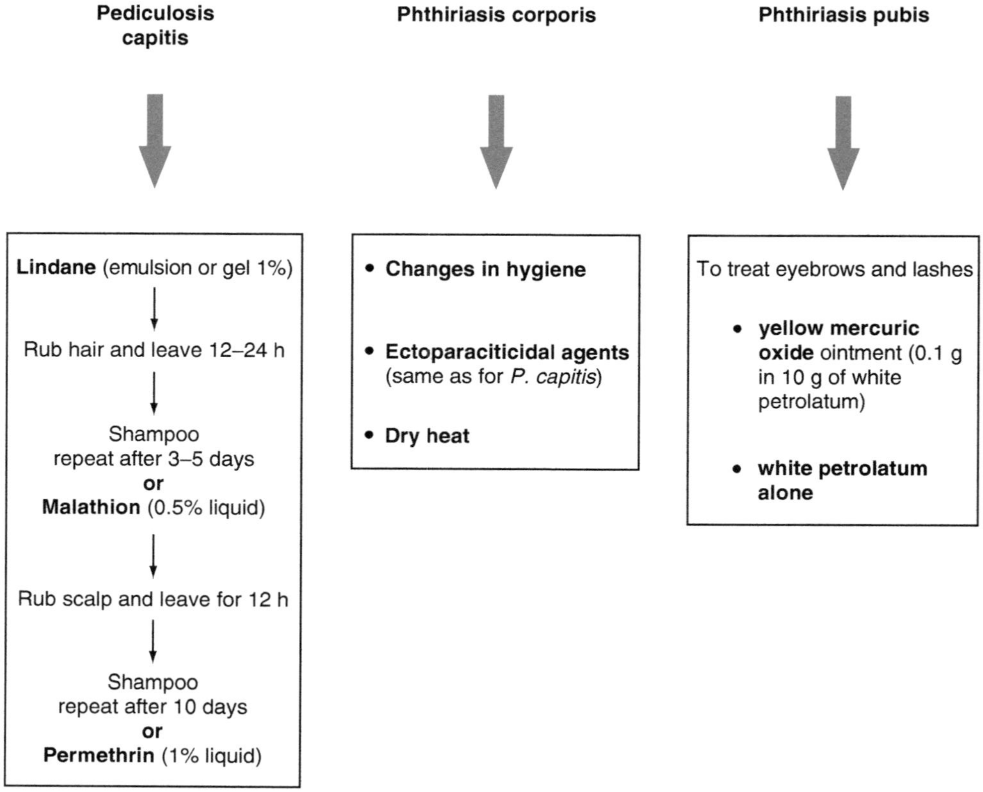

Pediculosis capitis
Phthiriasis corporis
Phthiriasis pubis
Lindane (emulsion or gel 1%)
Rub hair and leave 12–24 h
Shampoo
repeat after 3–5 days
or
Malathion (0.5% liquid)
Rub scalp and leave for 12 h
Shampoo
repeat after 10 days
or
Permethrin (1% liquid)
• Changes in hygiene
• Ectoparaciticidal agents (same as for P. capitis)
• Dry heat
To treat eyebrows and lashes
• yellow mercuric oxide ointment (0.1 g in 10 g of white petrolatum)
• white petrolatum alone

Figure 1

treatment of choice for head lice, because of its residual effect and minimal absorption and toxicity. Ivermectin, should be reserved in cases where permethrin fails.

Shampoos are usually the most convenient pediculocidal vehicles to use in children. Removing the dead ova may be psychologically important as some patients believe that the infestation has not been treated successfully if they remain. In general, if the ova are 1.0–1.5 cm from the scalp after adequate treatment, no active infestation is present.

Pediculosis corporis

Treatment for the non-sensitized person consists of changes in hygiene (if appropriate) and clothes, and use of the ectoparasiticidal agents noted above. Dry heat is equally effective in killing the lice and their ova in clothing.

Phthiriasis pubis

Treatment of phthiriasis pubis is the same as for pediculosis capitis with special attention paid to clothing and bedding infestation. Reinfestation after successful initial therapy is commonly due to reexposure to untreated sexual partners. Allergic and systemic reactions can develop in some patients. The treatment of infested eyebrows and lashes of infants presents more of a problem, as a toxic effect of the preparation is a possibility. The agents normally used are yellow mercuric oxide ointment (0.1 g in 10 g of white petrolatum) or white petrolatum alone. Lice and nits lodged in the eyelashes should be individually removed with forceps.

All specimens brought by patients should be carefully examined for organisms since delusions of parasitosis and parasitophobia are not uncommon.

It is very important to recognize and treat pediculosis in elderly people living together. However, one must be aware that the geriatric population may present difficulty regarding the diagnosis, because history taking may be more difficult or because the clinical manifestations may not appear classical, being overshadowed by other medical problems. The pruritus caused by the infestation will make the elderly people sick who, most of the time, have a set of other diseases. The treatment does not differ very much from that of younger patients. Malathione, lindane or permethrin are used and the dosages may require particular adjustments for this population.

Further reading

Blondell RD. Parasites of the skin and hair. *Prim Care* 1991; 18 (1): 167–83.

Buntin DM. The 1993 sexually transmitted disease treatment guidelines. *Semin Derm* 1994; 13 (4): 269–74.

Buntin DM, Roser T, Lesher JL Jr, Plotnick H, Brademas ME, Berger TG. Sexually transmitted diseases: viruses and ectoparasites, Committee on Sexually Transmitted Diseases of the American Academy of Dermatology. *J Am Acad Dermatol* 1991; 25 (3): 527–34.

Burns DA. The treatment of human ectoparasite infection *Br J Dermatol* 1991; 125 (2): 89–93.

Chosidow O. Scabies and pediculosis. *Lancet* 2000; 4: 355: 819–26.

Colven RM, Prose NS. Parasitic infestations of the skin. *Pediatr Ann* 1994; 23 (8): 436–42.

Di Napoli JB, Austin RD, Englender SJ. Eradication of head lice with a single treatment. *Am J Publ Health* 1988; 78: 978–80.

Elgart ML. Current treatments for scabies and pediculosis. *Skin Ther Lett* 1999; 5(1): 1–3.

Tan HH, Goh CL. Parasitic skin infections in the elderly: recognition and treatment. *Drugs Aging* 2001; 18(3): 165–76.

Pemphigus erythematosus

S. Albert, K.E. Harman and M.M. Black

Synonym

Senear–Usher syndrome.

Definition and epidemiology

Pemphigus erythematosus (PE) is a rare subtype of pemphigus foliaceus (PF) which has some clinical and immunological overlap with lupus erythematosus, although ultrastructurally lesions of PE are similar to PF. There is controversy regarding the diagnostic criteria in the literature. Senear and Usher first described this condition based on the lupus-like appearance of the malar eruption in patients with PF. Later, patients with a similar appearance but with immunological features of lupus erythematosus have been described and this subgroup in now considered to be PE. It is well documented that patients with sporadic or endemic forms of PF can have clinically similar involvement of the face and should not be considered as PE.

Aetiology and pathophysiology

Little is known of the pathophysiology of PE. It is unclear whether there is a genuine association between PF and lupus erythematosus in these patients. Antibodies bind to the intercellular substance of the epidermis in pemphigus and to the basement membrane zone in lupus erythematosus. The full identity of these antigens is not known although recently antibodies to desmoglein 1, the PF antigen, have been demonstrated.

Clinical characteristics and course

The incidence in almost equal in both sexes, and patients of all ages have been described. They often present with an erythematous to hyperpigmented scaly rash over the 'butterfly' or malar area of the face and superficial blisters with moist crusted lesions over the trunk, especially the seborrhoeic areas of the body. As with PF, mucosal involvement is rare and generalized involvement may occur. Most patients have only subclinical features of lupus, with often only a positive antinuclear antibody (ANA) result. PE rarely progresses to systemic lupus erythematosus. However a few fulfil the diagnostic criteria for SLE either before or after onset of PE. Some patients may experience worsening with sun exposure.

Limited long-term follow-up data are available but PE is considered to be a more benign disease than pemphigus vulgaris or PF with a high remission rate and excellent prognosis. Thymoma and myasthenia gravis have been reported to be associated in some of these patients.

Diagnosis

A skin biopsy of both truncal and facial lesions shows histological findings consistent with PF with an acantholytic split in the subcorneal or granular layer of the upper epidermis. Direct immunofluorescence (IF) shows both epidermal intercellular antibodies (immunoglobulin G (IgG), C3) and a 'lupus band' of immunoreactants (IgG, IgM, C3) along the basement membrane in the perilesional skin, more so in sun-exposed sites. Indirect IF will reveal the presence of circulating intercellular antibodies in the majority of cases but never a lupus band. Circulating ANA may be detected.

Differential diagnosis

- PF: direct and indirect IF.
- Lupus erythematosus: histology, ARA criteria, lupus band on direct IF
- Seborrhoeic dermatitis: negative IF studies.
- Photosensitive eczema: negative IF studies.

- Polymorphic light eruption: negative IF studies.
- Rosacea: negative IF studies.

Treatment

Treatment guidelines are similar to those for PF, a majority respond well to moderate doses of systemic steroids (20–40 mg) but some may require higher doses of steroids with adjuvant immunosuppressants such as azathioprine or cyclophosphamide. Dapsone 100–300 mg daily has been used successfully in several patients alone or in combination with steroids. Photoprotective measures and sunscreens are advised in those with a history of photoaggravation. Topical corticosteroids may be adequate in very mild or localized disease, and can even be used as an adjunct to systemic drugs. Very potent formulations should be used initially, e.g. clobetasol propionate 0.05%, and subsequently tapered to lower potency products.

Further reading

Amerian ML, Ahmed AR. Pemphigus erythematosus. Senear–Usher syndrome. *Int J Dermatol* 1985; 24(1): 16–25.

Gomi H, Kawada A, Amagai M, Matsuo I. Pemphigus erythematosus: detection of anti-desmoglein-1 antibodies by ELISA. *Dermatology* 1999; 199(2): 188–9.

Huilgol SC, Black MM. Management of the immunobullous disorders. II. Pemphigus. *Clin Exp Dermatol* 1995; 20(4): 283–93.

Piamphongsant T, Ophaswongse S. Treatment of pemphigus. *Int J Dermatol* 1991; 30(2): 139–46.

Pemphigus foliaceus

S. Albert, K.E. Harman and M.M. Black

Synonyms

Cazenave's pemphigus, endemic pemphigus, Brazilian pemphigus, fogo selvagem.

Definition and epidemiology

Pemphigus foliaceus (PF) is a rare autoimmune blistering disease of the skin. As with all forms of pemphigus, it is characterized by antibodies which bind to the cell surface of epidermal keratinocytes resulting in their separation from one another (acantholysis). The sporadic form affects all ethnic groups around the world but an endemic form (fogo selvagem = wild fire) is fairly common in the rural, tropical regions of Brazil, along major rivers and their tributaries.

Aetiology and pathophysiology

The PF antigen is a 160 Kd transmembrane desmosomal glycoprotein called desmoglein 1, an adhesion molecule belonging to the cadherin family of cell adhesion molecules. The gene for desmoglein 1 is localized on band q12 of chromosome 18. Immunoglobulin G (IgG) autoantibodies which bind to the intercellular spaces of the epidermis can be demonstrated in the skin and serum using direct and indirect immunofluorescence (IF), respectively. Their pathogenicity is supported by the observation that they can produce acantholysis both *in vitro* and *in vivo*, after passive transfer of sera to neonatal mice. It is not known what triggers the production of the PF antibody in sporadic cases but the geographical clustering of endemic cases in Brazil strongly suggests an environmental agent and the blackfly of *Simulium* species has been proposed as a likely vector. An increased incidence of the HLA allele DRBI*0404 in patients with fogo selvagem suggests that genetic susceptibility is also important. Drugs such as penicillamine can also precipitate sporadic PF.

Clinical characteristics and course

Sporadic PF can occur at any age but frequently the onset is in middle age. In contrast, endemic PF tends to occur in children and young adults. Both forms typically affect the seborrhoeic areas of the face, scalp, upper back and chest. Blisters occur at a high level in the epidermis and are thus very fragile and rarely remain intact. Localized and generalized forms have been described. In the localized type, lesions on the face often resemble those of lupus erythematosus. Circular erosions up to 2 cm in diameter are more commonly seen which become crusted and heal without scarring, although post-inflammatory hyperpigmentation is typical. Some lesions become heaped up and hyperkeratotic. Disease progression tends to be slow but erythroderma may occur and is common in fogo selvagem, the clinical appearance resembling an exfoliative dermatitis. In chronic cases, generalized hyperpigmentation and hyperkeratosis are predominant features. In both forms of PF, mucosal ulceration is uncommon in contrast to pemphigus vulgaris.

Sporadic PF follows a chronic benign course but the mortality of untreated fogo selvagem was 40%. Both forms respond well to treatment with long-standing remissions. Spontaneous remission is said to be between 10 and 20% in fogo selvagam and moving away from endemic areas increases the chances of remission.

Diagnosis

Intraepidermal clefting and acantholysis in the subcorneal region of the epidermis is the classical finding in a skin biopsy. However, the gold standard investigation is direct immunofluorescence or IF which will reveal IgG autoantibodies that bind to the surface of epidermal keratinocytes in almost all active cases. A biopsy of perilesional skin gives the highest diagnostic sensitivity for direct immunofluorescence.

Differential diagnosis

- Pemphigus vulgaris: mucosal lesions often present, histology—suprabasal clefting.
- Seborrhoeic dermatitis: negative direct immunofluorescence and IF.
- Staphylococcal scalded skin syndrome: negative IF studies.
- Impetigo: microbiology.
- Pustular psoriasis: negative IF studies.
- Subcorneal pustular dermatosis: negative IF studies.

Treatment

General therapeutic guidelines

Spontaneous remission is very rare and systemic treatment with corticosteroids and adjuvant drugs (often immunosuppressive agents) is usually required to induce and maintain remission. The successful management of pemphigus lies in achieving a balance between adequate disease control and minimizing the side-effects of treatment. It is common practice to commence treatment with systemic corticosteroids (often prednisolone), which have a rapid therapeutic onset and then combine with an adjuvant drug. The rationale behind this approach is that lower doses of each are ultimately required, thus minimizing the side-effects. However, in comparison to pemphigus vulgaris, it is often possible to use lower doses of corticosteroids to treat PF and less potent steroid-sparing drugs with lower side-effects. In milder cases with a low titre of intercellular antibodies it may be possible to avoid using systemic corticosteroids in preference to other adjuvant drugs, e.g. dapsone. Fortunately, all forms of pemphigus are rare but as a consequence there is a lack of controlled trial data to support the use of individual drugs.

PF can be exacerbated by sun exposure. Thus avoidance of bright sunlight and use of broad-spectrum sunscreens is recommended.

Recommended therapies

1 Sunscreens.
2 Antiseptics. These reduce the incidence of secondary infections in eroded skin, e.g. 0.01% potassium permanganate baths or chlorhexidine cleansing solutions.
3 Topical corticosteroids. These may be adequate in very mild or localized disease and can also be used as an adjunct to systemic drugs, allowing lower doses to be used. Very potent formulations should be used initially, e.g. clobetasol propionate 0.05%, and subsequently tapered to lower potency products.
4 Systemic corticosteroids. Low to moderate doses may be adequate to induce remission, particularly in mild cases. A starting dose of 40 mg of prednisolone daily, increasing by 50% every 4–7 days if necessary, until disease control is achieved is recommended. Once remission is maintained and the majority of lesions have healed, the dose of prednisolone may be slowly reduced to the minimum required to maintain remission. If adjuvant drugs are used, it may be possible to stop prednisolone altogether. In Brazil systemic triamcinolone in starting doses of 48 mg/day is preferred.
5 High-dose corticosteroids, e.g. 1000 mg methylprednisolone or 100 mg dexamethasone may be given as intravenous pulsed (monthly intervals) form in more severe or treatment-resistant disease.

6 Sulfone drugs. Dapsone has been used most commonly, both as monotherapy and in combination with systemic steroids. A starting dose of 25–50 mg daily, titrating upwards in 25-mg increments until disease control is achieved or to a maximum of 3 mg/kg may be used. Clinical improvement is often seen within 15 days once on an adequate dose of dapsone. The full blood count should be checked after each dose increment because haemolytic anaemia is a fairly common side-effect. Alternatives to dapsone are sulfapyridine and sulfamethoxypyridazine, 1.5–2.5 g daily.

7 Antimalarials. Hydroxychloroquine, 200 mg twice daily, has been successfully used in small numbers of patients with PF and may be used as monotherapy or in combination with systemic steroids. The maximum recommended daily dose is 6.5 mg/kg.

8 Tetracyclines and nicotinamide. This combination of oxytetracycline 500 mg four times daily and nicotinamide 500 mg four times daily has been successfully used to treat PF and is worth trying as monotherapy in milder cases. Nicotinamide 500 mg daily with increase by 500 mg increments every 7–14 days to reduce the incidence of vasodilator side effects can be used. Minocycline 100 mg daily may be used as an alternative to tetracycline but hyperpigmentation, which can occur as a side effect of long-term therapy, may be more likely to occur in older patients.

9 Immunosuppressants. These may be used as adjuvant drugs and as steroid-sparing agents:
- azathioprine 1.5–2.5 mg/kg per day or cyclophosphamide 1–3 mg/kg per day are widely used especially as steroid-sparing agents. Cyclophosphamide is also administered as a once monthly bolus i.v. dose of 500 mg along with high dose i.v. corticosteroids as a pulse therapy, followed by 50 mg oral cyclophosphamide daily in the intervening days;
- cyclosporin although initially reported to be effective, was found to be an ineffective adjuvant to corticosteroids in a recent controlled clinical trial;
- mycophenolate mofetil, the 2–morpholinoethyl ester prodrug of mycophenolic acid, is a relatively new agent which has been tried, and appears to be effective in doses of 1–2 g/day.

10 Plasmapheresis, intravenous immunoglobulin. PF is rarely life-threatening but if rapid disease control is required, it is worth considering these options. By plasmapheresis 1.5–3 L of plasma is removed from the patient and replaced with human albumin, isotonic citrate ACD and isotonic saline, thus removing circulating autoantibodies, but it must be combined with immunosuppressive drugs to prevent a rebound rise in antibody levels. This technique requires central venous access and there is thus a significant risk of sepsis in patients with ulcerated skin at the site of access. The administration of intravenous immunoglobulin (0.4 g/kg per day on 5 consecutive days) is less invasive and preliminary data suggest it has a rapid therapeutic onset.

Further reading

Amagai M. Pemphigus: autoimmunity to epidermal cell adhesion molecules. *Adv Dermatol* 1996; 11: 319–52.

Basset N, Guillot B, Michel B *et al.* Dapsone as initial treatment in superficial pemphigus. *Arch Dermatol* 1987; 123: 783–5.

Bystryn J-C, Steinman NM. The adjuvant therapy of pemphigus. *Arch Dermatol* 1996; 132: 203–12.

Chaffins ML, Collison D, Fivenson DP. Treatment of pemphigus and linear IgA dermatosis with nicotinamide and tetracycline: a review of 13 cases. *J Am Acad Dermatol* 1993; 28: 998–1000.

Hans-Filho G, Aoki V, Rivitti E, Eaton DP, Lin MS, Diaz LA. Endemic pemphigus foliaceus (fogo selvagem)—1998. The Cooperative Group on Fogo Selvagem Research. *Clin Dermatol* 1999; 17(2): 225–35.

Harman KE, Black MM. High-dose intravenous immune globulin for the treatment of autoimmune blistering diseases: an evaluation of its use in 14 cases. *Br J Dermatol* 1999; 140(5): 865–74.

Huilgol SC, Black MM. Management of the immunobullous disorders. II. Pemphigus. *Clin Exp Dermatol* 1995; 20: 283–93.

Hymes SR, Jordan RE. Pemphigus foliaceus: use of antimalarial agents as adjuvant therapy. *Arch Dermatol* 1992; 128: 1462–4.

Ioannides D, Chrysomallis F, Bystryn JC. Ineffectiveness of cyclosporine as an adjuvant to corticosteroids in the treatment of pemphigus. *Arch Dermatol* 2000; 136(7): 868–72.

Nousari HC, Sragovich A, Kimyai-Asadi A, Orlinsky D, Anhalt GJ. Mycophenolate mofetil in autoimmune and inflammatory skin disorders. *J Am Acad Dermatol* 1999; 40: 265–8.

Ohata Y, Amagai M, Ishii K, Hashimoto T. Immunoreactivity against intracellular domains of desmogleins in pemphigus. *J Dermatol Sci* 2001; 25(1): 64–71

Pasricha JS, Khaitan BK, Raman RS, Chandra M. Dexamethasone-cyclophosphamide pulse therapy for pemphigus. *Int J Dermatol* 1995; 34(12): 875–82.

Pemphigus vegetans

K.E. Harman, S. Albert and M.M. Black

Definition and epidemiology

Pemphigus vegetans is an uncommon variant of pemphigus vulgaris characterized clinically by verrucous plaques which occur predominantly in the body folds. There are two forms which differ slightly in their clinical appearance and behaviour, the Neumann and the Hallopeau subtypes.

Aetiology and pathophysiology

The epidermal intercellular immunoglobulin G (IgG) autoantibodies are presumed to be pathogenic but their target antigens are poorly characterized. Immunoblotting studies have shown that these patients have antibodies which bind to desmoglein 3, the pemphigus vulgaris antigen. Some studies have suggested that there are additional antibodies, which bind to other desmosomal proteins such as desmocollins and it is a possible explanation for the differences in clinical appearance with pemphigus vulgaris.

Clinical characteristics and course

The early presentation of the Neumann type is similar to pemphigus vulgaris with erosions and rarely intact bullae on the face, scalp, trunk, body folds and mucosal surfaces. In contrast, the primary lesions in the Hallopeau type are pustules rather than bullae. In both cases, the affected areas become hypertrophic and verrucous, particularly in the intertriginous areas and on the scalp. The vegetations may become fissured and exude serum. Oral vegetations are rare but occasionally the tongue develops a 'cerebriform' appearance which is typical of this condition. The Hallopeau type is said to follow a benign course and to show a better response to treatment than the Neumann type whose clinical course is more similar to pemphigus vulgaris.

Diagnosis

A skin biopsy may show acantholytic suprabasilar clefts, as seen in pemphigus vulgaris, but in contrast there is often a pronounced inflammatory infiltrate of eosinophils and neutrophils in the upper dermis and epidermis. A characteristic finding is the presence of intraepidermal abscesses filled predominantly with eosinophils and epidermal papillomatosis and hyperkeratosis are also seen. Direct and indirect immunofluorescence (IF) reveal intercellular IgG in the epidermis.

Differential diagnosis

- Tinea capitis with kerion formation: mycology.
- Hailey–Hailey disease: negative IF studies.
- Darier's disease: negative IF studies.
- Pyodermatitis–pyostomatitis vegetans: non-specific IF.

Treatment

General therapeutic guidelines

The treatment of pemphigus vegetans does not significantly differ from that of pemphigus vulgaris. However the use of topical agents may help in healing the resistant, verrucous lesions. In addition, systemic retinoids may be helpful. In view of the prominent inflammatory cell infiltrate in this variant of pemphigus, drugs with anti-inflammatory actions may be useful and there are a few case reports to support this approach.

Recommended therapies

Corticosteroids

A potent steroid cream/ointment, e.g. clobetasol propionate 0.05%, is worth using in addition to systemic drugs. Alternatively, intralesional corticosteroid may be used. Triamcinolone acetonide 5–10 mg/mL (0.1 mL per site) may be injected superficially in individual lesions with the bevel of the needle facing upwards. Lesions are reinjected every 1–2 weeks until healed but if no improvement is noted after three injections, this approach should be discontinued because of the risk of steroid-induced atrophy.

Retinoids

Etretinate 75 mg daily resulted in remission of pemphigus vegetans in a patient with concurrent psoriasis and 50 mg daily in combination with oral prednisolone led to remission in a second patient, while a third patient required only 10 mg/day.

Sulfone drugs

Their inhibitory actions on inflammatory cells may be particularly useful in this variant of pemphigus. Use as instructed for pemphigus foliaceus.

Tetracyclines and nicotinamide

The anti-inflammatory actions of this combination may also be particularly useful for the treatment of this variant of pemphigus. The combination was successfully used to treat one patient with pemphigus vegetans who had oesophageal involvement. Minocycline 100 mg daily was used rather than tetracycline. Prescribe as instructed for pemphigus foliaceus.

Further reading

Huilgol SC, Black MM. Management of the immunobullous disorders. II. Pemphigus. *Clin Exp Dermatol* 1995; 20: 283–93.

Ichimiya M, Yamamoto K, Muto M. Successful treatment of pemphigus vegetans by addition of etretinate to systemic steroids. *Clin Exp Dermatol* 1998; 23(4): 178–80.

Ohata Y, Amagai M, Ishii K, Hashimoto T. Immunoreactivity against intracellular domains of desmogleins in pemphigus. *J Dermatol Sci* 2001; 25(1): 64–71.

Sawai T *et al*. Pemphigus vegetans with oesophageal involvement: successful treatment with minocycline and nicotinamide. *Br J Dermatol* 1995; 132: 668–70.

Pemphigus vulgaris

V. Ruocco, S. Brenner and E. Ruocco

Definition and epidemiology

Pemphigus (from the Greek *pemphix* = blister) vulgaris (from the Latin for common) (PV) is the most frequent form of a group of mucocutaneous diseases (autoimmune pemphigus) characterized by intraepithelial blister formation.

PV is a potentially life-threatening blistering disorder caused by autoantibody formation against a desmosomal adhesion protein characteristic of epidermis and other stratified squamous epithelia. It is a rare disease, the incidence varying from 0.1 to 0.5 per 100 000 population, being higher among Jews and Indians. The disease is not related to sex and usually affects people between the ages of 30 and 60 years, but it can also occur in adolescence or even in childhood (especially in India) and in old age. There is a well-established HLA association with DR4, DR14, DQ1 and DQ3 antigens.

Aetiology and pathophysiology

The disease results from autoimmunity to the PV antigen, desmoglein 3, a normal component of keratinocyte cell membranes with a molecular weight of 130 kDa and belonging to the cadherin supergene family. Genetic factors alone are essential but not enough to initiate the autoimmune response. In several cases the outbreak of PV is facilitated by exogenous triggering factors, such as drugs (penicillin, pyrazolone or their derivatives, and interferons), physical agents (burns, ionizing radiations), viruses (Herpesviridae family), hormones (pregnancy, Graves' disease) and even foods (garlic, leek) or emotional stress. In the majority of patients no inducing agent can be detected, so the cause of the disease, leading to the production of pathogenic pemphigus antibodies (immunoglobulin G (IgG), occasionally IgA), usually remains unknown. These autoantibodies, probably aided by complement components and mediators such as plasminogen activator, bind PV antigens on squamous epithelial cell membranes and provoke cell–cell dyshesion, or detachment, namely acantholysis. It has also been speculated that pemphigus autoantibodies directly interfere with the molecules and peculiar enzyme activities (transglutaminase) responsible for cell–cell adhesion, thereby leading to acantholysis.

Clinical characteristics and course

The primary lesion in PV is a flaccid bulla that usually arises on apparently normal skin or mucosa. The bullae are fragile and break readily, leaving eroded areas which gradually heal.

In nearly two-thirds of cases, the oral mucosa is the site of onset and the disease may remain localized there for several months (oral pemphigus). Intact bullae are quite an uncommon finding in the mouth, where painful and poorly healing erosions represent the hallmark lesions.

Subsequently, the disease affects the skin with a certain predilection for the trunk, intertriginous areas (axillae, submammary and inguinal regions) and scalp, but every site may be involved. Pruritus and the degree of pain are variable. Other stratified squamous epithelial mucosal surfaces (pharynx, larynx, oesophagus, conjunctiva, urethra, cervix and anal mucosa) may also be affected in patients with more severe disease.

If left untreated, the disease becomes generalized (new crops of bullae appear everywhere, more and more areas of skin present eroded and crusted), the outcome being almost always fatal within 1–3 years due to uncontrolled fluid and protein loss or opportunistic infection. The use of systemic glucocorticoids and immunosuppressive therapy has completely modified the natural course and dramatically improved the prognosis of the disease. Currently, mortality from PV is low, but deaths from treatment complications are not a rare event.

Diagnosis

Diagnosis is based on the typical clinical patterns, clinical signs and laboratory tests.

Nikolski's sign I is produced when lateral pressure is applied to the edge of a bulla or to normal-appearing skin, with resultant separation of the upper layers of the epidermis. Nikolski's sign II (or Asboe–Hansen sign) shows extension of the bulla when direct pressure is exerted over it.

By scraping the floor of a bulla or an erosion, typical acantholytic cells may be observed under light microscopy (Tzanck test). Standard histology of a fresh bulla reveals extensive suprabasilar splitting with formation of one or more intraepithelial cavities. Direct immunofluorescence shows the intercellular deposition of IgG and C3 in the epidermis of the perilesional skin. Indirect immunofluorescence (using monkey oesophagus as substrate) is the classic method for detecting and determining the titre for pemphigus autoantibodies in the serum. This test is also important for evaluating treatment, because antibody titres usually parallel disease activity, and their abrupt change may herald a forthcoming alteration in the clinical state. When the diagnosis remains uncertain, immunoprecipitation and immunoblotting studies on the serum are needed.

Differential diagnosis

Recurrent aphthous stomatitis, Behçet's disease, erosive lichen planus, Stevens–Johnson syndrome or cicatrical pemphigoid can simulate the oral erosions of pemphigus, but Tzanck test is constantly negative in all these conditions. Widespread skin erosions may suggest bullous pemphigoid, glucagonoma syndrome or epidermolysis bullosa. In all doubtful cases, the histological examination of a fresh bulla, direct immunofluorescence on the perilesional skin, indirect immunofluorescence and, in particular circumstances (e.g. suspicion of paraneoplastic pemphigus), immunoprecipitation or immunoblotting establish the diagnosis.

Treatment

PV may present with wide clinical variations, ranging from the paucilesional oral pemphigus, to extensive erosions in the mouth and scattered blisters on the trunk, and ultimately the most severe forms, where the involvement of nearly all the Malpighian mucosae and the numerous large bullae together with vast eroded areas on most parts of the body threaten the patient's life. In addition, the patients with PV may also suffer from other diseases (diabetes, hypertension, peptic ulcer) that cannot be overlooked by the clinician who plans the therapy. Therefore, to indicate a standard treatment, tailored to all forms of PV and each patient's needs, is a Utopian task. Therapeutic guidelines for cases of average severity are given here. Indications for the management of problem cases as well as supportive measures and suggestions for all pemphigus sufferers are also outlined.

General therapeutic guidelines

The cornerstone therapy for PV is a combination of systemic corticosteroids and immunosuppressive drugs. As a rule, the impact of initial treatment determines therapeutic effectiveness, so that a full-dosage regimen should be started even in less severe cases. The combination can be given in continuous high dosage (conventional therapy), as suggested for patients with mild to moderate forms of disease, or at exceedingly high but intermittent doses (pulse therapy), in severe and especially in life-threatening cases, for some of which the adjunct of periodical plasma exchanges (plasmapheresis) may prove to be the winning move. Topical treatment is only supplementary treatment and is aimed at avoiding local infection and stimulating re-epithelialization of eroded areas.

Conventional therapy

In our experience combined deflazacort and azathioprine, given orally, is the most effective and safe management for the majority of patients with PV. This has lately been confirmed also for oral pemphigus. The schedule of treatment is organized in stages (Table 1).

Attack treatment

Therapy starts with daily doses of 120–150 mg of deflazacort (about 2 mg/kg) combined with 100 mg of azathioprine (about 1.5 mg/kg). This regimen is usually maintained until all active lesions disappear, which on average requires 4 weeks.

Decreasing steroid dosage on alternate days

The dosage of deflazacort is lowered by 6 mg every other day (e.g. even number days), progressively down to zero. On the other alternate days (e.g. odd number days), the initial dose of deflazacort remains unchanged (e.g. 120 or 150 mg). The daily dosage of azathioprine (e.g. 100 mg) is not modified during this period. When the corticosteroid has been suppressed on alternate days, which requires 6 (starting from 120 mg) to 7 (from 150 mg) weeks, the patient's condition is assessed, in particular by means of an oesophagoscopic monitoring and a titration of intercellular antibodies in the serum.

Decreasing steroid dosage weekly

If the therapeutical response is good (no mucosal lesions, antibody titre reduced or also unmodified), the alternate day administration of deflazacort will be lowered by 15 mg every week until it reaches 45 mg.

Table 1 Stages of conventional therapy for PV

I Attack treatment for 4 weeks

- Deflazacort 120 mg daily
- Azathioprine 100 mg daily

IIa Alternate day decrease in steroid dosage

Days	1	2	3	4	//	39	40
Deflazacort (mg)	120	114	120	108		120	0
Azathioprine		100 mg daily				100 mg daily	

IIb Weekly decrease in steroid dosage

Weeks	I							II							//	VI						
Days	1	2	3	4	5	6	7	1	2	3	4	5	6	7	//	1	2	3	4	5	6	7
Deflazacort (mg)	120	0	120	0	120	0	120	105	0	105	0	105	0	105		45	0	45	0	45	0	45
Azathioprine								100 mg daily										100 mg daily				

III Maintenance treatment: spacing steroid administration

- Deflazacort 45 mg every other day for 2 months
  45 mg every third day for 2 months
  45 mg on Tuesday and Friday for 2 months
  45 mg weekly for 6 months to 2 years
- Azathioprine 100 mg daily

Should mucosal lesions still persist or the antibody titre rise, the alternate day full-dose deflazacort has to be maintained and the daily dosage of azathioprine can be increased to 150 or 200 mg. The duration of this last schedule strictly depends on the course of the disease. When all signs of active PV have gone, the progressive reduction of the deflazacort dosage may be accomplished as indicated above. It seems wise not to reduce the dose of azathioprine at the same time; it may be lowered later; in any case, this reduction should not go lower than the initial 100 mg per day regimen.

Maintenance treatment: distancing steroid dosage

Once 45 mg dosage is reached, deflazacort is continued on alternate days for 2 months, then spaced out to every third day (for a further 2 months), twice a week (for another 2 months), and subsequently once a week for a variable period (6 months to 2 years). In the meantime the daily dose of azathioprine is maintained at 100 mg. There are no absolute criteria for when treatment can be stopped. If remission lasts 2 years, the weekly administration of deflazacort at 45 mg can be discontinued and the patient given only the immunosuppressive drug. One year later, the azathioprine treatment could also be terminated. In case of recurrence, the high-dosed combination of deflazacort and azathioprine should be reconsidered, but in less severe forms, a curative attempt with the immunosuppressive drug alone may reasonably be made.

Side-effects of deflazacort and azathioprine rarely raise serious problems. Gastric hyperacidity, changes in blood glucose levels and serum electrolytes, osteoporosis, menses alteration, cataracts, infections, mild and usually transient haematological abnormalities are the most common drawbacks to face. In particular, the patients who are homozygotes for the low-activity allele for thiopurine methyltransferase (TMT) are at risk for myelosuppression when treated long term with azathioprine. Therefore, before commencing this treatment, TMT levels should be measured.

If contraindicated, azathioprine can be replaced by other immunosuppressants with steroid-sparing effects that proved to be effective in controlling PV patients. Cyclophosphamide (1–3 mg/kg daily in two or three divided doses), chlorambucil (4–6 mg once daily), methotrexate (2.5 mg every 12 h × 3 doses each week) or mycophenolate mofetil (1 g twice daily) are the immunosuppressive drugs that can be added to the basic steroid treatment with good evidence-based results. Interestingly, with mycophenolate mofetil, which is characterized by a low toxicity profile and proved to be effective also in monotherapy, circulating pemphigus autoantibodies disappear by 2 months. Ciclosporin (5 mg/kg daily), in association with corticosteroids, offers no advantage over treatment with corticosteroids alone in PV patients, while it seems effective if combined with cyclophosphamide. A combination of systemic corticosteroids and dapsone may be used in childhood PV.

Pulse therapy

Pulse therapy (also named 'big shot' therapy) refers to discontinuous intravenous infusion of very high doses (megadoses) of drugs over a short time. With PV, the largest experience with pulse corticosteroid-immunosuppressive therapy has been made using daily megadoses of dexamethasone or methylprednisolone and cyclophosphamide. The standard regimen (Fig. 1) consists of administering 100 mg dexamethasone (or 500 mg methylprednisolone), dissolved in 500 mL of 5% dextrose, by a slow intravenous infusion over 1–2 h, on 3 consecutive days, along with 500 mg cyclophosphamide in the same infusion on the first day only. Such

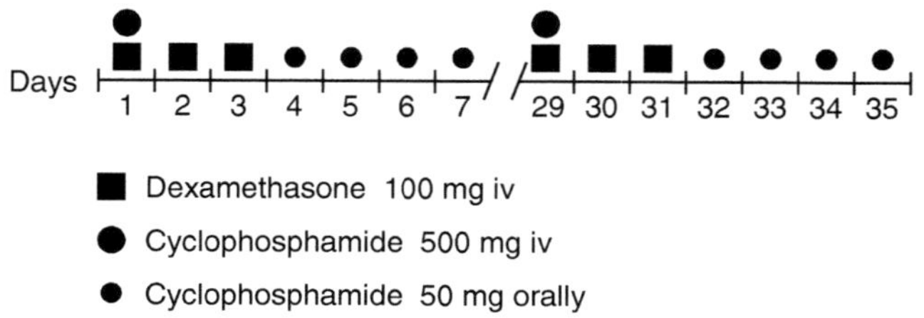

Figure 1 Pulse therapy: iv megadoses of corticosteroid and immunosuppressive drugs are given over a short time (3 and 1 days, respectively) every fourth week; in between these pulses a low-dosed immunosuppressive treatment is given orally.

corticosteroid-immunosuppressive pulses are repeated at 28-day intervals (in most severe cases at 14-day intervals).

In between the pulses, the patient is only given oral low-dose cyclophosphamide (50 mg/day). This treatment is continued for 4–6 months after complete clinical remission. The number of pulses required to induce complete clinical remission vary between 6 (about 50% of cases) and 30 (about 10% of cases). Then the pulses are stopped but a maintenance treatment of daily, oral 50 mg cyclophosphamide is continued for at least a year.

Lately, higher and repeated megadoses of cyclophosphamide (up to 50 mg/kg per day for 4 days) have been used successfully in patients with PV recalcitrant to standard therapy.

Side-effects of pulse therapy encompass mild acute events (nausea, facial flushing, mood change, sleep disturbance) and severe drawbacks (aseptic osteonecrosis, seizures, cardiac arrythmias, and even sudden deaths), the latter ones being rare and mostly occurring in patients with other risk factors. Long-term treatment with cyclophosphamide may cause sterility with azoospermia (so its use should be avoided in young patients), haematological abnormalities (depression in leukocytes and platelets), haemorrhagic cystitis, and hair loss, a transient side-effect especially disliked by women. Paradoxically, toxicities frequently noted with the use of oral cyclophosphamide therapy may be significantly less common with pulse intravenous administration of cyclophosphamide.

Plasmapheresis

Plasmapheresis was introduced in 1978 for treating patients with PV as a logical consequence of proven pathogenicity of the intercellular antibodies. The goal of periodic plasma exchanges in PV patients is to remove these circulating autoantibodies, which are known to be the cause of acantholytic lesions. However, a feedback mechanism regulates the antibody level in the circulation, so that a massive antibody depletion triggers a burst of new antibody production ('rebound'). Synchronization of plasmapheresis and pulse corticosteroid-immunosuppressive therapy can induce long-lasting remission of PV by selectively destroying the B-cell clones that produce pathogenic autoantibodies. This can best be achieved if the pulse treatment is given on the days immediately following large-volume plasma exchanges, when the antibody-producing cell clones reach the maximum rebound proliferation (Fig. 2). The regimen is scheduled with daily large-volume (60 mL/kg) plasmaphereses on days 1, 2, 3 and 7, i.v. prednisolone (2 mg/kg per day) and cyclophosphamide (12 mg/kg per day) on days 4, 5, 6 during the first week. Subsequently, the corticosteroid dosage is gradually reduced to zero within 11 months, while oral cyclophosphamide (100–150 mg/day) is given for 6 months, then tapered to 50 mg/day for a further 4 months.

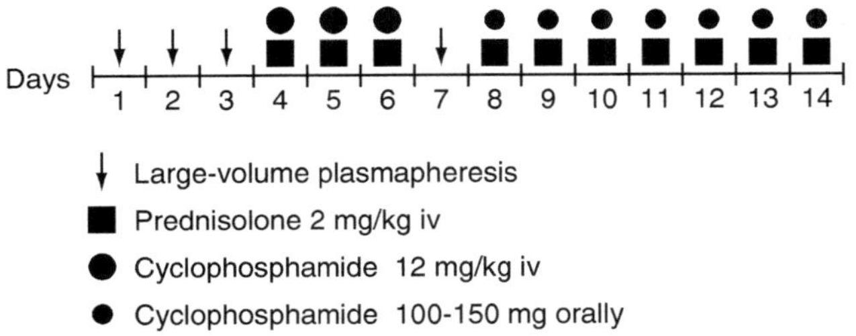

Figure 2 Synchronization of plasmapheresis and pulse corticosteroid-immunosuppressive therapy: the pharmacological treatment is given soon after the antibody depletion caused by plasma exchanges to best hinder the 'rebound' antibody production.

Plasmapheresis is a useful intervention in PV patients who are not responding to standard therapy or who require unacceptably high doses of corticosteroids or immunosuppressants. Severe exacerbation of PV in pregnancy specifically calls for plasmapheresis, as this treatment reduces the risk of intrauterine or neonatal pemphigus and obviates the serious side-effects that conventional immunosuppressive therapy may cause to the fetus. By comparing two techniques of plasma exchanges, single filtration plasmapheresis proved to be superior over double filtration plasmapheresis.

Minor complications of plasmapheresis include chills, fever, allergic reactions and transient hypotension. More serious complications are fluid and electrolyte imbalance (rarely resulting in pulmonary oedema or shock), depletion of platelets or clotting factor with consequent bleeding diathesis, and infections (pneumonia). High-dose intravenous IgG (IVIG) (daily 400 mg/kg for 5 days), used instead of cyclophosphamide to face the 'rebound' antibody burst subsequent to each plasma exchange, works better to prevent the risk of opportunistic infections. In fact, the administration of IVIG can partly compensate (instead of enhancing as cyclophosphamide does) the global immunosuppression provoked by plasmapheresis.

Topical treatment

Bullae should be incised and erosions treated with sprays or creams containing corticosteroids and antibiotics or nonirritant antiseptics. Painful oral lesions may require the use of topical anaesthetics, especially before eating, and of potent aerosolized steroids.

Intralesional corticosteroids (triamcinolone acetonide diluted to 10 mg/mL) can be used to speed the resolution of individual lesions. This modality is especially useful for treating recalcitrant oral erosions as well as new lesions in patients receiving tapering doses of conventional medication without intensifying systemic therapy.

In selected cases, the re-epithelialization of vast eroded areas can be hastened by means of hyperbaric oxygen treatment, which also has antiseptic and possibly immunosuppressive properties.

Patients with PV confined to the oral mucosa (so-called oral pemphigus) may respond to potent topical corticosteroids. Clobetasol propionate 0.05% ointment can be applied directly or under soft plastic or silicone rubber occlusive dental devices (trays) for 20 min twice daily, or inside a soft dental impression carrier, held in place four times daily for 1 h, or in an easy-to-spread bioadhesive polymer cream (Corega fit), which is very useful where a dental support is not available (e.g. buccal mucosa). Clobetasol propionate 0.05% cream can be useful to maintain remission in patients with mild PV. Topical ciclosporin (5 mL of a solution of 100 mg/mL swished in the mouth for 5 min, three times daily for 2 months) can enhance the efficacy of systemic therapy in patients with debilitating oral pemphigus. It can also be used to mantain remission.

Alternative and experimental treatments

The high doses and prolonged administration of corticosteroid and immunosuppressive drugs required to treat PV result in numerous side-effects, some of which may be fatal in the long run. This has spurred on a continued search for other therapies that might be used alone as sole systemic alternative treatment, or in combination with a low-dose conventional cure, as an adjuvant management. Plasmapheresis is such a good example of cure fitting both necessities that it is presently included among the standard treatments for life-threatening cases of PV. In problem patients, other alternative or adjunctive therapies are gold salts, gammaglobulins, the combination of tetracycline and niacinamide, and photopheresis.

Gold salts

Intramuscular injections of either gold sodium thiomalate or aurothioglucose are given once weekly, in single doses of 50 mg to a total dose of 1 g. The treatment can be continued with fortnightly doses to 2 g, then monthly doses up to 3 g. Adverse side-effects, such as pruritus, cutaneous allergic reactions, renal toxicity and bone marrow suppression, are frequent. Auranofin is an oral preparation (3 mg twice daily) which seems to be less toxic but also less effective. We do not favour the use of gold compounds in PV because of the reported onset of pemphigus lesions in patients treated with chrysotherapy for rheumatoid arthritis.

Gammaglobulins

High-dose IVIG treatment, which has been used in some autoimmune disorders, may be useful in PV, albeit experience is limited and the results are conflicting in the patients treated with it so far. The rationale for this promising, though expensive, treatment hinges upon its interaction with immune-mediated mechanisms. In fact, massive intravenous doses of IgG neutralize circulating autoantibodies and indirectly slow down their production.

IgG is given as a daily dose of 250–600 mg/kg for 3–5 consecutive days. Serious side-effects have not been reported. Minor complications, such as dyspnoea, abdominal pain, headache, hyperhidrosis and tachycardia, may occur. Conversely, local or systemic infections, facilitated by conventional immunosuppressive therapy for PV, may be better controlled by the use of polyclonal IgG in high concentrations.

IVIG treatment is indicated for immediate control of severe PV because of the rapid clinical remission it can induce in patients with recalcitrant PV.

Tetracycline and niacinamide

The association of oral tetracycline (2 g/day) or minocycline (200 mg/day) with niacinamide (1.5 g/day), in conjunction with topical steroids, has proven to be a beneficial adjunct to the conventional treatment, permitting a reduction in steroid or immunosuppressive doses required to maintain remission. Being a combination of relatively safe drugs, this therapeutic approach is worthy of further investigation. A reversible minocycline-induced hyperpigmentation seems to be a peculiar mucocutaneous side-effect in patients with immunobullous disorders.

Photophoresis

This sophisticated and still experimental treatment, consisting of extracorporeal UV radiation of blood following the ingestion of photosensitiving drugs (psoralens), has also been used in managing PV and given good results. Precautions and some side-effects are similar to those for plasmapheresis.

Innovative potential therapies

Understanding of the pathophysiology of PV suggests innovative therapeutic approaches for this disease. They point to either extracorporeal immunoadsorption of the pathogenic autoantibodies or the use of a chimeric autoantigen–toxin molecule capable of selectively destroying the autoantibody producing B cells.

Clinical precautions and useful suggestions

Patients with PV should be discouraged from over-indulging in unnecessary drugs (e.g. common analgesics, mucolytic drugs, laxatives), even in the stages of clinical remission, because of the risk for a drug-induced relapse of their disease (drug-induced pemphigus). In particular, the drugs implicated in inducing or triggering pemphigus (Table 2) should possibly be avoided and, if necessary, replaced by others with similar therapeutic action but not being considered at risk of pemphigus induction. For example, in the case of respiratory or cutaneous infections, macrolides can substitute penicillin, its derivatives and cephalosporins; in some cases of hypertension, β-blockers or calcium antagonists (except nifedipine) may take the place of angiotensin-converting enzyme (ACE) inhibitors.

Exposure to the sun and other UV sources requires special caution, since these physical agents may facilitate the outbreak of pemphigus or its relapses. The same can be said for intensive and prolonged emotional stress.

Patients with PV should be advised to have a balanced diet and avoid foods spiced with garlic, onion and leek; these culinary plants (belonging to the genus *Allium*) contain allyl compounds with proven acantholytic potential. As nicotine may improve pemphigus lesions, cigarette smoking is not contraindicated in patients with PV.

Table 2 Some drugs implicated in inducing or triggering PV

Antibiotics
Penicillin and its derivatives
Cephalosporins
Rifampicin
NSAIDs
Pyrazolone derivatives
Oxicam derivatives
Diclofenac
ACE inhibitors
Captopril
Enalapril
Fosinopril
Cytokines
α-Interferon
β-Interferon
Interleukin-2

Further reading

Amagai M, Hashimoto T, Shimizu N *et al.* Absorption of pathogenic autoantibodies by the extracellular domain of pemphigus vulgaris antigen (Dsg3) produced by baculovirus. *J Clin Invest* 1994; 94: 59–67.

Bjarnason B, Skoglund C, Flosattodir E. Childhood pemphigus vulgaris treated with dapsone: a case report. *Pediatr Dermatol* 1998; 15: 381–3.

Calebotta A, Sáenz AM, Gonzáles F *et al.* Pemphigus vulgaris: benefits of tetracycline as adjuvant therapy in a series of thirteen patients. *Int J Dermatol* 1999, 38: 217–21.

Ciompi ML, Marchetti G, Bazzichi L *et al.* D-penicillamine and gold salt treatments were complicated by myasthenia and pemphigus, respectively, in the same patient with rheumatoid arthritis. *Rheumatol Int* 1995; 15: 95–7.

Colonna L, Cianchini G, Frezzolini A *et al.* Intravenous immunoglobulins for pemphigus vulgaris: adjuvant or first choice therapy? *Br J Dermatol* 1998; 138: 1102–3.

Dumas V, Roujeau JC, Wolkenstein P *et al.* The treatment of mild pemphigus vulgaris and pemphigus foliaceus with a topical corticosteroid. *Br J Dermatol* 1999; 140: 1127–9.

Engineer L, Bhol KC, Ahmed AR. Analysis of current data on the use of intravenous immunoglobulins in management of pemphigus vulgaris. *J Am Acad Dermatol* 2000; 43: 1049–57.

Enk A, Knop J. Adjuvante Therapie von Pemphigus vulgaris und Pemphigus foliaceus mit intravenösen Immunoglobulinen. *Hautarzt* 1998; 49: 774–6.

Enk AH, Knop J. Mycophenolate is effective in the treatment of pemphigus vulgaris. *Arch Dermatol* 1999; 135: 54–6.

Euler HH, Loeffler H, Christophers E. Synchronization of plasmapheresis and pulse cyclophosphamide therapy in pemphigus vulgaris. *Arch Dermatol* 1987; 123: 1205–10.

Fleischli ME, Valek RH, Pandya AG. Pulse intravenous cyclophosphamide therapy in pemphigus. *Arch Dermatol* 1999; 135: 57–61.

Fox LP, Pandya AG. Pulse intravenous cyclophosphamide therapy for dermatologic disorders. *Dermatol Clin* 2000; 18: 459–73.

Gooptu C, Staughton RCD. Use of topical cyclosporin in oral pemphigus. *J Am Acad Dermatol* 1998; 38: 860–1.

Grando SA, Dahl MV. Nicotine and pemphigus. *Arch Dermatol* 2000; 136: 1269.

Grundmann-Kollmann M, Kaskel P, Leiter U *et al.* Treatment of pemphigus vulgaris and bullous pemphigoid with mycophenolate mofetil monotherapy. *Arch Dermatol* 1999; 135: 724–5.

Harman KE, Black MM. High-dose intravenous immune globulin for the treatment of autoimmune blistering diseases: an evaluation of its use in 14 cases. *Br J Dermatol* 1999; 140: 865–74.

Hayag MV, Cohen JA, Kerdel FA. Immunoablative high-dose cyclophosphamide without stem cell rescue in a patient with pemphigus vulgaris. *J Am Acad Dermatol* 2000; 43: 1065–9.

Ioannides D, Chrysomallis F, Bystryn JC. Ineffectiveness of cyclosporine as an adjuvant to corticosteroids in the treatment of pemphigus. *Arch Dermatol* 2000; 136: 868–72.

Jackson AP, Hall AG, McLelland J. Thiopurine methyltransferase levels should be measured before commencing patients on azathioprine. *Br J Dermatol* 1997; 136: 133–4.

Jolles S, Hughes J, Rustin M. Therapeutic failure of high-dose intravenous immunoglobulin in pemphigus vulgaris. *J Am Acad Dermatol* 1999; 40: 499–500.

Mehta JN, Martin AG. A case of pemphigus vulgaris improved by cigarette smoking. *Arch Dermatol* 2000; 136: 15–17.

Mignogna MD, Lo Muzio L, Mignogna RE *et al.* Oral pemphigus: long term behaviour and clinical response to treatment with deflazacort in sixteen cases. *J Oral Pathol Med* 2000; 29: 145–52.

Ogata K, Yasuda K, Matsushita M, Kodama H. Successful treatment of adolescent pemphigus vulgaris by immunoadsorption method. *J Dermatol* 1999; 26: 236–9.

Ozog DM, Gogstetter DS, Scott G, Gaspari AA. Minocycline-induced hyperpigmentation in patients with pemphigus and pemphigoid. *Arch Dermatol* 2000; 136: 1133–8.

Pacor ML, Biasi D, Carletto A *et al.* Ciclosporina topica nel trattamento del pemfigo orale. *Minerva Stomatol* 1998; 47: 183–6.

Pandya AG, Dyke C. Treatment of pemphigus with gold. *Arch Dermatol* 1998; 134: 1104–7.

Pasricha JS, Khaitan BK, Raman S, Chandra M. Dexamethasone-cyclophosphamide pulse therapy for pemphigus. *Int J Dermatol* 1995; 34: 875–82.

Piontek JO, Borberg H, Sollberg S *et al.* Severe exacerbation of pemphigus vulgaris in pregnancy: successful treatment with plasma exchange. *Br J Dermatol* 2000; 143: 455–6.

Proby CM, Ota T, Suzuki H *et al.* Development of chimeric molecules for recognition and targeting of antigen-specific B cells in pemphigus vulgaris. *Br J Dermatol* 2000; 142: 321–30.

Roujeau JC. Pulse glucocorticoid therapy. The 'big shot' revisited. *Arch Dermatol* 1996; 132: 1499–502.

Ruocco E, Aurilia A, Ruocco V. Precautions and suggestions for pemphigus patients. *Dermatology* 2001; 203: 201–7.

Ruocco V, Astarita, Pisani M. Plasmapheresis as an alternative or adjunctive therapy in problem cases of pemphigus. *Dermatologica* 1984; 168: 219–23.

Ruocco V, Brenner S, Ruocco E. Pemphigus and diet: does a link exist? *Int J Dermatol* 2001; 40: 161–3.

Ruocco V, Rossi A, Argenziano G, *et al.* Pathogenicity of the intercellular antibodies of pemphigus and their periodic removal from the circulation by plasmapheresis. *Br J Dermatol* 1978; 98: 237–41.

Ruocco V, Guerrera V, Lo Schiavo A, Pinto F. Il trattamento del pemfigo oggi. *G It Dermatol Venereol* 1997; 132: 259–69.

Ruocco V, Ruocco E, Wolf R. Bullous diseases: unapproved treatments or indications. *Clin Dermatol* 2000; 18: 191–5.

Sami N, Qureshi A, Ruocco E, Ahmed RA. Corticosteroid-sparing effect of intravenous immunoglobulin therapy in patients with pemphigus vulgaris. *Arch Dermatol* 2002; 138: 1158–62.

Sato N, Satake S, Fujiwara S *et al.* Pemphigus vulgaris treated with combined oral cyclosporin and cyclophosphamide. *Clin Exp Dermatol* 1998; 23: 92–6.

Shah N, Green AR, Elgart GW, Kerdel F. The use of chlorambucil with prednisone in the treatment of pemphigus. *J Am Acad Dermatol* 2000; 42: 85–8.

Sibaud V, Beylot-Barry M, Doutre MS, Beylot C. Pemphigus corticorésistant traité avec succès par immunoglobulines intraveineuses. *Ann Dermatol Venereol* 2000; 127: 408–10.

Smith TJ, Bystryn JC. Methotrexate as an adjuvant treatment for pemphigus vulgaris. *Arch Dermatol* 1999; 135: 1275–6.

Stanley JR. Therapy of pemphigus vulgaris. *Arch Dermatol* 1999; 135: 76–7.

Stanley JR. Understanding of the pathophysiology of pemphigus suggests innovative therapeutic approaches. *Br J Dermatol* 2000; 142: 208–9.

Turner MS, Sutton D, Sauder DN. The use of plasmapheresis and immunosuppression in the treatment of pemphigus vulgaris. *J Am Acad Dermatol* 2000; 43: 1058–64.

Wollina U, Lange D, Looks A. Short-time extracorporeal photochemotherapy in the treatment of drug-resistant autoimmune bullous diseases. *Dermatology* 1999; 198: 140–4.

Yano C, Ishiji T, Kamide R, Niimura M. A case of pemphigus vulgaris successfully treated with single filtration plasmapheresis: a correlation of clinical disease activity with serum antibody levels. *J Dermatol* 2000; 27: 380–5.

Photoageing

N.M. Craven and C.E.M. Griffiths

Definition and epidemiology

The term photoageing is used to describe the constellation of signs that distinguish skin which has endured prolonged exposure to the ultraviolet radiation (UVR) from that which has been largely protected from exposure. Although there are no data on prevalence, it is common in all races, and more severe changes are seen in those with fair skin, outdoor lifestyles and those living in areas of high incident UVR.

Aetiology and pathophysiology

It is generally accepted that most of the changes occurring in photoaged skin are due to the effects of ultraviolet A (UVA, 320–400 nm) and UVB (290–320 nm) radiation. Recent work has demonstrated that even low levels of UVB can increase dermal metalloproteinase expression in human skin leading to degradation of collagen, elastin and other dermal matrix proteins. By comparing changes in photoaged skin with those in photoprotected sites of the same patient (which controls for the effects of chronological ageing), it has been demonstrated that levels of collagens I and III are reduced within the dermis of photoaged skin, and at the dermal–epidermal junction (DEJ) there is a reduction in the number of anchoring fibrils and disruption of the fibrillin microfibril network.

Clinical characteristics and course

The cardinal features of photageing are coarse and fine wrinkles, laxity of the skin, mottled hyperpigmentation, a yellowish or 'sallow' appearance, a dry leathery texture to the skin and prominent telangiectases. These features are most prominent on areas such as the face (e.g. 'crow's feet' lines around the eyes), dorsal aspect of the neck (cutis rhomboidalis nuchae) and dorsal forearms. Such photoaged skin is susceptible to the development of neoplasia such as actinic keratoses and basal cell and squamous cell carcinomas. In contrast, sun-protected areas (such as buttock skin) remain pale and smooth, with fine wrinkles developing only in advanced age.

Photoaged skin demonstrates histological changes in both epidermis and dermis. Within the epidermis, keratinocyte atypia and dysplasia are seen, with increased numbers of melanocytes and decreased numbers of Langerhans' cells. The dermis contains a disorganized mass of thickened and degraded elastic fibres, decreased levels of collagen, and increased quantities of proteoglycans and glycosaminoglycans. Dermal blood vessels are dilated and tortuous with a perivascular infiltrate of neutrophils, lymphocytes and degranulating mast cells seen in the early evolving stages of photodamage. At least some of these histological changes occur in young adults before clinical evidence of photoageing is apparent.

Without treatment and adequate protection from further UVR exposure, the changes are slowly progressive, giving the erroneous impression of 'premature ageing'.

Differential diagnosis

The diagnosis is clinical and rarely poses a problem. Similar changes of wrinkling and laxity can be seen with widespread elastolysis of any cause, but in such cases the changes are not limited to areas of chronically sun-exposed skin and do not show the other typical features of photoageing.

Treatment

General therapeutic guidelines

Photoageing is a common condition and not all patients will require treatment. However, all such patients should be offered sun-protection advice in an attempt to reduce the risk of development of cutaneous malignancies. Treatment, for those who require it, must be continued on a long-term basis for sustained benefit.

Smoking should be discouraged. In addition to its well-known risks to general health, it also promotes the development of wrinkles.

Dryness of the skin is a feature of photoageing and can be ameliorated by the regular use of moisturizers.

Recommended therapies

Sun-protection measures

Patients wishing to improve the appearance of photoaged skin must be instructed in adequate sun protection in order to halt ongoing damage by UVR:

- avoid sunlight between 11 a.m. and 2 p.m. when UVR intensity is at its greatest
- when outdoors on bright days:

wear protective clothing and headgear: the fabric must be closely woven to provide an adequate barrier against UVR;

use a broad-spectrum sun block of SPF-15 or greater, applied every 2 h to exposed areas.

Topical all-trans retinoic acid

The ability of topical *all-trans* retinoic acid to improve features of photoageing has been demonstrated in vehicle-controlled double-blind studies. *All-trans* retinoic acid 0.05% in an emollient cream base is applied nightly to the affected areas of the skin. Treatment is continued on this basis for 4–6 months, followed by maintenance with applications either daily or once to three times weekly. Side-effects of dryness, peeling, erythema and irritation are common but diminish with continued treatment. Regular application of emollients may also alleviate these symptoms.

Smoothing of the skin occurs early, often within the first 4 weeks of treatment and is probably due to epidermal hyperproliferation, compaction of the stratum corneum and an increase in epidermal glycosaminoglycans. Lightening of hyperpigmented lesions is due to reduction in epidermal melanin content. Improvement in wrinkling occurs later and is probably related to changes at the DEJ and deposition of new collagen within the dermis itself. Histological features or epidermal atypia and dysplasia also improve.

All-trans retinoic acid binds with cytoplasmic binding proteins and specific nuclear receptors. Within the nucleus, the retinoid–receptor complex binds to specific DNA sequences situated in specific retinoid target genes, regulating transcription of these genes. Nuclear receptors and cytoplasmic binding proteins for retinoic acid have been demonstrated in human skin and gene expression of these proteins are induced by application of retinoic acid. Thus, it is probable that clinical improvement of photoageing is attributable to regulation of retinoid-specific gene expression.

Alternative and experimental treatments

Other topical retinoids

Topical 13-*cis* retinoic acid (isotretinoin), an isomer of *all-trans* retinoic acid, more often used systemically in the treatment of severe acne, has also been demonstrated to be effective in the treatment of photoageing. It is reported as being well tolerated, with less than 5% of patients experiencing severe reactions. *All-trans* retinoic acid is formed from retinal (vitamin A) by oxidation. Topical application of retinal in concentrations up to 1.6% produces biological changes characteristic of *all-trans* retinoic acid, but without significant erythema. This holds promise for topical retinoid therapy with fewer adverse reactions, but as yet retinal has not been formally evaluated for the treatment of photoageing.

Alpha hydroxy acids

Alpha hydroxy acids (AHA) such as glycolic acid or lactic acid, in low concentration (5–15% in water, ethanol or propylene glycol) applied twice daily to photoaged skin have been reported to diminish wrinkles. The mechanism seems to involve reduced corneocyte adhesion in the lower stratum corneum. Effects on wrinkles and other manifestations of photoageing may be enhanced by concomitant use of higher concentration AHA as a superficial chemical peel (see below).

Chemical peels

Chemical peeling involves controlled wounding of the skin, with subsequent regeneration. Peels may be deep (producing damage down to reticular dermis), medium depth (papillary dermis) or superficial (stratum corneum and epidermis). Deep peels produce better results but carry more risk of scarring, pigmentary change and if phenol is used as the peeling agent, systemic toxicity. Patient selection is important and experience is required in performing the technique safely.

Surgical treatments

Blepharoplasty and rhytidectomy (facelift) can reduce the appearance of wrinkles and remove excess skin, but will not affect other manifestations of photoageing. Dermabrasion involves the mechanical removal of epidermis and papillary dermis, with subsequent regeneration; a similar effect can be produced with an ultrapulse CO_2 laser. Collagen or silicone can be injected into wrinkles that do not respond to other therapeutic approaches.

Further reading

Kang S, Duell EA, Fischer GJ *et al.* Application of retinal to human skin *in vivo* induces epidermal hyperplasia and cellular retinoid binding proteins characteristic of retinoic acid but without measurable retinoic acid levels or irritation. *J Invest Dermatol* 1995; 105: 549–56.

Leyden JJ, Grove GL, Grove MJ *et al.* Treatment of photodamaged facial skin with topical tretinoin. *J Am Acad Dermatol* 1989; 21: 638–44.

Olsen EA, Katz HI, Levine N *et al.* Tretinoin emollient cream: A new therapy for photodamaged skin. *J Am Acad Dermatol* 1992; 26: 215–24.

Rafal ES, Griffiths CEM, Ditre CM *et al.* Topical tretinoin (retinoic acid) treatment for liver spots associated with photodamage. *NEJM* 1992; 326: 368–74.

Senagorta E, Lesiewicz J, Armstrong RB. Topical isotretinoin for photodamaged skin. *J Am Acad Dermatol* 1992; 27: S15–S18.

Van Scott EJ, Yu RJ. Alpha hydroxy acids: procedures for use in clinical practice. *Cutis* 1989; 43: 222–8.

Weinstein GD, Nigra TP, Pochi PE *et al.* Topical Tretinoin for the treatment of photodamaged skin. A Multicenter Study. *Arch Dermatol* 1991; 127: 659–65.

Weiss JS, Ellis CN, Headington JT *et al.* Topical tretinoin improves photoaged skin: a double-blind vehicle-controlled study. *JAMA* 1988; 259: 527–32. (Errata: *JAMA* 1988; 259: 3274 and 260: 926.)

Pityriasis lichenoides acuta

A. Andreassi and L. Andreassi

Synonyms

Mucha–Haberman disease, pityriasis lichenoides et varioliformis acuta.

Definition and epidemiology

Pityriasis lichenoides et varioliformis acuta (PLEVA) is the acute form of a papulosquamous cutaneous disorder, whose chronic form is also known as guttate parapsoriasis. A rare severe febrile ulceronecrotic variant is well known, whereas the exact nosological classification of lymphomatoid papulosis, a possible persistent variant of PLEVA, remains to be determined. The disease has been reported mainly in adolescents and in young adults, rarely in infancy or in old age.

Aetiology and pathophysiology

Pityriasis lichenoides acuta is a disease of unknown aetiology. It is debated if PLEVA is an immune complex-mediated hypersensitivity vasculitis triggered by various infectious agents, or a genuine lymphoproliferative process that is part of the cutaneous T-cell lymphoproliferative spectrum, possibly related to lymphomatoid papulosis. Although the attempts to isolate bacterial or viral agents have failed, the hypothesis of a reaction to an infective organism is accepted. The elevated incidence in young patients and the self-limited course support such a hypothesis.

Histological examination of early lesions shows individual cell necrosis in the epidermis, oedema in the papillary dermis and perivascular lymphocytic infiltrate. In evoluted lesions exocytosis of lymphocytes and erythrocytes and superficial and mid-dermal infiltrate are evident. In the epidermis exocytosis and vesiculation may be present before the entire epidermis becomes necrotic The dermal infiltrate is mainly represented by CD8+ suppressor/cytotoxic lymphocytes with a T-cell clonality, and this finding supports the hypothesis that PLEVA could be a lymphoproliferative disorder.

Clinical characteristics and course

The lesions of PLEVA usually appear on the anterior trunk and flexor surfaces of the extremities. The onset is sudden with reddish-brown macules and oedematous pink papules that undergo central vesiculation and haemorrhagic necrosis. Occasionally headache, malaise and fever may precede or accompany the onset of the disease. Lesions tend to be more numerous on the proximal than the distal parts of the extremities. The face, scalp and palmoplantar surfaces are usually spared but in some cases the lesions may involve the entire body surface.

In the febrile ulceronecrotic variant of PLEVA the disease begins with high fever, asthenia, malaise, intense myalgias, neuropsychiatric alterations and multiple cutaneous lesions. Older lesions progress to large painful ulcers with central necrosis and raised borders.

In most cases PLEVA is a self-healing process that resolves in a few months. Sometimes, however, the disease changes to pityriasis lichenoides chronica and may persist for years with a course characterized by remissions and exacerbation. The course of febrile ulceronecrotic variant can last from 1 month to 2 years with recurrent acute episodes.

Diagnosis

A number of laboratory abnormalities have been shown in patients with PLEVA, but they are not significant for the diagnosis. Skin biopsy showing the above described data is the only important finding. A malignant lymphoma mimicking PLEVA or related conditions, such as lymphomatoid papulosis, has to be considered.

Differential diagnosis

- Pityriasis lichenoides chronica: discrete papules and macules with micaceous scales.
- Guttate psoriasis: monomorphic lesions with stratified scales.
- Lymphomatoid papulosis: larger and less numerous lesions; lymphoma-like infiltrate.
- Secondary syphilis: palmoplantar involvement; positive serological tests.
- Varicella: involvement of scalp; multinucleate giant cells at cytological examination.
- Giannotti–Crosti disease: lack of necrosis; acral distribution of the lesions.
- Erythema multiforme: involvement of mucous membranes; target lesions.

Treatment

General therapeutic guidelines

Although PLEVA displays similar characteristics in adults and children, these latter cannot benefit by all available therapeutic procedures; among them methotrexate and psoralen and ultraviolet A (PUVA) therapy.

Most patients with PLEVA are in good general health and symptom free except low-grade fever and mild pruritus. For these subjects, considering that the disease is often a self-healing process, treatment is not always necessary. In any case therapy is required in more severe forms, particularly in febrile patients with ulceronecrotic nodules and plaques evolving in ulcerated lesions. In such subjects systemic administration of steroids is necessary.

Since clinical evidence suggests that PLEVA may be a reaction of hypersensitivity to an infectious agent, antibiotic treatment is recommended at least at the onset of the disease. Penicillin at standard doses is generally used, whereas oral erythromycin is the antibiotic of choice in children.

Recommended therapies

Topical steroid creams and systemic antihistamines

These are the most common and safe treatments and can be used both in adults and children. They may relieve pruritus but have little influence on the course of the disease.

Systemically administered steroids

These induce regression of the lesions only in sporadic cases, however in most patients they are able to reduce the intensity of the disease. In our experience a short treatment with prednisolone at 0.5 mg/kg daily induces the regression of general symptoms, permitting other treatments to be performed, particularly phototherapy in patients with severe clinical lesions.

UV radiation

This is the most powerful tool for the treatment of PLEVA. It has been used as simple solar exposure, PUVA, UVA without psoralen, UVB and UVAB. All these procedures, except PUVA, can be used in adults and children. Particularly recommended is phototherapy with UVB or UVAB.

Treatment with UVB is performed 2 or 3 times a week, starting with doses of 20–40 mJ/cm^2 in relation to skin type. Twenty to thirty sessions are usually required to obtain clearance of the lesions. UVAB therapy is performed with modalities similar to those used for UVB alone. Narrow-band UVB therapy with TL01 lamps should provide further advantages, but no data on the treatment of PLEVA are available.

Regression of PLEVA after UV radiation is not always permanent. Possible recurrences can be treated with further UV treatments. How UV radiation works in the treatment of PLEVA is not known. A possible hypothesis is that UV radiation inhibits the release of some inflammation mediators and therefore is able to interfere with lymphocyte infiltrate.

Alternative and experimental treatments

Tetracycline

Some patients with PLEVA are responsive to tetracycline given at the initial dose of 2 g daily for 2–4 weeks, followed by maintenance treatment of 1 g daily. Alternatively, minocyline or doxycycline can be used at dosage of 100 mg daily. Since tetracyclines are effective even if no infection signs are evident, a possible inhibition of neutrophil chemotaxis is hypothesized.

Dapsone

This may be helpful in some cases of PLEVA. Also this drug is thought to have an anti-inflammatory effect not related to its antibacterial activity.

Oral gold (auranofin)

This has been indicated as another possible avenue of therapy of Mucha–Habermann disease.

Methotrexate

At low doses (7.5–20 mg weekly) methotrexate is effective in many patients with PLEVA, but its potential side-effects, as well as the tendency of the disease to recur after treatment, suggest restricting the use of this drug to very selected patients.

Ciclosporin

This is an immunosuppressive agent that has provided a new approach to therapy in autoimmune diseases and has produced good therapeutic responses in a number of dermatoses including pityriasis lichenoides chronica, but no data concerning the treatment of PLEVA have been reported.

Further reading

Cornelison RL Jr, Knox JM, Everett MA. Methotrexate for the treatment of Mucha–Habermann disease. *Arch Dermatol* 1972; 106: 507–8.

Dereure O, Levi E, Kadin ME. T-cell clonality in pityriasis lichenoides et varioliformis acuta: a heteroduplex analysis of 20 cases. *Arch Dermatol* 2000; 136: 1483–6.

Groisser DS, Griffiths CE, Ellis CN *et al*. A review and update of the clinical uses of cyclosporine in dermatology. *Dermatol Clin* 1991; 9: 805–17.

Nakamura S, Nishihara S, Nakayama K *et al*. Febrile ulcero-necrotic Mucha Habermann's disease and its successful therapy with DDS. *J Dermatol (Tokyo)* 1986; 13: 381–4.

Piamphongsant T. Tetracycline for the treatment of pityriasis lichenoides. *Br J Dermatol* 1974; 91: 319–22.

Romani J, Puig L, Fernandez-Figueras MT *et al*. Pityriasis lichenoides in children: clinicopathologic review of 22 patients. *Pediatr Dermatol* 1998; 15: 1–6.

Shelley WB, Shelley ED. *Advanced Dermatologic Therapy*. Philadelphia: Saunders, 1987.

Tay Y-K, Morelli JG, Weston WL. Experience with UVB phototherapy in children. *Pediatr Dermatol* 1996; 13: 406–9.

Tsuji T, Kasamatsu M, Yokota M *et al*. Mucha-Habermann disease and its febrile ulceronecrotic variant. *Cutis* 1996; 58: 123–31.

Van Neer FJ, Toonstra J, Van Voorst Vader PC *et al*. Lymphomatoid papulosis in children: a study of 10 children registered by the Dutch Cutaneous Lymphoma Working Group. *Br J Dermatol* 2001; 144: 351–4.

Pityriasis lichenoides chronica

L. Rauch and T. Ruzicka

Definition and epidemiology

Pityriasis lichenoides is a benign, uncommon, acquired chronic immunoreactive or lymphoproliferative dermatosis. An acute form, commoner in the young—pityriasis lichenoides et varioliformis acuta (PLEVA, or Mucha–Habermann disease)—and a chronic form (Juliusberg) can be distinguished. Pityriasis lichenoides chronica (PLC) has no apparent geographical or racial predilection. This dermatosis occurs mainly in adolescents and young adults and is rare in old age and infancy. It shows a prevalence in men (approximately 70%).

Aetiology and pathophysiology

Some data postulate that the pathogenesis may be due to a hypersensitivity reaction to infectious agents. It belongs to the benign T-cell diseases.

Clinical characteristics and course

In PLC, the spots are less angry-looking compared to PLEVA and are covered with a firm scale. The papules are small erythematous to reddish brown, although with increased numbers compared to PLEVA. The eruption is often polymorphic, with lesions at different stages of evolution. The spots fade within 3–4 weeks but new spots may then occur. Lesions may appear on the palms, soles, face and scalp, and may be distributed symmetrically or asymmetrically on the trunk, buttocks and proximal extremities, with occasional acral involvement. Erosions and haemorrhagic crusts may be found. Mucosal lesions consisting of irregular erythema and superficial ulcerations on the buccal mucosa and palate have been reported. In dark-skinned people, PLC rarely may present with widespread macular hypopigmentation rather than the typical papular morphology, especially common in children.

Differential diagnosis

This chronic form should be differentiated from guttate psoriasis and lichen planus. In psoriasis they are pink with adherent silver scales; in lichen they are flat and violaceous and in the more acute forms, not scaly. PLC can also mimic secondary syphilis but the diagnosis can be excluded serologically. Less frequently, PLC may simulate insect bites and drug eruptions. The detachable, single mica-like scale on the red–brown papule is a pathognomonic sign, which along with histological examination provide the diagnosis. The lesions of lymphomatoid papulosis are sometimes mistaken for PLC, but they are less vesicular and more necrotic than those of PLC and histopathology reveals the correct diagnosis.

Treatment

General therapeutic guidelines

PLC is a self-limiting disease and may regress spontaneously after months or rarely persist for years. The low frequency of the disease, the unknown aetiology and the unpredictability of its course are limiting factors in the evaluation of the effectiveness of different treatments.

Nonetheless, the unsightly appearance, and the tendency to provoke pigment alterations leading to significant emotional, social and physical consequences favour treatment.

Recommended therapies

Topical steroids

To decrease the inflammatory process and itching component topical steroids are frequently prescribed, though they do not significantly influence the course of the disease.

Systemic steroids

To control the systemic and cutaneous symptoms in the ulceronecrotic variant of PLC the systemic application of glucocorticoids such as prednisone 0.5–1.0 mg/kg of bodyweight per day can be beneficial.

Antihistamines

Antihistamines may reduce the symptom of itching though they do not influence the course of the disease. Due to reduction of pruritus they may reduce scratching and secondary infection which can lead to scarring and pigment alterations.

Antibiotics

The idea that PLC may be a hypersensitivity reaction to infectious agents prompts the usage of antibiotics. Especially in the treatment of children a long-term (minimum 4–8 weeks) high-dose treatment with erythromycin (30–50 mg/kg per day) can be effective. Depending on the response the dosage can be tapered over the course of several months. Erythromycin should be preferred over tetracycline in patients younger than 12 years of age to avoid possible adverse effects in dentition.

For adults tetracyclines in high doses of about 2 g/day for at least 4 weeks have shown favourable results. Here also it seems to be reasonable to reduce the antibiotics slowly at the end of the treatment to minimize the risk of relapses.

As antibiotics have few side-effects, they should be considered as first-choice medication before other, possibly more toxic measures are instituted.

Photo(chemo)therapy

Good therapeutic results are described for phototherapy. Broadband ultraviolet B (UVB) and narrowband or selective UVB (UVB 311 nm) and UV radiation from fluorescent sunlamps seem to be useful options. Three to five sessions a week over a period of about 2 months usually lead to a good response. The therapeutic mechanism probably is a local alteration of cell-mediated immunity in the treated skin, notably T-cell apoptosis.

There are also descriptions of oral psoralen and ultraviolet A (PUVA) photochemotherapy with 8-methoxypsoralen (0.6 mg/kg) which shows a remarkable therapeutic effect after about 20 treatments 4 times a week with an average cumulative dose of 70 J/cm^2.

Nonetheless, relapses often follow after discontinuation of photo(chemo)therapy. Maintenance applications of UVB (broadband, narrowband or selective) irradiation with fluorescent lamps or PUVA therefore should be considered—the interval ranging from once a week to once every 3 weeks.

UVA treatments and natural sun exposure may also be helpful for the patient in accelerating the resolution of the disease.

Ciclosporin

In refractory cases oral ciclosporins may be considered as an alternative treatment. Ciclosporin has been shown to be effective in many T-cell mediated diseases by its inhibitory effect on the activation of helper/inducer T cells and on the subsequent production of inflammatory cytokines. Different authors favour a treatment with oral ciclosporin with an initial dose of 5 mg/kg per day over a period of about 6–8 weeks. After a sufficient response is achieved the dose should be slowly tapered. As ciclosporin can lead to hypertension and renal dysfunction these parameters have to be monitored every 2–4 weeks. After discontinuation of ciclosporin therapy these side-effects usually normalize within 1 month.

Regarding the benign nature of this self-limited disease we favour an initial dose of about 4 mg/kg per day which can be adapted according to effects and side-effects.

Methotrexate

Oral or intravenous methotrexate seem to be effective in the more severe forms of PLC. Recommended doses vary between an initial test dose of of 5–10 mg/week and can gradually be increased by 2.5–5 mg/week. The effective dose ranges between 7.5 and 20 mg/week. Methotrexate can be given as a single weekly oral or intravenous application. Reduction of the dose often leads to recurrence. Before treatment renal, hepatic and bone marrow function have to be monitored and should lie within the normal range. Laboratory control of the treatment is essential. As methotrexate is an antimetabolic drug its use in PLC in children cannot be recommended.

Alternative and experimental treatments

Topical immunosuppressants

Topical immunosuppressants like pimecrolimus or tacrolimus may be beneficial in the treatment of PLC. As these substances are known to be effective in other T-cell mediated diseases such as atopic eczema and the disease responds to different systemic immunosuppressants their use may be beneficial. However, lack of scientific data renders these drugs experimental.

High-dose UVA treatment

High-dose UVA treatment has shown to be effective in T-cell mediated diseases like atopic eczema and mycosis fungoides. No sufficient data exists on the use in pityriasis lichenoides.

Further reading

Assman T, Homey B, Ruzicka T. Application of tacrolimus for the treatment of skin disorders. *Immunopharmacology* 2000; 2–3: 203–13.

Gelmetti C, Rigoni C, Alessi E *et al.* Pityriasis lichenoides in children: A long term follow-up of eighty-nine cases. *J Am Acad Dermatol* 1990; 23: 473–8.

Gupta AK *et al.* Oral cyclosporine in the treatment of inflammatory and noninflammatory dermatoses. *Arch Dermatol* 1990; 126: 339–40.

Klein PA, Callen JP. Pityriasis lichenoides. www.emedicine.com

Michel G, Ruzicka T *et al.* FK 506 in the treatment of inflammatory skin disease: promises and perspectives. *Immunol Today* 1996; 17: 116–28.

Morita A *et al.* Evidence that singlet oxygen-induced human T helper cell apoptosis is the basic mechanism of ultraviolet-A radiation phototherapy. *J Exp Med* 1997; 186: 1763–8.

Plettenberg H *et al.* Ultraviolet A1 (340–400nm) phototherapy for cutaneous T-cell lymphoma. *J Am Acad Dermatol* 1999; 41: 47–50.

Romani J *et al.* Pityriasis lichenoides in children: Clinicopathologic review of 22 patients. *Pediatr Dermatol* 1998; 15: 1–6.

Shieh S, Mikkola DL, Wood GS. Differentiation and clonality of lesional lymphocytes in pityriasis lichenoides chronica. *Arch Dermatol* 2001; 137: 305–8.

Pityriasis rosea

H. Degreef

Synonym

Gibert's disease.

Definition and epidemiology

Pityriasis rosea is an acute, inflammatory, self-limiting dermatosis characterized by typical oval to coin-sized maculopapular and erythematosquamous lesions, located primarily on the trunk and the proximal portion of the extremities. The disorder mostly affects adolescents and young adults, rarely the elderly or young children. Approximately 1–2% of new dermatology patients consult for this disorder. Generally, only one disease period occurs; rarely do we see two or more periods. The lesions are seen mostly in the spring and autumn.

Aetiology and pathophysiology

The cause of this disease is still unknown. Many causes have been suggested, such as stress, irritation by clothing, insect bites, medications and an isomorphic response.

An infectious origin, primarily a viral infection, is the most widely accepted hypothesis, but a specific causal virus has yet to be demonstrated. In recent years a lot of attention has been given to the role of human herpes virus-6 and herpes virus-7. Some authors were able to identify by nested PCR and *in situ* hybridization to detect and isolate these viruses in skin and other organs; others were unable to confirm these findings. It has also been suggested that pityriasis rosea may be caused by a reactivation of these viruses by certain factors, as most people acquire HHV-6 virus in early infancy (6–24 months, exanthema subitum). HHV-7 could cause the same clinical symptoms. Circumstantial evidence suggestive that it is an infectious disease includes its seasonal variation, the presence of prodromal symptoms in some patients, the occurrence of minor epidemics in small, closed communities and the course of the disease. Although some immunohistochemical findings are suggestive of a humoral immunological reaction (including immunoglobulin M (IgM) antibodies against the cytoplasm of the keratinocytes in serum and in lesional skin), more elements are suggestive of a cell-mediated immune mechanism (including either perivascular aggregates or predominantly CD4 T-helper cells in the superficial dermis and an increased level of the antigen-presenting Langerhans' cells).

Clinical characteristics and course

In some patients (about 5%), the skin lesions are preceded by flu-like symptoms.

Herald patch (plaque mère, mother patch)

The initial lesion is often a solitary, round or oval erythematosquamous patch, 2–5 cm in diameter, generally on the trunk. The centre is mostly salmon red with a colorette of scales attached at the margin. This gives it the medallion appearance. Stretching the medallion across the long axis demonstrates the 'hanging curtain' sign. The herald patch, however, is not always present.

Pityriasis rosea eruption

After 5–15 days, an eruption appears, primarily on the trunk and the proximal portions of the extremities. However the disorder can be more extensive and even affect the face. Exceptionally, there is oral involvement.

The eruption consists of oval erythematous maculae or papules, sometimes covered with a fine scaling, a few millimetres in size, or of medallions, but smaller (1–2 cm) than the mother patch. Sometimes one of the clinical forms dominates. The number of lesions can vary considerably. They tend to occur with their longest axis along the skin-tension lines to produce the 'Christmas-tree' distribution.

Sometimes, there are abnormal skin lesions (vesicular, purpuric or even pustular).

Generally, there is no itching. A slight itching can be present, sometimes caused by excessively irritant treatments with antiseptics or antimycotics. Rarely are there serious complaints of itching.

Spontaneous healing generally occurs in 4–6 weeks, sometimes sooner and sometimes later. Seldom are there any residual lesions. Hypo- or hyperpigmentation occurs sometimes. It can be aggravated or elicited by exposure to the sun or ultraviolet B (UVB) therapy.

Diagnosis

The clinical picture will generally enable the diagnosis to be made. A potassium hydroxide (KOH) preparation and fungal culture may be necessary to differentiate the herald patch from tinea corporis.

The histopathological picture varies from subacute to chronic dermatitis, often difficult to distinguish from eczema dermatitis. Dyskeratotic cells with a homogenous eosinophilic aspect in the upper dermis have been found in about half of the histological preparations taken from patients and are quite characteristic.

Differential diagnosis

- Widespread tinea corporis: KOH, culture.
- Pityriasis versicolor: KOH, culture.
- Psoriasis, parapsoriasis guttata: biopsy, if necessary.
- Lichen planus: typical mucosal lesions, biopsy if necessary.
- Secondary syphilis: serology.
- Nummular eczema (dry variant = pityriasiforme eczématides): this differential diagnosis can be difficult to make. The lesions can persist for longer periods.
- Drugs: pityriasis rosea-like eruptions have been reported for several drugs (barbiturates, captopril, clonidine, gold, isotretinoin, metronidazole, penicillamine, omeprazole, bacille Calmette–Guérin (BCG) therapy for bladder cancer, non-steroidal anti-inflammatory drugs (NSAIDs), codeine etc.); the lesions are generally less typical, both in aspect and in distribution and duration of evolution.

Treatment

General therapeutic guidelines

Since the cause of pityriasis rosea is still unknown and since it is generally asymptomatic and self-limiting, treatment is generally not needed when the clinical diagnosis is certain.

Assuring the patient together with providing information about the expected course will generally suffice.

It is important not to irritate the skin (excessive use of soap and water, excessive sweating, occlusive clothing of wool or synthetics).

Less typical courses (pityriasis rosea-like eruptions) can be caused by underlying infections or by medications.

When complaints of itching or forms that take a serious course appear, treatment can be considered.

Recommended therapy

Topical therapy

Topical steroids, usually of moderate strength, are generally used when there is serious itching or when the lesions are very extensive. Often, however, the itching can be eased by antipruritic lotions (0.5–1% menthol), oatmeal baths or bath oils, or even bland emollients (for dryness of the skin).

Physical therapy

UVB, usually with five to 10 daily erythematogenic exposures starting at 80% of the minimal erythematogenic dose and increasing by 20% each treatment, can substantially decrease the severity of the disease. A favourable effect on serious itching is not constant, and the duration of the disease is not shortened. There is an increased chance of postinflammatory hyperpigmentation.

Systemic therapy

As with many dermatoses, antihistamines are given for the itching. No results from controlled studies are available. Comparative studies between sedating and nonsedating antihistamines are also lacking.

With very serious forms, oral corticosteroids (15–40 mg oral prednisolone) are given. The itching and exanthema are quickly suppressed, but the total disease duration is not reduced.

Occasionally, an aggravation of the disorder has been observed with this medication.

For the treatment of serious vesiculobullous forms, a single course of dapsone (2×100 mg/day) over a brief period has been advised.

Further reading

Allen RA, Janniger CK, Schwartz RA. Pityriasis rosea. *Cutis* 1995; 56: 198–202.

Arndt KA, Paul BS, Stern RS *et al.* Treatment of pityriasis rosea with UV radiation. *Arch Dermatol* 1983; 119: 381–2.

Breese Hall C. The human herpesviruses and pityriasis rosea: Curious covert companions? *J Invest Dermatol* 2002; 119: 793–7.

Chuh AA, Peiris JS. Lack of evidence of active human herpes virus 7 (HHV-7) infection in three cases of pityriasis rosea in children. *Pediatr Dermatol* 2001; 18: 381–3.

Karabulut AA, Kocak M, Yilmaz N, Eksioglu M. Detection of human herpesvirus 7 in pityriasis rosea by nested PCR. *Int J Dermatol* 2002; **41**: 563–7.

Katsambas A. Quality of life in dermatology and the EADV. *JEADV* 1994; 3: 211–14.

Leenutaphong V, Jiamton S. UVB phototherapy for pityriasis rosea: a bilateral comparison study. *J Am Acad Dermatol* 1995; 33: 996–9.

Leonforte VF. Pityriasis rosea: exacerbation with corticosteroid treatment. *Dermatologica* 1981; 163: 480–81.

Parsons JM. Pityriasis rosea update 1986. *J Am Acad Dermatol* 1986; 15: 159–67.

Watanabe T, Kawamura T, Jacob SE *et al.* Pityriasis rosea is associated with systemic active infection with both human herpesvirus-7 and human herpesvirus-6. *J Invest Dermatol* 2002; 119: 779–80.

Pityriasis rubra pilaris

N. Cammarota, J. Hergocova and T.M. Lotti

Definition and epidemiology

Pityriasis rubra pilaris (PRP) is a rare, idiopathic inflammatory and hyperproliferative dermatosis of juvenile or adult onset characterized by varying degrees of erythema and scaling.

PRP was described initially by Claudius Tarral in 1828, although the name was coined by Besnier in 1889.

PRP occurs with equal frequency in males and females. The age distribution is bimodal, with peaks in the first and fifth to sixth decades, or trimodal, with peaks in the first, second and sixth decades. Most cases are acquired, although a familial form has been described.

Classification and prognosis

In 1980 Griffiths described five types of PRP, two of which, the adult type (II) and the atypical juvenile type (V), may be variants of ichthyotic disorder (Tables 1 and 2). The classic adult type (I) and classic juvenile type (III) may appear clinically the same, except for the subject's age.

Table 1 Traditional Griffith's classification.

Classic adult type (type I)
Atypical adult type (type II)
Classic juvenile type (type III)
Circumscribed juvenile type (type IV)
Atypical juvenile type (type V)

Table 2 Current classification.

Classic adult and classic juvenile type (differ only in patient's age)
Circumscribed juvenile type (different aetiology?)
HIV-related type (recently introduced)

The circumscribed juvenile type (IV) consists of localized plaques, usually on the elbows and knees, that are sharply demarcated areas of follicular hyperkeratosis and erythema. This type does not progress to the widespread classic form, suggesting a different aetiology.

Recently, it has been suggested that PRP associated with human immunodeficiency virus (HIV) infection should be considered an additional type VI PRP, characterized by papulonodular and lichen spinulosus-like lesions, poor prognosis and refractoriness to treatment.

According to Griffiths, the classic adult type has the best prognosis usually showing remission after several years. Type III was initially thought to have a worse prognosis than type I, but it is now considered to be prognostically favourable. The prognosis of the inherited form of PRP is often chronic skin inflammation throughout life.

Clinical data

The diagnosis of PRP is based essentially on characteristic clinical features.

The classic form of PRP is characterized by follicular hyperkeratotic papules, perifollicular erythema tending towards confluency and palmoplantar keratoderma and furfuraceous scaling of the scalp. The subject usually first notices redness and then scaling of the face and scalp which may be accompained by extreme itching. When the lesions coalesce, the characteristic individual papules may have disappeared or be found only on the dorsal aspect of phalanges, and on extensor aspects of the wrists, arms and thighs. The eruption spreads in a cephalocaudal direction sometimes resulting in total erythroderma within 6 months. However, in juvenile subjects, the disease usually begins on the lower half of the body. Even individuals with generalized erythroderma present characteristic patches (about 1 cm in size) of normal-appearing skin ('islands of sparing'). Almost all subjects present palmar and plantar keratoderma, that may be the first manifestation of the affection, and the distinctively orange or yellowish erythema is best seen on the palms and soles. In cases of extensive disease, ectropion is frequent.

Approximately 20% of subjects experience pruritus or burning sensation. The nails may show longitudinal ridging, subungual hyperkeratosis and splinter haemorrhages.

The condition remains static for about 12 months and then begins to fade with more islands of sparing appearing scattered in the erythematous area. The eruption fades in a reverse direction from its onset and clearance usually occurs (80% of cases) within 3 years. In the remaining 20% of cases the eruption continues indefinitely, but in certain individual cases spontaneous clearance may begin even after many years.

Albeit rarely, PRP has presented as the initial manifestation of a previously undiagnosed malignancy.

Differential diagnosis

This must be distinguished from psoriasis, generalized hypersensivity reaction, cutaneous T-cell lymphoma, lichen planopilaris, seborrhoeic dermatitis and subacute cutaneous lupus erythematosus.

Distinguishing features of PRP include islands of spared skin in generalized erythroderma, follicular keratotic plugs and the orange hue of involved skin.

Histology

Although a diagnosis of PRP cannot be made solely on the basis of histological criteria because the histological features are not pathognomonic, a microscopic evaluation can be helpful to rule out other papulosquamous and erythematous disorders.

The microscopic features of PRP include hyperkeratosis, perifollicular parakeratosis, acanthosis and a perivascular lymphocytic dermal infiltrate.

Table 3 Topical agents.

Emollients
Tar and keratolytic agents
Calcipotriol cream 50 μg/g
Capsaicin (0.05–0.1%) cream (if oral antihistamines have been unsuccessful)

Treatment

Evaluation of treatment for PRP can be difficult because of low incidence and the fact that the affection often resolves spontaneously.

Local treatments (Table 3)

A regular and copious application of emollients is generally helpful. Many different moisturizers are appropriate, but lighter body creams and milky preparations are not suitable. A mixture of equal parts of liquid paraffin and white soft paraffin generally helps remove the scales and provides good protection for the skin, with the advantage that it is easily spread.

Conservative management is usually recommended for juvenile cases because of the overall good prognosis and frequent limited involvement. Topical treatments, such as tar and keratolytic agents, may produce moderate improvement and also topical calcipotriol may be effective in children.

In cases of pityriasis capitis, topical steroids and imidazole preparations are often used but are not generally effective.

The keratoderma is very difficult to treat effectively. The aim of treatment is to soften the keratin and aid dehiscence using a keratolytic and the preparation is applied at night under polythene occlusion. The following is a suitable formula:

Salicylic acid	2%	5%	10%	20%
Petrolatum jelly	2 g	5 g	10 g	20 g
up to 100 g				

The gross thickening of the nails makes them difficult to cut. If chiropody services are available, regular treatment at 1–2-week intervals is ideal. If this is not possible, calliper-type nail cutters with a vertical side action are to be preferred to the usual laterally acting nail clippers.

The prolonged erythema on the face results in tension in the skin of the upper malar region, which pulls the lower eyelids down, resulting in ectropion and epiphora. In the milder stages this can be treated with 10 min applications of a cold compress of normal saline to the upper malar region, followed by the application of white, soft paraffin to maintain skin hydration.

Systemic and anti-itching therapy

Although PRP does not represent a vitamin A deficiency state, general administration of isotretinoin, etretinate and vitamin A play a significant role in therapy for many affected subjects. In all likelihood the effects of vitamin A and the newer synthetic retinoids depends on non-specific actions of these agents.

Vitamin A

Vitamin A therapy is often successful, but may be toxic because of the necessarily high doses (150 000–300 000 IU/day oral vitamin A). It is worth noting that the recommended dietary allowance of vitamin A is 5000 IU/day.

Hypervitaminosis A has been reported in adults reciving prolonged daily administration of 50 000 IU of vitamin A. High doses of oral vitamin A result in a relatively high incidence of side-effects, in particular headache, nausea, chills and hypertriglyceridaemia.

Table 4 Systemic retinoids (first-choice treatment for PRP).

Isotretinoin (first choice)
dosage: 1.0–1.5 mg/kg per day
median duration of treatment: 4–6 months
half-life: 6–36 h
Etretinate
dosage: 1.0 mg/kg per day
median duration of treatment: 3 months
half-life: ~100 days

Isotretinoin and etretinate (Table 4)
Isotretinoin and etretinate are synthetic vitamin A derivates. Synthetic retinoids are currently the treatment of choice for PRP and have largely replaced vitamin A therapy because they confer the same pharmacological action without the toxic effects. Furthermore, they appear to be more effective than vitamin A.

Isotretinoin can be effective at dosages of 1.0–1.5 mg/kg per day. Symptomatic improvement of erythema, pruritus, scaling and ectropion may occur within 1 month, although significant improvement or clearing may take 4–6 months. During this period of treatment with isotretinoin, daily skin care is important, especially moisturization. Isotretinoin should be the first choice of systemic therapy for most subjects with PRP because of its therapeutic efficacy and safety. Since isotretinoin has a shorter half-life than etretinate, it is the more recommended of the two drugs.

Etretinate is an aromatic retinoid that is stored in adipose tissue and can be detected in the blood more than 2 years after discontinuation of therapy. The initial etretinate dosage is usually 1.0 mg/kg per day. Depending on the clinical response, the maintenance dose remains the same or is tapered during therapy. In both children and adults the median duration of treatment is 4 months.

Hyperlipidaemia or hepatic dysfunction may result not only from treatment with high doses of vitamin A, but also from systemic retinoids. Serum triglyceride and cholesterol levels and liver function tests should be monitored during treatment. Teratogenicity and bone changes, such as hyperostosis, are other possible adverse effects of systemic retinoids. Because of its long half-life, etretinate therapy is avoided in women of childbearing age.

Methotrexate and azathioprine

Treatment with cytotoxic or immunosuppressive agents have shown varying success.

Methotrexate given orally 15–25 mg/week should be regarded as a second-choice treatment.

In general, once methotrexate therapy is initiated, improvement manifests after approximately 6 weeks, with complete response after 3–4 months.

Although most subjects respond to methotrexate, many relapse when therapy is discontinued; reinstitution of the drug usually results in rapid clinical improvement.

Subjects must be followed carefully when on methotrexate due to the drug's possible adverse effects, including hepatotoxicity, myelosuppression, teratogenicity and defective spermatogenesis.

Combined oral retinoid and methotrexate therapy has been used for treating psoriasis, but this combination therapy should be administered with caution because of the risk of toxic hepatitis.

Azathioprine is an alternative agent for refractory PRP, but it does not seem to be as effective as methotrexate.

There have been sporadic reports of PRP responding to ciclosporin A. However, ciclosporin is generally considered ineffective in the treatment of PRP.

Phototherapy

The results of phototherapy in cases of PRP are much less dramatic than in psoriasis and the poor response to phototherapy is supportive of the diagnosis of PRP.

PUVA (systemic psoralens with long-wavelength ultraviolet light) is an established therapy used for patients with psoriasis vulgaris, mycosis fungoides and therapy resistant cases of atopic dermatitis.

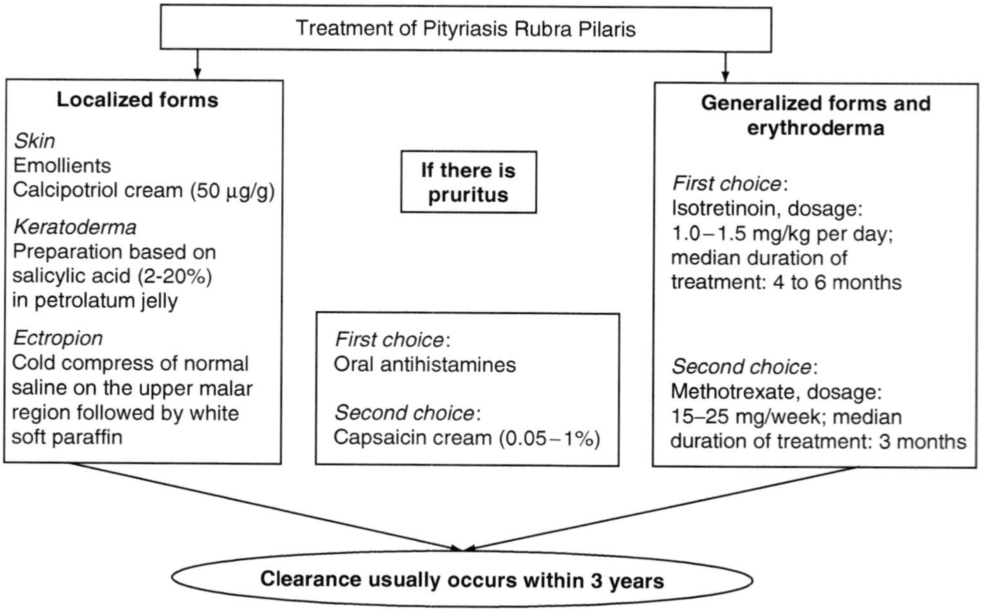

Figure 1 Treatment of pityriasis rubra pilaris

Most investigators have found that neither PUVA nor the Goeckerman regimen (ultraviolet B and crude coal tar) is beneficial.

The combination of PUVA and etretinate therapy (Re-PUVA) has also been used to treat PRP, but the disease recurred when the retinoid was stopped.

Ultraviolet B (UVB) treatment seems to be ineffective.

Antihistamines and capsaicin

The severity of PRP-related pruritus is variable. When treatment with oral antihistamines is unsuccessful, the pruritus can be treated with applications of topical capsaicin solution (0.03%).

Capsaicin is a substance derived from the plants of the Solanacae family. Topical application of this substance depletes and prevents reaccumulation of different neuropeptides, including substance P, which may be involved in the transmission of pain and itch sensations in peripheral sensory neurones.

Capsaicin cream (0.05–0.1%) is applied to itchy skin areas once a day for 4 weeks. Capsaicin cream can also be used to treat severe cases of PRP-related pruritus.

Further reading

Besnier E. Observation pour servir a l'historie clinique du pityriasis rubra pilaire. *Ann Dermatol Syphiligr* 1889; 10: 253–87.

Borok M, Lowe NJ. Pityriasis rubra pilaris. Further observations of systemic retinoid therapy. *J Am Acad Dermatol* 1990; 22: 792–5.

Cohen PR, Prystowsky JH. Pityriasis rubra pilaris: a review of diagnosis and treatment. *J Am Acad Dermatol* 1989; 20: 801–7.

Dicken CH. Isotretinoin treatment of pityriasis rubra pilaris. *J Am Acad Dermatol* 1987; 16: 297–301.

Dicken CH. Treatment of classic pityriasis rubra pilaris. *J Am Acad Dermatol* 1994; 31: 997–9.

Griffiths A. Pityriasis rubra pilaris: etiologic considerations. *J Am Acad Dermatol* 1984; 10: 1086–8.

Griffiths WAD. Pityriasis rubra pilaris. *Clin Exp Dermatol* 1980; 5: 105–12.

Griffiths WAD. Vitamin A and pityriasis rubra pilaris. *J Am Acad Dermatol* 1982; 7: 555.

Griffiths WAD. Pityriasis rubra pilaris: the problem of its classification. *J Am Acad Dermatol* 1992; 26: 140–2.

Lambert DG, Dalac S. Nail changes in type 5 pityriasis rubra pilaris. *J Am Acad Dermatol* 1989; 21: 811–12.

Marks R, Finlay AY, Holt PJA. Severe disorders of keratinization: effects of treatment with tigason (etretinate). *Br J Dermatol* 1981; 104: 667–73.

Miralles ES, Nunez M, De Las Heras ME. Pityriasis rubra pilaris and human immunodeficiency virus. *Br J Dermatol* 1995; 133: 990–3.

Reinhardt LA, Rosen T. Pityriasis rubra pilaris as the initial manifestation of leukemia. *Cutis* 1983; 31: 100–2.

Sanchez-Regana M, Lopez-Gil F, Salleras M, Umbert P. Pityriasis rubra pilaris as the initial manifestation of internal neoplasia. *Clin Exp Dermatol* 1995; 20: 436–8.

Sonnex TS, Dawber RPR, Zachary CB. The nails in adult type I pityriasis rubra pilaris. *J Am Acad Dermatol* 1986; 15: 956–60.

Tarral C. General psoriasis. Desquamation from the parts covered with hair. In: Rayer PA, ed. *Theoretical and Practical Treatise on the Diseases of the Skin*, 2nd edn. London: Bailliere, 1835: 648–9.

Thiers BH. The use of topical calcipotriene/calcipotriol in conditions other than plaque-type psoriasis. *J Am Acad Dermatol* 1997; 37: 69–71.

Usuki K, Sekiyama M, Shimada T, Shimada S, Kauzaki T. Three cases of pityriasis rubra pilaris successfully treated with ciclosporin A. *Dermatology* 2000; 200: 324–7.

Wells RS. In discussion on Borrie P. Pityriasis rubra pilaris treated with methotrexate. *Br J Dermatol* 1967; 79: 115–16.

Winkelmann RK, Thomas JR, Randle HW. Further experience with toxic vitamin A therapy in pityriasis rubra pilaris. *Cutis* 1983; 31: 621–9.

Polymorphic light eruption

J. Ferguson

Synonym

Polymorphous light eruption.

Definition and epidemiology

Polymorphic light eruption (PLE) is an inflammatory photosensitive skin disorder characterized by pruritic papules and/or vesicles occurring on photoexposed sites. North European females seem particularly affected with an incidence of 10–20%. Although the condition occurs in all races, it does appear that as the latitude shortens the incidence increases. The condition, which most commonly appears during the first three decades of life, can arise at any time. A range of familial incidence is reported (10–60%).

Aetiology and pathophysiology

PLE is a member of the idiopathic photodermatoses. Although evidence of immunological abnormality does exist and is centred on the delayed allergic concept, studies as yet have failed to disclose the precise nature of the disorder. While some PLE cases spontaneously improve, the majority have a chronic course.

Clinical characteristics and course

Although likely to be a group of closely related conditions, the great majority report a history of a pruritic burning or tingling, erythematopapular/vesicular eruption of sunlight-exposed skin arising particularly during the spring and summer months but not in the winter. The typical history of a severely affected individual is that 15 min of spring or summer sunlight results in pruritus with papules either immediately or several days later. These clear over the following 2–3 days. The itch often demands scratching. Patients frequently describe a hardening phenomenon, reporting that as the summer advances increasing amounts of sunlight are required to induce the eruption.

Diagnosis

Histology of affected skin shows a range of non-specific features. Phototesting, including provocation testing, may provoke papules in up to 50% of cases.

Differential diagnosis

- Actinic prurigo: nodules, eczematized perennial lesions, early age of onset, lower lip, eye and covered site involvement.
- Systemic lupus erythematosus: papular form may mimic PLE; biopsy with immunofluorescence, antinuclear antibody (ANA), anti-Ro and La.
- Solar urticaria: phototesting reveals urticaria.
- Photosensitive psoriasis: psoriasis morphology/histology.
- Lymphocytoma cutis: translucent miliary or nodular forms; histology.
- Jessner's lymphocytic infiltrate: dermal erythema and oedema; persistent duration; histology.
- Hydroa vacciniforme: larger blisters and crusting and chickenpox-like scars.
- Cutaneous porphyrias: check porphyrins.
- Chronic actinic dermatitis: phototest; dermatitis response; severe broad-spectrum photosensitivity.

Treatment

- No cure for this condition is available. Regardless of treatment used, the condition will tend to recur year on year.
- For active PLE lesions, potent topical steroid may provide improvement.

- For many, PLE is a minor problem appearing only on vacation in sunny climes. In the main, these patients can be successfully treated by emphasizing the need to gradually increase sunlight exposure (hardening).
- Behavioural avoidance involves emphasis on minimizing ultraviolet (UV) exposure during the maximum hours of insolation (10 a.m. to 3 p.m). Use of a broad-spectrum (total sun block) sunscreen is recommended.

Recommended therapies

Recommended therapies include desensitization, artificial hardening with phototherapy (UVB) or photochemotherapy (PUVA) (Table 1).

For PLE sufferers who find simple measures unsatisfactory, whether they report natural hardening or not, UVB phototherapy or PUVA early in the sunshine season can be tried. Initial impressions of benefit have been confirmed by study work. While there is evidence that PUVA gives better results than UVB, the recently used TL01 narrow-band UVB source has proved an effective and probably safer alternative. When preparing a patient for such a course, it is important to emphasize that each PLE sufferer is different and that the first desensitization course is exploratory requiring information on the increment steps that can be tolerated without PLE induction. Frequently, second and subsequent courses are less hazardous as the individualized patient treatment is established. It may be difficult to advise on the degree of 'top up' from natural sunlight that is required after each course to maintain photoprotection throughout subsequent summer months. If the need for this controlled sunlight exposure is not explained and postdesensitization sunlight exposure is avoided, the artificially gained protection will quickly be lost.

As the phototherapy-induced photoprotection is localized at therapy site, a decision must be made to treat either the whole body or limited areas. One policy for milder cases is to treat the whole body and those more severely affected with the reduced body area approach, i.e. only exposing limited areas of arms, legs and face. This latter group are asked to choose clothing items of thick cotton to wear at each desensitization treatment. The clothing must be worn in exactly the same position on each treatment day, for exposure towards the end of the course, when the treatment dose is highest may result in a burn or severe PLE induction of a site not exposed to the earlier desensitization treatments.

Table 1 PLE desensitization: a protocol for UVB–PUVA

Patient attends early in spring three times weekly for 5 weeks
Before starting treatment:
1 Check ANF, anti-Ro, anti-La antibodies to exclude lupus erythematosus
2 Determine either
minimal erythemal dose (MED) for UVB
minimal phototoxic dose (MPD) for PUVA
Start treatment use dose equivalent to 70% of MED or MPD
Thereafter the standard incremental step at each treatment is a 20% increase of previous dose adjusting for adverse effects
UV increments
PLE or erythema
none or mild 20%
mild 15%
moderate 10%
Treatment is omitted if symptoms are severe, and restarted at preceding dose

For a few exquisitely sensitive PLE subjects, the use of topical or systemic steroids during a desensitization course can be considered although objective data to support this practice is needed. Patients often value a written source of information not only about their PLE but also what to expect and what is expected of them during and after a desensitization course.

For oral photochemotherapy using 8-methoxypsoralen (8-MOP) or

5-methoxypsoralen (5-MOP), a standard regimen can be followed. Oral PUVA is not usually recommended for children under 12 years of age. For patients who may be pregnant or have abnormal liver function phototherapy is recommended. Treatment can be used daily or three times weekly for 10–15 treatments.

With treatment repeated yearly, the cumulative dose and number of treatments may cause concern. With a strict annual course of, say, 10–15 treatments of UVB, one can ask what additional risk are we exposing our patients to, particularly as many PLE cases have had less sun exposure than average? In addition, postdesensitization, patients are encouraged to be cautious regarding exposure to sunlight and not convert to 'sun soaking'.

Alternative and experimental treatments

For the minority who have failed to respond to prophylactic phototherapy or PUVA, or who find such treatment inconvenient or unavailable, a range of other treatments has been used, although there is a lack of confirmed evidence that such treatments are indeed indicated. It is therefore fortunate that the great majority of patients can be successfully managed by simple first-line therapy or a careful desensitization programme with UVB or PUVA.

Further reading

Ferguson J. Polymorphic light eruption and actinic prurigo. *Curr Prob Dermatol* 1990; 11: 127–47.

Ferguson J. The management of photodermatoses with phototherapy. In: Hönigsmann H, Jori G, Young AR, eds. *Fundamental Bases of Phototherapy.* Milano: OEMF Spa, 1996: 171–9.

Ferguson J, Katsambas A. Photosensitivity disorders. *Medicine* 1997; 25: 34–6.

Hölzle E, Plewig G, von Kries R, Lehmann P. Polymorphous light eruption. *J Invest Dermatol* 1987; 88: 32s–38s.

van Pragg MCG, Boom BW, Vermeer BJ. Diagnosis and treatment of polymorphic light eruption. *Int J Dermatol* 1994; 33: 233–9.

Young AR. Carcinogenicity of UVB phototherapy assessed. *Lancet* 1995; 345: 1431–2.

Porphyrias

M. Lecha, C. Herrero and D. Ozalla

Porphyrias are a group of diseases caused by partial enzyme deficiencies in the biosynthetic pathway of haem (Table 1). These enzyme deficiencies are usually inherited defects or acquired and result in characteristic patterns of accumulation and increased elimination of intermediate metabolites in the metabolic pathway to haem, the porphyrins and their precursors. The study of this group of diseases, has progressed step by step from the description of the different clinical forms to the biochemical investigation of the different accumulation and excretion patterns of precursors and porphyrins, the defective enzyme activity evaluation and the molecular genetic studies to establish the gene mutations resulting in a defective enzyme protein synthesis.

Epidemiologically, the frequency of the different clinical forms of porphyria depends upon racial prevalence of the genetic alteration that leads to enzyme deficiency. The most frequent forms are porphyria cutanea tarda (PCT), erythropoietic protoprophyria (EPP), acute intermittent porphyria (AIP) and porphyria variegata (VP). Other forms such as congenital erythropoietic porphyria (CEP), hepatoerythropoietic porphyria (HEP), hereditary coproporphyria (HCP) and aminolevulinic acid (ALA), dehydratase deficiency porphyria (ADP) are less frequent. PCT occurs usually as an acquired disease (PCT type I) but there is also an autosomal dominant hereditary familial form (PCT type II).

Aetiology and pathophysiology

Porphyrias are mainly hereditary diseases, either autosomal dominant or autosomal recessive (Table 1) with EPP presenting a peculiar inheritance pattern. Genetic defects are relatively frequent and heterogeneous but with a very low penetrance. Therefore approximately 80% of carriers of genetic defects will not show clinical or biochemical alterations. However, the appearance of homozygous forms without consanguinity and coincidence of two types of porphyria in the same patient, dual porphyrias, is possible.

The accumulated intermediate metabolites are reactive molecules which may act on several cell types (mast cells, neutrophils, fibroblasts, endothelial cells) and produce reactive oxygen species, trigger the secretion of soluble mediator substances and activate the complement system. These reactions explain the pathophysiology of the clinical picture of the different forms of porphyria.

Clinical aspects

Clinical manifestations result from deposition and accumulation of intermediate metabolites. There are three main types of clinical syndromes.

1 Cutaneous acute photosensitivity syndrome related to the accumulation and deposition of hydrophobic protoporphyrin.
2 Chronic bullous erosive cutaneous manifestations with skin fragility syndrome related to the accumulation of hydrophylic porphyrins mainly uroporphyrin, hepta-carboxyl-porphyrin and coproporphyrin (isomers I or III)
3 Neurological symptoms and abdominal pain syndrome related to porphyrin precursors ALA and porphobilinogen accumulation or to neuronal haem deficiency.

The different forms of porphyria may either be manifested by cutaneous symptoms (cutaneous porphyrias with acute photosensitivity as EPP or with chronic bullous erosive skin fragility symptoms as in CEP, PCT, HEP) or neurological symptoms and acute attacks (AIP, ADP), or as

Table 1 The Porphyrias

Haem biosynthesis pathway	Deficient enzyme	Porphyria	Inheritance
Glycine + Succinyl CoA	ALA-synthase		
Aminolevulinic acid	ALA-dehydrase	**ALA dehydrase deficiency porphyria (ADP)**	Autosomal recessive
Porphobilinogen	PBG-deaminase	**Acute intermittent porphyria (AIP)**	Autosomal dominant
Hydroxymethylbilane			
Uroporphyrinogen I	Urogencosynthetase	**Congenital erythropoietic porphyria (CEP)**	Autosomal recessive
Coproporphyrinogen I	Urogendecarboxylase	**Sporadic PCT**	Acquired
Uroporphyrinogen III		**Familial PCT**	Autosomal dominant
7-COOH porphyrin		**Hepatoerythropoietic porphyria (HEP)**	Autosomal recessive
6-COOH porphyrin			
5-COOH porphyrin			Autosomal dominant
Isocoproporphyrin	Coproporphyrinogen oxidase	**Hereditary coproporphyria (HCP)**	
Coproporphyrinogen III		**Harderoporphyria**	
Harderoporphyrinogen			Autosomal dominant
	Protoporphyrinogen oxidase	**Variegate porphyria (VP)**	
Protoporphyrinogen			Autosomal (dominant/ recessive tri-allelic)
	Ferrochelatase	**Erythropoietic protoporphyria (EPP)**	
Protoporphyrin IX			
Haem			

mixed porphyrias with cutaneous and neurological symptoms as in VP and HCP.

Hepatic disease is an important feature in PCT and EPP. On the other hand a higher frequency of hepatic tumours—hepatocarcinomas—has been reported in porphyric patients. PCT patients usually show altered hepatic function tests—elevated transaminases, sideraemia and ferritin levels. Liver biopsies may reveal the presence of various hepatic lesions (siderosis, steatosis, portal and periportal inflammatory reaction, portal fibrosis, and cirrhosis or hepatocarcinoma). Hepatic lesions were initially supposed to be a consequence of the hepatic deposition of uroporphyrin and hepta-carboxyl-porphyrin. But viral hepatitis infection may also have a prominent role in the development of hepatic inflammation in PCT associated with viral hepatitis.

In approximately 5% of EPP patients cholelithiasis and hepatic changes may be expected. Deposition of lipophylic protoporphyrin in the liver may produce intrahepatic biliary obstruction and hepatocellular lesions with a variable degree of inflammation and fibrosis. Acute hepatic failure may rarely occur. Haematological changes such as haemolytic anaemia and splenomegaly are usually present in CEP and are thought to be related to photohaemolysis.

Photoinduced ocular lesions—scleromalacia—have been reported in PCT, HEP and CEP.

Diagnosis

Clinical suspicion of a patient suffering from porphyria can be easily confirmed by biochemical analysis. It is known that each type of human porphyria is characterized by a specific pattern of accumulation and excretion of haem precursors, which reflects the intracellular accumulation of the substrate of the defective enzyme. The recognition of these patterns by appropriate laboratory measurements is essential for the differentiation of the porphyrias because different types can have the same clinical features (Table 2). This biochemical differentiation resides in the measurements of porphyrins and their metabolites in urine, faeces and blood (Fig. 1). The acute porphyric attacks are associated to an increase of urinary excretion of porphobilinogen (PBG), which can be detected in first-line by the Hoesch test. If the test is positive quantitation of PBG and ALA is performed by ion-exchange column. In porphyrias associated with skin lesions, screening tests are widely used to detect increase of porphyrin concentration in blood, urine and faeces. Individual porphyrin profiles are obtained by reversed phase high-performance liquid chromatography.

Enzyme measurements in erythrocytes or leucocytes, although technically difficult, are a useful tool for detecting cases of so-called latent porphyria. Except for the erythrocyte porphobilinogen deaminase determination, deficient in acute intermittent porphyria, the enzymatic measurements are only used by a few research laboratories.

The genetic investigation of the molecular defects in genes which encode enzymes involved in haem biosynthesis is a complementary analysis to the biochemical methods. Genetic analysis allow the establishment with certainty of the presence of porphyria, whether manifest or asymptomatic and also prenatal diagnosis in cases where a severe prognosis is suspected.

Treatment

Recommended therapies

ALA dehydratase deficiency porphyria

This form of porphyria, very unusual, is manifested by the same symptoms of AIP. Only six cases have been reported. No specific treatment has been described. Genetic studies have shown that patients are compound heterozygotes.

These individuals may be at high risk of toxic effects from chemicals or metals, such as lead, which are known to alter the activity of ALA dehydratase, the defective enzyme in this form of porphyria. Treatment of the acute attacks and prevention should be performed in the same way as for AIP.

Table 2 Laboratory diagnosis of porphyrias

	Excess intermediate metabolites				
	Urine		Faeces	Blood	
Porphyria	Precursors	Porphyrins	Porphyrins	Plasma	Erythrocytes
ALA dehydratase deficiency porphyria[a]	ALA	–	CP/PP	ALA	Zn–PP
Acute intermittent porphyria[a]	ALA > PBG	UP I/III	–	–	–
Congenital erythropoietic porphyria[b]	–	UP I > CP I	CP I > UP I	UP I > CP I	Zn–PP, UP I > CP I
Porphyria cutanea tarda[b]	–	UP I/III 7COOH-P III	IsoCP 7COOH-P-III	UP III CP III	–
Hepatoerythro-poietic porphyria[b]	–	UP I/III CP III	CP III IsoCP	Uro III Copro III	Zn–PP
Hereditary coproporphyria[c]	PBG > ALA	Copro III	Copro III	–	–
Hardero porphyria[c]	–	CP III	Hadero-P CP III	–	–
Variegate porphyria[c]	ALA > PBG (acute attacks)	CP III > UP III	PPIX > CPIII	CP III PP IX	–
Erythropoietic protoporphyria[d]	–	–	PP IX	PP IX	PP IX

[a]Acute porphyrias.
[b]Cutaneous porphyrias with chronic bullous erosive syndrome.
[c]Mixed porphyrias.
[d]Cutaneous porphyria with acute photosensitivity syndrome.
7-COOH-P III, seven carboxyl porphyrinogen isomer III;
ALA, aminolevulinic acid;
CP I/CP III, coproporphyrinogen isomer I or III;
Hardero-P, harderoporphyrin;
IsoCP, isocoproporphyrinogen;
PBG, porphobilinogen;
PP IX, protoporphyrinogen isomer IX;
UP I/UP III, uroporphyrinogen isomer I or III;
Zn–PP, zinc–protoporphyrin.

Acute intermittent porphyria

The goal in the treatment of AIP is the suppression of ALA synthase, the rate-controlling enzyme in the metabolic biosynthesis pathway of haem. This is achieved by avoiding precipitating factors, administration of carbohydrates and infusion of haem arginate.

Symptoms of the acute attack include abdominal pain, vomiting, constipation, hypertension, tachycardia, cranial nerve palsies, convulsions and epileptic seizures, respiratory distress and abnormal sphincter function.

Avoiding precipitating factors is a basic therapeutic measure. Precipitating factors include drugs, alcohol, fasting, smoking, infection, emotional and physical stress, and changes in the sex hormone balance (premenstrual phase). Acute attacks have a 1% mortality risk.

Pharmacological treatment may be performed by administration of carbohydrate (carbohydrate loading) or haem arginate infusion. Carbohydrate loading is performed by administration of 300–500 g/daily. Haem arginate is administered at a dose of 3 mg/kg per day for 4 days. These treatments result in normalization of clinical and biochemical manifestations reducing the synthesis of ALA and normalizing the excretion of excess ALA and PBG.

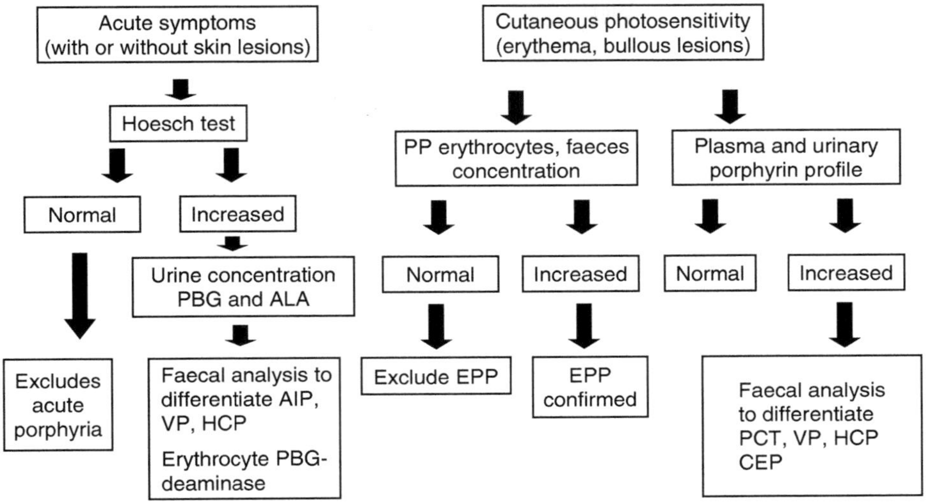

Figure 1 Algorithm for the diagnosis of porphyrias

Tin protoporphyrin has been reported to prolong remission after haem arginate treatment by inhibiting haem oxygenase.

Complementary preventive measures may include the administration of the contraceptive pill to those females who show tendency to acute attacks during the premenstrual phase. Induction of chemical menopause has also been suggested with luteinizing hormone releasing hormone agonists (GnRH) since 1984, initially in short-term treatments, but also on a long-term basis with encouraging results and gaining experience on side-effects. Acute attacks may also occur during pregnancy and haem arginate can be used normally.

Congenital erythropoietic porphyria

This severe form of cutaneous porphyria requires as first-line measures a preventive therapy with skin photoprotection, ocular photoprotection and avoidance of cutaneous mechanical trauma. Otherwise, cutaneous lesions may become extremely severe and mutilating. Protective clothing and broad-band sunscreens containing physical sun-screening agents should be prescribed because photosensitizing wavelengths include the Soret band in the visible radiation range. The administration of oral β-carotene has proved ineffective.

Several treatments directed to the biochemical normalization have been performed with variable results. High-level transfusions have been used to reduce erythropoiesis and porphyrin levels. The risk of this treatment is iron overload. The use of oral charcoal or cholestiramine has been reported to be of success in some cases. Oral activated charcoal has been claimed to be more effective than cholestiramine and Pimstone, Gandhi and Mukerji have suggested a dose of 60 g three times daily.

Splenectomy is performed in these patients with transient improvement of haemolysis and reduction of porphyrin levels.

Recently promising results have been obtained in three cases treated with bone marrow transplantation.

Porphyria cutanea tarda

This is the most frequent form of cutaneous porphyria and the only one in which the available treatments usually produce clinical and biochemical remission. As in other forms of cutaneous porphyria, preventative measures have to be also considered with photoprotection, cutaneous and ocular, and avoidance of mechanical skin trauma. Certain cutaneous manifestations, such as hyperpigmentation, hypertrichosis and scleroderma, if already present, will not show complete recovery.

The second preventive measure, as in AIP, is the avoidance of precipitating or triggering factors such as alcohol, oestrogens, iron overload and chlorinated hydrocarbons (role and required levels of different compounds may vary). Other risk factors for the development of PCT are viral infections—viral hepatitis, human immunodeficiency virus (HIV)—and the presence of hereditary haemochromatosis gene mutations.

Biochemical porphyrin alteration may be reversed by two proven treatment modalities:

1 Phlebotomy—performed as weekly or biweekly in a volume of 250–500 mL to reach a blood haemoglobin concentration of 100–110 g/L or an urinary excretion of porphyrin under 500 nmol/24 h. Improvement of clinical symptoms appears within 6 months of treatment and biochemical normalization within a year.
2 Low-dose chloroquine is also effective at 125–250 mg twice a week. Clinical improvement and biochemical remission appears with the same delay as with phlebotomy. This treatment modality is preferred when there is a possible contraindication for phlebotomy.

Both treatment modalities can be used in a combined form.

PCT associated with haemodialysis/chronic renal failure is usually treated with a different approach. In this setting, the administration of deferoxamine for iron removal or erythropoietin for treatment of anaemia in end-stage renal disease are the elective measures. Standard or low-volume phlebotomies and combined treatments have also been performed. Treatment protocols may vary. Deferoxamine is administered at doses ranging from 1.5 to 4 g with haemodialysis; erythropoietin 20–50 U/kg after haemodialysis, and low-volume phlebotomies from 50 to 100 mL/once or twice weekly. Treatment of PCT in this setting is still a challenge. There is no critical figure below which phlebotomies are contraindicated, but Shieh, Cohen and Lim suggest that above 10 g/dL haemoglobin, phlebotomy can be performed. Under 8 g/dL haemoglobin, erythropoietin should be preferred at a dose of 20–50 U/kg three times per week. Failure of either modality is an indication for combined therapy. Deferoxamine should be considered now as a second-line option. Plasma exchange or renal transplantation should be the elective therapy only in specific cases.

Cases of PCT related to hepatitis C virus infection have become extremely frequent in certain countries such as Spain, France, Italy, and Hungary. Treatment of hepatitis with interferon (IFN)-α has proved to have a beneficial effect on PCT associated with viral hepatitis C but reports published allow no definite conclusions.

Hepatoerythropoietic porphyria

This homozygous or compound heterozygous form of familial PCT presents with severe cutaneous manifestations similar to the features of CEP. Treatment is based on preventive sun-screening measures. A therapeutic approach as in PCT is absolutely ineffective in producing any clinical or biochemical improvement.

Hereditary coproporphyria–Harderoporphyria

The management of this form of mixed porphyria and the homozygous variant harderoporphyria consists of preventive measures with avoidance of sunlight exposure for cutaneous lesions and avoidance of precipitating factors for acute attacks, which may be treated in the same way as in AIP.

Variegate porphyria

This mixed porphyria is manifested with cutaneous lesions as in PCT and acute attacks as in AIP and has no specific treatment. Cutaneous symptoms have to be prevented by photoprotection in the same way as PCT. Due to the fact that cutaneous manifestations may not correlate with acute attacks, cases may be misdiagnosed clinically as PCT and no advice given against acute attack-precipitating factors. Biochemical diagnosis is therefore imperative before any treatment modalities for PCT are prescribed which however will be ineffective.

Erythropoietic protoporphyria

EPP is clinically characterized by a specific acute photosensitive syndrome, is usually manifested in early infancy but can also appear from the second decade of life and beyond. The severity of symptoms is variable and may be limited to a subjective sensation of stinging or burning during sun exposure, to mild erythema, urticarial or severe 'phototoxic' reactions with pruritic erythema or marked and persistent painful erythema and oedema with petechial and blistering lesions. Chronic lesions may also develop as a consequence of repeated acute episodes, with waxy thickening of exposed skin areas, face and hands. Cutaneous lesions of EPP are usually clearly distinct from those of other cutaneous porphyrias and have to be differentiated from polymorphous light eruption or solar urticaria outbreaks.

Liver alteration may also be a manifestation of EPP. Cholelithiasis is a possible complication in patients with EPP. In fortunately very few cases, patients with EPP may develop life-threatening acute liver failure. Some changes in the pattern of excess excretion of porphyrins have been supposed to herald imminent liver impairment: (a) extremely high levels of erythrocyte protoporphyrin; (b) simultaneous decline of fecal protoporphyrin excretion; and (c) increase in coproporphyrin levels in urine with isomer I in excess of isomer III.

In EPP patients, photoprotection is essential. This goal may be achieved by using broad-band sunscreens and by the oral administration of β-carotene, at a dose of 30–90 mg/daily for children and 60–180 mg/daily for adults to reach a maximum plasma level of 600 μg/dL. These measures reduce photosensitivity to allow normal outdoor activities, as has been confirmed after a long experience since 1970 and controlled trials. A similar therapeutic approach has been performed with the oral administration of cysteine. Phototherapy with narrow-band UVB has been tried with encouraging results.

On the other hand hepatic complications such as cholelithiasis may be surgically treated and acute liver failure should be considered an indication for liver transplantation. This latter therapeutic approach has already been successfully performed. To prevent these hepatic complications two treatment modalities have been tried: oral administration of cholestiramine (to interfere with entero-hepatic circulation of protoporphyrin) or iron overloaad (to enhance the conversion of protoporphyrin to haem) although this latter approach may have contradictory results. Other therapeutic measures have been reported with the aim of achieving biochemical normalization in EPP: oral vitamin C, avoidance of alcohol and cholestatic or hepatotoxic drugs, and chenodeoxycholic acid to increase protoprophyrin fecal elimination.

In extremely photosensitive EPP patients specific perioperative measures are advisable if they have to undergo any invasive surgical procedure, because illumination of the operative areas may produce a severe internal photosensitivity reaction.

Family studies

The possibility of performing genetic family studies is of special interest in the global management of porphyrias. Genetic defects should be studied in patients with acute and severe cutaneous forms. With the results of these studies, screening of all relatives of the patient is advisable to protect the asymptomatic carriers of the defect from the action of common precipitating factors. On the other hand exclusion of carrier status enables us to stop studies in unaffected family branches.

Further reading

Blake D, Poulos V, Rossi R. Diagnosis of porphyria. Recommended methods for peripheral laboratories. *Clin Biochem Rev* 1992; 13 (suppl): 2.13.

Corbett MF, Herxheimer A, Magnus IA *et al.* The longterm treatment with beta-carotene in erythropoietic protoporphyria: a controlled trial. *Br J Dermatol* 1977; 97: 655–62.

Cox TM, Graeme JM, Alexander MD, Sarkany RPE. Protoporphyria. *Semin Liver Dis* 1998; 18: 85–93.

Dower SB, Moore MR, Fitzsimmons EJ, Graham A, McCall KE. Tin protoporphyrin prolongs the biochemical remission produced by heme arginate in acute hepatic porphyria. *Gastroenterology* 1993; 153: 2004–8.

Elder GH. Molecular genetics of disorders of haem biosynthesis. *J Clin Pathol* 1993; 46: 977–81.

Elder GH. Porphyria cutanea tarda. *Semin Liver Dis* 1998; 18: 67–76.

Kauppinen R, Timonen K, Mustajoki P. Treatment of the porphyrias. *Ann Med* 1994; 263: 1–38.

Lim HW, Cohen JL. The cutaneous porphyrias. *Semin Cutan Med Surg* 1999; 18 (4): 285–92.

Lim HW, Sassa S. The porphyrias. In: Lim HW, Soter NA, eds. *Clinical Photomedicine*. New York: Marcel Dekker, 1993: 241–67.

Mascaro JM. Management of the erythropoietic porphyrias. *Photodermatol Photoimmunol Photomed* 1998; 14: 44–5.

Mascaro JM, Herrero C, Lecha M, Muniesa MA. Uroporphyrinogen-decarboxylase deficiencies: porphyria cutanea tarda and related conditions. *Seminars in Dermatology* 1986; 5: 115–24.

Mathews-Roth MM, Rosner B, Benfell K *et al.* A double-blind study of cysteine photoprotection in erythropoietic protoporphyria. *Photodermatol Photimmunol Photomed* 1994; 10: 244–8

McNulty SJ, Hardy KJ. Two patients with acute intermittent porphyria treated with nafarelin to prevent menstrual exacerbations. *J Roy Soc Med* 2000; 93: 429–30.

Meerman L, Verwer R, Slooff MJ *et al.* Perioperative measures during liver transplantation for erythropoietic protoporphyria. *Transplantation* 1994; 57: 155–8

Meyer UA, Schuurmansn MM, Lindberg RLP. Acute Porphyrias: pathogenesis of neurological manifestations. *Semin Liver Dis* 1998; 18: 43–52.

Okano J, Horie Y, Kawasaki H. Kondo M. Interferon treatment of porphyria cutanea tarda associated with chronic hepatitis type C. *Hepato-Gastroenterology* 1997; 44: 525–8.

Shieh S, Cohen JL, Lim HW. Management of porphyria cutanea tarda in the setting of chronic renal failure: A case report and review. *J Am Acad Dermatol* 2000; 42: 645–52.

Thadami H, Deacon A, Peters T. Diagnosis and management of porphyria. *Br Med J* 2000; 320: 1647–51.

Thoas C, Ged C, Nordman Y *et al.* Correction of congenital erythropietic porphyria by bone marrow transplantation. *J Pediatr* 1996; 18: 217–20.

Thunell S. Porphyrins, porphyrin metabolism and porphyrias. I. Update. *Scan J Clin Lab Invest* 2000; 60: 509–40.

Todd DJ. Therapeutic options for erythropoietic protoporphyria. *Br J Dermatol* 2000; 142: 826 (letter).

Pruritus

D. Ioannides

Synonyms

Itching is sometimes used to denote pruritus with visible skin lesions. Although some distinctions can be made pruritus and itch are synonymous.

Definition and pathophysiology

Pruritus can be defined as the sensation that provokes the desire to scratch. It is almost always a very unpleasant sensation, although sometimes it may be pleasurable.

The pathophysiology of pruritus is not very well understood. The sensation of itch seems to be mediated by C nerve fibres which enter the spinal cord and transmit impulses to the thalamus and hypothalamus and finally to the cerebral cortex. It has been suggested that A-delta nerve fibres may also be involved in the transmission.

Pruritus and pain share similar pathways. It has been thought that itching is a minor form of pain. However, there is experimental evidence to support the view that itching and pain are two separate sensory modalities.

Histamine is the most extensively studied mediator of pruritus. Other mediators, however, may also play a role. Various amines like serotonin and adrenaline, proteases like kallikrein, neuropeptides like substance P, opioids, eicosanoids and several growth factors and cytokines may also be primary mediators of pruritus.

Clinical characteristics

Pruritus can be observed in almost any disease associated with inflammation, infection, tumour or metabolic abnormalities. Rarely, it is idiopathic but a thorough investigation should be made to exclude any possible cause before itching is assigned to idiopathic reasons. Pruritus may be burning, prickling, tingling, deep or superficial. It is either localized or generalized.

Every area of the body can itch. Localized itch usually points to specific local causes, such as:

- atopic, contact and seborrhoeic dermatitis
- photodermatitis
- eczema
- psoriasis
- lichen planus
- dermatophytosis
- scabies
- pediculosis
- schistosomes, jellyfishes and anemones in fresh and salt water.

In the anal and vulvar region pruritus may be secondary to an underlying disorder, in addition to local causes. Pruritus ani may be caused by:

- haemorrhoids
- rhagades
- proctitis due to inflammatory bowel disease
- tumours.

Pruritus vulvae may be the result of:

- cystitis
- cervicitis
- proctitis neoplastic disease.

Persistent itching in both sites can be of psychological origin. Persistent pruritus along the medial border of the shoulder blades is called notalgia paraesthetica and is probably an isolated sensory neuropathy.

Generalized pruritus is a prominent feature of many cutaneous diseases or a manifestation of numerous systemic disorders. Most of the systematic causes of generalized pruritus are as follows:

- pregnancy
- drug reactions
  barbiturates,
  antibiotics,

contraceptives,
psoralen and ultraviolet A (PUVA), etc.
- parasitic infestations
  trichinosis,
  onchocerciasis,
  echinococcosis, etc.
- infective disorders
  varicella
  roseola
- chronic renal failure/uraemic pruritus
- obstructive disease of the bile ducts
- haematological
  leukaemias
  myeloproliferative disorders
  paraproteinaemia/myeloma
  hypereosinophilic syndrome
  iron deficiency
- endocrine
  hyper-, hypothyroidism
  diabetes
  hyper-, hypoparathyroidism
- neurological
  cerebrovascular disease
  multiple sclerosis
  neurosis/psychosis
  peripheral nerve injuries
  post-herpes zoster
- Sjögren's syndrome
- mastocytosis
- human immunodeficiency virus (HIV) infection
- internal malignant tumours
  carcinoid syndrome, etc.
- aquagenic pruritus
- psychological reasons.

Diagnosis

The clinical approach to a patient with pruritus includes a thorough physical examination and history. Laboratory evaluation may be helpful in some cases.

During physical examination it is crucial to differentiate primary skin lesions pointing to a skin disease from the secondary lesions caused by scratching. Lymphadenopathy, hepatomegaly or splenomegaly suggest systemic disease.

The history of pruritus is decisive in making a diagnosis. It is useful to know if pruritus is:
- localized or generalized
- how long it has been present
- if it is acute or chronic
- the relationship to activities (occupation, hobbies)
- the time relation (night-time or not)
- the provoking factors (water, exercise, pets, etc.)
- the existence of allergy and/or atopy
- the medications taken or applied
- the travel and sexual history.

It is better to know the patient's opinion about the condition.

The suggested screening includes:
- complete blood cell count
- haematocrit
- haemoglobin
- serum iron
- sedimentation rate
- glucose
- alkaline phosphatase and bilirubin
- blood urea nitrogen and creatinine
- T3, T4 and thyroid-stimulating hormone
- Stool for occult blood, ova and parasites.

Treatment

General therapeutic guidelines

If an underlying disorder is diagnosed and corrected, the pruritus may spontaneously subside. Negative findings on initial evaluation do not necessarily exclude associated systemic disease. Reassessment and re-evaluation is essential for these patients.

When the pruritus is localized I use topical therapy. Generally, my treatment of the patient progresses from topical to systemic therapy.

The diagnosis and the factors affecting itching should be clearly explained to the patient. It is essential to break the itch–scratch cycle, especially in disorders such as atopic dermatitis.

Dryness of the skin should be avoided, because it provokes itching. Excessive bathing and low ambient humidity in winter within heated households or in summer because of air conditioning dry the skin.

Contact with wool and animal products, ingestion of alcohol or other causes of vasodilation such as hot food should be taken into account.

Recommended therapies

Topical treatment

Emollients and cooling agents

The application of an emollient immediately after bathing is recommended to all patients with localized or generalized pruritus. The emollients range from vaseline to a wide variety of elegant products. It is better to advise the patient to try different products and select which one feels more comfortable.

Ice or cold compresses with water, milk, Burrow's solution or potassium permanganate (0.1 g in 1 L water) can be used locally. Medicated baths (40–44°C) can help in generalized pruritus. I recommend oatmeal baths or baths with potassium permanganate (6–8 g in a full bathtub of water), which I found very helpful, especially in renal pruritus. Tub stains may be removed with sodium thiosulphate solution or household vinegar, and nail stains with 3% hydrogen peroxide. Bath oils are not recommended often because they tend to make the tub slippery with the possibility of injury. Tar baths and baths with baking soda may also be helpful in alleviating itching.

Lotions or creams containing 0.5–2% menthol, 0.2–5% camphor, 0.2–5% phenol (use with care in children; do not use in pregnant women), 1–2% salicylic acid, 3–10% tar, 2–5% resorcinol, 5–10% urea, 6–20% ammonium lactate, lactic acid and other α-hydroxy acids and 5–10% precipitated sulphur have soothing and antipruritic effects and can be used in combination with wet dressings or baths. I found Castellani's paint (0.5% menthol and 5% salicylic acid in alcohol 70°) an effective preparation for pruritus of intertriginous and anal areas.

Corticosteroids

I tend to prescribe topical steroids only in localized pruritus and in cases where the cause of itch is a dermatosis, which justifies their use. I always start with low-potency corticosteroids in children, and on the face, genital and intertriginous areas of adults. In other areas of the body I may start with a high-potency product for 1–2 weeks and then switch to a moderately potent preparation. Chronic use of topical corticosteroids may be accompanied by application of 0.0025–0.005% tretinoin or of 12% ammonium lactate to counteract the atrophy which may be caused by the continuous steroid use.

Corticosteroid creams or lotions can be added to emollients or preparations containing other antipruritic agents. It should be noted that corticosteroid strength may not be reduced by being diluted to various preparations and that the stability of the corticosteroid molecule may be altered by being mixed with other agents.

Antihistamines, anaesthetics

The use of topical antihistamines is limited because they are relatively ineffective and because of the risk of allergic sensitization. It is expected that newer preparations may overcome those concerns. Doxepin, a tricyclic medication, in a 5% cream has been found to reduce itching significantly in patients with atopic dermatitis, lichen simplex chronicus, nummular eczema and contact dermatitis.

Topical anaesthetics do not seem to be effective in reducing itching and can cause allergic reactions. EMLA, a slow-onset anaesthetic which contains 2.5% lidocaine (lignocaine) and 2.5% prilocaine, pramoxine, or capsaicin cream may be effective for localized pruritus such as prurigo nodularis, notalgia paraesthetica or pruritus related to haemodialysis. Capsaicin diluted in topical corticosteroids may be used in pruritus ani.

A recently developed preparation of liquid aspirin was found to decrease itching significantly in comparison to placebo. Tacrolimus ointment is a non-steroidal topical immunomodulator which seems to be safe and effective for long-term treatment of atopic dermatitis in children

Systemic treatment

Antihistamines, tricyclic antidepressants

Antihistamines are among the most widely used medications in the world. They may be useful in itching disorders that are mediated primarily by histamine release, such as urticaria. These agents can be divided into the classic sedating histamine-blocking agents, the newer non-sedating histamine-blocking agents and the tricyclic antidepressants.

Of the traditional H_1-antihistamines in general, the ethanolamine class, including diphenydramine, is considered more sedating than agents of the piperazine class, such as hydroxyzine and cyproeptadine. New-generation antihistamines have the added action to inhibit the release of a variety of inflammatory mast cell mediators, while causing no more sedation than placebo. Of these antihistamines cetirizine and acrivastine are more likely to result in sedation than loratadine and fexofenadine. New antihistamines also possess a longer duration of action than the classic H_1-blockers.

Astemizole and terfenadine are no longer in use due to severe side-effects, which could be caused by their administration. The old compounds chlorpheniramine, tripelennamine, and diphenydramine appear to be safe in pregnancy. Hydroxyzine, cyproeptadine and tripolidine need further evaluation. Bromopheniramine appears to be teratogenic. The effects of the newer non-sedating drugs given during pregnancy have not been sufficiently studied.

I usually start with one of the new-generation antihistamines in the morning to avoid sedation and, if these drugs are not adequate to control pruritus, I add hydroxyzine at bedtime. Hydroxyzine may perhaps be more effective than the other sedating antihistamines in suppressing pruritus. However, several antihistamines and various combinations may have to be tried, because very often individuals respond differently to these preparations.

Cyproheptadine is also a serotonin antagonist and has been used in polycythaemia vera and cholinergic urticaria. Ketotifen has been successfully administered in mastocytosis. Finally, the addition of an H_2-antagonist, cimetidine or ranitidine, may be helpful in some cases of generalized pruritus.

Corticosteroids

Steroids should rarely be given and their use should be restricted to cases where a dermatosis or other disease justifies their administration. I usually start with 20–40 mg of prednisone equivalent daily until itching subsides and then taper the dose by 25% every 3 days. Antihistamines may also be given concurrently.

Phototherapy

Phototherapy with UVB, UVA combined UVB and UVA, and PUVA has been successfully used to treat generalized pruritus. Patients usually have a response within seven treatments of suberythemogenic doses. If no response is observed after 15 treatments, therapy is discontinued.

This mode of treatment is primarily used in renal pruritus and in pruritus associated with biliary cirrhosis, atopic dermatitis, photosensitive disorders, lichen planus and aquagenic pruritus. However, it has also been used in a number of other

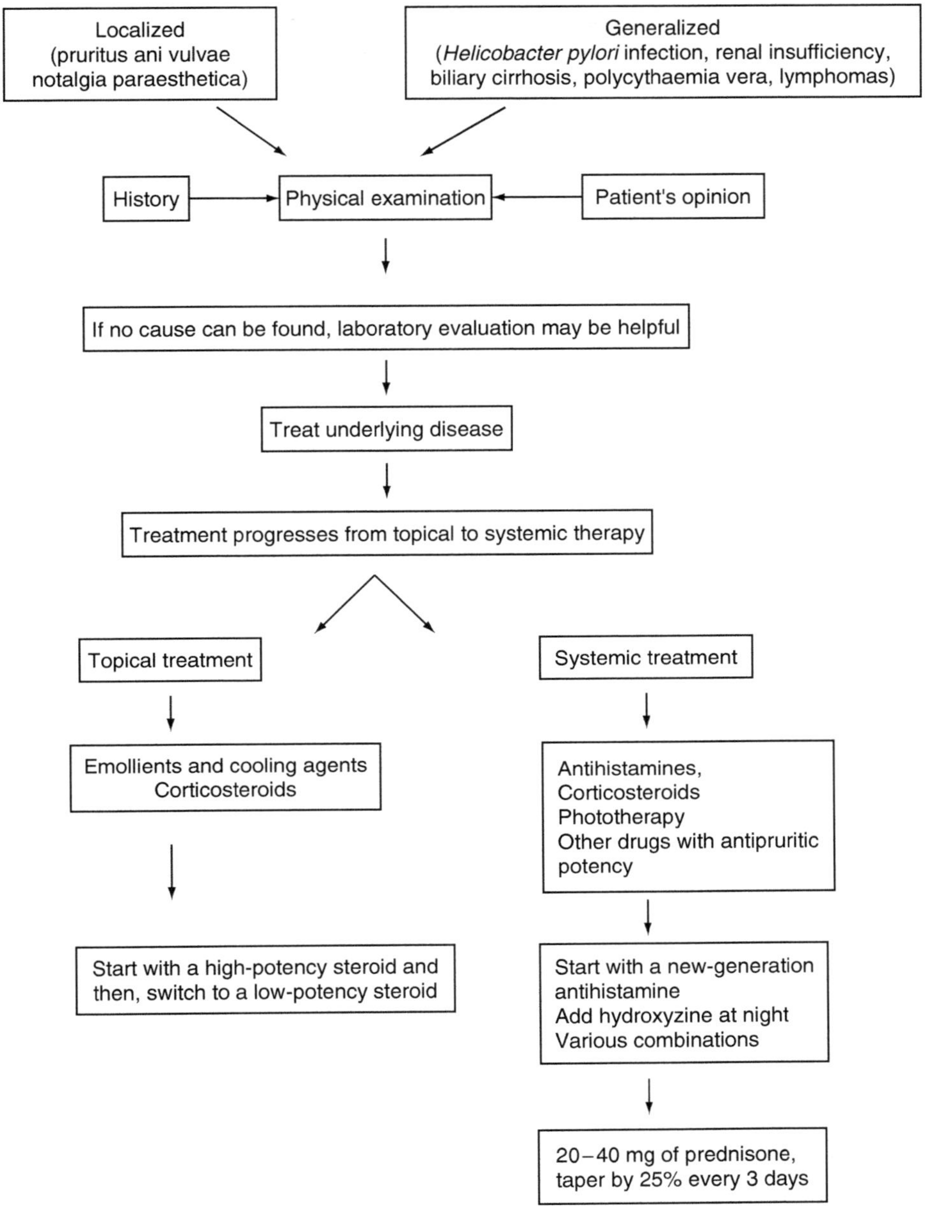

Figure 1 Algorithm of treatment for pruritus

pruritic conditions. Idiopathic pruritus is more resistant to treatment than symptomatic itching.

It should be noted that PUVA itself can cause pruritus in the early phases of therapy.

Other drugs with antipruritic potency

Cholestyramine given orally at a dose of 4 g, 1–3 times daily, may be helpful in decreasing pruritus associated with renal failure, cholestasis and polycythaemia vera. Phenobarbital (3–4 mg/kg per day p.o.), rifampin (10 mg/kg per day), oral hydroxyethylrutosides and ondansetron, a serotonin receptor antagonist, can reduce cholestatic pruritus. Erythropoietin and ondansetron may be useful in patients with uraemia on haemodialysis.

The tranquillizers, such as haloperidol, alprazolam and buspirone and other neurotropic and psychotropic drugs like pimozide and gabapentin have been given to treat pruritus with variable results. Opiate antagonists, naloxone, naltrexone, nalmefene, nalbuphine and droperidol, in injections and orally, have been found effective in cholestasis, atopic dermatitis and urticaria.

Ciclosporin seems to be effective in controlling severe pruritus caused by psoriasis, prurigo and dermatitis of any type. Ascomycin derivatives, a new class of compounds with immunomodulating properties that can only penetrate the damaged skin, have been used for the treatment of inflammatory skin diseases, especially atopic dermatitis.

A relationship between skin diseases and *Helicobacter pylori* infection has been suggested. In a recent study it has been proposed that it may be prudent to test patients with generalized pruritus for *H. pylori* infection and to eradicate the infection in those whose test is positive.

Aspirin has been successfully given to patients with polycythaemia vera and oral cromalyn to patients with systemic mastocytosis and Hodgkin's disease. Encouraging results in generalized pruritus have also been obtained with thalidomide. Resenfertoxin, an ultrapotent analogue of capsaicin, is now being tested as a systemic treatment for generalized pruritus. Intravenous propofol, a new hypnotic used in anaesthesiology, has been found to be effective in relieving both motor and sensory components of pruritus.

Alternative and experimental treatments

Thermal stimulation with heat, vibration, transcutaneous electrical nerve stimulation, acupuncture and electroacupuncture have been found to be effective in reducing itching in both clinical and experimental settings.

Plasmapheresis and partial external diversion of bile have been tried and have been effective in certain extreme situations.

Further reading

Arndt K, Bowers K, Chuttani A. *Manual of Dermatologic Therapeutics*. Boston: Little, Brown, 1995.

Bernhard F. *Itch. Mechanisms and Management of Pruritus*. New York: McGraw Hill, 1994.

Denman ST. A review of pruritus. *J Am Acad Dermatol* 1986; 14: 375–92.

Gatti S, Serri F. *Pruritus in Clinical Medicine*. London: Martin Dunitz, 1991.

Katsambas A. Quality of life in dermatology and the EADV. *J Eur Acad Dermatovener* 1994; 3: 211–14.

Katsambas A, Goula M. In: Larry Millikan, ed. *Antihistamines. Drug Therapy in Dermatology*. Marcel Dekker, 2000: 243–51.

Lorette G, Vaillant L. Pruritus: Current concepts in pathogenesis and treatment. *Drugs* 1990; 39: 2188–23.

Shiotani A, Okada K, Yanaoka K *et al*. Beneficial effect of *Helicobacter pylori* eradication in dermatologic diseases. *Helicobacter* 2001; 6: 60–5.

Weisshaar E, Gollnick H. Systemic drugs with antipruritic potency. *Skin Ther Lett* 2000; 5: 1–25.

Yosipovitch G, David M. The diagnostic and therapeutic approach to idiopathic generalized pruritus. *Int J Dermatol* 1999; 38: 881–7.

Psoriasis

B. Bonnekoh and H. Gollnick

Epidemiology and pathogenesis

Psoriasis is a frequent disease with prevalence around 2–3% in most European countries. Nowadays, there is agreement in the scientific community about psoriasis being an autoimmune disease mediated by T cells. A putative autoantigen or even a spectrum of various autoantigens are thought to exist with highly skin-specific expression in the epidermopapillary compartment (Fig. 1). It seems that the degree of expression and/or accessibility, respectively, of these autoantigen structures correlate positively with the degree of inflammation and hyperproliferation, in the sense of a positive feedback mechanism. Through the local activation of autoreactive T lymphocytes—possibly mediated by dedicated antigen-presenting cells (APC)—and subsequent secretion of proinflammatory cytokines the vicious circle of disease is completed.

This model would sufficiently explain the clinically well-recognized features of (a) self-perpetuation of the psoriatic lesion; (b) its inducibility in terms of the Köbner phenomenon; and (c) its curability with the restoration of a completely normal, non-inflammatory, low-proliferative local skin state, although lasting mostly for only a limited time in the range of weeks and months until relapse. The familiarity of the disease and the well-documented associations with distinct HLA patterns are due to the known immunogenetic principle of major histocompatibility complex (MHC) restrictions of autoantigen peptide epitopes. The assumption of their cross-reactivity with microbial determinants, such as streptococcal proteins or tissue components of the joint compartments, provides a clue for understanding the trigger function of microbial foci as well as the relationship to psoriatic osteoarthritis. Superantigen-related activation of the immune system might further lead to more specific autoantigen-related reactions in terms of a 'superantigen/autoantigen switch'.

It has to be emphasized that it is still a matter of debate if CD4- or CD8-positive T cells represent the pivotal autoantigen reactive lymphocyte population. In the current and ongoing discussion it will have to be kept in mind that psoriasis most probably represents a spectrum of microheterogeneic disease subentities defined by various autoantigens and various antigen-recognizing types of T cells, as well as combinations thereof. There are also some arguments that dysregulation of innate, i.e. antigen-independent, immune functions could play a central pathogenetic role in at least some variants of psoriasis.

Clinical characteristics

For clinical treatment decisions (Fig. 2) the subclassification systems that are most helpful are those which allow some estimate of eruption pressure and irritability occurring in a spectrum of more or less stable and unstable variants (Fig. 3). In general antipsoriatics with known irritation potential should be avoided in case of an unstable, irritable psoriasis subtype.

One well-established subclassification discerns type I and type II psoriasis. About 75% of patients belong to type I with an early first manifestation of the disease, i.e. before the age of 40 years. This group of patients is characterized by a strong linkage to defined HLA types, such as Cw6, A30, B13 or B57/17, a substantial familial involvement, an increased resistance to microbial skin infections and a highly frequent elicitability of the Köbner phenomenon. In contrast, the latter is only rarely positive in type II psoriasis showing its first manifestation after the age of 40 years with a background of

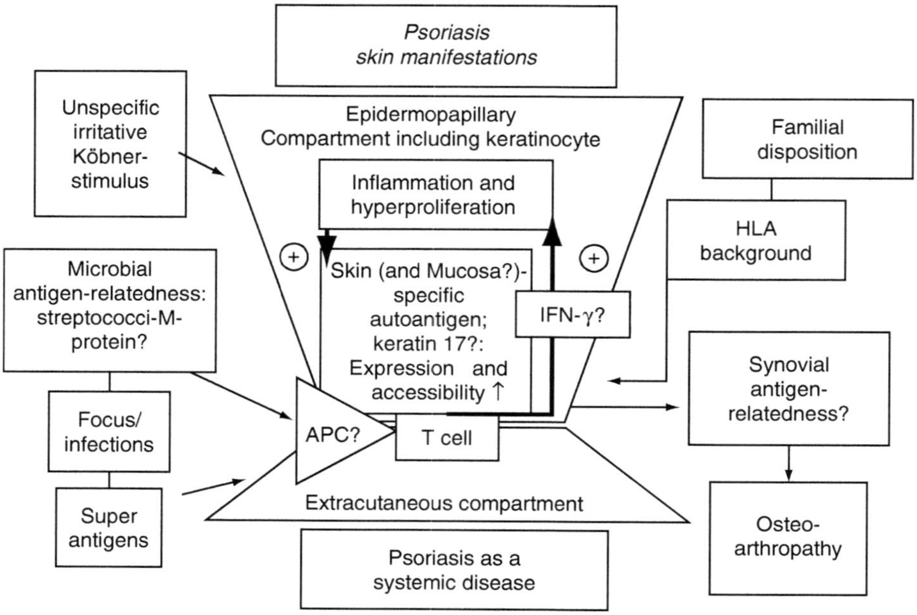

Figure 1 Aetiopathogenic scenario of psoriasis as an autoimmune disease driven by T cells. An 'IFN-γ/ keratin 17 autoimmune loop' may be postulated as the decisive vicious circle in a subgroup of psorasis patients.

A Present findings

Clinical psoriasis manifestation
Severity and affected body area (PASI)
eruption pressure and irritability
possible exudative character
localization
Possibility of joint and bone involvement
Endogenous and exogenous provocation factors

B History with regard to preceding antipsoriatic treatments

C Overall situation of the patient
Gender, age
Associated diseases (medication)
Personality, subjective affliction (life quality): psychosomatic and somatopsychic aspects
Stress and social surrounding (family, friends, profession, etc.)
Compliance

Figure 2 Decisive factors for the choice of appropriate antipsoriatic treatment: an 'holistic' view.

low expression of familial disease and HLA association.

Another more clinicomorphologically orientated subclassification (Fig. 3) discerns (a) psoriasis vulgaris as the 'typical psoriasis' found in about 95% of all patients; and (b) in the remaining 5% a mixture of various so-called exudative (erythrodermic and/or pustular) psoriasis variants known to be highly irritable.

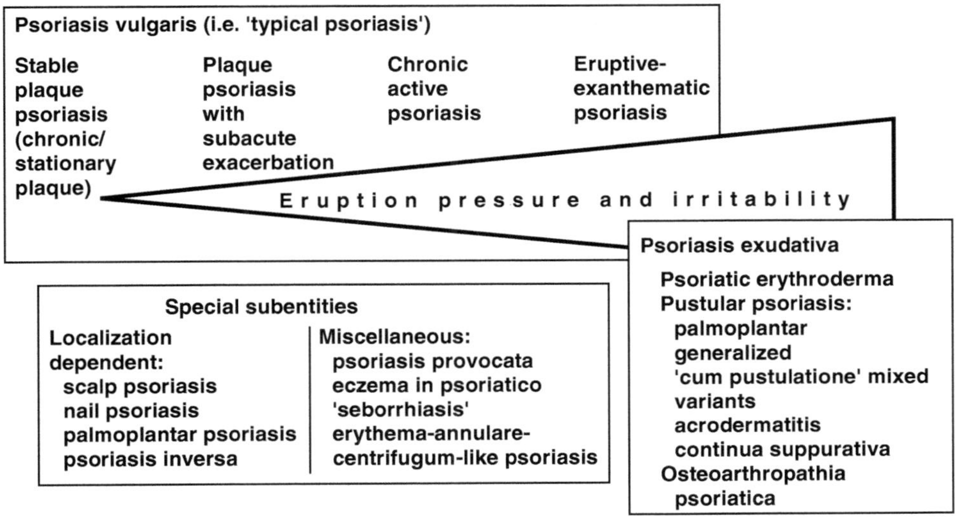

Figure 3 Clinicomorphological subclassification of psoriasis.

Psoriasis vulgaris may be considered as a subspectrum flanked by stable plaque psoriasis and the more instable and irritable eruptive–exanthematic type which is especially frequently in children and adolescents as the first manifestation.

Given the multifactorial immunogenetic pathogenesis of psoriasis, the first step of any treatment approach will always be the identification and elimination of specific and non-specific trigger mechanisms. The careful recording of patient history is of vital importance.

Exogenous triggers comprise physical provocation factors, such as skin friction and pressure (e.g. by clothing, shoes, various mechanical forces) as well as trauma (insect bites, tattoos, surgery, ultraviolet (UV) burning). A chemical Köbner factor may be present in detergents leading to delipidization and irritation of the skin. Various dermatoses are known to provoke psoriasis, e.g. allergic contact dermatitis, resulting in 'eczema in psoriatico' in particular on the hands and feet.

Endogenous triggers may be summarized into five categories: (a) infectious diseases (e.g. tonsillitis, pharyngitis, osteomyelitis; human immunodeficiency virus (HIV) infection); (b) metabolic disorders (obesity, hyperlipidaemia, hypocalcaemia); (c) drugs (β-receptor antagonists, lithium salts, chloroquin, interferons, angiotensin-converting enzyme (ACE) antagonists); (d) consumed substances (alcohol, nicotine); and (e) special local factors (oedema of the lower legs).

Given the continuously increasing knowlege about psychoneural/immunological implications, there is no doubt that psychic stress factors are able to precipitate psoriasis outbreaks or aggravate the disease. Therefore the psychosomatic as well as somatopsychic aspects of psoriasis have to be noted in each individual case. Stress relaxation (e.g. through reorganization of the patient's daily life activities accompanied by autogenic training) may be a highly supportive measure.

Treatment

General therapeutic guidelines

Any treatment decision will have to consider the following: (a) some basic aspects of the pathogenesis; (b) the disease's subclassification; and (c) possible trigger factors. Treatment modalities may be divided into three major categories: (a) topical drugs; (b) systemic medications; and (c) UV irradiations including balneo applications. The principles of simultaneously combining and successively rotating these modalities offer significant advantages in terms of an additive efficacy and a minimizing of unwanted side-effects.

Topical treatment

Adjuvants

Emollients and bath applications

In the psoriatic lesion the stratum corneum barrier is highly disturbed with much increased transepidermal water loss. It is well established that occlusion—with lipidizing, rehydrating emollients and bath applications or even hydrocolloid dressings—by itself exerts an antipsoriatic efficacy, mainly through restoration of the stratum corneum barrier function. Emollients also have an important protective function, especially in the context of skin challenges due to occupational strain.

Salicylic acid

Salicylic acid is used primarily as a keratolytic agent, especially at the start of treatment in order to eliminate squames and hyperkeratoses allowing the penetration of antipsoriatics. Salicylic acid will usually be applied in concentrations of 3% in vaselinum album for larger skin areas and up to 10% for palm, sole and scalp hyperkeratoses. In the scalp an oily vehicle preparation is preferred. Salicylic acid is resorbed percutaneously with the potential risk of intoxication, which is pronounced in children as well as in patients suffering from renal function impairment.

Urea

Urea exerts keratolytic, penetration-enhancing, antipruritic as well as mildly antiproliferative effects. The agent is typically applied in subirritative concentrations of 10% in adults and 5% in children.

Tar

Tar counteracts the disturbances found in the psoriatic lesion by its strong antiproliferative and anti-inflammatory effects, thus representing an efficacious antipsoriatic monotherapy. However, the application of tar is impractical because of its messiness, and consequent discoloration of the skin and unpleasant odour. More important is the experimentally proven potential mutagenic, carcinogenic and teratogenic risk linked to any use of tar preparations due to the genotoxic polyaromatic hydrocarbon (PHC) content. Therefore tar preparations should be avoided as far as possible. However, careful risk/benefit evaluation considering the latency of chemocarcinogenesis can still justify its use in selected and specially controlled individuals—the adjuvant use of relatively PHC-poor tar preparations, such as 5% liquor carbonis detergens (LCD), seems justifiable.

Miscellaneous

Agents such as selendisulfide, pyrithion zinc, tioxolon and natrium bituminosulfonate are used as antipsoriatic adjuvants especially in the scalp. In cases with proven colonization of scalp psoriasis by *Malassezia furfur* (a decisive cofactor) the following antimycotics are recommended as shampoo-like lotions: clotrimazole, ketoconazole, ciclopirox and bifonazole.

Vitamin D and analogues

During the last decade the topical treatment of psoriasis by vitamin D analogues has been established as highly effective. Up to now calcipotriol has been used most widely, followed by tacalcitol and calcitriol, the latter as the naturally occurring 1,25-dihydroxy vitamin D3. These compounds are assumed to target specific vitamin D receptors, thereby exerting antiproliferative and prodifferentiating effects upon the keratinocytes as well as anti-inflammatory and immunosuppressive effects.

Calcipotriol, tacalcitol and calcitriol are resorbed percutaneously with the dose-dependent potential sequellae of interference with systemic calcium metabolism resulting in hypercalcaemia and hypercalciuria. Therefore dose limitations must be strictly considered as shown in Table 1. Calcipotriol lotion has been proven as a valuable treatment of scalp and nail psoriasis, especially in combination with topical corticosteroids (see below).

Dithranol

The successful application of dithranol for the treatment of psoriasis has been reported since 1916. In a lipophilic vehicle, such as vaselinum album, dithranol is relatively stable. However the compound becomes rather unstable in contact with oxygen in an aqueous environment, with light exposure and at basic pH. Dithranol is assumed to exert its antipsoriatic efficacy through a cascade of molecular events initiated by entering the lipid compartments of the stratum corneum and the underlying living cell layers. The dithranol molecule decays leading to highly reactive products and oxygen species interfering with various cellular and subcellular mechanisms thus resulting in a reversal of the psoriatic process. Thereby, dithranol is completely inactivated to compounds such as monomeric danthrone within the upper skin layers.

Dithranol is considered a very effective and safe antipsoriatic. Its application is however, hampered by a skin-irritative potential as well as staining of skin, clothes and sanitary equipment (such as baths and showers). Thus dithranol should be used for the treatment of stable psoriasis types as inpatients.

The classical administration of dithranol is in vaselinum album (with 2% salicylic acid as an antioxidant) applied once or twice daily and left for 12 or 24 h. Depending on individual sensitivity, dithranol application is started with a concentration of 0.05% which is about doubled every 3–4 days. This regimen implies incremental concentrations of 0.1, 0.25, 0.5 and 1.0%. In certain well-adapted patients maximum concentrations of 2.0 and 3.0 may be reached. In a minority of particularly dithranol-sensitive patients an initial pretreatment should be performed very carefully starting at a concentration as low as 0.005% with a step-wise escalation over 0.01 and 0.02%.

For outpatients the short contact protocol is considered attractive. This protocol uses dithranol at incremental concentrations of 0.5, 1, 2 and 3% for application times of 10–30 min. Meta-analyses demonstrated average healing times of 30 days for classical dithranol treatment as compared to 37 days for short contact

Table 1 Dose limitations for topical vitamin D, its analogues and tazarotene as a topical retinoid in adult psoriasis patients.

Compund (concentration related to vehicle)	Application form	Daily application frequency	Maximum body area	Maximum weekly dosage
Calcipotriol (50 μg/1 g)	Ointment, cream	2×	30%	100 g
Tacalcitol (4.17 μg/1 g)	Ointment	1×	15–20%	70 g
Calcitriol (3 μg/1 g)	Ointment	2×	35%	210 g
Tazarotene (0.5 and 1 mg/1 g)	Aqueous gel	1×	10 (–20)%	Not specified

therapy. Dithranol sticks have proved valuable, allowing highly accurate treatment of the involved skin and sparing the healthy surrounding skin.

An innovative alternative is dithranol in a lipid-crystalline microencapsulation (Crystalip, Micanol). At temperatures above the 30°C reached on the skin surface, the dithranol is released. In this way the staining of clothes and bathroom items is minimized.

Corticosteroids

Psoriasis is a corticosteroid-sensitive dermatosis. The antipsoriatic action of corticosteroids relates to their antiproliferative, immunosuppressive, anti-inflammatory and vasoconstrictive effects mediated by many different cytomolecular mechanisms. However, corticosteroids show a general antianabolic (protein-catabolic) function, simultaneously stimulating glucose synthesis, thus potentially producing some adverse effects (see below).

Topical corticosteroids represent the most frequently used treatment modality for psoriasis worldwide. However, given the nature of psoriasis as a lifelong, relapsing disease mostly affecting larger parts of the body surface, corticosteroids should be used in a highly responsible, restrictive manner. This warning is emphasized by the fact, that topical corticosteroids, depending upon the potency and time of application, may lead to well-known, severe local and even systemic unwanted side-effects. These include various types of skin atrophy (skin thinning, hypopigmentation, pseudoscars, ulcerations, delayed wound healing, teleangiectasias), acne reactions, hypertrichosis, immunosuppression (leading to microbial skin infections), cataract, glaucoma and diabetogenic as well as cushingoid reactions. The percutaneous resorption of corticosteroids depends on the anatomical localization, being worse on the face and scrotal area. However, topical long-term application of corticosteroids on the scalp is usually not linked to any atrophogenic potential which may make it a good treatment for psoriasis capillitii.

A systemic corticosteroid treatment for psoriasis should generally be strictly avoided for the following reasons: the variety of possible substantial adverse effects, tachyphylaxis (i.e. progressive decrease of corticosteroid sensitivity), rebound phenomena (i.e. shortly after drug withdrawal occurrence of relapse characterized by severity above the baseline), aggravation of the disease's character (e.g. change from non-pustular to pustular psoriasis) and 'steroid addiction'.

Experienced dermatologists mostly do not use corticosteroids as a topical monotherapy but only in combination with dithranol, vitamin D analogues or tazarotene. Topical corticosteroids may be especially indicated at the beginning of a treatment course when psoriatic lesions appear overlaid by eczematous irritation.

Topical corticosteroid preparations are classified with regard to the potency, which is influenced by (a) the relative efficacy of the compound compared to a reference; (b) its concentration; and (c) the formulation (vehicle) chosen. For a highly effective treatment of plaque psoriasis potent World Health Organization (WHO) group III corticosteroids are needed, such as betamethasone 17, 21-dipropionate 0.05% or mometasone furoate 0.1%. Many studies have been published using the superpotent clobetasol 17 propionate 0.05% (group IV corticosteroid)—this should, however, be restricted to short-term applications because of adverse reactions. Under well-selected conditions we prefer combination treatment modalities including medium-potent group II corticosteroids, e.g. methyprednisolone aceponate 0.1%.

The use of corticosteroids may be especially advantageous for psoriasis manifestations in the following areas:

intertriginous and palmoplantar areas, scalp (alcoholic vehicle, see above) and nails. Any abrupt withdrawal of corticosteroid monotherapy in psoriasis is almost inevitably succeeded by a quickly occurring relapse. This is why corticosteroids should be used in combination protocols (see above) and slowly tapered off in a potency/concentration step- or interval-wise manner.

At the beginning of the corticosteroid era many patients felt enthusiastic about the high efficacy and practical convenience of this treatment. Today, in contrast, a high percentage of patients are afflicted by a 'cortisone-phobia' which is partly due to the uncritical prescription of corticosteroids. It is a challenging task to regain patient confidence by giving careful explanations and adequate information explaining the value of corticosteroids in psoriasis.

Tazarotene

Tazarotene is a member of a new generation of retinoids characterized by a selective affinity for retinoid acid receptors (RAR). The compound is marketed in a 0.01 and 0.05% concentration as an aqueous gel. It is recommended to use the gel once daily with the restriction, not to exceed 10 (to 20)% of the body surface area (Table 1). Given the known teratogenicity of retinoids, tazarotene is contraindicated during pregnancy.

There is still limited experience for this relatively new antipsoriatic treatment. Its effectiveness has been proven in plaque psoriasis. Given its mild irritative potential, the treatment should be started with the lower concentrated gel, applied only to the lesion, preferably with the surrounding skin protected by a barrier emollient. Controlled studies have demonstrated that the antipsoriatic efficacy of tazarotene was significantly increased by combination with a potent group III corticosteroid (fluocinonide 0.05% or mometasone furoate 0.1%) or UVB treatment, respectively. Under the latter conditions daily UVB exposure should be given before the topical tazarotene treatment.

Additionally, tazarotene shows promise for the treatment of psoriasis in special areas such as the scalp and paronychial areas.

Systemic medications

Ciclosporin

In 1979 Mueller and Herrmann reported in a letter to the *New England Journal of Medicine* about the favourable efficacy of ciclosporin in a cohort of rheumatoid arthritis patients including four cases of psoriatic arthritis with a simultaneous response of their skin symptoms. In subsequent years ciclosporin, as a lipophilic cyclic undecapeptide isolated from the fungus *Tolypocladium inflatum Gans*, not only revolutionized transplantation medicine but also the understanding of the aetiopathogenesis of psoriasis as a T-cell mediated autoimmune disease. Ciclosporin acts mainly through the inhibition of T-cellular interleukin (IL)-2 production via binding to cytoplasmic cyclophilin and subsequent suppression of the calcium-dependent signal transduction downstream to T-cell receptor activation.

For the treatment of psoriasis ciclosporin is administered orally in a standard starting dosage of 2.5–3.5 mg/kg body weight divided over two daily doses in the morning and evening. Depending upon the severity of the disease and the intended response, the initial daily dosage may be chosen up to a maximum of 5 mg/kg body weight.

From the literature, we have differentiated the following four ciclosporin regimens.

- Crisis intervention with ciclosporin for 2–6 weeks followed by another initially overlapping treatment modality, e.g. bath psoralen and ultraviolet A (bath PUVA).

- Short-interval treatment with ciclosporin for 1.5–4 months, a subsequent ciclosporin-free interval and repetition(s) of ciclosporin if needed.
- 'Six-month block treatment'.
- Continuous long-term treatment over 1 (up to 2) years.

Experience of treating psoriasis continuously with ciclosporin over more than 2 years is still very limited.

A substantial response of psoriatic skin manifestations is observed in most patients at 2–4 weeks after onset of ciclosporin, sometimes in the first few days. In most cases the psoriasis area and severity index (PASI) is reduced by more than 85% after 16 weeks of ciclosporin monotherapy.

The safe handling of ciclosporin requires careful consideration, especially of the potential of a variety of mostly dose-dependent frequent and rare adverse effects, as well as drug interferences which have varying degrees of severity. Up-to-date specialist pharmacological literature is available for dermatologists prescribing ciclosporin: it is important to be aware of the long list of possible adverse events and drug interferences. Any symptom and patient complaints should be analysed for the possibilities of adverse events or drug interferences.

The most frequent and therefore important adverse reactions to ciclosporin concern the induction of renal dysfunction and arterial hypertension (Table 2). This is why treatment guidelines recommend strict monitoring of these parameters. Diastolic arterial pressure >95 mmHg requires antihypertensive medication and, if that fails, a reduction in the ciclosporin dose. The individual serum creatinine level of each patient should always be determined before ciclosporin medication and set to 100% as a reference level. An increase of serum creatinine by more than 30% would mean a reduction in ciclosporin. At the beginning of ciclosporin medication the above-mentioned monitoring should be performed every 2 weeks. Successful ciclosporin treatment of psoriasis depends very much upon fine tuning of the dosage adaptation in relation to individual drug tolerability and efficacy.

Retinoids

The second-generation, monoaromatic retinoids, i.e. etretinate and its first metabolite acitretin, are characterized by a systemic, broad antipsoriatic efficacy. Today, acitretin is in use worldwide not only for the treatment of psoriasis but also for ichthyoses, palmoplantar keratoses, Darier's disease, pityriasis rubra pilaris, hyperkeratotic hand eczema, keratosis lichenoides chronica and lichen ruber. Mediated by specialized retinoid receptors, acitretin exerts its pleiotropic influence on proliferation, keratinization and differentiation of epithelial cells, additional effects on cellular and humoral immune responses, and anti-inflammatory actions, partly related to

Table 2 Most frequent and relevant adverse events of low-dose ciclosporin in the treatment of psoriasis (≤ 2.5–5 mg/kg per day). Drug-induced neuromuscular disturbances including the gastrointestinal tract may be due to hypomagnesaemia necessitating an adequate Mg substitution.

Renal impairments	Viral infections
Arterial hypertension	Muscle pains
Hypertrichosis	Cramps and oedema of lower legs
Tremor	Gastrointestinal complaints
Gingiva hyperplasia	Hypomagnesaemia
Paraesthesias	Hyperlipedaemia: triglycerides ↑, cholesterol ↑
Headache, fatigue	Transaminases ↑

the arachidonic acid cascade and migration of polymorphonuclear leucocytes.

In chronic plaque psoriasis acitretin, and etretinate (where it is still available), can be used for combination therapy with topical antipsoriatic agents such as dithranol, vitamin D analogues, PUVA or UVB (see Table 5). However, in the erythrodermic variants of psoriasis or in severe pustular psoriasis, including acrodermatitis continua suppurativa (Hallopeau's disease), oral monotherapy with retinoids still represents the therapy of choice. In addition, etretinate and acitretin show good efficacy as maintenance drugs for chronic plaque psoriasis after clinical remission.

Standard dosage of acitretin is about 0.25–0.6 mg/kg daily, but it has to be adapted in terms of indication and individual response. Maximum acitretin dosages of 1.0 mg/kg may be administered in the first few days of starting the treatment of severe pustular or recalcitrant hyperkeratotic palmoplantar types of psoriasis. Absence of severe diseases of the liver and kidney or other metabolic diseases, including severe diabetes and impairment of lipid metabolism, are preconditions for oral treatment with retinoids. The dynamics of the clinical response depends on the clinical type of psoriasis to be treated: relatively slowly occurring in chronic stable plaque type, but fast in the pustular and even the erythrodermic variant.

Maximal therapeutic efficiency can be achieved after 2–3 months of treatment. For further stabilization after clearing the acute disease, a constant maintenance dose of 0.125–0.4 mg/kg daily is advisable for about 3–6 months. Due to its non-immunosuppressive but immunomodulating properties, oral application of acitretin is also adequate in the treatment of the severe types of psoriasis found in immunosuppressed and human immunodeficiency virus (HIV)-positive patients.

Acitretin has a characteristic spectrum of side-effects similar to chronic hypervitaminosis A syndrome. Retinoid-induced cheilitis is almost unavoidable and occurs more or less rapidly, depending on the dose administered. It is also a parameter for drug absorption and patient compliance. In addition, 'retinoid dermatitis' (skin xerosis, irritation and pruritus), mucosal dryness and the feeling of burning or sticky skin is a common side-effect. Hair loss and brittle nails are observed quite frequently, depending on the dose. All these effects are reversible after cessation of acitretin treatment.

Increased serum triglycerides is a common side-effect under retinoid treatment; increased serum cholesterol and liver enzymes are observed less frequently. In most cases the changes in laboratory parameters are transient. The increase in serum lipids can be prevented by a low-fat and low-carbohydrate diet. Less frequently combinations with serum lipid-reducing drugs are necessary.

In some patients, especially in chronic and frequently relapsing pustular psoriasis, retinoid therapy may be needed long term, perhaps for several years. In these cases it is particularly important to pay attention to retinoid-induced side-effects on the bones. It is advisable to take X-rays of the spine before starting the therapy and to carefully document possible skeletal pain and mobility restrictions. If there is any clinical doubt, radiographic control of symptomatic parts of the skeleton is necessary. After long-term acitretin application the so-called diffuse idiopathic skeletal hyperostosis (DISH syndrome) has been observed.

The teratogenicity of retinoids is an unresolved problem. Although the plasma half-life of acitretin is only about 50–60 h, its re-esterification to etretinate requires very safe contraceptive measures for women of childbearing age. Contraception should be started about 1 month before application and continued for at least 2 years after cessation of therapy depending on local regulations. As an alternative isotretinoin may be tried provided that appropriate contraception during and 2 months after treatment is ensured.

Interaction of retinoids is possible with tetracyclines, phenytoin, barbiturates, non-steroidal anti-inflammatory drugs (NSAIDs), ketoconazole and ciclosporin. Combination therapy with methotrexate is contraindicated because of additional hepatotoxic side-effects.

Fumaric acid derivatives

In 1994 a team of clinical researchers headed by Altmeyer reported on the significant antipsoriatic efficacy of an oral medication consisting of a mixture of fumarates in a large case, double-blind, placebo-controlled study. These data led to the approval of a fumarate preparation (Fumaderm) first appearing in Germany. The preparation is available in two strengths as indicated in Table 3.

It is recommended to initiate the fumarate treatment by a slow escalation of the dosage in step-wise increments over several weeks as outlined in Table 4. The escalation of the dosage depends on therapeutic efficacy and the limitations of individual tolerance. Following this recommendation a maximum daily dosage of 1290 mg total fumarate may be reached divided over 3 single administrations per day, i.e. in the morning, at noon and in the evening. In most cases the maximum dose of 3 × 2 tablets of Fumaderm per day is not necessary to treat the disease, but this dosage represents an absolute maximum. The individually tailored dose is then administered as maintenance therapy. The drug manufacturer recommends a limit on the cycle of continuous fumarate administration to a duration of 6 months. Continuous intake of fumarates over longer time spans, even up to several years as seen in many patients, has not been investigated in controlled clinical studies.

Oral fumarate treatment is indicated in severe psoriasis cases with (a) 10 (–25)% affected body surface; (b) high tendency for relapsing; and (c) in exceptional treatment recalcitrance. A substantial clinical response becomes evident from the 4th to 6th week. About 50–80% of psoriasis patients experience a significant benefit from fumarate treatment. In the remaining, about 25% of patients find this treatment is not efficacious or impossible because of unacceptable side-effects. Fumarates also proved to be effective in nail psoriasis and psoriatic arthritis.

Systemic fumarate treatment is contraindicated under the following circumstances: severe diseases of the

Table 3 Composition of the fumarate preparation as approved for the treatment of psoriasis in Germany.

	Fumaderm Initial: mg/1 tablet	Fumaderm: mg/1 tablet
Dimethylfumarate	30	120
Ethylhydrogen-fumarate		
–Ca	67	87
–Mg	5	5
–Zn	3	3

Table 4 Recommended schedule for the incremental initiation of fumarate treatment depending upon individual tolerance and antipsoriatic efficacy.

	Fumaderm Initial			Fumaderm					
Week	**1**	**2**	**3**	**4**	**5**	**6**	**7**	**8**	**9**
Morning		1	1		1	1	1	2	2
Noon			1			1	1	1	2
Evening	1	1	1	1	1	1	2	2	2

gastrointestinal tract including the liver, all cases of renal impairment, malignancies, haematological diseases, age below 18 years, pregnancy, nursing and the topical application of fumaric acid and derivatives (generally regarded as ineffective).

Side-effects include flush reactions (in about 30–50% of patients), gastrointestinal complaints (in about 30%: nausea, tenesmus, diarrhoea), headache, fatigue and dizziness. The flush reactions occur about 30 min to 6 h after drug intake and last for up to 30 min. Flush reactions are especially prominent during the first couple of weeks (the initiation phase of fumarate treatment) and fade away later. The pharmacokinetic and biochemical bases of flush reactions and the corresponding adaptation mechanism are unknown. In a minority of cases reversible nephrogenic side-effects, i.e. tubular impairments, with proteinuria and an increase of serum creatinine have been reported. The possible fumarate-related impact on kidney function leads to the precautionary recommendation of fluid intake of at least 1.5–2 L/day.

Fumarate treatment necessitates regular laboratory control of the following parameters: serum creatinine, urine sedimentation and protein, white blood cell count and differentiation, thrombocyte count and liver enzymes (serum glutamate oxaloacetate transaminase, serum glutamate pyruvate transaminase, γ-glutamyl transferase and alkaline phosphatase). These should be performed at least every 14 days during the first 3 months, and then every 4 weeks.

Termination of fumarate treatment or at least dose reduction should be considered in the following conditions:

- increase of serum creatinine by more than 30% from pretreatment level
- proteinuria
- decrease of leucocytes to <3000/μL
- decrease of lymphocytes to <500/μL
- persistent eosinophilia = 25%.

The exact mode of fumarate's antipsoriatic action is a current objective of international research. *In vitro* studies indicate that dimethylfumarate may be the most active single compound. Clinical data point to a mainly immunomodulatory profile as indicated by the significant decrease of T and B lymphocytes, natural killer (NK) cells and total leucocytes in the peripheral blood under oral fumarate administration lasting several months. Moreover, a fumarate-dependent shift from Th1 to Th2 predominance as well as dimethylfumarate-induced suppression of a putative psoriasis autoantigen have been observed.

Systemic co-medication with retinoids, ciclosporin, methotrexate, psoralen as well as otherwise immunosuppressive, cytostatic or potentially nephrotoxic drugs is contraindicated.

Methotrexate

Methotrexate is a classical, well-established systemic treatment modality for severe cases of psoriasis including erythrodermic and pustular types as well as psoriatic osteoarthritis. The drug is a folic acid analogue and inhibits dihydrofolate reductase, thereby dose-dependently and successively inhibiting thymidine, purine, DNA, RNA and protein synthesis. This cytostatic mode of action is assumed to hit hyperproliferative keratinocytes as well as lymphocytes as decisive cellular targets in psoriasis.

The drug is characterized by hepatotoxic potential. Contraindications to be considered include: severe impairment of hepatic and renal function (e.g. active virus hepatitis, liver cirrhosis, alcohol addiction), leucopenia, thrombocytopenia, immunodeficiency (HIV infection), pregnancy, intended reproduction and non-compliance. Methotrexate may interfere with a variety of drugs, such as NSAIDs, phenytoin, barbiturates, tetracyclines, chloramphenicol, sulphonamides and metamizole.

Before starting methotrexate treatment the following tests should be checked: blood cell count including differential leucocyte count, liver-related parameters (serum glutamate oxaloacetate transaminase, serum glutamate pyruvate transaminase, γ-glutamyl transferase, alkaline phosphatase, bilirubin, albumin), kidney-related parameters (S-creatinine, creatinine clearance, urea, urine status), hepatitis serology and HIV infection diagnostics.

During the last decades three methotrexate regimens have been successfully established for psoriasis:

- triple weekly administration: methotrexate is administered 3 times a week with 12-h intervals (according to Weinstein and Frost); the cumulative dosage is 15–22.5 mg/week
- single weekly oral administration: methotrexate is given once a week in a dosage of 10–25 mg (up to a maximum of 30 mg)
- single weekly intramuscular administration: methotrexate is injected once a week in a dosage of 12.5–15 mg (up to a maximum of 25 mg).

During the course of treatment the dose must be carefully adjusted with regard to individual clinical efficacy, in order to minimize drug toxicity. The above-mentioned liver, blood cell and kidney-related laboratory parameters must be carefully monitored. Methotrexate medication should remain under the direct control of a dermatologist: in the past severe life-threatening intoxications have been observed due to overdosage, especially in cases where the intended weekly dosage was falsely applied on a daily basis. Under such circumstances calcium folinate is the appropriate antidote.

In high-risk patients a pretreatment liver biopsy is recommended by the American Academy of Dermatology (Psoriasis Task Force 1996) and the American College of Rheumatology. In the other cases a first liver biopsy may be performed after a cumulative methotrexate dosage of 1.5 g. Given unsuspicious liver histology, the methotrexate treatment can be continued up to a cumulative dosage of 3–4 g, when another control liver biopsy is recommended. Dynamic liver scintigraphy and determination of serum aminoterminal procollagen propeptide have been proposed as additional helpful parameters to assess possible liver damage.

A good treatment response to methotrexate can be expected in 75–80% of patients. In the remaining patients the response is only moderate with a low percentage of almost complete failure. Usually increasing clinical improvement is noticed from weeks 2–8 after onset of treatment, with near to complete healing after 8–12 weeks. Typical side-effects of long-term methotrexate treatment in psoriasis comprise elevated liver-related laboratory parameters, nausea, abdominal complaints, fatigue, headache, vertigo, haematopoietic suppression, effluvium and increased susceptibility to infections.

UV treatment

Heliotherapy of dermatoses has been known since antiquity. The UV spectrum is divided into UVC (110–280 nm), UVB (280–315 nm), UVA2 (315–340 nm) and UVA1 (340–400 nm). In Western Europe the natural solar global spectrum of electromagnetic irradiation reaching the earth ranges from about 304 to 5000 nm.

In order to perform safe UV treatment of psoriasis, it is mandatory that (a) the skin type, the present degree of tanning as well as the minimal erythema dose (MED for UVB and UVB/A) and minimal phototoxicity dose (MPD for PUVA), respectively, are determined before starting the irradiation; and (b) the patient is visited each day to ensure an appropriate dose escalation.

The simultaneous administration of photodynamic drugs (e.g. tetracyclines) or ingestion of photodynamic foods and additives (celery, certain herbs, cyclamate) has to be ruled out.

UVB

In systematic trials Parrish and Jaenicke demonstrated that UV irradiation in the spectrum between 254 and 290 nm did not improve psoriasis, while healing was induced at wavelengths ranging from 296 to 313 nm. Thus there is a rather erythematogenic, photocarcinogenic spectral range which is discernible from the antipsoriatic effective spectrum.

The closest approximation to the most effective antipsoriatic spectral range may be achieved by using the Philips TL01 light source, which emits nearly monochromatic light with a maximum of 311 $\pm$ 3 nm. TL01 narrow-spectrum treatment proved to be advantageous over TL12 broad-spectrum treatment especially with regard to erythematogenic, irritative side-effects.

UVA/B

Treatment of psoriasis by an UVA/B overlapping spectrum in the range 295–366 nm is very well established (e.g. Saalmann SUP (selective ultraviolet phototherapy) light source). Usually such UVA/B irradiations are performed 3–5 times per week. UVB erythema is known to reach its maximum after 24 h which allows increases in dosage in a daily rhythm. UVA/B irradiation is initiated at 70–80% of MED.

Balneophototherapy

There is convincing experience from many patients worldwide that therapy in the Dead Sea is a very effective treatment for psoriasis. This geographical phenomenon is characterized by (a) a cut-off of the most erythematogenic short-wave UVB bands at 300 m below sea-level; and (b) a high salt concentration of more than 30% in the Dead Sea water. Such a high salt concentration is considered to have a topical effect by itself, e.g. through extraction of leucocyte elastase activity from psoriatic lesions and anti-inflammatory effects of magnesium ions. These conditions may be successfully artificially mimicked in so-called 'balneophototherapy', which is the combination of bathing in synthetically generated Dead Sea salt (5–15%) and UV(A)B irradiation. Corresponding technical challenges of such high salt concentrations are (a) corrosion of bath tubs and sewage pipes; and (b) environmental aspects—these have to a certain extent been resolved by foil bath strategies (drastically reducing the required bath fluid volume) and the development of very effective water recycling systems.

Photochemotherapy (PUVA)

Photochemotherapy combines UVA irradiation with the systemic or topical application of a photosensitizing agent, i.e. a psoralen compound.

Systemic PUVA

The standard procedure is to ingest 8-methoxypsoralen (8-MOP) in dosages according to the body weight (0.3–0.6 mg/kg) at 1–2 h before UVA treatment. In some countries 5-MOP is approved. UVA broad-spectrum emission sources are used peaking at 360–365 nm with an action spectrum around 335 nm. Initial dosing is adapted for skin type and pretesting of MPD. Depending upon the individual MPD the starting UVA dose lies around 1 J/cm^2. Treatments are performed 2–4 times a week on not more than 2 consecutive days with a dose increment at about every third session by 0.5–1.0 J/cm^2. Clearance is achieved in the majority of patients after 19–25 treatments with a cumulative UVA dose ranging from 100 to 245 J/cm^2. The male genitalia should not be exposed to UVA to control for locality-dependent increased risk of PUVA-induced skin carcinogenesis. The eyes must be protected by special UVA-absorbing glasses until dusk on the day that psoralen was ingested.

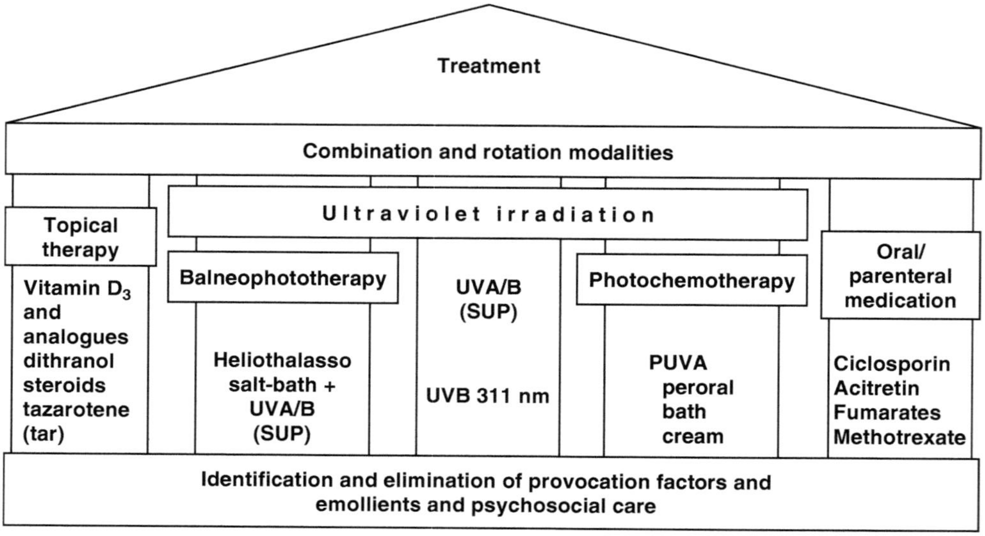

Figure 4 The 'skilful architecture' of psoriasis treatment.

The recognition that systemic PUVA was correlated with an increased skin cancer risk led to the following conclusions: (a) less aggressive systemic PUVA protocols are preferred with regard to UV dosage; (b) combination treatment protocols should be used to reduce the impact of systemic PUVA and its related adverse events (see below); (c) maintenance treatment by systemic PUVA should be stopped after clearing; and (d) systemic PUVA should be replaced by topical PUVA wherever possible.

Bath PUVA

This treatment modality has been especially developed in Scandinavian countries. A bath is taken in an 8-MOP, 5-MOP or trimethylpsoralen aqueous solution, after which UVA irradiation is performed.

An example of bath PUVA treatment is a 15 mL solution containing 0.5% 8-MOP in 96% ethanol added to bath water at 50°C to a final volume of 150 L at 37°C. The bath is taken for 20 min with subsequent UVA irradiation. The starting UVA dosage is 30% of MPD which is usually 0.2–0.3 J/cm^2. A maximum of 4 exposures is performed per week on not more than 2 subsequent days. The UVA dose is increased at every third session by 0.2–0.3 J/cm^2 steps to a maximum dose around 5 J/cm^2. Risk of carcinogenicity is assumed to be significantly lower as compared to classical PUVA.

PUVA modifications

Topical PUVA may also be applied with psoralen application in the shower in cream or solution.

Principle of combination and rotation treatment

The rationale for the treatment of psoriasis by combining various antipsoriatic modalities is based upon the following.

- Treatment modalities are characterized by special profiles of efficacy, each targeting different points and subsystems of the pathogenetic cascade (i.e. proliferation, differentiation and activation of various cell types in a microenvironment of soluble factors/mediators, cell–cell interactions and tissue matrix determinants, etc.).
- Combining of individual treatment modalities offers the advantage of

Table 5 The established antipsoriatic treatment modalities are grouped into four categories ('poles'), i.e. (I) topical drugs, (II) systemically administrated drugs, (III) non-PUVA UV treatment procedures and (IV) PUVA. Efficacious, safe and frequently chosen combinations are indicated by dashed lines connecting the 'coordinate-alike' corresponding modalities.

	(II) Systemic medications				
	Ciclosporin	Acitretin	Fumarates	Methotrexate	
(I) Topicals					**(IV) PUVA**
Vitamin D and derivatives (± corticoid)					Topical: bath, shower, cream, solution
Dithranol (± corticoid)			**1** (1st column)		
Tazarotene (± corticoid)			**2** (3rd column)	**3** (4th column)	Peroral/systemic
	(III) Non-PUVA UV modalities				
	UVB (± salt-water bath)		UVB/A – SUP(± salt-water bath)		
Basics: identification and elimination of provocation factors and psychosocial care and emollients					

1, A potential risk of cumulative kidney toxicity may derive from percutaneous absorption of salicylic acid from dithranol preparations in coincidence with systemic fumarates.
2, The experience with combining systemic fumarates and UV is still limited.
3, The combination of methotrexate and UV light may implicate an increased carcinogenic risk.

additive and synergistic efficacy resulting in higher clearance rates and longer disease-free intervals.

- Minimizing of side-effects by dose reduction.

Furthermore, rotating the patient successively through the spectrum of different antipsoriatic treatment modalities reduces the cumulative side-effects and long-term risks of each treatment (Fig. 4).

Topical antipsoriatics like vitamin D and derivatives, dithranol, tazarotene and tar may be used in combination with topical corticosteroids. It is contraindicated to combine systemic antipsoriatic treatment modalities such as ciclosporin, acitretine, fumarates and methotrexate. The variety of possible combinations investigated in clinical studies and approved in everyday practice is listed in Table 5.

The well-known combination regimens inaugurated by Goeckerman (tar plus UV) and Ingram (tar plus UV plus anthralin) are being increasingly abandoned because of the potential carcinogenic risk due to the tar component (see above).

Table 6 Selection of innovative drugs, so-called biologicals and non-pharmaceutical treatment approaches, explored during the last few years for their therapeutic potential in psoriasis (for details of the favourable, but partly also unfavourable, outcomes see the original references listed). All listed modalities are characterized by a clinicoexperimental status lacking official approval for the treatment of psoriasis.

Treatment	Authors	Reference
Anti-CD4 antibody	P. Morel *et al.*	*J Autoimmun* 1992; 5: 465–77
Anti-CD11a/LFA-1 antibody	J.G. Krueger *et al.*	*Br J Dermatol* 1999; 141: 994
Anti-E-selectin antibody	M. Bhusban *et al.*	*Br J Dermatol* 1999; 141: 988
Anti-IL8 antibody	M.E. Lohner *et al.*	*Br J Dermatol* 1999; 141: 989
Anti-TNF-αantibody	E. Proksch *et al.*	*Arch Dermatol Res* 2001; 293: 101
	A.L.J. Ogilvie *et al.*	*Br J Dermatol* 2001; 144: 587–9
Ascomycine derivative SDZ ASM 981	U. Mrowietz *et al.*	*Br J Dermatol* 1998; 139: 992–6
Basiliximab (Simulect): anti-CD25 monoclonal antibody	A. Salim *et al.*	*Br J Dermatol* 2000; 143: 1121–2
Bexaroten (Targretin)	J.V. Smit *et al.*	*Br J Dermatol* 1999; 141: 992–3
CO_2 laser resurfacing of plaque psoriasis	M.B. Alora *et al.*	*Lasers Surg Med* 1998; 22: 165–70
CTLA41g	J.R. Abrams *et al.*	*J Exp Med* 2000; 192: 681–93
DAB_{389} fusion protein	J. Bagel *et al.*	*J Am Acad Dermatol* 1998; 38: 938–44
Daclizumab (Zenapax): anti-CD25 antibody	J.G. Krueger *et al.*	*J Am Acad Dermatol* 2000; 43: 448–58
Etanercept (Enbrel): TNF-αblockade	P.J. Mease *et al.*	*Lancet* 2000; 356: 385–90
Interferential current	A. Philipp *et al.*	*Eur J Dermatol* 2000; 10: 195–8
Interleukin-10	K. Asadullah *et al.*	*J Clin Invest* 1998; 101: 783–94
Interleukin-11	W.L. Trepicchio *et al.*	*J Clin Invest* 1999; 104: 1527–37
LFA3TIP (Amevive): recombinant fusion protein out of the extracellular domain of LFA-3 and the hinge/C_H2/C_H3–IgG1 sequence	G. Krueger	*Br J Dermatol* 1999; 141: 979–80
Liarozol	J.P. van Pelt *et al.*	*Skin Pharmacol Appl Skin Physiol* 1998; 11: 70–9
Maxacalcitol	J.N.W.N. Barker *et al.*	*Br J Dermatol* 1999; 141: 274–8
Mycophenolate mofetil	M.G. Haufs *et al.*	*Br J Dermatol* 1998; 138: 179–81
Peptide T	S.K. Raychaudhuri *et al.*	*Int J Immunopharmacol* 1998; 20: 661–7
Photodynamic therapy	W.H. Boehncke *et al.*	*Lancet* 1994; 343: 801
Sirolimus (syn. rapamycine)	M.J. Kaplan *et al.*	*Arch Dermatol* 1999; 135: 553–7
Tacrolimus (FK506)	A. Remitz *et al.*	*Br J Dermatol* 1999; 141: 103–7
Tioguanin (syn. 6-thioguanine, 2-amino-6(1H)-purinthione)	F.P. Murphy	*Arch Dermatol* 1999; 135: 1495–502

Miscellaneous aspects

With regard to the specialities of treatment of psoriasis during childhood, pregnancy and HIV infection the reader is referred to the psoriasis textbooks listed in the further reading. This also applies to further information concerning nail, scalp and pustular psoriasis, psoriatic erythroderma and osteoarthropathica psoriatica.

Experimental treatment modalities and perspectives

A selection of innovative antipsoriatic treatments have been recently explored which have a clinico-experimental status as summarized briefly in Table 6.

Further reading

Altmeyer PJ, Matthes U, Pawlak F *et al.* Antipsoriatic effect of fumaric acid derivatives: results of a multicentre double-blind study in 100 patients. *J Am Acad Dermatol* 1994; 30: 977–81.

Ashcroft DM, Li Wan Po A, Williams HC, Griffiths CEM. Quality of life measures in psoriasis: a critical appraisal of their quality. *J Clin Pharm Ther* 1998; 23: 391–8.

Bonnekoh B, Böckelmann R, Ambach A, Gollnick H. Dithranol and dimethylfumarate suppress interferon-γ induced up-regulation of cytokeratin 17 as a putative psoriasis autoantigen. *Skin Pharmacol Appl Skin Physiol* 2001; 14: 217–25.

Bonnekoh B, Huerkamp C, Wevers A *et al.* Upregulation of keratin 17 expression in human HaCaT keratinocytes by interferon-γ. *J Invest Dermatol* 1995; 104: 58–61.

British Photodermatology Group. British Photodermatology Group guidelines for PUVA. *Br J Dermatol* 1994; 130: 246–55.

Camisa C. *Handbook of Psoriasis.* Oxford: Blackwell Science, 1998.

De Jong EMGJ, van Vlijmen IMMJ, van Erp PEJ *et al.* Keratin 17. A useful marker in antipsoriatic therapies. *Arch Dermatol Res* 1991; 283: 480–2.

Geilen CC, Tebbe B, Bartels CG, Krengel S, Orfanos CE. Successful treatment of erythrodermic psoriasis with mycophenolate mofetil. *Br J Dermatol* 1998; 138: 1101–2.

Gollnick H, Bonnekoh B. *Psoriasis—Pathogenese, Klinik und Therapie.* Bremen: Uni-Med Verlag AG/London: International Medical Publishers, 2001.

Gollnick H, Dümmler: U. Retinoids. *Clin Dermatol* 1997; 15: 799–810.

Gollnick H, Finzi AF, Marks R *et al.* Optimising the use of tazarotene in clinical practice: consensus statement from the European advisory panel for tazarotene (Zorac TM). *Dermatology* 1999; 199: 40–6.

Gollnick H, Menke T. Current experience with tacalcitol ointment in the treatment of psoriasis. *Curr Med Res Opinion* 1998; 14: 213–18.

Gollnick HPM. The psoriatic patient and the use of topical antipsoriatics. *J Dermatol Treat* 1998; 9: 7–11.

Gollnick HR, Bauer C *et al.* Acitretin versus etretinate in psoriasis. Clinical and pharmacokinetic results of a German multicenter study. *J Am Acad Dermatol* 1988; 19: 458–69.

Griffiths CEM, Kirby B. *Psoriasis.* London: Martin Dunitz, 1999.

Gudmundsdottir AS, Sigmundsdottir H, Sigurgeirsson B *et al.* Is an epitope on keratin 17 a major target for autreactive T lymphocytes in psoriasis? *Clin Exp Immunol* 1999; 117: 580–6.

Haustein UF, Ryter M. Methotrexate in psoriasis: 26 years experience with low-dose long-term treatment. *J Eur Acad Dermatol Venereol* 2000; 14: 382–8.

Henseler T, Christophers E, Hönigsmann H, Wolff K. Skin tumors in the European PUVA study. Eight year follow-up of 1643 patients treated with PUVA for psoriasis. *J Am Acad Dermatol* 1987; 16: 108–16.

Ho VCCEM, Griffiths G, Albrecht F *et al.* The PISCES study group: Intermittent short courses of cyclosporin (Neoral) for psoriasis unresponsive to topical therapy: a 1-year multicentre, randomized study. *Br J Dermatol* 1999; 141: 283–91.

Hutchinsonm PE, Marks R, White J. The efficacy, safety and tolerance of calcitriol 3 μg/g ointment in the treatment of plaque psoriasis: a comparison with short-contact dithranol. *Dermatology* 2000; 201: 139–45.

Jenisch S, Henseler T, Nair RP *et al.* Linkage analysis of human leukocyte antigen (HLA) markers in familial psoriasis: strong disequilibrium effects provide evidence for a major determinant in the HLA-B/-C region. *Am J Hum Genet* 1998; 63: 191–9.

Karrer S, Eholzer C, Ackermann G, Landthaler M, Szeimies R-M. Phototherapy of psoriasis: comparative experience of different phototherapeutic approaches. *Dermatology* 2001; 202: 108–15.

Kirby B, Fortune DG, Bhushan M, Chalmers RJG, Griffiths, CEM. The Salford Psoriasis Index. an holistic measure of psoriasis severity. *Br J Dermatol* 2000; 142: 728–32.

Koo J, Lebwohl M. Duration of remission of psoriasis therapies. *J Am Acad Dermatol* 1999; 41: 51–9.

Koo JY. Current consensus and update on psoriasis therapy: a perspective from the US. *J Dermatol* 1999; 26: 723–33.

Kragballe K. Treatment of psoriasis by the topical application of the novel cholecalciferol analogue calcipotriol (MC 903). *Arch Dermatol* 1989; 125: 1647–52.

Lebwohl M, Ellis C, Gottlieb A *et al.* Cyclosporine consensus conference with emphasis on the treatment of psoriasis. *J Am Acad Dermatol* 1998; 39: 464–75.

Mahrle G. Dithranol. *Clin Dermatol* 1997; 15: 723–37.

Menter MA, See J-A, Amend WJC *et al.* Proceedings of the psoriasis combination and rotation therapy conference. *J Am Acad Dermatol* 1996; 34: 315–21.

Merk HF, Bickers DR. *Dermatopharmakologie und Dermatotherapie*. Oxford: Blackwell Science, 1992.

Mrowietz U, Christophers E, Altmeyer P for the German Fumaric Acid Ester Consensus Conference. Treatment of severe psoriasis with fumaric acid esters: scientific background and guidelines for therapeutic use. *Br J Dermatol* 1999; 141: 424–9.

Nickoloff BJ, Wrone-Smith T. Superantigens, autoantigens, and pathogenic T cells in psoriasis. *J Invest Dermatol* 1998; 110: 459–60.

Orfanos CE, Ehlert R, Gollnick H. The retinoids.A review of their clinical pharmacology and therapeutic use. *Drugs* 1987; 34: 459–503.

Roenigk HH Jr, Maibach HI, eds. *Psoriasis*, 3rd edn. New York: Marcel Dekker, 1998.

Van de Kerkhof P, ed. *Textbook of Psoriasis*. Oxford: Blackwell Science, 1999.

Weinstein G, Frost P. Methotrexate for psoriasis: a new therapeutic schedule. *Arch Dermatol* 1971; 103: 33–8.

Wollina U, Hein G, Knopf B, eds. *Psoriasis und Gelenkerkrankungen*. Zena, Stuttgart: Gustav Fischer Verlag, 1996.

Purpuras

T.M. Lotti, C. Comacchi and I. Ghersetich

Definition

Purpura is the discoloration of the skin due to extravasation of red blood cells. Pressure by fingers or diascopy fails to blanch the purpuric lesion, thus distinguishing it from erythema and telangiectasia. Purpuric lesions vary in colour from purple to bluish-red to brown with evolution (due to chemical degradation of haemoglobin) through a greenish-yellow or a brownish-yellow hue.

Clinically purpuras may be subdivided into three main types: palpable purpura and non-palpable purpura and capillaritis of unknown cause.

Palpable purpura—aetiology and pathophysiology

This clinical condition is mainly related to cutaneous necrotizing vasculitis (CNV), characterized by angiocentric segmental inflammation, endothelial cell swelling and fibrinoid necrosis of blood vessel walls. The skin is often the only organ apparently involved, but clinically relevant systemic involvement usually occurs and skin lesions may just represent the initial sign of a systemic disease. CNV may also represent the cutaneous sign of any systemic vasculitis.

Although blood vessels of any size may be affected in systemic vasculitis, CNV usually occurs in the small venules (postcapillary venules), being characterized by two main histological patterns: a leukocytoclastic form with a presumed pathogenesis mediated by immune complexes and a lymphomonocytic form, in which a cell-mediated pathogenesis is proposed.

More recent data seem also to suggest the participation of a secondary cell-mediated immune response in the late phase of the leukocytoclastic form.

Palpable purpura is the major clinical presentation of CNV, whereas erythematous macules, wheals, papules, blisters, large palpable nodules, ecchymoses, pustules, haemorrhagic vesicles, ulcers and a net-like pattern of the skin (livedo reticularis) are less common manifestations. The eruption most often appears on the legs, persisting for 1–4 weeks, leaving hyperpigmentation and/or atrophic scars, and may be recurrent for years.

The fibrinolytic system is responsible for the degradation of fibrin into fibrin degradation products. This is a consequence of the activity of inhibitors and activators of fibrinolysis. Cutaneous fibrinolytic activity is usually increased in the early form of CNV (characterized clinically by urticarial wheals), while it is reduced or absent in the late phase (clinically manifested by palpable purpura). This may lead to microvascular thrombosis, because of excessive intraperivascular deposition of fibrin, with consequent tissue hypoxia and necrosis.

Gamma/delta T lymphocytes and heat shock proteins have been widely represented in cases of CNV with documented infective aetiology. This aspect might furnish, if supported by further studies, a clue to the infective aetiology of CNV.

The disorder occurs equally in both sexes and at all ages, approximately 10% of the cases occurs in children. No genetic factors are recognized. Many incidental factors, especially drugs (insulin, penicillin, sulfonamides, etc.), chemicals (insecticides, petroleum products), foods (milk proteins, etc.) and infections (viral, bacterial, fungal, protozoan, helminthic) should be considered as causes of CNV.

CNV has been reported in association with coexistent diseases (i.e. collagen–vascular diseases, hyperglobulinaemic purpura, cryoglobulinaemia, inflammatory bowel disease, malignant neoplasm, cystic fibrosis, etc.).

In many cases the cause of CNV remains unknown (i.e. in Henoch–Schönlein purpura, urticarial vasculitis, erythema elevatum diutinum, nodular vasculitis, atrophie blanche, cutaneous polyarteritis nodosa).

Non-palpable purpura—aetiology and pathophysiology

Non-palpable purpura is characterized by the distinctive clinical feature of cutaneous non-infiltrated haemorrhagic spots. Non-palpable purpura is more frequently observed in relation to platelet and vascular tissue alterations (often coexistent) and in such cases it is frequently characterized by simultaneous gingival bleeding and microhaematuria. Coagulation disturbances, instead, are manifested more frequently in cases with internal haemorrhage (i.e. visceral, intra-articular) that usually lasts for a long time. In dermatological clinical practice, platelet and vascular tissue disorders are often associated and the patient commonly presents with petechiae, generally without relationship to previous trauma, often accompained by gingival bleeding and/or micro- or macrohaematuria of recent onset. Coagulative disorders are manifested by deep haematomas and gastrointestinal or intra-articular haemorrhage that generally last for several days. In these cases family history and the report of prolonged bleeding after tonsillectomy or dental extraction may be helpful for the diagnosis; however, the family history is usually non-contributory in one-third of haemophiliacs and in all patients with acquired coagulation disorders. The 'vascular' purpuras, clinically polymorphous, are not usually associated with extracutaneous bleeding, with the exception of the pattern of 'relapsing juvenile epistaxis' (with nasal bleeding) and the pattern of 'hereditary haemorrhagic telangiectasia' (with possible visceral bleeding). Careful physical examination may be important for the diagnosis on the basis of the criteria summarized in Table 1, together with the information obtained from the diagnostic tests listed in Table 2.

Capillaritis of unknown cause—aetiology and pathophysiology

Capillaritis of unknown cause (CUC) is a group of dermatoses whose aetiology is unknown. The fundamental clinical characteristics of CUC consist of red-brownish pigmentation particularly on the lower extremities. These disorders are much more common in males. Familial incidence has been reported. Histologically the CUC are all similar, the histological examination revealing lymphomonocytic perivascular infiltrate confined to the vessels in the upper dermis with endothelial swelling, extravasation of red blood

Table 1 Clinical criteria for differential diagnosis among purpuras related to platelet, vascular tissue and coagulative alterations.

	Platelet alterations	Vascular tissue alterations	Coagulative disturbances
Sex	Both	Generally women	Generally men
Family history	Generally negative	Often positive	Generally positive
Past history (bleeding)	Generally negative	Often positive	Generally positive
Outbreak	Spontaneous or microtrauma	Spontaneous or microtrauma	Traumatic or spontaneous
Systemic manifestations	Gums, gastrointestinal or genitourinary apparatus	Nasal mucous membrane (males)	Large joints, muscles, visceral organs
Kind of bleeding	Sudden, short duration	Short duration	Long duration (days)

Table 2 Principal diagnostic tests in cutaneous and systemic haemorrhagic diseases.

Tests	Platelet alterations	Vascular tissue alterations	Coagulative disturbances
Bleeding time	Lengthened	Normal or lengthened	Normal
Platelet count	Sometimes decreased	Normal	Normal
Functional platelet deficiency	Possible	Absent	Absent
Negative pressure test	Positive	Positive	Negative
Hammer test	Positive	Positive	Negative
Hess test	Negative	Often positive	Negative
Partial thromboplastin time	Normal	Normal	Altered
Prothrombin time	Normal	Normal	Altered

cells and, in old lesions, haemosiderin deposits in macrophages. Recent histochemical and ultrastructural studies have suggested that a lymphocyte-mediated immune reaction evoked by unknown circulating antigens might play an important role in the pathogenic mechanism.

The group of CUC includes some clinically autonomic varieties, such as Schamberg's disease, eczematide-like purpura of Doucas and Kapetanakis, pigmented purpuric lichenoid dermatosis of Gougerot and Blum, lichen aureus, purpura annularis telangiectoides and purpura telangiectasia arciformis.

Other purpuras of dermatological interest

Amyloidosis purpura

In amyloidosis, purpura may occur because of amyloid deposits within vessel walls, platelet changes or liver disease.

Contact purpura

A list of substances capable of causing contact purpura includes khaki clothing, azoydes in clothing, various rubber additives and optical whiteners. In contact purpura the lesions may involve areas wider than those of actual contact.

Gravitational purpura

This purpura is often a consequence of chronic venous hypertension of the legs. It occurs most frequently in adult men. The characteristic clinical feature of the dermatosis is the presence of yellowish-brown, brownish or bluish-violet spots on the lower legs. The lesion may extend to the dorsa of the feet and toes. Oedema, ulceration and sclerosis may be associated.

Neonatal purpura

Neonatal purpura may be due to an accentuation of the normal fall of prothrombin within the first week of life. Nowadays the widespread use of vitamin K has reduced the incidence. Purpura also may be associated with the Wiskott–Aldrich syndrome or with the neonatal rubella syndrome. It may also occur in a child whose mother has systemic lupus erythematosus.

Gardner–Diamond syndrome

In the Gardner–Diamond syndrome (psychogenic purpura, painful bruising syndrome, autoerythrocyte sensitization syndrome) there is onset of painful ecchymotic lesions usually in middle-aged women with hysterical personality after acute psychoemotional stress, often in areas subjected to microtrauma. The patients may experience concomitant recurrent epistaxis and visceral bleeding. Initially it was thought that extravasated red blood cells might stimulate the formation of skin-sensitizing antibodies, but more recent studies gave negative results. Skin tests with autologous blood cells have been reported to reproduce clinical lesions, but only when the patient had been previously informed about the expected reaction, suggesting a psychogenic origin of this disease. Recent research has shown that this purpuric condition may be caused by systemic or, more often, local (cutaneous) abnormal activation of the fibrinolytic system due to excessive release of tissue-type plasminogen activator from endothelial cells, finally leading to cutaneous haemorrhage.

Main investigations in palpable purpura (CNV)

In patients with CNV a laboratory screening is always required for confirmation of the diagnosis and pathogenesis and to determine the extent of involvement of systemic vasculitis and/or the existence of underlying associated diseases. Laboratory evaluation includes histopathological and immunofluorescence studies, blood tests and urinalysis.

In the leukocytoclastic form, direct immunofluorescence of the lesional skin may show immunoglobulins, complement components and fibrin deposits in and around the blood vessels; immunoglobulin G (IgG) rather than IgM are more likely to be present when there is an underlying collagen vascular disease, and IgA may be indicative of the Schönlein–Henoch purpura. Decreased levels of complement components are often noted in leukocytoclastic CNV associated with rheumatoid arthritis (C1, C4, C2), systemic lupus erythematous (C1q, C4, C2, C3, factor B, C9), cryoglobulinaemia and Sjögren's syndrome. Circulating immune complexes, rheumatoid factor, antinuclear antibodies, antiphospholipid antibodies and cryoglobulins can be detected with antistreptolysin antibodies and hepatitis B (C and A) surface antigens. Also, in patients in whom systemic syndromes are being considered, tests such as antineutrophil cytoplasm antibody (ANCA) for Wegener's granulomatosis may be diagnostically helpful. Urine analysis may reveal proteinuria, haematuria and cylindruria caused by a possible renal involvement.

In the lymphocytic form of CNV these laboratory tests are usually normal or negative.

Treatment

Different treatments are reserved for palpable, non-palpable purpuras and capillaritis of unknown cause (Table 3).

Treatment of palpable purpura

In patients with CNV, when possible, identification and removal of causative agents (drugs, chemicals, infections, foods), represents the best aetiological treatment, followed by rapid clearance of the skin lesions, so that no other treatment is necessary. In the remaining cases, local and systemic therapies are recommended.

Local treatments

Topical therapy (corticosteroid creams) may be helpful in some cases. Gradient support stockings may be useful for lesions on the legs if coexistent with chronic venous hypertension.

General treatments

These treatments include: corticosteroids, non-steroidal anti-inflammatory drugs, colchicine, dapsone, potassium iodide, fibrinolytic agents, aminocaproic acid, immunosuppressive agents, drugs reducing platelet aggregation and antihistamines.

Systemic treatment with corticosteroids (prednisone 60–80 mg/day) is advised in the majority of patients for 7–15 days in the acute phase (especially in Schönlein–Henoch purpura, urticarial vasculitis, Behçet's disease).

Non-steroidal anti-inflammatory drugs, such as acetylsalicylic acid (150–1000 mg/day) and indometacin (25–150 mg/day),

Table 3 Different treatments are reserved for palpable and non-palpable purpuras, and capillaritis of unknown cause.

Palpable purpura	Non-palpable purpura	Capillaritis of unknown cause
In the acute phase (especially in Schönlein–Henoch purpura, urticarial vasculitis, Behçet's disease) Oral prednisone (60–80 mg/day) for 7–15 days *Vasculitis with more persistent or necrotic lesions* Acetylsalicylic acid (150–1000 mg/day) and indometacin (25–150 mg/day) *In the chronic forms* Oral colchicine (0.6 mg twice daily) *Erythema elevatum diutinum* Dapsone (50–200 mg day) *Nodular vasculitis* Potassium iodide (0.3–1.5 g four times daily) *In various types of hypofibrinolytic vasculitis* Stanozolol (5 mg twice daily) or phenformin hydrochloride (50 mg twice daily) plus ethylestrenol (2 mg four times daily) or heparin (5000 units twice daily), mesoglycans (50–100 mg/day) or defibrotide (700 mg i.m./day) *In the vasculitis associated with livedo reticularis and the livedoid vasculitis* Low molecular weight dextran (500 ml i.v./day) *In the hyperfibrinolytic states of vasculitis* Aminocaproic acid (8–16 g/day for many months) *In patients with CNV with a rapidly progressive course or with systemic involvement which is not controlled with corticosteroids* Immunosuppressive agents: cyclophosphamide (2 mg/kg per day), methotrexate (5–25 mg/week), azathioprine (50–200 mg/day) and ciclosporin A (3–5 mg/kg per day) *In the course of vasculitis induced by immune complexes with concomitant arterial disease* Drugs reducing platelet aggregation: dipyridamole (400–800 mg/day), acetylsalicylic acid (100–300 mg/day) ticlopidine hydrochloride (250–500 mg/day) and plasmapheresis	***In drug-induced purpura***: a short treatment (3–7 days) of oral prednisone (0.5–1 mg/kg per day). ***When bleeding is observed in cases with severe thrombocytopenia***: platelet transfusion. ***Disseminated intravascular coagulation***: high doses of intravenous heparin (20000–30000 U/day) plus antithrombin III (500–1000 UI/day). ***Hyperfibrinolytic conditions:*** aprotinin (500000 U) or oral ϵ-aminocaproic acid preparations (4–6 g/day). ***Thrombocytosis-dependent purpuras***: anti-aggregating agents [(acetylsalicylic acid (100–300 mg/day), ticlopidine hydrochloride (250–500 mg/day), dipyridamole (400–800 mg/day)]. ***Purpuras due to microvascular defects both of microangiopsathyrotic and angiophylic***: systemic and/or local corticosterids and administration of vitamin PP (100–500 mg/day) or vitamin C (1–2 g/day), etamsilate (1–1.5 g/day), calcium dobesilate (1–2 g/day).	Hydrocortisone creams PUVA treatment *In selected cases with reduced cutaneous and plasma fibrinolytic activity* stanozolol (3–6 mg/day) for 1–3 months *or* pentoxifylline (300 mg day) for 8 weeks.

have been used for vasculitis with more persistent or necrotic lesions. Some cases of urticarial vasculitis have responded to indometacin. Phenylbutazone (400–600 mg/day), oxyphenbutazone (300–600 mg/day) and ibuprofen (600–900 mg/day) are indicated for thrombophlebitis in the course of nodular vasculitis.

Oral colchicine, which inhibits neutrophil chemotaxis, in doses of 0.6 mg twice daily may be helpful in the chronic forms of the disease.

Dapsone (50–200 mg/day) has also been used, usually in patients with skin involvement alone (especially in patients with erythema elevatum diutinum).

Potassium iodide (0.3–1.5 g four times daily) is useful for nodular vasculitis.

Fibrinolytic agents can be used in patients with reduction of plasma and/or cutaneous fibrinolytic activity. Stanozolol (5 mg twice daily) or phenformin hydrochloride (50 mg twice daily) plus ethylestrenol (2 mg four times daily) can be used for about a year. Other fibrinolytic agents as heparin (5000 U twice daily), mesoglycans (50–100 mg/day) and defibrotide (700 mg i.m./day) seem beneficial in various types of hypofibrinolytic vasculitis.

Low molecular weight dextran (500 mL i.v./day) because of fibrinolytic effect, is also indicated in the hypofibrinolytic phase of disease. This seems to produce beneficial effects in the vasculitis associated both with livedo reticularis and the livedoid vasculitis.

Aminocaproic acid (8–16 g/day for many months) can be used in the hyperfibrinolytic states of CNV.

Immunosuppressive agents such as cyclophosphamide (2 mg/kg per day or as a monthly intravenous pulse), methotrexate (5–25 mg/week), azathioprine (50–200 mg/day) and ciclosporin A (3–5 mg/kg per day) are effective, especially in patients with CNV with a rapidly progressive course or with systemic involvement which is not controlled with corticosteroids.

In the course of vasculitis induced by immune complexes with concomitant arterial disease, drugs reducing platelet aggregation—dipyridamole (400–800 mg/day), acetylsalicylic acid (100–300 mg/day) and ticlopidine hydrochloride (250–500 mg/day)—and plasmapheresis can be used.

H_1-antihistamines alone or in combination with H_2-antihistamines are used to alleviate itch and to block histamine-induced venular endothelial gap formation with resultant trapping of immune complexes.

The correction of local factors such as trauma, cold stasis and lymphoedema may also be important.

Experimental treatments

Recently a patient with intractable systemic vasculitis has been treated with two monoclonal antibodies, Campath-1H and rat CD4.

Treatment of non-palpable purpura

The treatment of the various forms of non-palpable purpura is strictly dependent on their aetiopathogenesis.

In drug-induced purpura it is necessary to stop the ingestion of the suspected drug(s). A short treatment (3–7 days) of oral prednisone (0.5–1 mg/kg per day) may be useful, above all in forms with immunological pathogenesis.

When bleeding is observed in cases with severe thrombocytopenia, platelet transfusion may be indicated.

Disseminated intravascular coagulation may be usefully treated with high doses of intravenous heparin (20 000–30 000 U/day) plus antithrombin III (500–1000 U/day).

Hyperfibrinolytic conditions can be corrected by administration of aprotinin (500 000 U) or oral ϵ-aminocaproic acid preparations (4–6 g/day).

Thrombocytosis-dependent purpuras may be advantageously treated with anti-aggregating agents—(acetylsalicylic acid

(100–300 mg/day), ticlopidine hydrochloride (250–500 mg/day) or dipyridamole (400–800 mg/day).

Purpuras due to microvascular defects both of microangiopsathyrotic and angiophylic origin require discontinuation of systemic and/or local corticosterids (or, rarely, other presumably responsible drugs) and administration of vitamin PP (100–500 mg/day) or vitamin C (1–2 g/day) (scurvy), etamsilate (1–1.5 g/day) or calcium dobesilate (1–2 g/day).

Treatment of capillaritis of unknown cause

Capillaritis of unknown cause may require hydrocortisone creams, or psoralen and ultraviolet A (PUVA) treatment. In selected cases with reduced cutaneous and plasma fibrinolytic activity, oral stanozolol (3–6 mg/day) for 1–3 months or pentoxifylline (300 mg/day) for 8 weeks may achieve complete clearance of the purpuric lesions.

Further reading

Burge S. The management of cutaneous vasculitis. In: Panconesi E, ed. *Dermatology in Europe*. Oxford: Blackwell Scientific Publications, 1991: 328–30.

Comacchi C, Ghersetich I, Lotti T. Le porpore pigmentarie croniche. *G Ital Dermatol Venereol* 1994; 129: 69–78.

Comacchi C, Ghersetich I, Lotti T. La vasculite necrotizzante cutanea. *G Ital Dermatol Venereol* 1998; 133: 23–49.

Ghersetich I, Lotti T, Bacci S, Comacchi C, Campanile G, Romagnoli P. Cell infiltrate in progressive pigmented purpura (Schamberg's disease): immunophenotype, adhesion receptors, and intercellular relationships. *Int J Dermatol* 1995; 34(12): 846–50.

Kano Y, Hirayama F, Orihara M. Successful treatment of Schamberg's disease with pentoxifylline. *J Am Acad Dermatol* 1997; 36: 827–30.

Lotti T. The management of systemic complications of vasculitis. In: Panconesi E, ed. *Dermatology in Europe*. Oxford: Blackwell Scientific Publications, 1991: 330–2.

Lotti T, Celasco G, Tsampau D *et al.* Mesoglycan treatment restores defective fibrinolytic potential in cutaneous necrotizing venulitis. *Int J Dermatol* 1993; 32 (5): 368–71.

Lotti T, Comacchi C, Ghersetich I. Cutaneous necrotizing vasculitis. *Int J Dermatol* 1996; 35: 457–74.

Lotti T, Ghersetich I, Comacchi C, Jorizzo JL. Cutaneous small vessel vasculitis. *J Am Acad Dermatol* 1998; 39(5): 667–87.

Lotti T, Ghersetich I, Comacchi C, Panconesi E. Purpuras and related conditions. *J Eur Acad Dermatol Venereol* 1996; 7: 1–25.

Lotti T, Ghersetich I, Panconesi E. The purpuras. *Int J Dermatol* 1994; 33(1): 1–10.

Lotti T, Ghersetich I, Panconesi E. Why should we use PUVA treatment in pigmented purpuric lichenoid dermatitis. *J Am Acad Dermatol* 1994; 30(1): 145.

Mathieson PW, Cobbold SP, Hale CG *et al.* Monoclonal-antibody therapy in systemic vasculitis. *N Engl J Med* 1990; 323: 250–4.

Ryan TJ. Cutaneous vasculitis. In: Rook A *et al.* eds. *Textbook of Dermatology*. Oxford: Blackwell Scientific Publications, 1992: 1893–961.

Soter AN. Cutaneous necrotizing vasculitis. In: Freedberg IM, Eisen AZ, Wolff K *et al.*, eds. *Dermatology in General Medicine*, 5th edn. New York: McGraw-Hill, 1999: 2044–53.

Pyoderma gangrenosum

M.J. Camilleri and J.L. Pace

Definition and epidemiology

Pyoderma gangrenosum (PG) is a reactive dermatosis characterized by chronic, non-infective, necrotic cutaneous lesions, which usually occur in association with a systemic disorder, in particular inflammatory bowel disease (IBD) and monoclonal gammopathies. PG is a neutrophilic dermatosis characterized histologically by an intense dermal neutrophilic infiltrate without primary vasculitis. PG is a rare condition, affecting males and females equally and with peak age incidence of 25–54 years. Although rare, it may also be seen in children.

Aetiology and pathogenesis

The exact aetiology and pathogenesis of PG is largely unknown, but it is thought to represent a manifestation of altered immunological reactivity, as evidenced by the numerous humoral and cell-mediated defects reported in association with PG (Table 1).

The pathergic response, which is the localization of PG at sites of trauma, represents an altered and uncontrolled inflammatory response seen in patients with altered immune reactivity.

Table 1 Immunological abnormalities associated with PG.

Humoral defects
Congenital and acquired hypogammaglobulinaemia
Selective IgA deficiency
Hyperimmunoglobulin E syndrome
Autoantibodies against skin and bowel
Various dermatonecrotic factors
Streaking leukocyte factor
Cell-mediated defects
Cutaneous anergy
Diminished lymphocytic ability to produce lymphokines
Defective neutrophilic function (decreased chemotaxis, decreased phagocytosis, decreased oxygen uptake, deficient leukocyte-adherence glycoprotein)
Abnormal T_4/T_8 ratio

Clinical characteristics and course

PG can be classified clinically into four variants:

- ulcerative PG
- pustular PG
- bullous PG
- vegetative PG (superficial granulomatous pyoderma).

The clinical features of PG are listed in Table 2.

Diagnosis

Diagnosis of PG

The diagnosis of PG depends mainly on the recognition of the evolving clinical features, since there are no pathognomonic histopathological features or specific serological or haematological markers.

The histological hallmark of PG is the presence of dermal neutrophilic abscess formation with other features that depend on the clinical type of PG—epidermal ulceration, follicular/perifollicular and lymphocytic vasculitis peripherally in ulcerative PG; subcorneal pustules and subepidermal oedema in pustular PG; subepidermal bulla in bullous PG; and pseudoepitheliomatous hyperplasia, sinus tracts and a palisading granulomatous reaction in vegetative PG.

The diagnosis of PG is a diagnosis of exclusion and most investigations are performed to rule out other conditions that may resemble PG clinically.

Investigations to exclude conditions that mimic PG are:

- cutaneous biopsy for: haematoxylin and eosin stain; stains and culture for microorganisms (bacteria, fungi and

Table 2 Clinical features suggesting a diagnosis of PG

Risk factors	Ulcerative	Pustular	Bullous	Vegetative
Onset	Rapid onset	Rapid onset	Rapid onset	Slow onset
Progression	Pus-filled blisters that break down into ulcers that enlarge, usually following trauma	Pus-filled blisters that do not ulcerate	Superficial large blister that breaks down into a large ulcer	Ulcerating lesion with a raised edge
Symptoms	Very painful	Very painful	Very painful	Usually painless
Site	Lower limbs and trunk	extensors and trunk	extensors	Trunk
Underlying systemic disease	IBD and monoclonal gammopathy	IBD	Haematological malignancies (50%)	None
Signs				
Lesions	Pustules with a red halo, and ulcers with an undermined violaceous border	Pustules with a red halo, with no ulcers	Superficial ulcer with a bulla at the edge	Superficial ulcer with a vegetative border
Site	Lower limbs and trunk	Extremities and trunk	Upper limbs	Trunk
Number	Single or multiple	Multiple	Single	Single

mycobacteria); and direct immunofluorescence to rule out vasculitis

- blood tests: iodide and bromide; calcium and phosphate; lupus anticoagulant/anticardiolipin antibodies; antineutrophil cytoplasmic antibody (C and perinuclear antineutrophilic cytoplasmic antibody (P-ANCA)); syphilis serology.

Investigations to diagnose an associated systemic disorder are:

- gastrointestinal studies: barium enema; proctosigmoidoscopy/colonoscopy
- haematological tests: complete blood count with differential and smear; serum protein electrophoresis; urine Bence-Jones proteins; bone marrow aspirate and biopsy; chest X-ray, computed tomography (CT) chest/abdomen/pelvis and lymph node biopsy
- other tests: joint radiographs; rheumatoid factor; antinuclear antibody; γ-globulin; and human immunodeficiency virus (HIV).

It is especially important to exclude the various infections that mimic PG, since these may worsen if immunosuppressive therapy is started for a presumptive diagnosis of PG.

Diagnosis of any associated systemic diseases

The systemic disorders that may be associated with PG are:

- IBD. PG is seen with both ulcerative colitis and Crohn's disease with equal frequency (1.5–5%) and may precede, follow or occur with IBD. It is usually of the ulcerative or pustular type.
- Arthritis. Thirty-seven per cent of the ulcerative type of PG is associated with arthritis. This arthritis is usually an asymmetric seronegative monoarthritis of the large joints. Also seen with the arthritis of IBD, rheumatoid arthritis, Felty's syndrome, osteoarthritis and sacroiliitis.
- Immunological disease: congenital and acquired hypogammaglobulinaemia;

selective immunoglobulin A (IgA) deficiency; hypoimmunoglobulin E syndrome; immunosuppression.
- Monoclonal gammopathy. This is seen in 10% of PG, usually of the ulcerative type. It is usually IgA secreting.
- Malignant disease. This is seen in 7% of PG, usually of the bullous type. The most common associated malignancies include: haematological malignancies—leukaemia (acute myeloid leukaemia; chronic myeloid leukaemia), IgA multiple myeloma and Waldenström's macroglobulinaemia, polycythaemia rubra vera, others (myelofibrosis, Hodgkin's and non-Hodgkin's lymphoma, cutaneous T-cell lymphoma); and solid tumours (uncommon)—carcinoid, carcinoma of the colon, bladder, prostate, breast, bronchus or ovary.
- Others: chronic active hepatitis, thyroid disease and possibly its treatment with propylthiouracil, autoimmune haemolytic anaemia, chronic obstructive pulmonary disease, hidradenitis suppurativa, acne conglobata, sarcoidosis, atrophic gastritis, diabetes mellitus, systemic lupus erythematosus (SLE) and Takayasu's disease.

Differential diagnosis

A number of conditions mimic PG clinically, thus making the diagnosis even more difficult. The differential diagnosis of PG can be summarized as follows.

Inflammatory disease

Infective

- Bacteria
  tuberculous and atypical mycobacteria
  tertiary gummatous syphilis
  synergistic gangrene
  blastomycosis-like pyoderma
- deep fungal infections
- amoebiasis
- viral infection—chronic varicella infection in the immunosuppressed.

Non-infective

- Systemic vasculitis
- antiphospholipid syndrome
- necrotizing arachnidism (spider bite).

Neoplasms

- Primary cutaneous malignancies
- secondary metastasis.

Drugs/toxins

- Halogenodermas—iodides or bromides
- granulocyte colony-stimulating factor (G-CSF)
- isotretinoin.

Trauma

Including factitial dermatoses.

Calciphylaxis

Treatment

General therapeutic guidelines

- PG is a rare condition and consequently none of the therapeutic modalities recommended have been studied in large, randomized, placebo-controlled trials. Most of the evidence of the efficacy of these therapeutic agents in PG is based on limited non-randomized studies and anecdotal reports.
- It is of utmost importance to treat any underlying systemic disease, since most of these are serious and require treatment. In addition, treating any underlying IBD will result in resolution of PG.
- Supportive therapy is important in PG and includes the following.

Wound care

The basic goal of wound care in PG is to provide the ideal conditions to promote wound re-epithelialization and closure, whilst the specific therapy controls the underlying inflammation that is causing the ulceration. The same basic principles of wound management apply to that of the ulcers of PG and include the following.

- Prevention and treatment of secondary wound infection: this involves daily wound cleaning with sterile saline and antiseptic solutions, hydrocolloid occlusive dressings that protect the wound and provide an acidic environment that inhibits microbial growth, constant wound monitoring for infection by culturing the wound surface fluid, and immediate use of topical or systemic antibiotics on the first sign of infection.
- Debridement of the wound base: aggressive surgical debridement is contraindicated in PG because of the pathergic response. Thus gentle debridement is necessary, usually achieved by the use of wet saline compresses, 0.5% silver nitrate, Burow's solution, dilute potassium permanganate, and whirlpool and hydrocolloid dressings or hydroactive gels.
- Promotion of wound re-epithelialization and closure: Besides keeping the wound free from infection and slough, one can also attempt to stimulate wound re-epithelialization by increasing growth factor levels on the wound surface. This can be achieved with hydrocolloid occlusive dressings which concentrate growth factors on the wound; cultured keratinocyte autografts or allografts; split-thickness skin grafting with concurrent specific immune therapy; and use of topical preparations of growth factors. In a recent report the use of bioengineered skin as an adjunct to concurrent immunosuppressive therapy with ciclosporin hastened the healing and diminished pain in a rapidly enlarging leg ulcer. Within 2 weeks, the ulcer was 30–40% healed, achieving 100% re-epithelialization within 6 weeks.

Pain control

PG lesions tend to be very painful, and although specific therapy relieves the pain, more often than not more immediate measures of pain control are needed. These include the usual stepwise use of analgesics (paracetamol, non-steroidal anti-inflammatory drugs, opioids, and combinations) and specifically in PG, hyperbaric oxygen therapy and possibly also cyproheptadine.

Other supportive measures

These include treating anaemia of chronic disease and control of any pyrexia.

Figure 1 provides a helpful working diagram on the management of PG according to extent and severity of onset.

Recommended therapies

Since PG is an immunological disorder, specific therapy mainly includes agents that suppress or modulate the immune system. Specific, recommended therapeutic agents used in PG include: corticosteroids, agents that inhibit neutrophilic action and immunosuppressants and immunomodulators

Corticosteroids (Table 3)

Corticosteroids in PG act via their anti-inflammatory and immunosuppressive properties, but one study suggests that corticosteroids may restore monocyte function in this condition. Corticosteroids may be administered in various ways, all of which may be used in PG.

Agents that inhibit neutrophilic function (Table 4)

Antineutrophilic agents are beneficial in PG as is expected from the fact that it is mainly characterized by a dermal neutrophilic infiltrate. The main indication of these agents include use as a steroid-sparing agent or in addition to a steroid when the latter gives a partial response or

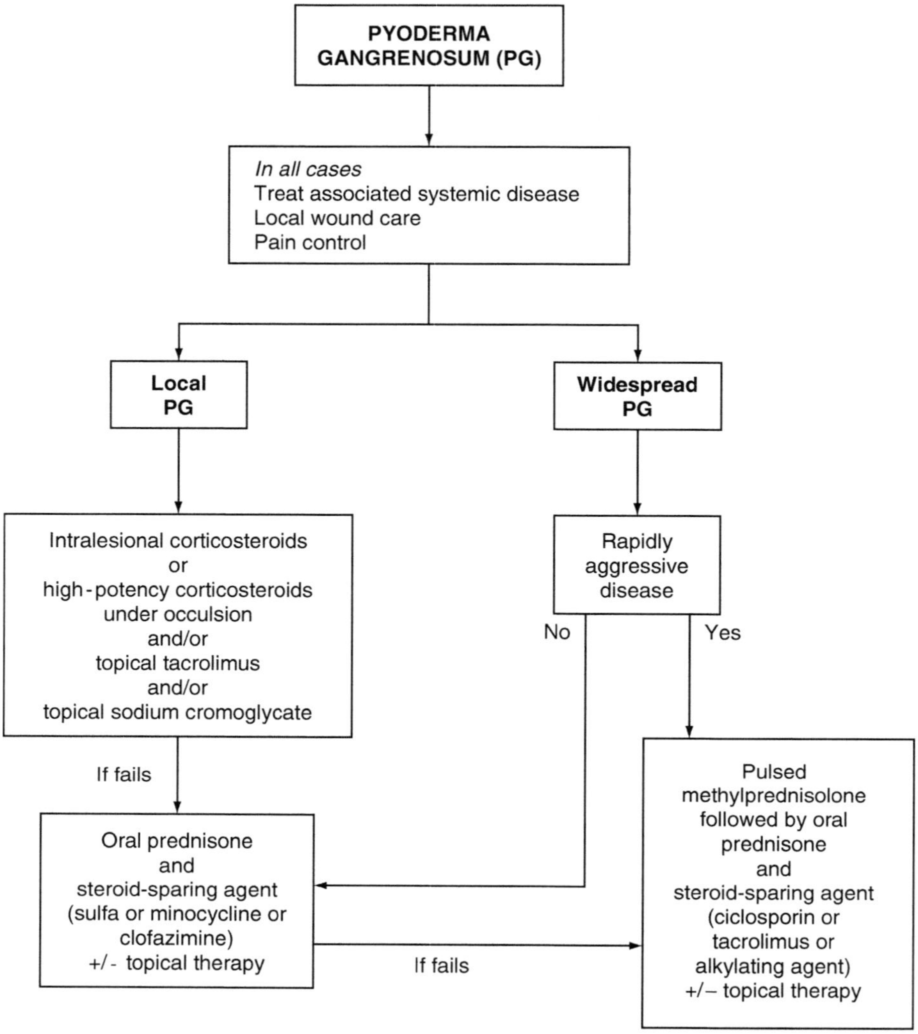

Figure 1 Treatment of PG

in non-aggressive widespread disease or when local therapy fails.

Immunosuppressants and immunomodulators (Table 5)
The mechanism of action of these agents in PG is by correcting or altering the immunological defects present in PG. The indications for use of immunosuppressants and immunomodulators in PG are either as an adjunctive or alternative therapy when systemic corticosteroids fail or as first-line therapy with systemic steroids in aggressive disease.

Alternative and experimental therapies

Sodium cromoglycate
This has also been found to be helpful when applied as a 1–4% solution three times a day, either as monotherapy in local disease or as an adjunctive therapy in widespread disease.

Table 3 Corticosteroid use in PG

Agent	Indications	Dosage	Adverse effects
Intralesional steroids	Early and local disease Adjunct to systemic therapy	Triamcinolone diacetate solution at a conc. < 10 mg/ml, injected in single or multiple doses per ulcer	Introducing infection Slow healing Skin atrophy
Topical steroids	As above, but not as effective	Strong topical steroid (e.g. clobetasol propionate) with or without occlusion	As above
Oral steroids	First line in severe, acute rapidly progressive and widespread disease If local treatment fails	Prednisone is started at a dosage of 40–120 mg daily, then tailed off when disease is controlled	Hypertension, Hyperglycaemia Electrolyte disturbance Cushingoid features if long-term use
Pulsed methyl-prednisolone	Cases not responding to oral steroids	Methylprednisolone 1 g in 150 ml of 5% dextrose for 5 days followed by tapering dose of prednisone	As above with more emphasis of acute metabolic effects

Table 4 Use of agents that inhibit neutrophilic function in PG

Agent	Indications	Dosage	Adverse effects
Sulpha drugs	As a steroid-sparing agent Added to steroid when it fails Non-aggressive widespread disease Failure of local therapy	Sulphasalazine: 1–4 mg/day initially, going down to maintenance dose of 0.5–1 g/day Dapsone: 100–200 mg/day Sulphapyridine: 4–8 mg/day Sulfoxone: 1–tab/day	Haemolysis, methaemoglobinaemia leukopenia/ agranulocytosis, crystalluria
Minocycline	As above	200–300 mg/day, long-term maintenance is needed	Vertigo, pigmentation?, intracranial pressure, liver toxicity, SLE
Clofazamine	As above	200–400 mg/day	Red pigmentation of skin, sweat, tears and urine, dry skin splenic infarcts
Thalidomide	As above	150–400 mg/day	Teratogenicity neuropathy
Potassium iodide	As above	300 mg twice or three times a day	May induce PG, metallic taste, athralgia

Thalidomide

This is given at a dose of 150–400 mg/day. The main side-effects are teratogenicity and neuropathy.

Potassium iodide

This is given at a dose of 300 mg two to three times a day. The main side-effects are metallic taste, arthralgia and occasionally may induce a neutrophilic dermatosis.

Plasma exchange

This is done once to three times a week for a total of 4–27 exchanges. The main side-effects are fluid and electrolyte disturbance, bleeding tendency and infections.

Table 5 Immunosuppressive/immunomodulator use in PG

Agent	Indications	Dosage	Adverse effect
Azathioprine/ mercaptopurine	Adjunct/alternative therapy in failure of systemic steroid First line with a steroid if aggressive	Azathioprine: 100–200 mg/day Mercaptopurine: 75 mg/day	BM suppression GI upset Liver damage Increase in infections Increase in neoplasia
Systemic cyclosporin	As above	4–6 mg/kg per day	Nephrotoxicity Hypertension Increase in neoplasia and infection Hypertrichosis GI upset
Tacrolimus	As above	0.15 mg/kg twice a day	Nephrotoxicity Neurotoxicity Diabetes
Alkylating agents	As above	Cyclophosphamide: Oral 100–150 mg/day i.v. 500 mg/m^2 pulses, then 100 mg/day orally Chlorambucil: 4 mg/day Melphalan: 5 mg/day of one dose then 2 mg/day	BM suppression Increase in neoplasia Haemorrhagic cystitis Sterility GI upset Aphthous ulcers Alopecia Liver and cardiac toxicity Lung fibrosis
Plasma exchange	As above	1–3 weekly for a total of 4–27 exchanges	Fluid and electrolyte disturbance Bleeding tendency Infections
Intravenous immuno-globulin G	As above	0.4 g/day × 5 days, then 0.1 g/day × 2 days after 2 weeks	High cost Headache Increase in infection
Topical ciclosporin	Early and local disease Adjunct to systemic therapy	35 mg in isotonic saline injected into the ulcer	Local irritation

Intravenous IgG

This is given at a dose of 0.4 g/day for 5 days followed by 0.1 g/day for 2 days after 2 weeks. The main side-effects are the high cost, headache, and increased infections.

5-aminosalicylic acid

This was found to be effective when applied topically as a 10% cream daily on the lesions of PG. The mode of action is possibly through suppression of leucocyte motility and cytotoxicity.

Nicotine gum

A beneficial effect has been noted at a dose of 6 g/day in clearing PG.

Nitrogen mustard

This has been found to be helpful when applied as a 20% solution.

Cytosine arabinoside and daunorubicin

Myophenolate mofetil

Chinese herbal treatment

This consists of oral *Tripterygium wilfordii* multiglycoside.

Surgery

In unstable patients with intractable multiple medical problems, surgical treatment of PG may be indicated by the existence of these life-threatening comorbidities. The recent literature suggests that surgical management of PG may also be appropriate in other special circumstances. Surgical management, including amputation, may have a role in the management of PG. Further research is needed to delineate precisely the circumstances and patient factors that are appropriate indications for such surgery.

Further reading

Albertazzi P, Di Micco R. Pyoderma gangrenosum of the cervix. *Obstet Gynecol* 2000; 96(5 Pt 2): 825–6.

Anstey AV. Treatment of pyoderma gangrenosum. *J Am Acad Dermatol* 1997; 38: 802.

Armstrong PM, Ilyas I, Pandey R, Berendt AR, Conlon CP, Simpson AH. Pyoderma gangrenosum. A diagnosis not to be missed. *J Bone Joint Surg Br* 1999; 81(5): 893–4.

Bennett ML, Jackson JM, Jorizzo JL, Fleischer AB, White WL, Callen JP. Pyoderma gangrenosum. A comparison of typical and atypical forms with an emphasis on time to remission. Case review of 86 patients from 2 institutions. *Medicine (Baltimore)* 2000; 79(1): 37–46.

Brady E. Severe peristomal pyoderma gangrenosum: a case study. *J Wound Ostomy Continence Nurs* 1999; 26(6): 306.

Chow RK, Ho VC. Treament of pyoderma gangrenosum. *J Am Acad Dermatol* 1996; 34: 1047–60.

Coors EA, von den Driesch P. Pyoderma gangrenosum in a patient with autoimmune haemolytic anaemia and complement deficiency. *Br J Dermatol* 2000; 143(1): 154–6.

Darben T, Savige J, Prentice R, Paspaliaris B, Chick J. Pyoderma gangrenosum with secondary pyarthrosis following propylthiouracil. *Australas J Dermatol* 1999; 40(3): 144–6.

de Imus G, Golomb C, Wilkel C, Tsoukas M, Nowak M, Falanga V. Accelerated healing of pyoderma gangrenosum treated with bioengineered skin and concomitant immunosuppression. *J Am Acad Dermatol* 2001; 44(1): 61–6.

Fearfield LA, Ross JR, Farrell AM, Costello C, Bunker CB, Staughton RC. Pyoderma gangrenosum associated with Takayasu's arteritis responding to cyclosporin. *Br J Dermatol* 1999; 141(2): 339–43.

Federman GL, Federman DG. Recalcitrant pyoderma gangrenosum treated with thalidomide. *Mayo Clin Proc* 2000; 75(8): 842–4.

Groves RW, Schmidt-Lucke JA. Recombinant human GM-CSF in the treatment of poorly healing wounds. *Adv Skin Wound Care* 2000; 13(3 Pt 1): 107–12.

Ho KK, Browne A, Fitzgibbons J, Carney D, Powell FC. Mycosis fungoides bullosa simulating pyoderma gangrenosum. *Br J Dermatol* 2000; 142(1): 124–7.

Hughes AP, Jackson JM. Clinical features and treatment of peristomal pyoderma gangrenosum. *JAMA* 2000; 27; 284(12): 1546–8.

Hughes AP, Jackson JM, Callen JP. Clinical features and treatment of peristomal pyoderma gangrenosum. *JAMA* 2000; 284(12): 1546–8.

Katsambas A. Quality of life in dermatology and the European Academy of Dermatology. *JEADV* 1994; 3: 211–14.

Koskinas J, Raptis I, Manika Z, Hadziyannis S. Overlapping syndrome of autoimmune hepatitis and primary sclerosing cholangitis associated with pyoderma gangrenosum and ulcerative colitis. *Eur J Gastroenterol Hepatol* 1999; 11(12): 1421–4.

Li LF. Treatment of pyoderma gangrenosum with oral *Tripterygium wilfordii* multiglycoside. *J Dermatol* 2000; 27(7): 478–81.

Litvak D, Kirsner RS, Pakdaman NN, Federman DG. Pyoderma gangrenosum and myelodysplastic syndrome. *South Med J* 2000; 93(9): 923–5.

Mrowietz U, Christophers E. Clearing of pyoderma gangrenosum with intralesional cyclosporin A. *Dermatology*1992; 184: 499.

Nasca MR, O'Toole EA, Palicharla P, West DP, Woodley DT. Thalidomide increases human keratinocyte migration and proliferation. *J Invest Dermatol* 1999; 113(5): 720–4.

Powell FC, Su WPD, Perry HO. Pyoderma gangrenosum: classification and management. *J Am Acad Dermatol* 1996; 34: 395–409.

Reynoso-von Drateln C *et al.* Intravenous cyclophosphamide pulses in pyoderma gangrenosum: an open trial. *J Rheumatol* 1997; 24: 4689–693.

Ronnau AC, von Schmiedeberg S, Bielfeld P, Ruzicka T, Schuppe HC. Pyoderma gangrenosum after cesarean delivery. *Am J Obstet Gynecol* 2000; 183(2): 502–4.

Shenefelt PD. Pyoderma gangrenosum associated with cystic acne and hidradenitis suppurativa controlled by adding minocycline and suphasalazine to the treatment regimen. *Cutis* 1996; 57: 5315–19.

Tamir A, Landau M, Brenner S. Topical treatment with 1% cromoglycate in pyoderma gangrenosum. *Dermatology* 1996; 192: 3252–4.

Teitel AD. Treatment of pyoderma gangrenosum with methotrexate. *Cutis* 1996; 57: 5326–8 B6.

Umezawa Y, Oyake S, Oh-i T, Nagae T, Ishimaru S. A case of pyoderma gangrenosum on the stump of an amputated right leg. *J Dermatol* 2000; 27(8): 529–32.

V'lckova-Laskoska MT, Laskoski DS, Caca-Biljanovska NG, Darkoska JS. Pyoderma gangrenosum successfully treated with cyclosporin A. *Adv Exp Med Biol* 1999; 455: 541–5.

Vadillo M, Jucgla A, Podzamczer D, Rufi G, Domingo A. Pyoderma gangrenosum with liver, spleen and bone involvement in a patient with chronic myelomonocytic leukaemia. *Br J Dermatol* 1999; 141(3): 541–3.

Wolf R. Nicotine for pyoderma gangrenosum *Arch Derm* 1998; 134(9): 1071–2.

Wollina U, Karamfilov T. Treatment of recalcitrant ulcers in pyoderma gangrenosum with mycophenolate mofetil and autologous keratinocyte transplantation on a hyaluronic acid matrix. *J Eur Acad Dermatol Venereol* 2000; 14(3): 187–90.

Rosacea

F.C. Powell

Synonyms

Rosacea, acne rosacea, papulopustular rosacea.

Definition and epidemiology

Rosacea is a chronic facial dermatosis characterized by non-transient erythema, and acute flares of papules and pustules, mainly on the convexities of the forehead, nose, cheeks and chin with concentration on the central face. Additional features of flushing and telangiectasia, oedema and rhinophyma and ocular symptoms are present in some patients. Rosacea affects both males and females in equal numbers, but male patients may develop more severe disease, and rhinophyma occurs almost exclusively in this sex. Peak onset is between 35 and 45 years. There may be accompanying seborrhoeic dermatitis and the orifices of the sebaceous glands especially around the nose, may be patulous in those prone to rhinophyma. The frequency of rosacea in populations vary from country to country and has not been accurately defined. Figures ranging from 0.09% to 10% of the population have been reported. It is uncommon in black-skinned individuals. About 15% of patients with rosacea give a positive family history of the disease.

Aetiology and pathophysiology

The aetiology of rosacea is unknown. There is probably a genetic susceptibility to the disease, manifested by its frequent occurrence in certain populations (people of Celtic origin seem to be particularly susceptible) and the positive family history of the condition in some patients. Fair sun-sensitive skin seems to be particularly susceptible to developing rosacea.

The vascular theory of pathogenesis is currently the most widely accepted. This proposes that the initiation of rosacea is with flushing and blushing which gradually becomes more frequent occurring at a lower threshold, and is more sustained, eventually leading to the appearance of fixed telangiectatic vessels on the face. The blood flow through these widened and damaged vessels is sluggish, and there is escape of fluid through the vessel walls into the surrounding connective tissue. This causes a secondary inflammatory reaction with the development of papules, pustules and oedema. Fibroblasts in the connective tissue are stimulated to proliferate, causing phymatous changes. The vascular pathogenesis is supported by the reported occurrence of rosacea in patients with the carcinoid syndrome. This theory, however, overlooks the fact that many patients who develop rosacea do not begin their disease with flushing, and does not explain the development of pustules. Although pustules are cardinal features of this disease, there is as yet no firm evidence to support a microbiological cause, and the role of the *Demodex* mite which is found in plentiful numbers on rosacea skin remains a mystery. The follicular orientation of the histological findings, the abundance of the 'follicle dweller' *Demodex*, the frequent involvement of the modified sebaceous glands in the eye (Meibomian glands) and the effectiveness of therapy which acts through anti-inflammatory mechanisms suggests that rosacea is an inflammatory disorder of the pilosebaceous unit rather than a vasodilatory disease of blood vessels.

Clinical characteristics and course

Contrary to the descriptions in many textbooks of dermatology, rosacea does not always start with flushing. In many patients the initial clinical presentation is of small dome-shaped erythematous papules with occasional surmounted central pinhead pustules. Rosacea is concentrated on the central facial skin and is most marked on the convex skin surfaces. The eruption is often accompanied by erythema in the surrounding skin, which may be exacerbated by heat/cold etc., some patients in addition have definite episodes of flushing which may also be provoked by temperature change, hot liquids, alcohol, etc., and a psychological overlay due to consciousness and embarrassment over the skin condition. Telangiectasias, small, fine and centrally located on the face, are present in some patients. Oedema may occur secondary to the inflammatory skin changes, or may present as an isolated feature without other manifestations of rosacea (Moybihan's disease). The oedema is often concentrated on the forehead, and is evident around the eyes and to a lesser degree on the central cheeks. Rhinophyma presents initially as large patulous follicles with mild thickening of the nose. This occurs almost exclusively in male patients, and in extreme cases can eventuate in grotesque overgrowths of nasal tissue due to sebaceous gland hyperplasia. Some patients who develop rhinophyma have no preceding inflammatory rosacea, and some with severe eruptions of papules and pustules do not develop rhinophyma.

Diagnosis

The diagnosis of rosacea is based on the clinical features described above. There is no diagnostic histological or serological marker of the disorder. Histology of a pustule shows follicular orientated inflammation, with lymphocytes and histiocytes, and neutrophils in the follicular ostium. Papules may show a similar picture with mild to marked perivasular inflammatory reaction. Oedematous rosacea shows prominent mast cells within the dermis while rhinophyma histologically is composed of hyperplasia of sebaceous glands and hypertrophied connective tissue. Serological tests are not important in the diagnosis of rosacea except in differentiating a diffuse telangiectatic erythema from systemic lupus erythematosus with positive antibody tests in the latter condition.

Differential diagnosis

- Acne vulgaris: comedones and scarring. Less erythema. Not limited to central face. Earlier age of onset. Deeper cystic lesions.
- Perioral dermatitis: distribution limited to below nose. Papules and pustules. Telangiectasias not prominent.
- Seborrhoeic dermatitis: may coexist with rosacea. Greasy scale, itch and distribution to alae nasi, eyebrows and scalp involvement.
- Carcinoid syndrome: dry flushing with systemic systems (diarrhoea, palpitations, wheezing etc.).
- Mastocytosis: dry flushing with palpitations, dyspnoea, nausea, pruritus etc.
- Menopausal symptoms: flushing with sweating.
- Systemic lupus erythematosus: butterfly erythema. Positive antibody tests. Discoid lesions cause scarring. Papules and pustules absent.
- Perniosis of nose (chilblains): uniform bluish red discoloration which is well defined and limited to the nose.
- Lupus pernio: firm erythematous/violaceous indurated swelling of the nose with non-caseating granulomas shown histologically.

Treatment

General therapeutic guidelines

Patients with rosacea often have inflamed, sensitive and irritable skin. About one-third of patients will have accompanying seborrhoeic dermatitis. Patients are advised to avoid provoking influences as listed below.

Alcohol

Many patients with rosacea do not drink alcoholic beverages, in spite of the popular misconception that the skin changes are consequent to alcohol abuse. However, the vasodilatory effect of alcohol on facial blood vessels heightens the pre-existing erythema (at least some of which is inflammatory in origin), and so should be avoided by patients. Red wines in particular can lead to histaminuria and are contraindicated in rosacea.

Hot drinks

The thermoregulatory mechanisms within the mouth initiate a heat-dispersing facial vasodilation in response to the ingestion of hot liquids. This is dictated solely by the heat of the liquid and is not related to the presence or absence of caffeine. Patients with rosacea should be advised to avoid ingestion of tea, coffee, soup etc. which is heated to a warm or hot temperature. Alternatively, sipping on iced cold drinks will have a cooling and vasoconstrictive effect on facial blood vessels and is recommended for rosacea sufferers.

Diet

The evidence linking dietary intake to the development or exacerbation of rosacea is less clear than alcohol or hot drinks. However, some patients note increased erythema after eating, particularly a large hot meal. In general it is advised to avoid spicy foods, curries, etc. and specifically spinach, aubergine, tomatoes, liver, yeast and some cheeses, especially parmesan cheese are thought to exacerbate rosacea, but the evidence for this is anecdotal. Dietary elements that may induce flushing are

- hot beverages
- large hot meals
- spicy foods
- pickled or marinated foods
- sometimes liver
  steak
  cheese
  yoghurt
  coffee
  tea
  chocolate
  soy sauce
  yeast extract
  tomatoes
  plums.

Sunlight

Exposure to sunlight may mask the erythema of rosacea temporarily giving an impression of improvement, but should be avoided by rosacea sufferers who are generally fair-skinned as it leads to increased telangiectasia, collagen dystrophy and in the long term heightens facial redness. Daily application of a high factor sun-block cream (factor 25 or more) for winter and summer is helpful.

Vasodilator drugs

These are contraindicated in patients with rosacea who have a tendency to flushing. Drugs to avoid include nicotine acid and its derivatives, amyl nitrite, mitramycin and nifedipine.

Cosmetic camouflage

Patients with rosacea suffer not only from an uncomfortable skin condition that is readily visible to other people, but also the stigma of the popular misconception that their condition is a consequence of alcohol abuse. Correction of the facial erythema by use of a cosmetic preparation containing brilliant green can be very effective when the inflammatory component of the rash is controlled. It must be remembered that these cosmetics do not protect against sunburn, and that patients with rosacea tend to have sensitive skin, poorly tolerant of skin care products which contain astringents/toners, strong soaps and exfoliating agents.

Cosmetic preparations which some patients with rosacea have reported to be helpful are

- Mint Cooling (Clinique)
- Tender Green No. 327 (Christian Dior)
- Controlling Green (Shiseido)
- Aqua-Tint lotion (Ultima II)
- Rosetone Colour Control (Boots)
- Colour Corrector (Yardley)
- Amazingly Light Moisturiser (Boots).

Recommended therapies

The treatment of rosacea should be customized according to the patient's most prominent clinical feature (Fig. 1). Thus, laser therapy might be the most appropriate for some patients, while others may require oral medications, ranging from β-blockers to antibiotics.

Systemic antibiotic therapy

This is the treatment of choice for acute papulopustular rosacea. Either oral tetracycline or erythromycin, both given 1 g/day in divided doses (500 mg twice a day—between meals for tetracycline) are equally effective. Treatment at full dosage should be continued for 3–6 weeks by which time 90% of patients will show a major clinical improvement in both skin and ocular disease. Minocycline is also effective and has the advantage of being a single dosage, which can be taken with food, but tends to be more expensive. Patients resistant to these antibiotics will often respond to oral metronidazole 200–400 mg three times a day. This medication can have an adverse reaction with

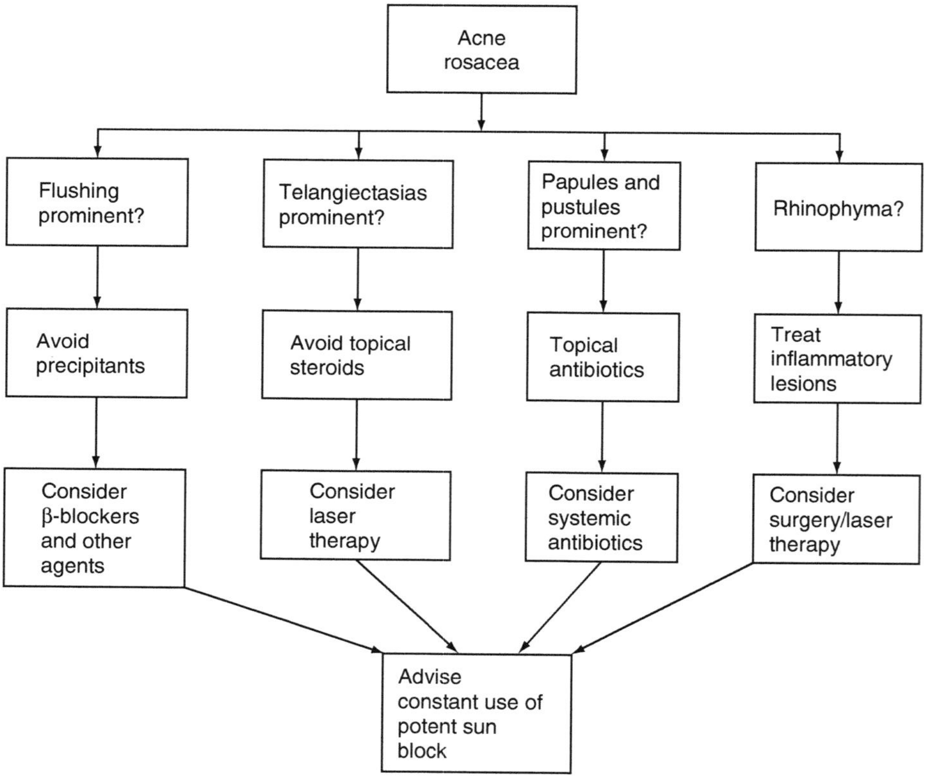

Figure 1 Spectrum of clinical features in rosacea

alcohol leading to gastrointestinal upset, vomiting, headache and flushing, and should not be continued long term as side-effects including peripheral neuropathy may occur. When rosacea goes into remission with systemic antibiotic therapy the dosage should be reduced to half for 2 weeks, then one-quarter for a further 2 weeks before stopping. If relapse is apparent during the reduction phase of therapy the dosage can be increased again. The majority of patients will clear with the above regimen, but many will tend to relapse with time, often within several weeks of stopping systemic antibiotics. Topical therapy (described below) will help to prolong remission and avoid relapse of rosacea controlled by systemic therapy. The PERT syndrome is the phenomenon of telangiectasias which are revealed posterythema therapy with systemic antibiotics. Patients should be warned that these vessels are often present in the initial stages, but are masked by inflammatory erythema and only become apparent after treatment.

Oral retinoids

Oral isotretinoin has been used successfully to treat rosacea. Most clinicians reserve this treatment for resistant or severe cases. The dosage should be half to quarter that used to treat patients with acne vulgaris, i.e. 0.25 mg/kg, as patients with rosacea are very intolerant of its drying effects, particularly on the eyes. A satisfactory clinical response will be obtained with this low dosage, but prolonged remission (as in acne vulgaris) is not typical. Concomitant ocular lubrication should be prescribed. Disappointingly, oral isotretinoin has little effect on the sebaceous hyperplasia that makes up rhinophyma.

Topical antibiotics

These are particularly useful in the management of mild rosacea or in the prolongation of remission induced by systemic antibiotics, or in the treatment of early relapses. Most effective and most widely used is topical metronidazole. Gel formulations tend to be somewhat irritant to the skin, particularly if the rosacea is active and inflammatory and creams seem to be better tolerated. Topical metronidazole should be applied twice daily to affected areas. Topical erythromycin and clindamycin have also been used with success to treat rosacea (again applied twice daily), but would probably be considered less effective than metronidazole. Topical erythromycin has the advantage of safety during pregnancy, a time that rosacea can flare actively in some female patients. A 10% sodium sulfaceramide with sulphur 5% in a lotion base has been marketed in the USA for rosacea. It is not as yet available on the European markets.

Topical steroids

Topical steroids are generally contraindicated in the treatment of rosacea. However mildly potent topical steroid preparations have a role to play in two different aspects of rosacea management. Firstly, a patient who has inappropriately applied potent steroids to facial rosacea will experience an initial improvement with reduction of erythema and inflammatory lesions, but this will be rapidly followed by a severe rebound and flare with discontinuation of therapy. In order to avoid this rebound effect a mild topical steroid preparation can be applied 3–4 times a day. Used in conjunction with systemic antibiotic therapy it can be gradually discontinued as the rosacea comes under control. The second situation in which topical steroids are helpful in rosacea is when it is acutely inflamed and active, or in the rare fulminating case. Mild to moderately potent agents are used in conjunction with systemic antibiotic therapy for a short period of time while the inflammation is being brought under control. Systemic steroid therapy is contraindicated in rosacea, with the exception of some rare cases of fulminating rosacea.

Topical retinoids

Topical tretinoin has been used successfully to treat patients with rosacea. Its main disadvantage is the drying effect it has on already dry skin, and its mild irritant qualities on the sensitive skin of the rosacea sufferer. In my experience many patients with active rosacea are intolerant of this treatment, but it may play a role in prolonging remission which has been induced by other agents.

Laser therapy

Lasers can be helpful in the management of rosacea in two clinical situations. The tuneable pulsed dye or argon laser in a condition mode can be used in the treatment of facial telangiectasia which can be a source of considerable cosmetic embarrassment and contribute to the erythema of this disease. Vascular lesions around the nose are particularly suited to this form of therapy. Prior to the advent of lasers, electrolysis was the treatment of choice for telangiectasias, and is still useful for the cauterization of isolated large vessels.

The carbon dioxide (CO_2) laser can be used successfully with vaporization alone (for mild disease) or sequentially by laser excision and then vaporization to treat rhinophyma, and is an alternative to the traditional surgical approach to this problem. Dermabrasion has also been used to treat the hypertrophic tissue of rhinophyma, and some investigators have combined the use of isotretinoin and dermabrasion with good results.

Treatments of flushing

Patients who experience profound and frequent flushing are very difficult to treat. Agents which have been reported to be successful in some patients include β-blockers (Nadolol), clonidine, naproxen, methyldopa, spironolactone, and in post-menopausal women hormone replacement therapy and venlafaxine. Selective sympathectomy has been reported to be helpful, but is not without serious side-effects and should only be considered for those with disabling flushing.

Alternative therapies

Treatment of rosacea by medical practitioners before the advent of antibiotics included the use of topical precipitated sulphur/salicylic acid preparations (still useful in concentrations of 2–5% combined in a moisturizing cream base). A topical therapy for rosacea accredited to a famous German dermatologist Dr Unna is:

- resorcinol 5%
- salicylic acid 2%
- ichthymol 5%
- white soft paraffin 80%.

This preparation was applied at night with apparently good results.

Early dermatologists associated rosacea with disturbance of the gastrointestinal tract and hydrochloric acid and pepsin were often prescribed. Recently *Helicobacter pylori* has been suggested as being of aetiological significance, and in some selected patients eradication of this infection with appropriate therapy has been paralleled by a clearing of the skin eruption. Oral antihistamines have been used in the management of oedematous rosacea because of the presence of numerous mast cells in the dermal infiltrate, but the results have been poor. β-blockers, especially nadolol may sometimes be helpful in the management of the patient with rosacea who experiences frequent and severe flushing and is usually given in a dosage of 20–80 mg daily over 3–4 months.

Some patients with oedematous rosacea have found facial massage helpful. Massage is initiated gently with the fingertips, started at the eyelids/central facial region, and moving outwards in a centrifugal fashion towards the ears. This is usually done in the mornings when oedema is often at its worst.

Traditional therapies

Cucumber (*Cucumis sativus*) preparations have been used for many years as a traditional treatment for facial redness. They are mentioned in Culpeper's *Herbal Remedies* published in 1649. It has been used as a natural remedy by some patients who have pureed several slices of peeled cucumber and combined it with several tablespoons of natural yoghurt. This is applied as a facemask and left on for approximately 10 min after which it is washed off with cool water. One patient with severe oedematous rosacea obtained benefit from placing whole chilled cucumber slices over the affected area each morning for 10–15 min with subsequent reduction in swelling and redness. Cucumber juice is an ingredient of many natural beauty creams and cosmetics and its irritancy potential to the skin seem to be low, but stomatitis from ingestion of cucumbers has been reported, so caution is needed with these preparations.

Ocular rosacea

The symptoms of ocular rosacea (burning/stinging/dry eyes) are usually relieved by the systemic antibiotic therapy used for cutaneous disease. If significant ocular disease is suspected, referral to an ophthalmologist is advisable.

Further reading

Bleicher PA, Charles JH, Sober AJ. Topical metronidazole therapy for rosacea. *Arch Dermatol* 1987; 123: 609.

Drott P, *et al.* Successful treatment of facial blushing by endoscopic transthoracic sympathicotomy. *Br J Dermatol* 1998; 138: 639.

El-Azhary RA, Roenigk RK, Wang TD. Spectrum of results after treatment of rhinophyma with the carbon dioxide laser. *Mayo Clin Proc* 1991; 66: 899–905.

Erlt GA, Levine N, Kligman AM. A comparison of the efficacy of topical tretinoin and low-dose oral isotretinoin in rosacea. *Arch Dermatol* 1994; 130: 319–24.

Knight AG, Vickers CFH. A follow-up of tetracycline-treated rosacea, with special reference to rosacea keratitis. *Br J Dermatol* 1975; 93; 577–80.

Marsden JR, Shuster S, Neugebauer M. Response of rosacea in isotretinoin. *Clin Exp Dermatol* 1984; 9: 484–8.

Sobye P. Treatment of rosacea by massage. *Acta Dermatovener* 1951; 31: 174–83.

Wilkin JK. Effect of nadolol on flushing reactions in rosacea. *J Am Acad Dermatol* 1989; 20: 202–5.

Wilkin JK, De Witt S. Treatment of rosacea: topical clindamycin versus oral tetracycline. *Int J Dermatol* 1993; 32: 65–7.

Sarcoidosis

S. Jablonska

Definition and epidemiology

Sarcoidosis is a multisystemic disease characterized by histological features of non-caseating granulomas, involving lungs, bones and joints, eyes, peripheral lymph nodes, liver and almost every organ. The skin is involved in 25–50% of cases.

The prevalence differs from country to country, in Europe it varies from 10 to 50/100 000 inhabitants, is higher in females, and highest in Northern parts of the continent. In the USA sarcoidosis is most frequent in blacks who have usually a more severe disease.

The immunogenetics is non-homogeneous. HLA association differs in various population groups.

Aetiology and pathogenesis

The aetiology is unknown. The data on the presence of *Mycobacterium* tuberculosis DNA in sarcoidosis are conflicting—positive in some cases in some studies, but negative in others. Thus the role of *Mycobacterium* tuberculosis complex or other mycobacteria in the pathogenesis is unclear and no antituberculous therapy is indicated for cases with no signs of coexisting tbc infection. The formation of granuloma appears to be due to immune response to unknown antigen processed and presented by macrophages to T lymphocytes. Activated T lymphocytes release several proinflammatory cytokines, i.e. interleukin (IL)-2, interferon (IFN)-γ, macrophage chemoattractive factor, IL-1 and others which also contribute to granuloma formation and development of fibrosis, especially in the lungs. The persistent antigen stimulation is responsible for macrophage-derived giant cell formation. Some T-helper lymphocytes are present in the non-caseating centre and mostly T-suppressor OKT8 lymphocytes at the periphery.

Clinical characteristics and course

Cutaneous sarcoidosis

The cutaneous lesions in sarcoidosis are non-specific or specific, and the course of the disease may be acute or chronic. In about 40% of cases seen by dermatologists the internal involvement is absent.

Non-specific lesions

Erythema nodosum is the most frequent non-specific manifestation in acute or subacute sarcoidosis. It presents a hypersensitivity reaction to unknown agents, and has the same characteristics as erythema nodosum associated with bacterial, fungal and other infectious agents or induced by chemical antigens. It may be accompanied by fever and arthralgia. Association of erythema nodosum with bilateral hilar lymphadenopathy and arthralgia is known as Lofgren syndrome, which, as a rule, regresses spontaneously. Other non-specific lesions—erythematous, scaly, ichthyotic and others—are non-characteristic, not long lasting and reversible.

Specific lesions

These are macular, papular, nodular, plaque-like or subcutaneous. The most severe subset is lupus pernio involving the nose, cheeks and ears, associated with pulmonary involvement (infiltrations and fibrosis), often also with uveitis and bone changes (especially finger bones). The patients are usually females, the course is chronic and the lesions tend to persist in spite of therapy.

The symmetrical plaques on the face and limbs, if purple, elevated and covered with telangiectasia, are referred to as angiolupid.

The nodular, papular, sometimes circinate lesions, subcutaneous nodules and tumours can be recognized as sarcoidosis if the biopsy shows non-caseating granulomas.

Ulcerative sarcoidosis is in Europe extremely rare, involves preferentially the legs and occurs mainly in black women. However, differentiation from other granulomatous ulcerative diseases, such as syphilis or leprosy, might be very difficult.

Scar sarcoidosis appears in predisposed individuals after trauma or surgery.

Systemic manifestations

- Lungs: characteristic are restrictive changes, reduced vital capacity, bilateral hilar lymphadenopathy in early stage, fibrosis in later stages.
- Musculoskeletal system: arthralgia may be present in all stages, in chronic disease the joints (mainly knees, elbows, small joints of the hands) could be swollen, tender, or painful. Multiple cysts in distal phalanges detected by radiography are referred to as ostitis cystica.
- Eyes: uveitis could be acute or chronic. Coexistence of iridocyclitis, swelling of parotis gland and facial nerve pulsy is known as Heerfordt syndrome.
- All organs can be involved in chronic sarcoidosis: liver, spleen, heart, larynx, nervous system, peripheral lymph nodes.

Sarcoidosis in children

Sarcoidosis is not a rare disease among children of various ages. Maculopapular skin eruption, uveitis, hilar lymphadenopathy and arthritis are characteristic features of childhood sarcoidosis. The articular changes and pulmonary involvement may be severe, long lasting and recurrent.

Course of sarcoidosis

The course depends on the extent of systemic involvement. The most severe manifestation is pulmonary fibrosis, and in children deforming arthritis and eye involvement. However, all involved visceral organs, nervous and musculoskeletal systems may show variously pronounced abnormalities.

Diagnosis

For cutaneous lesions the only significant examination is skin biopsy showing non-caseating granulomas by negative staining for acid-fast bacilli and no characteristics of foreign body granuloma.

Laboratory examinations

These should include a chest and finger bone X-ray and tuberculin testing (usually anergy to tuberculin and other standard test for delayed-type hypersensitivity, however the positive test does not exclude sarcoidosis).

Examination for calcium serum level (hypercalcaemia is a characteristic finding due to increased intestinal absorption of calcium), and evaluation of serum angiotensin-converting enzyme (ACE) levels, found to be increased in fibrotic processes, especially in lungs. This test has a limited diagnostic value since it may be positive in various fibrotic processes (in liver, skin etc.). However the levels of ACE might be useful in monitoring the therapy. In our experience, if sarcoidosis is exclusively cutaneous, ACE level is often not increased. Routine laboratory investigations show not infrequently a moderate increase in erythrocyte sedimentation rate, leukopenia, thrombocytopenia, and hypergammaglobulinaemia (B-cell activation).

Differential diagnosis of cutaneous manifestations

Tuberculosis (tbc luposa) differs by admixture of lymphocytes at the periphery of granuloma, strongly positive tuberculin reaction, a possible detection of mycobacteria tuberculosis in culture and their DNA in polymerase chain reaction (PCR).

Late syphilis should be differentiated especially in cases of ulcerative sarcoidosis; it differs mainly by plasma cell infiltrates, and positive serology.

Lupoid rosacea differs by clinical presentation of rosaceiform eruption and the course.

Lymphoma differs by systemic involvement, histology, and characteristic immunohistochemical markers.

Treatment

General therapeutic guidelines

The treatment of sarcoidosis is in general reserved for the cases with systemic involvement.

Topical corticosteroids of high potency are usually sufficient to control cutaneous manifestations.

In cases displaying exclusively cutaneous non-specific and/or specific changes therapy is, in general, not needed since in the majority of patients spontaneous resolution occurs. Lofgren syndrome, both in children and adults, is no indication for therapy since all lesions regress spontaneously within several months

In all cases investigations for systemic involvement should be performed which is a determining factor for the choice of therapy.

In cutaneous sarcoidosis the therapy should be introduced if hypercalcaemia or hypercalciuria or some cardiac or neurological symptoms are detected. Pulmonary functional abnormalities or some radiological chest changes with no respiratory dysfunction do not present indications for systemic therapy. The patients should be followed up for 6–12 months, and the therapy installed in cases of aggravation.

In children the therapy should be introduced after the presence of eye changes, severe pulmonary, renal, or neurological involvement is established since the course of the disease might be less favourable than in adults.

In pregnant women the only regimen is application of corticosteroids. The pregnancy itself has no unfavourable effect, however it is necessary to control the calcium metabolism for a possible hypercalcaemia.

Recommended therapies

Topical corticotherapy

The treatment should start with low-potency topical corticosteroids, indicated mostly for cosmetic reasons.

Topical therapy with high-potency corticosteroids is recommended for specific papular and nodular lesions, for scalp and scar sarcoidosis (for nodular lesions under occlusion).

Intralesional corticosteroids (triamcinolone 5–10 mg/mL) are applied once monthly for nodular and subcutaneous changes.

Systemic corticotherapy

Oral corticosteroids are the first-line therapy for sarcoidosis with systemic involvement.

The second-line therapy in these cases is methotrexate and synthetic antimalarials. Only these three regimens were proved to be effective in cutaneous sarcoidosis.

Systemic corticotherapy is recommended only in severe cutaneous disfiguring forms (lupus pernio, ulcerative sarcoidosis) non-responsive to topical corticotherapy, for eye involvement, painful arthritis with fever, severe pulmonary changes, cardiac, central nervous and liver dysfunctions.

The dosages are moderate or small: 40 mg/day, progressively reduced by 5 mg/per week; maintenance dose 10–15 mg/day. Duration of therapy—several months depending on the extent of extracutaneous involvement and the control of clinical symptoms. Sensitive marker for the disease activity is hypercalcaemia and, in cases of lung involvement, ACE serum levels and repeated functional respiratory tests. Corticosteroids are very effective in controlling hypercalcaemia.

Synthetic antimalarials

Chloroquine or hydroxychloroquine 250–500 mg/day for several months. The indications are mainly limited to cutaneous sarcoidosis (progressive widespread lesions by contraindications for systemic corticotherapy) or as corticosteroid-sparing agent. Some effect was also shown in pulmonary involvement (relapse after treatment withdrawal, and clearance after reintroduction of therapy). Antimalarials may be used jointly with corticosteroids. Ophthalmological examination should be repeatedly performed (prevention of irreversible retinopathy).

Immunosuppressive drugs

Methotrexate is applied in small dosages 10–25 mg/week in intramuscular injections or perorally for several months, often combined with oral prednisone. Favourable effects have been obtained in cutaneous sarcoidosis. Indications are aggressive cutaneous changes (e.g. lupus pernio) with systemic involvement. The limitation of the use of methotrexate is its hepatotoxicity and a possible risk of hepatic fibrosis.

Chlorambucil (4.0 mg/day), cyclophosphamide (2–2.5 mg/kg/day), azathioprine (100–200 mg/day) is used mainly in lung disease, for cases non-responsive to corticosteroids. The evaluation of effects is difficult.

Ciclosporin (in doses up to 6 mg/kg per day) had a moderate, transient effect in patients with severe pulmonary, ocular and neurological involvement, in some cases was ineffective.

Alternative and experimental treatments

Drug treatments non-verified in controlled studies but found effective in a few cases are as follows:

- Allopurinol (100–300 mg/day): favourable effects were reported in the treatment of cutaneous sarcoidosis with lung involvement resistant to corticosteroids. The therapy was applied for many months, side-effects were minimal.
- Thalidomide (100–200 mg/day) applied for 3 weeks, followed by 50–100 mg/day for several weeks, and 50 mg every other day for several months, was found effective in a few cases of extensive cutaneous sarcoidosis with pulmonary involvement, resistant to other therapies. The drug should be used with a great precaution in women of child-bearing age.
- Tetracyclines: minocycline 200 mg/day, for about 12 months and doxyciclin 200 mg/day as a maintenance therapy, in non-controlled study were found beneficial in cases of cutaneous sarcoidosis.
- Transilat (antihistamine and antifibrotic action) was found effective for cutaneous sarcoidosis in a dose of 300 mg/day, applied for 3 months.

Further reading

Bachelez H, Senet P, Cadranel J, Kaounkhov A, Dubertret L. The use of tetracyclines for the treatment of sarcoidosis. *Arch Dermatol* 2001; 137: 69–73.

Baughman RP. Can tuberculosis cause sarcoidosis? New techniques try to answer an old question. *Chest* 1998; 114: 626–9.

Carlesimo M, Giustini S, Rossi A, Bonaccorsi P, Calvieri S. Treatment of cutaneous and pulmonary sarcoidosis with thalidomide. *J Am Acad Dermatol* 1995; 32: 866–9.

Kleman H, Husain AN, Cagle PT, Garrity ER, Popper HH. Mycobacterial DNA in recurrent sarcoidosis in the transplanted lung: a PCR based study of four cases. *Virchows Arch* 2000; 436: 365–9.

Li N, Bajoghli A, Kubba A, Bhawan J. Identification of mycobacterial DNA in cutaneous lesions of sarcoidosis. *J Cutan Pathol* 1999; 26: 271–8.

Lower EE, Baughman RP. Prolonged use of methotrexate for sarcoidosis. *Arch Intern Med* 1995; 155: 846–51.

Newman L, Rose C, Maier L. Sarcoidosis. *N Engl J Med* 1997; 336: 1224–34.

Pfau A, Stolz W, Karrer S, Szeimies RM, Landthaler M. Allopurinol in der Behandlung der kutanen Sarkoidose. *Hautarzt* 1998; 49: 216–18.

Russo G, Millikan LE. Cutaneous sarcoidosis: diagnosis and treatment. *Compr Therapy* 1994; 20: 418–21.

Sassolas B, Castanet J. Sarcoidose. *Ann Dermatol Venereol* 1997; 124: 102–11.

York EL, Kovithavons T, Man SF, Rebuck AS, Sproule BJ. Cyclosporine and chronic sarcoidosis. *Chest* 1990; 98: 1026–9.

Zic JA, Horowitz DH, Arzubiaga C, King LE. Treatment of cutaneous sarcoidosis with chloroquine. Review of the literature. *Arch Dermatol* 1991; 127: 1034–40.

Scabies

A. Górkiewicz-Petkow

Definition

Scabies is an ectoparasite skin infection. The role of mites as a cause of ectoparasite skin infections in man has often been underestimated. In the presence of a pleomorphic, pruritic, papular eruption the possibility of mite infestation should be taken into account. Scabies has been recognized for thousands of years. The causative mite was discovered in the 17th century.

Aetiology and epidemiology

The causative mite is *Sarcoptes scabiei* var. *hominis*. The increase in scabies infestations is independent of socioeconomic situation (although in underdeveloped countries prevalence has been higher), age or sex. Epidemics of scabies still occur in schools, hospitals, and nursing homes, within families and between immunosuppressed patients. Frequently, inadequate epidemiological recognition, and consequent inadequate treatment, is the cause of the spread of disease. Scabies is easily transmitted by skin-to-skin contact or through contaminated environments (dust, chairs, curtains, sheets, pillow, toys). Adult female mites can survive 24–36 h at ambient room temperature. The incubation period varies from 4 days to 6 weeks. The number of mites living on an infected host varies from 50 to several million in crusted scabies and human immunodeficiency virus (HIV)-positive patients.

Clinical characteristics and course

The skin disease associated with scabies results from a type IV immunological reaction to the mite or its faecal pellets. Skin lesions are various, depending on local and general immunological response.

The primary complaint of a patient with scabies is itching, particularly at night (it has been suggested that it may be connected with increased activity of the female mite in warmer and darker conditions, or as an immune response to the mite and its products). The onset of symptoms is gradual. Pruritus begins slowly; the patient is unable to pinpoint the exact date of symptoms or rash. Symptomatic pruritus can persist for 2–4 weeks after treatment, while the dead mites in the outer layers of stratum corneum are sloughed off with normal exfoliation. Conversely in reinfestation symptoms reappear almost immediately. The most characteristic features of scabies are burrows and vesicles; less characteristic are papules, pustules, excoriations, nodules and bullae. Affected areas include the hands (interdigital areas and palms), lateral borders of feet, ankles, elbows, breasts, periumbilical area, genitals (particularly penis and scrotum) and buttocks. In children under 2 years of age possible involvement of the face and soles is observed. In severe cases or in immunosuppressed patients scabies can involve the entire skin surface. There have been reports on subungual and nail involvement in persons with crusted scabies or in neonatal scabies. Scabies can coexist as an additional infection with different skin diseases especially with sexually transmitted diseases.

Complications of scabies

These include urticarial reactions, persisting dermatitis and pruritus after treatment, nodular lesions, and psychological problems (parasitophobia). There are reports on pemphigoid-like eruption and histiocytosis-like lesions in patients treated for scabies.

Clinical variants of scabies

Crusted (keratotic, Norwegian) scabies

This is a distinctive form of scabies with a predilection for the physically disabled, mentally ill individuals and immunosuppressed patients, and can, although seldom, also occur in healthy individuals. Keratotic scabies is not very rare, and can mimic other skin conditions such a psoriasis, exfoliative dermatitis and T-cell lymphoma, and therefore is often misdiagnosed. The most characteristic lesions are hyperkeratotic plaques involving scalp, ears, knees, palms and soles. The lesions are heavily infested with mites, which can be detected also in the patient's environment (bed, linen, floor, carpets). Pruritus is rare but occasionally may be severe. These patients are often a source for scabies epidemics in nursing homes and hospitals.

Neonatal scabies

Neonatal scabies differs from that seen in older patients by its generalized character involving all body areas. Lesions consist of papules, vesicles, and crusts. It often occurs secondary to infection with weeping and desquamation. The itch is not always present.

Diagnosis

Scabies should be suspected in patients with nocturnal itch, erosions and pleomorphic lesions in typical distribution. A definite diagnosis requires identification of the mite or eggs in the presence of burrows. Burrows may appear as elevated lines or erythematous or oedematous linear lesions, sometimes with vesicle formation at the top. The brownish to black discoloration of the burrows is due to the presence of faeces, eggs or the mite itself. Burrows may be better seen by applying mineral oil on the skin, liquid tetracycline preparations or by burrow ink test. The next step is to demonstrate the scabies mite by extracting the mite with a sterile needle, by shaving or stripping the lesion with cellophane tape and examining the obtained material under the microscope.

Differential diagnosis

Skin eruption caused by different mites

Domestic animals (birds, dogs, cats, rabbits), dust, or grain may be the source of infestation. The main difference in the clinical picture is lack of burrows. The eruption consists mainly of papules, urticarial lesions and vesicles with no characteristic distribution. The itch persists all day. To confirm the diagnosis a detailed history about work conditions, hobbies, domestic animals and detection of mites in the environment may be helpful.

Differentiation from other skin diseases

These include allergic dermatitis, pyoderma, ecthymatosis, Darier's disease, and dermatitis herpetiformis.

Problems in the diagnosis

- Proper diagnosis and choice of adequate treatment of scabies is vital.
- Treatment of endemic disease in nursing homes and schools.
- Diagnosis of crusted scabies.

Treatment

General therapeutic guidelines

There are a variety of scabicides so the choice of treatment depends often on the personal preferences, availability of the drug or economic situation of the patient. In each case it is necessary to confirm diagnosis and source of infestation, which relates also to non-human mite infestations. There are several questions which should be explained to the patient before starting the treatment. Because the use of scabicides can cause irritation, patients should be warned against over treatment, and physicians, in cases of persistent infestation or reinfestation, should only administer repeated applications. If secondary infection is present antibiotics should be prescribed. Sometimes pruritus persists for several weeks after completion of the treatment. In these patients antihistamines and emollients may be helpful. Treatment should always be carefully supervised since most failures are due to inadequate application of scabicide. All members of the family and all contacts should be treated, even where there is no evidence of infection. The environment should be decontaminated, especially in cases of Norwegian scabies. All personal clothing and bed linen should be changed and washed. In large-scale epidemics it is advisable to establish treatment centres.

Remember:

- to start treatment after confirmation of diagnosis
- to give all instructions and explanations to the patient
- to treat all contacts
- to treat the whole body including intertriginous areas, toenails, subungueal areas
- to follow strictly the instructions of the manufacturer
- to choose adequate medication for children, pregnant women or immunocompromised patients
- to be aware of the greater permeability of scabicides in patients with impaired skin barriers.

Recommended therapies

Pyrethrins

Commercial preparation—Lyclear dermal cream 5% permethrine

Permethrins, synthetic pyrethroids, are well tolerated, adverse reactions are rare, and irritation of the skin is infrequent. For the treatment of scabies in adults a single application, after a bath, for 8–12 h is sufficient. This could be repeated, if necessary. Permethrin can be used in neonates and children under 2 years of age in reduced amounts and in pregnant women with caution.

Chlorinated insecticides

- Gammahexachlorocyclohexane—Lindane 1% emulsion.
- Commercial preparations—Jacutin, Quellade lotion, Aphtiria.

Adverse reactions are possible. Central nervous system (CNS) toxicity occurs only if not properly used, or ingested. It is not recommended for neonates, small children under 4 years of age, or for pregnant women. The following recommendations have been proposed to minimize the potential risk of lindane treatment: it should not be applied after a hot bath which can enhance absorption, in very slim, cachectic patients (atrophy of fat tissue is facilitating absorption), or in patients with massive excoriations or dysfunction of epidermal barrier. Lindane should be washed off the skin after 8–12 h, with only 2 applications possible during 1 month. Treatment schedule: one or two applications on two consecutive nights.

Benzyl benzoate

- Commercial preparations—ascabiol 10% solution for children, 25% for adults.
- Adverse reactions—locally irritant.
- Treatment schedules (not unified) after bath 2–3 applications with 12-h intervals. May be used in children, excluding neonates and those under 4 months of age, and pregnant women in lower concentration.

Anticholinesterase inhibitors

- Commercial preparation—Derbac-M (malathion 0.5% aqueous sol.).
- Treatment schedule: single application for 12 h, not preceded by a hot bath. May be used with caution in children and in pregnant women.

Sulphur

- 5%, 10% in petrolatum base, 25% in zinc base.
- Adverse reactions: locally irritation.
- Treatment schedules: after bath 3–4 applications with 12-h intervals. For children lower concentration indicated. The major disadvantages of sulphur are its unpleasant smell and messy consistency.

Crotamitone

- Commercial preparations—Eurax, Euraxil.
- Crotamitone has lower potential as scabicide but has in addition some antipruritic activities.
- Treatment schedule: after a bath on 4–5 consecutive nights. May be used in children and pregnant women. Also used for the treatment of postscabietic pruritus or pruritus of other origin.

Alternative treatments

Ivermectin

- Commercial preparation—ivermectin (Stromectole).
- Ivermectin is an antiparasitic agent with a structure similar to the macrolide antibiotics, but without antibacterial activity. It is a synthetic derivative of abamectin. The drug has an endectocidal effect causing paralysis by suppressing the conduction of the nervous impulses in the interneuronic synapses of parasites. Ivermectin is widely used for the treatment of onchocerciasis.

Since 1992 there have been reports on systemic administration of this drug for uncomplicated scabies infestations in humans (Polynesia, India, Sierra-Leone, Mexico, USA) or scabies in HIV-positive patients. The patients received a single oral dose of 100 or 200 fg of ivermectin/kg or two repeated doses in weekly inter-

Table 1 Recommended topical treatment for scabies and pediculosis*

Scabies		Pediculosis	
Adults	Permethrin 5% cream Malathion 0.5% aqueous sol. Lindane 1% emulsion Benzyl benzoate 25% sol. Sulphur 6–15%	Head lice Pubic lice	Permethrin 5% conditioner Carbaryl 0.5% alc. lotion Carbaryl 0.5%, 1% aqueous sol. Carbaryl 0.5%, 1% shampoo Malathion 0.5% alc. lotion Lindane 1% shampoo (in older children) All preparations should be used with caution in children under 6 months
Pregnant women	Sulphur 6–10%, crotamitone, (permethrine 5% cream, malathion 0.5% aqueous sol., benzyl benzoate 10%—with caution)	Infestation of eyelashes	Physostigmine eye ointment, malathion and carbaryl aqueous sol. with caution. Petrolatum, mercuric oxid eye ointment, mechanical removal of lice
Children	Sulphur 6%, crotamitone Permethrin 5% cream after 2 months of age in reduced amounts Malathion 0.5% aqueous sol. and benzyl benzoate with caution after 4 years of age Lindane 1% emulsion after 4 years of age with caution (not to be ingested)		

*Treatment schedules in the chapter on scabicides and pediculicides.

val in HIV-positive patients, crusted scabies or epidemics in nursing homes. Sometimes the use of concomitant topical treatment is recommended, e.g. benzyl benzoate. The benefits of oral ivermectin are high therapeutic efficacy (quick relief of pruritus), good tolerance, administration once a week, lack of local irritation and action on the whole body surface.

Further clinical studies are necessary to evaluate optimal regimen of treatment, to exclude possible interactions with topical treatments (e.g. lindane), and to assess the incidence of serious adverse reactions.

Thiabendazole cream

Thiabendazole has a broad spectrum of antihelminthic action (strongyloidiasis, cutaneous larva migrans). In South America there are reports of oral administration of thiabendazole in the treatment of scabies (25 mg/kg for 10 days), and on thiabendazole 5% cream for topical treatment of scabies applied for 5 consecutive nights.

Further reading

Alberici F, Pagani L, Ratti G, Viale P. Ivermectin alone or in combination with benzyl benzoate in the treatment of human immunodeficiency virus-associated scabies. *Br J Dermatol* 2000; 142: 969–72.

Almond DS, Green CJ, Geurin DM, Evans S. Lesson of the week: Norwegian scabies misdiagnosed as an adverse drug reaction. *BMJ* 2000; 320: 35–6.

Andersen BM, Haugen H, Rasch M, Heldal-Haugen A, Tageson A. Outbreak of scabies in Norwegian nursing homes and home care patients: control and prevention. *J Hosp Infect* 2000; 45: 160–4.

Barkwell R, Shields S. Deaths associated with ivermectin treatment of scabies. *Lancet* 1997; 349: 1140–5.

Becheral PA, Barete S, Frances C, Chosidow O. Ectoparasitoses (pediculosis et gale): strategie therapeutique actuelle. *Ann Dermatol Venereol* 1999; 126: 755–61.

Burkhart CG, Burkhart CN, Burkhart KM. An epidemiologic and therapeutic reassessment of scabies. *Cutis* 2000; 65: 233–40.

Dannaoui E, Kiazand A, Piens M, Picot S. Use of ivermectin for the management of scabies in a nursing home. *Eur J Dermatol* 1999; 9: 443–5.

Dourmishev A, Serafimova D, Dourmishev L. Efficacy and tolerance of oral ivermectin in scabies. *J Eur Acad Dermatol Venereol* 1998; 11: 247–51.

Estes SA. *The Diagnosis and Management of Scabies*. Reed and Carrnick, 1988: 4–28.

Folster-Holst R, Ruffi T, Christophers E. Die Skabiestherapie unter besonderer Berucksichtigung des fruhen Kindesalters, der Scwangerschaft und Stillzeit. *Hautzarzt* 2000; 5: 7–13.

Gach JE, Heagerty A. Crusted scabies looking like psoriasis. *Lancet* 2000; 356: 650.

Hashimoto K, Fujiwara K, Punwaney J *et al*. Postscabetic nodules: a lymphohistiocyte reaction rich in indeterminate cells. *J Dermatol* 2000; 27: 181–94.

Judge MR, Kobza-Black A. Crusted scabies in pregnancy. *Br J Dermatol* 1995; 132: 116–19.

Marliere V, Roul S, Labreze C, Taieb A. Crusted (Norwegian) scabies induced by use of topical corticosteroids and treated successfully with ivermectin. *J Pediatr* 1999; 135: 122–4.

Meinking TL, Taplin D. Safety of permethrin vs lindane for the treatment of scabies. *Arch Dermatol* 1996; 132: 959–62.

Meinking TL, Taplin D, Hermida JL, Pardo R, Kerdel FA. The treatment of scabies with ivermectin. *N Engl J Med* 1995; 333: 26–30.

Nordt SP, Chew G. Acute lindane poisoning in three children. *J Emerg Med* 2000; 18: 51–3.

Schuster O, Menke G, Czichowsky H, Loew D. Pharmacokinetics of crotamiton following topical application to healthy male volunteers. *J Dermatol Treat* 1992; 3: 57–60.

Sirera G, Rius F, Romev J *et al*. Hospital outbreak of scabies stemming from two AIDS patients with Norwegian scabies. *Lancet* 1990; 335: 1227.

Sterling GB, Janniger CK, Kihiczak G. Neonatal scabies. *Cutis* 1990; 45: 229–31.

Talanin NY, Smith SS, Shelley D, Moores WB. Cutaneous histicytosis with Langerhans cell features induced by scabies: a case report. *Pediatr Dermatol* 1994; 11: 327–30.

Taplin D, Menking TL, Chen JA, Sanchez R. Comparison of crotamiton 10% cream (Eurax) and permethrin 5% cream (Elimite) for the treatment of scabies in children. *Pediatr Dermatol* 1990; 7: 67–73.

Seborrhoeic dermatitis

J. Faergemann

Definition and epidemiology

Seborrhoeic dermatitis is characterized by inflammation and desquamation in areas with a rich supply of sebaceous glands, namely the scalp, face and upper trunk. Dandruff is the mildest manifestation of the disease. Seborrhoeic dermatitis is a common disease, and the prevalence ranges from 2 to 5% in different studies. It is more common in males than in females. The disease usually starts during puberty and is more common around 40 years of age.

Aetiology and pathophysiology

There are now many studies indicating that the lipophilic yeast *Malassezia* (formerly *Pityrosporum ovale*) plays an important role in seborrhoeic dermatitis. Many of these are treatment studies which describe effectiveness of antimycotics, paralleled by a reduction in number of *Malassezia*, and recolonization leading to a recurrence of seborrhoeic dermatitis. The increased incidence of seborrhoeic dermatitis in patients with immunosuppressive disorders suggests that the relationship between *Malassezia* and the immune system is of importance.

Studies in the literature on both humoral and cellular immune responses in peripheral blood as well as lymphocyte stimulation and transformation tests are conflicting. The discrepancy may be due to the presence of lipids in the cell wall. However, there are studies that show that patients with seborrhoeic dermatitis have an impaired immune response with increased frequencies of natural killer cells and subnormal mitogen stimulation responses. Other studies have found a reduced lymphocyte stimulation reaction when lymphocytes from patients with seborrhoeic dermatitis were stimulated with a *Malassezia* extract. Additionally, interleukin (IL)-2 and interferon (IFN) production by lymphocytes from patients was markedly depressed and IL-10 synthesis were increased after stimulation with *Malassezia* extract.

The immune response in the skin may be of greater importance. In a recently published study we found that the immune response in the skin showed an irritant non-immunogenic response in combination with both a stimulation of interleukins for both Th1 and Th2 function indicating a response similar to that found in cutaneous *Candida* infections. The lipid amount on the skin in patients with seborrhoeic dermatitis was significantly higher than in controls. In conclusion impaired cell-mediated immunity may facilitate fungal survival in the skin. The inflammatory response to *Malassezia* products would not be downregulated, and therefore an increased inflammatory response would occur and the dermatitis triggered.

Clinical characteristics and course

Seborrhoeic dermatitis is one of the most common skin diseases. The disease is characterized by red scaly lesions predominantly located on the scalp, face and upper trunk. It is more common in males than in females. The disease usually starts during puberty and is most common around 40 years of age. The skin lesions are distributed on the scalp, eyebrows, nasolabial folds, cheeks, ears, presternal and interscapular regions, axillae and groins. Around 90–95% of all patients have scalp lesions and lesions on glabrous skin are found in approximately 60% of the patients. The lesions are red and covered with greasy scales. Itching is common in the scalp. Complications include lichenification, secondary bacterial infection and otitis externa. The course of seborrhoeic dermatitis tends to be chronic with recurrent flare-up. A seasonal variation is observed with the majority of patients being better during the summertime. Mental stress and dry air are factors that may aggravate the disease. A genetic predisposition is also of importance in the disease. Seborrhoeic dermatitis is seen more frequently than expected in patients with pityriasis versicolor, *Pityrosporum* folliculitis, Parkinson's disease, major truncal paralysis, mood depression and acquired immunodeficiency syndrome.

Diagnosis

The diagnosis is primarily based on the clinical picture. Although the *Malassezia* yeasts are necessary for the development of seborrhoeic dermatitis the number of yeast cells are within the normal range and direct microscopy or culture of skin scales are therefore of no benefit for the diagnosis. The histological picture of seborrhoeic dermatitis is said to be half way between eczema and psoriasis and it is not diagnostic.

Differential diagnosis

- Psoriasis: typical distribution; colour of scales.
- Atopic dermatitis: history; distribution; itch; elevated IgE.
- Pityriasis versicolor: microscopy.

Treatment

General therapeutic guidelines

Seborrhoeic dermatitis is a chronic disease and to inform the patients about the risk for relapse and predisposing factors is very important.

Stress and winter climate have a negative effect on the majority of patients and summer and sunshine have a positive effect.

In patients with neurological diseases and especially in patients with immunosuppressive disorders seborrhoeic dermatitis is more resistant to therapy. In a young individual with resistant lesions always think of human immunodeficiency virus (HIV) infection.

Mild corticosteroids are effective in the treatment of seborrhoeic dermatitis. However the disease recurs quickly often within a few days.

Antifungal therapy is effective in the treatment of seborrhoeic dermatitis and, because it reduces the number of the *Malassezia* yeasts, the time to recurrence is increased compared to corticosteroids. Antifungal therapy should be the primary treatment of this disease.

Recommended therapies

Antifungal treatment

Antifungal therapy against *Malassezia* is effective in treating most cases of seborrhoeic dermatitis and prophylactic treatment with antifungal drugs reduces the recurrence rate much more than corticosteroids. In one study the combination of hydrocortisone and miconazole in an alcoholic solution was significantly more effective than hydrocortisone alone in reducing the number of *Malassezia* and the recurrence rate was also significantly lower with the combination therapy; 16% with the combination compared to 82% for hydrocortisone alone.

Ketoconazole is very effective *in vitro* against the *Malassezia* yeasts with minimum inhibitory concentrations (MICs) in the range of 0.02–0.5 μg/mL. Oral ketoconazole has been effective in a double-blind placebo-controlled trial in patients with seborrhoeic dermatitis of the scalp and other areas. Itraconazole 200 mg daily for 2 weeks is also effective and will be the preferred drug today compared with ketoconazole. However oral therapy should be reserved for patients not responding to topical therapy. In another double-blind, placebo-controlled study ketoconazole 2% cream has been effective in the treatment of seborrhoeic dermatitis of the scalp and face, and in a comparative study between ketoconazole and hydrocortisone cream no difference was seen in effectiveness.

Ketoconazole shampoo used twice weekly is very effective in treating seborrhoeic dermatitis of the scalp. In a double-blind placebo-controlled study of ketoconazole shampoo used twice weekly for 4 weeks, 89% in the ketoconazole group was cured, compared with only 14% in the placebo group. Ketoconazole used once weekly has also been effective in preventing recurrence of dandruff in previously treated patients.

Other topical antimycotics are effective in the treatment of seborrhoeic dermatitis. Shampoos containing zinc pyrithione or selenium sulfide are effective and widely used. Propylene glycol solutions has also been used successfully.

Corticosteroids

Mild corticosteroid solutions, creams or ointments are effective in the treatment of seborrhoeic dermatitis due to a nonspecific anti-inflammatory activity. However, they apparently have no effect on *Malassezia* because seborrhoeic dermatitis recurs quickly when corticosteroids are used, often within a few days after treatment has ended.

Combination therapy with antifungals and corticosteroids

In severe inflammatory seborrhoeic dermatitis topical treatment with antifungal therapy alone may not be so effective. Some of these patients respond well to oral ketoconazole or itraconazole. Another therapy that can be effective is to combine potent topical corticosteroids with topical antifungal therapy. After clearance many of these patients will remain free of lesions on prophylactic topical antifungal treatment.

Keratolytic therapy

When lesions are covered with thick adherent scales keratolytic therapy, especially in the scalp, is necessary.

Antibiotics

Seborrhoeic dermatitis especially in the scalp and external ear canal may be secondarily infected with bacteria. In these patients topical or oral antibacterial therapy in combination with regular treatment are indicated.

Further reading

Faergemann J. Seborrhoeic dermatitis and *Pityrosporum orbiculare*: Treatment of seborrhoeic dermatitis of the scalp with miconazole-hydrocortisone (Daktacort), miconazole and hydrocortisone. *Br J Dermatol* 1986; 114: 695–700.

Faergemann J. Propylene glycol in the treatment of seborrhoeic dermatitis of the scalp: A double-blind study. *Cutis* 1988; 42: 69–71.

Faergemann J. Treatment of seborrhoeic dermatitis with bifonazole. *Mycoses* 1989; 32: 309–11.

Faergemann J. Treatment of seborrhoeic dermatitis of the scalp with ketoconazole shampoo. *Acta Dermato-Vener (Stockh)* 1990; 70: 171–2.

Ford GP, Farr PM, Ive FA *et al*. The response of seborrhoeic dermatitis to ketoconazole. *Br J Dermatol* 1984; 111: 603–7.

Marks R, Pears AD, Walker AP. The effects of a shampoo containing zinc pyrithione on the control of dandruff. *Br J Dermatol* 1985; 112: 415–22.

Shuster S. The aetiology of dandruff and the mode of action of therapeutic agents. *Br J Dermatol* 1984; 111: 235–42.

Skinner RB, Noah PW, Taylor RM *et al*. Double-blind treatment of seborrhoeic dermatitis with 2% ketoconazole cream. *J Am Acad Dermatol* 1985; 12: 852–7.

Stratigos ID, Katamboas A, Antoniu CH *et al*. Ketoconazole 2% cream versus 1% hydrocortisone cream in the treatment of seborrhoeic dermatitis: A double-blind comparative study. *J Am Acad Dermatol* 1988; 19: 850–3.

Seborrhoeic keratosis

A. Picoto

Synonyms

Seborrhoeic wart, verruca seborrhoeica senilis, basal cell papilloma.

Definition and epidemiology

Seborrhoeic keratosis appears as macules and papules, brownish to grey or black. They are sometimes polypoid with a 'stuck on' appearance and greasy surface with plugged horns, predominantly on the face, chest and back of adult whites.

They are common in whites (third decade onwards), uncommon in black people and Indians; probably many cases are dominantly inherited. Males and females are equally affected. Black and Asian patients can develop a variant of seborrhoeic keratosis called dermatosis papulosa nigra. This consists of heavily pigmented papules, some pedunculated, on the face, developing as early as adolescence.

Aetiology and pathophysiology

While the aetiology is unknown, there are many clinopathological variants:

- reticulated seborrhoeic keratosis
- stucco keratosis
- clonal seborrhoeic keratosis
- irritated seborrhoeic keratosis
- melanoacanthoma
- dermatosis papulosa nigra.

Clinical characteristics and course

Seborrhoeic keratosis appears exclusively on hair-bearing skin, often in a 'Christmas tree' pattern, and mainly on skin rich in sebaceous glands.

It begins as flat brown macules that slowly transform into greasy papules, with multiple grey or black plugged follicles. The lesions are often located bilaterally and are symmetrical, predominantly on the face, trunk and extremities.

The sudden appearance of a large number of lesions with pruritus may be associated with internal malignancy (adenocarcinoma) and this is the so-called Leser–Trélat sign. This sign is still not accepted by all authors and is very rare. The lesions are benign. There is no evolution towards malignancy and they become symptomatic when irritated. There is a possible association with basal cell carcinoma so when they present signs of inflammation, histological examination is mandatory.

They are of cosmetic concern and may cause difficulties when dressing and undressing. There is no spontaneous resolution.

Diagnosis

Clinical diagnosis is usually not difficult after analysing the characteristics of the lesions and their distribution. One can press the surface of the papules or macules with the fingernail and confirm their 'greasy' nature. Dermatoscopy or epiluminescence microscopy can be helpful in establishing the diagnosis.

Differential diagnosis

This includes:

- pigmented naevi
- melanoma
- pigmented basal cell carcinoma
- verruca vulgaris
- lentigo and lentigo maligna
- actinic keratosis
- acanthosis nigricans.

Clinical inspection, better done with the help of a dermatoscope is usually sufficient to establish a firm diagnosis. Freezing with liquid nitrogen is said to intensify the appearance of the multiple comedo-like openings of the typical cases. When doubt persists there should be no hesitation to biopsy for a histological examination, before a therapeutic decision is taken.

Treatment

General therapeutic guidelines

It has been mentioned already that seborrhoeic keratosis is only of cosmetic concern, so treatment should provide a satisfactory or preferably very good cosmetic result. The treatment should be explained to the patient, and in particular the time necessary for healing. Recommendations for the home treatment of the wounds should also be given in a very precise manner, preferably in writing to avoid complications and anxiety for the patient and family.

The aim of the treatment will be to destroy the lesions completely, avoiding recurrence, without much pain and leave no scar or a cosmetically acceptable scar.

Recommended therapies

Curettage

This is the mainstay of therapy. A sharp curette and local anaesthesia should be used. I always use EMLA cream before injecting lidocaine (lignocaine) buffered with potassium bicarbonate. EMLA cream should be put over and around the lesions under occlusion by tape and remain there for at least 20 min. Local injection of ansesthesia with lidocaine should be performed using a 30-gauge needle slowly injecting into the dermis. If seborrhoeic keratosis is multiple, which is normally the case, a treatment plan should be established with the patient and be carried out in several sessions. In the first session one should not be too ambitious and treat only a few lesions, preferably the more conspicuous or inconvenient to the patient according to his/her opinion.

After curettage there is the problem of stopping the bleeding, and for this cautery or diathermy is usually applied. The risk of scarring is great. If instead of cautery or diathermy a CO_2 laser is used either in a classical or superpulse mode, the risk of scarring remains.

Some authors recommend the use of aluminium chloride or Monsel's solution for haemostasis but there is a risk of permanent brown staining.

There are many varieties of curette available. Diameters vary from 4 to 12 mm. Disposable curettes are also available but in my opinion, being so sharp they need great expertise in their use. I consider the best method the so-called 'fast method' that consists of holding the skin taut and with a firm grasp of the instrument, sweeping the lesion off the skin with a single motion. When I use the curette, I do not follow with any coagulation except mild pressure with a gauze impregnated with peroxide for a few minutes. Then the wound is dressed with an antibiotic ointment. If the lesion is very thick, like the papillomatous varieties, then the lesion can be 'cooked' first either by electrodesiccation or CO_2 laser, followed by curettage.

Liquid nitrogen

It is also possible to do the same with liquid nitrogen, freezing followed by curettage. Freezing with liquid nitrogen is also a treatment modality useful for multiple lesions. The lesions and a 1-mm border around this should be frozen with liquid nitrogen. There is a risk of hypopigmentation surrounded by a ring of hyperpigmentation secondary to the inflammatory response to the cryosurgery particularly in darker skinned patients.

Shaving

Shaving excision with scalpel or Gillette blue razor is another possible technique mainly for thick lesions.

Chemical peeling

Chemical peeling with trichloroacetic acid (TCA) either pure or from 25% to

50% can be tested. It is necessary to protect the skin around the lesions being treated with petrolatum and avoid spilling of the TCA (it will produce a 'tattoo'). Frequently the procedure has to be repeated and is very slow. We do not recommend it for everyday use. Chemical peeling with α-hydroxy acid compounds can flatten and lighten the lesions, but it is not a definitive treatment. Dermabrasion can be used in special cases.

In conclusion, there is not at the moment a perfect treatment for this vexing problem. Perhaps a new laser technique will provide a better tool.

Further reading

Braun-Falco O, Plewig G, Wolff HH, Winkelmann RK. *Dermatology.* Berlin: Springer, 1991: 987–89.

Grob JJ, Rava MC, Gouvernet J *et al.* The relation between seborrhoeic keratoses and malignant solid tumours. A case-control study. *Acta Derm Venereol* 1991; 71 (2): 166–9.

Grossin M, Picard C, Tousignant J *et al.* Aspects evolutifs particuliers dés verrues seborrheiques: hyperplasie pseudoepitheliomateuse et transformation maligne. A propos de 2 cas. *Ann Dermatol Venereol* 1990; 117 (11): 875–6.

Kenet RO, Kang S, Kenet BJ, Fitzpatrick GB, Sober AJ, Barnhill RL. Clinical diagnosis of pigmented lesions using digital epiluminescence microscopy. Protocol and atlas. *Arch Dermatol* 1993; 129 (2): 157–74.

Lindelof B, Sigurgeirsson B, Melander S. Seborrhoeic keratoses and cancer. *J Am Acad Dermatol* 1992; 26 (6): 947–50.

Peooer E. Dermabrasion for the treatment of a giant seborrhoeic keratosis. *J Dermatol Surg Oncol* 1985; 11: 646–7.

Poo BK, Freeman RG, Paulos FG, Arberfeld L, Rendon M. The relationship between basal cell epithelioma and seborrhoeic keratosis. A study of 60 cases. *J Dermatol Surg Oncol* 1994; 20 (11): 761–4.

Schwartz RA. Sign of Leser-Trélat. *J Am Acad Dermatol* 1996; 35 (1): 88–95.

Smoller BR, Graham G. In: Arndt, Leboit, Robinson, Wintroub, eds. *Cutaneous Medicine and Surgery.* Saunders, 1996: 1444–9.

Soyer HP, Kerl H. Microscopie de surface dés tumeurs cutanées pigmentées. *Ann Dermatol Venereol* 1993; 120 (1): 15–20.

Vincent CY, Mclean DI. In: Fitzpatrick TB *et al.*, eds. *Dermatology in General Medicine.* McGraw-Hill, 1993: 855–958.

Sjögren's syndrome

A.G. Tzioufas and
H.M. Moutsopoulos

Synonyms

Sicca syndrome, autoimmune epithelitis, Gougerot disease, Mikulicz's disease.

Definition and epidemiology

Sjögren's syndrome (SS) is a chronic autoimmune disease of unknown aetiology, characterized by lymphocyte infiltration of exocrine glands resulting in xerostomia and keratoconjunctivitis sicca. In more than one-third of patients, extraglandular manifestations, such as skin, lung, kidney, liver, muscle and blood vessel involvement, can occur. SS can be found alone (primary SS) or in association with other autoimmune diseases, such as rheumatoid arthritis, systemic lupus erythematosus and scleroderma (secondary SS). Five per cent of patients may develop B-cell lymphoma.

SS primarily affects women (nine women to every man), mainly in the fourth and fifth decades of life. However, it can occur in people of all ages including children and elderly persons. Epidemiological studies performed in the general population has shown that SS is a rather common disease since it affects approximately 0.5% of the total population. SS is a disorder of unknown aetiology. It seems likely that the disease may develop in three stages: autoimmunity can be triggered by a given environmental factor, acting on the given genetic background, perpetuation of the autoimmune reactivity becomes chronic through normal imune regulatory mechanisms, the lesions occur as a consequence of the ongoing inflammatory process.

The two major autoimmune phenomena observed in SS, are lymphocytic infiltration, around the affected epithelial tissues and a remarkable poly- and oligomonoclonal B-cell hyperactivity, which is manifested by the presence of hypergammaglobulinaemia (80% of patients) and autoantibodies to organ-specific autoantigens such as the cytoskeletal protein α-fodrin and non-organ-specific autoantigens such as the ribonucleoproteins Ro/SSA and LaSSB.

Clinical characteristics and course

In the majority of primary SS patients, it runs a rather benign course. The initial manifestations can be non-specific and usually 8–10 years elapse from the initial symptoms to the full-blown development of the disease.

Glandular manifestations

The principal oral symptom of SS is dryness. Patients describe this as difficulty in swallowing dry food, inability to speak continuously, and a burning sensation. Examination shows a dry, erythematous, sticky oral mucosa and on the dorsum of the tongue, atrophy of the filliform papillae. Enlargement of the parotids or other major salivary glands can be seen in 70% of patients.

Ocular involvement is a major glandular manifestation of SS. Diminished tear secretion leads to the destruction of the corneal and bulbar conjunctival epithelium termed keratoconjunctivitis sicca. The patients usually complain of a burning, foreign-body sensation, a sandy or scratchy sensation under the lids, itchiness, redness and photosensitivity. Clinical signs include dilatation of the bulbar conjunctival vessels, pericorneal injection, irregularity of the corneal image and sometimes enlargement of the lacrimal glands.

Extraglandular manifestations

Extraglandular manifestations are seen in one-third of patients with primary SS.

These include easy fatigue, low-grade fever, myalgias and arthralgias. Arthritis is seen in 70% of patients. Pulmonary involvement includes dryness of the tracheobronchial mucosa (xerotrachea) and small airways obstruction. Interstitial disease or pleurisy are uncommon. Acute or chronic pancreatitis are rarely reported. Chronic liver disease, resembling stage I of primary billiary cirrhosis is seen in 2–3% of patients. Renal involvement includes interstitial renal disease and occasionally glomerulonephritis. Vasculitis is found in approximately 5% of patients with SS. It affects small and medium sized vessels. The skin is most commonly affected, but cases with visceral organ involvement such as kidney, lungs, and gastrointestinal tract have been described. Neurological manifestations of SS include peripheral sensory or sensorimotor neuropathy as a consequence of vascular involvement.

Skin involvement

Apart from the eyes and mouth, other mucous membranes as well as the skin may exhibit dryness. Nasal dryness with crusting, vaginal dryness with dyspareunia, cheilitis and xerosis (dry skin) have been described. Patients with dry skin frequently experience dermal stinging and itching.

A distinct epidermal direct immunofluorescence (DIF) pattern in primary SS, consisting of IgG deposits in the basal and suprabasal layers of the epithelium, widespread in the intercellular space and demarcating cell surface membranes has been described. Of more than 100 patients studies, 68% had this feature.

Purpura is a rather common finding in primary SS patients. Flat purpura are usually seen in hypergammaglobulinaemic patients, while palpable purpura is a manifestation of dermal vasculitis.

In recent years, numerous reports from Japan claimed hitherto unreported skin lesions in patients with SS. Annular erythemas consisting of wide elevated erythematous borders with central pallor are located on the face (especially cheek and preauricular skin), upper extremities and back, occasionally coalescing to form polycyclin patterns. The erythema fades within a few months, leaving no scars or pigmentary changes. There is a striking clinical resemblance to Sweet's syndrome. The most conspicuous histological finding is the lymphocytic infiltration throughout the dermis around blood vessels and appendices. Annular erythema in primary SS is significantly associated with the presence of serum antibodies against Ro/SSA (100%) and La/SSB (75%). The annular erythema in SS differs clinically from the polycyclic annular and papulosquamous erythemas in subacute cutaneous lupus erythematosus (SCLE), especially in its oedematous borders without significant scaling.

Raynaud's phenomenon occurs in about 35% of patients with primary SS and usually precedes the sicca manifestations by many years. SS patients with Raynaud's phenomenon present with swollen hands, but in contrast to scleroderma they do not experience digital ulcers and telangiectasias.

Pernio-like lesions (chilblain) on the distal extremities were noted in Japanese patients. Reports on other skin disorders are rare: one case in which SS and Sweet's syndrome developed simultaneously, and one in which a woman developed vascular poikiloderma atrophicans after 12 years of SS. Two cases of lipodystrophy, have also been reported in patients with SS.

Diagnosis/differential diagnosis

The diagnosis of definite SS is based on the presence of four out of six criteria established by the European Union SS concerted action:

- patient has dry mouth
- patient has dry eyes
- objective findings of xerostomia (i.e. diminished parotid flow rate)

- objective findings of keratoconjunctivitis sicca (KCS) (i.e. positive Schirmer's test or rose bengal staining)
- positive minor salivary gland biopsy (lymphocytic focus score > 1 mm^2)
- positive serum autoantibodies (rheumatoid factor, antinuclear antibodies, anti-Ro/SSA or anti-La/SSB).

Differential diagnosis must include other diseases responsible for KCS, xerostomia and parotid gland enlargement. Sarcoidosis in one of the diseases can mimic the clinical picture of SS. However, there is a lack of autoantibodies to Ro/SSA or La/SB, and sometimes the minor salivary gland biopsy reveals non-caseating granulomas. Other medical conditions which can mimic SS are lipoproteinaemias (types IV and V), chronic graft-vs.-host disease, amyloidosis and more recently human immunodeficiency virus (HIV) infection, as well as hepatitis C infection.

Treatment

General therapeutics guidelines

Glandular and extraglandular manifestations

SS remains an incurable disease, since no therapeutic modality that can alter the course of the disease has been identified. Careful follow-up of patients, including regular outpatient visits, close collaboration with rheumatology, ophthalmology and oral medicine, outpatient clinics and concentration on simple measures to relieve desiccation, give the most satisfactory results in the therapy of SS.

Treatment of patients with SS is divided into two parts: treatment of glandular manifestations and their consequences and treatment of the extraglandular manifestations.

Treatment of glandular manifestations

The principal goal in treating the impaired lacrimal and salivary production associated with SS is the successful replacement of glandular secretions. Therapeutic measures for dry eyes include local stimulators of tear secretion, protective bicarbonate-buffered solutions, artificial lubricants and supportive operative procedures. Ciclosporin A 2% in olive solution in the form of eye drops, has been shown to be relatively effective in placebo-controlled clinical trials. The choice of therapeutic procedure used, depends on the experience the ophthalmologist may have of the disease.

The treatment of xerostomia should accomplish the following:

- maintain oral hygiene to prevent dental caries
- careful examination to diagnose and treat oral candidiasis
- systemic therapy to stimulate glandular secretions
- use of saliva substitutes.

Systemic therapy to stimulate glandular secretions includes the use of cholinergic agonist pilocarpine hydrochloride (5 mg four times daily). Contraindications of pilocarpine include pregnancy, history of gastrointestinal ulcer, arrhythmias and severe, poorly-controlled hypertension. New-generation agonists such as cevimeline 'evoxac' have been shown to improve symptoms of dry mouth. The recommended dose is 30 mg three times a day and the drug should be used with caution in patients with cardiovascular disease. Systemic corticosteroids (0.5 mg/kg daily) and immunosuppressive drugs (i.e. cyclophosphamide) are used in severe extraglandular disease such as diffuse interstitial pneumonitis, glomerulonephritis, vasculitis and peripheral neuropathy.

Treatment and skin manifestations

Patients with dry skin should refrain from daily use of soap, except for skin creases, and from too frequent bathing, especially in hot water. Bath oils and frequent use of emollients (i.e greases based on lanolin, lanolin/paraffin mixtures, or creams based on emulsifying wax, macrogel) are beneficial. Increasing the humidity of the environment may also be helful. Vasculitis limited to the skin (leukoclastic vasculitis), which manifests as palpable purpura, does not require specific therapy. Avoidance of cold exposure or emotional stress, together with nifedipine 5–10 mg three times daily are indicated for decreasing the severity and frequency of Raynaud's phenomenon. Vaginal dryness is a cause of painful intercourse. Vaginal lubricants such as K-Y jelly or the recently available vaginal inserts are helpful. Patients should avoid cortisone creams. In postmenopausal women, oestrogen preparations are recommended.

Further reading

Fox PC, Atkinson JC, Naynski AA *et al.* Pilocarpine treatment of salivary gland hypofunction and dry mouth (xerostomia). *Arch Intern Med* 1991; 151: 1149–52.

Haneji N, Nakamura T, Takiok *et al.* Identification of α fodrin as a candidate autoantigen in primary Sjögren's syndrome. *Science* 1997; 276: 604–7.

Moutsopoulos HM. Sjögren's syndrome—autoimmune epithelitis. *Clin Immunol Immunopathol* 1994; 72: 162–5.

Moutsopoulos HM, Velthuis PJ, DeWide PCM, Kater L. Sjögren's syndrome. In: Kater L, de la Faille HB, eds. *Multisystemic Autoimmune Diseases.* Amsterdam: Elsevier Science, 1995: 173–205.

Talal N, Moutsopoulos HM, Kassan SS. *Sjögren's Syndrome. Clinical and Immunological Aspects.* Berlin: Springer, 1987.

Tzioufas AG, Moutsopoulos HM. Sjögren's syndrome. In: Klippel JH, Dieppe PA, eds. *Rheumatology.* London: Mosby, 1993, 6:32.1–12.

Vivino FB, Al-Hashimi I, Khan Z *et al.* Pilocarpine tablets for the treatment of dry mouth and dry eyes symptoms in patients with Sjögren's syndrome: a randomized, placebo-controlled, fixed-dose, multicenter trial. P92–01 Study group. *Arch Intern Med* 1999; 159: 174–81.

Vlachoyiannopoulos PG, Moutsopoulos HM. Therapy of Sjögren's syndrome. In: van de Putte LBA, Furst DE, Williams WJ, van Riel PLCM, eds. *Therapy of Systemic Rheumatic Disorders.* New York: Marcel Dekker, 1998: 615–28.

Skin diseases from the marine environment

G. Monfrecola and G. Posteraro

Definition and epidemiology

Many aquatic organisms are able to produce skin eruptions and occasionally systemic reactions. No data are available about the prevalence of marine-related diseases, but it is likely that they are very common in view of the number of people in the sea for recreational or working activities.

Aetiology and pathophysiology

Excluding aquatic dermatological conditions such as infections (i.e. mycobacteriosis), aquagenic urticaria or pruritus, irritant or allergic dermatitis (i.e. from diving gear) and barotrauma, cutaneous lesions can be caused by accidental contact with the following organisms.

Cnidarians (or coelenterates)

Jellyfish (Scyphozoa), anemones and corals (Anthozoa), the Portuguese man-of-war and fire corals (Hydrozoa) belong to this phylum. Note that the Portuguese man-of-war (Physalia) is wrongly regarded as a jellyfish as it is actually a colonial hydroid. Jellyfish, anemones, corals and hydroids are characterized by the presence on their tentacles of thousands of stinging organelles (nematocysts) filled with poison. Nematocysts are sac-like structures (3–100 f) containing a spirally-coiled thread tube that can be everted in about 100th of a second with an ejection force of 2–5 p.s.i.; the discharged thread, like a harpoon, sticks into the enemy tegument and releases its venom. The nematocist discharge can be stimulated by mechanical and chemical mechanisms. The cnidarian venoms are mixtures of peptides or proteins (enzymes) with inflammatory, necrotic, haemolitic and neurological activities. The human skin can be affected by contact with the whole organism or parts of them (detached tentacles) and also by contact with other marine species using the cnidarian nematocysts as a weapon, i.e. in sea slugs (Nudibranchs) or the Mediterranean octopus (*Tremoctopus violaceous*). Besides the type of nematocysts depending on the species of cnidarians, other factors can influence the intensity of human reaction: the sensitivity of the patient, the size of the involved body surface, the anatomical site of contact and the behaviour of the patient after the contact. The reaction usually has a toxic nature, but immune-mediated mechanisms have been described.

Sea urchins and starfish (echinodermata)

The discomfort results from the penetration of the sea urchin spine through the skin but also from active compounds lining the spine. Investigations on granulomatous reaction failed to demonstrate the presence of substances or organisms able to induce cutaneous granulomas. Pain and granulomas can also be induced by contact with the thorns of some starfish.

Bristle worms (anellida)

The bristles, locomotor and defensive organelles of the *Hermodice carunculata*, can penetrate the skin during accidental or voluntary contact.

Venomous fish stings

The envenomation from fish spines are defined as ichthyoacanthotoxicosis. Many fish, not only in tropical or subtropical areas of the oceans but also in temperate climates (i.e. the Mediterranean sea), can induce severe injuries because the injection of the venom secreted by their cutaneous glands, e.g. weeverfish (*Trachinus* spp.), scorpionfish (*Scorpaena* spp.), zebrafish (*Pterois* spp.), stonefish (*Synanceja* spp.), stargazers (*Uranoscopus* scaber), stingrays, catfish, toadfish (*Thalassophryne* spp.), leatherbacks (*Scomberoides sanctipetri*), moray (*Murenidi* spp.) and boxfish (*Ostraciontidae* spp.).

Sea snake, blue-ringed octopus bites and conidi stings

Sea snakes and blue-ringed octopus (the only cephalopods characterized by two blue rings on a yellow–brown mantle, really dangerous to man) inhabit tropical and subtropical regions of the Indo-Pacific ocean. Both are able to inject potent neurotoxins. Depending on the absorbed dose of venom, their bites can cause death from respiratory arrest (25% of cases). *Conus aulicus* and *Conus geographus* are tropical bivalves with very beautiful shells whose stings have led to dermatological and systemic symptoms leading to death from cardiac paralysis.

Sponges

When brushed against the skin some sponges (*Tedania ignis, Fibula nolitangere*) can produce irritation, similar to the microtraumatic irritative 'glass wool' dermatitis, due to the fine spicules on their surfaces. Moreover, through the spicules, some sponges inject toxic mixtures able to induce skin reactions.

Seaweed and sea moss

Classified as vegetables, these differ in size, colour and shape, and are widely present in both salt and fresh water. A few species of seaweeds (i.e. *Lyngbya majuscola*) can release and spread toxins in the sea causing dermatitis for the bather, in particular on the swimsuit covered body areas. *Alcyonidium gelatinosum* and *Electra pilosa* (sea moss) can cause contact dermatitis in fishermen handling fishing nets.

Clinical characteristics and course

The intensity of both cutaneous and systemic signs and symptoms induced by the interaction between marine inhabitants and man depends on: (i) the duration of contact; (ii) the part of the body involved; (iii) the size of the involved skin area; (iv) the skin rectivity to irritants or allergens; and (v) the general state of health.

Contact with cnidarians is characterized immediately by a burning and painful sensation, followed by an urticarial, papular, vesicular, haemorrhagic or ulceronecrotic eruption. The tentacles can provoke typical lesions showing a linear pattern. In severe cases toxic systemic symptoms can occur such as headache, weakness and fever, and sometimes nausea, vomiting, respiratory and cardiovascular impairment. Injuries from sea urchins and starfish generally cause a severe pain beginning only several minutes after the punctures; several months later, some patients observe the appearance of round papular granulomas. While the chitinous tin spines of the bristle worms provoke a mild erythematopapular itching eruption, the stings from venomous fish result in immediate intense pain radiating from the wound which becomes hot, swollen and reddened. In severe cases fever, nausea, headache, vomiting, convulsions, cardiac and respiratory failure occur. Sea snake or blue-ringed octopus bites and conidi stings cause systemic symptoms such as nausea, vomiting, peripheral muscle weakness or paresis, vision alterations and respiratory failure. Sponges, seaweed and sea moss usually provoke cutaneous lesions such as erythema and oedema with marked itch; in severe cases, vesicobullous reactions with pain and stiffness of the affected body areas can also occur.

Diagnosis

The diagnosis is mainly based on the anamnestic data. Radioallergosorbent test

(RAST) and enzyme-linked immunosorbent assay (ELISA) tests can be utilized in cases of allergic reaction. The sea snake bite is asymptomatic; this means that sometimes the victim can be unaware of the risk. A sea snake bite must be suspected in patients with a paresis occurring hours after swimming in a possibly infested tropical area.

Treatment

Cnidarians

The treatment of cnidarian stings depends on the extension and site of the lesions and on the type of coelenterate. Therefore, when possible, the capture of the cnidarians or part of them can help to establish the correct management. The application of an adhesive tape represents a simple method for collecting from the skin and indicating by microscopy the type of nematocyst involved. Most cnidarian stings produce only moderate cutaneous reactions—the contact with the tentacles may initially cause the discharge of relatively few nematocysts. Therefore, the first measure is to avoid further discharge of nematocysts from the tentacles still adhering to the skin: do not rub the affected area, remember that fresh water, alcohol and human urine cause worsening of the eruption because of a massive discharge of nematocysts. Before gently removing the tentacles, applications of acetic acid (3–10%) or vinegar (in case of contact with *Physalia, Chironex* or *Pelagia* spp.) or sodium bicarbonate mixed with water to obtain a powder slurry (for *Crysaora* spp.) can prevent further nematocyst envenomation and reduce skin reaction and pain. The immersion of the affected body part in heated sea water (45–50°C) denatures the venom's proteins, and can help to minimize the effect of the venom. The oral administration of phenacetine, aspirin, indometacin, ibuprofen or the i.m. or i.v. injection of meperidine and morphine can be useful for severe pain. Systemic corticosteroids, antihistamines and epinephrine (adrenaline) are indicated for allergic reactions. A specific antivenom is available against *Chironex fleckeri* stings (Commonwealth Serum Laboratories, Parkville, Australia). The serum i.v. (20 000 U) or i.m. (60 000 U) injected during the early stages of envenomation reduces the pain and the cutaneous reaction. Cardiac involvement after *Chironex fleckeri* contact can be treated with i.v. verapamil.

Sea urchin punctures

Treatment is based on the extraction of the spines and on cleansing the involved parts to avoid secondary infection. Granulomatous lesions can be treated with cryosurgery or, in severe cases, with surgical excision.

Bristle worm punctures

Treatment consists of removing the bristles with small forceps or adhesive tape.

Venomous fish stings

Fish spines can produce dot-like wounds but also deep lacerations of the tissues. In any case the first step is to irrigate the wounded part with salt water or sterile saline solution to remove the poison; in order to inactivate the venom it has been proposed soaking the wound promptly in hot water (45–50°C) for 30–60 min. After washing it is important to debride surgically and clean the wound using antiseptic solutions. Specific therapy should be used to reduce the pain: phenacetin, aspirin, naloxone-reversible opiates or infiltration of lidocaine (lignocaine; 1–2%) around the wound can help during follow-up. Antibiotic therapy is recommended only if there are evident signs of secondary infection and it should be guided by the isolation of the responsible microorganism. Few severe cases require hospitalization for cardiovascular or respiratory complications. The Australian

Commonwealth Serum Laboratories have developed an antivenin (2000 U per ampoule) against scorpionfish venom; the dose depends on the quantity of the injected venom which is related to the number of inflicted punctures: one ampoule for every two punctures.

Sea snake and blue-ringed octopus bites and conidi stings

Taking into account that there is time (hours) before the systemic symptoms appear, transfer to a hospital is mandatory. However, the prognosis is strongly influenced by the manoeuvres carried out during first aid which consists of the avoidance of venom spread from the wounded area (usually a limb), through the lymphatics to the circulatory system. The incision of the bitten area or any attempts at cleansing the wound can only increase the absorpion of the venom. The most effective measure is to apply immediately a compression bandage starting over the bitten site and covering the whole limb. The compression must allow regular arterial and deep venous flow. Moreover to reduce the muscular pump it is important to immobilize and splint the limb. Care at the medical centre includes the following:

- clinical examination with emphasis on neurological signs
- support of the respiratory and cardiocirculatory functions (if necessary)
- laboratory studies including blood count, creatinine, electrolytes, muscle enzymes, blood gases and urine (myoglobinuria)
- venom detection in blood and urine or from the wounded area
- remove the compressive bandage and control the patient for respiratory or cardiovascular insufficiences.

No specific antidote is available against the potent tetrodotoxin present in the salivary glands of the blue-ringed octopus. For sea snake bite the Commonwealth Serum Laboratories have prepared an antivenin (Australian Sea Snake Antivenom) indicated in cases with systemic neuromuscular signs. Subcutaneous injection of 0.25–0.5 mg epinephrine and i.v. injection of 10 mg promethazine are recommended before the i.v. injection of the antivenin.

Sponges

In order to remove the stings from the skin, the application of scotch tape can represent an immediate cure. This measure must be followed by medication with isoprophilic alcohol.

Seaweed and sea moss

Treatment is with topical or systemic steroids (depending on the intensity of the skin reaction).

Further reading

Burnett JW, Calton GJ, Burnett HW. Jellyfish envenomation syndromes. *J Am Acad Dermatol* 1986; 14: 100–6.

Burnett JW, Calton GJ, Burnett HW, Mandojana RM. Local and systemic reactions from jellyfish stings. In: Mandojana RM, ed. *Clinics in Dermatology: Aquatic Dermatology*. Philadelphia: Lippincott, 1987.

Solar urticaria

M. Jeanmougin

Definition

Solar urticaria (SU) is a rare photosensitivity disorder, characterized by itching, erythema and whealing immediatly after exposure to sunlight or artificial radiation. It is an acquired condition, without familial incidence. There is a slight preponderance in females (60%). The peak age is between 20 and 30 years.

Aetiology and pathophysiology

In the majority of cases, the cause is unknown. Some exogenous substances can induce solar urticarial reactions such as tar, chlorpromazine, repirinast and tetracycline.

Although its exact mechanism remains unknown, evidence supports the immunological nature of SU. From a chromophore, present in the skin or in the circulation, irradiation-induced chemical changes to form a photoproduct (photoallergen) that elicits urticaria. Depending on the results of the *in vitro* serum test and passive and reverse passive transfer tests, two types of SU are distinguished:

- type I, immunoglobulin E (IgE)-mediated hypersensitivity to specific photoallergens, which are generated only in patients with SU
- type II, induction of IgE-mediated hypersensitivity to a non-specific photoallergen, which is generated both in patients with SU and in normal persons.

The wavelengths responsible for SU usually fall between 290 and 700 nm, essentially visible light in 60% of cases.

Clinical characteristics and course

Within 5–10 min of exposure to sunlight (occasionally to an artificial light source), patients experience itching, erythma and patchy or confluent whealing, fading spontaneously within about 1 h.

Urticaria develops only in irradiated skin, although clinical lesions may appear under clothing if it transmits an adequate amount of light. Chronically exposed skin (face, arms) is generally less likely to be involved than areas normally covered. Fixed SU is a peculiar type, strictly limited to the same circumscribed skin areas.

In some cases, serious complications exist such as systemic symptoms (nausea, anxiety, abdominal cramps), loss of consciousness, and severe anaphylactic shock.

SU may remit spontaneously, but it generally persists for years, and some patients continue to react after decades of photosensitivity.

Diagnosis

- Phototesting is the most certain means of reproducing the clinical features and thus asserting the diagnosis of SU. Irradiation using a solar simulator equipped with a monochromator determine the action spectrum and the minimal urticarial dose (MUD) for each triggering spectral band. Lasers may be useful tools in performing visible phototesting, especially at longer wavelengths.
- All solar wavelengths can be effective for SU induction: rarely ultraviolet (UV) B (290–320 mn) alone, frequently UVA (320–400 nm) or mainly blue–violet range of visible light (400–500 nm). The urticarial reaction may be inhibited by immediate reirradiation with UVA or visible light (inhibition spectrum). The diversity of the action spectra reported in the literature can be attributed to differences in photoallergens.

Differential diagnosis

- Protoporphyria: erythrocyte protoporphyrin levels.
- Polymorphous light eruption: the eruption starts a few hours to several days after sun exposure and may last a week or more; phototesting.
- Photocontact dermatitis: the acute aspects, from erythema to bullae, resolve in days to weeks.

Treatment

General therapeutic guidelines

It will not be possible to approach treatment at the level of a fundamental mechanism until the aetiological photoantigens are known. No specific therapy is currently available for SU.

Avoidance of all sun exposure is effective but impractical for most patients.

Treatment is difficult, but some techniques have afforded some patients substantial or total relief, even if only temporarily.

Recommended therapies

Sun protective measures

Avoidance of the sun and use of high-protective clothing fabrics are highly recommended. For patients whose sensitivity is primarily in the UV range, some commercial broad-spectrum sunscreens increase MUDs. However, these sunscreens must provide highly efficient filtering properties, not only in the UVB but also in the UVA range of the solar spectrum. Unfortunately, the amount of increase of MUD is generally too little to be of practical significance. A patient reacting to other wavelengths than UV, such as visible light, will not benefit at all.

H1-blocking antihistamines

High doses of non-sedating H1-blocking antihistamines are our first-line treatment, with a success rate of 70%. The therapeutic effect seems to vary considerably from one patient to another. Terfenadine (240 mg/day) has been prescribed widely but has been withdrawn from Europe, and replaced by fexofenadine. Thirty minutes prior to sun exposure, high doses of cetirizine (20 mg/day) or loratadine (10 mg/day) may be of benefit. After irradiation, erythema may appear immediately, but without wheal formation.

Hardening phenomenon

Light hardening by phototherapy, using repeated exposure to UVA or visible light, or repeated exposures to sunlight are established methods to induce tolerance, possibly due to the exhaustion of chemical mediators. However, this hardening phenomenon is short-lived, lasting up to 48 h, so maintenance treatment is required.

Oral photochemotherapy

The combination of psoralen and UVA radiation (PUVA) can be helpful in SU. Experimentally, PUVA treatment inhibits mast cell degranulation and the release of chemical mediators. Three treatments weekly for 8 weeks are used in a clearing phase, followed by a maintenance phase of one PUVA treatment weekly. The recommended 8-methoxypsoralen dose is 0.6 mg/kg and should be taken orally 2 h before UVA exposure. The initial dose is given according to skin type or at 80% of the MUD in those persons sensitive to UVA radiation. Low-dose UVA 0.1–0.25 J/cm^2 is initially necessary to avoid causing a rash.

PUVA is our second-line treatment, but maintenance therapy is required. Whereas patients can tolerate less than 15 min of sun exposure before therapy, they are able to tolerate more than 2 h of exposure after PUVA. They are advised to have 1 h of sun exposure three times weekly during the summer months to maintain tolerance.

When a patient is sensitive in the UVA range, UVB phototherapy may be effective, using narrow-band UVB or broadband UVB. Pre-PUVA UVA desensitization may be tried.

Alternative and experimental treatments

Plasmapheresis

Plasmapheresis is known to reduce the symptoms of SU in those patients with detectable levels of circulating photoallergen. However, it has potentially severe side-effects, such as inducing anaphylactoid reactions. In exceptional cases, when conventional treatments have failed for highly debilitating SU, plasmapheresis has been tried and resulted in decreasing patient photosensitivity to such an extent that PUVA treatment was successful and a long period of remission was enjoyed.

Miscellaneous agents

There are sporadic reports of patients being helped by treatment with antimalarial drugs, betacarotene, cimetidine and doxepin. In our experience, synthetic antimalarials, carotenoids, nicotinamide or gammaglobulins are ineffective.

Very severe cases could be treated with ciclosporin or intravenous immunoglobulins.

Further reading

Bilsland D, Ferguson J. A comparison of cetirizine and terfenadine in the management of solar urticaria. *Photodermatol Photoimmunol Photomed* 1991; 8: 62–4.

Collins P, Ahamat R, Green C, Ferguson J. Plasma exchange therapy for solar urtacaria. *Br J Dermatol* 1996; 134: 1093–7.

Collins P, Ferguson J. Narrow-band UVB (TL-01) phototherapy: an effective preventative treatment for the photodermatoses. *Br J Dermatol* 1995; 132: 956–63.

Dawe RS, Fergusson J. Prolonged benefit following ultra-violet A phototherapy for solar urticaria. *Br J Dermatol* 1997; 137: 144–8.

Edström DW, Ros AM. Cyclosporin A therapy for severe solar urticaria. *Photodermatol Photoimmunol Photomed* 1997; 13: 61–3.

Harris A, Burge SM, George SA. Solar urticaria in an infant. *Br J Dermatol* 1997; 136: 105–7.

Hudson-Peacock MJ, Farr PM, Diffey BL, Goodship THJ. Combined treatment of solar urticaria with plasmapheresis and PUVA. *Br J Dermatol* 1993; 128: 440–2.

Kobza A, Ramsay CA, Magnus IA. Oral betacarotene therapy in actinic reticuloid and solar urticaria. *Br J Dermatol* 1973; 88: 157–66.

Machet L, Vaillant L, Muller C *et al.* Traitement par UVB thérapie d'une urticaire solaire induite par les UVA. *Ann Dermatol Venereol* 1991; 118: 535–7.

Monfrecola G, Masturzo E, Riccardo AM, del Sorbo M. Cetirizine for solar urticaria in the visible spectrum. *Dermatology* 2000; 200: 334–5.

Monfrecola G, Masturzo E *et al.* Solar urticaria: a report on 57 cases. *Am J Cont Dermatol* 2000; 11: 89–94.

Neittaanmaki M, Jaaskelainen T, Harvima RJ, Fraki JE. Solar urticaria: demonstration of histamine release and effective treatment with doxepin. *Photodermatology* 1989; 6: 52–5.

Nocera T, Peyron JL, Moyal D *et al.* Protection contre l'urticaire solaire par les filtres: une méthode de détermination du coefficient de protection UVA. *Nouv Dermatol* 1998; 17: 301–4.

Puech-Plottova I, Michel JL, Rouchouse B *et al.* Urticaire solaire: un cas traité par immunoglobulines polyvalentes. *Ann Dermatol Venereol* 2000; 127: 831–5.

Roelandts R, Ryckaert S. Solar urticaria: the annoying photodermatosis. *Int J Dermatol* 1999; 38: 411–18.

Sams WM. Chloroquine: its use in photosensitive eruptions. *Int J Dermatol* 1986; 15: 99–111.

Schwarze HP, Marguery MC, Journe F *et al.* Fixed solar urticaria to visible light successfully treated with fexofenadine. *Photodermatol Photoimmunol Photomed* 2001; 17: 39–41.

Uetsu N, Miyauchi-Hashimoto H, Okamoto H, Horio T. The clinical and photobiological characteristics of solar urticaria in 40 patients. *Br J Dermatol* 2000; 142: 32–8.

Squamous cell carcinoma

B. Giannotti and V. De Giorgi

Synonyms

Epithelioma spinocellulare, spinocellular carcinoma, spinalioma.

Definition and epidemiology

Cutaneous squamous cell carcinoma (SCC) is a malignant tumour arising from epidermal keratinocytes, that grows in a destructive way and metastasizes mainly via the lymphatic system.

It is less common than basal cell carcinoma (ratio about 1 : 5) and the overall incidence among white Caucasians is 20–200 per 100 000/year, with great variations from one geographical area to another.

Aetiology and pathophysiology

Several predisposing and/or pathogenic factors for the occurrence of this tumour are known, including ultraviolet (UV) radiation, chronic inflammatory skin changes, chemical carcinogens, immunosuppression and viral infections.

Descriptive studies show that the incidence of SCC is maximal in populations in which sun exposure and skin (epidermal) transmission of solar radiation are high, and doubles with each 8–10 degree decrement in geographical latitude, being highest at the equator. Fair-skinned populations, particularly those who sunburn easily and tan poorly, are definitely at higher risk. This suggests a strong association of SCC with chronic, repeated sun exposure.

Analytical epidemiological studies confirm that exposure to the UV component of sunlight is the major environmental determinant of skin cancers and associated skin alterations, and evidence of a causal association between cumulative sun exposure and SCC, actinic keratoses and photodamage is relatively straightforward. Complementary to epidemiological data is the molecular evidence of UV-related mechanisms of carcinogenesis, such as UV-specific mutations in the DNA of tumour-suppressor genes. With increased UV irradiation resulting from the thinning of the ozone layer, skin cancer incidence rates are predicted to increase unless, as is hoped, human behaviour to reduce sun exposure can offset this predicted rise.

An increased risk of SCC in patients who have received long-term PUVA therapy has been reported in USA. The spontaneous course of PUVA-induced malignancies has not been documented, to the best of our knowledge. However, the principles of UV-induced carcinogenesis clearly indicate that damage is permanent and that repeated UV exposure exerts its biological effect in accordance with a cumulative dose–response curve.

The incidence of SCC, like that of other malignant neoplasms, is significantly increased in immunosuppressed patients. In organ-transplant recipients (kidney, heart, etc.), a higher frequency of malignant tumours, including SCC, is observed.

Ciclosporin A, the prototype immunosuppressive drug, may result in an increased occurrence of SCC, especially when associated with PUVA treatment.

SCC may develop *de novo*, although this is not at all frequent. Indeed, chronic skin injury is an important cofactor in its development. SCC occurs almost exclusively on chronically injured skin, either directly or via precancerous lesions: actinic keratoses (more frequently, although with a relatively low malignant potential, estimated to be about 5–10%), burn scars and chronic radiodermatitis, the latter especially via radiation-induced keratoses (the potential of malignant transformation increases to 30%); sinus tracts;

lupus vulgaris or chronic discoid lupus erythematosus scars; lichen sclerosus et atrophicus; and chronic leg ulcers.

Exposure to chemical carcinogens (arsenic, polycyclic aromatic hydrocarbons) predisposes to the development of SCC in the skin. In this case, *in situ* carcinomas (Bowen's disease, erythroplasia of Queyrat, malignant leukoplakia) generally precede invasive SCC. Viruses of the human papillomavirus group possibly play a role in the aetiology of some SCCs.

Clinical characteristics and course

The most common sites are the face, neck, dorsum of the hands and lower lip. The typical lesion is an indurated, firm, raised, skin-coloured or pink to red nodule, whose growth can progress rapidly when extensive ulcerative necrosis occurs. On the lips or genitalia, the presenting sign may be a fissure or small erosion or ulcer which fails to heal and bleeds recurrently. As the ulceration proceeds, the lesion may be covered by a crust, or merely present a raw granular surface which bleeds readily. The margins of induration are usually poorly defined.

In general, these lesions pursue one of two clinical courses: either they develop as an exuberant cauliflower-like growth or they progress as an invasive tumour with infiltration of adjacent tissues. The former tends to be more differentiated with less tendency to metastasize, the latter less differentiated with more tendency to metastasize. Well-differentiated tumours may have a hyperkeratotic cap.

SCC mainly spread first into the regional lymph nodes, and only later into distant nodes and/or visceral organs. The lymph nodes are enlarged and hard; then, the tumour invades the surroundings, and becomes fixed.

The frequency of metastases in SCC ranges substantially between 5% and 40%, depending on the degree of differentiation, site (mucosal SCCs have a worse prognosis), histological type, size, depth, and associated immunosuppression. Locally recurrent tumours have a higher metastatic rate.

The 5-year rate of recurrence after excision of low-risk primary cutaneous lesions is 8%, but large lesions (> 2 cm in diameter) recur at a rate of 15% (which is twice that of smaller lesions) and have a three times higher likelihood of metastatic spread.

To define the extent of invasion of the tumour (local, regional or distant) staging procedures are needed: clinical examination, X-rays, ultrasound, computed tomography (CT) scan, or magnetic resonance imaging (MRI).

Diagnosis/laboratory examinations

The diagnosis of SCC, although easily made in typical cases, may sometimes be difficult. Histological examination is mandatory to confirm the clinical diagnosis, and may give useful information for the choice of proper treatment: e.g. surgery or electrodesiccation plus curettage for well-differentiated tumours, surgery or radiotherapy for poorly differentiated ones.

Histologically, SCC consists of irregular masses of epidermal cells that proliferate downward into the dermis. The invading tumour masses are composed in varying proportions of normal to anaplastic, eosinophilic squamous cells. The more the tumour is malignant, the lower is keratinization and the higher is the number of atypical squamous cells. Atypicality of squamous cells expresses itself as a great variability in size and shape of the cells, hyperplasia and hyperchromasia of the nuclei, keratinization of individual cells, and presence of atypical mitotic figures. The prognosis of perineural and/or lymphatic invasion is poor.

Differential diagnosis

The SCC must be differentiated from keratoacanthoma, basal cell carcinoma, actinic keratosis, seborrhoeic keratoses, warty dyskeratoma, pseudoepitheliomatous epidermal hyperplasia, amelanotic malignant melanoma, and Merkel cell tumours.

Treatment

General therapeutic guidelines

The aim of the treatment of SCC can be stated simply, as follows: to eliminate the disease and to secure the best functional and cosmetic result. The main accepted modes of treatment are: surgery, radiotherapy, electrosurgery, cryosurgery and chemotherapy. All these modalities of treatment have their place. The choice depends on tumour features, i.e. location, shape, size, invasion into deeper tissues, histologic pattern of differentiation, as well as on individual familiarity and skill of the clinician with the technique. Five-year recurrence rates from 2 to 53% are reported in the literature with different modalities of treatment.

Surgery is probably the most suitable treatment of SCC at present. In many countries, however, radiotherapy is widely used to treat SCC.

Electrodesiccation and curettage are used alternatively to destroy the tumour and an extra margin of clinically unaffected skin. This process may be repeated several times. In this way, however, no specimen of surrounding tissue is available for histological examination in order to judge the complete removal of the tumour. This modality is best suited for small (less than 1 cm) low-risk superficial tumours.

Cryosurgery may be used in small SCC when other surgical treatments are refused by the patient or contraindicated, particularly in patients with bleeding disorders.

Systemic chemotherapy (most often with Bleomycin) can be used when radical excision is not possible, or preoperatively to reduce tumour mass, and of course in metastasized tumours. Polychemotherapy is currently used in selected cases.

Treatment of metastasis may involve radiation, lymph-node dissection, or both.

Recommended therapies

At present, there is no agreement on the optimal procedure to treat SCC. Generally, the position is that SCC should be treated by surgery.

Surgical excision is useful for both primary and recurrent lesions. It is the treatment of choice when cartilage or bone are invaded. Its advantages are the histological assessment of surgical margins and rapid healing. It is difficult to define precise limits for the margin of normal tissue to be included in the excision. Experienced surgeons develop a sensitivity in this decision based on their knowledge of this particular tumour and previous experience with such excisions (when their assessment of a safe margin has been confirmed or proved wrong by the pathologist's report or by local recurrence). In addition, the limits for the margin of normal tissue are influenced by the anatomical site: it is obvious that one can include the wider limits where ample tissue is available, but one may need to stay within the lower limits where a more radical excision would sacrifice vital structures and impose serious disability or disfigurement. However, a margin of 4–6 mm (depending on the site, size and depth of the tumour) around the clinical border of the lesion is recommended.

Mohs' surgery has established itself as the optimal technique for a high cure rate of SCC occurring on the face. However, after resection carried out with Mohs' technique, the defects, when extensive, require careful planned reconstruction in order to produce a good cosmetic result. While flap reconstruction is available for smaller lesions, larger defects are often covered by expansion techniques. However, recurrence rates following Mohs' surgery are lower than after non-Mohs' surgery. Mohs' micrographic surgery should be the first choice for incompletely excised or recurrent SCC and primary SCC at high risk because of clinical and/or histological factors: size >2 cm, ulceration, poor differentiation, anatomic location, rapid growth, invasion into deeper tissues, perineural and/or lympathic invasion.

Even if SCC is a radiosensitive tumour, radiotherapy is usually preferred when other techniques cannot be performed for definitive treatment of selected cases (elderly patients, location on head and neck, poorly differentiated histological pattern) and for palliation of inoperable tumours. Fractionation of radiation is preferred to a simple high dose.

Alternative and experimental treatments

Cutaneous SCC is not as sensitive as basal cell carcinoma to photodynamic therapy (PDT) with 5-aminolevulinic acid (ALA) or haematoporphyrin derivative (HPD). The average rate of complete response is around 70%. This could be explained not just by tumour insensitivity to PDT, but rather by insufficient concentration of sensitizer in the target tissue and by poor penetration of light. In this regard, new compounds such as benzoporphyrin derivative-monoacid ring A (BPD-MA), tin ethyl etiopurpurin (SnET2) and N-aspartyl-chlorine-6 (NPe6) could yield promising results since they show good tumour selectivity and are activated by deeper penetrating wavelengths (660–690 nm). So far PDT is considered a new approach. The high number of recently created photosensitizers clearly points to forthcoming practical applications. The penetration of topically applied substances can be improved with better vehicles, liposomal formulations, esterified derivatives. The combination of PDT with surgery could improve cure rates and cosmetic results. All the above-mentioned considerations show PDT to be a promising treatment modality for SCC with a good potential for future development.

Further reading

Alam M, Ratner D. Cutaneous squamous-cell carcinoma. *N Engl J Med* 2001; 344: 975–83.

Bernstein SC, Lim KK, Brodland DG *et al.* The many faces of squamous cell carcinoma. *Dermatol Surg* 1996; 22(3): 243–54.

Braun-Falco O, Plewig G, Wolff HH *et al. Dermatology.* Berlin: Springer-Verlag, 1991.

Ceburkov O, Gollnickc H. Photodynamic therapy in dermatology. *Eur J Dermatol* 2000; 10: 568–76.

Green A, Whiteman D, Frost C *et al.* Sun exposure, skin cancers and related skin conditions. *J Epidemiol* 1999; 9 (6 Suppl.): S7–13.

Hodgkinson DJ, Lam Q. Expansion techniques after Mohs'surgery on the face. *Australas J Dermatol* 2001; 42(1): 9–14.

Lever WF, Schaumburg-Lever G. *Histopathology of the Skin.* Philadelphia: Lippincott, 1983.

Peng Q, Warloe T, Berg K *et al.* 5-Amino-levulinic acid-based photodynamic therapy. *Cancer* 1997; 79: 2282–308.

Roseeuw D, Katsambas AD. Squamous cell carcinoma. In: Katsambas AD, Lotti TM, eds. *European Handbook of Dermatological Treatments.* Berlin: Springer, 1999.

Stern RS, Laid N, Melski J *et al.* Cutaneous squamous-cell carcinoma in patients treated with PUVA. *N Engl J Med* 1984; 310: 1156–61.

Van De Kerkhof PCM, De Rooij MJM. Multiple squamous cell carcinomas in a psoriatic patient following high-dose photochemotherapy and cyclosporin treatment: response to long-term acitrein maintenance. *Br J Dermatol* 1997; 136: 275–8

Subacute cutaneous lupus erythematosus

M.N. Manoussakis and H.M. Moutsopoulos

Definition and epidemiology

Subacute cutaneous lupus erythematosus (SCLE) represents a relatively distinct and homogeneous subset of lupus erythematosus (LE) identified by chronic and recurrent development of characteristic erythematous, non-scarring and mostly photosensitive skin lesions associated with particular clinical, immunological and genetic features. SCLE-specific cutaneous lesions include the papulosquamous–psoriasiform eruption and the annular-polycyclic erythema. These are found in approximately 10% of total LE patients and affect predominantly white Caucasian women of all ages. In addition, a significant proportion of patients with SCLE eruptions may have Sjögren's syndrome (SS). Extracutaneous manifestations are usually, but not always, mild. Serum autoantibodies to Ro (SSA) cellular antigen that occur in approximately 25–30% of total systemic lupus erythematosus (SLE) patients, are more common in SCLE (found in 60–70%) suggesting that SCLE comprises roughly 30–40% of all anti-Ro (SSA) positive patients. Approximately 50% of anti-Ro (SSA) positive SCLE patients display also serum anti-La (SSB) antibodies. Associations of SCLE with HLA-DR3, HLA-DR2 as well as C4 null alleles have been also reported. Finally, besides SLE and SS, a number of other systemic diseases that have been described to precede, to coincide with or to follow the onset of SCLE include rheumatoid arthritis (RA), porphyria cutanea tarda, Sweet's syndrome, malabsorption, gluten-sensitive enteropathy, hereditary angioedema and various malignancies, including malignant melanoma, lung, breast and gastric cancer.

Aetiology and pathophysiology

The majority of SCLE patients are photosensitive. Coincidental exposure to ultraviolet (UV) radiation, including both UVB and psoralen–UVA photochemotherapy has been reportedly associated with the development of SCLE. In addition, several drugs have been incriminated for the development of SCLE-specific lesions, including hydrochlorothiazide, procainamide, d-penicillamine, gold salts, sulfonylureas, spironolactone, piroxicam, naproxen, oxyprenolol, griseofulvin, diltiazem, and cilizapril. Although humoral mechanisms, typically represented by anti-Ro (SSA) antibody, are likely important, keratinocytes from SCLE patients reportedly show enhanced cytotoxicity to ultraviolet radiation and to antibody-mediated cytotoxicity. UV light as well as distinct genetic polymorphisms are thought to contribute to the accumulation of inflammatory cells in lesions by the *in situ* upregulation of cytokines and the induction of expression of selectins, adhesion and costimulatory molecules.

Clinical characteristics and course

SCLE lesions often evolve from erythematous macules or papules that eventually present as either the papulosquamous–psoriasiform or the annular–polycyclic type of eruptions. A few patients may have a combination of them. In addition, a pityriasiform rash has also been described. The analysis of clinical and serological features of patients presenting with papulosquamous and of those with annular lesions had not reveal significant or consistent differences between these two subtypes of SCLE. The distribution of SCLE eruptions is predominantly in sun-exposed regions but often extend to photoprotected areas as well. Regions most frequently involved are the upper back, the shoulders, the V-area of the neck, the dorsal arms and forearms, whereas face, scalp and lower extremities are usually, but not always, spared. Morphologically, in contrast to typical discoid lupus erythematosus (DLE) lesions, scales in SCLE eruptions are superficial and non-atrophic, with minimal or absent follicular plugging or adherent hyperkeratosis. Papulosquamous eruptions usually evolve to form psoriasiform plaques. Annular erythematous lesions of SCLE tend to coalesce with frequent formation of polycyclic patterns consisted of borders with significant basal cell degeneration generating crusting and vesiculation that leave less active central areas with subtle greyish hypopigmentation and telangiectasia. Despite their tendency to exacerbate and remit for many years, SCLE lesions have an indolent course and generally, scarring does not occur. Most lesions often resolve leaving hypopigmentation that may fade or remain as vitiligo-like changes, whereas telangiectasias may persist indefinitely. Progression of annular SCLE lesions to morphoea-like plaques has been also reported. Rarely, more severe SCLE has been observed manifesting toxic epidermal necrolysis-like lesions and exfoliative erythroderma.

Patients with SCLE eruptions may also manifest other types of LE-specific lesions. Approximately 20% of SCLE patients also have typical DLE lesions that often predate the onset of SCLE lesions. In addition, 15% of SCLE patients may also present acute cutaneous LE (ACLE) rushes, such as malar erythema. In addition, a variety of LE non-specific skin lesions may coincide with SCLE eruptions, including mucosal ulcers, alopecia, livedo reticularis, periungual telangiectasia, vasculitic lesions and Raynaud's phenomenon. Approximately half of SCLE patients fulfil the American College of Rheumatology criteria for SLE, however, features of systemic disease are usually mild, most frequently illustrated by musculoskeletal complaints and serological abnormalities. Serious central nervous system (CNS) or kidney involvement are relatively uncommon. Nevertheless, severe extracutaneous involvement, such as nephritis, may develop in a few patients during disease course, particularly in those with coexisting ACLE lesions. Distal renal tubular acidosis with hypokalaemia may be encountered, often as a manifestation of associated SS.

Diagnosis

The diagnosis of SCLE is mainly established on clinical grounds by the identification of either of the two typically non-scarring and mostly photosensitive types of eruptions.

Supportive tests

- Given their high incidence among patients with SCLE lesions, assessment should include tests for serum antinuclear antibodies (ANA, by indirect immunofluorescence on human epithelial cell substrate) and for anti-Ro (SSA) and anti-La (SSB) antibodies (by counterimmunoelectrophoresis or double immunodiffusion using extracted cellular antigens as substrate).
- Skin biopsies from SCLE lesions (usually unnecessary) show histopathology specific for LE, but largely indistiguishable from ACLE or DLE. Findings include variable degrees of hyperkeratosis, basal cell degeneration, dermal oedema and mononuclear infiltrates usually limited to the perivascular and adnexal structures of the upper dermis. Approximately 70% of patients display immune deposits (IgM, IgG and/or IgA and complement components) in a granular band-pattern along dermal–epidermal junctions at both lesional and non-lesional areas. 'Dust-like particle' IgG deposits in and around

epidermal keratinocytes have been also described in some patients, possibly associated with *in vivo* anti-Ro (SSA) antibody deposition.

Differential diagnosis

- DLE lesions: atrophic, with heavy follicular plugging and hyperkeratosis.
- Psoriasis: distribution, non-photosensitive, negative serology.
- Lichen planus: distribution, non-photosensitive, negative serology.
- Associated systemic disease: history, symptoms and physical findings.
- Drug eruptions: history, reversibility upon drug discontinuation, usually negative serology.

Treatment

General therapeutic guidelines

Education of patients to employ photoprotective measures is of paramount importance. Exposure to sun, particularly during midday hours, as well as to artificial UV light exposure should be generally avoided on a reasonable basis. Patients should be advised to use sun-protective clothing in conjunction with broad-spectrum sunscreens with high sun-protective factor (SPF, of 15 or greater), whenever they go outdoors, even on cloudy days. Broadest range of UV protection is offered by preparations that contain avobenzone and titanium dioxide. Several commercially available cosmetics provide both highly effective photoprotection and suitable masking results. Additional measures may include the application of UV-blocking films in house and car windows and rational avoidance of UV radiation-emitting appliances such as fluorescent light bulbs and photocopiers. Patients should be also instructed to avoid UV light exposure reflected by surfaces such as sand, water, snow or pavements. Finally, the potentially photosensitizing drugs mentioned above should be avoided as possible.

Recommended therapies

Local and oral corticosteroids

In most patients, topical corticosteroid preparations (fluocinonide tape, clobetasole propionate 0.05%, betamethasone dipropionate 0.05%, diflorasone diacetate 0.05% or amcinonide 0.01%) given alone may provide some benefit, however this is often proven inadequate. In addition, local application of corticosteroids carries the risk of regional atrophy, telangiectasia, striae and acne that are more frequent upon prolonged usage and particularly on sensitive areas such as the face. Therefore, whenever prescribed, patients should be directed to use them in a cyclical fashion, twice daily for no more than a 2-week period, followed by 2 weeks of rest from application. Ointments are generally preferred for dry skin and creams for oily skin. Fluorinated forms are stronger and more prone to induce atrophic changes, and thus should be avoided for the face. Intralesional application of potent topical steroids (such as triamcinolone acetonide 2.5–5.0 mg/mL), although effective and particularly helpful for a resistant lesion, may be also complicated by local atrophy and hypopigmentation and it is generally impractical for most patients with multiple lesions.

Oral corticosteroids should be generally avoided for the treatment of SCLE lesions. Exception to this rule is an occasional patient with widespread SCLE lesions where more immediate relief is required. In that case, a short 'burst' of oral steroids can be prescribed as an adjunct to other forms of therapy instituted. A scheme proposed involves the administration of 30 mg/day of prednisone for one week followed by 20 mg/day for 7 days and then 10 mg/day for additional 10 days before complete discontinuation.

Antimalarials

The orally administered aminoquinoline antimalarial drugs (hydroxychloroquine sulfate, chloroquine phosphate and quinacrine hydrochloride) currently represent the first-line systemic drugs and the mainstay of treatment of SCLE lesions. Approximately 80% of patients respond promptly to a single agent or combined antimalarial therapy. The slow-acting anti-inflammatory effects of these drugs are believed to be associated with their accumulation in the epidermis. In general, hydroxychloroquine appears the best tolerated with least side-effects, whereas some patients may show more adequate response to one antimalarial drug over the others. Therapy is usually started with hydroxychloroquine at 400 mg/day in two divided doses. Maximum effect of the antimalarial is usually delayed by approximately 1 month, therefore a combination of hydroxychloroquine with a short 'burst' with oral steroids (as described above) may be applied whenever a more immediate therapeutic benefit is needed. If significant improvement has occurred by the end of 1–2 months of treatment, the dose of hydroxychloroquine can be reduced to 200 mg once daily. After 2–3 years with remission, slow tapering to 200 or 400 mg/week may be justified. Alternatively, if lesions are still resistant after a 2-month period of treatment with 400 mg hydroxychloroquine/day, quinacrine 100 mg/day can be added in the regimen. If response is not attained by 4–6 weeks of hydroxychloroquine plus quinacrine, hydroxychloroquine can be substituted by chloroquine 250 mg/day, while continuing quinacrine. Smoking has been shown to interfere with the efficacy of antimalarial therapy.

Hydroxychloroquine and chloroquine (but reportedly not quinacrine) have been associated with a risk for retinal toxicity. However, doses up to 6 mg/kg per day of hydroxychloroquine (or 4 mg/kg per day of chloroquine) are associated with minimal risk for retinopathy. Nevertheless, a baseline ophthalmological evaluation prior to the institution of therapy and regularly thereof at 6-month intervals during treatment, is advised. Evaluation should include fundoscopy, visual fields (including central field testing with a red object) and visual acuity testing. Prior to antimalarial therapy, patients (particularly those with African or Mediterranean ancestry) should be tested for glucose-6-phosphate dehydrogenase (G6PD) deficiency. It has been shown that quinacrine hydrochloride more frequently induces haemolysis in G6PD-deficient individuals than hydroxychloroquine or chloroquine. Blue–black pigmentation of the skin (particularly in sun-exposed regions) as well as on the palatal mucosa and nails can be induced by antimalarial therapy. Rarely, hair-bleaching may occur. The use of quinacrine is associated with a diffuse yellowish appearance of the skin, sclerae and bodily secretions that are fully reversible upon discontinuation of the drug. Severe bone marrow toxicity preceded by lichenoid eruption has been described with administration of quinacrine. In patients receiving antimalarials, haematological and hepatic function tests should be obtained periodically for occasional idiosyncratic reactions. Neurotoxic and proximal myopathic reactions to antimalarials seen more often in the past (when significantly higher doses were administered) are infrequently occurring.

Dapsone

Dapsone (diaminodiphenylsulfone) has been successfully employed in the treatment of SCLE lesions unresponsive to antimalarials. Significant improvement is seen in approximately 50% of SCLE patients within a few weeks of treatment, but relapses are not uncommon and rashes may occasionaly worsen, possibly due to its sulfa component. Initial dosage is 25–50 mg/day that can be increased up to 150 mg/day, whereas higher doses may precipitate a mononucleosis-like syndrome. A compensated haemolytic anaemia is regularly seen, that can be improved by concurrent administration of 800 U of vitamin E daily. Prior to the administration of the drug, patients should be assessed for G6PD deficiency for the avoidance of significant haemolytic anaemia. Because of the risk of pancytopenia and resulting aplastic anaemia complete blood counts should be obtained every 2–3 weeks for the first 6 months of therapy. In addition, patients should be regularly monitored for potential renal and hepatic toxicity.

Retinoids

Synthetic vitamin A analogues such as isotretinoin, etretinate and acitretin (in a dosage of 1 mg/kg per day) have been also demonstrated to be highly effective in the treatment of refractory SCLE lesions. Dose-related mucosal dryness is common to all of these drugs, as well as phototoxic reactions that necessitate regular photoprotective measures. Temporary hair loss and peeling of the palms and soles are also frequently seen with administration of etretinate. Retinoids are known to cross readily the placenta and may lead to serious teratogenic effects, particularly in the first trimester of pregnancy. Therefore, the practice of strict birth-control strategies is recommended. Other potential adverse effects from retinoids include a risk for hypercholesterolaemia, hypertriglyceridaemia and drug-induced hepatitis that require periodic laboratory evaluation (every 6–8 weeks). Finally, long-term use of these drugs has been also incriminated for the development of diffuse skeletal hyperostosis (DISH) syndrome.

Thalidomide

Patients with resistant SCLE eruptions have been shown to be highly responsive to thalidomide (100–200 mg/day) and its usage even as a first-line therapy has been advocated by certain centres. However, relapses are common. Adverse reactions include a significantly high incidence of sensory neuropathies (up to 25% in some studies), whereas potential teratogenicity renders birth-control compulsory during treatment of women of child-bearing age. Thrombotic events have been also described.

Alternative and experimental treatments

Clofazimine

Although experience is relatively limited, this drug (at a dose of 100 mg/day) has been reportedly successful and well tolerated in the treatment of annular forms of SCLE lesions. Administration of higher doses should be avoided as they have been associated with the development of severe adverse effects such as splenic infarction and mesenteric artery inclusion. Gastrointestinal intolerance and discoloration of bodily secretions are common side effects, whereas long-term administration of clofazimine often result in hyperpigmentary changes that may ultimately resolve after months or years following discontinuation of the drug.

Gold salts

Gold salts in the form of oral (auranofin) as well as parenteral preparations (aurothiomaleate and aurothioglucose) have been shown beneficial in the treatment of various cutaneous forms of LE resistant to other less toxic therapies. Adverse reactions include haematological, renal, pulmonary as well as mucocutaneous (lichenoid drug eruptions and exfoliative erythroderma) toxicities that obligate regular monitoring of patients. Indirect evidence from treated RA patients indicates that the presence of anti-Ro (SSA) antibodies may be associated with an increased risk for intolerance to the drug.

Systemic corticosteroids and cytotoxic agents

Aggressive systemic therapy with corticosteroids and cytotoxic agents is generally reserved for patients with serious disease that is resistant to other forms of therapy. Occasionally, severe and widespread cutaneous eruptions (e.g. toxic epidermal necrolysis or blistering eruptions) may dictate their usage even as an initial modality. Pulse intravenous methylprednisolone therapy (1 g infused slowly over a 4-h period of time, for 3 consecutive days) has been shown effective in patients with SCLE and systemic manifestations. In addition, azathioprine, cyclophosphamide and methotrexate have been also successfully employed in the treatment of refractory SCLE. Nevertheless, due to potential risks for immunosuppression, cancer induction, bone marrow suppression and other severe adverse effects, decision for application of these agents should always be made on the basis of patient's risk-to-benefit ratio.

Interferon-α

Recombinant interferon α_2 has been employed in the treatment of four SCLE patients ($18–120 \times 10^6$ units injected weekly for 4–13 weeks). Two patients showed complete response, one patient partial response and one patient did not

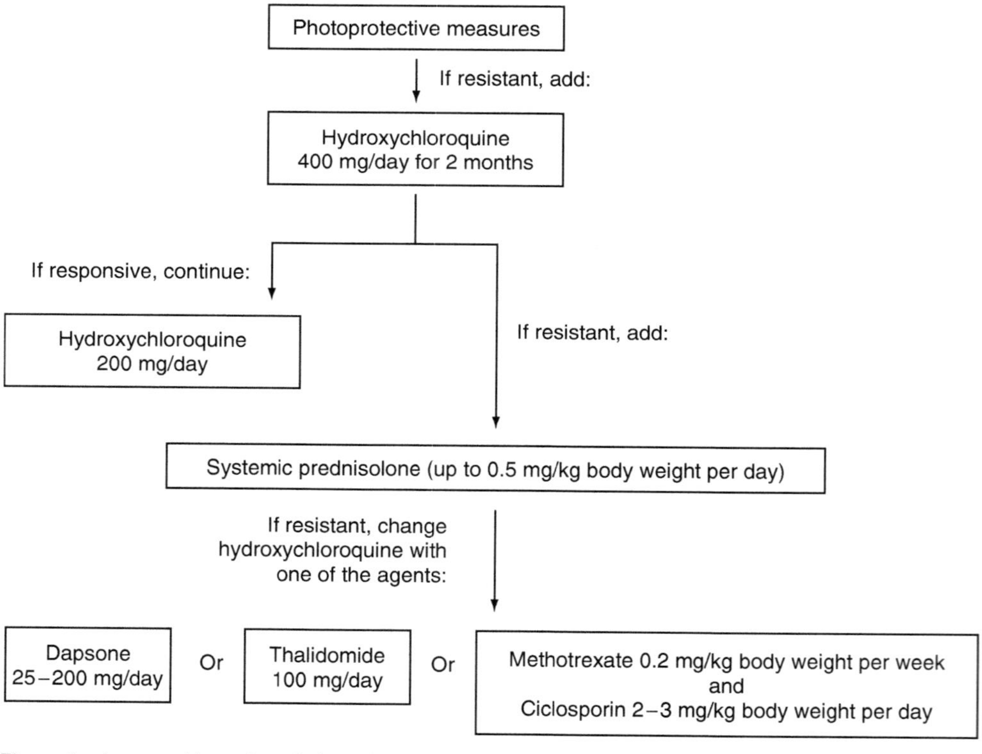

Figure 1 A non-evidence based algorithm that we currently use for the treatment of patients with SCLE. Patients are advised to take sun-protective measures always. If these measures are not adequate, hydroxychloroquine should be started. Since the beneficial effects of this drug may be delayed, it is appropriate to continue treatment for at least 2 months. Patients who fail to respond to antimalarial therapy alone may require the addition of low-dose prednisolone. Finally, in resistant cases, prednisolone in combination with another agent may be also tried, as outlined.

respond at all. All patients who responded to treatment relapsed 4–12 weeks following discontinuation of the drug.

UVA-I phototherapy

Studies in experimental animal models of SLE have indicated a putative immunosuppressive effect of UVA irradiation. Preliminary evidence suggests that patients with SCLE may be improved by irradiation with very low doses of whole-body UVA-I (340–400 nm). Due to the often extreme photosensitivity of SCLE lesions, these results require cautious interpretation and should be confirmed in controlled studies.

Further reading

Chlebus E, Wolska H, Blaszczyk M, Jablonska S. Subacute cutaneous lupus erythematosus versus systemic lupus erythematosus: diagnostic criteria and therapeutic implications. *J Am Acad Dermatol* 1998; 38: 405–12.

Duna GF, Cash JM. Treatment of refractory cutaneous lupus erythematosus. *Rheum Dis Clin N Am* 1995; 21: 99–115.

Fenton DA, Black MM. Low-dose dapsone in the treatment of subacute cutaneous lupus erythematosus. *Clin Exp Dermatol* 1986; 11: 102–3.

Furner BB. Treatment of subacute cutaneous lupus erythematosus. *Int J Dermatol* 1990; 29: 542–7.

Maddison PJ. Nature and nurture in systemic lupus erythematosus. *Adv Exp Med Biol* 1999; 455: 7–13.

Naafs B, Bakkers EJM, Flinterman J, Faber WR. Thalidomide treatment of subacute cutaneous lupus erythematosus. *Br J Dermatol* 1982; 107: 83–6.

Ruzicka T, Sommerburg C, Goerz G, Kind P, Mensing H. Treatment of cutaneous lupus erythematosus with acitretin and hydroxychloroquine. *Br J Dermatol* 1992; 127: 513–18.

Sontheimer RD, Provost TT. Cutaneous manifestations of lupus erythematosus. In: Wallace DJ, Hahn BH, eds. *Dubois' Lupus Erythematosus*, 5th edn. Baltimore: Williams and Wilkins, 1997: 569–623.

Wallace DJ. Occasional, innovative and experimental therapies. In: Wallace DJ, Hahn BH, eds. *Dubois' Lupus Erythematosus*, 5th edn. Baltimore: Williams and Wilkins, 1997: 1191–1202.

Syphilis

M.A. Waugh

Definition and epidemiology

Syphilis is an infectious disease caused by *Treponema pallidum*. If it is not treated, it may run a chronic course, systemic from the outset, capable of involving most organs, and able to simulate many other diseases. It is distinguished by florid manifestations and periods of asymptomatic latency. The majority of cases in adults are venereally acquired, but it can be endemic or sporadic. It may be acquired by congenital transmission. It is transmissible to certain laboratory animals.

The incidence of syphilis in developed countries with adequate health-care systems has declined much in the last 100 years. It is associated with many factors: poorly organized health care, civilian and military unrest, prostitution and poverty, and homosexuality. In recent years in the USA, the incidence has been high in poorer black and Hispanic populations, often associated with crack cocaine. There is much evidence in industrialized countries that since 1996 and the introduction of highly active antiretroviral therapy (HAART) for human immunodeficiency virus (HIV) disease, some groups of male homosexuals have reverted to unsafe sexual practices with the result that sporadic outbreaks of infectious syphilis have been reported in these groups from North America and North Western Europe. In Russia and neighbouring countries, there have been increasing cases of syphilis in the last 12 years. In Asia and Africa sexually transmitted diseases (STDs) and especially those characterized by genital ulceration are epidemiologically associated with HIV infection, with high prevalence rates for both, reported from commercial sex workers (CSW) in African countries and India. Although prostitution is still illegal in China, increasing industrialization has meant that the incidence of syphilis in CSWs has risen there as well.

Aetiology and pathophysiology

T. pallidum is a corkscrew-shaped prokaryotic microorganism, a spirochaete, a class of bacteria with flexible helically coiled cell walls. It cannot be distinguished from *T. carateum* causing pinta or *T. pertenue* causing yaws. Replication is by fission every 30–33 h.

T. pallidum invades mucosal surfaces and abraded skin in humans, colonization taking place at the site of entry, the chancre, or via the lymphatic system to the regional lymph nodes and systemic dissemination. Treponemes attract lymphocytes and plasma cells causing a proliferative endarteritis at blood vessels. Later fibroblasts replace lymphocytes and plasma cells causing fibrosis and scarring.

Although local immune processes appear to bring primary infection under control, secondary syphilis indicates that the host response remains incompletely understood. Altered states of immunity i.e. in HIV infection, may well lead to different responses to *T. pallidum* in the human host, with clinical and therapeutic consequences.

Clinical characteristics and course

Primary syphilis

The incubation period is usually 2–6 weeks occasionally lasting up to 3 months. A chancre develops at the site of entry, together with regional lymphadenopathy. It may be in the anogenital area or mouth.

Secondary syphilis

This may occur 1–6 months after primary syphilis in the untreated person. There are many manifestations, a generalized papulosquamous non-itchy rash being the commonest, often involving the palms and soles. Atypical rashes are found. Other features are patchy alopecia, mucous patches, condylomata lata, lymphadenopathy, fever, headaches, malaise and infrequently, signs of systemic involvement, meningitis, cranial nerve lesions, hepatitis, nephritis and arthralgia.

Latency

Divided into disease ensuing early (<1 year) and late (>1 year).

Tertiary syphilis

This is uncommon where patients are treated or receive by chance antitreponemal antibiotic therapy for other diseases. There has been some evidence recently that in severely immunocompromised individuals with HIV infection, late stages of syphilis such as neurosyphilis either asymptomatic or symptomatic may be more rapid in onset.

In tertiary (late) syphilis, the most common features are gummas involving the liver, skin or bones, late neurosyphilis (tabes dorsalis or general paresis) and cardiovascular syphilis (aortic aneurysm and aortic incompetence).

Congenital syphilis

Transplacental infection results in spontaneous abortion, stillbirth or presentations at or after birth. It is as though an infant often small for dates had severe secondary syphilis. Manifestations may include encephalitis, skin rash, snuffles (osteochondritis of the nasal bones), failure to thrive, pneumonia, hepatomegaly, and later cranial nerve defects. Late congenital syphilis has many skeletal abnormalities. Hutchinson's triad classically occurs—interstitial keratitis, 8th cranial nerve deafness, and Hutchinson's teeth (incisors).

Endemic syphilis

This occurs in conditions of poor hygiene and is rare in Europe, being transmitted in childhood. Examples are being seen again in Eastern Europe, but it is still found in Africa on the fringes of the Tropics and was seen as bejel in the Middle East.

Diagnosis

It is impossible to culture *T. pallidum in vitro*.

In many cases in primary and secondary syphilis, Darkfield microscopy demonstrating *T. pallidum* in lesion exudates may be performed. It has limitations. It requires not inconsiderable practice, and it may be potentially dangerous to operators when the patient is HIV infected. If antiseptics have been used or spirochaetal antibiotics have been taken, demonstration is limited. Oral lesions abound with commensal treponemes, causing confusion.

Serological tests for syphilis

Specific anti-*T. pallidum* immunoglobulin M (IgM) is detectable in the second week of infection, and production of specific antitreponemal IgG begins around the fourth week of infection and reaches higher levels than those for IgM. Serological tests are for screening such as Venereal Disease Research Laboratory (VDRL), standard non-treponemal antigen serological test (VDRL) or rapid plasma region (RPR), cardiolipin antigen tests, or using a *T. pallidum* antigen test—*T. pallidum* haemagglutination assay (TPHA) or enzyme-linked immunosorbent assay (ELISA). Confirmation is with the increasingly rarely used *T. pallidum* immobilization (TPI) test or fluorescent treponemal antibody absorption (FTA-ABS) test, a positive FTA-IgM usually indicating fresh infection.

There are some difficulties in the serological diagnosis of syphilis.

False and true negative syphilis serology

Prozone phenomenon—a false negative reaginic test—may occur in secondary syphilis due to the use of undiluted serum.

In patients with concomitant HIV infection a temporary negative reaginic test may occur in secondary syphilis.

Other causes of positive syphilis serology and biological false positive (bfp) reactions

The endemic treponematoses, endemic syphilis, yaws (framboesia), pinta all give similar results to the antibody responses of *T. pallidum*.

False positive results may occasionally be encountered in borreliosis when very high antibody titres against *B. burgdorferi* occur.

BFP results may occur in reagin tests.

- Acute—under 6 months may occur in pregnancy, after immunization, after recent myocardial infarction and during fevers.
- Chronic—may be seen in injecting drug users, autoimmune diseases, leprosy, chronic liver pathology and old age.

Serological tests do not preclude good history taking, examination or treatment data. Response to treatment is often difficult to interpret. In the author's experience, a fall in the VDRL titre at least fourfold in the first year after infection is a useful clinical pointer of response.

Diagnostic requirements in neurosyphilis

All patients with positive syphilis serology who have neurological symptoms or signs should undergo cerebrospinal fluid (CSF) examination. Most will have a positive non-treponemal (VDRL or RPR) CSF test and a raised CSF white cell count (> 5 cells $\times 10^6$/L).

Some hold the view that the FTA test should be performed on the CSF which although it has a lower specificity for a diagnosis for neurosyphilis than VDRL/RPR may be more sensitive and if negative would usually exclude a diagnosis of neurosyphilis. However, CSF abnormalities may be muted in HIV infection. In adequately treated patients with early syphilis who are not immunocompromised, there is no need to perform lumbar puncture after treatment if there is a satisfactory clinical progress.

Differential diagnosis

In the early stages, a good sexual history is important. Primary syphilis on the penis or vulva may be mistaken with genital herpes, chancroid or donovanosis, all requiring specific confirmatory tests. Drug eruptions, trauma and neoplasia may be mimicked. Secondary syphilis may simulate any other dermatological condition. In adults it is said not to be bullous. It can itch.

In late syphilis, the disease has to be considered for any neurological or cardiovascular presentation.

Treatment

Intramuscular penicillin remains the antimicrobial treatment of choice for all stages of syphilis in patients who are not hypersensitive to it.

There is no evidence of the development of *T. pallidum* resistance to penicillin.

While the aim is to maintain a prolonged low concentration of penicillin within the tissues, this must be continuous. Some workers have criticized the use of benzathine penicillin stating that it is not adequately taken into the central nervous system, but nevertheless it is most useful especially when there is doubt that the patient may return for follow-up.

Alternative antibiotics for those allergic to penicillin are tetracycline, doxycycline or erythromycin. There is a little work recently performed which shows that azithromycin may have potential. Cephalosporins may show cross-sensitivity with penicillin in allergic patients.

There are several guidelines for the treatment of syphilis all of which follow similar patterns. In the USA, the Centers for Disease Control and Prevention publishes and updates its advice frequently. In Europe national guidelines have been published in several countries, those of the UK (Clinical Effectiveness Group) being published in 1999. A pan-European group guidelines project has advised on treatment (Radcliffe *et al.* 2001). World Health Organisation Guidelines (2001) are most useful as worldwide practical advice and are followed here.

Early syphilis

This is defined as primary, secondary, or latent syphilis of not more than 2 years' duration.

Recommended regimen

Benzathine penicillin G, 2.4 million IU, by intramuscular injection, at a single session. Because of the volume involved this dose is usually given as two injections at separate sites.

Alternative regimen

Aqueous procaine benzathine penicillin G, 1.2 million IU daily, by intramuscular injection, for 10 consecutive days.

There are few data on the optimal treatment of syphilis, and there is consequently considerable disagreement among experts regarding therapeutic recommendations. Some recommend treating secondary and latent syphilis with regimens of longer duration.

Either benzathine penicillin G, 2.4 IU by intramuscular injection, once weekly for 3 consecutive weeks or aqueous procaine benzathine penicillin G, 1.2 IU, by intramuscular injection, once daily for 15 consecutive days.

Anecdotal evidence suggests that therapy with benzathine penicillin G may be ineffective in HIV-infected patients with abnormalities of the CSF. Some experts recommend the use of daily procaine benzathine penicillin G for at least 10 days when HIV infection is considered likely.

Alternative regimen for penicillin-allergic non-pregnant patients

Tetracycline 500 mg orally, four times daily for 15 days or doxycycline 100 mg orally, twice daily for 15 days.

Late latent and benign syphilis

This is defined as latent syphilis of more than 2 years duration or of indeterminate duration.

Recommended regimen

Benzathine penicillin G, 2.4 million IU by intramuscular injection, once weekly for 3 consecutive weeks.

Alternative regimen

Aqueous procaine benzathine penicillin G, 1.2 million IU, by intramuscular injection, once daily for 20 consecutive days.

Cardiovascular syphilis

Recommended regimen

Aqueous procaine benzathine penicillin G, 1.2 million IU by intramuscular injection, once daily for 20 consecutive days.

Consultation with a cardiologist is recommended when caring for a patient with cardiovascular syphilis.

Alternative regimen for penicillin-allergic non-pregnant patients

- Tetracycline, 500 mg orally, four times daily for 30 days or
- Doxycycline, 100 mg orally, twice daily for 30 days
- Penicillin is the preferred therapy and should be given whenever possible. The evidence supporting the use of tetracycline is stronger than for doxycycline. It should be emphasized that antibiotic treatment is less well defined for late syphilis than it is for early syphilis. In general, late syphilis requires longer therapy.

Neurosyphilis

Recommended regimen

Aqueous crystalline benzathine penicillin G, 12–24 million IU by intravenous injection, administered daily in doses of 2–4 million IU every 4 h for 14 days.

Alternative regimen

Aqueous procaine benzathine penicillin G, 1.2 million IU by intramuscular injection, once daily, and probenecid 500 mg orally, 4 times daily, both for 10–14 days.

This regimen should be used only for patients whose outpatient compliance can be assured.

Note. Some authorities recommend adding benzathine penicillin G, 2.4 million IU, by intramuscular injection, in 3 consecutive doses once weekly, after completing these regimens, but there is no data to support this approach. Benzathine penicillin G, 2.4 million IU by intramuscular injection does not give therapeutic levels in the cerebrospinal fluid.

Alternative regimens for penicillin-allergic, non-pregnant patients

- Tetracycline, 500 mg orally, four times daily for 30 days or
- **Doxycycline, 200 mg orally, twice daily for 30 days**
- *Note.* The above alternatives to penicillin for the treatment of neurosyphilis have not been evaluated in systematic studies. Although their efficacy is not yet well defined, third-generation cephalosporins may be useful in the treatment of neurosyphilis.

The central nervous system may be involved during any stage of syphilis. Clinical evidence of neurological involvement (e.g. optic or auditory symptoms, cranial nerve palsies) warrants examination of the CSF. However, this is also highly desirable in all patients with syphilis of more than 2 years duration, or of uncertain duration, in order to evaluate the possible presence of asymptomatic neurosyphilis. Some experts recommend consulting a neurologist when caring for a patient with neurosyphilis, and careful follow-up is essential.

Syphilis and HIV infection

All patients with syphilis should be encouraged to undergo testing for HIV because of the high frequency of dual infection and its implications for clinical assessment and management. Neurosyphilis should be considered in the differential diagnosis of neurological disease in HIV-infected individuals. When clinical findings suggest that syphilis is present, but serological tests are negative or inconclusive, alternative tests, such as biopsy of lesions, dark-field examination, and direct fluorescent antibody staining of lesion material should be used. In cases of congenital syphilis, the mother should be encouraged to undergo testing for HIV; if her test is positive, the infant should be referred for follow-up.

Recommended therapy for early syphilis in HIV-infected patient is no different from that in non-HIV-infected patients. However, some authorities advise examination of the cerebrospinal fluid and/or more intensive treatment with a regimen appropriate for all patients dually infected with *T. pallidum* and HIV, regardless of the clinical stage of syphilis. In all cases, careful follow-up is necessary to ensure adequacy of treatment.

Syphilis in pregnancy

Pregnant women should be regarded as a separate group requiring close surveillance, in particular to detect possible reinfection after treatment has been given. It is also important to treat the sexual partner(s).

Recommended regimens

Pregnant patients at all stages of pregnancy, who are not allergic to penicillin, should be treated with penicillin according to the dosage schedules recommended for the treatment of non-pregnant patients at a similar stage of the disease.

Alternative regimens for penicillin-allergic pregnant patients

- Early syphilis (i.e. primary, secondary, or latent syphilis of not more than 2 years duration) erythromycin, 500 mg orally, four times daily for 15 days.
- Late syphilis (i.e. late latent syphilis of more than 2 years duration or of indeterminate duration, late benign syphilis, cardiovascular syphilis, or neurosyphilis) erythromycin, 500 mg orally, four times daily for 30 days.
- *Note.* The effectiveness of erythromycin in all stages of syphilis and its ability to prevent the stigmata of congenital syphilis are highly questionable, and many failures have been reported. Its efficacy in neurosyphilis is probably low. Although data is lacking consideration should probably be given to using an extended course of a third-generation cephalosporin in pregnant women whose allergy is not manifested by anaphylaxis.

All infants born to seroreactive mothers should be treated with a single intramuscular dose of benzathine penicillin G, 50 000 IU/kg by intramuscular injection as a single dose, whether or not the mothers were treated during pregnancy (with or without penicillin).

Follow-up

Following treatment, quantitated non-treponemal serological tests should be performed at monthly intervals until delivery, retreatment being undertaken if there is serological evidence of reinfection or relapse. Subsequent follow-up of the mother is the same as for non-pregnant patients.

Congenital syphilis

Recommended regimens

- Early congenital syphilis (up to 2 years of age). (a) Infants with abnormal CSF: aqueous crystalline benzathine penicillin G, 50 000 IU/kg by intramuscular or intravenous injection, daily in 2 divided doses for a minimum of 10 days or aqueous procaine benzathine penicillin G, 50 000 IU/kg by intramuscular injection, as a single daily dose for 10 days. (b) Infants with normal CSF: Benzathine penicillin G, 50 000 IU/kg by intramuscular injection, at a single session.
- *Note.* Some experts treat all infants with congenital syphilis as if the CSF findings were abnormal. Antibiotics other than penicillin (i.e. erythromycin) are not indicated for congenital syphilis except in cases of severe allergy to penicillin. Tetracyclines should not be used in young children.
- Congenital syphilis of 2 or more years duration. Aqueous crystalline benzathine penicillin G, 200 000–300 000 IU/kg per day by intravenous or intramuscular injection, in divided doses for 10–14 days. Dosage should be adapted to patient's weight, but should not exceed that used for late acquired syphilis.

Alternative regimen for penicillin-allergic patients, after the first month of life

Erythromycin, 7.5–12.5 mg/kg orally, 4 times daily for 30 days.

Congenital syphilis may occur if the expectant mother has syphilis, but the risk is minimal if she has been given penicillin during pregnancy. All infants of seropositive mothers should be examined at birth and at monthly intervals for 3 months until it is confirmed that serological tests are, and remain, negative. Any antibody carried over from mother to baby usually disappears within 3 months of birth. Where available, IgM-specific serology may aid diagnosis.

Infected babies of untreated syphilitic mothers can be asymptomatic at birth and can also be seronegative if the mother was infected late in pregnancy.

However, some experts recommend that treatment should be given (a) in the presence of clear serological evidence/and or clinical, radiological sign of disease; (b) if the treatment of the mother was inadequate or is unknown; (c) if antibiotics other than penicillin were used; or (d) if clinical and serological follow-up of the infant cannot be ensured.

Early congenital syphilis generally responds well, both clinically and serologically, to adequate doses of penicillin. Recovery may be slow in seriously ill children with extensive skin, mucous membrane, bone or visceral involvement. Those in poor nutritional conditions may succumb to intercurrent infections, e.g. pneumonia. In such cases, admission to a hospital is advised.

Follow-up

The follow-up of patients treated for early syphilis should be based on available medical services and resources. The clinical condition of the patients should be assessed and attempts made to detect reinfection during the first year after therapy. Patients whose early syphilis has been clinically treated with appropriate doses and preparations of benzathine penicillin G, should be evaluated clinically and serologically, using a non-treponemal test, after 3 months to assess the results at 6 months, again after 12 months, to reassess the condition of the patient and detect possible reinfection.

All patients with cardiovascular syphilis and neurosyphilis should be followed for many years.

The follow-up should include clinical, serological cerebrospinal fluid and, where necessary, radiological examinations based on the clinician's assessment of the individual patient's condition and evaluation of the illness.

At all stages of the disease, retreatment should be considered when:

- clinical signs or symptoms of active syphilis persist or recur
- there is a confirmed fourfold increase in the titre of a non-treponemal test
- an initially high titre non-treponemal test (e.g. VDRL 1 : 8 or above) persists for over a year.

Examination of the CSF should be undertaken before retreatment, unless reinfection and a diagnosis of early syphilis can be established.

Patients should be retreated with the schedules recommended for syphilis of more than 2 years' duration. In general, only one retreatment course is indicated because adequately treated patients may maintain stable, low titres in non-treponemal tests.

Further reading

Centers for Disease Control and Prevention. *Guidelines on Sexually Transmitted Diseases*. Atlanta: CDC, 2001.

Clinical Effectiveness Group. National Guideline for the Management of Early Syphilis. *Sex Transm Infect* 1999; 75 (Suppl. 1) S29–S33.

Clinical Effectiveness Group. National Guideline for the Management of Late Syphilis. *Sex Transm Infect* 1999; 75 (Suppl.): S34–S37.

Hooshmand H, Escobar MR, Kopf SW. Neurosyphilis: a study of 241 patients. *JAMA* 1972; 219: 726–9.

Radcliffe KK, Gomberg MA, Patel R, Poder A, Ross JDC, Van Voorst Vader PC. European STD (Sexually Transmitted Diseases) Guidelines Project. *Int J STD and AIDS* 2001: 12 (Suppl. 2) 45–7.

World Health Organisation. *Management of Sexually Transmitted Diseases*. Geneva, WHO: 2001.

Systemic sclerosis: scleroderma

U.-F. Haustein

Definition and epidemiology

Systemic sclerosis is a chronic progressive disease in which features of Raynaud's phenomenon and vascular occlusion are followed by sclerotic and fibrotic changes in the skin and internal organs. The average incidence is 8–12 patients per million population with a predominance of 3–4 females to one male.

Aetiology and pathophysiology

The aetiology of systemic sclerosis is still unknown. In the pathophysiology three systems—the blood vessels, immune system and the fibroblast—are discussed.

The microvasculature (endothelial cells, platelets, capillaries) is one of the first affected compartments, sometimes preceding the outbreak of the disease even for years, e.g. Raynaud's phenomenon.

There is evidence that the disease may be immunologically triggered. Perivascular inflammatory infiltrates in the skin are represented by activated T lymphocytes and the disturbed immune reactivity is reflected by abnormal cytokine production and polyclonal B-cell stimulation with antitopoisomerase and anticentromere antibodies specific for systemic sclerosis. Disturbances of the microvasculature and the immune system may dysregulate the fibroblast through mediators (cytokines and growth factors) leading to progressive fibrosis of skin and internal organs. In addition, cell–cell and cell–matrix interactions of fibroblasts are impaired.

Finally some clones of fibroblasts escape the physiological control mechanisms and produce the abundant amounts of collagen type I as determined at the protein as well as at the mRNA expression level. Such fibroblasts behave autonomously via autocrine loops of stimulation by transforming growth factor-β (TGF-β), interleukin-6 (IL-6) and others. Furthermore as in various autoimmune diseases the pathogenesis is partly based on a genetic background and modulated by environmental factors. Skin changes are characterized by abundant accumulation of homogeneous, densely packed collagen fibres, septae penetrating into the subcutaneous tissue, loss of appendages, perivascular lymphocytic infiltrates, and thickening of the vessel wall with subsequent devascularization. The 5-year survival is about 50–70%. It is determined by the involvement of kidney (uraemia, malignant hypertension), heart and lung (pulmonary fibrosis, pneumonia).

Clinical characteristics and course

In the majority of cases the disease starts with Raynaud's phenomenon and arthralgias followed by cutaneous sclerosis and involvement of various internal organs such as gastrointestinal tract, lung, heart, kidney and musculature. Systemic sclerosis is defined by one major criterion (proximal scleroderma) and three minor criteria (sclerodactyly, digital pitting scars or loss of substance on the distal finger pad and bibasilar pulmonary fibrosis). Based on the clinical features, the course of the disease and its prognosis two subsets can be distinguished:

- Limited scleroderma:
  Raynaud's phenomenon for years at presentation
  skin sclerosis limited to hands, feet, face, and forearms, or absent
  significant late incidence of pulmonary hypertension, trigeminal neuralgia, calcinosis, and telangiectasia
  dilated nailfold capillary loops, usually without capillary dropouts

- Diffuse scleroderma:
  onset of Raynaud's phenomenon within 1 year of onset of skin changes
  truncal and acral skin involvement
  presence of tendon friction rubs
  early and significant incidence of interstitial lung disease, oliguric renal failure, diffuse gastrointestinal disease and myocardial involvement
  presence of anti-DNA topoisomerase I (anti-Scl-70) antibodies
  absence of anticentromere antibodies
  nailfold capillary dilatation and destruction.

CREST syndrome is defined as calcinosis, Raynaud's phenomenon, oesophagus dysmotility, sclerodactyly and teleangiectasias. Overlap syndromes include features of systemic lupus erythematosus, Sjögren's syndrome and dermatomyositis and are associated with U_1 RNP, La, Ro and Pm-Scl antibodies, respectively.

Diagnosis (laboratory examination)

Early diagnosis is difficult to make. Antinuclear antibodies are found in 97% of cases using Hep 2 cells as substrate. Centromere antibodies occur in 50–70% of limited subset (CREST syndrome), antitopoisomerase antibodies (Scl-70) in about 36% of cases with diffuse subset. β-galactosidase and N-terminal procollagen III propeptide are elevated as a sign of increased collagen metabolism due to activated fibroblasts. Skin biopsy may be helpful for diagnosis.

Differential diagnosis

- Raynaud's phenomenon: primary or symptomatic in other diseases.
- Generalized morphoea: plaques, rare visceral involvement.
- Systemic lupus erythematosus: overlapping.
- Dermatomyositis: overlapping.
- Sclerodermiform porphyria cutanea tarda: porphyrins.
- Scleromyxoedema: paraproteins, light chains.
- Acrogeria: genetic.
- Scleroderma-like lesions: solvents, vinyl chloride, drugs.
- Scleroedema adultorum (Buschke's disease): acute onset, postinfectious event.
- Graft-versus-host disease: late form after transplantation.

Treatment

General therapeutic guidelines

- Scleroderma is incurable, but not untreatable.
- Randomized double-blind placebo-controlled (multicentre) trials are needed, in particular in patients with diffuse scleroderma of less than 24 months duration.
- Therapy is to be adjusted to stage, severity and progression of the disease (extent of internal organ involvement).
- Quantitative measurement of skin score and severity of organ involvement is desirable for follow-up studies.
- Therapy is targeted in the limited form primarily vascular, in the early stage immunomodulatory and later antifibrotic.
- General recommendations include:
  nutrition: easily chewed and swallowed, high content of proteins and vitamins
  avoidance of nicotine
  personal behaviour: keep warm, warm protective clothing
  lubrication of skin with emollients.
- Physical therapy comprises:
  heat: warm compresses, bath, infrared, hot paraffin
  massage: regular, underwater, lymph drainage
  active exercises.
- Psychological guidance is very helpful. Psychotherapy includes interview counselling and autogeneous training.

Recommended therapies

Symptomatic treatment

- Arthralgia and arthritis, tendon friction are treated with non-steroidal antiphlogistics, cyclooxigenase (COX) II inhibitors (Vioxx, Celebrex) or small doses of glucocorticosteroids.
- Dryness (sicca syndrome): artificial tears and saliva substitutes are available.
- Gastrointestinal tract: reflux oesophagitis can be successfully treated with the proton pump inhibitor omeprazole (20–40 mg/day per os), antacids and H_2-antagonists (cimetidine, ranitidine). Metoclopramide (Paspertin), 3×10 mg/day per os, acts as gastroprokinetic. Small bowel bacterial overgrowth (diarrhoea) can be inhibited by tetracycline, ampicillin and metronidazole.

Vasoactive substances

- Calcium channel blockers are the therapy of choice in Raynaud's phenomenon. Nifedipine is applied 3×5–10 mg/day p.o. Alternatives are nitrendipine, verapamil and nicardipine. Beware of hypotension.
- Pentoxyphylline, 0.4–0.8 g/day acts as a vasodilator and exerts, in addition, immunomodulatory and antifibrotic effects.
- Prostacyclins inhibit platelet aggregation and mediate vasodilatation. Intravenous infusions of prostaglandin E1, e.g. 0.5–2.0 ng/kg per min are more effective and better tolerated than oral doses of the prostacyclin analogue Iloprost (100–300 μg/day). Beware of headache, flush and hypotension.
- Angiotensin-converting enzyme inhibitors, e.g. captopril (4 × 12.5 mg/day) or enalapril (10 mg/day) are applied in hypertension. They represent a considerable advance in preventing or treating acute renal crisis.
- In digital ulcers we usually recommend flexible hydroactive dressings such as Duoderm, Sorbsan and antimicrobial creams or solutions such as povidone-iodine solution (Betadine), hydrogen peroxide solution (1.5–3%) or silver sulfadiazine cream.
- Digital sympathectomy and radial microarteriolysis for a critically ischaemic digit are the last resort in therapy.

Alternatives

- Antagonist of angiotensin II receptor type I (Losartan) exerts clinical benefit in Raynaud's phenomenon after 12 weeks.
- As an antihypertensive agent clonidine (3 × 0.15–0.3 mg/day p.o.) is to be considered.
- As an α-receptor blocker prazosin (1–4 mg/day p.o.) can be used.
- Of less relevance is ketanserin (60–120 mg/day p.o.) as a serotonin antagonist.
- Fibrinolysis enhancing drugs such as dextran, tissue plasminogen activator, urokinase and stanozolol can be tried.

Immunomodulatory substances

- Prednisolone is the most effective drug in the early inflammatory stages or episodes of the disease (with significant immunological activity). At the onset 40–80 mg/day are tapered off to a maintenance dose (about 10 mg/day). Prednisolone can be combined with other immunosuppressants, in particular with cyclophosphamide (2 mg/kg body weight per day per os maximum) against lung fibrosis. Chlorambucil and azathioprine are less effective.
- In a double-blind study methotrexate, 15–25 mg/week showed 53% responders versus 10% in the controls in terms of skin score and lung function.
- Immunosuppression with ciclosporin A (1.5–5 mg/kg of body weight per day) is more selectively directed against T cells, IL-2 release and other

cytokines. However, nephrotoxicity and renal crisis is to be taken into account.

- Photopheresis (extracorporal photochemotherapy) inhibits activated T cells. In general it did not fulfil expectations. However, long-term treatment for more than 18–36 months in cycles every 4 weeks, has shown beneficial effect on disabling symptoms such as fingertip ulcus, hand motility, Raynaud's phenomenon and skin stiffness.

Alternatives and experimental therapeutics

- Controlled clinical trials with methotrexate are in progress.
- Antilymphocyte globulins are of little if any benefit.
- Plasmapheresis removes cytokines, antibodies and immune complexes. It is only of possible benefit, if combined with other immunosuppressants.
- Oral administration of bovine type I collagen (0.1–0.5 mg daily) for 12 months reduced the T-cell reactivity to human collagen I, appears to be well tolerated and improves the skin score.
- Autologous stem cell transplantation: 66 patients have been treated worldwide. However, the mortality rate is still 9%.
- CD4 antibodies, anti-intercellular adhesion molecule (ICAM) and antisense oligonucleotides belong to experimental therapy.

Antifibrotic substances

- Penicillin G (10 million IU/day intraveneously within 30 min for 14 days) acts as prolyl hydroxylase inhibitor with beneficial effects.
- D-Penicillamine inhibits the cross-link formation of collagen fibrils. In higher doses, side-effects such as bone marrow depression, proteinuria, gastrointestinal ulcer, dysgeusia, pemphigus, myositis and rash are significant. Recently it has been shown that high-dose therapy (750–1000 mg/day) is not superior to low-dose therapy (125 mg every other day) and similar to placebo. Therefore, it can no longer be recommended, the more so as 80% of the adverse event-related withdrawals occurred in the high-dose patients.
- Psoralen and ultraviolet A (PUVA) bath photochemotherapy enhances collagenase activity of fibroblasts and improves skin sclerosis, in particular in generalized morphoea.
- UVA1 high-dose therapy not only depletes skin-infiltrating T cells through the induction of apoptosis, but it also upregulates the expression of matrix metalloproteinase-1 (collagenase-1). UVA1 phototherapy-treated skin lesions were markedly softened after 9–29 exposures.
- Minocycline (50–100 mg/twice daily) is worth trying in early diffuse systemic sclerosis.

Alternatives and experimental treatment

- Treatment with interferon-γ ($3 \times 50\,\mu g$/week s.c.) is associated with stabilization of the skin score and lack of worsening of internal organs. Improvement could not be observed.
- Planned studies with recombinant human relaxin were cancelled due to ineffectivity, although in a previous study 25 mg/kg per day were associated with reduced skin thickening, improved mobility and improved function after 24 weeks.
- Retinoids, vitamin D analogue, colchizine, griseofulvin, potassium para-aminobenzoate (Potaba) and cyclophenyl cannot definitely be recommended.

In general, therapy has to be tailored individually in each patient.

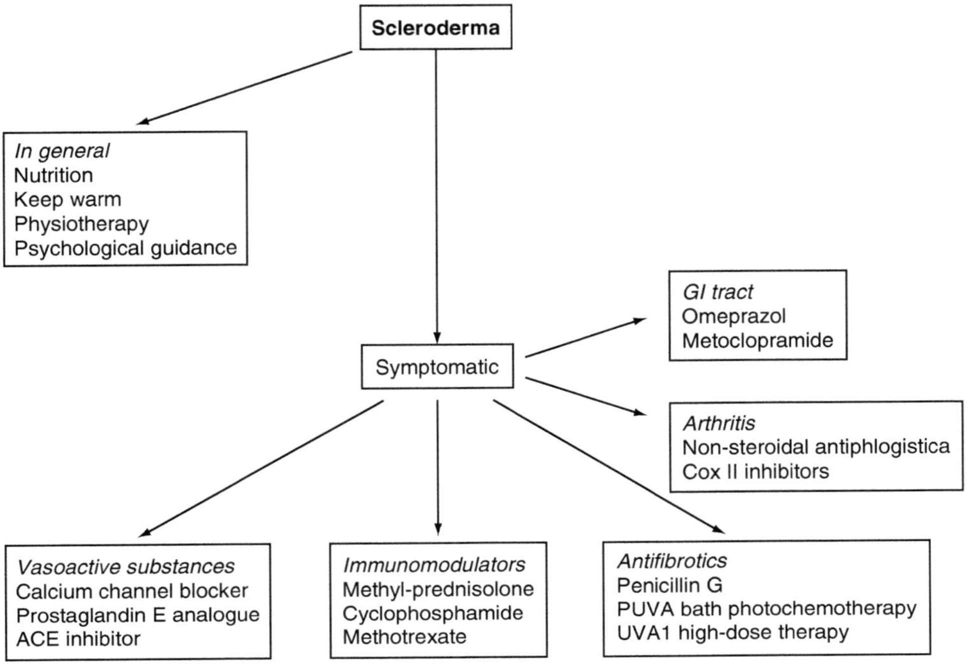

Figure 1 Treatment of scleroderma

Further reading

Clements PJ, Furst DE, Wong W-K *et al.* High-dose versus low-dose D-penicillamine in early diffuse systemic sclerosis. *Arthritis Rheum* 1999; 42: 1194–203.

Dziadzio M, Denton CP, Smith R *et al.* Losartan therapy for Raynaud's phenomenon and scleroderma. *Arthritis Rheum* 1999; 42: 2646–55.

Haustein U-F, Anderegg U. Pathophysiology of scleroderma: an update. *J Eur Acad Dermatol Venereol* 1998; 11: 1–8.

Haustein U-F, Mittag M. Zur Behandlung der systemischen Sklerodermie. *Akt Dermatol* 2000; 26: 271–7.

Hunzelmann N, Anders S, Fierlbeck G *et al.* Systemic scleroderma—multicenter trial of 1 year of treatment with recombinant interferon gamma. *Arch Dermatol* 1997; 133: 609–13.

Kerscher M, Meurer M, Sander C *et al.* PUVA Bath photochemotherapy for localized scleroderma. *Arch Dermatol* 1996; 132: 1280–2.

Le CH, Morales A, Trentham DE. Minocycline in early diffuse scleroderma. *Lancet* 1998; 352: 1755–6.

McKown KM, Carbone LD *et al.* Induction of immune tolerance to human type I collagen in patients with systemic sclerosis by oral administration of bovine type I collagen. *Arthritis Rheum* 2000; 43: 1054–61.

Morita A, Kobayashi K, Isomura I, Tsuji T, Krutmann J. Ultraviolet A1 (340–400 nm) phototherapy for scleroderma in systemic sclerosis. *J Am Acad Dermatol* 2000; 43: 670–4.

Pope JE. Treatment of systemic sclerosis. *Rheum Dis Clin* 1996; 2: 893–907.

Rook AH, Freundlich B, Nahass GT *et al.* Treatment of autoimmune disease with extracorporal photochemotherapy: progressive systemic sclerosis. *Yale J Bio Med* 1989; 62: 639–45.

Seibold JR, Korn JH, Simms R *et al.* Recombinant human relaxin in the treatment of scleroderma. *Ann Intern Med* 2000; 132: 871–9.

Sollberg S, Hunzelmann N, Roux M, Krieg T. Therapie der systemischen Sklerodermie. *Z Haut Geschl Krankh* 1994; 69: 6–14.

Steen VD, Medsger RA, Rodnan GP. D-penicillamine therapy in progressive systemic sclerosis (scleroderma). A retrospective analysis. *Ann Intern Med* 1982; 97: 652–9.

Stege H, Bernburg M, Humke S *et al.* High-dose UVA_1 radiation therapy for localized scleroderma. *J Am Acad Dermatol* 1997; 36: 939–44.

Tick dermatoses

G. Leigheb

Definition and epidemiology

Ticks are very widespread cosmopolitan arachnid arthropods, haematophagous parasites to mammals, birds and reptiles. There are about 650 species of hard ticks (family Ixodidae) and about 150 species of soft ticks (family Argasidae). Besides their usual hosts, which represent the real reservoir of these parasites, they can adapt themselves to alternative hosts, including man. Ticks cause cutaneous lesions (granulomas and necrosis) at the site of the bite, and often provoke allergic reactions especially in previously sensitized people. They are also carriers of many bacterial and viral infections (borreliosis, rickettsiosis, tularaemia), some of which have not yet been studied fully (e.g. arboviruses). The most common dermatoses due to tick bites are described briefly below. The most common species of hard ticks in Europe are *Ixodes ricinus* (sheep tick) and *Rhipicephalus sanguineus* (dog tick).

Clinical characteristics and course

Tick granuloma results from an erythemato-oedematous lesion which appears at the site of the bite. At first the lesion causes very little itching, so that the patient often remains unaware of the presence of the parasite which can remain attached to the skin for several days. Subsequently, the tick may drop off spontaneously having gorged on blood, or the hypostoma (buccal apparatus) may remain fixed into the skin after unsuccessful attempts to detach the parasite. In the latter case, a foreign-body granuloma appears. Thereafter, a delayed sensitization reaction may develop. Itching is considerable and the lesion may persist for many months. In the case of further bites, common in farmers, gardeners, shepherds, sportspeople and hikers for example, the local and systemic symptoms (eczematous patches, or diffuse papulonodular lesions simulating the initial granuloma) become more serious and chronic.

Diagnosis and differential diagnosis

The diagnosis is easily made when the tick is seen and bedded in the skin. After the parasite has dropped off, the presence of a small hole in the centre of the granuloma is pathognomonic. The delayed onset of itching and the history can also suggest the diagnosis. The differential diagnosis involves granulomas due to insect stings and foreign-body granulomas.

Treatment

General therapeutic guidelines

Besides adopting suitable preventive measures such as the use of boots and repellants (dimethylphthalate, pyrethrum, permethrin) it is important to treat the infestation of affected animals and the infested areas, and to remove the parasites embedded in the skin correctly.

Recommended therapies

The most effective method is to apply a cotton-wool pad soaked with ether or petrol over the tick for 15 min. This causes paralysis of the parasite's muscles and subsequent spontaneous detachment. Alternatively, oil or liquid paraffin can be applied to suffocate the tick. The granulomas are treated with antibiotic and corticoid creams or with galenic preparations containing 5–10% coaltar. Systemic corticosteroids are useful in the presence of disseminated secondary nodular or eczematous lesions due to sensitization to the tick. Antihistamines are used as symptomatic measures to alleviate the pruritus. In the case of lesions due to *Argas reflexus* (pigeon tick), which are becoming increasingly common on account of the presence of these birds in urban areas, suitable preventive measures are essential: the elimination of the pigeons, disinfestation of the windows, balconies, mouldings and roof gutters with chlorhexidine and pyrethrum preparations. The cutaneous lesions are treated with antibiotic-corticoid creams. There remains the problem of the serious systemic complications that may arise in sensitized patients who, after being bitten, may develop serious, even fatal, anaphylactic reactions. Such cases require emergency medical treatments consisting of the administration of epinephrine, intravenous corticoids and antihistamines.

Many insecticidal formulations can be applied to domestic pets to rid them of their ticks: 0.5% malathion, 1% carbaryl, 0.1% dioxathion or 1% Conmaphos; or 5% carbaryl, 0.5% conmaphos or 1% trichlorphon dusts applied to the coats of pets. Floors of dog houses, porches and balconies where infected animals sleep should be sprayed with oil solutions or emulsions of 1% propoxur, 0.5% diazinon or 2% malathion.

Further reading

Basset-Stheme D, Couturier P, Sainte-Laudy J. Giant urticaria caused by *Argus reflexus* bites: a propos of a case. *Allerg Immunol* 1999; 31: 61–2.

Leigheb G. *Terapia Galenica in dermatologia*. Rome: Lombardo, 1987.

Leigheb G. Entomodermatosi. Dermatosi da acari. In: A. Giannetti. *Trattato di Dermatologia*, Vol. II. Padova: Piccin, 2001.

Taplin D, Meinkig TL. Pyrethrins and pyrethroids in dermatology. *Arch Derm* 1990; 126: 213–21.

Tinea versicolor: pityriasis versicolor

M. Le Maître and A. Dompmartin

Definition and epidemiology

Known since the middle of the 18th century tinea versicolor is a superficial fungal infection, very common throughout the world. The causal agent is a lipophilid yeast. It occurs in young adults of both sexes. Among all tinea versicolor, 4–11.4% cases are in children. Tinea versicolor is characterized by slightly scaling and discolored patches. It is highly recurrent.

Aetiology and pathophysiology

The causal agent is *Malassezia*. The genus *Malassezia* comprises seven different species; *M. furfur* and *M. globosa* are involved in tinea versicolor. The mycelial phase predominates in the lesions of tinea versicolor. *Malassezia* belongs to the physiological skin flora. In tinea versicolor, there is a transformation of the yeast phase into mycelial phase. Mycelia invade the keratinocytes of the stratum corneum. *Malassezia* can induce a depigmentation by tyrosinase inhibition.

Some circumstances are important to *Malassezia* pathogenesis:

- High sebum production.
- Humidity: this explains the prevalence in warm climates and the increase in hyperhidrosis and occlusive clothes. A familial factor has also been reported. Tinea versicolor is more prevalent in tropical and subtropical countries. In temperate climates, it occurs more often in summer.
- Immunological factors may be involved in the pathogenesis, but these are unknown. Investigations show that the host is sensitized by *Malassezia* (IgG response). Patients with tinea versicolor do not have a cell-mediated immune deficiency to *Malassezia* mycelial antigens.

Clinical characteristics and course

The primary lesion is a light brown slightly scaling macule. Macules are well demarcated and commonly multiple. Children often present with lesions of the face. Their size varies from a few millimetres to several centimetres. They are confluent in large areas with polycyclic outlines. The common sites of eruption are the upper trunk, neck and proximal arms. In tropical countries, the face is commonly affected. Tinea versicolor is not found on palms, soles, and mucosae. Scales can be removed easily with fingernail 'coup d'ongle of Besnier'. The name 'versicolor' is due to the numerous variation in colour of the macules: brown, red or depigmented.

Sometimes pruritus may be present, but it rarely disturbs the patient. The visible and non-aesthetic lesions are more disturbing for patients.

Tinea versicolor alba is very frequent. Depigmentation may be complete, without any scaling.

Without treatment, tinea versicolor has a chronic evolution. The lesions grow in number. Sun exposure deepens the colour of the lesions. After treatment, recurrences are very frequent, and consecutive treatments are necessary.

Diagnosis

- Clinical diagnosis is often easy because of the characteristic macules and the distribution of the lesions.
- Yellow fluorescence of the scaled lesions under Wood's lamp may be useful.
- Direct examination of scale, treated by 30% KOH solution and coloured with black ink, show hyphae and round or ovale spores (like spaghetti and meatballs)

- Direct microscopy may be facilitated by the use of scotch tape. The adhesive rubber is pressed against the skin and mounted on a slide. It is a reliable method to assess the value of treatment.
- Culture or anatomopathological examination are not necessary for the diagnosis.
- When skin biopsy is performed, periodic acid–Schiff (PAS) stain shows fungal elements in the stratum corneum.

Differential diagnosis

- Pityriasiform disease: seborrhoeic dermatitis (different location of the lesions which are more inflammatory; both can coexist). Pityriasis rosea (macules and course are different). Eczematids (imprecise outline, no 'coup d'ongle'). Epidermomycosis (mycological examination). Erythrasma (in axilla; red fluorescence under Wood's lamp).
- In hyperpigmented forms: Becker's naevus (stability, hairs).
- Tinea versicolor alba: vitiligo (may be difficult; hyperpigmentation on the margin of the lesions, Wood's lamp, electron microscopy, mycological examination).
- Other depigmented disease: leprous, idiopathic guttata leucodermae, depigmented eczematids.

Treatment (Fig. 1)

General therapeutic guideliness

- Tinea versicolor is a benign disease therefore topical treatment is mainly prescribed. Oral treatment may be used to treat large eruptions, or when the lesions resist well-managed local treatment. Only topical treatment is used for childhood disease.
- It is necessary to apply on all the skin surface (hair and face included).

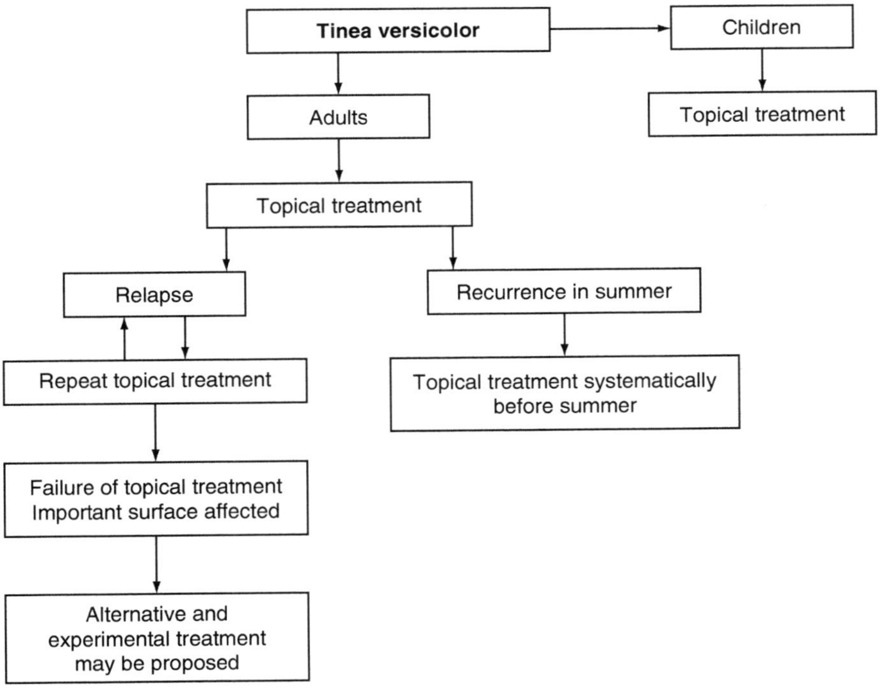

Figure 1 Treatment of tinea versicolor

- Ideally topical treatment must not be expensive, cosmetically pleasant, easy and rapid to apply, and without side-effects.
- After the treatment depigmented lesions are persistent for several weeks. Repigmentation of the patches will occur after sun exposure.
- As *Malassezia* is a saprophyte, tinea versicolor can always relapse, and it is not possible to avoid recurrence.
- Tinea versicolor is not contagious, so hygienic measures are useless to prevent familial transmission.

Recommended therapies

Classical treatment

Propylene glycol
At 50% in water twice daily for 2 weeks.

Zinc pyrithione shampoo
Use once a day for 2 weeks.

Selenium sulfide
In a 2.5% suspension this is applied three times a week. This treatment is efficient but it has to stay for 15 min on the skin, before being washed off. Sulfide smells badly and dries out the skin.

Cyclopiroxolamine
Use twice a day for 2 weeks. Available in cream (not easy) or spray.

Terbinafine
Use once a day for 1 or 2 weeks. Available in cream and solution (spray) 1% which is easy to apply. Propylene glycol/terbinafine is a synthetic antifungal agent (cellylamine class). One week of topical treatment is sufficient. The spray remains active for several weeks after application (highly lipophilic and keratophile). However, oral treatment with terbinafine is not effective.

Imidazole derivatives
These include miconazole, econazole, isoconazole, clotrimazole, triconazole, sulconazole, voriconazole, bifonazole and ketoconazole. They are active against most pathogenic yeasts, by inhibiting the synthesis of ergosterol through a selective interaction with cytochrome P450. They are available in spray or shampoo form. One application per day for 2 weeks is usually sufficient.

Ultrashort topical treatment
Short treatment of 3 consecutive days with bifonazole cream is efficient.

The best treatment seems to be an application of ketoconazole emulsion 2% on all skin surfaces (including hair and face) for 5 min. After 1 month 84% of patients have a negative scotch test, and after 1 year 80% have no recurrence. To increase the efficacy of this treatment, ketoconazole can be applied three times every 8 or 10 days. The side-effects of the emulsion are very few: some patients report smarting on the skin. The smell is acceptable and emulsion is easy to apply.

Prophylactic treatment
With the good results obtainable with ultra-short therapeutic treatment prophylactic treatment is becoming obsolete. Nevertheless regular use of pirithion zinc-based soap or selenium sulfate-based soap can be useful.

Some patients have recurrence in summer (warm weather, perspiration). We recommend systematically one application of ketoconazole emulsion before summer.

We advise our patients not to use oil for solar protection, but gel formulation.

Alternative and experimental treatments
When topical treatment fails oral treatment may be tried. Some patients have

frequent relapses, and compliance is better with oral medication.

The newer azoles (itraconazole and fluconazole) seem to be safer than ketoconazole.

Ketoconazole per os

Use one tablet (200 mg) per day for 10 days, taken in the middle of a meal. Some hepatotoxicity may occur. Transaminase observation is necessary. Prophylactic treatment for very recurrent tinea versicolor with 200 mg of ketoconazole every month has been proposed.

Itraconazole per os

Itraconazole is given as 200 mg/day for 1 week. Itraconazole persists for several weeks in the epidermis. The treatment is very efficient.

Fluconazole per os

Also efficient; 300 mg (one single dose) seems to be the more effective regimen. The absorption of fluconazole is very good and penetration in the skin rapid. Elimination is very slow. No side-effects were reported in the different studies.

A prophylactic treatment has also been suggested with these latter two substances.

It is important to note that all these antifungal substances are expensive. According to the different legislations with Europe, insurance companies may not accept the prescription for tinea versicolor.

Other oral antifungal molecules (griseofulvine and terbinafine) are ineffective.

Further reading

Bouassida S, Boudaya S, Ghorbel R *et al.* Pityriasis versicolor in children a retrospective series of 164 cases. *Ann Dermatol-Venereol* 1998; 37: 581–4.

Crespo Erchiga V, Ojeda Martos A, Vera Casano *et al. Malassezia globosa* as the causative agent of pityriasis versicolor. *Br J Dermatol* 2000; 143: 799–803.

El Euch D, Mnajja N, Mokni M *et al.* Le pityriasis versicolor. Etude prospective de 126 cas. *Ann Dermatol-Venereol* 2000; 127: 45–200.

Faergemann J. Treatment of pityriasis versicolor with a single dose of fluconazole. *Acta Derm Venereol* 1992; 72: 74–5.

Faergemann J, Bratel AT. The *in-vitro* effect of fluconazole on the filament form of *Pityrosporum ovale*. *Acta Derm Venereol* 1996; 76: 444–6.

Faergemann J, Frediksson T. Tinea versicolor. Some new aspects on etiology, pathogenesis and treatment. *Int J Dermatol* 1982; 21: 8–10.

Galimberti RL. Ultra-short topical treatment of pityriasis versicolor with 2.5% bifonazole cream. *Clin Exp Dermatol* 1993; 18: 25–9.

Gupta AK, Kohli Y, Li A, Faergemann J, Summerbell RC. *In vitro* susceptibility of the seven *Malassezia* species to ketoconazole, voriconazole, itraconazole and terbinafine. *Br J Dermatol* 2000; 142: 758–65.

Katsambas A, Stratigos J. Econazole 1% shampoo versus selenium in the treatment of tinea versicolor. *Int J Dermatol* 1996; 35: 604–5

Lange DS, Richards HM, Guarnieri J *et al.* Ketoconazol 2% shampoo in the treatment of tinea versicolor: A multicenter, randomized, double-blind, placebo-controlled trial. *J Am Acad Dermatol* 1998; 39: 944–50.

Meisel C. Treatment of tinea versicolor emulsion vs. climbazole and placebo. A double blind study. *Zeitschr Hautkr* 1991; 66: 415–18.

Montero-Gei F, Robles ME, Suchil P. Fluconazole vs. Itraconazole in the treatment of tinea versicolor. *Int J Dermatol* 1999; 38: 601–3.

Rekacewicz I, Revuz J. Etude en double insu contre excipient du ketoconazole lotion moussante à 2%. *Ann Dermatol-Venereol* 1990; 117: 709–11.

Saadatzadeh MR, Ashbee HR, Cunliffe WJ, Ingham E. Cell-mediated immunity to the mycelial phase of *Malassezia* spp. in patients with pityriasis versicolor and controls. *Br J Dermatol* 2001; 144: 77–84.

Savin R, Eisen D, Fradin M. Tinea versicolor treated with terbinafine 1% solution. *Int J Dermatol* 1999; 38: 863–5.

Silva V, Fischman O, Pires de Camargo Z. Humoral immune response to *Malassezia furfur* in patients with pityriasis versicolor and seborrheic dermatitis. *Mycopathologica* 1997; 139: 79–85.

Sunenshine PJ, Schwartz RA, Janniger CK. Tinea versicolor. *Int J Dermatol* 1998; 21: 648–55.

Toxic epidermal necrolysis (Lyell's syndrome)

A. Minas

Definition and epidemiology

Toxic epidermal necrolysis (TEN) is an acute, severe, often life-threatening skin reaction, which is characterized by extensive necrosis and detachment of the epidermis and mucous membranes. It has been observed worldwide and affects people of both sexes and all ages. It occurs more often in the elderly and women and its incidence is about 0.4–1.3 cases per million per year.

Aetiology and pathophysiology

The aetiology of the disease remains unknown. Factors that have been suspected as possible causes are:

- Drugs: frequently implicated are sulfonamides, antiepileptic drugs, nonsteroidal anti-inflammatory agents, allopurinol, antibacterials and others. However, laboratory or other definite evidence for such an association is usually lacking.
- Non drug-related factors: viruses, bacteria, fungi, vaccinations or systemic diseases. On the whole, the reported cases are few and it is only clinical experience that confirms this aetiological association.

The discrepancy in the aetiology of TEN substantiates the notion of the idiopathic form of the disorder.

The pathophysiology of the disease is unclear. Several hypotheses have been postulated:

- Immunological processes: coexistence of TEN with systemic lupus erythematosus (SLE), graft-versus-host disease (GVHD) or other autoimmune disorders, occasional development of post-TEN Sjögren's syndrome.
- Toxic effect of the responsible drugs and/or their metabolites: genetically determined predisposition of certain drugs to hepatotoxicity.
- Combination of the two hypotheses: the existence of a genetic background that regulates the immune function and presence of transient, unexpected factors, such as viruses, abnormal immune responses or drugs, result either in the release of autocytotoxic cells or in a specific immune effect against keratinocytes, which is very intense and modified by drugs or their metabolites.

Clinical characteristics and course

A prodrome of 2–3 days duration, with fever, malaise, headache, myalgia, arthralgia, as well as nausea or vomiting with or without diarrhoea.

Acute phase of 8–12 days duration, with persistence of fever and a rapidly spreading necrosis, detachment of the mucous membranes at first, 1–3 days prior to the epidermis, in one third of the patients. The skin becomes denuded in 2–3 days to a great extent or almost completely and the appearance is like that of a second-degree thermal burn. The re-epithelialization period starts after a few days, while the lesions are still spreading, and lasts for 2–3 weeks. The duration of the disease is 3–4 weeks, when the evolution is uncomplicated. Usually, there is multisystemic involvement with manifestations from the gastrointestinal tract and the respiratory system, as well as several haematological abnormalities and disorders of kidney function. There is a great loss of fluid, proteins and electrolytes, due to the extensive epidermolysis. Endogenous or exogenous infections, impaired thermoregulation, immune disorders and hypercatabolism may develop as well. The disease mortality ranges from 25% to 70%.

Diagnosis

Not easy. It is based on the clinical picture and confirmed by histology. Histological examination demonstrates a full-thickness epidermal necrosis with detachment from the dermis. Electron microscopy reveals a split between the lamina densa and the epidermis.

Differential diagnosis

- Staphylococcal scalded skin syndrome (SSSS): mostly infants and children, more erythrodermic skin than slough, intact mucous membranes, positive Nikolsky sign even in normal skin (in TEN, positive only in lesions); Tzanck: acantholysis, histological examination: subcorneal split, intercellular intraepidermal immunofluorescence.
- Stevens–Johnson syndrome (SJS): typical target lesions, percentage of total body surface area involved estimated by the rule of nines or burn unit area charts, more bullae than sloughing.

TEN should be sometimes differentiated from:

- The toxic shock syndrome: erythroderma, hand–foot desquamation, menstruating women.
- Kawasaki disease: erythroderma, children less than 5 years of age.
- A generalized bullous fixed drug eruption: absence of target lesions, a history of a similar episode with typical fixed macules or plaques.
- The generalized acute pustular psoriasis of von Zumbusch: lakes of pus, erosions–crusts in Tzanck neutrophilic polymorphonuclear leucocytes, histologically intraepidermal microabscesses.

Treatment

General therapeutic guidelines

- Expeditious referral of the patient to an intensive care or burn unit, under the care of a group of doctors of many if not all specialties.
- During the transfer to the unit, aseptic handling, sterile fields, avoidance of adhesive materials.
- Before admission to the hospital, the immediate patient care is dictated by certain principles, that do not differ from the fundamental and classic principles of general surgery.

These are as follows:

- Placing the patient in a warm environment, avoidance of any skin trauma.
- Administration of macromolecular solutions through a peripheral venous line.
- Evaluation of the patient's general condition (pulse, blood pressure, central venous pressure, heart rate, respiratory rate, body temperature, hourly urine output, chest auscultatory and X-ray findings, total plasma proteins, serum K^+ and Na^+, urine-specific gravity, state of consciousness).
- Estimation of the extent of necrolysis by the rule of nines or burn tables.
- Set a limit to corticosteroid administration.
- Withdrawal of most if not all drugs.
- Obtain skin biopsies (immediate examination of frozen sections, when SSSS is suspected).
- Instillation of a bland ophthalmic solution.
- Reassurance of the patient, use of tranquillizers if necessary.

Recommended therapies

Symptomatic treatment

Replacement of fluids

On the first few days fluid replacement should be conducted intravenously, preferably through peripheral veins, away from affected areas. The amount of fluid administered is proportional to the extent of lesions and covers two-thirds to three-quarters of the fluid amount given during the first 24 h, in burns of similar extent. Macromolecular substitutes (albumin solution, dextranes) are given concurrently, over the first 24 h, as well as phosphate salts, that are considered to be necessary for the prevention of hypophosphoraemia and their consequences (rises in insulin resistance, changes in the neurological status, impairment of the function of the diaphragm). The rate and quantity of fluids administered are reassessed daily. The abrupt restoration of hypovolaemia and the following haemodynamic instability should be avoided, because of the especially great danger of overloading the circulatory system, mainly during the absorption of oedema. Over the following days, oral fluids are gradually increased, so that by the second week, and a while before the re-epithelialization of lesions, the patient is supported exclusively by a nasogastric tube.

Nutritional support

This should begin as early as possible, is intensive and is preferably accomplished by a nasogastric tube. Daily, 2–3 and 3–4 g/kg body weight of protein are administered in adults and children, respectively.

Antibacterial treatment

Patients with TEN are extremely susceptible to hospital infections. Great attention is required to potential sources, like the nasogastric and Foley catheters. Topical use of antiseptics, like povidone-iodine (ointment 10%), chlorhexidine (solution 0.05%), cetrimide (cream 0.5%), silver nitrate (solution 0.5%), or dyes (methylene blue, eosin, crystal violet), helps in preventing infection of lesions. Prophylactic use of systemic antibiotics is not recommended, especially when all other measures regarding the care and therapy of TEN patients are taken.

Criteria for the initiation of systemic antibiotics could be:

- the rapid increase in bacterial flora in certain, preselected areas, that are cultured every 2 days
- a sudden drop in fever and blood pressure
- worsening of the patient's general condition.

Unfortunately, no antibiotic is absolutely indicated, because the pharmacokinetics of all drugs are modified due to the hypoproteinaemia, renal and hepatic dysfunction and constant loss of fluid and proteins through the skin. Usually, a broad-spectrum antibiotic is chosen and administered in high doses, so that it can reach its therapeutic serum levels quickly. Drug serum levels are frequently measured.

Environmental temperature

This is maintained stable between 30° and 32°C with the help of heat shields, infrared lamps and air-fluidized beds, that have a drying, antiseptic effect on the skin's bacterial flora, are comfortable and act in a relaxing way on the patient's mood.

Other supportive treatment modalities

These include, if necessary, anticoagulation, action against pseudodiabetes and adrenocortical insufficiency, prevention of the appearance of an acute peptic ulcer, gastroplegia or paralytic ileus, pharmaceutic or other support of the cardiovascular system, administration of immunoglobulins and blood, and lastly, emotional and psychiatric support.

Surgical care and rehabilitation

As with burns, some authors advocate the debridement of the necrotic epidermis and immediate cover of the erosions with heterografts, homografts and synthetic allografts.

Specific treatment

There is no specific treatment for the disease.

Corticosteroids

These have been used for 30 years and are still administered in various dose regimens, with no evidence, however, of their efficacy. Several studies of a sufficient or great number of cases confirm that TEN may even occur during treatment with steroids for pre-existing diseases and that their administration greatly increases the disease mortality. Moreover, the concept that long-term therapy with steroids may delay the onset or halt the progression of TEN is questioned. Nevertheless, if their administration is decided, then this should be done as soon as possible (first to second 24 h of the acute phase), in high doses (180–200 mg prednisone per day, according to the extent of the exanthem and severity of the patient's general condition) and for a short time period (4–5 days only). If there are no signs of improvement, steroids should be withdrawn and another treatment modality should be chosen.

Plasmapheresis

This has been used on certain occasions since 1984, with beneficial and promising results. The lack of controlled studies, even regarding the mechanism of action of plasmapheresis, make it difficult to determine its true efficacy. Some authors believe that plasma exchange does not have a significant treatment effect in TEN. However, plasmapheresis is the best therapeutic modality, in some extremely ill TEN patients, more so, when the quick and controlled administration of steroids is unsuccessful during the first few days.

The use of ciclosporin could be a good candidate to reverse TEN progression, because of its antiapoptotic properties, whereas the use of cyclophosphamide does not allow us to draw any conclusions.

Lastly, pentoxifylline and high-dose intravenous immunoglobulins have been used in the treatment of TEN. I believe that prospective studies are needed to further define their usefulness.

The role of any specific treatment for TEN, other than symptomatic, is still debatable.

Long-term care of patients

Scar tissue sequelae, like phimosis and oesophageal stricture, sometimes require surgical procedures. Post-TEN ocular syndrome requires constant ophthalmological follow-up. Often artificial tears and lubricants are needed. Surgical procedures like punctal occlusion, lysis of synechiae and the use of conjunctival flaps offer little improvement, and tarsorrhaphy may be required. Topical use of tretinoin helps significantly in the treatment of conjunctival keratinization, which is incriminated for most corneal complications.

Further reading

Arevalo JM, Lorente JA. Skin coverage with Biobrane biomaterial for the treatment of patients with toxic epidermal necrolysis. *J Burn Care Rehabil* 1999; 20: 406–10.

Chaidemenos G, Chrysomallis F, Sombolos K *et al.* Plasmapheresis in toxic epidermal necrolysis. *Int J Dermatol* 1997; 36: 218–21.

Egan CA, Grant WJ, Morris SE, Saffle JR, Zone JJ. Plasmapheresis as an adjunct treatment in toxic epidermal necrolysis. *J Am Acad Dermatol* 1999; 40: 458–61.

Furubacke A, Berlin G, Anderson C, Sjoberg F. Lack of significant treatment effect of plasma exchange in the treatment of drug-induced toxic epidermal necrolysis? *Intensive Care Med* 1999; 25: 1307–10.

Green D, Law E, Still JM. An approach to the management of toxic epidermal necrolysis in a burn centre. *Burns* 1997; 19 (5): 411–14.

Guibal F, Bastuji-Garin S, Chosidow O *et al.* Characteristics of toxic epidermal necrolysis in patients undergoing long-term glucocorticoid therapy. *Arch Dermatol* 1995; 131: 669–72.

Heng MCY, Allen SG. Efficacy of cyclophosphamide in toxic epidermal necrolysis. *J Am Acad Dermatol* 1991; 25: 778–86.

Ioannides D, Vakali G, Chrysomallis F *et al.* Toxic epidermal necrolysis: a study of 22 cases. *JEADV* 1994; 3: 266–75.

Kelemen JJ III, Cioffi WG, McManus WF *et al.* Burn center care for patients with toxic epidermal necrolysis. *J Am Coll Surg* 1995; 180 (3): 273–8.

Magina S, Lisboa C, Goncalves E *et al.* A case of toxic epidermal necrolysis treated with intravenous immunoglobin. *Br J Dermatol* 2000; 142: 191–2.

Paquet P, Pierard GE. Would cyclosporin A be beneficial to mitigate drug-induced toxic epidermal necrolysis? *Dermatology* 1999; 198: 198–202.

Renfro L, Grant-Krels JM, Daman LA. Drug-induced toxic epidermal necrolysis treated with cyclosporin. *Int J Dermatol* 1989; 28: 441–4.

Roujeau JC. Treatment of severe drug eruptions. *J Dermatol* 1999; 26: 718–22.

Roujeau J-C, Chosidow O, Saiag P, Guillaume J-C. Toxic epidermal necrolysis (Lyell syndrome). *J Am Acad Dermatol* 1990; 23: 1039–58.

Yamada H, Takamori K, Yaguchi H, Ogawa H. A study of the efficacy of plasmapheresis for the treatment of drug induced toxic epidermal necrolysis. *Ther Apher* 1998; 2: 153–6.

Urethritis: gonococcal

D. Freedman

Definition
Urethritis, specifically caused by the bacterium *Neisseria gonorrhoea.*

Epidemiology
Recent resurgence in Western Europe and North America, especially in particular risk groups or in areas of socioeconomic deprivation. Epidemics in Eastern Europe and the Russian Republics have now plateaued. Pandemic in parts of Africa and South-East Asia, where antibiotic-resistant strains, especially to penicillin and more recently quinalones, are very common.

Pathophysiology
Infection of the columnar epithelium of the urethra induces a vigorous polymorphonuclear leucocytic response resulting in an acute purulent urethritis in over 90% of cases. However may be asymptomatic, particularly if masked by inappropriate antibiotic usage.

Clinical presentation
Typically an acute purulent urethritis with a short incubation period of 2–14 days (median 3–4) from sexual contact. Profuse purulent discharge, sometimes blood stained (80%), dysuria (50%) and distal urethral discomfort. *Analogous to a running tap*! Acquisition from vaginal and insertive anal and oral sex. In the case of the latter the patients are frequently surprised at the occurrence as they feel they have been following *safe sex practices*. Patients identified by contact tracing are more frequently asymptomatic.

Complications
These are rare.

- Local
  acute: lymphangitis, periurethral abscesses epididymitis, orchitis
  late: stricture of the urethra.
- Distal
  disseminated gonococcal infection, septic arthritis, septic dermatitis, major organ focal infection.

Diagnosis
Acute urethritis, clinically obvious in the majority of cases, but not diagnostic. Some cases may only have a microscopic urethritis. Examination of the initial voided urine will show *threads* or *beads of pus* and have a positive leucocyte esterase dipstick test. Diagnosis is by investigations.

Investigations
- Gram stain: a thinly spread smear of urethral exudate; the finding of pus cells with Gram-negative intracellular diplococci under $\times 1000$ oil immersion microscopy is highly suggestive, but not definitive, of infection with *N. gonorrhoea*. Sensitivity 90–95% in symptomatic, and 50–75% in asymptomatic cases. Methylene blue stain is sometimes used, but lacks sensitivity and specificity.
- Culture: definitive diagnosis requires cultures using a specific medium such as modified Thayer–Martin or New York City medium to support the fastidious *N. gonorrhoea*. The culture plate should be fresh, moist and at room temperature. It should be inoculated directly from the clinical specimen and incubated rapidly at 35–37°C in a 5% CO_2 enriched atmosphere. Commercial culture/transport kits such as the JEMBEC allow simplification of the procedure. Definitive identification of the *Neisseria* species requires a

specific set of carbohydrate fermentation reactions showing the ability to metabolize glucose, but not maltose, sucrose, fructose, or lactose. Coagglutination kits are also available which are rapid, easily performed and specific in urethral specimens, but may not be so in specimens from other sites. Precise and specific identification of the *N. gonorrhoea* infection is essential if one is requested to give evidence for medicolegal purposes in matrimonial or 'palimony' cases.

- Molecular identification: nucleic acid amplification techniques are available for the identification of *N. gonorrhoea*. These have not yet reached routine clinical practice. They initially appeared to have the potential to provide a syndromic test kit to identify multiple organisms from one specimen, or to be used for epidemiological screening using non-invasive specimens, such as initial voided urine. However, they have not provided any significant improvement over the conventional culture system in sensitivity or specificity, are more expensive, and do not allow the antibiotic sensitivity pattern of the organism to be determined.

Differential diagnosis

The finding of Gram-negative intracellular diplococci with confirmation of *N. gonorrhoea* by culture, together with fermentation reaction or agglutination reaction is specific.

However, *N. gonorrhoea* may coexist with other causes of urethritis, especially *Chlamydia trachomatis* (see chapter on urethritis: non-gonococcal).

Definitive diagnosis is essential as a specific diagnosis will improve treatment compliance and partner notification and referral.

Treatment

General guidelines

As with all sexually transmitted infections, the management of urethritis due to *N. gonorrhoea* involves:

- Full routine sexually transmitted disease screen to rule out other concomitant infections.
- Appropriate antibiotic therapy.
- Patient counselling and education.
- Avoidance of unprotected sex until patient and partner(s) have completed treatment.
- Partner/contact tracing.
- Review for test of cure.

Exclude other sexually transmitted diseases

Chlamydia trachomatis has been described as occurring concurrently with *N. gonorrhoea* in 15–25% of cases. Failure to identify and treat *C. trachomatis* or other causes of non-specific urethritis will result in postgonococcal urethritis. Prophylactic treatment for *C. trachomatis* and other causes of non-gonococcal urethritis are usually incorporated into treatment schedules for gonococcal urethritis in most centres (see below).

Patients must have a full routine screening examination to rule out other concomitant infections. As gonorrhoea is essentially an acute infection, a repeat serological screen should be carried out 3 months later to cover the 'window period' for the detection of syphilis, hepatitis B and human immunodeficiency virus. Patients should be warned that certain infections, such as human papilloma virus or herpes viruses, may only manifest themselves after a prolonged period, are frequently carried asymptomatically and are not detected by a routine sexually transmitted disease screen.

Antibiotic therapy

The chosen treatment regime should eradicate more than 95% of uncomplicated anogenital gonococcal infections. The choice of antibiotic will depend on local prevalence of resistant strains if the infection was acquired locally, or knowledge of likely antibiotic resistance if acquired abroad. In general, resistance with penicillin producing neisseria gonorrhoea (PPNG) strains can be assumed if acquisition occurred in South-East Asia or Africa, or from a person from those regions. Urethral gonorrhoea responds rapidly to a *stat.** dose of an appropriate antibiotic allowing *one shot* and *directly observed therapy* to ensure compliance. Because of the potential for concurrent incubating syphilis in areas of acquisition of gonorrhoea, a regime that is also effective for incubating syphilis is preferred. Allergic reactions or sensitivity to antibiotics should be ascertained before administration, and emergency supplies to deal with an anaphylactic reaction should be readily available.

Regimens

With increasing prevalence of penicillin resistance, most guidelines have adopted a first-line treatment with this expectation.

N. gonorrhoea *isolate resistant to penicillin and derivatives, or presumptive gonorrhoea acquired in areas where penicillin resistance is common (penicillinase producing* N. gonorrhoea $\geq$ *5%) is treated as follows.*

Oral regimens

- Ciprofloxacin 500 mg *stat.*
- Cefixime 2 × 200 mg *stat.*

*Resistant strains isolated in South-East Asia, Pacific areas and west coast USA. Likely to become more commonplace. Sporadically isolated in Europe and Australia.

Parenteral regimens

- Spectinomycin 2 g *stat.*
- Ceftriaxone 150 mg i.m. *stat.*

To date resistance to ceftriaxone has not been reported and the *Gonococcus* remains very sensitive at all sites. Ceftriaxone is a first treatment of choice in the American Centers for Disease Control (CDC) Guidelines (2002).

In areas where penicillin resistance is unlikely, and there is almost certainty that the patient will return for test of cure and results of culture and antibiotic sensitivity testing, amoxycillin offers an effective and economical therapy.

N. gonorrhoea *isolated sensitive to penicillin and derivatives, or presumptive gonorrhoea acquired in areas where penicillin resistance is uncommon.*

- Amoxycillin 3 g stat. together with 1 g probenecid.

Note: if there is a likelihood of *N. gonorrhoea* infection at other sites, such as the anal canal or pharynx, a 5-day course of amoxycillin 500 mg q.i.d. is recommended in addition to the above.

Treatment of gonorrhoea in special circumstances

Penicillin allergy

- Ciprofloxacin 500 mg *stat.*
- Co-trimoxazole 480 mg twice daily × 4 days.
- Doxycycline 100 mg b.d. for 7 days.

Pregnancy

- Amoxycillin 3 g together with probenecid 1 g *stat.*
- Ceftriaxone 150 mg i.m. *stat.*
- Erythromycin: 500 mg q.i.d. for 7 days.

Allow evolution of syphilis

That is, the effective treatment of gonorrhoea which will not mask incubating syphilis.

- Ciprofloxacin 250 mg *stat.*
- Co-trimoxazole 480 mg b.d. for 3 days.
- Azithromycin has been used in the treatment of *N. gonorrhoea*, but the oral dose of 1 g, used for the treatment of *C. trachomatis*, has only a 93% cure rate, insufficient for reliable clinical usage.

Dual therapy for gonococcal and chlamydial infections

These regimens should all be followed by an effective treatment for *C. trachomatis* and other causes of non-gonococcal urethritis, either administered shortly afterwards (6 h) or at attendance for the first test of cure.

Suggested regimens

- Azithromycin 1 g *stat.*
- Doxycycline 100 mg b.d. × 7–10 days.
- Oxytetracycline 500 mg q.i.d. × 7–10 days.

Azithromycin has the advantage of a *stat.* dose permitting 'directly observed therapy' and is best administered at the visit for the initial test of cure.

Poor compliance with treatment and follow-up may be seen with migrant or disadvantaged populations with erratic health-care seeking behaviour: directly observed therapy is to be preferred.

Pharmacoeconomics

This becomes of relevance where there is a larger caseload. In areas of low penicillin resistance, amoxycillin offers an economical treatment. In areas where PPNG prevalence is > 5%, policy decisions should be made in conjunction with the microbiological service and relate to local costings. Economical antichlamydial therapy is achieved with oxytetracycline, but the advantages of compliance and directly observed therapy may make the additional expenditure of azithromycin worthwhile.

Partner/contact tracing

Gonorrhoea does not occur in isolation. It is an infection occurring in two or more people, often involved in sexual networks. It is an essential component of management and treatment to ascertain the recent sexual contacts and provide means for their treatment. Patients are frequently embarrassed to reveal the full extent of their sexual athleticism. An expert, knowledgeable and non-judgmental attitude on the part of the attending physician will help overcome this.

It is important to explain to the patient that their contact is most likely to be asymptomatic and to have no knowledge of the infection. This is particularly the case in cervical, anal and pharyngeal sources. One has to emphasize that the symptomatic patient may be the only source of information for the contact that an infection is present. One may put it in the context that if the contact was *good enough to have sex with the patient, the patient should be good enough to go back and tell them.* It is most advantageous for the contact(s) to attend the same physician as the source patient, who can then deal with any other problem that may be revealed through the full sexually transmitted disease screen. The doctor's card or contact slip with the diagnosis (coded if required) and source patient reference number is given to the patient for each contact.

All sexual contacts of patients with urethritis due to *N. gonorrhoea* should be screened and treated for *N. gonorrhoea* and *C. trachomatis* if their last sexual exposure with the contact(s) was within 60 days before symptom onset or diagnosis, or if the last sexual exposure was more than 60 days before the onset of symptoms or diagnosis, the most recent sex partner should be screened and treated.

Review-test of cure

Traditionally, patients should return for review and test of cure at least once. Whilst this may be deemed unnecessary by some due to the efficacy of current regimens, it does ensure eradication of the infection and to deal with any further problems that may emerge from screening. It permits further discussion and exploration of partner/contact tracing and giving information on safe sex guidelines at a more receptive period, when the patient is less focused on the acute infection. Current reports indicate that it is the time spent and quality of counselling that most impacts on patient compliance with safe sex guidelines.

Finally, gonococcal urethritis is an acute infection, usually symptomatic within 10 days of acquisition. Patients must return 3 months later for 3-month serology to rule out incipient syphilis, hepatitis B or human immunodeficiency virus.

Gonorrhoea may be only a simple acute bacterial infection, easily diagnosed, easily treated, but its acquisition indicates risk-taking behaviour and perhaps an underlying personal and emotional need that would warrant exploration and counselling for proper management in the complete sense of the word.

Notification

Most European countries require notification of cases of *N. gonorrhoea* to public health authorities (Table 1).

Table 1 Treatment schedules for gonococcal urethritis

Drug	Dose			Cost
Low expectation of penicillin resistance				
Amoxycillin	3.0 g	*Stat.*	Together with probenecid 1.0 g *stat.*	€
Expectation of penicillin resistance				
Oral regimens				
Ciprofloxacin	500 mg	*Stat.*	Resistance reported: rare	€€
Ofloxacin	400 mg	*Stat.*		€€
Cefixime	400 mg	*Stat.*		€€
Parenteral regimens				
Spectinomycin	2.0 g	*Stat.*	Resistance reported: rare	€€€
Ceftriaxone	150 mg	*Stat.*	Reliable for all sites	€€€
Special circumstances				
Penicillin allergy				
Ciprofloxin	500 mg	*Stat.*		€€
Cotrimoxazole	480 mg	4	b.d. × 4 days	€
Doxycycline	100 mg	1	b.d. × 7 days	€€
Pregnancy				
Amoxycillin	3.0 g	*Stat.*	Together with probenecid 1.0 g *stat.*	€
Ceftriaxone	150 mg	*Stat.*	Reliable for all sites	€€€
Erythromycinbase	500 mg	1	q.i.d. × 7 days	€
Allow evolution of syphilis				
Ciprofloxin	250 mg	2 *stat.*		€€
Cotrimoxazole	480 mg	4	b.d. X 4 days	€

Patients should also receive therapy for potential *C. trachomatis* co-infection

€Cheap; €€mid-price; €€€expensive.

Further reading

Centers for Disease Control and Prevention. Sexually transmitted diseases treatment guidelines 2002. *Morbid Mortal Wkly Rep* 2002; 51(RR6): 36–41.

European Guidelines for the Management of Gonorrhoea. *Int J STD and AIDS* 2001; 12, (Suppl. 3): 27–9.

UK National Guidelines on Sexually Transmitted Infections and closely related conditions. *Sex Transm Infect* 1999; 75 (Suppl. 7): S13–15.

Urethritis: non-gonococcal

D. Freedman

Definition

Urethritis *not* caused by the bacterium *Neisseria gonorrhoea*. Also known as Non-Specific Urethritis.

Epidemiology

There is a worldwide prevalence, and it is the commonest form of male urethritis in Western Europe, North America and Australia, with millions of cases per annum. Increasing incidence is being recognized in Eastern Europe and the Russian Republics. It is probably equally common in parts of Africa and South-East Asia, but masked by the high prevalence of acute urethritis caused by gonorrhoea.

Pathophysiology

It is caused by a variety of microorganisms infecting the columnar epithelium of the urethra causing a mild inflammatory response, and resulting in the common clinical spectrum of a mild to moderate urethritis, with a delayed incubation period. Frequently it is asymptomatic. Polymorphonuclear response may show initially, but may be succeeded by mononuclear response in recurrent or long-standing infections. The role of hypersensitivity reaction or pathogen sensitization has also been considered.

Chlamydia trachomatis is the microorganism most closely associated with non-gonococcal urethritis, due to the ready availability of diagnostic and screening tests over the past two decades, and knowledge of the complications of the infection. More recently, attention is being paid to the role of *Mycoplasma genitalium* in the aetiology of urethritis, especially non-gonococcal, non-chlamydial urethritis (Table 1).

In some cases, especially with infection by *C. trachomatis*, healing occurs by fibrosis causing damage to the delicate reproductive structures, and having the potential to cause infertility.

Clinical presentation

Typically minimal to mild urethritis presents with a longer incubation period of 10–30 days from sexual contact. Minimal discharge and dysuria with some distal urethral discomfort may be evident. There is often only a little secretion or crusting noted in the morning, the so-called 'gleet': analogous to a dripping tap! It is frequently completely asymptomatic, and only found on routine screening. Acquisition is most commonly from vaginal sex, but may also be acquired from insertive anal and oral sex.

Table 1 Major aetiological agents for non-gonococcal urethritis (NGU)

Agent	Cases NGU as causal agent (%)	Type of agent
Chlamydia trachomatis	20–40	Pathogen
Ureaplasma urelyticum	15–25	?Commensal
Mycoplasma genitalium	12–50	?Pathogen
Candida species	?5	?Pathogen
Anaerobes	?Underestimated	?Pathogen
Trichomonas vaginalis	?5–10	Pathogen
Herpes genitalis	?5–10	Pathogen
Urethral/meatal warts	?Underestimated	Pathogen
Unidentified/idiopathic	25–30	?Pathogen ?Hypersensitivity

Some cases (5–15%) of non-gonococcal urethritis, especially those caused by *C. trachomatis*, will spontaneously recur. These cases cause considerable frustration, and frequently no causative organism is found: they may relate to a hypersensitivity reaction. However, when *C. trachomatis* is identified, it may be due to reacquisition of the infection, as reported from centres that serve a large adolescent population, or may represent treatment failure with persistence of latent forms of *C. trachomatis*. They all require rescreening to rule out acquisition of a fresh infection.

Complications

- Local:
  acute: epididymitis, orchitis
  late: infertility.
- Distal: follicular conjunctivitis, Reiter's syndrome.

Diagnosis

Urethritis may be clinically obvious in some cases, but not diagnostic. Many cases may only have a microscopic urethritis. Examination of the first catch urine may show threads or 'beads of pus' and have a positive leucocyte esterase test.

Investigations

Testing to obtain a specific diagnosis is mandatory to ensure treatment compliance and partner notification, as well as reporting to public health authorities.

Gram stain

- A thinly spread smear of urethral exudate stained by Grams method: the finding of >4 pus cells per high power field and the absence of Gram-negative intracellular diplococci under ×1000 oil immersion microscopy. Methelyne blue stain is sometimes used, but lacks sensitivity.
  and/or
- Gram stain of a first catch urine showing >10 pus cells per high power field ×1000 oil immersion microscopy.

Recent micturition renders these investigations less sensitive: urine should be held for at least 1 h before testing, with 4 h being conventional.

Screening for *Chlamydia trachomatis*

This should be performed as part of routine examination. Culture for *C. trachomatis* is highly specific, but lacks sensitivity. Antigen detection techniques, either by direct fluorescent antibody or enzyme-linked immunosorbent assay (ELISA), are commonly used and allow higher sensitivity with some loss of specificity.

The newer techniques of nucleic acid amplification tests, such as polymerase chain reaction and ligase chain reaction have enabled highly specific and sensitive tests to be evolved. These have now reached routine clinical practice, and have highlighted the lack of sensitivity of the older methods. They provide the ability to give reliable results from non-invasive sampling, using specimens such as initial voided urine, and consequently open up opportunities for epidemiological screening. They may also be incorporated in a syndromic test kit to identify multiple organisms from one specimen.

Trichomonas vaginalis

This may be sought on occasions by suspending a drop of exudate in saline and microscopic examination for motile flagellated organisms, as well as culture.

Fungi

Fungi may be excluded by examination of a drop of exudate suspended in 10% potassium hydroxide.

Herpes simplex virus

Herpes simplex virus may be identified by viral culture in cases where there is clinical suspicion.

Identification of other organisms

Testing for organisms such as mycoplasmas or ureaplasmas, which may cause non-gonococcal urethritis, is not routinely performed in normal clinical practice.

Serological testing

Complement fixation or more specific serological testing for *C. trachomatis* or *Mycoplasma* has no place in the diagnosis of urethritis.

Differential diagnosis

The signs and symptoms of non-gonococcal urethritis may be caused by other local infections such as meatal herpes simplex virus infection, urethral or meatal warts: other causes include fixed drug eruption, or physical or chemical trauma, which could arise from unusual sexual practices. In addition, some cases of balanitis result in sufficient local irritation as to induce a meatitis indistinguishable from non-gonococcal urethritis. Urethral foreign bodies, periurethral fistula and abscesses should be excluded by palpation. Bacterial urethritis may occur with predisposing factors such as phimosis, stricture, postinstrumentation, and following more traumatic sexual practices, such as insertive anal sex, where the urethra is also exposed to a wider variety of organisms, as well as subject to trauma. Self-examination and manipulation of the penis in those with a sexually transmitted disease anxiety may provoke a local reaction and produce symptoms to reinforce their worst fears. On occasions, men present with an anxiety over physiological secretions, such as a pre-ejaculation mucous, especially when there is remorse after a real or imagined sexual indiscretion.

Upper urinary tract problems, such as renal lithiasis or anatomical abnormalities, may manifest as an urethral discharge, as may tuberculosis of the urinary tract, which is now uncommon, but should not be forgotten. Urinary tract infections occasionally present as an acute urethritis, with a purulent discharge: they are more likely in those over the age of 35 years. Their occurrence in a male should prompt a full renal tract investigation to rule out any underlying cause.

Prostatitis, either acute or chronic, may result in an urethral discharge. The discomfort is frequently felt at the meatus and the perineum, and has a diffuse quality.

Treatment

General guidelines

As with all sexually transmitted diseases, the management of non-gonococcal urethritis involves:

- Full routine sexually transmitted disease screen to rule out other concomitant infections.
- Appropriate antibiotic therapy.
- Patient counselling and education.
- Avoidance of unprotected sex until patient and partner(s) have completed treatment.
- Partner/contact tracing.
- Review for test of cure.

Rule out other sexually transmitted diseases

Patients must have a full routine screening examination to rule out other concomitant infections. A repeat serological screen should be carried out 3 months later to cover the 'window period' for the detection of syphilis, hepatitis B and human immunodeficiency virus. Patients should be warned that certain infections, such as human papilloma virus or herpes viruses, may only manifest themselves after a prolonged period, are frequently carried asymptomatically and are not detected by a routine sexually transmitted disease screen.

Antibiotic therapy

Chlamydia trachomatis has a relatively long lifecycle of around 36 h and requires prolonged exposure to an antibiotic for its elimination. Cure rates of >95% have been achieved with a 7-day course of tetracycline or its derivatives. The development of a novel azalide, azithromycin, with an extremely long half-life and concentration in inflamed tissues has allowed the development of an effective *stat.* or 'one shot' therapy for *C. trachomatis*, which is also equally efficacious for non-identified other causes of non-gonococcal urethritis. Compliance, through 'directly observed therapy' is thought to contribute greatly to its effectiveness. Additionally, it is the treatment of choice for *Mycoplasma genitalium*. Antibiotic resistance is not an apparent problem to date with *C. trachomatis*, although its detection is technically very demanding. *In-vitro* studies and case reports have suggested that amoxycillin sometimes renders chlamydial infection latent, rather than eradicating it. Although multifactorial, non-gonococcal urethritis seems to respond uniformly to a range of antibiotics with antichlamydial and antimycoplasmic activity.

Recommended regimens:
- Azithromycin 250 mg × 4 *stat.*
- Doxycycline 100 mg b.d. × 7 days.
- Oxytetracycline 500 mg q.i.d. × 7 days.
- Erythromycin: 500 mg q.i.d. × 7 days
- Erythromycin: 500 mg b.d. × 14 days
- Ofloxacin 200 mg b.d. × 7 days.

Treatment of non-gonococcal urethritis in special circumstances

Tetracycline allergy
- Azithromycin 250 mg × 4 *stat.*
- Erythromycin: 500 mg q.i.d. × 7 days;
- Erythromycin: 500 mg b.d. × 14 days
- Ofloxacin 200 mg b.d. × 7 days.

Pregnancy
- Erythromycin: 500 mg q.i.d. × 7 days
- Erythromycin: 500 mg b.d. × 14 days
- Amoxycillin 500 mg t.i.d. for 7 days (risk of latency: potential for neonatal *Chlamydia* infection).

Allow evolution of syphilis
This is, effective treatment of gonorrhoea which will not mask incubating syphilis.
- Ofloxacin 200 mg b.d. × 7 days.

Persistent/recurrent non-gonococcal urethritis
This is frustrating to patient and physician alike; it occurs in 20–30% of patients with non-gonococcal urethritis. Controversy as to whether it represents inadequate treatment compliance by patient and partner(s), reactivation of latent infection, reacquisition of infection or merely a hypersensitivity reaction. Same diagnostic criteria.

Management

Symptomatic
- Repeat azithromycin or doxycycline.
- Erythromycin 500 mg q.i.d. for 2 weeks with metronidazole 400 mg b.d. for 5 days.

Asymptomatic
- Repeat azithromycin or doxycycline.
- Erythromycin 500 mg 4 times a day for 2 weeks.
- No treatment.

There is no evidence that female partners of men with persistent/recurrent *Chlamydia*-negative non-gonococcal urethritis are at any increased risk of pelvic inflammatory disease provided they have been appropriately treated initially.

Prolonged urethritis
Limited evidence or consensus on best management of patients with prolonged symptomatology or ongoing recurrences. Multiple treatment courses are commonly administered, but there is no evidence that these patients are persistently infected. Urological assessment may be considered. The prostate should be investigated to exclude prostatitis. Psychosexual assessment may be considered. On occasions, recurrent or persistent com-

Table 2 Treatment schedules for non-gonococcal urethritis uncomplicated

Drug	Dose	Frequency	Duration
Azithromycin	250 mg	4 stat	Directly observed therapy
Doxycycline	100 mg	b.d.	× 7 days
Oxytetracycline	500 mg	q.i.d.	× 7 days
Erythromycin	500 mg	q.i.d.	× 7 days
Erythromycin	500 mg	b.d.	× 14 days
Ofloxacin	200 mg	b.d.	× 7 days
	SPECIAL CIRCUMSTANCES		
Tetracycline Allergy			
Azithromycin	250 mg	4 stat	Directly observed therapy
Erythromycin	500 mg	q.i.d.	× 7 days
Erythromycin	500 mg	b.d.	× 14 days
Pregnancy			
Erythromycin	500 mg	q.i.d.	× 7 days
Erythromycin	500 mg	b.d.	× 14 days
Allow evolution of Syphilis			
Ofloxacin	200 mg	b.d.	× 7 days
Persistent / Recurrent NGU			
Symptomatic:			
Repeat initial therapy: particularly if compliance with the initial course is doubtful			
Erythromycin	500 mg	q.i.d.	× 14 days
Plus Metronidazole	400 mg	b.d.	× 5 days
Asymptomatic:			
Repeat initial therapy: particularly if compliance with the initial course is doubtful			
Erythromycin	500 mg	q.i.d.	× 14 days
No treatment			Re-assurance

plaints of urethritis may be a manifestation of depression or other psychiatric disorders, especially when there is remorse over a sexual indiscretion.

Azithromycin has the advantage of a *stat.* dose permitting 'directly observed therapy', guaranteeing compliance. This is especially important in populations with erratic health seeking behaviour.

Allergic reactions or sensitivity to antibiotics should be ascertained before administration, and emergency supplies to deal with an anaphylactic reaction should be readily accessible.

Pharmacoeconomics

Economical antichlamydial therapy is achieved with oxytetracycline, but the advantages of compliance with directly observed therapy and reduction of costs for additional clinic visits may make the additional expenditure of azithromycin worthwhile.

Partner/contact tracing

This is an essential component of management and treatment to ascertain the recent sexual contacts and provide means for their treatment.

It is important to explain to the patient that their contact is most likely to be asymptomatic and to have no knowledge of the infection. This is particularly the case in cervical, anal and pharyngeal sources. One has to emphasize that the symptomatic patient may be the only source of information for the contact that an infection is present. It is most advantageous for the contact(s) to attend the same physician as the source patient, who can then deal with any other problem that may be revealed through the full sexually transmitted disease screen. The doctor's card or contact slip with the diagnosis (coded if required) and source patient reference number is given to the patient for each contact.

As an arbitrary guide, all sexual contacts of patients with urethritis should be screened and treated if their last sexual exposure with the contact(s) was within 60 days before symptom onset or diagnosis, or if the last sexual exposure was more than 60 days before the onset of symptoms or diagnosis, then the most recent sex partner should be screened and treated.

Review-test of cure

Traditionally, patients should return for review and test of cure at least once. Whilst this may be deemed unnecessary by some due to the efficacy of current regimens, it does ensure eradication of the infection and gives an opportunity to deal with any further problems that may emerge from screening. It permits sexual health promotion with further discussion and exploration of partner/contact tracing and giving information on safe sex guidelines at a more receptive period, when the patient is less focused on the acute infection. Current reports indicate that it is the time spent and quality of counselling that most impacts on patient compliance with safe sex guidelines.

Patients must return 3 months after the last sexual contact for 3-month serology to rule out incipient syphilis, hepatitis B or human immunodeficiency virus.

Recent recognition of high prevalence of chlamydia in women with previous chlamydial infection has resulted in recommendation of re-screening for chlamydia, 3–4 months after treatment of the initial infection. Additionally, annual screening is recommended for sexually active adolescents and young adults, as well as for those over 25 years with a risk factor for chlamydial acquisition, such as partner change.

Non-gonococcal urethritis may be only a simple acute bacterial infection, easily diagnosed, easily treated. But its acquisition indicates risk-taking behaviour and perhaps an underlying personal and emotional need that would warrant exploration and counselling for proper management in the complete sense of the word. Additionally, it has the potential to cause ascending infection in the female partner, leading to pelvic inflammatory disease, with the risk of infertility or ectopic pregnancy in the future.

Notification

Most European countries require notification of cases of non-gonococcal urethritis and *Chlamydia trachomatis* to public health authorities.

Further reading

Byrne GI. Chlamydial treatment failures: a persistent problem? *JEADV* 2001; 14: 381.

Carlin EM, Barton SE. Azithromycin as the first-line treatment of non-gonococcal urethritis (NGU): a study of follow up rates, contact attendance and patients' treatment preference. *Int J STD AIDS* 1996; 7: 185–9.

Centers for Disease Control and Prevention. Sexually transmitted diseases treatment guidelines 2002. *Morbid Mortal Wkly Rep* 2002; 51(RR6): 30–36.

Drug treatment of genital chlamydial infection. *Drugs Ther Bull* 2001; 39: 27–30.

European Guidelines for the Management of Gonorrhoea. *Int J STD AIDS* 2001; 12 (Suppl. 3), 27–9.

Morton RS, Kinghorn GR. Genitourinary chlamydial infection: a reappraisal and hypothesis. *Int J STD AIDS* 1999; 10: 765–75.

Stamm WE, Hicks CB, Martin DH *et al.* Azithromycin for empirical treatment of the nongonococcal urethritis syndrome in men. *JAMA* 1995; 274: 545–9.

Taylor-Robinson D. *Mycoplasma genitalium*—an update. *Int J STD AIDS* 2002; 13: 145–51.

UK National Guidelines on Sexually Transmitted Infections and closely related conditions. *Sex Transm Infect* 1999; 75 (Suppl. 7), S13–15.

Urticaria

F. Lawlor and A. Kobza Black

Synonyms

Urticaria has been variably described as nettle rash (the lesions resembling those induced by nettle stings), weals or hives.

Definition and epidemiology

Urticaria appears on the skin as multiple short-lived erythematous, macular, annular and wealing lesions which usually itch. Each lesion lasts less than 24 h. The lesions change continually and weals vary in size from tiny (1–2 mm) to very large (several centimetres). Angioedema is considered to be a deeper form of urticaria, presenting as swellings of the eyes, lips, ears, and other areas. It originates in subcutaneous or submucosal tissues. These swellings may last between 24 h and 72 h, are less likely to be itchy and also leave normal skin. Angioedema may occur alone or concurrently with the urticaria.

A physical urticaria is one which occurs in response to a specific physical stimulus. The physical stimuli which produce lesions are divided into mechanical trauma (friction and pressure), change in temperature (cold and heat), light and water. Physical urticarias often occur in association with ordinary urticaria and with each other.

Any urticaria, which remits up to 6 weeks after onset, is arbitrarily deemed to be acute urticaria. Urticaria with episodes, which last longer than 6 weeks, is considered chronic urticaria.

There are no data relating specifically to the incidence of acute urticaria in the population. Chronic urticaria comprises 70% of all urticaria patients seen at dermatology clinics. Women are affected twice as frequently as men. Twenty per cent of patients seen in dermatology clinics have physical urticarias.

Aetiology and pathogenesis

Acute urticaria

The most dramatic urticaria, acute allergic urticaria is an immunoglobulin E (IgE)-mediated allergic reaction which may be associated with systemic anaphylaxis. Many of these patients are atopic subjects. A minor IgE-mediated reaction may present solely as urticaria without systemic symptoms. This response may be provoked by insect stings, drugs, blood products, latex and by various foods for example fish, milk, nuts, beans, shellfish, eggs, potatoes, celery, parsley or spices. Acute urticaria may be associated with viral or bacterial infections, ingestion of medication such as antibiotics or non-steroidal anti-inflammatory drugs, or with the onset of thyroid disease but frequently no cause is found. Aspirin is the sole cause of urticaria in some people and worsens the disease in 50% of patients. The mechanism is non-immunological but the precise mechanism has not been defined. Other non-steroidal anti-inflammatory medication may behave in the same way. Codeine and morphine release histamine from mast cells.

Angiotensin-converting enzyme inhibitors may cause severe angioedema and are best avoided in patients with urticaria and angioedema. In very rare cases dyes (including tartrazine, sunset yellow, red and blue dyes), and preservatives (including benzoic acid, salicylates and ascorbic acid) have been reported to cause acute urticaria.

Chronic urticaria

In the absence of a physical provoking factor, no underlying cause is found in most cases. However in patients presenting with predominantly angioedema it is necessary to consider a deficiency of C1 esterase inhibitor (C1 INH). The deficiency may be inherited as an autosomal dominant trait and usually presents in the first two decades of life. An acquired form has occurred in lymphoproliferative disease, for example B-cell lymphoma as well as systemic lupus erythematous and both rectal adenocarcinoma and thyroid carcinoma.

Recently, functionally significant histamine-releasing IgG autoantibodies have been demonstrated in up to 50% of patients with ordinary chronic urticaria. These are directed usually against the high affinity IgE receptor (FcεRI) but less frequently against IgE. The subclasses are usually IgG1 and IgG3, which bind complement, and participation of complement in enhancing histamine release is probable in some patients. Histamine-releasing high-affinity IgE receptor (FcεRI) autoantibodies appear to be specific for ordinary chronic urticaria. The suggestion of an autoimmune pathogenesis of the disease in these patients is supported by increased association of thyroid autoimmunity, a strong association with HLADRB1* (DR4), and by the response to treatments designed to remove, reduce or neutralize autoantibodies.

There is no easy or commercially available test to detect the autoantibodies directed against high-affinity IgE receptor (FcεRI) and IgE. A screening test is the use of the autologous serum skin test, to detect a weal-inducing factor in the serum of patients with active chronic urticaria, and further identification is the measurement of differential histamine release from normal basophils of low and high IgE occupancy. It would be useful to develop an enzyme-linked immunosorbent assay (ELISA) assay, but this is proving difficult because of the low levels of the antibodies and also would not prove histamine-releasing functionality.

However although autoimmune urticaria is more severe, the treatment is similar, except for the most resistant cases when immunomodulating medication may be tried.

Clinical characteristics and course

The clinical characteristics of the lesions have been described above. It is generally not appreciated how severely the condition affects the quality of life because of the itching, occasional pain, the disfigurement and unpredictability of the lesions. Patients who attended a hospital urticaria clinic had a similar quality of life in many aspects as those waiting for a triple coronary bypass.

Although 50% of patients with urticaria had cleared in 6 months to a year, up to 25% of those with urticaria with or without angioedema still had lesions 20 years later. The clinical course in any patient is impossible to predict, although there is often a gradual tendency towards improvement. However some patients have intermittent episodes, and may develop exacerbations during infections.

Diagnosis and laboratory examinations

The diagnosis is clinical as patients may not have visible lesions when assessed. The initial interview with the patient will give nearly all available useful information. If there are no specific indicators in the history, the only routine investigation suggested is a full blood count, erythrocyte, sedimentation rate and urine analysis. If the history is suggestive of physical urticaria challenge tests should be performed if possible to confirm the diagnosis.

Routine tests for immediate food allergy (e.g. prick tests) are not indicated, but may be performed to investigate a suspected food allergen in the history.

If patients strongly suspect a dietary factor, a placebo-controlled challenge testing to food additives may be carried out, and a positive result confirmed by rechallenge.

If C1 INH inhibitor deficiency is suspected, the plasma level of C4 is a useful screening test for hereditary angioedema. Treatment of this is not covered, readers are advised to consult specialist publications. A skin biopsy is necessary to demonstrate a suspected urticarial vasculitis or may be helpful to confirm delayed pressure urticaria.

Differential diagnosis

The main differential diagnosis of urticaria is urticarial vasculitis. Here weals last 3–7 days, are burning, painful or itchy, purpuric, urticarial and very occasionally bullous. Bruised looking angioedema is suggestive of urticarial vasculitis which is generally poorly responsive to antihistamines. An autoimmune disorder such as lupus erythematosus should be considered in patients with confirmed urticarial vasculitis. Other differential diagnoses include acute inflammatory skin conditions in the early phase, such as acute contact dermatitis, erythema multiforme and prebullous eruptions. In the early stages of inflammatory diseases when the swellings may fluctuate, conditions such as acute contact dermatitis and collagen vascular diseases including lupus erythematosus and dermatomyositis and granulomatous cheilitis may be confused with angioedema.

Treatment

General therapeutic guidelines

Patient education

Where this is no obvious cause of urticaria from the history and clinical examination, it is important for the patient to understand that the condition is not allergic in origin, except in certain acute cases. Ordinary urticaria is not associated with any underlying diseases, not fatal, not malignant, not contagious and not curable. However there is usually a tendency to improvement, it can be emphasized at the onset of urticaria, most will remit spontaneously within weeks. Once chronic, having lasted for more than 6 weeks, in 50% of patients the disease will remit within 6 months. However, no promises can be made as in some it will last years. Patients should understand that an exhaustive series of tests will not be helpful. Patients should be requested to avoid the drugs, which exacerbate urticaria including non-steroidal anti-inflammatory drugs especially aspirin, histamine liberators such as codeine, but paracetamol can usually be tolerated. Exclusion diets are rarely helpful and diets should only exclude substances proven to be a problem.

Keeping cool, cool baths and soothing topical applications, e.g. calamine cream or 1% menthol in a moisturizing base, minimizing stress and alcohol are helpful in some people.

Drug treatment

H_1-receptor blockade

The condition can usually be controlled with H_1-antihistamines taken in adequate dosage.

The aim of drug treatment for urticaria with antihistamines is to decrease the itch and the number and size of duration of the weals. It may not be possible to completely control the condition without an unacceptable level of side-effects. Since each individual patient responds uniquely, it may be necessary to change and combine antihistamines and try doses higher than those recommended by the manufacturer. This may be the case because higher doses have additional antiallergic properties *in vitro*, but such additional benefit has not been proved clinically. A combination of antihistamines of a different chemical group such as loratadine 10 mg in the morning and cetirizine 10 mg in the evening appear to be useful in practice, but there are no trials confirming the benefit of combinations of antihistamines.

Antihistamines are well absorbed when taken orally and absorption is not related to the ingestion of food. The timing of tablet taking is important and should be related both to the time of day when the urticaria is at its worst and to the half-life of the drug or its active metabolite. The half-life is longer in the elderly so the drug may accumulate and the half-life is shorter in children who tolerate higher doses.

The first two available second-generation antihistamines terfenadine and astemizole have been withdrawn in many countries due to the ability of the parent compounds rarely to cause cardiac arrhythmias particularly irregular ventricular tachycardias, in special circumstances. This included accumulation of the drugs by exceeding the recommended dose, inhibition of degradation by cytochrome P450 by drugs metabolized by the same pathway (azoles, macrolide antibiotics), liver disease and a predisposition to cardiac arrhythmias. This would include congenital QT prolongation and concomittant use of tricyclic antidepressants, antipsychotics, antiarrythmic drugs and electrolyte imbalance.

No antihistamine has been shown to be devoid of the risk of the teratogenicity but the older antihistamines, e.g. chlorpheniramine are traditionally used in pregnancy. It is important to remember that any antihistamine has the potential to worsen urticaria. The mechanism is not determined but it is suggested that this may be due to a direct toxic effect on the mast cell membrane.

Recommended treatments

Second-generation H_1-receptor antagonists

Second-generation antihistamines are the first-line drug treatment for urticaria and have been proven by double-blind trials to improve urticaria, generally by the order of two-thirds. This group of drugs include cetirizine, loratadine, acrivastine, mizolastine and ebastine. These drugs are H_1-receptor antagonists and block the H_1-receptor by competitive inhibition. Generally, if the manufacturers' recommended doses are used, they do not cause significant drowsiness, psychomotor impairment or anticholinergic side-effects. However there is individual variation, and patients should be warned of these rare possibilities, and also that excess alcohol should be avoided. Generally all these antihistamines are as effective as each other in clinical trials. It should be emphasized to the patient that the antihistamine is not a cure, but is best taken regularly as a prophylactic, until the urticaria resolves.

Second-generation H_1-antihistamines

Cetirizine is derived from hydroxyzine. The manufacturers recommended dose is 10 mg over 24 h. It is excreted by the kidneys and may cause problems in the elderly where it should be monitored carefully. The recommended dose is 10 mg per 24 h. The drug rarely cause drowsiness, but does more frequently if this dose is exceeded. So far there have not been any major adverse effects with this drug.

Loratadine 10 mg daily is an effective antihistamine with no significant sedation or interaction with other medications.

Mizolastine is also an effective antihistamine in a dose of 10 mg/day. Prolongation of the QT interval has occurred in a few patients, so the dose should not be increased and it has the same precautions that applied to astemizole and terfenadine above.

Acrivastine is not usually potent enough alone to control urticaria. The recommended dose is 8 mg three times a day. It is helpful if a rapid response to treatment is sought and as an adjunct to treatment with other antihistamines as it has a fast onset and a short duration of action.

Ebastine at a dose of 10 mg daily is an effective antihistamine with no significant sedation or side-effects or interactions with other medications.

Third-generation H_1-receptor antagonists

Some authorities describe a third generation of antihistamines which are the active metabolites of the second generation, as having fewer side-effects and some antiallergic properties, but the distinction is arbitrary.

Fexofenadine hydrochloride is an active metabolite of terfenadine and without the cardiotoxic effects of terfenadine. To date, few adverse effects and no drowsiness have been reported. The recommended daily dose is 180 mg in the evening.

Desloratadine is an active metabolite of loratadine with powerful antihistaminic properties and also antiallergic activity *in vitro*. There are studies to show that it improves urticaria compared to placebo, but licensing for this indication is awaited. The recommended dose is 5 mg daily.

Classical antihistamines

If necessary and if sedation might be helpful a first-generation antihistamine would be used especially for night-time sedation. The group includes chlorpheniramine maleate, hydroxyzine hydrochloride and diphenhydramine hydrochloride. Doxepin, a tricyclic antidepressant with a powerful antihistaminic activity can control urticaria used on its own, but is best for night-time sedation of the anxious patient. With the exception of hydroxyzine these drugs tend to be less effective than the second-generation antihistamines.

Combining H_1- and H_2-receptor antagonists

The results of trials combining H_1- and H_2-receptor antagonists are conflicting, though some show a significant improvement compared to either medication alone, in practice the combination is disappointing and does not usually produce a clinically significant improvement. However an H_1-antagonist in full dose can be given in conjunction with ranitidine 150 mg 12 hourly for a trial period.

Medication stabilizing mast cells

Although there are some controlled studies, which demonstrate that the addition of medication with *in vitro* mast cell stabilizing properties, such as nifedipine and theophylline to antihistamines leads to improved control of urticaria, this has not been the experience of the authors.

Systemic steroids

Systemic steroids are best avoided for the treatment of chronic urticaria except in special circumstances and for very short periods. In the longer term, they may be ineffective and the side-effects are unacceptable.

They can be used short term (for a few days to weeks) for acute urticaria, or for an acute exacerbation of chronic urticaria. A starting dose of 30–40 mg would be appropriate. Longer-term therapy may be necessary for severe urticarial vasculitis and delayed pressure urticaria not responding to other therapy.

Treatment of angioedema

Acquired ordinary angioedema should be treated in the same way as urticaria with a dosage of H_1-antihistamine designed to suppress the disease. If angioedema occurs in the mouth and causes moderately severe problems, this can be treated with adrenaline inhaler, four puffs into the oral mucosa in hospital or the surgery. This is available in the USA and can be prescribed on a named basis (Primatene Mist, Whitehall Laboratories, USA). Severe angioedema is treated with epinephrine (adrenaline) (0.5 mg to 1.0 mL of 1 : 1000 mg/mL solution intramuscular or subcutaneous injection) then by hydrocortisone (100–200 mg i.m). Adrenaline is available for self-administration by patients as a mini-jet (0.5 mL) or as an adrenaline Epipen (0.3 mL for an adult or 0.15 mL for paediatric use). Patients should be taught how to self administer and in what circumstances, e.g. for difficulty breathing. Patients with a history of severe oropharyngeal and laryngeal angioedema or anaphylaxis, should have two in-date ones available for emergency use, as a repeat dose should be administered after 10 min if the initial response is not satisfactory.

Treatments for the physical urticarias

Symptomatic dermographism

This usually responds well to treatment with H_1-antihistamines, but in severe cases a larger than recommended dose may need to be used. Ultraviolet B therapy at suberythrogenic doses 2–3 times/week for 8 weeks may provide additional improvement.

Delayed pressure urticaria

This nearly always occurs in conjunction with chronic urticaria, but the pressure urticaria may be the major problem. Treat the chronic urticaria with H_1-antihistamines and minimize pressure on the skin. Large doses of cetirizine may have a marginal effect on pressure-induced weals. Topical benzydamine cream occasionally helps. In very severe disease, short course of prednisolone (30 mg daily) can be given but side-effects are troublesome if long-term use is contemplated.

Cholinergic urticaria

Cholinergic urticaria responds partially to conventional antihistamines.

Danazol (200–800 mg) or Stanozolol (2.5–10 mg daily) may be used in resistant disease, with adequate precautions. It is hoped that it will be for a short-term only, in contrast to their use in hereditary angiodema.

Cold urticaria, localized heat urticaria, vibratory angioedema

In these conditions H_1-antagonists are partially effective. Induction of tolerance by repeated graduated exposure to the physical precipitant can be helpful in all of these conditions, but is cumbersome to perform, and needs to be maintained regularly.

It is important to warn patients with cold urticaria against cold water bathing due to the risk of anaphylaxis and potential drowning.

Aquagenic urticaria

This rare physical urticaria usually responds at least partially to conventional H_1-antihistamines.

New experimental treatments for ordinary 'idiopathic chronic' urticaria

Medication reported to be effective in case reports

Medications that have been reported to be effective in case reports or open trials include anabolic steroids, tranexamic acid (for angioedema) and leukotriene antagonists. In extremely severely affected suitably selected patients these can be tried before considering immunotherapy.

Immunomodulating agents

These have been mainly used in severely affected patients with disease suggestive of autoimmune urticaria unresponsive to conventional treatment.

Ciclosporin

There are several open trials of the efficacy of ciclosporin in severe urticaria. A recent placebo-controlled trial of ciclosporin at a dose of 4 mg/kg for 1 month was performed in patients with a positive autologous serum skin test, while continuing on cetirizine 10 mg twice a day. Non-responders were offered ciclosporin for another month. At the end of the study, two third of patients showed greater than 75% improvement, which was maintained in 26% at 6 months. Side-effects were common, but not severe. In a previous study a similar improvement was shown in patients who had a negative autologous serum skin test, so ciclosporin may also be effective in this group of patients, but further studies are needed.

Intravenous immunoglobulin (IVIG)

In an open trial, of 10 patients with autoimmune urticaria given 0.4 g/kg per day of immunoglobulin intravenously for 5 days, improvement was induced in nine patients, three of whom were in remission 3 years later. Although headache, pyrexia and superficial thrombophlebitis were common during treatment, there were no serious side-effects.

Plasmapheresis

The treatment is expensive and potentially hazardous. It is reserved for the most recalcitrant, extremely severely affected autoimmune urticaria patients. In one open study, plasma exchange carried out in eight patients over a 5-day period produced temporary improvement in six patients.

Further reading

Greaves M. Chronic urticaria. *N Engl J Med* 1995; 332 (25): 1767.

Kobza Black A, Grattan CEH. Advances in the management of urticaria. In: Marks R, Leyden, eds. *Dermatological Therapy in Current Practice.* London: Martin Dunitz, 2001.

Lawlor F, Greaves MW. Chronic urticaria. In: Lichtenstein FM, Fauci AS, eds. *Current Therapy in Allergy, Immunology and Rheumatology.* Philadelphia: Mosby, 1997.

Simons FER, Simons KJ. The pharmacology and use of H_1-receptor antagonist drugs. *N Engl J Med* 1994; 330 (23): 1667.

Varicella

S. Georgala

Synonyms

Chickenpox.

Definition and epidemiology

Varicella is a highly communicable acute primary infection caused by the varicella-zoster virus (VZV). It is characterized by a rapidly progressing pruritic eruption that appears in successive crops and consists of intermingled papules, vesicles, pustules and crusts. Although commonly occurring as a benign disease of childhood, it may be associated with life-threatening complications when it affects adults, pregnant women, newborns or immunocompromised patients.

Varicella is more prevalent in temperate climates, where it shows peaks in winter and spring. In the USA, there are 3–4 million cases annually. Of the cases, 90% involve children younger than 10 years of age and fewer than 5% involve individuals older than 15 years. In the UK, chickenpox increasingly affects preschool children compared with other age groups.

Varicella is highly contagious, as indicated by the very high (> 90%) secondary attack rate in household contacts. It is transmitted mainly by airborne droplets or, less commonly, by direct contact with varicella or herpes zoster lesions. A patient is infectious for 1–2 days before the onset of the rash until all lesions have crusted, usually by day 6.

One attack of varicella usually confers lasting immunity. However, clinical recurrence occurs more frequently than it is generally recognized.

Aetiology and pathophysiology

Varicella is caused by herpes virus varicellae, also referred to as VZV, an enveloped, double-stranded DNA, α-herpes virus.

The virus enters through the mucosa of the upper respiratory tract, the oropharynx and, less often, the conjuctivae. Local multiplication results in primary viraemia. The virus is removed by cells of the reticuloendothelial system, which represent the major site of viral replication. During secondary viraemia that follows, peripheral mononuclear cells disseminate the virus throughout the body, especially to the skin and the respiratory mucosa, permitting spread to susceptible contacts. Specific humoral and cellular immune response to VZV terminates viraemia. It appears that cell-mediated immunity plays a central role in the disease control. Therefore, patients with defective cell-mediated immunity experience more severe varicella, compared to those with impaired humoral immunity. VZV may become latent in the dorsal root or other sensory ganglia. If reactivated, it causes herpes zoster.

Clinical characteristics and course

After an incubation period averaging 14–17 days (range 7–23 days), the illness commences with prodromal symptoms (fever, chills, malaise, anorexia, headache, back or abdominal pain), usually mild or absent in children, but more prominent and prolonged in adults. Temperature elevation is usually moderate, but occasionally may reach 40–41°C. The eruption first appears on the scalp or the trunk, exhibiting a centripetal distribution on the face, the trunk and the proximal part of the extremities. It is usually more profuse in protected parts, as well as at sites of chronic cutaneous inflammation. Lesions initially appear as discrete erythematous macules that quickly evolve to papules and then to clear, thin-walled vesicles surrounded by an irregular erythematous areola that gives the classic appearance of 'dew-drops on a rose petal'. Clouding and umbilication of vesicles results in evolution to pustules and finally to crusts that fall off in 1–3 weeks without residual scarring. The progression from macule to crust lasts approximately 8–12 h. A characteristic feature of varicella is that lesions appear in successive crops. As a result, lesions at different stages of development can be observed in any one part of the body. This is pathognomonic for varicella. Lesions (vesicles evolving to ulcers) may develop also on mucous membranes, especially of the oral cavity (palate) or of the genitals. Moderate to intense pruritus is most often present throughout the vesicular stage.

In normal children, varicella almost invariably runs a mild, self-limited course. Complications are rare and can be divided into viral and bacterial. Of them, bacterial skin and soft-tissue infections (impetigo, furuncles, cellulitis, erysipelas, necrotizing fasciitis/pyomyositis), most commonly due to *Staphylococcus aureus* or *Streptococcus pyogenes*, are the most frequent. These are inflicted by scratching and may produce crater-like pockmark scars.

On the other hand, the following groups are at high risk of severe disease associated with life-threatening complications:

- otherwise healthy adults and adolescents
- pregnant women
- newborns
- patients with immunosuppressive malignancy or patients with leukaemia or cancer under immunosuppressive chemotherapy or radiotherapy
- patients with iatrogenic immunosuppression due to treatment with cytotoxic or immunosuppressive agents or corticosteroids (systemic or intranasal).
- transplant recipients under immunosuppression, particularly bone marrow transplant recipients
- human immunodeficiency virus (HIV) infected individuals

In adults and in immunocompromised patients, primary varicella pneumonia (PVP) is the major complication. In a study, radiographic evidence of PVP was found in 16% of healthy adult males, while clinical signs were present in 4%. PVP usually occurs 1–6 days after the onset of the rash and it is manifested by cough, dyspnea, cyanosis and pleuritic chest pain, or it may be asymptomatic. Physical signs are minimal and chest X-rays reveal diffuse bilateral nodular densities. Mortality rate is 10–30%.

Neurological complications, including encephalitis, acute cerebellar ataxia, acute ascending or transverse myelitis, Guillain–Barré syndrome, etc., occur in fewer than 1 in 1000 cases. Complete recovery is the rule. In contrast, adult encephalitis has a mortality rate of up to 35%. Reye's syndrome is an acute encephalopathy associated with fatty degeneration of the viscera, especially of the liver. Salicylates have been incriminated in its obscure pathogenesis. Although it is an uncommon complication of normal children, its mortality is as high as 40%.

Mild chemical hepatitis is common. Other visceral complications include nephritis, orchitis, pericarditis, myocarditis and pancreatitis. Involvement of multiple organs is particularly likely in those with defective host defence. Haemorrhagic complications range from transient thrombocytopenia to haemorrhagic varicella (purpura fulminans).

In HIV+ patients atypical forms of varicella have been described (such as verrucous varicella) and the most frequent complications are recurrent and persistent varicella.

Varicella during pregnancy poses a threat for both mother and the fetus.

The reported incidence of gestational varicella is 1–7 per 10 000 pregnancies. The mother is at increased risk for disseminated varicella or serious PVP. Maternal viraemia may result in intrauterine infection. Early infection of the embryo may lead to abortion. The risk for fetopathy is 2% or less, reaching its peak between the seventh and 20th week. Maternal chickenpox during the first two trimesters of pregnancy may cause congenital varicella syndrome. This is manifested by limb hypoplasia and skeletal anomalies, neurological or ocular defects, cicatricial skin scarring and low birth weight. Vertical transmission in late pregnancy may result in preterm delivery or stillbirth. Maternal chickenpox around the time of delivery can cause severe and even fatal disease in the newborn. When the rash in the mother occurs less than 5 days before, or within 2 days after delivery, the onset of varicella in the newborn occurs between the fifth to 10th day of life. At this stage, the infant's immune system is immature and the infant is born before sufficient protective maternal antibody has crossed the placenta to modify the infection. Perinatal varicella is associated with 20% mortality due to progressive visceral disease.

Diagnosis

Varicella diagnosis is made chiefly by history and clinical examination. Laboratory confirmation is important to establish diagnosis in atypical cases.

- Routine laboratory investigation is non-contributory. Asymptomatic elevation of alanine aminotransferase (ALT) and aspartate aminotransferase (AST) may be noted. Chest X-ray is necessary in adult patients.
- Tzanck test: cytological examination of material scraped from the base of an early vesicle demonstrates the presence of multinucleated giant cells and epithelial cells containing acidophilic intranuclear bodies. It can not distinguish between herpes simplex virus and VZV infection.
- Electron microscopy: identification of herpes virus particles in biopsy material or vesicle fluid.
- Viral culture: isolation of VZV in cell cultures (human fibroblast monolayers) inoculated with vesicle fluid, blood or infected tissue.
- Identification of VZV antigens in vesicle fluid, biopsy material, etc., by immunofluorescence or other techniques.
- Identification of VZV-DNA by polymerase chain reaction (PCR).
- Serology offers retrospective diagnosis of varicella by comparing antibody titres in acute and convalescent sera. Presence of immunoglobulin M (IgM) antibody or four-fold increase (or greater) in paired sera IgG titres, is indicative of varicella. Serological tests are also useful to determine the immune status to VZV and to identify susceptible individuals.

IgG, IgM and IgA to VZV are detectable within 2–5 days after the onset of varicella and reach their peak during second to third week. IgM and IgA titres decline rapidly, while IgG persists at low levels for life.

For varicella histology see chapter on herpes zoster.

Differential diagnosis

Other generalized vesicular eruptions should be excluded:

- Smallpox or generalized vaccinia (eradication of smallpox and cessation of vaccination has diminished the diagnostic problem).
- Disseminated herpes simplex or disseminated herpes zoster (concentration of lesions at the site of primary infection/isolation of virus in tissue cultures or identification of viral antigens or nucleic acid).

- Bullous impetigo (usually larger, more purulent and crusted lesions/bacterial culture).
- Eczema herpeticum.
- Vesicular exanthems caused by Coxsackie viruses, echoviruses or ricketsial pox.
- Drug eruption, erythema multiform.
- Dermatitis herpetiformis.
- Insect bites, scabies, papular urticaria.

Treatment

General therapeutic guidelines

Treatment of varicella can be divided into symptomatic and aetiological (antiviral).

Symptomatic therapy is directed mainly towards pruritus and fever. All patients may benefit from symptomatic therapy.

Itching may be alleviated by application of a drying antipruritic lotion, e.g. calamine alone or with 0.25% menthol and/or 1.0% phenol. Cool water compresses or tepid baths with baking soda (1/4 cup per tub of water) may also offer relief. Oral antihistamines may prove effective in controlling generalized pruritus.

To avoid scratching nails should be kept short and clean.

To control fever, antipyretics may be necessary. Aspirin is contraindicated due to the suggested association with Reye's syndrome.

Mouth and perineal lesions can be treated with rinses or compresses with 1.5% hydrogen peroxide, saline or other agents.

Topical corticosteroids should be avoided.

To treat bacterial superinfections of skin lesions, topical antibiotics, e.g. mupirocin ointment or bacitracin-polymyxin, should be applied. If the infection is widespread, systemic antibiotics, such as erythromycin, dicloxacillin or cephalexin, should be administered.

Hygiene is important. Bathing, stringent soaks, isolation in a well-ventilated room with regular change of bedding and light diet should be provided.

Aetiological therapy is directed against VZV. The range of antiviral agents available includes several chemotherapeutic agents, mostly nucleoside analogues, that interfere with viral replication by inhibiting specific steps of this process. Antiviral agents have only a virostatic effect on replicating virus. Consequently, viral latency is not eradicated.

Recommended therapies

Aciclovir (ACV)

ACV is the drug of choice. ACV (guanosine analogue) is selectively phosphorylated by VZV thymidine kinase to ACV monophosphate and by cellular enzymes to ACV triphosphate that inhibits viral DNA polymerase and halts viral DNA synthesis. ACV has been used safely and effectively in the treatment of herpes virus infections for over 10 years. ACV must be initiated within 24–48 h from the onset of rash. It may be administered orally (20 mg/kg, maximum 800 mg, 4 times daily for 5 days in children, or 800 mg 5 times daily for 5 days in adults) or, in cases of disseminated or complicated varicella, intravenously (500 mg/m^2 or 10 mg/kg, every 8 h for 7–10 days or until no new lesions have appeared for 48 h). Randomized placebo-controlled studies have shown that oral ACV in normal children, adolescents and adults, reduces the severity and duration of cutaneous and systemic signs and symptoms, with an excellent safety profile. In addition, intravenous ACV has proved effective in preventing dissemination of varicella and has markedly decreased the incidence of visceral complications, the viral shedding time and the length of healing in patients of the high-risk groups. Good hydration and adjustment for decreased creatinine clearance levels is necessary in patients with renal insufficiency.

Guidelines for the use of ACV for varicella (modified from the recommendations of the American Academy of Pediatrics—1993) are as follows:

1 Based on marginal therapeutic effect, cost and feasibility of drug delivery, oral ACV is not recommended routinely for the treatment of uncomplicated varicella in otherwise healthy children. These patients require only symptomatic therapy.
2 In the following groups at increased risk for severe varicella, the use of oral ACV is optional:
   - otherwise healthy non-pregnant individuals 13 years of age or older
   - secondary household contacts
   - children older than 12 months with chronic cutaneous, or pulmonary disorders (e.g. cystic fibrosis), or diabetes mellitus, or patients requiring long-term salicylate therapy or intermittent steroid therapy.
3 In the following groups of previously ill patients, ACV must be initiated as soon as possible and should be given intravenously:
   - patients with malignancy (leukaemia, lymphoproliferative disorders, metastatic cancer, etc.)
   - patients with congenital T-cell immunodeficiency or HIV infection
   - patients receiving high doses of steroids
   - bone marrow or organ transplant recipients
   - neonates with varicella that follows maternal disease beginning within 5 days before and 2 days after delivery
   - patients with visceral complications, such as primary varicella pneumonia or encephalitis.

For patients receiving cytotoxic or immunosuppressive chemotherapy, the latter should be temporarily discontinued, if possible, and resumed 7 days after complete crusting of lesions. Accordingly, steroids should be tapered during incubation period.

4 Pregnant women with varicella may benefit from oral ACV, but it is still controversial if this is safe for the fetus.

Resistance to ACV is very rare among immunocompetent individuals. However, increasing clinical use of ACV has been associated with the emergence of drug resistant VZV strains, particularly among immunocompromised patients. Resistance results from mutations at the level of thymidine kinase (TK). In these cases, antiviral treatment with foscarnet (40 mg/kg i.v. every 8 h) is indicated. Foscarnet is a direct inhibitor of viral DNA polymerase and does not require activation by the viral TK. Recently, emergence of foscarnet-resistant strains has also been reported, which are sensitive to the acyclic nucleoside phosphonate cidofovir. The latter depends only on cellular enzymes for its conversion to the diphosphoryl derivative, which inhibits the viral DNA polymerase.

Vidarabine and interferon-α

Vidarabine intravenously (10 mg/kg over 12 h for 5 days) represents an alternative antiviral treatment for severe varicella. It is as effective as ACV, but is far more toxic. Human interferon-α (3.5×10^5 U/kg daily for 2 days, followed by 1.75×10^5 U/kg daily for 3 days) or infusion of irradiated lymphocytes from healthy donors recovering from VZV infection, have been employed with satisfactory results.

Alternative and experimental treatments

Several new antiviral agents have been developed, some of which are still under clinical evaluation. Oral penciclovir (and its prodrug famciclovir) and oral valaciclovir are particularly effective against VZV, but their indication for varicella has not been approved as yet. They both have high oral bioavailability which permits less frequent dosing and avoidance of intravenous therapy in many cases. Oral sorivudine (BV-AraU) is a nucleoside analogue with enhanced *in vitro* and *in vivo* efficacy against VZV and enhanced oral bioavailability, as compared to existing antivirals. It is administered once daily at a dose of 40 mg for 5 days. In controlled studies, it has proved to be superior to ACV. In the USA, sorivudine has been licensed for treatment of varicella in adults. Other promising agents include brivudin, brovavir, desciclovir, cidofovir, valganciclovir, etc.

Bacterial focal infections should be treated with antibiotics, guided by the results of Gram-stained smears and cultures.

Primary varicella pneumonia necessitates antiviral chemotherapy with intravenous ACV, combined or not with corticosteroids. Assisted ventilation or extracorporeal membrane oxygenation is employed in cases of respiratory insufficiency.

Central nervous system and haemorrhagic complications are treated with antiviral chemotherapy combined with corticosteroids.

Prevention

Prevention of varicella is difficult because it is communicable during the end of the incubation period. Isolation of patients with clinically evident disease until all lesions have crusted, is justified.

No preventive measures are recommended for a normal child who has been exposed to varicella. However, every effort should be made to keep high risk susceptible individuals away from contact with varicella or herpes zoster patients and to offer passive immunization in case of exposure.

Passive immunization can be achieved with standard human serum globulin (ISG), zoster immunoglobulin (ZIG), or varicella-zoster immunoglobulin (VZIG). Early administration, preferably within 3 days of exposure, can prevent varicella in normal children or modify varicella in immunocompromised patients (subclinical or mild infection). The duration of the protection is estimated to be 3 weeks. In the immunocompromised, ACV prophylaxis as adjuvant to VZIG is warranted. The use of VZIG after exposure during pregnancy does not appear to prevent primary varicella pneumonia of the mother, but there are preliminary indications that it could lower the risk for congenital varicella syndrome. Neonates of mothers who developed varicella within 7 days before and after delivery, should receive VZIG or a combination of intravenous immunoglobulin and intravenous ACV, to prevent or modify potentially fatal disease.

Active immunization with live attenuated VZV vaccine (Oka/Merck strain) is now available in some countries. It can be applied to all susceptible persons 12 months of age or older. The vaccine is recommended, first of all, for seronegative immunodeficient persons. However, the indication for vaccination of healthy children and normal susceptible adults remains controversial. Some authorities recommend serotesting rather than presumptive vaccination. A single dose is necessary for routine vaccination of 12–18-month-old infants or for catch-up immunity of children aged 18 months to 12 years. Two doses are given to immunize susceptible adolescents and adults. A 96% and 94% seroconversion rate has been reported for children and adults, respectively. The immunity induced by the vaccine is not as solid as that induced by the wild-type VZV infection, although there is evidence of long-term immunity (6–10 years). The vaccine reduces the incidence and morbidity of varicella, but it does not affect the incidence of herpes zoster. The vaccine was found immunogenic also in immunocompromised patients and can be safely administered to susceptible high risk individuals. Adverse reactions include fever, papulovesicular rash and reactions at the injection site.

There is no available chemoprophylaxis for varicella. Long-term prophylaxis with oral ACV (40 mg/kg daily) in the early

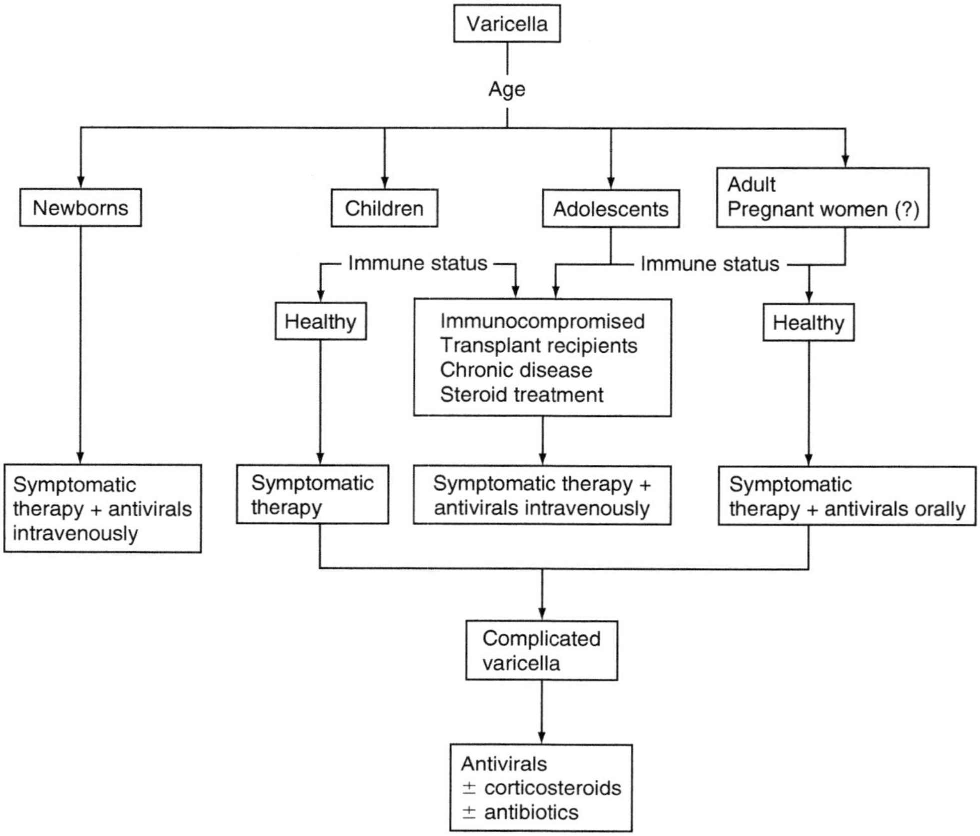

Figure 1 Varicella

months following bone marrow transplantation or in leukaemic children has shown satisfactory results.

Further reading

Alrabiah FA, Sacks SL. New antiherpesvirus agents. Their targets and therapeutic potential. *Drugs* 1996; 52 (1): 17–32.

American Academy of Pediatrics Committee of Infectious Diseases. The use of oral acyclovir in otherwise healthy children with varicella. *Pediatrics* 1993; 91 (3): 674–6.

Balfour HH Jr, Benson C, Braun J *et al.* Management of acyclovir-resistant herpes simplex and varicella-zoster virus infections. *J Acquir Immune Defic Syndr* 1994; 7 (3): 254–60.

De Clercq E. Antivirals for the treatment of herpesvirus infections. *J Antimicrob Chemother* 1993; 32 (Suppl. A): 121–32.

Drwal Klein LA, O'Donovan CA. Varicella in pediatric patients. *Am Pharmacother* 1993; 27 (7–8): 938–49.

Kesson AM, Grimwood K, Burgess MA *et al.* Acyclovir for the prevention and treatment of varicella zoster in children, adolescents and pregnancy. *J Paediatr Child Health* 1996; 32 (2): 211–17.

Snoeck R, Andrei G, Clercq ED. Novel agents for the therapy of varicella-zoster virus infections. *Expert Opin Invest Drugs* 2000; 9: 1743–51.

Vasquez M, LaRussa PM, Gershon AA *et al.* The effectiveness of the varicella vaccine in clinical practice. *N Engl J Med* 2001; 344: 955–60.

Wallace MR, Bowler WA, Murray NB *et al.* Treatment of adult varicella with oral acyclovir. A randomized, placebo-controlled trial. *Ann Intern Med* 1992; 117 (5): 358–63.

Wallace MR, Chamberlain CJ, Sawyer MH *et al.* Treatment of adult varicella with sorivudine: a randomized placebo-controlled trial. *J Infect Dis* 1996; 174 (2): 249–55.

Whitley RJ. Therapeutic approaches to varicella-zoster virus infections. *J Infect Dis* 1992; 166 (Suppl. 1): 851–7.

Whitley RJ. Sorivudine: a potent inhibitor of varicella-zoster virus replication. *Adv Exp Med Biol* 1996; 394: 41–4.

Vascular birthmarks: vascular malformations and haemangiomas

X.-H. Gao and G.W. Cherry

Definition, classification and epidemiology

Vascular birthmarks (superficial vascular anomalies, vascular neavi) are skin lesions that are mostly first noticed at birth or during the first weeks of life as a red, blue or purple blemish. The currently widely accepted classification for this group of diseases was initiated by the International Society for the Study of Vascular Anomalies (ISSVA) in 1992 and modified slightly in 1996. They are classified, based on clinical, histopathological manifestations and biological behaviours, as either vascular tumours (most of which are haemangiomas) or vascular malformations.

Haemangiomas of infancy are benign vascular tumours exhibiting cellular proliferation with typical developmental pattern; a period of active growth followed by a period of inactivity and subsequent involution. Based on their clinical appearances and histological involvements, haemangiomas of infancy can be classified into superficial (so-called 'strawberry haemangiomas', constituting about 50–60%), deep (formerly called 'cavernous haemangiomas', constituting 15%) or mixed types (constituting about 25–35%), all of which undergo the same maturation sequence. They are the most common benign tumours of infancy, present in 1.0% and 2.6% of newborns. The incidence by 1 year of age is approximately as high as 10–12% among white people. They are especially common among those infants born prematurely; there seems to be a strong correlation of incidences with birth weight (approximately one of every four newborns weighing less than 1000 g will develop a haemangioma), although a possible correlation with gestational age cannot be ruled out. The incidence of haemangiomas is about 4–6 times higher in females than males.

Vascular malformations, however, are structural anomalies of the vascular system and can be composed of capillaries, veins, lymphatics, arteries, or combinations of these. These lesions do not exhibit endothelial cell proliferation and they mostly do not tend to regress. They are divided into fast-flow vascular malformations and slow-flow vascular malformations, based on rheology and channel morphology. The former may be either arterial or arteriovenous—arterial malformation, arteriovenous fistula or arterial venous malformation. The latter may be venous, lymphatic and capillary malformations. There are also complex combined vascular malformations among arterial, venous, capillary and lymphatic structures, including capillary lymphatic malformations, capillary venous malformations, lymphatic venous malformations, arterial capillary malformations, capillary arteriovenous malformations and capillary arteriovenous lymphatic malformations. In addition, cutaneous vascular malformations can be a part of multiorgan involvement, the so-called syndromic vascular malformations. Among these various forms of vascular malformations, the most relevant entities to dermatologists are port-wine stains and salmon patches. Port-wine stains are characterized pathologically by ectasia of dermal capillaries and clinically by persistent macular erythema. The reported incidence in the newborn has been from 0.1% to 2%. They usually present at birth and rarely disappear in later life. Salmon patches have similar clinical and histological appearance with port-wine stains, while more than half of them have a dramatically different outcome—they tend to disappear 1 year after birth. They have been observed in the neonatal period in 20–60% of children of all races.

Caution should be taken about the above classification, as there are a small minority of patients who have an association of vascular malformations and haemangiomas.

Aetiology, pathogenesis and histopathology

Haemangiomas

The exact aetiology and pathogenesis of haemangiomas is not clear as many cellular or molecular components might be involved. Some molecules including proliferating cell nuclear antigen, type IV collagenase, vascular endothelial growth factor (VEGF) and basic fibroblast growth factor (bFGF) are highly expressed on endothelial cells. These molecules in part mediate endothelial cell differentiation and in turn evoke an influx of mast cells during the rapid growth phase of haemangiomas. Later expression of a potent inhibitor of new blood vessel formation—tissue inhibitor of metalloproteinase type 1 (TIMP-1)—might be an important factor to induce the involutional phase of haemangiomas.

Histopathological profiles of both superficial and deep haemangiomas are the same. In the proliferative stage they are comprised of syncytial aggregates of plump endothelial cells and pericytes, some of which form lumina and others solid cords; abundant pericytes, fibroblasts and mast cells are also characteristic. During the involutional phase the endothelial cells flatten and the vascular channels become more ectatic producing large thin-walled vessels. Islands of fatty tissue and fibrous strands gradually replace the tumour cells. Multilaminated basement membrane is persistent throughout the entire cycle of haemangiomas.

Vascular malformations

Vascular malformations are congenital lesions that have normal endothelial cell turnover and lack of excessive proliferation. They are structural anomalies of the vascular system and may be composed of capillaries, veins, lymphatics and arteries. Aberrant development during the retiform plexus stage might cause malformations. Dilated dermal capillary vessels can be seen in port-wine stains and salmon patches, and sometimes even no apparent histological abnormalities can be observed, especially at birth.

Clinical features and course

Haemangiomas

Early lesions may be clinically subtle and resemble a scratch, a bruise, a small patch of telangiectasias or hypopigmentation. Superficial haemangiomas evolve into circumscribed, vivid red, elevated, dome-shaped nodules or plaques of a rubbery consistency that can be partially blanched with pressure. Deep haemangiomas are skin-coloured or bluish and are an easily compressible mass that may fluctuate in size and deepen in colour with crying, activity or dependency of the affected part. The mixed haemangiomas usually have a deep mass with a central superficial component. The regression stage of superficial haemangiomas is heralded by softening of the lesion and by the appearance of opaque, pinkish grey areas in the centre of the surface; these foci gradually become confluent and extend towards the periphery of the lesion. Regression of deeper lesions is more difficult to visualize; however, the timing and progression are equivalent. About 40% of patients leave residual permanent skin changes after involution completed, including scarring, atrophy, redundant skin, discoloration and telangiectasias. About 50% of lesions occur on the head and neck, 25% on the trunk; perianal area is also a favoured site in both sexes. There can be single or multiple lesions in haemangiomas of infancy.

Approximately half of haemangiomas are present at birth; the remainder usually become evident within the first month of life. A characteristic growth phase follows the initial presentation for about 6–10 months, though an occasional deep haemangioma continues to enlarge slowly for another few months. Maximum size is usually reached by the end of the first year. Most of them undergo spontaneous regression for an average of 2–6 years. However, haemangiomas over the lip, parotid gland or distal nose appear more likely to persist or involute only partially.

Vascular malformations

Some types of vascular malformations, particularly venous or arteriovenous malformations, are quite similar clinically to haemangiomas of infancy. They usually present at birth, but lack the tendency to spontaneous resolution, and generally grow in proportion to the child. Salmon patch lesions usually take the form of irregular, dull, pinkish red, macular areas, often featuring fine, linear telangiectasia. The nape of the neck is the commonest site; followed by lesions on glabella, forehead, upper eyelids, tip of the nose or upper lip. Lesions on the face tend to fade quickly within a year, though some of them might be visible again; nuchal lesions tend to be much more persistent with about half of them visible in adult life.

Port-wine stains are almost always present at birth. They vary in colour from a fairly pale pink to a deep red or purple, and in size from a few millimetres to many centimetres in diameter. The face is the commonest site, usually with a fairly sharp midline cut-off. Generally, the surface area remains unchanged relative to body size. Lesions on the face tend to darken progressively throughout life, and tend to become raised and thickened, while lesions on trunk and limbs tend to fade over the years.

Complications

Haemangiomas

Bleeding tends to happen on eroded or traumatized lesions, especially large ones.

Ulceration tends to develop during the phase of rapid proliferation, in anogenital area or sites which are vulnerable to trauma, such as ears, nose or the lips.

Infection often develops secondary to ulceration, either localized to skin or can spread to the deeper tissues.

Heart failure is a rare complication usually associated with large or numerous haemangiomas.

Systemic haemangiomas are featured by multiple organ involvement of the tumours; extensive systemic lesions cause high mortality.

Kasabach–Merritt syndrome is featured by consumption coagulopathy, coupled with single deep haemangioma of larger size, or rarely multiple small haemangiomas, or visceral angiomas.

Impairment of vision happens when the haemangiomas involves the eyelids, possibly leading to obstructive amblyopia or astigmatism.

Airway obstruction may occur when there is a subglottic haemangioma, the situation is most likely when the cutaneous lesion is in the neck. Involvement of the nose in the neonatal period may also interfere with respiration as well as feeding.

Obstruction of the external auditory canal by haemangiomas might interfere with hearing in the short term.

Deformation of bone might develop due to direct pressure of the tumour.

Vascular malformations

Severe complications are noted when a vascular malformation is syndromic to anomalies of various organs. Manifestation of complications depends on the organs involved as well as the lesion itself.

Ocular problems may be associated with port-wine stains, the most significant of which is glaucoma.

Sturge–Weber syndrome is characterized by ocular anomalies, pial vascular malformations, and ipsilateral facial port-wine stain. Patients may develop contralateral seizures, neurological deficits, hemiparesis or hemiplegia, glaucoma, retinal detachment and even blindness.

Underlying soft-tissue swelling and/or bony overgrowth sometimes complicate with port-wine stains.

Diagnosis and differential diagnosis

Haemangiomas

In 95% of cases diagnosis can be established on the basis of history and physical examination alone. The diagnosis is confirmed by the presence of typical-appearing vascular tumours in conjunction with a history of a lesion at birth or developing shortly thereafter, and with characteristic proliferation in early infancy and involution phases usually a year later.

Haemangiomas should be differentiated from several cutaneous neoplasms and anomalies, including several types of vascular malformations, pyogenic granuloma, myofibromatosis, spindle and epithelioid naevus, dermoid cysts, etc.

Vascular malformations

Vascular malformations often share similar clinical features with haemangiomas. Key points for their diagnosis include: (i) the history of a lesion present since birth; (ii) the lack of any tendency to spontaneous resolve; and (iii) the frequent presence in the area of the lesion of other elements such as port-wine staining, eccrine angiomatous naevus and lymphangioma circumscriptum. Ultrasound and computed tomography and magnetic resonance imaging might help in some situations.

Port-wine stains should be well differentiated from salmon patches for their significant difference in outcome. The key points are clinical manifestations and their clinical courses.

Treatment

Haemangiomas

Because of their benign nature and self-limiting course, non-intervention might be the best policy for most of the haemangiomas. Parents must be reassured of the outcome and advised to visit regularly. It is best to take photographs at regular intervals to document the change of the lesions during the observation course. Local care should be taken to prevent ulceration and secondary infection, especially those lesions in anogenital area. Commonly employed therapies include antibiotics, barrier creams, and bio-occlusive dressings.

In a minority of patients, treatment should be indicated:

- Life- and function-threatening haemangiomas (e.g. those causing impairment of vision and feeding, airway obstruction, Kasabach–Merritt syndrome, heart failure).
- Haemangiomas in certain anatomical locations that tend to leave permanent scars or deformity (e.g. those lesions on nose, lip, ear and glabellar area).
- Large facial haemangiomas, especially those with a prominent dermal component that tend to leave permanent scarring.
- Small haemangiomas in exposed areas that are unlikely to leave scarring or significant side-effects when treated.
- Ulceration.
- Pedunculated haemangiomas that are likely to leave significant fibrofatty tissue after involution.

Treatment options include:

- Corticosteroids (systemic, intralesional and topical)
- Interferon-α therapy

- Laser
- Cryosurgery
- Surgical excision
- Pressure occlusion
- Sclerosant injection
- Embolization
- Radiotherapy.

Selection of treatment options should be based on careful evaluation on a number of factors such as anatomical location, lesional profiles, phase of the lesions, presence of functional impairment, etc. The listed treatments may be used singly, or in combination with each other.

Corticosteroids

Systemic corticosteroids

These are the first-line therapy for the high-risk lesions (i.e. large, prognostically poor location, likely to leave permanent disfigurement, causing functional impairment, or involving extracutaneous structures). Corticosteroids treatment should be initiated during the proliferative phase as early as possible.

Prednisone (or equivalent dose of prednisolone) of 2–4 mg/kg per day should be maintained for 4–8 weeks, before tapering the dose off by 1 year.

Response rates vary from 30 to 90%. This approach should be abandoned if no response is seen after 3–4 weeks of treatment.

Common side-effects are cushingoid, personality changes, and reversible growth impairment.

Intralesional corticosteroids

Often applied to lesions on the eye, other well-localized area, or the low-risk haemangiomas (small, causing no functional impairment and unlikely to leave permanent disfigurement).

Triamcinolone acetonide 10–40 mg/mL, sometimes mixed with dexamethasome sodium phosphate 4 mg/mL can be given at 6-week intervals for 3–5 times. Caution should be taken to avoid damaging the adjacent organs.

Topical corticosteroids under occlusion

Potent topical steroids under occlusion are reported to be effective for small superficial haemangiomas.

Interferon-α therapy

This option is generally reserved for those life-threatening haemangiomas that are corticosteroid resistant.

Initial dose 1 million U/m^2 per day, which is increased to 3 million U/m^2 per day if tolerated. Treatment is gradually discontinued over a 3-month period when good results have been achieved.

Common side-effects include flu-like symptoms, neutropenia, anaemia, increased transaminases (reversible). The most alarming side-effect is central nervous system toxicity that caused permanent spastic diplegia in as many as 20% of treated infants.

Laser therapy

585-nm pulsed-dye laser treatment is mainly indicated either to slow or to arrest proliferation in early haemangiomas, to correct or minimize complications (i.e. bleeding and ulceration), or to improve cosmetically residual telangiectatic lesions.

Fluences of 5.5–6 J/cm^2 with a 5-mm spot are generally used, with treatment intervals reduced to every few weeks to achieve satisfactory results. In small infants, anaesthesia with amethocaine gel may be adequate, although general anaesthesia is sometimes necessary.

The deeper component of the haemangiomas may still develop, despite successful treatment of the superficial component, due to the low penetration nature of the laser (1.2 mm).

Lasers that penetrate more deeply, such as the argon and Nd : YAG may have a role in the treatment of deeper and complicated haemangiomas; however, they have a greater risk for scarring or pigmentary change.

CO_2 laser can be useful for excisional purposes, particularly lesions in the mouth, although a degree of scarring is inevitable.

Cryosurgery

Traditional cryosurgery with temperatures from −70°C to −196°C is no longer in widespread use for its unfavourable sequelae as scarring, pigmentary changes. A recent study showed that superficial or mixed type haemangiomas respond well to −32°C contact tip without leaving side-effects such as scarring or hypopigmentation.

Surgical excision

Mainly indicated for emergent situations such as Kasabach–Merritt syndrome or haemangiomatosis of the liver unresponsive to corticosteroids or interferon therapy, for lesions on upper eyelid, distal nose, or for the redundant folds of atrophic skin that persist after involution of large haemangiomas.

Pressure occlusion

Mainly indicated for large lesions on extremities. Effects have not been well evaluated. A recent trial showed healing and pain relieving effects on ulcerative haemangiomas with polyurethane film.

Sclerosant injection

Indicated for deep haemangiomas that had incomplete involution or no sign of further involution over a period of at least a year.

0.5–5.0 mL of solutions such as sodium citrate 30%, monoethanolamine oleate 5%, glucose 30% or saturated saline is injected at fortnightly or monthly intervals.

Embolization

Particularly indicated for hepatic haemangiomas, high-output cardiac failure, or Kasabach–Merritt syndrome.

Radiotherapy

Mainly used in the treatment of function or life threatening haemangiomas when other approaches have failed. Long-term undesirable sequelaes are carotid artery occlusion, disturbed bone growth, hypoplasia of soft tissues, and increased risk of malignancies.

Vascular malformations

The management of arterial, arteriovenous, venous, lymphatic or complex-combined malformations requires a multidisciplinary approach. Mainstay of treatment options includes sclerotherapy, surgical resection, embolization, or combination of various methods.

Port-wine stains, or persistent salmon patches, particularly when they occur on the face, pose a strong influence on a child's psychological development. A great variety of options have been tried to treat port-wine stains in the past. These include excision and grafting, tattooing, Grenz rays, cryotherapy, etc. All of these showed limited effects or nasty side-effects such as scarring, pigmentary change, and have been gradually abandoned. By far, the most widely accepted choices of treatment are lasers.

The pulsed-dye laser was the first laser specifically designed for the selective photothermolysis of cutaneous blood vessels. The laser is set at a wavelength of 585 nm, pulse duration of 450 ms after setting up the fluence, treatment can be initiated and usually repeated at intervals of 8 weeks. The fluences of the laser is determined by a test treatment over a range of fluences and reviewing the patient 8 weeks later; the lower range of fluences should be used at delicate skin sites in children. Most patients will experience satisfactory lightening of their port-wine stain in the first four to 10 treatments. Gradually, through a course of treatment, the lightening after each treatment gets smaller until no further progress can be seen. Topical anaesthetic agents or general anaesthesia should be applied to relieve pain.

Only a minority of patients achieve clearance, while most of them show lightening effect of various degrees. The incidence of side-effects is rather low. They include hyperpigmentation and scarring.

A recent study showed that potassium titanyl phosphate (KTP) laser (wavelength at 532 nm) with fluences ranging from 18 to 24 J/cm^2 and pulse width of 9–14 ms can further lighten pulsed-dye laser resistant port-wine stains. KTP is also beneficial to port-wine stains of older patients with more raised or nodular lesions.

Argon laser, which was the first laser used successively to treat large numbers of port-wine stains, has been limited to carefully selected adult patients with telangiectasias, small vascular lesions, or small, dark, nodular port-wine stains, due to its severe disfiguring side-effects. Copper vapour laser has an efficacy between PDL and argon laser.

Lasers with different wavelength, fluences have also been tried in different clinical or histological situations. Individualized laser treatment option might be the future trends.

Further reading

Atherton DJ. Naevi and other developmental defects. In: Champion H, Burton JI, Ebling FJG, eds. *Textbook of Dermatology*. Blackwell Science, 1998: 551–616.

Chowdhury MMU, Harris S, Lanigan SW. Potassium titanyl phosphate laser treatment of resistant port-wine stains. *Br J Dermatol* 2001; 144: 814–17.

Enjolras O. Classification and management of the various superficial vascular anomalies: Hemangiomas and vascular malformations. *J Dermatol* 1997; 24: 701–10.

Enjolras O, Mulliken JB. Vascular malformations. In: Happer J, Oranje A, Prose N eds. *Textbook of Pediatric Dermatology*. Oxford: Blackwell Science, 2000: 975–96.

Esterly NB. Haemangiomas. In: Happer J, Oranje A, Prose N eds. *Textbook of Pediatric Dermatology*. Oxford: Blackwell Science, 2000: 997–1034.

Frieden IJ, Eichenfield LF, Esterly NB, Geronemus R, Mallory SB and the Guidelines/Outcomes Committee. Guidelines of care for haemangiomas of infancy. *J Am Acad Dermatol* 1997; 37: 631–7.

Garzon MC, Enjolras O, Frieden IJ. Vascular tumours and vascular malformations: Evidence for an association. *J Am Acad Dermatol* 2000; 42: 275–9.

Hedersdal M. cutaneous side effects from laser treatment of the skin: Skin cancer, scars, wounds, pigmentary changes, and purpura. *Acta Derm Venereol (Suppl) (Stockh)* 1999; 207: 1–32.

Lamberg L. New and emerging dermatologic therapies presented at conference. *JAMA* 2000; 283: 2377–8.

Lanigan SW. Treatment of vascular naevi in children. *Hosp Med* 2001; 62: 144–7.

Metry DW, Hebert AA. Benign cutaneous vascular tumors of infancy: when to worry, what to do. *Arch Dermatol* 2000; 136: 905–14.

Oranje AP, de Waard-van der Spek FB, Devillers AC, de Laat PC, Madern GC. Treatment and pain relief of ulcerative hemangiomas with polyurethane film. *Dermatology* 2000; 200: 31–4.

Reischle S, Schuller-Petrovic S. Treatment of capillary hemangiomas of early childhood with a new method of cryosurgery. *J Am Acad Dermatol* 2000; 42: 809–13.

van der Horst CM, Koster PH, de Borgie CA, Bossuyt PM, van Gemert MJ. Effect of the timing of treatment of port-wine stains with the flashlamp-pumped pulsed–dye laser. *N Eng J Med* 1998; 338: 1028–33.

Vitiligo

A.D. Katsambas, T.M. Lotti and J.P. Ortonne

Definition and epidemiology

Vitiligo is an acquired chronic disease characterized by macular patches lacking completely cutaneous pigmentation. It affects about 0.5–1% of the population and it occurs in all races and both sexes. In 20% of vitiligo cases, a family history can be detected. Inheritance may be determined by an autosomal dominant gene with variable penetrance or it may be polygenic and probably caused by four sets of alleles that make the individual more prone to developing vitiligo under the influence of the various environmental factors.

Aetiology and pathophysiology

Vitiligo is an idiopathic disorder, with selective destruction of the melanocytes in the depigmented patches.

Autoimmune processes (i.e. presence of circulating organ-specific autoantibodies, evidence of autoantibodies to normal human melanocytes, decrease of T-helper cells), deficiency of melanocyte growth factor, enzymatic self-destruct mechanism and abnormal neurogenic stimulus leading to dermatomal melanocyte destruction, have been postulated as pathogenetic factors. The question is raised whether vitiligo is a syndrome or a single disease. It is likely that vitiligo vulgaris in humans represents a multitude of pathophysiological mechanisms, i.e. a variety of different diseases. A 'convergence theory' in which different causal factors may act independently or synergistically to induce disappearance of melanocytes is a reasonable possibility. In some patients, vitiligo is associated with other diseases, mainly of autoimmune nature, like alopecia areata, thyroiditis, pernicious anaemia, diabetes and Addison's disease. Appropriate studies for these conditions are recommended when there is clinical suspicion.

Clinical characteristics and course

Lesions are round or oval macules, sharply demarcated and pure white. They are distributed, usually symmetrically, around orifices (lips, eyes, anogenital areas) over bony prominences such as the wrists and in interdiginous areas. In affected areas, the hair usually is also white. Margins of the lesions may become hyperpigmented. At times, the pure white patches are surrounded by an area of the skin that is intermediate in colour before merging in the normal coloured skin. This is known as trichome vitiligo and is mostly seen in black people. Vitiligo can be classified into two major clinical types, segmental and non-segmental. The course of vitiligo is unpredictable. In some cases, the lesions remain stable over many years (mostly segmental vitiligo) but in others they can enlarge in size while new patches appear to involve large portions of the skin surface (mostly non-segmental type). However, spontaneous repigmentation may occur in 10–20% of patients, mainly in sun-exposed areas. Repigmentation usually begins perifollicularly creating pigmented spots that gradually may enlarge and coalesce.

Diagnosis (laboratory examinations)

Skin biopsy with special staining for melanocytes is the only significant examination but usually is not necessary. Histology reveals the absence of melanocytes which appear to be replaced by Langherans' cells in the lesions. A lymphomonocytic infiltrate is sometimes present in the marginal areas.

Differential diagnosis

Wood's light examination should be part of the evaluation of every patient with vitiligo. It is most useful to differentiate the pure white appearance of the amelanotic vitiligo macules from the tan-white of grey-white colour of the relatively hypomelanotic disorders.

- Pityriasis alba: fine scales on the lesions.
- Postinflammatory leucoderma: irregular mottling of hyperpigmented and hypopigmented blotches.
- Tinea versilocor: microbiology, Wood's lamp.
- Piebaldism: hyperpigmented macules within the depigmented areas.
- Naevus depigmentosus: present at birth; unilateral; stable.
- Morphoea: speckled appearance; palpable induration, scleroatrophy.
- Hypomelanocytic leprosy: anaesthetic macules.
- Chemical leukoderma: history of repeated exposure to phenols and sulfhydryls.
- Idiopathic guttate hypomelanosis: numerous, small, white macules mainly distributed on the legs of dark skinned individuals.
- Tuberous sclerosis: congenital, dull to off-white confetti macules; seizures and mental retardation.

Treatment

General therapeutic guidelines

- At present, no entirely effective treatment is available. Regardless of the treatment used, repigmentation may be slow and never be complete.
- Many patients will require only reassurance and advice on the use of the sunscreens and cosmetic camouflage. Active treatment is indicated in patients who have a marked cosmetic disability, particularly those whose life style, self-esteem and productivity have been altered by the disease.
- New patches are possibly triggered by physical trauma (Koebner phenomenon) especially during spreading phases. It is recommended to avoid medical or surgical cosmetic procedures which can traumatize skin like deep peeling, lifting, etc.
- With the existing treatment methods, different results are obtained at different sites of involvement, i.e. vitiliginous patches over bony prominences respond poorly while lesions on the face and body respond much better.
- If the involved site has no hair follicles, therapy usually fails because hair follicles seem to be necessary to supply new melanocytes.
- Treatment method should be chosen after consideration of the age of the patient, the areas involved and the extent of the disease.
- Spontaneous repigmentation occurs in about 10–20% of the patients and usually is only partial.
- Avoidance of the sun is highly recommended. Broad-spectrum sunscreens (SPF-15 or greater) should be applied to all exposed skin, 30–60 min prior to sun exposure to decrease the short- and long-term effects of UV radiation and to reduce the contrast between the normal skin and the vitiliginous areas.

Recommended therapies

- Cosmetic camouflage.
- Repigmentation.
- Depigmentation (extremely widespread disease—greater than 50% of the body surface area).

Cosmetic camouflage

Cosmetic cover-up is quite acceptable to some patients with vitiligo. Camouflage may be achieved with various cosmetics and stains containing mainly aniline dyes and dihydroxyacetone (DHA). 'Quick Tan' preparations containing dihydroxyacetone (3–5%) are produced by many cosmetic firms. DHA is a sugar that binds with the amino acids of the corneum layer inducing the production of coloured components that change from yellow to brown giving the skin a tanned effect. DHA dyes are easy to apply; they are neither dirty nor greasy. The pigmentation appears a few hours later and the application has to be repeated until the desired result is obtained, and more times in a week, because the DHA-induced pigment reduces with normal epidermis exfoliation. These dyes do not provide protection against sunburn and psoralen phototherapy can be used. When cosmetics and make-up are used, the attention of a professional cosmetician is of great help in demonstrating how to choose and apply the appropriate product.

Repigmentation

Psoralen photochemotherapy

Oral and topical psoralen photochemotherapy is currently the most efficacious treatment.

Topical photochemotherapy

Topical psoralen photochemotherapy is often considered for patients with limited involvement (less than 20% of the body surface), or localized disease. It can be used to treat both children over 2 years old and adults. Dilutions of 1% 8-methoxypsoralen are made with alcohol, or lotions for final concentrations of 0.01% to 0.1% in order to minimize adverse phototoxic reactions. The preparation is applied to the vitiliginous areas 30 min prior to exposure to ultraviolet A light (UVA). The initial UVA dose is 0.12 or 0.25 J/cm^2 and is increased by increments of 0.12 or 0.25 J/cm^2 weekly according to the patient's skin type. After a moderate asymptomatic erythema is achieved, the UVA and psoralen dosage should be maintained at a constant level to retain the minimal degree of erythema. Treated areas should be washed with soap and covered with broad-spectrum sunscreen before the patient leaves the physician's office. Treatments are given once or twice per week. The psoralen should be applied by hospital or medical personnel, and not by the patient.

The major side-effects of topical photochemotherapy are a severe phototoxic reaction and blistering, and patients should be warned of this before the treatment begins. If erythema and blistering develop, treatments are stopped until the reaction subsides. On reinstitution of therapy, the UVA exposure is usually decreased to half the previous dosage. For 6–8 h after the treatment, unnecessary exposure to sunlight must be avoided because of the high potential of developing severe phototoxic reactions.

Hyperpigmentation may develop in perilesional normal skin during treatment; this is a temporary phenomenon that resolves after the treatment stops. Topical PUVA cannot be considered a first choice treatment for any kind of vitiligo. However, topical PUVA is preferable to oral PUVA in patients with hepatic and gastrointestinal (uncertain absorption) disorders, cataracts, poor eye protection, poor compliance and when shorter irradiation times are necessary (children and claustrophobic individuals).

Oral photochemotherapy

Oral photochemotherapy is considered one of the treatments of choice for vitiligo. Oral photochemotherapy is used for patients with more than 20% of the skin surface involvement and for individuals who are recalcitrant to topical photochemotherapy. Oral psoralens are not usually recommended for children under 12 years of age. Contraindications for oral photochemotherapy include abnormal liver function, ocular defects including cataracts and pregnancy. In addition, the presence of photosensitivity disorders contraindicates the use of both oral and topical PUVA. Before therapy is begun, the following tests are required:

- blood count
- sedimentation rate determination

- test for antinuclear antibodies
- liver function
- a baseline ophthalmological examination.

All these examinations should be repeated yearly. The maximum recommended 8-methoxysporalen dose is 0.6 mg/kg. It should be taken orally 2 h before UVA exposure. Patients may occasionally experience some gastrointestinal irritation (nausea, vomiting, abdominal pains) with psoralen, which becomes less frequent when the drug is taken after food. An initial dose of 1–2 J/cm^2 is generally given, with subsequent increments of 1 J/cm^2 every other visit until moderate asymptomatic erythema is observed. The dose of UVA must be adjusted, depending on the sensitivity of the individual patient. Treatments are given twice weekly but never on 2 consecutive days.

Protective UVA glasses should be worn for 24 h after oral psoralen intake. As a UVA source, PUVA cabinets are usually used (320–400 nm-emitting fluorescent tubes).

If the patient is unable to come to the physician's office for treatment, trioxysalen (4,5,8-trimethylpsoralen) and sunlight is suggested, in a dose of 0.6 mg/kg. An initial sun exposure of 5 min is recommended. The best time for sun exposure is from 10 a.m. to 2 p.m. Subsequent exposures are increased in increments of 5 min with each treatment until a mild erythema is attained, after which the exposure times are held constant until an increase is necessary to maintain the erythema. Treatments are given three times weekly but not on 2 consecutive days.

Trioxysalen, is less phototoxic than 8-methoxypsoralen and less effective as a repigmenting agent. Patients should apply broad-spectrum sunscreens to the treated areas immediately after the treatment, and limit further both sun and UVA exposure.

PUVA-induced repigmentation is permanent in the majority of patients, but some may require maintenance treatment. Psoralen photochemotherapy induces maximal repigmentation of the face and neck, intermediate responses on the trunk, arms and legs, and minimal responses on the hands and feet. Treatment should be continued for at least 6 months to a year before the patient is classified as recalcitrant. Often as many as 200–300 treatments are required to produce a uniform repigmentation of the vitiliginous areas.

UVB Phototherapy

There are three main types of UVB treatments:

- broadband UVB
- narrowband UVB
- narrowband focused UVB microphototherapy.

The differences that exist are related to the spectrum used and to the skin surface treated, whether whole body surface (broadband and narrowband) is treated or only the vitiligo patches (narrowband focused UVB microphototherapy). No oral (systemic) drug are required and that are safe for children and pregnant women.

Broadband UVB

The device is a bed or a cabinet with UVB broadband fluorescent tubes (e.g. Philips TL-12) with a spectrum range from 290 to 320 nm. The start dose is 20 mJ/cm^2 (for all skin types) and should be increased by 20% until minimal erythema occurs. After that the dose must be kept 20% lower than the minimal erythematous dose (MED). Patients must be treated two or three times a week, with an interval of more than 1 day.

Narrowband UVB (selective UVB)

Narrowband UVB treatment is more efficient to treat vitiligo than broadband and has the same carcinogenic risk. The starting dose is 250 mJ/cm^2 (for all skin types) and it is increased by 10–20% until minimal erythema is achieved in the vitiligous areas. The exposition is made two three times a week, not in 2 consecutive days.

Narrowband focused microphototherapy

It is possible to treat exclusively vitiligo patches avoiding normally tanned skin especially in children and if the surface affected does not exceed the 20% of the total body surface. A new phototherapy device (Bioskin) allows selective narrow band UVB (311 nm) treatment limited to the white patches. The main characteristics of the Bioskin generator are that it produces UVB rays, in a spectrum of 300–320 nm, with maximum emission at 311 nm; the energy displayed by the UVB generator is 10–100 mJ/cm^2 per second and the diameter of the light spot is 1 cm. This new device has been particularly efficient in the treatment of limited affected areas and segmental vitiligo. This new technique has several advantages: it does not increase the colour contrast between normal pigmented skin and affected skin, and the total irradiation dose is minimal depending on the percentage of body surface affected. The method consists in weekly sessions of irradiation of all vitiligo patches. The dose is 20% lower than MED, which is measured before the beginning of the treatment. This phototherapy treatment permits a differentiated irradiation. Thus, it is possible to irradiate hands and feet with a dose five or six times higher than the dose used for eyelids.

Corticosteroids (CCS)

Topical CCS

These are sometimes effective repigmenting agents, in early localized forms of vitiligo especially in children. High-potency steroids i.e. 0.1% betamethasone valerate and 0.05% clobetasol propionate, applied twice daily for a period of 3–5 months is recommended. Lower potency preparations must be used for the face, eyelids or intertriginous areas. Patients should be followed up for side-effects of topical steroids use, particularly atrophy and glaucoma (if used around the eyes).

Systemic CCS

The use of systemic CCS for therapy of vitiligo is useful, considering the relationship between benefits and side-effects, mainly for the treatment of active, rapidly progressive generalized vitiligo. In these patients, oral mini-pulse therapy (betamethasone/dexamethasone 5 mg for 2 consecutive days for 6 months to 2 years) has shown the ability to arrest the progression of the disease. The dose of CCS in children under 16 years of age must be halved.

Depigmentation

Depigmentation should be considered when vitiligo patients have >80% cutaneous involvement and are recalcitrant to repigmentation. The process is permanent and irreversible, and the patient will be permanently photosensitive. For these reasons this form of therapy should be considered for patients over 40 years old who have had an adequate trial of PUVA and have failed or are unwilling to undergo repigmentation therapy. The dermatologist must feel confident that complete depigmentation will be not only cosmetically satisfactory but also psychologically acceptable, especially in black patients.

Monobenzyl ether of hydroquinone (MBEHQ)

MBEHQ is used as a depigmenting agent. It destroys melanocytes. The treatment starts with 10% concentration of MBEHQ by diluting the full-strength preparation with any water-soluble vehicle. The preparation is then applied to the pigmented areas twice daily. The concentration is increased by 5% every 1 or 2 months until the patient is using 20% MBEHQ.

Patients should be advised that effective treatment may require several months to

1–2 years of therapy. The major side-effect of MBEHQ therapy is dermatitis, which usually responds rapidly to topical applications of steroids. Other common side-effects include contact dermatitis, pruritis, xerosis, conjunctival melanosis, corneal pigment deposition and greying of the hair.

Laser depigmentation

The Q-switched ruby laser beam is capable of destroying selectively melanin and melanocyte (694 nm). The established method consists of a previous test session to evaluate the safety and efficacy of this technique in the patient. The response to this test is evaluated 2 months after the test and if there is no response, laser depigmentation should be discouraged.

If the depigmentation test has caused significant depigmentation, the treatment can be continued until the desired bleaching effect has been achieved. This technique is safe (no drug is required). The contraindications are the same as those for depigmentation with bleaching agents.

Alternative and experimental treatments

L-Phenylalanine

When taken orally (1–3 g/day for 12–36 weeks) and followed by UVA irradiation it is a promising agent for the treatment of childhood vitiligo.

Topical khellin

Khellin is a furochrome chemically related to psoralens. Khellin has been used in combination with sunlight or in combination with UVA (KUVA). Khellin was administered either topically (2% solution in 90% acetone and 10% propylene glycole) or systematically UVA was delivered 1–2 h later, three times a week. The results were variable. Regular monitoring of liver enzyme should be performed and the treatment should be stopped if the liver enzyme levels increase.

Melagenina I and II

Melagenina is an alcoholic extract of human placenta. The active ingredient is an α-lipoprotein of low molecular weight. Melagenina is applied topically three times a day. One of the daily applications is followed by a 15-min solar infrared exposure. The results are rather conflicting and the use of melagenina still remains experimental until random double-blind studies are done for both efficacy and safety.

Traditional Chinese medication

Although some Chinese physicians believe that the administration of some Chinese medicinal herbs may be beneficial for vitiligo, lack of scientific data renders these treatments experimental.

Pseudocatalase

Due to the report that patients with vitiligo have very low catalase activity, a group of investigators applied a vehicle with pseudocatalase twice daily, followed by a twice-weekly total body suberythema UVB radiation for 1 h. Excellent repigmentation was noted in 90% of patients after almost 15 months. Further studies are needed to determine the effectiveness of this method.

Permanent tattooing

Permanent dermal micropigmentation using a non-allergic iron oxide pigment can permanently tattoo recalcitrant areas of vitiligo (i.e. hands, perioral region, and the hairline).

New surgical techniques

A number of surgical techniques to transplant autologous melanocytes from pigmented skin to non-pigmenting areas using grafting and autologous cultured melanocytes have been found promising in cases of stable unilateral or stable bilateral vitiligo. All these methods at present should be regarded as experimental.

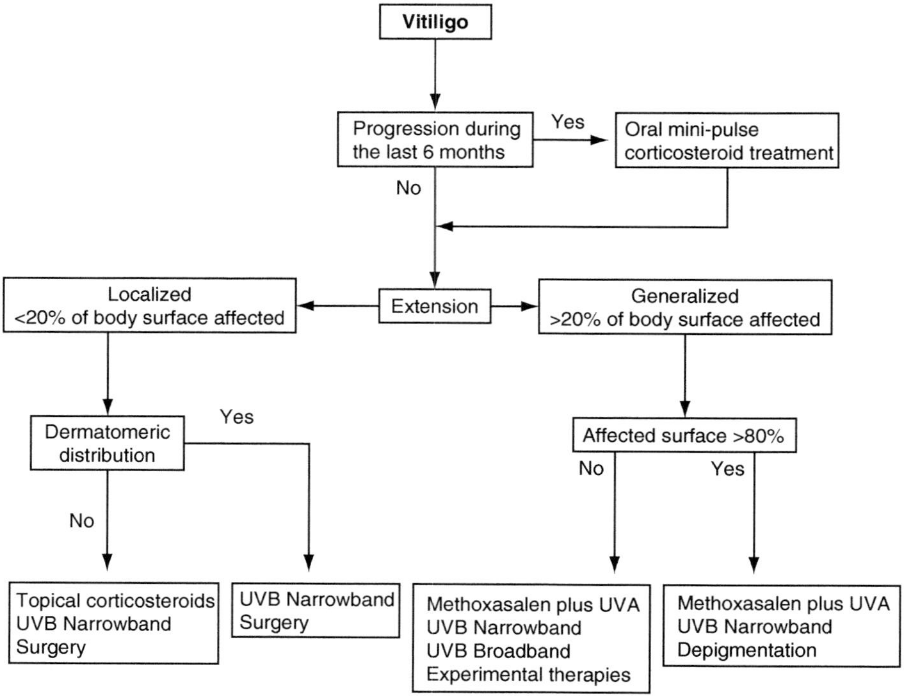

Figure 1 Vitiligo

Further reading

Andreassi L, Pianigiani E, Andreassi A, Taddeucci P, Biagioli M. A new model of epidermal culture for the surgical treatment of vitiligo. *Int J Dermatol* 1998; 37: 595–8.

Antoniou C, Katsambas A. Guidelines for the treatment of vitiligo. *Drugs* 1992; 43: 490–8.

Camacho F, Mazuecos J. Treatment of vitiligo with oral and topical phenylalanine: 6 years of experience. *Arch Dermatol* 1999; 135: 216–17.

Castanet J, Cortonne JP. Pathophysiology of vitiligo. *Clin Dermatol* 1997; 15: 845–51.

Falabella R, Arrunategui A, Barona MI, Alzate A. The minigrafting test for vitiligo. Detection of stable lesions for melanocyte transplantation. *J Am Acad Dermatol* 1995; 32 (2 Part 1): 228–32.

Gupta S, Jain VK, Saraswat PK. Suction blister epidermal grafting versus punch skin grafting in recalcitrant and stable vitiligo. *Dermatol Surg* 1999; 25 (12): 955–8.

Halpern SM, Anstey AV, Dawe RS *et al.* Guidelines for topical PUVA. A report of a workshop of the British Photodermatology Group. *Br J Dermatol* 2000; 142: 22–31.

Hann SK, Chen D, Bystryn JC. Systemic steroid suppress antimelanocyte antibodies in vitiligo. *J Cut Med Surg* 1997; 14: 193–5.

Koester W, Wiskemann A. Phototherapy with UV-B in vitiligo. *Zeitschr Hautkrank* 1999; 65: 1022–4.

Lotti TM, Menchini G, Andreassi L. UV-B radiation microphototherapy. An elective treatment for segmental vitiligo. *J Eur Acad Dermatol Venereol* 1999; 113 (2): 102–8.

Morliere P, Honigsmann H, Averbeck D *et al.* Phototherapeutic, photobiologic and photosensitizing properties of khellin. *J Invest Dermatol* 1988; 90: 720–4.

Njoo MD, Bossuyt PMM, Westerhof W. Management of vitiligo. Results of a questionaire among dermatologists in The Netherlands. *Int J Dermatol* 1999; 38: 866–72.

Njoo MD, Westerhof W, Bos JD, Bossuyt PM. The development of guidelines for the treatment of vitiligo. Clinical Epidemiology Unit of the Istituto Dermopatico dell'Immacolata-Istituto diRecovero e Cura a Carattere Scientifico (IDI-IRCCS) and the Archives of Dermatology. *Arch Dermatol* 1999; 135 (12): 1514–21.

Thissen M, Westerhof W. Laser treatment for further depigmentation in vitiligo. *Int J Dermatol* 1997; 36 (5): 386–8.

Westerhof W, Nieuweboer-Krobotova L. Treatment of vitiligo with UVB 311 nm versus topical PUVA. *Arch Dermatol* 1997; 133: 1525–8.

Westerhof W, Nieuweboer-Krobotova L, Mulder PGH, Glazenburg EJ. Left-right comparison study of the combination of fluticasone propinate and UVA vs either fluticasone propinate or UVA alone for the long-term treatment of vitiligo. *Arch Dermatol* 1999; 135: 1061–6.

Warts and condylomas

J.M. Mascaró and J.M. Mascaró Jr

Definition and epidemiology

Warts and condylomas are pseudotumoral proliferations of skin and mucous membranes resulting from the infection of keratinocytes by human papilloma viruses (HPV). Both conditions are extremely common and may appear clinically as common viral warts, frequent in children, especially on the hands; verruca planae (flat warts), also more frequent in children and adolescents; plantar warts, that may be seen in all age groups, but more commonly in young people; and genital warts (condyloma), which develop usually in sexually active individuals. Both sexes and all races are equally affected.

Aetiology and pathophysiology

Warts and condyloma represent tumoral growths of terminally differentiated keratinocytes from the epithelia of the skin and mucous membranes infected by HPV. These are small, non-enveloped, double-stranded DNA viruses that possess approximately 8000 nucleotide base pairs. The viral DNA is packed in a protein capsid forming virions, that are icosahedral, 50–55 nm in diameter. Few enzymes are encoded by HPV DNA, and they do not possess polymerases, kinases, or proteases which could act as targets for already established antiviral substances currently used against herpesviruses or the human immunodeficiency virus (HIV). HPV capsids are not surrounded by any lipoprotein envelope and this feature confers a great stability to HPV, being highly resistant to environmental stresses such as heat, soaps, and desiccation. HPV are highly host specific, and humans are not infected by other animal papilloma virus.

Up to now, more than 80 different HPV types have been isolated based on differences in DNA sequence. There is a clear correlation between HPV type and clinical manifestations. Common warts are mainly due to HPV types 2 and 4; plantar warts to type 1; flat warts to 3 and 10; and anogenital condyloma to 6 and 11. There are also some HPV types (HPV 6 and 11) able to produce laryngeal papillomas in children, by vertical transmision from mothers during delivery. HPV types 16, 18, 31, 33–35, 39, 41, 51, 52, 56, 58, 59, 68 and 70 are oncogenic and may induce genital dysplasia that progresses to squamous cell carcinoma. The expression of some genes (E6 and E7) of high-risk HPV would be important for malignant transformation of the epithelium of the cervix. Finally, there is a large group of HPV usually considered non-pathogenic (3, 5, 8, 9, 12, 14, 15, 17, 19–25, 36, 47, 49 and 50) that may infect genetically predisposed individuals producing a rare disease named epidermodysplasia verruciformis. In this condition patients present with multiple flat warts on the sun-exposed areas and tinea versicolor-like lesions of the trunk. Many patients develop skin cancers on sun-exposed areas some years after the onset. Immunocompromised patients, most commonly renal transplant recipients, are also frequently infected by the same HPV types seen in immunocompetent individuals as well as by HPV types usually seen in patients with epidermodysplasia verruciformis. These patients have a substantial increase in warts and HPV-related skin cancers.

Clinical characteristics and course

Common warts appear as single or multiple keratotic papules or tumours. They are usually located on the hands and limbs. Plantar warts present as hyperkeratotic papules or plaques on the soles. Characteristically, pressure over plantar warts produces pain of variable intensity, and it may be disabling in some patients.

Paring of the surface of these lesions with a scalpel demonstrates multiple small bleeding points, the consequence of microscopic bleeding of dermal papillae blood capillaries. Flat warts present as multiple small yellow or red flat papules located on the face; the lesions may develop over a superficial erosion due to scratch (Koebner phenomenon). Filiform and digitate warts may also appear on the skin as small, often multiple, exophytic papilloma with a vegetating keratotic top; they occur commonly in males on the beard region, and on the scalp and nares in both sexes. Warts may also develop on the mouth and conjunctiva as exophytic reddish papillomas that may have a whitish keratotic centre.

Condyloma is the traditional name for genital warts. These lesions can be flat, and almost invisible, but more often appear as multiple exophytic and cauliflower-like growths on the external genitalia of both sexes. Condyloma may also appear in the anus and perianal area, usually but not always due to venereal contagion. Although condyloma on the external genitalia and perianal region may be easily detected, gynecological and rectal examination will be necessary to detect cervical and intra-anal or rectal condyloma, respectively. Acetic acid test, colposcopy and rectoscopy may be of interest (see section on diagnosis).

Warts and condylomas may initially grow and multiply. However spontaneous regression is possible, especially for common and flat warts and it has been reported that 60–70% disappear spontaneously within 2 years.

Diagnosis

The acetic acid test is useful in diagnosing flat condyloma of the genitalia. Application of diluted acetic acid produces a characteristic whitening of the wart surface 10–15 min after applying the solution. However, this test is not highly specific or sensitive for condyloma (there are false positive and negative results), but it can be useful.

Anogenital condyloma may necessitate further investigations. In women, a gynecological examination with colposcopy should be done to rule out cervical condyloma, dysplasia or neoplasia. In the presence of perianal condyloma rectal examination can detect intra-anal and rectal condyloma. Sexual partners of patients with anogenital warts should also be investigated because of the high infectivity of these lesions.

Although most lesions are diagnosed clinically, histopathology of cutaneous warts usually shows the presence of vacuolated cells in the granular cell layer containing typical multiple basophilic inclusions. Genital exophytic and flat warts have characteristic large epithelial cells with clear optically empty cytoplasm and pycnotic nucleus ('koilocytes').

Immunohistochemical techniques have been used in the past to detect HPV structural proteins in biopsy specimens and confirm the presence of virus in a lesion. However, they are not sensitive and are not able to assign HPV types.

Electron microscopy can detect viral particles in infected tissue but it has a low sensitivity and is not used for routine diagnosis.

Serological assays are currently being developed for the diagnosis of HPV infection. The establishment of assays for the detection of HPV type-specific antibodies is very interesting. Nowadays those assays are not sensitive enough and are not type-specific.

Assays using nucleic acid hybridization (dot blot, Southern blot, *in situ* hybridization and the polymerase chain reaction) can also be performed. Those assays are highly sensitive and specific for HPV infection. They allow HPV typing and are useful in identifying oncogenic types. Commercial kits are available for some of these assays, although in others the technique is labour-intensive and therefore not suitable for clinical practice.

Differential diagnosis

Cutaneous warts are usually easily differentiated from other benign tumours and inflammatory conditions such as actinic and seborrhoeic keratosis, achrocordons, dermatofibroma, molluscum contagiosum, lichen planus and granuloma annulare. Flat warts may be confused with lesions of lichen planus and both may present with the Koebner phenomenon. Plantar warts must be differentiated from callosities (clavus) which mainly develop in pressure points. In clavus, pain can only be induced when pressure in applied just over the centre, while in plantar warts it also appears when pressure is applied on the borders of the lesion. In addition, in plantar warts the epithelial ridges of the skin are not continued over the surface of the lesion and paring with a scalpel will show the characteristic black dots (bleeding of dermal papillae blood capillaries, see clinical characteristics). Genital warts must be distinguished from lesions of secondary syphilis, seborrhoeic keratosis, psoriasis, lichen planus, pearly penile papules, and vulvar papillae.

- Common warts from molluscum contagiosum: molluscum have a central umbilication.
- Plantar warts from clavus: central pressure provokes pain in both. Lateral pressure provokes pain in warts only. Central small dark dots (haemorrhages) in warts.
- Flat warts from lichen planus: lichen more bluish or reddish. Flat warts more yellowish.
- Flat warts from freckles: reticulate pattern of pigment in freckles (more visible with dermatoscopy). Freckles darken with sun exposure.
- Genital warts from condyloma latum: warts are pedunculated. Condyloma latum have large base.

Treatment

There is currently no fully satisfactory therapy for warts and condyloma. This is supported by the existence of multiple treatment methods described. All available therapies are suboptimal because HPV is not eradicated by treatment. All methods, at the present time, are more or less effective in treating the warts (i.e. the epidermal growth) but there is no effective method to treat HPV infection. As mentioned above, HPV are not sensitive to antiviral drugs used in other viral infections.

Treatment options for cutaneous warts

There are diverse possibilities.

Topical agents

- Keratolytic and caustic agents: salicylic, lactic acid, trichloroacetic acid.
- Vesicants: cantharidine.
- Cytotoxic agents: podophyllin, podophyllotoxin.
- DNA inhibitors: 5-fluorouracil, bleomycin (intralesional or bleopuncture), cidofovir.
- Other methods: glutharaldehyde, formalin, occlusion (tape), heat.

The problem with this group of substances is that in many cases we do not know if they are really effective or act as a placebo. Recent reports of 1% cidofovir efficacy are encouraging.

Destruction or excision

- Electrosurgery.
- Cryotherapy (liquid nitrogen): destruction, superficial freezing and curettage or repeated short freezing.
- Selective photothermolysis with laser or intense pulsed light.
- CO_2 laser.
- Surgical excision.

The problem with these methods is that they are often painful, some may induce permanent scarring, and do not prevent from recurrences. Further, infectious HPV has been demonstrated in the vapour both with electrosurgery and CO_2 laser therapy of warts; therefore preventive measures (use of protective masks and smoke vacuum aspirator) must be taken. Selective photothermolysis with pulsed dye laser 585 nm, Q-switched Nd: YAG 532 nm, photoderm 570–590 nm, or Nd: YAG 1064 nm is able to produce thrombosis of subepithelial blood capillaries of the wart and it can be used as treatment for recurrent warts.

Cellular modifying agents
Oral retinoids.

Immunotherapies
- Immunomodulators: glycophosphopeptides, cimetidine, inosine pranobex.
- Sensitization with DNCB, diphenciprone, squaric acid dibutylester.
- Immune response modifiers: topical imiquimod.

Antivirals
- Interferons (intralesional or systemic)

The problem with all these methods is, again, that their efficacy (i.e. comparison with placebo therapy) has not been proved. On the other hand, sensitization with DNCB may be mutagenic and, finally interferon therapy is expensive. Recently it has been reported that systemic protease inhibitor antiretroviral therapy may be beneficial for the course of recalcitrant warts in HIV-infected patients.

Miscellaneous treatments
- Photodynamic therapy with topical 5-aminolevulinic acid and white light irradiation.
- Oral betacarotene.
- Behavioural techniques: hypnosis.

Treatment options for genital condyloma

There are different potential treatments.

Topical agents
- Caustic and cytotoxic agents: trichloroacetic acid, podophyllin, podophyllotoxin.
- DNA inhibitors: 5-fluorouracil.

Podophyllotoxin has many advantages over podophyllin: It is non-mutagenic, easy to store and to apply (the patient can do it himself), does not produce local nor systemic side-effects and a lower dose is needed (6 times lower than podophyllin).

Destruction
- Electrosurgery.
- Cryosurgery with liquid nitrogen.
- CO_2 laser.
- Selective photothermolysis with lasers or intense pulsed light.

Cellular modifying agents
Oral retinoids.

Antivirals and immune response modifiers
- Interferons (intralesional or systemic).
- Topical imiquimod.

Immunotherapies
- Vaccines.

In animal models vaccinations against HPV L1 or L2 viral capsid proteins provide protection against infection. Therapeutic vaccines based on recombinant HPV E6 and/or E7, fusion proteins or E7 peptides able to be recognized by cytotoxic T-cell epitopes are in phase I/II trials in patients with cervical carcinomas. Intramuscular administration of the HPV E7gene, transfected to dendritic cells, generates antitumour immunity in murine models. These results are a hope for an effective vaccine in humans in the near future.

General schedule for cutaneous warts

Any method can be useful as a first choice for single or a few warts. For multiple warts a topical treatment (keratolytic, vesicant, caustic or cytotoxic agent) can be used, sometimes in association with one of the oral immunomodulatory agents. Cimetidine has been reported to be effective as monotherapy in children. Topical retinoids are often prescribed for plane warts, alone or in combination with an immunomodulatory agent. Most of these methods are simple, non-expensive and non-aggressive.

In case of recurrences bleopuncture is a good choice in many cases. After extemporaneous preparation of a bleomycin solution, some drops are disposed over the wart surface with a syringe (the surface of the wart must be horizontal to permit the solution to remain over the wart). After that the wart surface is punctured with the needle of an empty syringe until a light bleeding appears. This procedure must be repeated many times until the entire wart is covered by a mixture of bleomycin solution and blood. The surface is then covered with plastic tape (better than tissue tape to avoid liquid absorption by the bandage) that is maintained with a bandage for 24–48 h. Three to five days later the wart becomes necrotic and a few days later falls off. Most patients are cured with this method but, if necessary, bleopuncture can be repeated at monthly intervals.

Selective photothermolysis of superficial blood capillaries with lasers (pulsed dye laser 585 nm, Q-switched Nd : YAG 532, Nd : YAG 1064 nm) or intense pulsed light (photoderm 570–590 nm) could be useful in resistant warts. The horny layer must first be removed and usually three to four sessions are needed.

General schedule for epidermodysplasia verruciformis

Cryotherapy and systemic retinoids (isotretinoin 0.5 mg/kg per day, and later lower maintenance doses) can give good results. Photoprotection is very important is these patients because the risk of malignant transformation of the lesions is increased in sun-exposed areas.

General schedule for genital warts

The first choice is destruction of the lesion by any method (cryotherapy, CO_2 laser) or application of podophyllin or podophyllotoxin. Topical 5% imiquimod can be beneficial for multiple lesions or recurrences. In case of continued recurrences after these therapeutic modalities, destruction of the lesions combined with systemic interferon can be tried. Our schedule consists of subcutaneous injections of interferon-α_2 in the thighs, 3 million units three times per week on 12 consecutive weeks. The dose is usually divided, and half-dose is administered to each thigh. To minimize flu-like side-effects, injections are scheduled at 7 p.m. and the patients receive 500 mg of paracetamol at the time of injection and 2 h later. Mild asthenia is not uncommon after the third week of treatment, but patients can usually continue their normal activity. In case of further recurrences, destruction of condyloma can be associated with systemic interferon and oral retinoids (isotretinoin 0.5 mg/day).

We can conclude that management of cutaneous warts and anogenital condyloma offer many possibilities but none of the treatments is uniformly effective. Each patient must be individually evaluated to select the best method. Education and control of sexual partners is important in anogenital warts.

Further reading

Androphy EJ, Beutner K, Olbritch S. Human papilloma virus infection. In: Arndt KA, Robinson JK, Leboit PE, Wintroub BU eds. *Cutaneous Medicine and Surgery: an Integrated Program in Dermatology.* Philadelphia: W.B. Saunders, 1996; 1100–22.

Berth-Jones J, Hutchinson PE. Modern treatment of warts: cure rates at 3 and 6 months. *Br J Dermatol* 1992; 127: 262–5.

Bonnez W, Elswick RK Jr, Bailey-Farchione A *et al.* Efficacy and safety of 0.5% podofilox solution in the treatment and suppression of anogenital warts. *Am J Med* 1994; 96: 420–5.

Breitburd F, Coursaget P. Human papillomavirus vaccines. *Semin Cancer Biol* 1999; 9: 431–44.

Calista D. Topical cidofovir for recalcitrant warts in two children. *Eur J Pediat Dermatol* 2000; 10: 9–12.

Cirelli R, Tyring SK. Interferons in human papillomavirus infections. *Antiviral Res* 1994; 24: 191–204.

Gollnick H, Barasso R, Jappe U *et al.* Safety and efficacy of imiquimod 5% cream in the treatment of penile genital warts in uncircumcised men when applied three times weekly or once per day. *Int J STD AIDS* 2001; 12: 22–8.

Gross G. Viral infections. human papilloma virus infections treated with immunostimulatory drugs and vaccination therapies. In: Burg G, Dummer RG. *Strategies for Immunointerventions in Dermatology.* Berlin: Springer, 1997: 293–305.

Hruza GJ. Laser treatment of warts and other epidermal and dermal. *Dermatol Clin* 1997; 15: 487–506.

Orlow SJ, Paller A. Cimetidine therapy for multiple warts in children. *J Am Acad Dermatol* 1993; 28: 794–6.

Shelley WB, Shelley DE. Intralesional bleomycin sulfate therapy for warts. *Arch Dermatol* 1991; 127: 234–6.

Spach DH, Colven R. Resolution of recalcitrant hand warts in an HIV-infected patient treated with potent antiretroviral therapy. *J Am Acad Dermatol* 1999; 40: 818–21.

Spiro JM. Technique for treatment of resistant warts using bleomycin. *Vaccination Cutis* 1996; 57: 180–2.

Stender MI, Lock-Andersen J, Wulf HC. Recalcitrant hand and foot warts succesfully treated with photodynamic therapy with topical 5-aminolevulinic acid: a pilot study. *Clin Exp Dermatol* 1999; 24: 154–9.

Wang TL, Ling M, Shih MI *et al.* Intramuscular administration of E7-transfected dendritic cells generates the most potent E7-specific anti-tumor immunity. *Gene Ther* 2000; 7: 726–33.

Xanthomas

A.D. Tosca and J.C. Katsantonis

Definition and pathogenesis

The term xanthomas has been applied to cutaneous lesions with various clinical appearances, which are characterized by the constant presence of 'xanthoma' or 'foam' cells. These cells are mainly macrophages containing a sudanophilic material 'lipid droplets' and they form large or small aggregates. The xanthoma cell accumulation, the admixture with other cells and the chemical composition of the intracellular lipid droplets are different in the various types of xanthomas. In most cases, xanthomas are due to hyperlipidaemia, either primary (resulting from a genetically determined dysfunction of lipid metabolism) or secondary (due to various internal disorders not directly connected to lipid metabolism).

The exact mechanisms responsible for the xanthoma formation are not quite known. It has been hypothesized that local inflammation, tissue trauma as well as the scavenger of acetyl low-density lipoprotein (LDL) receptors on skin macrophages and the increased *in situ* lipid formation are the possible pathways which lead to the specific skin lesions. Table 1 depicts the clinical types of xanthomas combined with the lipid metabolic disturbances, which may underlie each type. Since dermatologists are usually the first to deal with these cutaneous manifestations, it is necessary to ascertain the prognostic significance of each xanthoma type in order to recommend subsequently the appropriate treatment. It should be stressed (Table 1) that besides xanthelasma palpebrarum, other xanthomas have also been thought to occur in otherwise normocholesterolaemic individuals. However, in most of these cases, after a close follow-up with detailed lipid and lipoprotein analysis, serious metabolic abnormalities have been shown. The family history has also to be seriously considered. In addition, the presence of xanthelasma palpebrarum in apparently normolipidaemic patients does not exclude the risk of atherosclerosis.

Classification

Xanthomas are classified as:

- xanthelasma palpebrarum
- tuberous xanthoma
- tendinous xanthoma
- eruptive xanthoma
- plane xanthomas (palmar plane and generalized plane).

Treatment regimens

Surgical procedures

Local treatment modalities

These have been tried mainly for xanthelasma palpebrarum. Mohs' micrographic surgery for atypical fibrous xanthomas or the removal of large periorbital xanthomas using blepharoplasty island musculocutaneous flaps, for the defect closure, have been used with remarkable cosmetic results. In addition, the surgical excision of skin contractions from xanthoma disseminatum with split-thickness skin grafting has also been reported. Xanthelasma palpebrarum, when stable and isolated, can also be destroyed either by cautery or by repeat applications (3–4 times over several weeks) of 35% trichloroacetic acid. Recently, various laser systems have been tried with success. Carbon dioxide as well as ultrapulsed carbon dioxide and argon lasers with local anaesthesia and some risk of scarring and pigmentation. More promising appear to be pulsed dye and pulsed erbium-YAG laser without anaesthesia and excellent cosmetic results. However, the main problem that still remains is the increased rate of local recurrence.

Table 1 Types of xanthomas and the common underlying disturbances

Xanthelasma palpebrarum	Tuberous xanthoma	Tendinous xanthoma
Localized phenomenon Primary systemic hyperlipidaemia Type II hyperlipoproteinaemia (FH) Type III hyperlipoproteinaemia (FH) Mixed hyperlipidaemia (type IV) Apolipoprotein E phenotypes	Primary systemic hyperlipidaemia Type II hyperlipoproteinaemia (FH) Type III hyperlipoproteinaemia (FH) (familial dysbetalipoproteinaemia)	Primary systemic hyperlipidaemia Type II hyperlipoproteinaemia (FH) Apolipoprotein E phenotypes
Chronic biliary obstruction	Secondary hyperlipidaemia Hypothyroidism Chronic biliary disease Nephrotic syndrome Monoclonal gammopathy	Secondary hyperlipidaemia with prolonged cholestasis
Cerebrotendinous xanthoma	Cerebrotendinous xanthoma	Cerebrotendinous xanthoma
β-sitosterolaemia	β-sitosterolaemia	β-sitosterolaemia

Eruptive xanthoma	Plane xanthoma		Other types
	Palmar plane	Generalized plane	Xanthomas in: Lymphoedema Inflammatory diseases Neoplastic diseases Histiocytoma Juvenile xanthogranuloma
Primary systemic hyperlipidaemia Type I hyperlipoproteinaemia (familial lipoprotein lipase deficiency) Type III hyperlipidaemia Type IV hyperlipidaemia (familial hypertriglyceridaemia) Type V hyperlipidaemia Type IIb hyperlipidaemia (combined hyperlipidaemia)	Type III hyperlipoproteinaemia Primary systemic hyperlipidaemia FH homozygotes	Primary systemic hyperlipidaemia Type III primary hyperlipidaemia Secondary hyperlipidaemia	
Secondary hyperlipidaemia Diabetes mellitus Alcoholism Oestrogens and contraceptives Retinoids Hypothyroidism Nephrotic syndrome	Secondary hyperlipidaemia Diabetes mellitus Chronic biliary obstruction Prolonged cholestasis Monoclonal gammopathy	Monoclonal gammopathy associated with: Myeloma (type III pattern) Macroglobulinaemia Lymphoma, leukaemia, rheumatoid arthritis IgA gammopathy with hypolipidaemia	

Therefore diet, drugs and/or other therapeutic measures have to be used in the vast majority of skin xanthoma treatments.

Generalized surgical approach

When there are indications of rapidly progressing coronary atherosclerosis, aggressive surgical use of arterial grafts combined with intensive drug therapy and in some cases with LDL apheresis, is recommended. Patients undergoing such treatment have shown good long-term outcome in spite of their severe hyperlipidaemia.

The end-to-side portacaval shunt had also notable results in some cases of homozygous familial hyperlipidaemia (FH). Although the precise mechanism for the postoperative decrease of cholesterol and LDL remains obscure, it has to be mentioned that these changes were associated with elevated concentrations of plasma glucagon and bile acids.

Diet

It seems that this therapeutic approach is quite effective when instituted early in life. It has been shown that dietary therapy in 2–7-year-old children heterozygous for FH has provided a mean overall reduction of total and LDL cholesterol levels. The diet should consist of food rich in polyunsaturates and lacking in cholesterol saturate lipid. Olive oil and legumin-enriched food (Mediterranean type of diet) seems to offer an alternative basis for a long-term hypocholesterolic diet. However, eventually, some children may require the addition of a drug to achieve a satisfactory decrease of the lipid level. Hypercholesterolaemic adults also need to follow such a diet, but not as the only therapeutic measure. A lot of dietary modalities have been tested trying to get the optimum metabolic balance. It has been referred that an oligocaloric high carbohydrate and low-fat diet (90.5% glucose oligosaccharides, 1.3% safflower oil, 8.2% crystalline amino acids) can normalize the blood lipid levels and softens the cutaneous xanthomas in patients with homozygous FH.

Drug therapy (primary hypercholesterolaemia)

The bile acid binding resins (cholestyramine and colestipol) do not act systemically. They actually bind the bile acids in the intestinal lumen, causing interruption of their enterohepatic circulation and in this way they increase the fecal steroid excretion. However, it has to be noticed that in some cases these drugs may promote increased hepatic production of very low-density lipoproteins (VLDL) and LDL and thereafter to exacerbate hypertriglyceridaemia instead of decreasing it. Besides, although cholestyramine has been found to be effective in reducing LDL cholesterol levels in children with inherited hyperlipidaemia, the majority of children did not comply due to the drug's adverse effects—constipation, foul taste and nausea with bloating being the most common. Folate deficiency may also occur and vitamin D supplements should be considered.

The hypocholesterolaemic effects of nicotinic acid are probably mediated through decreased hepatic synthesis of VLDL and LDL and they are well documented. However, the increased hypolipidaemic effects of high doses of nicotinic acid have to be balanced against the increased incidence of side-effects, which may result in intolerance to the drug. Cutaneous flushing, nausea, discomfort, skin dryness and in some cases blurred vision may occur. Active liver disease, hyperuricaemia, diabetes or peptic ulcer, are contraindications for the nicotinic acid administration.

It should be mentioned that nicotinic acid and bile acid sequestrants, although they seem to offer a sufficient solution for patients with other primary causes of hypercholesterolaemia, do not seem able to control hyperlipidaemia and xanthomas in patients with heterozygous FH.

Lovastatin is a widely used inhibitor of 3-hydroxy-3methyl glutaryl coenzyme A (HMG-CoA) reductase, an enzyme that facilitates the intracellular synthesis of cholesterol. The inhibition of the HMG-CoA reductace action may lead to increased activity of the LDL receptors which subsequently may stimulate the LDL catabolism rate. Thus, the ability of this drug to reduce LDL concentrations is primarily due to increased LDL catabolism and secondarily to reduction of VLDL and LDL production.

Lovastatin is a well-tolerated drug. The known side-effects are headaches, nausea, fatigue, insomnia, skin exanthems, bowel dysfunction and in extremely rare cases myositis. It is an effective drug in patients with heterozygous FH, familial combined hyperlipidaemia or other not well-characterized lipid metabolism disorders. However, the use of lovastatin is not indicated in children and it should be administered with caution in women of childbearing potential. Combination therapy with lovastatin and LDL apheresis has been tried with remarkable results. In some extremely severe cases the drug has been combined also with liver transplantation.

In the class of HMG-CoA reductase inhibitors, several other drugs are included. Simvastatin and pravastatin are the most common ones. Like lovastatin, simvastatin has also been given in combination with LDL apheresis. In some cases, therapy with simvastatin alone, did not prevent progression of carotid or aortotibial vascular disease, but when combined with LDL apheresis, a remarkable decrease in the intima-media thickness of the carotid artery was observed, without any increase in the lower limb, of haemodynamically significant stenoses.

The fibric acid derivatives seem also to be effective in hyperlipidaemias and they can be used as first-line drugs. Clofibrate, gemfibrozil, bezafibrate, fenofibrate and ciprofibrate are the most common among them. The last three seem to have the most potent hypocholesterolaemic effects. Increased activity of lipoprotein lipase, enhanced LDL catabolism and reduced VLDL synthesis are the mechanisms of action. These drugs can also be used in children. The combination of sitosterol with bezafibrate was proven to be acceptable, safe and effective for children with high-risk familial hypercholesterolaemia.

Probucol, although a modestly effective drug for primary hypercholesterolaemia, seems to interfere with cholesterol synthesis and transport in human tissues, which might explain the observed benefical effects of this drug on cutaneous xanthomas. Probucol has been found to cause regression of tendon xanthomas and xanthelasmas. As a general rule, the use of two or more hypolipidaemic drugs with different mechanisms of action, which may act additively or synergistically, has been commonly instituted in many patients, particularly those with heterozygous FH.

LDL apheresis

The most severe forms of hypercholesterolaemia scarcely respond to diet and drug administration. Therefore they need alternative treatment. Besides, surgical methods (ileal bypass, liver transplantation, for example) are not always feasible.

Therapeutic plasma exchange has been shown to result in a remarkable amelioration in patients with FH. Semiselective and selective techniques have consequently been developed using secondary membrane filtration in order to remove LDL cholesterol alone. The side-effects have been reported to be rare and not serious (i.e the maintenance of serum albumin and vitamin E levels during LDL apheresis, the reduced blood pressure and the alteration of blood viscosity).

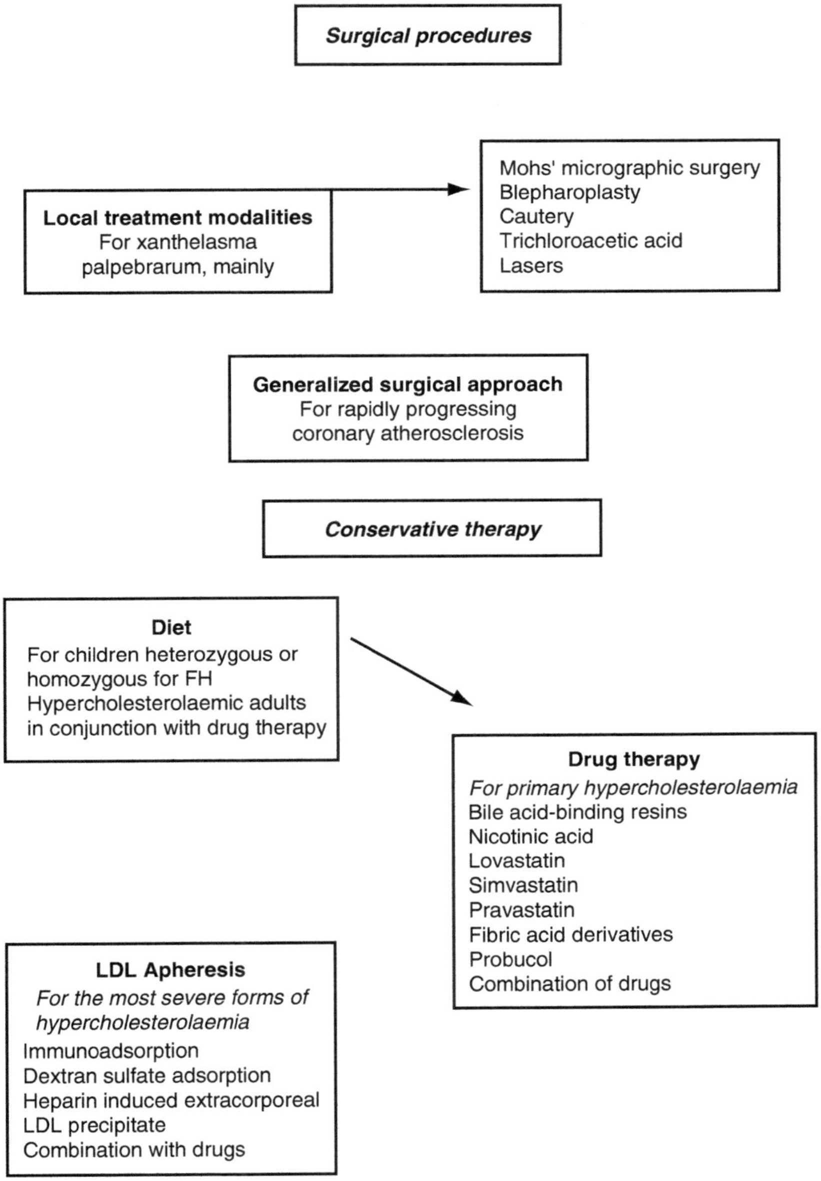

Figure 1 Treatment of xanthomas

Three major LDL apheresis methods have been developed: immunoadsorption (IMAC), dextran sulphate adsorption (DSAL) and heparin-induced extracorporeal LDL precipitate (HELP). The effectiveness of these methods is similar, but selectivity and biocompatibility are different. The therapeutic relevance of these differences for long-term treatment has not yet been completely elucidated.

Furthermore, it has been shown that LDL apheresis methods can be safely combined with HMG-CoA reductase inhibitors for the duration of a year without serious side-effects. Such therapies have been proved to lead to regression of skin and tendon xanthomas and of vascular atherosclerosis. In homozygotes with FH, LDL alpheresis alone leads to prolongation and improved quality of life. In heterozygotes, a combination of LDL apheresis, hypolipidaemic drugs and dietary provisions seems to be the most effective therapeutic schedule. A further advantage of LDL apheresis is that it does not interfere with physiological adaptation of lipoprotein metabolism in pregnancy; therefore it has been used with excellent results in pregnant women.

Further reading

Glueck CJ, Tsang RC, Fallat RW, Mellies MJ. Diet in children heterozygous for familial hypercholesterolemia. *Am J Dis Child* 1977; 131 (2): 162–6.

Hosokawa K, Susuki T, Kikui TA, Tahara S. Treatment of large xanthomas by the use of blepharoplasty island musculocutaneous flaps. *Ann Plast Surg* 1987; 18 (3): 238–40.

Illingworth DR. Drug therapy of hypercholesterolamia. *Clin Chem* 1988; 34 (8): 123–32.

Kawasuji M, Sakakibara N, Takemura H, Matsumoto Y, Mabuchi H, Watanabe Y. Coronary artery bypass grafting in familial hypercholesterolemia. *J Thorac Cardiovasc Surg* 1995; 109 (2): 364–9.

Kroon AA, Van Asten WN, Stalenhoef AF. Effect of apheresis of low density lipoprotein on peripheral vascular disease in hypercholesterolemic patients with coronary artery disease. *Ann Intern Med* 1996; 125 (12): 945–54.

Liacouras CA, Coates PM, Galagher PR, Cortner JA. Use of cholestyramine in the treatment of children with familial combined hyperlipidemia. *J Pediatr* 1993; 122 (3): 477–82.

Raulin C, Schoenermark MP, Werner S, Greve B. Xanthelasma palpebrarum: treatment with the ultrapulsed CO_2 laser. *Lasers Surg Med* 1999; 24 (2): 122–7.

Schaumann D, Welch-Wichary M, Voss A, Schmidt H, Olbricht CJ. Prospective cross-over comparisons of three low-density lipoprotein (LDL)-apheresis methods in patients with familial hypercholesterolaemia. *Eur J Clin Invest* 1996; 26 (11): 1033–8.

Schonermark MP, Raulin C. Treatment of xanthelasma palpebrarum with the pulsed dye laser. *Lasers Surg Med* 1996; 19 (3): 336–9.

Teikemeier G, Stein E. Controlled dermabrasion with a newly developed erbium-Yag laser system. Report of preliminary experiences. *Hautarzt* 1996; 47 (7): 530–2.

Teruel JL, Lasuncion MA, Navarro JF, Carrero P, Ortuno J. Pregnancy in a patient with homozygous familial hypercholesterolemia undergoing low density lipoprotein apheresis by dextran sulfate adsorption. *Metabolism* 1995; 44 (7): 929–33.

Thompson GR, Barbin M, Okabayashi K, Trayner I, Larkin S. Plasmapheresis in familial hypercholesterolemia. *Arteriosclerosis* 1989; 9: 1152–7.

Methods

Acne scar treatment

L. Rusciani

Acne is a chronic inflammatory disease that affects approximately 90% of those aged between 14 and 16 years, and usually disappears by the age of 25–27 years. In some cases, acne persists during adulthood.

Almost 5% of patients exhibit acne in a severe form: in these cases, acne usually leads to permanent scars that are often a cause of severe social discomfort and loss of self-esteem.

Therapeutic approach to acne scars

Several therapeutic techniques are available for the treatment of acne scars. Virtually all scars can be optimally treated with the correct method, obtaining satisfactory results. Nevertheless, treatment of acne scars is often difficult and requires expert physicians.

Patient selection

To choose the most suitable treatment, one must distinguish patients with active acne from patients with past acne.

Patients with active acne present both 'active' (comedones, pustules, papules) and cicatricial lesions. An effective treatment must be undertaken in these patients to minimize existing scars and to prevent the development of new ones. Surgical treatment is not indicated. Patients with past acne present only permanent scars. These patients can be successfully treated with surgical techniques.

Other important factors to be evaluated are a past history of hypertrophic scar or keloid formation, or recent therapy with isotretinoin.

Types of scars

Acne scars can be atrophic or hypertrophic. They vary widely in shape, length, depth and dimensions, and often coexist on the same patient.

Atrophic acne scars

These are depressed and differ in their shape and size: they can be wide and shallow ('boxcar' scars), or narrow and deep ('ice-pick' scars). When subcutaneous tissue is severely damaged, the result can be subcutaneous tunnels or large retractions that significantly alter facial contours.

- Boxcar scars: these are usually wide and superficial. The treatments of choice are: filling, peeling, dermabrasion and laser abrasion.
- Ice-pick scars: these have a 'punctate' aspect, sharp walls and extend vertically and deeply (> 2 mm). The surface opening is usually larger than the infundibulum.

These two types can be treated with dermabrasion, laser abrasion, base elevation or transplant, but often appreciable results can be obtained with only surgical excision.

- Subcutaneous tunnels and retractions: these lesions usually modify facial contour. The only possible treatments are surgical excision and, in the case of large retractions, facial lifting.

Elevated scars

A patient with acne may present mature hypertrophic scars or keloids.

- Hypertrophic scars: these are nodular with a small, bumpy surface, and can be treated with intralesional infiltration of steroids or with dermabrasion
- Keloid scars: these are less common but more difficult to treat. Some physicians do not treat them because of the possibility of recurrence or of worsening of the lesion. The treatments

of choice are cryotherapy, intralesional steroids and compressive dressings.

Treatment of acne scars

Minor surgical treatments

Peeling

Peeling causes epidermal exfoliation by the use of chemical agents, and permits good results in the treatment of superficial scars (superficial boxcar scars). Many acid derivatives can be used: our favourites are phenol and trichloroacetic acid (TCA). Skin is cleaned with alcohol, and then acid is applied with cotton tampons. Ice packs or cold water applied after the peeling may diminish unpleasant burning and pain.

Phenol is usually employed at a concentration of 50%, according to Baker's formula. Unfortunately, it can cause renal, cardiac or hepatic damage.

Peeling with TCA is a simpler and safer technique, free from systemic adverse effects. TCA can be used at different concentrations, in order to obtain different results.

- 20% TCA: this concentration causes only superficial exfoliation, and is not indicated for acne scars
- 35% TCA: this is employed to obtain a medium depth peeling on small and superficial scars. After the treatment, lesions are not wrapped, and patients must avoid sun exposure for 3 months by applying a sun-block daily.
- 50% TCA: indicated for the treatment of large, superficial scars. During the first week after the treatment, patients must wear a bandage. The peeling causes a deep exfoliation and the formation of crusts that detach leaving a translucent, bright pink epidermis. This is the maximum employable concentration. Higher than 50% concentrations may cause atrophic scarring and hypopigmentation.

Compressive dressings

External compression with silicone sheets (Silastic, Epi-derm) or occlusive dressing (SIL-K) may be adopted to treat recent (< 6 months) keloids. They must be applied on the lesion without compression for 12–20 h, then removed, washed with soap and reapplied. This kind of bandage is also useful in the post-treatment phase, to prevent the recurrence of keloids. Occlusive bandage must not be applied on hairy regions, because they can precipitate folliculitis. Silicone sheets must be substituted every 1–2 weeks, occlusive bandages every 1–2 months.

Cryotherapy

Cryotherapy is useful in the treatment of keloids, alone or combined with other techniques.

Lidocaine (lignocaine) 1–2% is infiltrated to achieve local anaesthesia, and then keloid is frozen with liquid nitrogen. Sometimes another treatment after 4–6 weeks is necessary for a good result. Generally, a necrotic crust develops after this treatment that usually heals in 2–3 weeks. Aggressive cryotherapy can destroy skin melanocytes, leaving hypopigmentation that can persist for 18 months or more especially in patients with darker complexions.

Intralesional steroids

Intralesional injections of steroids (usually triamcinolone acetonide) can be a valid therapeutic option for hypertrophic scars and keloids, especially if they are performed on recent scars, when they are still immature. Steroids acts on the growing lesions interfering with their bulking mechanisms, making them recede.

The treatment usually is performed with triamcinolone acetonide 40 mg in 3–4 mL saline solution.

Possible adverse local effects include atrophy. Systemic steroid-related effects (such as hirsutism, striae distensae, Cushing's syndrome) are usually not observed.

Fillers

Fillers are natural or synthetic substances that are injected into depressed scars to raise the bottom of pits towards the top. They are indicated for soft and shallow lesions but are not so useful for ice-pick scars, especially when intradermal pits are firm and adherent to the underlying surface. Most fillers are composed of the following.

- Collagen is a biomaterial, compatible with skin tissue, but it is very expensive and gives only temporary results.
- Silicon is a synthetic material that gives definitive correction. Despite its low cost, it can be used with satisfactory results, but it can induce granulomatous or fibrotic reactions. Sometimes it can migrate from the point of injection, and correction is very difficult. Silicon is used mainly for small scars.
- Autologous fat implants are used for correction of large scars and are less expensive. Fat is harvested with a large needle from a patient donor area, then washed with saline solution and re-injected into the recipient site. With this technique, rejection is almost non-existent, but the results are often unsatisfactory, and several treatments are necessary.

Major surgical treatments

Laser abrasion

Resurfacing with a laser can guarantee a considerable improvement of acne scarring. This procedure can be extremely exact in sculpturing the border of scars, evaporating a greater quantity of tissue only in the areas of interest, and carrying out only superficial resurfacing in the remainder.

Tissue retraction can result in remarkable improvements in moderate atrophic scars with sloping planes. Some ice-pick scars must be removed with excision, then laser resurfaced after 6–12 weeks for optimal results. Scars that have not been previously treated with excision can be improved, but the degree of improvement depends on the depth of the lesion and on the ability of the surgeon. The lasers used most often for acne scarring are the CO_2 and the Er : YAG.

The regulation of the lasers depends upon the depth of the scar. For superficial scars we usually use the erbium laser only; for medium and deep scars we use the CO_2 laser alone or in combination with the erbium laser.

Dermabrasion

Dermabrasion is a technique that was first described during World War I. It is a surgical procedure that, by removing the epithelium and thinning the dermis, makes the scar less evident.

Dermabrasion is performed with a rotatory motor that transmits the movement to a pin that carries different metallic brushes or abrasive diamond material. The skin surface is lowered towards the level of the bottom of the scar. Best results are obtained with wide and superficial scars, but elevated scars can also be successfully treated.

When treating acne scars, the entire exposed region must be dermabraded, degrading towards the line of demarcation with the adjacent feature to achieve a homogeneous surface. Dermabrasion may be associated with peeling of other facial regions, for better aesthetic results.

Best results are obtained with one treatment every 5 or 6 months; two or three treatments are usually required. Best results are obtained in fair Caucasian patients. For olive Caucasian complexion or darker skin types (black, oriental) dermabrasion is contraindicated, because of the possibility of hyperpigmentation.

Microsurgery

Microsurgery for the treatment of acne scarring is continuously evolving. Two types of microsurgery exist as follows.

- Punch microsurgery: punches of 1.5–2 mm are used depending on the scar's diameter. After local anaesthesia, the scar is punched out to its entire thickness and the loss of substance is sutured with a reabsorbable suture 5/0–6/0 or with intradermic suture nylon 6/0 or external suture with nylon 7/0. Skin implant is a variation of surgery with punch microsurgery.
- Microsurgery with blade: classic surgery with local anaesthesia with a No. 15 blade. Usually used for scars with an extended shape but not those which are round because it is very difficult to attack them with a punch. The type of suture is the same as above.

Further reading

Ellis AFE. Surgical treatment of acne scarring: non-linear scar revision. *J Otolaryngol* 1987; 16 (2): 116–19.

Goodman GJ. Post-acne scarring. A short review of pathophysiology. *Aust J Dermatol* 2001; 42: 84–90.

Robinson *et al. Atlante di Chirurgia Cutanea.* EdiSES 1999.

Biopsy

E. Haneke

Histopathology is the most important method in dermatology which requires good biopsy specimens for diagnosis. In most European countries, biopsies are daily routine procedures for virtually all dermatologists. Poor biopsy specimens hinder the diagnostic process and there are many pitfalls in performing biopsies.

Indications for biopsy

Each piece of tissue that is removed should be examined histopathologically. However, multiple benign lesions such as acrochordons, seborrhoeic keratoses or mollusca contagiosa may not require histopathology although one representative lesion should be sent for histopathological examination. The extent of a biopsy is governed by the suspected clinical diagnosis: whereas benign lesions may be partially or serially excised, a diagnostic therapeutic excisional biopsy is indicated for a malignant lesion such as melanoma.

The most important reasons for biopsies are:

- to make or confirm the diagnosis
- tumour grading and staging
- follow-up
- scientific documentation.

Biopsies can be divided according to the:

- instrument used to perform them
- depth of biopsy
- tissue biopsy.

Biopsy treatment

Punch biopsy

The punch is a cylindrical knife that cuts into the tissue while turning it on its longitudinal axis. Disposable punches are commonly used because they are usually sharper and less traumatizing. Punch diameters range from 1 to 8 mm, with 4 and 6 mm punches used most often for diagnostic purposes. They are held vertically on the skin surface and the tissue cylinder is cut with turning motions under slight pressure. The tissue is then gently lifted, either with a forceps or with the tip of an injection needle that has been bent to 90°, and it is cut at the level of the superficial subcutaneous fat. Extreme caution is necessary not to squeeze the tissue specimen because this will give rise to hourglass deformation of the tissue cylinder with serious crush artefacts of inflammatory infiltrate cells rendering the biopsy more or less useless.

Punch biopsies are not adequate for lesions of or extending into the subcutaneous tissue, or for bullous lesions because the blister roof will inevitably be sheared off.

Small punch biopsies may be left for second-intention healing whereas those of 4 or more millimetres in diameter usually require a suture. Monofil suture material, most frequently 5-0 or 6-0, gives good cosmetic results. A modified cross-stitch with the stitches over the skin running parallel ensures excellent defect closure.

Scalpel biopsy

The scalpel is the universal instrument for any type of biopsy of almost all tissues. Most diagnostic biopsies are performed as fusiform or elliptical excisions of tissue. Although many different types of scalpel blades may be used the no. 11 usually gives the best results, especially for smaller biopsies. Its sharp tip is vertically stabbed into the skin and the desired biopsy is sectioned with either a straight cut through the entire skin down to the subcutaneous fat or with gentle stabbing motions, carefully avoiding 'carving motions'. Depending on the type of lesion the biopsy should either include the whole lesion, a representative piece from one side to the other or the margin with both central lesional skin and normal surrounding skin. A small drawing showing the lesion, the biopsy and how it is supposed to be cut in the laboratory should accompany the biopsy so that the histopathology laboratory can see how the biopsy was performed and how it should be sectioned to yield adequate histological section for diagnosis.

The defect is usually closed with simple interrupted sutures, 5-0 for most localizations, 6-0 for the face, 7-0 for eyelids and 4-0 for back and lower extremities. Buried dermal sutures using monofil absorbable threads give the best cosmetic results. For particularly delicate locations, the suture should be secured with suture strips. Tissue glue is adequate for narrow defects that can be closed without tension. However, scar dehiscence remains a common problem, particularly on the back. Tiny 'dog-ear' scars may develop if the biopsy's length-to-width ratio was too small which may be particularly disturbing on the face.

Electrical scalpel and laser

These modalities may be used for larger excisional biopsies when there is no risk that the biopsy margins might be damaged by heat; this might mean that they cannot be properly evaluated histopathologically. The CO_2 laser, particularly when used in the ultrapulse mode, and high-frequency electrosurgery ('radiosurgery') devices are much less tissue damaging than the older electrosurgery machines. They have the advantage of leaving an almost bloodless field due to the heat generated by these procedures. The disadvantages are heat artefacts of the biopsy specimen margins and prolonged healing with inferior cosmesis of the biopsy scar.

The suture technique depends on the site, size and depth of the wound.

Curette biopsy

Even though the curette is useful to remove superficial lesions (see chapter on curettage) it is too coarse an instrument for almost all diagnostic biopsies. It leaves tissue debris that no longer allows the architecture of a lesion to be evaluated. The tissue is less seriously damaged when a so-called sharp ring-scalpel is used. This allows strips of tissue to be cut from the surface of the skin.

The resulting defect is left for secondary intention healing. Use of a haemostyptic solution or electrocautery to stop the bleeding etches the biopsy wound and prolongs the healing time and often causes a whitish scar. It is therefore recommended to apply a thick padded dressing to absorb the blood. Plenty of ointment avoids its sticking to the wound. This dressing may be removed after 24–48 h and only an antibiotic ointment is then used, usually several times a day in order to prevent the scab from drying out. Healing is twice to three times faster with moist wound healing.

Depth of biopsy

Shave biopsy

Shave biopsy is a simple, inexpensive and time-honoured procedure. It should only be used for superficial lesions involving the epidermis and papillary dermis. The lesion is slightly raised, either by gently pressing it up with the fingers of the non-dominant hand or by injecting local anaesthetic directly under the lesion thus producing a wheal. A scalpel with a no. 23, or for very small lesions no. 15, blade is pressed lightly to the surface of the surrounding skin and the lesion biopsied with back-and-forth sawing movements parallel to the skin surface. Depending on the size of the scalpel blade, relatively large superficial biopsies can be taken that resemble split-thickness skin grafts.

The biopsy specimen is transferred with the scalpel upside down onto wet gauze and gently spread. A small piece of filter paper is laid on its undersurface where it sticks and the perfectly spread specimen is immersed into 4% formalin solution for fixation. This technique guarantees excellent histological sections.

The wound is left for epithelialization by second intention. We favour not cauterizing it for haemostasis because this would delay wound healing (see section on curette biopsy above).

Shave biopsies are ideal for seborrhoeic keratoses, actinic keratoses and other lesions sitting on the skin or only affecting the uppermost layers. They are not adequate for most inflammatory alterations, lesions extending into the hair follicles and most tumours.

Incisional and excisional skin biopsies

Biopsies including the epidermis and entire dermis down to, but not including, the subcutaneous fat can be performed with a punch. The tissue specimen is a round cylinder, which cannot be further orientated in the histopathology laboratory. Due to the shearing forces when rotating it the punch is not useful for bullous lesions. The defect is round and a perfect closure is not always possible by suturing.

Scalpel biopsies are universally applicable and can reach down to the subcutaneous tissue, fascia and even muscle. Fascia and dermis are sutured, whereas approximation of the subcutaneous adipose tissue is usually not necessary. The surgical specimen can be marked so that secure orientation is possible in the laboratory.

Biopsies of subcutaneous tissue

These biopsies require scalpel surgery. Whether or not a piece of overlying skin is included in the biopsy depends on the suspected diagnosis. However, inflammatory dermatoses should always be biopsied with the overlying dermis and epidermis.

Tissue for biopsy

Scalp

Two neighbouring punch biopsies yielding a figure-of-eight defect are ideal for scalp biopsies. One of the specimens is cut vertically, the other horizontally for histopathology. The margins of the figure-of-eight defect are advanced against each other so that a tongue-in-groove picture results. Two stitches keep the wound together yielding a lazy S scar line.

Ear

A biopsy including ear cartilage may be indicated for the diagnosis of relapsing polychondritis. Local anaesthesia is performed in the retroauricular fold and a narrow spindle of skin with underlying cartilage is taken from the back of the pinna. The skin is closed usually with a running suture, but the cartilage is not touched.

Vermilion of the lip

Biopsies of the vermilion of the lip are indicated for precancerous lesions and carcinomas as well as for rare isolated labial involvement of psoriasis and other dermatoses. The incisional biopsy should be a narrow spindle with the long axis perpendicular to the mouth. Biopsies along the border of the vermilion of the lip would invariably distort this important cosmetic structure. Benign and precancerous lesions need not include parts of the underlying orbicularis oris muscle, though this is necessary in cases of suspected malignancy.

Oral mucosa

Biopsies of the labial and buccal mucosa do not pose any particular problem. However, infiltration local anaesthesia causes an instream of plasma into the epithelium with vacuolization of keratinocytes, crescentic deformation of nuclei as well as intra- and intercellular deposition of immunoglobulins and other proteins. For suspected immunodermatoses, a regional block of the mental or infraorbital nerve should be used if possible. Suture is either intramucosal or with other soft threads.

Both the hard palate and the attached gingiva are rarely biopsied. Because of their firm attachment to the bone, biopsies should be small and are not sutured but may be sealed with a dental silicone paste.

Biopsies of the dorsum of the tongue usually also involve the lingual musculature which is intimately connected with the epithelium. A narrow spindle of tissue is excised and the wound sutured without tying the knots too tight.

Minor salivary gland biopsy is a valuable adjunct for the diagnosis of Sjögren's syndrome. Mental nerve block anaesthesia is performed and a 2-cm horizontal incision is made in between the vermilion and the fornix inferior opposite the 2nd incisor. The mucosa is gently spread exposing greyish, glassy, round peppercorn-sized glands, which are separated from the underlying submucosa using blunt-tipped curved scissors. Six to eight glands should be collected. Infiltrates of more than 50 lymphocytes are typical, but epithelial islands are rare in minor salivary glands.

Axilla and other apocrine regions

Both inflammatory lesions and carcinomas may occur in these regions. Biopsy site and size are chosen according to the particular lesion. Since these are intertriginous areas with maceration due to eccrine sweat and often heavy bacterial and sometimes fungal colonization, airtight dressings must be avoided and dry sterile dressings reapplied every 24–48 h.

Breast and nipple

Punch and scalpel biopsies are commonly orientated along the relaxed skin tension lines, but those of the nipple always in a radial manner. A vasoconstrictor in addition to the local anaesthetic would cause the nipple to contract and is therefore not recommended. A layered suture is used to prevent scar spread and the patient is asked to wear a tight-fitting bra for the next few days.

Penis and scrotum

The glans penis often presents plaque-like red lesions, which are difficult to diagnose on clinical grounds alone. Superficial infiltration anaesthesia elevates the epithelium and subepithelial connective tissue separating it from the corpus cavernosum thus facilitating a superficial scalpel biopsy. The defect is sutured with simple stitches.

Prepuce and penis shaft are biopsied like skin of any other region.

Biopsies of scrotal lesions should be fusiform and include skin and immediate subepithelial tissue. Sutures are only lightly tied to avoid them cutting through scrotal skin.

Vulva

The labia majora are similar to scrotal skin. However, biopsies for suspected malignant lesions must reach the deep fascia.

Labia minora lesions are best biopsied by removing a full-thickness wedge of tissue and a two-layered suture is used for repair.

Palms and soles

Both inflammatory and malignant lesions may have to be biopsied. For small lesions, a 3–4 mm punch is ideal. If possible, the handedness of the patient is respected: the left palm is chosen for right-handers, and vice versa.

Biopsies from the sole of the foot have to be kept as small as possible, preferably using a punch. Local anaesthesia is usually very painful, and infiltration may have begun from the side of the foot. The subcutaneous tissue with its elastic cushion function is unique and cannot be repaired. Biopsies over callous regions must be avoided because the scar may remain tender and painful for life. Sutures must be left for 2 weeks at a minimum.

Nail

Biopsies of the lateral and proximal nail folds may be tangential for superficial lesions.

Nail bed lesions require a punch, maximum diameter 4 mm, or a narrow longitudinal fusiform biopsy after (partial) nail avulsion. Gentle undermining at the level of the bone, extending to the fibroadipose tissue of the lateral nail folds permits suture without tension.

Matrix lesions located on one side of the nail are best treated using the lateral longitudinal nail biopsy yielding a 2-mm wide tissue bloc containing proximal nail fold, matrix, nail bed and hyponychium. The first incision is started at the distal dorsal crease of the distal interphalangeal joint and carried straight through the nail down to the bone to the tip of the digit about 2 mm central from the lateral nail edge. The second incision is performed in parallel and through the lateral nail groove. The bloc is dissected from the bone with curved iris scissors. The central margin is marked for the histopathology laboratory. The defect is sutured with simple stitches through the proximal nail fold and hyponychium, but backstitches are used for the nail bed in order to recreate the lateral nail fold. Small biopsies from the more medial part of the matrix may be performed with a 3-mm punch and the defect left open. Larger lesions require a transverse fusiform or crescentic biopsy. Its distal margin should run parallel to the lunula margin. Sutures must not cut through the fragile matrix.

Large melanocytic foci in the matrix may be treated with excisional biopsy. The proximal nail fold is reflected and part of the proximal third of the nail plate is separated and lifted to allow access to the lesion. A superficial incision is carried all around the lesion with an adequate safety margin and the lesion horizontally excised with back-and-forth movements of the no. 15 scalpel. The nail plate is laid back and stitched to the lateral nail fold, and then the proximal nail fold is sutured. Healing is without scarring.

Artery

Arterial biopsy is indicated to confirm the diagnosis of arteritis cranialis. A 15–20 mm segment of the hard temporal artery is marked; the skin is anaesthetized and incised. The artery is atraumatically dissected and a segment of the organized artery taken out for histopathology. Ligation is usually unnecessary.

Skeletal muscle

Muscle biopsy for the diagnosis of dermatomyositis is either performed according to electromyogram (EMG) findings or from the deltoid muscle, which is most commonly affected. After generous infiltration anaesthesia, a 5-cm skin incision is carried down to the fascia, which is then carefully incised. A few fibres of the bulging muscle are atraumatically isolated and ligated on both sides about 2 cm apart. They are cut distal from these ligations and the muscle is spread on a piece of firm cardboard using the sutures in order to avoid muscle contraction. During the entire procedure, the muscle to be examined histopathologically must not be touched with the pincer since this will produce crush artefacts and render the biopsy useless.

Nerve

In leprosy, the ulnar nerve is often seen and palpated as a narrow string subcutaneously. It can be biopsied for histopathology.

Similarly, string-like lesions on the thorax may be biopsied for the diagnosis of Mondor's thrombotic lymphangitis.

Further reading

Haneke E. Über die diagnostische Aussage von Biopsien der kleinen Lippenspeicheldrüsen bei Mundtrockenheit. *Dtsch Z Mund Kiefer-Gesichtschir* 1981; 5: 26–9.

Haneke E. Exzisions-und Biopsieverfahren. *Z Hautkr* 1988; 63 (Suppl.): 17–19.

Haneke E. Reconstruction of the lateral nail fold after lateral longitudinal nail biopsy. In: Robins P, ed. *Surgical Gems in Dermatology.* New York: Journal Publishing Group, 1988: 91–3.

Haneke E. Variationen der Flaschenzugnaht. In: Mahrle G, Schulze H-J, Krieg T, eds. *Fortschritte der Operativen und Onkologischen Dermatologie 8: Wundheilung–Wundverschluß.* Heidelberg: Springer, 1994: 158–64.

Haneke E. Developments and techniques in general cutaneous surgery. In: Dahl MV, Lynch PJ, eds. *Current Opinion in Dermatology*, Vol. 2. Philadelphia: Current Science, 1995: 129–36.

Haneke E. Flachexzision von Nävuszellnävi. In: Garbe C, Rassner G, eds. *Dermatologie—Leitlinien und Qualitätssicherung für Diagnostik und Therapie.* Berlin: Springer, 1998: 523–5.

Haneke E. Operative Therapie akraler und subungualer Melanome. In: Rompel R, Petres J, eds. *Operative und Onkologische Dermatologie. Fortschritte der Operativen und Onkologischen Dermatologie 15.* Berlin: Springer, 1999: 210–14.

Haneke E, Bübl R. Demonstration of immunoglobulins in the normal epithelium of the lip mucosa. *Arch Dermatol Res* 1983; 275: 266.

Krull EA, Zook EG, Baran R, Haneke E. *Nail Surgery. A Text and Atlas.* Philadelphia: Lippincott, Williams & Wilkins, 2001.

Chemical peeling

I. Ghersetich, B. Brazzini and T. Lotti

Chemical peeling involves the application of an exfoliating chemical agent on the skin to produce a controlled, partial-thickness injury with subsequent removal of superficial skin lesions, regeneration of new tissue with improvement of skin texture and long-lasting therapeutic and cosmetic benefits.

Chemical peelings are commonly used in dermatological practice for the treatment of sun-damaged skin with actinic elastosis, facial wrinkles and actinic keratoses, sun-related pigmentary dyschromias (especially lentigo simplex), postinflammatory hyperpigmentation and melasma, acne and acne scars, warts and rough oily skin with enlarged pores.

Classification of chemical peeling

On the basis of wound depth, chemical peeling is classified as follows.

Superficial chemical peels

These penetrate the epidermis down to the dermal–epidermal interface. Examples of superficial peeling agents are listed in Table 1. The peeling agent used is one of the most important determining factors for peeling depth but many other factors should be considered including length of application, Fitzpatrick skin type, prepeeling treatments and repeeling.

Although the procedure is standardized as much as possible, a 'light' peeling agent can sometimes result in a deeper peel.

Medium-depth peels

These are obtained with agents or a combination of agents (Table 2) that produce an injury depth down to the upper reticular dermis. The application of medium-depth peeling agents induces both full-thickness dermal necrosis and partial-thickness dermal necrosis.

Trichloroacetic acid (TCA) alone or in combination with other agents is the mainstay of medium-depth chemical peels. Combination chemical peels attempt to maximize the therapeutic effects of different agents while minimizing adverse reactions and side-effects through decreased concentrations of caustic agents. In general, a combination chemical peel consists of two wounding agents: the first causes epidermal thinning or necrosis (Jessner's solution (JS), glycolic acid (GA), salicylic acid (SA)), while the second (TCA 35%), that penetrates easily and deeper, accomplishes dermal necrosis.

These peelings are relatively simple and associated with a favourable risk/benefit ratio. However, proper patient selection, with attention to both medical and psychological factors, requires sound experience.

The indications for these peelings are both medical and cosmetic conditions. Primary medical conditions include diffuse actinic keratosis, and cosmetic conditions include mild to moderate wrinkles, dyschromias, solar elastosis, solar lentigines, melasma and postinflammatory hyperpigmentation.

Deep chemical peels

These involve the use of chemoexfoliants that penetrate to the mid-reticular dermis. Deep chemical peels entail longer healing times and increase the potential for complications. Baker–Gordon's formula (Table 3) is the most commonly used deep chemical peeling agent. Deep phenol peeling can lead to irreversible hypopigmentation because of the melanotoxicity of phenol and, thus, is not advised for dark skin types. Cardiac arrhythmia and hepatorenal toxicity may occur with systemic absorption, therefore this peel must be performed with very slow application of

Table 1 Superficial chemical peeling agents

Jessner's solution
Glycolic acid 50–70%
Salicylic acid
Modified Unna's resorcinol paste
Trichloroacetic acid, 10–20%
Pyruvic acid 40–50%

Table 2 Medium-depth chemical peeling agents

Trichloroacetic acid 35–50%
Jessner's solution + TCA 35%
Glycolic acid 25–70% + TCA 35%
Salicylic acid + TCA 35%
Pyruvic acid 70%
Salicylic acid + Pyruvic acid 50–70%

Table 3 Baker–Gordon's phenol formula

Phenol USP 88%	3 mL
Distilled water	2 mL
Septisol soap	8 drops
Croton oil	3 drops

the solution in an operating theatre with the assistance of an anaesthetist to monitor eventual cardiac arrhythmia. Physical parameters that should discourage deep chemical peels are a history of aberrant wound healing evidenced by a paucity of adnexal structures or hypertrophic scarring and poor health.

An 88% concentration of phenol causes immediate coagulation of epidermal keratin and penetrates only to the level of the upper reticular dermis. However, when diluted to 45–55%, phenol becomes a keratolytic, disrupting sulphur bonds, with the capability of deeper penetration, to the mid-reticular dermis; therefore it is considered a deep peeling agent. In addition, phenol has bactericidal and bacteriostatic effects.

Peeling agents

Jessner's solution

This is used as a keratolytic peeling agent since its application in a triple-layer produces only stratum corneum separation with upper epidermal intraepithelial and intercellular oedema, but it does not affect the dermis (Table 4). JS is used mainly alone for the treatment of acne or dyschromic skin changes and in combination with 35% TCA for improving moderate photodamaged skin and actinic keratosis.

Table 4 Jessner's solution

Resorcinol	14 g
Salicylic acid	14 g
Lactic acid (85%)	14 g
Ethanol (95%)	100 cm^3

The solution is clear and sensitive to light and air; it must be stored in a dark container and can be kept for up to 2 years. It is faintly amber coloured, and becomes darker with time and exposure to light. This formulation avoids the syncopal and thyroid-depressing effects of resorcinol and the tinnitus of salicylism.

The JS peel rarely causes 'overpeel' and therefore is at low risk of complications. The principal disadvantages are the great variability in the manufacturing process and the fact that it causes an intense burning sensation during application and noteworthly exfoliation, that is sometimes unpleasant for the patient.

Salicylic acid

SA has recently been formulated in a hydroethanolic vehicle at concentrations between 20% and 30% for use as a superficial peeling agent. SA is a hydroxyl derivative of benzoic acid and represents a carboxylic acid attached to an aromatic alcohol, phenol. It is a lipophilic agent that produces desquamation and fast thinning of the upper, lipophilic layers of the stratum corneum and induces rapid turnover of the keratinocytes in the lower layers. Its effects are limited to the epidermis.

SA can be used as a single peeling agent on rough, oily skin with enlarged pores, comedonal and inflammatory acne, papular and pustular rosacea, early to moderate photoageing, postinflammatory hyperpigmentation and melasma. An important advantage of SA over other superficial peeling agents is that it is a safe and efficacious treatment for acne and dyschromias in subjects with skin types V and VI (Fitzpatrick's classification).

SA can also be used in combined peelings to achieve thinning of the epidermis that permits better penetration of other caustic agents, such as TCA or pyruvic acid (PA).

Resorcinol peeling

Currently the resorcinol formula most often used is modified Unna's paste (Table 5). Resorcinol (*m*-dihydroxybenzene) is structurally and chemically related to phenol. It is soluble in water, alcohol and ether, and acts as a potent reducing agent. Application of resorcinol induces a split at the granular cell layer, vasodilatation, increased mitosis of the basal cell layers, fibroblast proliferation and formation of a thickened dermal band. It has bactericidal and keratolytic properties.

This type of peel is quite easy to handle and has a low risk of side-effects (temporary hyperpigmentation and occasional contact allergy).

Resorcinol peeling is recommended especially for subjects with acne, including comedonic acne, and is successful in clearing pigmentary acneic outcome and very superficial scars. Melasma usually responds favourably.

Pyruvic acid ($CH_3-CO-COOH$)

This is an α-keto acid that converts physiologically to lactic acid, and its additional properties make it a particularly effective topical peeling agent. This very

Table 5 Modified Unna's paste

Resorcinol	40 g
Zinc oxide	10 g
Benzoinated axungia	28 g
Ceyssatite	20 g

potent acid can be used as a peeling agent, without risks of scarring, in concentrations between 40% and 70% in a well-balanced proportion between water and ethanol. The application of PA in the above-mentioned concentrations induces keratinocyte detachment with thinning of the upper layers of the epidermis. PA penetrates down to the upper papillary dermis and causes dermal–epidermal separation and increased production of collagen, elastic fibres and glycoproteins. In addition to its keratolytic and desmoplastic properties, PA has also demonstrated antimicrobial activity.

Thus, PA can be employed as a superficial–medium peeling agent in subjects with inflammatory acne, moderate acne scars, greasy skin, actinic keratosis and warts. We have also achieved good results in the treatment of photodamaged skin (fine wrinkles and localized superficial hyperpigmentations—colour mismatch).

Glycolic acid

GA, an α-hydroxy acid (AHA), at concentrations of 50–70% has been the most popular peeling agent over the past 10–15 years. We use solutions of 50–70% GA made with water or a combination of water, alcohol and propylene glycol. These solutions are clear, not sensitive to light and are highly stable (more than 2 years), but evaporate easily (the bottle must be kept tightly closed).

Application of high concentrations of GA reduce corneocyte cohesion (interacting with ionic bonds on the cellular surface) immediately above the granular layer and induce complete epidermolysis, epidermal and dermal thickening, reversal of basal cell atypia, dispersal of melanin, increased synthesis of glycosaminoglycans and collagen; it may also improve the quantity and quality of elastic fibres. Clinically these effects on the epidermis and dermis result in an improvement in skin surface irregularities, dyschromias, minor wrinkles and moderate acne.

An *in vivo* preliminary study by our group showed an increase of epidermal Langerhans' cells in three subjects treated for 1 month with GA (70% peeling once a week and daily home therapy with a 10% lotion). In the same subjects we also demonstrated an increase in the mRNA of transforming growth factor-β (TGF-β), a cytokine that is critically involved in dermal matrix remodelling.

Interestingly, all these effects occurred without any evident inflammatory outcome. In keeping with this, there is one report showing that GA has anti-inflammatory activity combined with antioxidant properties. This strengthens the hypothesis that the mechanism of action of the AHAs and related substances is a specific direct effect on the skin, one that goes beyond the irritating effect.

It is very important to note that the effect of a GA peel depends on the length of time it is left on the skin and, thus, the peel needs to be neutralized with water or sodium bicarbonate with perfect timing to prevent deeper dermal penetration that would lead to variable healing, crusting and even scarring.

Trichloroacetic acid

TCA can be used at different concentrations (10–20% for superficial peels, 30–50% for medium-depth peels), that lead to different peeling depths. In all cases the peeling is easy to control and predictable because it is neutralized by serum in superficial dermal blood vessels. This acid is non-toxic systemically. The solution is clear and transparent with no precipitates, is not sensitive to light and no refrigeration is necessary; it is stable for at least 2–3 weeks.

TCA causes necrosis and exfoliation of normal and actinically damaged cells and also precipitates epidermal proteins. Histological and ultrastructural studies have demonstrated that TCA peeling can renovate epidermal polarity, reducing epidermal intracytoplasmic bodies, increasing the number of fibroblasts and increasing the deposition of collagen type I. Generally these effects become visible after 1 month of treatment.

The main indications for TCA peeling are moderate photoageing with sun elastosis, slight wrinkles, superficial localized hyperpigmentations and actinic keratoses.

Clinical uses of chemical peels

The first step in treating a subject with a chemical peel is to determine any possible contraindications for peeling. For instance, a subject with recurrent herpetic lesions on the face may need either to avoid medium and deep chemical peels or require preprocedural oral antiviral therapy (aciclovir). Prior to a superficial peel we do not administer prophylaxis for herpes simplex unless the patient has had herpetic lesions within 2 weeks prior to the chemical peel procedure. Other contraindications (Table 6) include oral therapy with retinoids that may alter post-peel healing (it is best, in our experience, to wait at least 6 months after cessation of the oral retinoid before medium and deep peelings).

As stated above there are many indications for chemical peels (Table 7). Each case requires a specific treatment depending on the severity of the disorder and the charac-

Table 6 Relative contraindications for chemical peels

Fitzpatrick skin type IV–VI
High degree of photoageing
Daily sun exposure
Past history of superficial X-ray treatment
Present or recent use of oral retinoids
Recent cosmetic surgery
Big smokers
Use of anticoagulants (warfarin)
Chemotherapy
HIV infection
History of recurrent herpes simplex
Hypertrophic scar or keloid formers
Unrealistic expectations

Table 7 Major indications for chemical peels

Facial skin rejuvenation
Dyschromias: melasma, postinflammatory hyperpigmentations, lentigo
Acne and acne scars
Greasy skin

teristics of the individual subject. Thus, each treatment must be personalized. However, we can propose general guidelines for the major disorders that can be treated with chemical peels.

Postpeel care is similar for all types of chemical peels; in particular all subjects must avoid sun exposure for at least 1 month after superficial peels and 6 months after medium-depth peels, use sunscreens and apply facial moisturisers daily. After superficial peels subjects can return to social life immediately, using cosmetic camouflage if necessary. For medium and deep peels a 7–10-day stay at home is necessary and the subject must follow a very careful postpeel care procedure (described below).

Facial rejuvenation

The wrinkles, textural alterations, diffuse dyschromia, yellowing and mottling characteristics of photodamaged skin can be significantly improved with chemical peels. Superficial peels are recommended for subjects with early photoageing, or those who do not want to experience the temporary discomfort following medium and deep peel treatments.

Before performing any kind of chemical facial peel it is advisable to treat the subjects for at least 2 weeks with topical tretinoin (0.025%), topical bleaching agents (4% hydrochinone, azelaic acid) and 1% hydrocortisone to decrease the risk of postinflammatory hyperpigmentation and promote wound healing. Subjects should also apply AHA creams (8–15% GA) or PA creams for long periods (remembering to interrupt the application for at least 1 week after each chemical peeling); this reduces the thickness of the stratum corneum and helps maintain the effect of the peeling.

Peeling with 70% GA is recommended for only mildly photodamaged skin with fine wrinkles. To improve fine wrinkles effectively, the peeling is done in a series of 4–6 repeated treatments, once every 3–4 weeks. Before each peeling the skin must be degreased with alcohol or acetone in order to remove surface debris, oils and portions of the stratum corneum to allow uniform penetration of the peeling agent. The acid can be applied with a special brush, cotton bud or gauze. Once the acid has been applied to the whole face (starting from the forehead and then spreading to the cheeks, chin, upper lip and nose), it is necessary to wait to see if erythema or 'frosting' occurs. Frosting may occur with GA peeling as a spotted pattern indicating epidermolysis, consisting in detachment of the epidermis from the papillary dermis. Generally, the aim of GA peeling is a slight exfoliation (without side-effects) to make the skin smoother. The occurance of 'frosting' presents no additional benefit, but rather discomfort for the individual with increased risk of postinflammatory hyperpigmentation and scarring. Therefore, the acid must be neutralized immediately if frosting appears. The length of time of the application varies extremely from one subject to another in an unpredictable manner. It is advisable to observe subjects carefully during applications to build expertise based on personal experience. There is a great difference in manufacturing methods for products from different companies and it is not advisable to use products you have not tested personally before performing a peeling.

The acid must be neutralized with water or sodium bicarbonate to prevent deep dermal penetration, 'overpeel'. Following the peeling, no cream containing AHA should be applied for 1 week; if the patient does not show signs of irritation, erythema or abrasion no specific postpeel care is necessary. In cases of significant erythema, topical non-halogenated steroids should be prescribed. If overpeel with abrasions occurs application of an antibiotic ointment is recommended for at least 1 week.

Peeling with PA is suggested for subjects with mild to moderate photoageing with numerous dyschromias and rough skin with dilated pores. If the skin appears particularly thickened a peeling with SA should be performed 1 week before beginning the series of PA peels in order to induce thinning of the epidermis that permits deeper, more uniform penetration of PA.

Before the application of SA the skin is degreased with alcohol or acetone. The peel solution is applied with a brush or a cotton-tipped applicator starting from the forehead and progressing down to the cheeks, chin, upper lip, nose and eyelids. Subjects experience a stinging and burning sensation that increases progressively and then decreases rapidly when the peeling agent is neutralized with water. A small fan will help the subjects tolerate this discomfort better. The hydroethanolic vehicle volatilizes, leaving a white precipitate of SA on the skin surface (Fig. 1). SA does not need to be neutralized, but a splash of water on the skin stops the burning sensation and the SA precipitate is removed very easily. If the SA is applied in multiple layers and left on the skin for a longer time (> 3 min) the skin turns greyish, meaning that frosting has occurred. Frosting is not required in this type of peel.

PA is applied after degreasing the skin with alcohol. Since PA causes very intense burning, we suggest applying it to small areas (forehead, one cheek at a time, chin, nose and upper lip) and neutralizing each area with sodium bicarbonate before progressing to the next one. It is best to apply PA with a gauze and scrub gently and continuously for about 1 min (Fig. 2). When PA vapours are inhaled they are pungent and irritating to the upper respiratory mucosa so a small fan should be used during the procedure. To achieve a satisfactory result, 4–6 peelings are required, to be done once every 3–4 weeks. Subjects will experience tightening of the skin and desquamation, and only rarely abrasions for a few days immediately after the peeling. Therefore, it is necessary to prescribe a moisturising cream that should be applied daily.

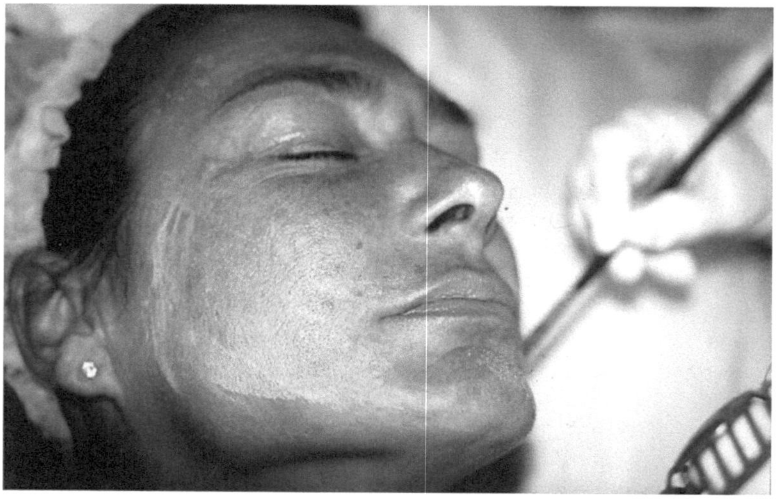

Figure 1 White precipitate of salicylic acid on the skin surface.

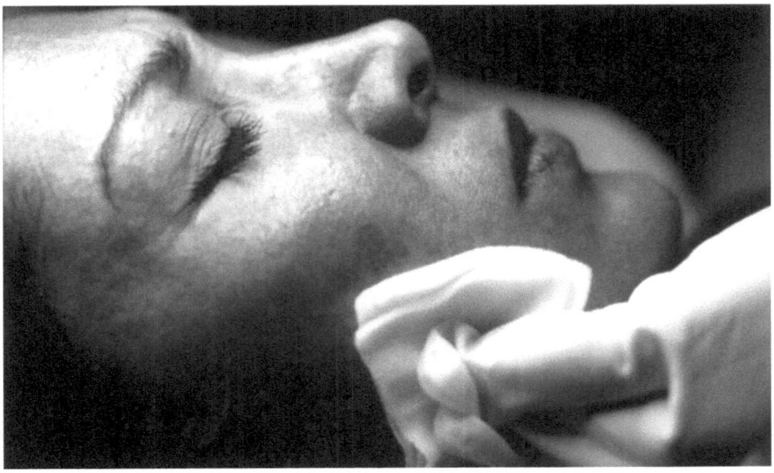

Figure 2 Application of pyruvic acid with a gauze on a small area of the face.

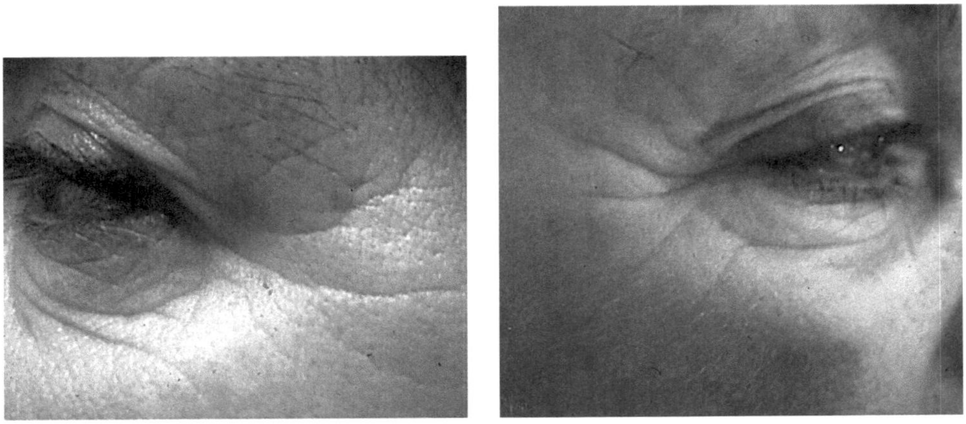

(a) (b)

Figure 3 (a) Moderate wrinkles of the periorbital area before treatment. (b) The same patient after 4 peelings with salicylic acid.

Some authors also suggest the use of multiple SA peels, at 4-week intervals, for the treatment of moderate photoageing (Fig. 3). This procedure presents several advantages over the other superficial chemical peels. Firstly the main benefit of SA compared to GA is its predictability. It is easy to achieve uniform application and there is no worry about timing or overpeeling: also, the peel causes superficial anaesthesia (burning ceases rapidly). This type of peeling causes significantly more desquamation than GA.

In cases of more advanced photoageing, with skin laxity and diffuse dyschromias peelings with 35% TCA alone or preceded by the application of JS or 70% GA are recommended.

The face is cleaned with a gauze pad soaked with acetone, alcohol or chlorhexidine gluconate until the sebaceous oils have been thoroughly removed. The eyes are protected with sterile ophthalmic ointment, gauze pads and hypoallergenic tape or goggles. Oral or intramuscular anxiolytics may be used. Local anaesthesia is not required.

A cotton-tipped applicator is moistened with TCA and rolled against the wall of the glass cup to remove excess fluid. The TCA is applied to the skin area to be treated by firmly rubbing the moistened applicator in a circular or linear fashion and the substance is allowed to penetrate for a few seconds, after which a further application is made, sometimes followed by a third application. Usually application is started from the forehead and progresses to the cheeks, chin, upper lip and nose. Once the skin has been treated, it slowly changes colour, becoming whitish-grey as a result of chemical coagulation of the epidermis (frosting). The frost appears more rapidly with high concentrations of TCA and may not appear with low concentrations, especially if the skin has not been adequately degreased. After the acid is applied, a dry gauze pad is used to blot (not wipe) excess TCA. Neutralization, as used for GA, is not necessary.

TCA stings when applied, and the severity depends on the concentration. The pain crescendos, normally peaking approximately halfway through the procedure. A hand-held fan may be helpful to soothe discomfort.

Often, anatomical facial subunits require different concentrations of TCA, i.e. forehead, cheeks, chin—40%; jaw line, perioral area—30%; periorbital regions—18%. TCA should not be passed directly over the eyes. When eyelids are treated, particular care must be used to avoid seepage of TCA onto the sclera.

Immediate postoperative care consists of application of an antibiotic ointment, sometimes followed by a hydrogel dressing. Subjects must be warned to expect various skin changes, such as: (a) itching; (b) transitory marked hyperpigmentation, possibly associated with oedema; and (c) exfoliation, that is never regularly distributed all over the treated areas but generally starts at the periorbital and perioral areas and ends at the forehead. It is very important not to remove the skin in this phase, to avoid postinflammatory hyperpigmentation.

Generally, during the days that follow the peeling subjects must avoid use of soaps and detergents, apply antibiotic creams or ointments twice a day and use total sun-block; direct sun exposure must be avoided for at least 4–5 months. In some cases the skin maintains a pinkish colour for 2–3 weeks following exfoliation. A non-halogenated corticosteroid cream or zinc oxide paste may accelerate the return to normal skin colour.

The final result of TCA peels can be appreciated 3–4 weeks after the treatment. The skin will appear tightened, with a general improvement in skin texture, rhytidosis will be much less evident and the skin colour will be more homogeneous.

For skin rejuvenation it is also possible to use two caustic agents to increase the depth of the peeling while reducing the side-effects. 70% GA–35% TCA and JS–35% TCA are the combined peelings most often performed.

70% GA is uniformly applied to the cutaneous surface (as formerly described) and then neutralized. Then, 35% TCA is applied on the same areas.

JS is applied evenly to the skin, after appropriate degreasing, with either cotton-tipped applicators or a 2×2 cm gauze, to achieve a light but even frosting. The frosting achieved with JS is much lighter than that with TCA and produces less discomfort to the patient. A mild erythema appears with a faint tinge of frost evenly all over the face. JS does not need to be neutralized. At this point the 35% TCA is applied evenly with a cotton-tipped applicator, and the acid is left on the skin for a few moments until a white frost appears. The peel is then neutralized with water. Combined peels usually require a longer time for the procedure, approximately 20 min, and this is sometimes unpleasant for the subjects being treated.

The effects of the these combined peels is comparable to that of 50% TCA, but with lower risk of complications, especially less risk of scarring.

Dyschromias

Melasma, postinflammatory hyperpigmentation and photo-induced dyschromia can be improved with PA, modified Unna's paste or 35% TCA peels. We find that 35% TCA gives the best results in dyschromia due to photoageing, while PA and resorcinol peels are more effective in cases of melasma and postinflammatory hyperpigmentation. However, chemical peels alone are not adequate in such cases. Simultaneous treatment with bleaching agents (4% hydrochinone, azelaic acid, kojic acid) and life-long use of sun-blocks is a must for these individuals.

Acne and acne scars

There are various peeling options for the treatment of greasy skin and acne.

Greasy skin is characterized by skin thickening and increased sebaceous secretion, giving the face a shiny appearance, especially on the nose and forehead. Superficial chemical peels with SA or PA can significantly improve this unpleasant situation. The same results are obtained with these two kinds of peelings, although SA peels require fewer applications. In particular, two peeling sessions with a 3-week interval are adequate with SA, while at least 3 sessions are necessary with PA.

The peeling procedures and postpeel care are the same as for facial rejuvenation.

Very satisfying results are also obtained using SA and PA in acne patients. These two peeling agents can be used in comedonal, inflammatory and nodular acne, and papular and pustular rosacea, because of their keratolytic and bactericidal properties. Repeated treatments, 1 peeling every 2–3 weeks for a total of 6–8 treatments, are necessary to achieve clinically significant benefits (Fig. 4).

Also 70% GA and JS have been reported to be efficient for the treatment of facial acne, but in our experience the best

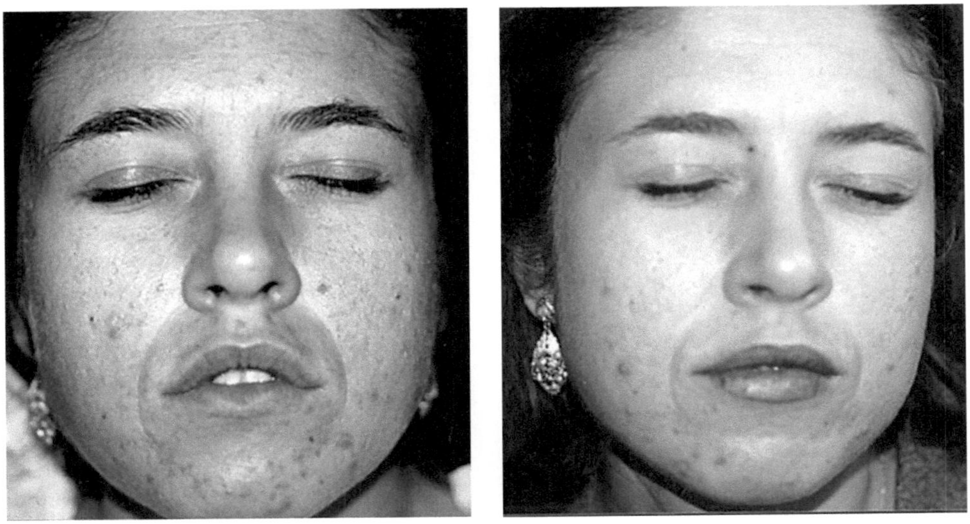

(a) (b)

Figure 4 (a) Inflammatory acne before treatment. (b) The same patient after 5 treatments with pyruvic acid.

results, with minimal discomfort for the subject and lowest risk of complications, are achieved with SA and PA peels. GA and JS should not be used in cases of inflammatory acne.

Moreover, modified Unna's paste is recommended in cases of comedonic acne and in clearing pigmentary acneic outcomes and very superficial acne scars. This paste is applied with a spatula to the area to be treated and left on for 1–2 h (Fig. 5). The postapplication reaction resembles that of a first-degree burn with further exfoliation of dark brown skin that generally lasts for 7–10 days. Postpeel care includes a 1-week home stay for cosmetological reasons, and the use of antibiotic and moisturising creams for 10 days, and total sunblock for at least 2 months. It is advisable to pretreat the patients (as for skin rejuvenation) with topical 0.025% tretinoin, topical bleaching agents (4% hydrochinone, azelaic acid) and 1% hydrocortisone.

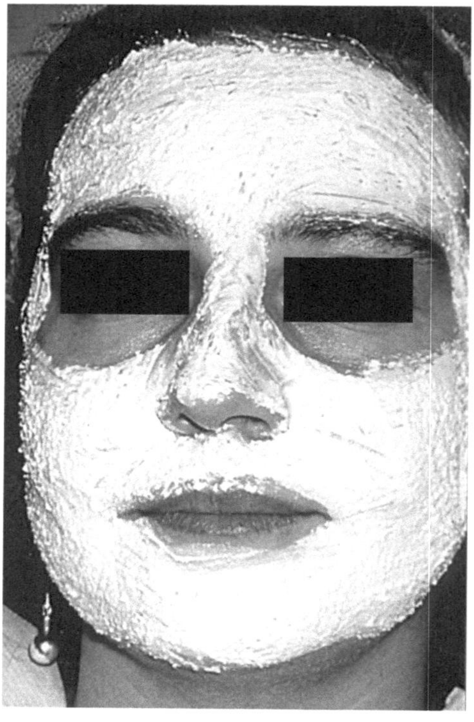

Figure 5 Unna's paste applied to the face and left on for 1 h.

In cases of acne scars, only moderate (partial) results are obtained with chemical peels; laser resurfacing is usually recommended. However, some good results can be obtained with 35–50% TCA peels or combined peels (GA–TCA or JS–TCA) (Figs 6 and 7).

Complications

Obviously, the deeper the peeling the higher the risk of complications. The most frequent complications are listed in Table 8. Most of the complications listed occur after phenol peeling; hyperpigmentation is the only true complication that occurs after superficial or medium-depth peel.

There is an evident difference in colour with clear boundary lines between the exfoliated and the non-treated areas. Generally this is temporary, and uniform skin colour will be observed within 1–2 months.

The most feared complication following chemical peels is hyperpigmentation. This is often due to even minimal sun exposure, but may occur without such exposure, especially in dark-skinned subjects (Fitzpatrick IV–V). Hyperpigmentation can be treated with bleaching agents, generally with good results. It sometimes disappears spontaneously after some months. It is more difficult to treat a hypopigmentary outcome caused by destruction of melanocytes. This may be a permanent side-effect, and it usually occurs with deep peelings (50% TCA or phenol).

Infections associated with peeling are very rare, but the frequency of this complication increases with the depth of the peeling and is more pronounced in case of formation of crusts allowing bacterial colonization. The most common pathogens are *Streptococcus* and *Staphylococcus* species. A small percentage of patients manifest *Streptococcus* and *Staphylococcus*

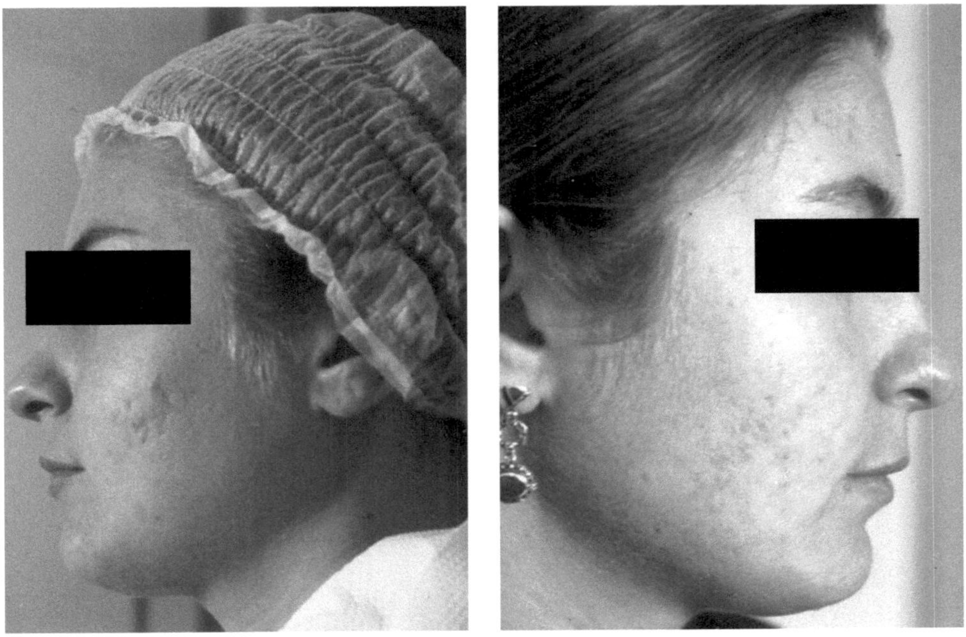

(a) (b)

Figure 6 (a) Acne scars. (b) Same patient after peeling with 35% TCA.

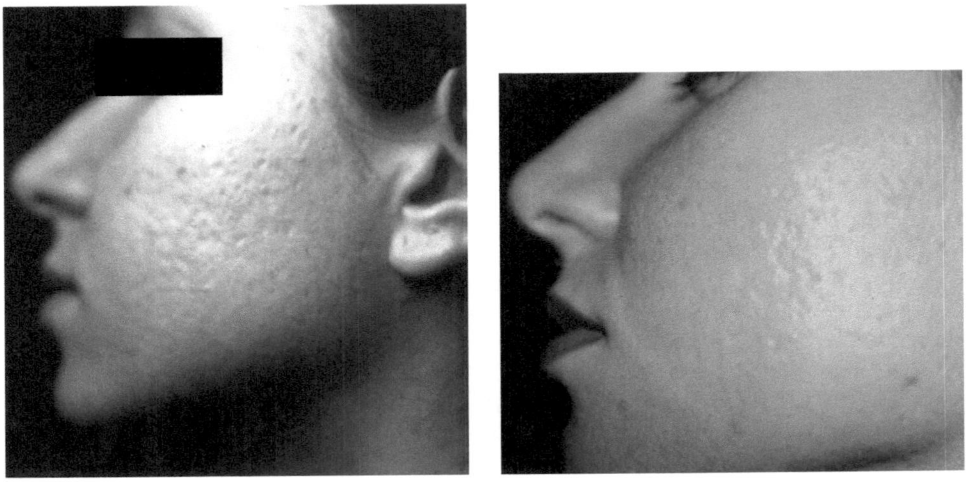

(a) (b)

Figure 7 (a) Acne scars. (b) Same patient after peeling with 35% TCA.

Table 8 Complications of chemical peels

Pigmentary changes	Hyperpigmentation Hypopigmentation Depigmentation (porcelain) Mixed combination pigmentation Lines of demarcation Naevi accentuation
Scarring	Atrophic Hypertrophic Keloidal
Infections	Streptococcal or staphylococcal folliculitis (acne-like eruptions) *Pseudomonas* infections Toxic shock syndrome Herpes simplex Epstein–Barr virus keratitis
Prolonged erythema or pruritus	
Textural changes	Uneven texture Enlarged pores
Atrophy	
Milia	
Cold sensitivity or cold urticaria	
Cardiac arrhythmias	
Laryngeal oedema	
Poor physician/patient relationship	
Allergic reactions	

infections as folliculitis or acne-like eruptions. Infections due to *Pseudomonas* are very rare. A herpes simplex infection may be reactivated by any peeling agent (superficial, medium and deep). Suitable local and/or systemic therapy with antibiotics or antiviral drugs provides quick relief and if well timed can prevent scar formation.

Allergic reactions are generally very rare, and most occur after resorcinol peels. An allergic reaction is often difficult to diagnose since the symptoms may be similar to alterations induced by the peeling itself (erythema and oedema). Identification and therapy of this complication is mandatory, since it drastically increases the likelihood of side-effects such as hyperpigmentation and scarring.

Persisting erythema lasting for 2–3 weeks is considered a normal event, especially after medium and deep peels. Erythema persisting more than 3 weeks may indicate hypertrophic scar formation.

Scarring is certainly the most dreadful complication. The risks of scars are greater in subjects who undergo deep peelings or overpeel with superficial and medium peels, those with a past history of hypertrophic scarring or keloid formation, and those who have recently undergone systemic treatment with isotretinoin, or in cases of postpeel infection or allergic reaction.

Different scarring reactions are possible, including flat, hypopigmented, depressed atrophic areas; thickened, elevated areas; and keloids. The treatment differs according to the type of scar and involves the use of intralesional steroids, silastic plasters, laser therapy, cryotherapy, and even excision and surgical revision of the scar in the most extreme cases.

Written informed consent to chemical peeling

Each individual to be treated by a cosmetic procedure that involves a risk of complications should provide signed written, informed consent. It is appropriate to give the subject written information on

The undersigned ____________________ herewith gives formal consent to the chemical peeling treatment at ____ .
The treatment has been explained to me and I have had the opportunity to ask questions. This procedure will cause a modification in the treated area of my face/ body which may be unpleasant. My face will become red and successively pigmented as if sunburnt. Exfoliation will then start and last about 10 days. An erythema may persist for 15–20 days. I have been informed that there is a minimum risk of side effects, such as hyperpigmentation and scarring (very rare). I agree that photographs of my treated area may be taken.

Date ________________

Patient's signature (or patient's parents if < 18 years old)

Figure 8 Shows a draft form of written informed consent.

side-effects and complications, discomfort and temporary skin changes that may or may not occur.

Figure 8 shows a draft form of written informed consent.

Conclusion

Chemical peeling is an efficacious and safe approach to the treatment of some cutaneous problems of an aesthetic nature. To avoid any undesired side-effects it should be performed by a specialist, and according to a standardized procedure, when possible.

Apart from the well-known chemical exfoliating effect, the stimulatory activity of some of the chemical peeling agents (GA and TCA) on fibroblasts has been described in numerous studies. For this reason, the use of these substances in photoageing can be recommended, and there is also a possibility that they can be used in other skin lesions. Further investigation of the exact molecular mechanism inducing fibroblast activation and subsequent collagen synthesis is definitely needed. Several studies document the benefit of combining chemical peeling with topical tretinoin, but comparative studies on the use of topical tretinoin and chemical peeling, mostly with GA, have not yielded fully satisfactory results to date. In any case the most successful chemical peeling agent seems to be TCA that can be used for superficial, medium and deep peelings. Depth of penetration is easily noted when frosting occurs; neutralization is not needed; and there is no systemic toxicity. The combined use of two substances to peel the skin has recently proved successful. Proper degreasing, use of GA or JS, and 35% TCA are steps that usually make peeling very effective. The amount of each agent applied governs the intensity and thus the efficacy of the peel. The variables can be adjusted according to the individual skin type and the area of the body being treated. Familiarity with the technique of single or, better, combination peeling, especially in subjects with moderate/severe signs of photodamage, is a prerequisite for expert use of this safe and inexpensive tool for effective chemical resurfacing of the skin.

Further reading

Brody HJ. Histology and classification. In: Brody HJ. *Chemical Peeling and Resurfacing*, 2nd edn. St. Louis: Mosby, 1997: 7–28.

Brody HJ. Histology and classification. In: Brody HJ. *Chemical Peeling and Resurfacing*, 2nd edn. St. Louis: Mosby, 1997: 73–108.

Ditre CM, Griffin TD, Murphy GF *et al.* Effects of α-hydroxy acids on photoaged skin: a pilot clinical, histologic, and ultrastructural study. *J Am Acad Dermatol* 1996; 34: 187–95.

Ghersetich I, Comacchi C, Teofoli P, Lotti T. Modificazioni delle cellule di Langerhans epidermiche (CD1a+) e del TGF-β nella cute foto-esposta di soggetti trattati con acido gli colico. *Abstract of the Giornate di Terapia in Dermatovenereologia*, Catania, Italy, 25–26 January 1997: 176.

Ghersetich I, Lotti T. Incremento delle cellule di Langerhans (CD1a+) nell'epidermide dopo trattamento con acido gli colico. *Current* 1995; 5: 30–3.

Ghersetich I, Teofoli P, Gantcheva M, Ribuffo M, Puddu P. Chemical peeling: how, when, why? *J Eur Acad Dermatol Venereol* 1997; 8: 1–11.

Grimes PE. The safety and efficacy of salicylic acid chemical peels in darker racial-ethnic groups. *Dermatol Surg* 1999; 25 (1): 18–22.

Halasz CL. Treatment of warts with topical pyruvic acid: with and without added 5-fluoruracil. *Cutis* 1998; 62 (6): 283–5.

Katsambas A. Chemical peeling: an overview. *Proceedings of the 19th World Congress of Dermatology*, 1997: 687–90.

Kim SW, Moon SE, Kim JA, Eun HE. Glycolic acid versus Jessner's solution: which is better for facial acne patients? *Dermatol Surg* 1999; 25 (4): 270–3.

Kligman D, Kligman AM. Salicylic acid as a peeling for the treatment of acne. *Cosmetic Dermatol* 1997; 10 (9): 44–7.

Kligman D, Kligman AM. Salicylic acid peels for the treatment of photoaging. *Dermatol Surg* 1998; 24: 325–8.

Letessier SM. Chemical peeling with resorcin. In: Roenigk RK, Roenigk HH, eds. *Dermatologic Surgery: Principles and Practice*. New York: Dekker, 1989: 1017–24.

LoVerme WE. Toxic shock syndrome after chemical face peel. *Plast Reconstr Surg* 1987; 80: 115–18.

Matarasso SL, Brody HJ. Deep chemical peeling. *Sem Cutaneous Med Surg* 1996; 15 (3): 155–61.

Monheit GD. The Jessner's–TCA peel: an enhanced medium-depth chemical peel. *Facial Plastic Surg Clin N Am* 1994; 2 (1): 21–7.

Moy LS, Peace S, Moy RL. Comparison of the effect of various chemical peeling agents in a mini pig model. *Dermatol Surg* 1996; 22: 429–32.

Otley CC, Roenigk RK. Medium-depth chemical peeling. *Sem Cutaneous Med Surg* 1996; 15 (3): 145–54.

Tse Y, Ostad A, Lee HS *et al.* A clinical and histologic evaluation of two medium-depth peels. *Dermatol Surg* 1996; 22: 781–6.

Cryosurgery

L. Marini

Human cells work better within a well-defined range of temperatures. Cellular malfunction and death are caused by increasing or decreasing microenvironmental temperatures beyond certain thresholds. Cryosurgery is a versatile surgical procedure which uses controlled freezing to produce local cellular destruction. Healing of any ensuing defects occurs by second intention.

Many terms have been used to identify this procedure, e.g. cryocautery, cryocoagulation, cryotherapy and cryogenic surgery. It is a widely used procedure, particularly common among dermatologists and dermatology surgeons. In recent reports, cryosurgery was the second most common in-office procedure after skin excision.

Cryosurgery has been used by dermatologists since the turn of the last century. After the development of the vacuum flask to store sub-zero liquid elements like nitrogen, oxygen and hydrogen, the number of cases treated with cryosurgery increased dramatically. Many different techniques have been proposed to deliver freezing temperatures to living tissue: cotton applicators, closed-system units with spraying capabilities and metal probes, all producing consistent therapeutic results in selective benign and malignant skin alterations.

By 1990, 87% of dermatologists worldwide were practising cryosurgical procedures in their practice. This incredible success is due to the relative ease of use, low cost and well-accepted cosmetic results.

History and principles

Cooling can be more appropriately described as withdrawal of heat from volumes of various size, filled with molecules at certain temperature. A so-called 'heat sink' is formed at the site of cryogen contact. One of the most important factors influencing the rate of heat removal is the proximity of the heat sink to the target surface. Slow cooling is not as harmful to living tissue as rapid cooling. Brain and heart surgery take good advantage of ultra-slow cooling of tissues to decrease overall cellular metabolism. Different cells organized in tissues belonging to different organisms show variable degrees of response to cold exposures.

Some viruses can survive for years at −196°C while non-melanocytic skin cells generally do not survive temperatures between −30 and −40°C. Before the era of scientific 'objectivity', many contributions to the knowledge of the effects of cold on living tissues were made by clinical observations reported by prominent physicians. John Hunter of London stated, in 1777, that living tissue exposed to cold temperatures developed necrotic changes, vascular stasis and excellent cosmetic second intention healing.

Knowledge of cryosurgery has progressively improved by measuring the effects of cold produced by natural sources, refrigerants colder than ice and clinical research on the effects of extreme cold on normal and diseased skin.

The anti-inflammatory and analgesic effects of natural cold were well known among the Egyptians and the Greeks. James Arnott of London, said to be the father of 'modern cryosurgery', described the effects on living tissue of temperatures as low as −24°C, achieved by adding salt solutions to crushed ice.

The birth of modern cryogenics goes back to 1877 with the work of a French scientist, Cailletet, and a Swiss engineer, Pictet. They described the possibility of liquefying small quantities of oxygen and carbon monoxide by expansion of gases from extremely high temperatures and by means of mechanical refrigeration cascade, employing sulphur dioxide and carbon dioxide boiled under reduced pressures. Wroblewski and Olszenski were able to convert oxygen and nitrogen into their liquid phases in a Polish laboratory in 1883.

Commercial production of liquid air from which liquid nitrogen could be extracted was started by von Linde in the last years of the 20th century. An English scientist, James Dewar developed a vacuum flask to store sub-zero fluids.

The term 'cryogenics' was coined by the Dutch physicist Kamerlingh Omnes, who liquified helium in 1908. The first medical use of liquid air is attributed to A. Campbell White in 1899. White was trained in dermatology and reported successful clinical results using cotton-tipped applicators to deliver liquid air to selected skin conditions like warts, naevi and premalignant skin alterations. In 1907, Whitehouse, a dermatologist practising in New York, invented a method to spray the active refrigerant directly onto the skin. He reported consistent clinical results on many patients affected by non-melanoma skin cancers. Another dermatologist practising in Chicago, William Pusey, promoted the use of carbon dioxide snow for the same skin conditions.

In the 1920s, liquid oxygen became commercially available but achieved only limited use in the treatment of skin diseses because of safety considerations. Carbonic acid (carbon dioxide snow) gained some popularity among the European dermatologists who used it in various forms until 1945. A mixture of carbonic acid and acetone, known as carbon dioxide 'slush', has been used to treat acne and postacneic scars.

After the availability of liquid nitrogen in 1945, the real 'modern' era of cryosurgery began. Liquid nitrogen was preferred to liquid oxygen because it did not support combustion. In 1950 Allington first described the cotton swab technique to treat warts, keratoses, leucoplakia, haemangiomas and keloids. The limitations of liquid nitrogen soaked cotton applicators were described in a report by Grimmett in 1961. He microscopically studied the levels of cryonecrosis reached by this technique several days after freezing. In the 1960s, Zacarian and Adham tried to achieve greater cryonecrotic depths through the use of solid copper cylinder disks dipped into liquid nitrogen prior to putting them in contact with the skin.

The introduction of automated cryosurgical systems by Cooper and Lee in 1961 began the era of modern cryosurgery. Cooper, a very active neurosurgeon, studied extensively the effects of cryosurgery on central nervous structures producing a large amont of literature which contributed to further diffusion of this technique to other specialties. Two American dermatologists, Douglas Torre and Setrag Zacarian further contributed to modern cryosurgery by developing an apparatus specifically designed for dermatological uses. Torre worked closely with George Garamy, an engineer at Union Carbide Company based in Connecticut, while Zacarian developed his liquid nitrogen spray unit with the help of Michael Bryne of Brymill Company based also in Connecticut.

Various pressurized spray units were then developed making cryosurgery progressively more popular among dermatologists and other specialist alike. Andrew Gage, a general surgeon, reported in 1965 on the efficacy of cryosurgery in oral cancers and on the treatment of inoperable rectal cancers. Contact cooling started to be effectively used in ophthalmology, gynaecology and oral surgery, but hand-held open spray devices were, and still remain, the most widely used units among dermatologists.

How cryosurgery works

The mechanism by which freezing temperatures destroy living cells is based on the fast transfer of heat from target tissues to the heat sink produced by selected cryosurgical instruments. The rate of heat transfer, and therefore the clinical efficacy of the cryosurgical procedure, is dependent on the temperature difference between the target tissue and the heat sink (Table 1).

When the spray technique is used, liquid nitrogen is directly applied upon the skin and evaporation (boiling heat transfer) occurs. This specific effect produces a very rapid heat transfer from the target tissue to the surface in direct contact with the boiling liquid nitrogen and the freeze progresses to a greater depth.

The cryoprobe technique produces a slower heat transfer through a conduction mechanism from the target tissue to the metal (usually copper) probe.

Every time we produce a heat-sink effect on living tissue a cryolesion of a well-defined volume and shape will be generated. Within depths equal or less than 6 mm the shape of the cryolesion is rounded, i.e. the lateral spread of the freezing front is approximately equal to its deeper edge. Beyond these depths the shape of the cryolesion becomes more triangular.

Keeping the peripheral borders of the cryolesion induced by the heat-sink constant for 30 s has been shown to produce a negative temperature variation of −40° at the periphery of a freezing circle of 2 cm in diameter; while −50° has been recorded 5 mm below the treated surface.

Table 1 Heat sink temperatures produced on tissues by various refrigerants

Refrigerant	Temperature (°C)
Ice	0°
Salt-ice	−20°
CO_2 snow	−79°
CO_2 slush	−20°
Nitrous oxide	−75°
Liquid nitrogen	−20° (Q-tip applicator); −196° (spray-probe)

Different cell lines show different thermal responses to freezing. Melanocytes are very sensitive to cold temperatures, much more than keratinocytes. The first are usually destroyed by temperatures reaching −5°, while keratinocytes require −50° for 'optimal' destruction. This different susceptibility to low temperatures explains the hypopigmentation usually noted after cryosurgical procedures on darker-skinned individuals.

Cell injury occurs during the postfreezing thaw time. Due to the hyperosmotic intracellular conditions, ice crystals do not form until −5 to −10°C are reached. The transformation of water into ice crystals, concentrates the extracellular solutes, resulting in an osmotic gradient across cell membranes causing further damage. Extracellular ice damages cell membranes. This phenomenon is particularly effective in densely packed cells in solid neoplasms. Intracellular ice also forms in many cells, especially after prolonged freezing, possibly producing irreversible damage to mitochondria and endoplasmic reticulum. Slow thawing is associated with recrystallization of ice thus producing much more destructive changes than rapid thawing. Exposure to cold has been known to induce capillary vasoconstriction followed by vasodilatation. Microthrombi have been observed to be fixed on the endothelium of affected vessels at temperatures of −15° and below. The resulting final effect is ischaemic necrosis directly dependent upon the depth of freeze and its lateral spread. Capillaries and venules are more easily occluded by the cooling achieved during cryosurgical procedures, producing 'venous gangrene'. Major arteries are extremely rarely blocked by this level of freezing. Vascular damage is more pronounced after rapid freeze and slow thaw and refreeze.

Technology has provided two main monitoring methods to assess the depth of freezing fronts during cryosurgical procedures: thermocouple/pyrometer systems and impedance/resistance systems. These instruments are useful in monitoring the freezing effect during oncological procedures.

Equipment and techniques

Liquid nitrogen has been preferred to other common refrigerants because of its lower boiling point, ease of use and relative safety. Other freezing sources, such as freon, carbon dioxide and nitrous oxide do exist but are not as efficient in destroying skin lesions due to their higher boiling point.

Liquid nitrogen is usually stored in vacuum containers of different capacities which are able to hold it for a certain number of days proportional to their volumes. Various treatment methods have been devised to treat skin lesions with cryosurgery. These include the spray freeze technique, the contact probe technique and the applicator technique.

Thick, hyperkeratotic lesions should be pared down to increase the efficiency of cryosurgery avoiding the formation of unnecessary large ice-balls. Keratin is an excellent insulator and might prevent subzero temperatures reaching the base of the target.

The spray equipment has become increasingly popular among dermatologists because of its very good cost-efficiency ratio, its versatility in effectively treating almost all skin lesions and its ease of use. The most common units found in office practice are relatively small metal or plastic vacuum flasks with a screw-on top with a spray release trigger and a valve providing a working pressure of 6 p.s.i. and a safety relief pressure of 70 p.s.i. (Fig. 1) Various spray attachments can be fitted on the delivery outlet. Benign lesions will usually require the horizontal freezing front to spread an average distance of 2 mm beyond their visible margins. Premalignant and malignant lesions will require a safety freezing belt of approximately 1 cm. In practice, the cryosurgeon may use the spot-freeze technique, the

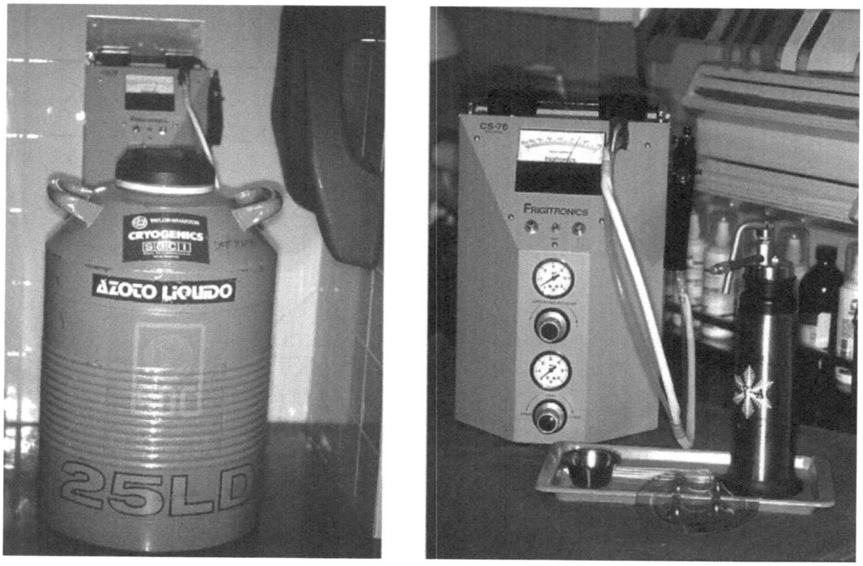

Figure 1 Common liquid nitrogen delivery systems used for in-office dermatological cryosurgery procedures.

paint-spray technique and the spiral technique to reach the freezing parameters necessary for treatment. Regardless of the spray technique selected, once the desired peripheral limits of the freezing front have been reached, this should be maintained for an adequate length of time (5–30 s, depending on the pathology of the lesion). Pulsing each spray avoids overexpansion of the freezing front and prevents complications. The nozzle tip of the spray gun is usually held 1 cm from the surface to be treated and liquid nitrogen is sprayed until a suitable ice-ball is formed. Some operators palpate the lesions to physically determine the size reached by the ice-ball interrupting the freezing. This process is repeated until an ice-ball of the requisite size is created. Once the ice-ball is produced the operator starts to count the freezing time previously planned to treat the lesion successfully. Due to the high chances of hypopigmentation after cryosurgery, lightly freezing the skin at the periphery of the ice-ball surface will prevent abrupt demarcation lines giving better cosmetic results.

Variations of the spray technique involve the use of various accessories which limit the involuntary 'scattering' of liquid nitrogen onto non-affected skin at the periphery of the lesions being treated. Neoprene or plastic cones of varying diameters allow liquid nitrogen to be concentrated on the contact surface, providing a more rapid freezing than that produced by the standard 'open' spray technique. The use of disposable speculas instead of non-disposable cone attachments offers several advantages. They can be cut with scissors to vary the size and shape of the aperture to match the shape and dimensions of the lesion to be treated. With the advent of human immunodeficiency virus (HIV) and other important communicable diseases, the use of disposable devices will minimize the chances of contamination. Open cylinders of different diameters have been used to 'recycle' liquid nitrogen droplets produced by scatter during spraying, further decreasing the freezing time of targets (Fig. 2).

The probe technique allows cryosurgeons to freeze target tissue through direct contact of metal probes of different diameters within which liquid nitrogen circulates in a closed system. Copper is usually chosen because of its high thermal conductivity. Probes vary from 1 mm up to several millimetres in diameter and are selected according to the clinical dimensions of the lesions being treated (Fig. 3). In practice, the probes must be perfectly dried before starting the freezing procedure to obtain adequate skin contact. A small quantity of lubricant jelly or petrolatum is applied to the skin. Once started, the probe will firmly adhere to the skin in 5–6 s. It will then gently retract towards the operator, thus surrounding tissue is protected from unnecessary thermal damage and subsequent inflammatory changes. Freezing will continue for a suitable amount of time (10–60 s) according to the diameter and the pathology of the lesions. Once finished, the probe cannot be removed immediately. This will usually be possible after 10–30 s, once the thawing process is sufficiently advanced.

The applicator technique is the simplest and easiest method of applying liquid nitrogen to the skin. The cryosurgeon will dip the cotton extremity of the applicator directly into a sterile metal container previously filled with liquid nitrogen. Containers should be changed and residual liquid nitrogen discarded when treating different patients to avoid cross-contamination with freeze-resistant viruses like HIV, the human papillomavirus family, the herpes virus family and the hepatitis virus family. This method is not easy to reproduce due to the many variables involved: the pressure applied onto tissue by the operator, the environmental temperature where the procedure takes

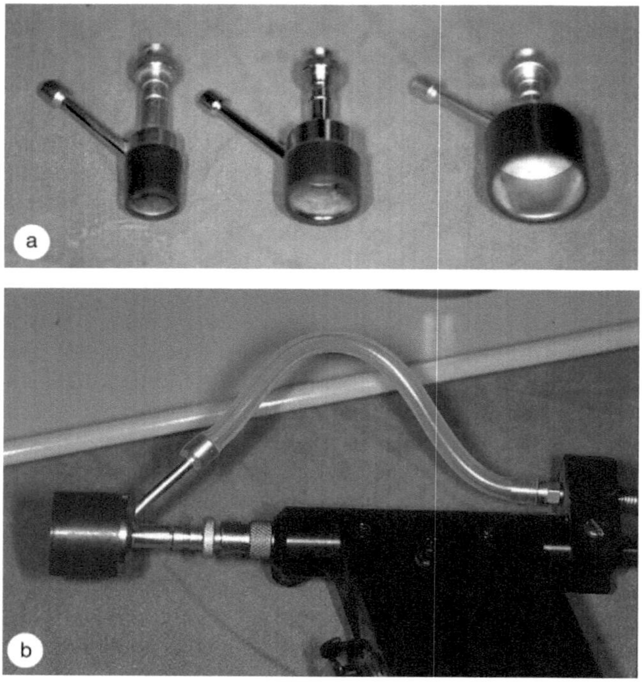

Figure 2 (a) Open-end liquid nitrogen recycling cylinders of different diameters; (b) and one open-end cylinder accessory mounted on a cryogun.

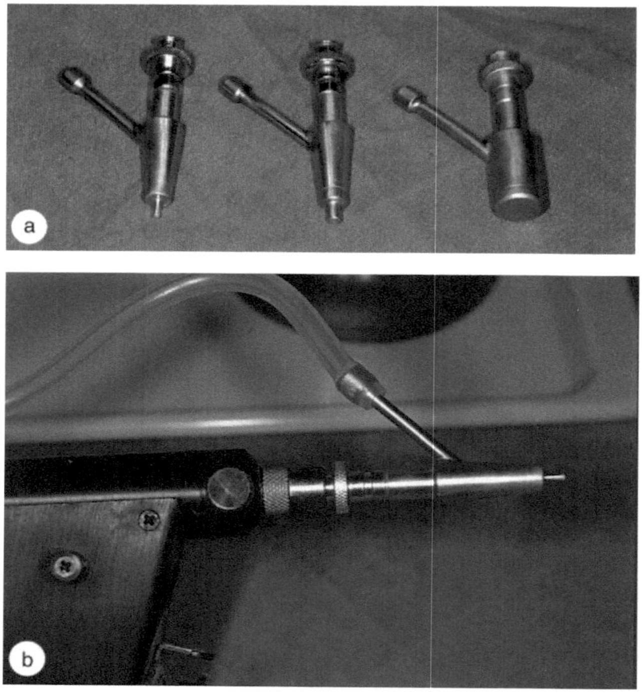

Figure 3 (a) Closed liquid nitrogen freezing copper probes with different contact diameters; (b) one cryoprobe mounted on a cryogun.

place and the time elapsed between the withdrawal of the Q-tip from the liquid nitrogen container and its actual contact with the target. This method is usually good only for small, superficial benign lesions.

Clinical applications

Various lesions have been successfully treated with cryosurgery. In cases of suspected malignant lesions to obtain complete destruction of the target lesion, preoperative clinical diagnosis, supported by dermatopathology, is crucial in selecting the proper freeze–thaw cycles to be used. For most of these lesions, cryosurgery is not the only, and often not the best, modality of treatment. It does, however, represent a valuable therapeutic alternative in selected patients. Furthermore, cryosurgery represents the standard first-line therapy for simple, benign lesions such as actinic keratoses, warts and seborrhoeic keratoses.

Benign lesions

A wide variety of benign lesions are amenable to treatment by cryosurgy (Table 2). For most high cure rates and low morbidity can be expected. Hyperkeratotic lesions must be surgically debulked prior to freezing and viral warts should be chemically treated with topical keratolitic agents (usually salicylic acid) before and in between cryosurgical sessions. If lesions are on the fingers, all rings must be removed before any cryosurgical procedure because of the swelling produced by the postoperative inflammatory process.

Table 2 Benign lesions for which cryosurgery might be indicated

Lesion	Cryosurgical technique	Average number of sessions
Acne—cysts	Probe or open spray	2–3
Acne—comedones	Open spray—peel	1
Acne—scars	Open spray—peel	1
Acne keloidalis	Probe	2–3
Adenoma sebaceum	Probe	2–3
Angiokeratoma	Probe or open spray	2–3
Angiolymphoid hyperplasia	Open spray	1
Capillary cherry angioma	Probe	1
Chondrodermatitis nodularis helicis	Open spray	3–4
Cutaneous horn	Open spray	1
Dermatofibroma	Probe	2–3
Epidermal naevus	Open spray or probe	2–3
Granuloma annulare	Open spray or probe	2–3
Granuloma faciale	Open spray or probe	2–3
Haemangioma	Probe	3–5
Keloid	Open spray or probe	2–3
Lentigines	Open spray	1
Lentigo simplex	Open spray or probe	1
Lymphangioma	Open spray or probe	2–3
Melasma	Open spray	1
Milia	Probe	1
Molluscum contagiosum	Probe or open spray	1
Mucocoele (lip)	Probe	1
Myxoid cyst	Open spray or probe	1
Pyogenic granuloma	Open spray or probe	1
Seborrhoeic keratosis	Open spray or probe	1
Skin tags	Open spray	1
Venous lakes	Probe	2–3
Warts (human papillomavirus)	Open spray	1–4
Xanthoma	Open spray or probe	1–2

Malignant lesions

Both intraepidermal and extraepidermal cutaneous malignancies of selected origin can be successfully treated with proper cryosurgical techniques. Cure rates are inversely proportional to tumour depth. Patient selection is extremely important since cryosurgery does not represent the first-line treatment in this group of skin lesions. When other, more effective and less morbidic procedures cannot be selected, cryosurgery can offer some advantages.

Elderly patients in poor general health can be treated with cryosurgery since the procedure is purely 'local' and does not involve aggressive and invasive surgical procedures. Fair-skinned types (Fitzpatrick phototype I–II) is very forgiving since hypopigmented scars are less noticeable. Patients on anticoagulant therapy or those allergic to local anaesthetic can be safely treated with cryosurgery. Recurrent lesions on previously irradiated sites might also be treated with cryosurgery.

There are some other obvious general advantages which might influence the surgeon to select the cryosurgical approach:

- it is a low-risk outpatient procedure
- it is performed without the need of general anaesthesia
- it is a relatively rapid procedure (which does, however, require strict aseptic technique)
- it allows multiple tumours to be treated during a single session
- its associated complications are relatively mild and rare
- cosmetic results are usually well accepted by patients
- cure rates are high in selected neoplasms.

When treating malignant skin neoplasms in their extraepidermal growth phase, adequate equipment and proper technique must be selected if cryosurgery is to be chosen (Tables 3 and 4). As with other treatment modalities, the aim when dealing with skin cancers, is the complete elimination or destruction of the lesion, ideally at the first treatment session. To achieve adequate depth of necrosis cryosurgeons should perform a double 30-s freeze–thaw cycle spaced by a minimum of 5-min thaw period between each freeze. Lesions not properly suitable for a cryosurgical approach include: tumours larger than 2 cm in diameter, recurrent lesions, tumours situated on critical anatomical regions for which a high rate of recurrence has been reported, lesions situated on the lower legs (extremely prolonged healing times after cryosurgery) and cancers with particularly aggressive histological behaviour (morphea-like or metatypical basal cell carcinoma).

Table 3 Intraepidermal growth phase malignant lesions for which cryosurgery might be indicated

Lesion	Technique	Average number of sessions
Actinic cheilitis	Open spray	1
Bowen's disease (skin, genital)	Open spray	1–2
Keratoacanthoma	Open spray	2–3
Leucoplakia	Open spray	1–2

Table 4 Extraepidermal growth phase malignant lesions for which cryosurgery might be indicated

Lesion	Technique	Average number of sessions
BCC	Open spray or probe	1
SCC	Open spray	1
Kaposi's sarcoma	Open spray	1

BCC, basal cell carcinoma; SCC, squamous cell carcinoma.

Complications, side-effects and contraindications

As with any procedure, complications and side-effects can occur. These can be divided into acute, delayed, prolonged–

Table 5 The most common complications and side-effects after cryosurgery

Category of complication or side-effect	Complications and side-effects
Acute	Pain
	Headache (after freezing lesion on scalp, temple, forehead)
	Insufflation of subcutaneous tissue (extremely rare)
	Haemorrhage
	Oedema
	Syncope
	Blister formation
Delayed	Postoperative infection
	Fever
	Haemorrhage
	Exuberant formation of granulation tissue
Prolonged–temporary	Hyperpigmentation
	Altered sensory nerve function
	Milia
	Hypertrophic scars
	Acral bone thermal necrosis
Prolonged–permanent	Hypopigmentation
	Alopecia
	Keloid scars
	Textural changes—skin atrophy
	Ectropion
	Skin depressions over cartilageneous structures

temporary and prolonged–permanent (Table 5). Patients should be properly informed before starting a cryosurgical procedure in order to obtain a valid informed consent to the treatment.

There are many concurrent diseases that may be considered as relative contraindications for a cryosurgical procedure (Table 6). These should be sought in every patients for which cryosurgery has been proposed as a treatment modality.

Conclusion

Cryosurgery is a safe and easy procedure that can be successfully used to destroy many benign and malignant lesions. Even if newer and more sophisticated techniques are available, which can effectively treat the same range of lesions, a good dermatology surgeon should not forget the therapeutic possibilities offered by the 'old classics'.

Cryosurgery is unique since it survived many alternative innovations and is still considered a valid option in a wide range of selected cases. It is a pity that modern training programmes and courses focus almost exclusively on current, very expensive, high-tech procedures. As experienced cryosurgeons like Stephen Chiarello prove, cryosurgery can be a very good alternative to full-face oncological laser resurfacing and can still compete effectively with more expensive laser units, producing almost similar clinical results in the treatment of solar lentigines, as reported in a recently published paper written by researchers at the University of Utah, Salt Lake City.

Table 6 Relative contraindications to be considerd before performing cryosurgery

Agammaglobulinaemia
Blood dyscrasias of unknown origin
Cold intolerance
Cold urticaria
Cryoglobulinaemia
History of pyoderma gangrenosum
Raynaud's disease

Further reading

Arnott J. *On the Treatment of Cancer by the Regulated Application of an Anesthetic Temperature*. London: Churchill, 1851.

Chiarello SE. Cryopeeling (extensive cryosurgery) for treatment of actinic keratoses: An update and comparison. *Dermatol Surg* 2000; 26 (8), 728–32.

Cooper IS, Lee A. Cryostatic congelation: a system for producing a limited controlled region of cooling or freezing of biologic tissues. *J Nerv Ment Dis* 1961; 133: 259–63.

Dawber R, Colver G, Jackson A. *Cutaneous Cryosurgery.* London: Martin Dunitz, 1997.

Gage AA. What temperature is lethal for cells? *J Dermatol Surg Oncol* 1979; 5: 459–64.

Gage AA. History of cryosurgery. *Semin Surg Oncol* 1998; 14: 99–109.

Gage AA, Koepf D, Wehrle D *et al.* Cryotherapy for cancer of the lip and oral cavity. *Cancer* 1965; 18: 1646–51.

Graham GF, Clark LC. Statistical analysis in cryosurgery of skin cancer. In: Breitbart EW, Dachow-Siwiec E eds. *Clinics in Dermatology: Advances in Cryosurgery.* New York: Elsevier, 1990: 191–7.

Kuflik EG. Monitoring treatment with tissue temperature measurement. *J Dermatol Surg Oncol* 1986; 12: 925–6.

Kuflik EG. Treatment of basal cell carcinoma with the open-spray technique. *J Dermatol Surg Oncol*1986; 12: 125–6.

Kuflik EG. Cryosurgery updated. *J Am Acad Dermatol* 1994; 31: 925–44.

Kuflik GK, Gage AA, Lubritz RR, Graham GF. History of dermatologic cryosurgery. *Dermatol Surg* 2000; 26 (8): 715–22.

Kuwahara RT, Craig SR, Amonette RA. Forceps and cotton applicator method of freezing benign lesions. *Dermatol Surg* 2001; 27 (2): 183–4.

Pusey W. The use of carbon dioxide snow in the treatment of nevi and other lesions of the skin. *J Am Med Assoc* 1907; 49: 1354–6.

Todd MM, Rallis TM, Gerwels JW, Hata TR. A comparison of 3 lasers and liquid nitrogen in the treatment of solar lentigines: a randomized, controlled, comparative trial. *Arch Dermatol* 2000; 136 (7): 841–6.

Torre D, Lubritz RR, Kuflik EG. *Practical Cutaneous Cryosurgery.* Norwalk: Appleton & Lange, 1988.

White AC. Liquid air: its applications in medicine and surgery. *Med Record* 1899; 56: 109–12.

Whitehouse H. Liquid air in dermatology: its indications and limitations. *J Am Med Assoc* 1907; 49: 371–7.

Zacarian SA. Cryosurgery of skin cancer and cryogenic techniques in dermatology. Springfield: C.C. Thomas, 1969: 71.

Curettage

E. Haneke

The curette is a useful instrument to remove superficial lesions, but it is too coarse an instrument for almost all diagnostic biopsies. It leaves tissue debris that no longer allows the architecture of a lesion to be evaluated. The tissue is less seriously damaged when a so-called sharp ring-scalpel is used. This allows strips of tissue to be cut from the surface of the skin producing longitudinal superficial tissue specimens. However, margin control is usually impossible. Fibrotic lesions are not an indication for curettage, but the curette is useful to shell out soft tumour masses from fibrotic stroma.

The technique of using a curette is crucial for a good result. The skin to both sides of the lesion is stretched between the thumb and the longer fingers of the non-dominant hand and the curette pressed tangentially on the skin about a millimetre from the lesion's margin. In mollusca contagiosa, the curette is quickly moved towards the little nodule, which is then snipped off the skin leaving a small depressed wound, which rapidly heals by epithelialization from the margins.

Seborrhoeic and actinic keratoses are also removed by stretching the lesion tensely. While pressing it to the skin surface the curette scrapes the lesion off in strips of tissue. Completely even capillary bleeding must be achieved, and no pigmented areas must remain.

Superficial basal cell carcinoma may be curetted but using a small curette is recommended because it penetrates better into the small depressions caused by the tumour cell nests sitting under the surface of the epidermis.

Bowen's disease is not a good candidate for curettage because it often extends into the follicles and these follicular extensions cannot be completely removed with the curette.

Paget's disease and *in situ* as well as superficial melanomas must not be curetted.

Curettage is also often used as an adjunct to other treatment modalities. In nodular basal cell carcinoma, the soft epithelial tumour portion can be removed by shelling it out from its capsule-like surrounding connective tissue and the resulting wound is then further treated with 40% zinc chloride solution or by electrocoagulation. The latter procedure is often referred to as curettage and electrodesiccation.

Curettage is also used to remove the outermost layers of keratotic debris and crusts of superficial basal cell carcinoma, actinic keratoses or Bowen's disease before applying 5-aminolaevulinic acid for photodynamic treatment.

Some dermatologists curette the nail matrix before applying liquefied phenol for the treatment of ingrown toenails.

The resulting defect after curettage is left for secondary intention healing. Using a haemostyptic solution or electrocautery to stop the bleeding etches or burns the biopsy wound, which prolongs the healing time and often causes a whitish scar. We therefore recommend applying a thick padded dressing able to absorb the blood. Plenty of ointment avoids its sticking to the wound. This dressing is removed after 24–48 h after which only an antibiotic ointment is used, usually several times a day in order to prevent the scab from drying out. Healing is twice to three times faster with moist wound healing.

Further reading

Haneke E. *Developments and Techniques in General Cutaneous Surgery.* In: Dahl MV, Lynch PJ, eds. *Current Opinion in Dermatology,* Vol. 2. Philadelphia: Current Science 1995: 129–36.

Haneke E. Exzisions-Biopsieverfahren. *Z Hautkr* 1988; 63 (Suppl.): 17–19.

Electrosurgery

E. Haneke

Electrosurgery comprises:

- hot electrocautery
- electrofulguration
- electrodesiccation
- electrocoagulation
- electrosection
- electrical epilation
- radiofrequency resurfacing.

The more modern, radio wave surgery allows cutting to be done almost without thermal damage. Electrosurgery is the destruction or removal of tissue using electrical energy and provides a rapid, cost-effective treatment for many skin lesions. There are now many different electrosurgical machines available worldwide. The modern devices generate several different electrical outputs each for specific use. Radiosurgery using a device with megahertz current competes with the carbon dioxide laser.

Terminology in electrosurgery is often incorrectly used. Monopolar means that the electrode has only one point whereas bipolar means that two tips are used to coagulate tissue in between. Monoterminal refers to the use of only one electrode, biterminal when two connections or electrodes, usually an active surgical and an indifferent ground plate electrode, are used.

The indications for electrosurgery are summarized in Table 1.

Electrocautery

Metal is heated by electric current from a battery or an outlet-dependent device. The tip of the unit consists of a wire with high electrical resistance. When the current is turned on the wire starts glowing. It is then gently held on to the anaesthetized lesion to be destroyed. Since the heat does not penetrate deeper than the papillary dermis, this method is best used for very superficial lesions or small pedunculated lesions, such as flat seborrhoeic keratoses or small acrochordons. When the glowing tip of the instrument touches the lesion, this starts bubbling until it becomes dry and carbonizes. A crust forms that is shed after a few days.

Since no electrical current flows through the patient this method can be used in patients with pacemakers. It is also useful for achieving haemostasis in a 'bloody field'. Its chief disadvantage is that larger lesions cannot be treated, in particular large tumours cannot be removed, and the treated lesion is destroyed so that histopathological examination is not possible.

Electrofulguration

An electrical spark is used to treat small superficial lesions resulting in carbonization of the skin surface.

Electrodesiccation

A high-voltage, low-amperage damped current from a spark gap unit is used in a monoterminal fashion for electrodesiccation. If the electrode is held at a slight distance from the tissue a spark is created causing very superficial destruction (electrofulguration) whereas direct tissue contact of the electrode is used for electrodesiccation. These techniques are suited for the treatment of very superficial lesions such as seborrhoeic and actinic keratoses, plane warts, acrochordons and xanthelasmas, and they also provide haemostasis for small capillary bleeding after curettage.

This technique requires local anaesthesia except for small skin tags. Alcoholic skin cleansers prior to electrosurgery must not be used because they may ignite with electrosurgery. Postoperative care includes a sterile dressing. Delayed bleeding may occur.

Table 1 Indications for electrosurgery

Electrodesiccation	Electrocoagulation	Electrosection
Molluscum contagiosum	Acrochordons	Condyloma acuminatum
Flat warts	Telangiectasia	Hidradenitis suppurativa/ Pyodermia fistulans sinifica
Epidermal naevi	Spider naevi	Rhinophyma
Flat seborrhoeic keratoses	Sun-burst veins	Incisions in skin and plastic surgery
Dermatosis papulosa nigra	Venous lake	
Sebaceous hyperplasia	Pyogenic granuloma	
Syringoma	Granulation tissue	
Xanthelasma	Bleeding vessels in surgery	
After curettage of basal cell carcinoma	Oozing lymph vessels in surgery	
	Hypertrichosis, hirsutism	
	Actinic keratosis	
	Nodular BCC	

Electrodesiccation is often used in conjunction with curettage for the treatment of basal cell carcinomas (BCC). This approach, often designated as curettage and electrodesiccation (C & D), has a high cure rate for small nodular BCCs but cannot be recommended for larger tumours.

Electrocoagulation

This technique uses moderately damped, partially rectified current with active concentrating and dispersing neutral electrodes. The voltage is lower and the amperage is higher than in electrodesiccation. It penetrates deeper thus causing more tissue destruction.

Indications for electrocoagulation are deep tissue destruction and surgical haemostatis.

- Tissue destruction: a ball electrode is directly applied to, and slowly moved over, the lesion. The charred tissue is removed with a gauze pad or a curette. This procedure is repeated until the lesion is completely destroyed. Usually three passes are necessary for malignant tumours.
- Haemostasis: the electrode may directly touch the bleeder vessel or the vessel may be grasped with a fine pincer or clamped with a haemostat which are touched with the electrode. The power of the instrument should be set as low as possible in order to achieve coagulation of several millimetres which reduces the risk of delayed bleeding. Bipolar electrocoagulation with special forceps is used for less traumatizing pinpoint haemostasis. However, it requires a dry operative field.

Electrocoagulation is the most effective means for treating spider naevi. A needle electrode is lightly held on and the nurse then slowly turns on the power. The needle sinks into the tissue gently coagulating the feeding vessel. No scarring is observed when using this technique cautiously.

Electrosection

Cutting is performed using slightly damped, fully rectified current in a biterminal fashion. High amperage and low voltage are further characteristics. Cutting and haemostasis are obtained by tissue vaporization. Lateral heat spread is low reducing peripheral tissue damage. The higher the power the easier is the cutting and the less is the coagulation, and vice versa.

The narrow electrode passes effortlessly through the tissue leaving an almost dry cut surface. If the electrode drags, the power setting is too low. If it sparks, it is too high. For incision, a needle or blade electrode may be used. A thin loop electrode is optimal for removing tissue slices such as in rhinophyma, of pedunculated or protruding lesions such as condylomata acuminata, or to excise small tumours with one stroke. We also use loop electrodes for removal of tissue in pyodermia fistulans sinifica (hidradenitis suppurativa), keloidal acne and other deep-seated infectious diseases not amenable to conservative therapy.

Radiowave electrosurgery uses higher frequency of 1.2 MHz. In the cut mode, fully filtered current is used. There is minimal heat generation, therefore (almost) no coagulation, and specimens thus excised can be submitted for histopathological control of margins. In fact, lateral tissue damage is even less than with the continuous wave surgical CO_2 laser. The instrument can also be set to fully rectified current for cutting and coagulating, and to partially rectified current for coagulation. This device is optimal for surgery of the face and for creating skin flaps.

Electroepilation

Removal of unwanted hair by electrical current is usually performed by cosmeticians. Two different techniques are available:

- electrolysis
- thermolysis.

Electrolysis uses direct current to induce a chemical reaction at the hair bulb. The anode is inserted into the follicle and the patient holds the cathode as a moist pad. When being switched on, the current produces an electrochemical reaction generating sodium hydroxide which is caustic. The procedure takes 30–60 s for each follicle to be destroyed.

Thermolysis is a much faster procedure causing heat destruction of the hair root. In the slower technique, lower heat is generated for 3–20 s. In the flash technique high temperatures are delivered for less than 1 s.

A combination of both methods ('blend') was developed to speed up treatment and increase efficacy.

For all techniques, a very fine needle is inserted into the follicle down to the hair bulb. The needle tip is rounded in order to avoid puncturing through the follicle wall, and its length is insulated (Kromayer needle) in order to avoid damage to the superficial follicular portion with the risk of scarring.

Side-effects are rare. Electrolysis is less painful and has probably a higher success rate when carried out by an experienced therapist. Post-treatment pigmentary disturbance depends on skin type.

Devices for home self-use are not effective. Hair shafts are not conductive for electrical current, therefore holding a hair with tweezers and applying electrical current cannot permanently destroy the hair root.

Radiofrequency resurfacing

The removal of superficial skin layers including skin resurfacing is a new electrosurgical technique. Whereas carbon dioxide laser resurfacing works by thermal damage this is replaced by a much cooler and more controlled ablation (hence the term 'coblation'). A fine layer of an electrically conductive solution, usually physiological saline, is sprayed on the skin. The hand-held bipolar electrode-tipped wand is set on this layer on the target. When the current is switched on the saline between the electrodes is converted into an ionized vapour layer, called plasma. Ions accelerate across this gradient toward the skin dissociating molecular bonds within tissue structures thus removing tissue layers and ultimately causing collagen neosynthesis and improved skin appearance. The process runs at only 80–90°C as compared to 300–600°C with the CO_2 laser. Heat damage to the surrounding tissue is considerably lower suggesting that the risk of persistent erythema and scarring is lower and wound healing is considerably faster.

Risks of electrosurgery

Preoperative discussion includes information about the procedure, healing time of at least 2 weeks for small wounds, scab formation and scarring. Preoperative evaluation discusses bleeding disorders, hepatitis, human immunodeficiency virus, immune defects, individual scarring, pacemaker and prosthesis.

There are some risks inherent in electrosurgery such as ignition of inflammable gases and fluids; therefore, preoperative preparation requires non-alcoholic disinfectants. Electrosurgical electrodes are not self-sterilizing and spread of infection is possible if they are not properly sterilized. Furthermore, the plume generated by the heat may contain intact virus particles and effective smoke evacuation is therefore mandatory. However, no case of transmission to the surgeon has been described. Smoke evacuation is also recommended for extensive procedures such as hidradenitis surgery. Postoperative management is disputed. We have seen that drying up the wound is easier for the patient but takes longer to heal than occlusive or semi-occlusive treatment.

Delayed postoperative bleeding is due to incomplete coagulation of vessels. Postoperative pain may be intense. Some reddening around the wound is frequently observed. Eschar formation and sloughing of necrotic tissue are obligatory. Electrosurgery carries the risk of delayed wound healing and hypertrophic scarring. They are dependent on the amount of tissue coagulation. Hyperpigmentation in dark-skinned and hypopigmentation in fair-skinned people is common. Electrosurgery is thought by many to be contraindicated on the soles of the feet. Improper contact with the ground plate electrode may cause burns. However, we have seen acute allergic contact dermatitis from the epoxy resin adhesive of the ground plate which was misinterpreted as a burn. Patients with sensitive electrical facilities such as demand-dependent pacemakers or implantable cardioverterdefibrillators are at risk. There may be interference with cardiac monitoring devices.

Further reading

Burns RL, Carruthers A, Langtry JA, Trotter MJ. Electrosurgical skin resurfacing: a new bipolar instrument. *Dermatol Surg* 1999; 25: 582–6.

Colver GB, Peutherer JR. Herpes simplex virus dispersal by Hyfrecator electrodes. *Br J Dermatol* 1987; 117: 627–9.

Hettinger DF. Soft tissue surgery using radiowave technique. *J Am Pediatr Med Ass* 1997; 87: 131–5.

Palmer SE, McGill LD. Thermal injury by *in vitro* incision of equine skin with electrosurgery, radiosurgery, and a carbon dioxide laser. *Vet Surg* 1992; 21: 348–50.

Pollack SV, Grekin RC. Electrosurgery and electroepilation. In: Roenigk RK, Roenigk HH Jr, eds. *Dermatologic Surgery. Principles and Practice*. New York: Dekker, 1989: 187–203.

Riordan AT, Gamache C, Fosko SW. Electrosurgery and cardiac devices. *J Am Acad Dermatol* 1997; 37: 250–5.

Sebben JE. The hazards of electrosurgery. *J Am Acad Dermatol* 1987; 16: 869–72.

Spencer JM, Tannenbaum A, Solan L, Amonette RA. Does inflammation contribute to the eradication of basal cell carcinoma following curettage and electrodesiccation? *Dermatol Surg* 1997; 23: 625–31.

Tope WD. Multi-electrode radio frequency resurfacing of human skin. *Dermatol Surg* 1999; 25: 348–52.

Wagner RF, Tomich JM, Grande DJ. Electrolysis and thermolysis for permanent hair removal. *J Am Acad Dermatol* 1985; 12: 441–9.

Epiluminescence microscopy of pigmented skin lesions

V. De Giorgi and P. Carli

Epiluminescence microscopy (ELM), also known as *in vivo* cutaneous surface microscopy, incident light microscopy, magnified oil immersion diascopy, dermatoscopy and dermoscopy, is an *in vivo*, non-invasive technique that has disclosed a new dimension of the clinical morphological features of pigmented skin lesions using incident light magnification systems with immersion oil at the skin–microscope interface.

The purpose of this method is to obtain the visualization of numerous morphological features, not visible with the naked eye, that enhance the clinical diagnosis of nearly all pigmented skin lesions.

These morphological features seen by ELM examination have specific, rather well-defined histopathological correlates. By knowing the histopathological equivalent of such structures, the investigators are able to understand the dermoscopic features better and also to increase the *in vivo* diagnostic accuracy of benign vs. malignant pigmented skin lesions.

Technique

ELM is performed by a surface microscope using incident light delivered from an acute angle and oil immersion. By covering the lesion with immersion oil together with a glass slide applied with a slight pressure, the surface reflection due to the different refractive index mismatch between air and skin is eliminated. This makes the stratum corneum translucent, enabling *in vivo* visualization of pigmented anatomical structures of the epidermis and, even beyond that, of the dermal–epidermal junction and superficial papillary dermis invisible with the naked eye.

Depending on the localization of the melanin pigment within the skin, different colours can be observed with ELM. Melanin pigment localized in the horny layers of the epidermis appears black; pigmentation of lower epidermal layers appears light to dark brown depending on its concentration. Pigment localized in the papillary dermis appears grey, whereas pigmentation of the reticular dermis is steel blue.

ELM can be performed with binocular stereomicroscopes, which provide a magnification range from 6× to 80×. These instruments can be equipped with additional optical systems for simultaneous viewing by a second investigator and a camera mounted on a side arm for instant photography. The stereomicroscopes permit high and variable magnification, a three-dimensional appearance of the lesion and the simultaneous viewing by a second investigator. Disadvantages are size, weight and costs of the instrument, space requirements and the long time needed for the examination.

ELM can also be performed with a hand-held microscope equipped with an achromatic lens that allows a fixed magnification of 10×; an incident light at an acute angle of 20° is delivered from a built-in light source powered by a battery in the shaft of the body. This relatively inexpensive equipment is adequate for use in daily clinical practice.

Modern advanced systems are presently based on advanced computer technology enabling image data to be processed (acquisition, storage and retrieval). These digital ELM camera systems are a powerful technology that can improve clinical visualization and facilitate a more detailed study of the subtle epidermal and superficial dermal pathology of pigmented lesions.

Digital ELM camera systems are now available in order to acquire, process, print and review clinical and ELM images thus facilitating the follow-up of doubtful pigmented skin lesions.

ELM criteria

The structures seen by ELM examination are very heterogeneous and can confuse an inexperienced investigator. Therefore, it has been necessary to define the terminology for these dermoscopic features—also called ELM criteria. Moreover, the diagnostic significance of these ELM criteria has been elaborated.

ELM criteria are defined by purely descriptive terms and have been correlated with the underlying histopathological substrates. For each criterion, additional descriptors are used to specify the architectural distribution thus contributing to the final diagnosis. For example, pigmented network represents a subtle network of brownish lines over a diffuse background tan, whose anatomical basis is melanin pigment in the epidermal basal cells.

The holes of the network correspond to the tips of the dermal papillae whereby the lines of the network result from the projection of the pigmented rete ridges to the skin surface. According to the size and configuration of the rete ridges—differently associated with the benign or malignant nature of the lesion—the pigment network can be regular or irregular (depending on the size and shape of the meshes of the network), narrow or wide (depending on the thickness of the lines), delicate or prominent (depending on the intensity of pigmentation), or well- or ill-defined at the margin of the lesion (depending on the cut-off at the borderlines). In evaluating these descriptors as well as the ELM features described below, the observer is able to recognize the nature—benign or malignant—of the given lesion. Major ELM criteria together with their histopathological correlates are summarized in Table 1.

In spite of many efforts in this direction, it remains difficult to define precisely the dermoscopic terminology. In fact, investigators are still using different names even for morphologically identical criteria.

Diagnosis of pigmented skin lesions

ELM pattern analysis

Austrian research groups introduced in 1987 a systematic analysis of these new morphological features that become apparent with ELM. They proposed a model of qualitative pattern analysis based on ELM criteria, in order to distinguish the different types of cutaneous pigmented lesions. So, the 'standard ELM pattern analysis' is based on the qualitative assessment of numerous individual ELM criteria recognized within a given pigmented skin lesion.

The features analysed in this diagnostic model include specific patterns, colours and intensities of pigmentation, as well as the configuration, regularity and other characteristics of both the margin and the surface of pigmented skin lesions. According to this, a dermoscopic diagnosis of a pigmented skin lesion must be based always on a critical, simultaneous evaluation of all available criteria.

According to Pehamberger, the assessment of ELM criteria is based on the following rules:

1 The presence of a criterion is more important than its absence. Because the frequency of each criterion in melanomas is far from 100%, it is inappropriate to reason that a given pigmented lesion is not considered to be a melanoma just because those criteria considered the most specific for melanoma diagnosis, i.e. pseudopods, radial streaming or grey–blue areas, are absent.

Table 1 ELM criteria and histological correlates for pigmented skin lesions

ELM criterion	Definition	Histological correlates
Pigment network	Network of brownish lines over a background tan	Pigmented rete ridges
Diffuse pigmentation (blotches)	Pigmentation that precludes recognition of other criteria	Melanin at all levels of the epidermis and/or the dermis
Brown globules	Round, oval or spherical bodies	Nests of pigmented melanocytes at the dermal–epidermal junction and/or in the papillary dermis; or clusters of melanophages in the papillary dermis
Black dots	Small, punctate and black structures	Focal collections of melanin in the stratum corneum
Radial streaming	Linear, brown to black streaks radiating from the border of the lesions	Radially arranged pigmented nests
Pseudopods	Bulbous, often kinked projections, directly connected to the body of the lesion or to the pigmented network	Radially arranged pigmented nests
Whitish veil	Whitish film overlying a more darkly pigmented area	Compact orthokeratosis and hypergranulosis
Grey–blue areas	Circumscribed zones that have a grey and/or blue hue	Fibrosis and pigmented melanophages or melanocytes in a thickened papillary or reticular dermis
White areas	Depigmented areas that appear as dead white or light pink patches	Lack of melanin and fibroplasia
Hypopigmented areas	Areas of relatively lighter pigmentation	Reduced amount of melanin
Vascular pattern	Linear, dotted or globular red structures	Neovascularization or vascularized nests of amelanocytic cells
Horny pseudocystis	Circular whitish-yellow areas	Intraepidermal horn globules underneath the surface
Pseudofollicular openings	Comedo-like openings	Intraepidermal horn globules reaching the surface
Red–blue areas	Red–blue, sharply demarcated areas	Dilated vascular spaces in the papillary dermis
Maple leaf-like areas	Maple leaf-like, light to dark brown areas with branching or bud-like arrangement	Pigmented epithelial nodules
Pseudopigment network	A grid of large, roundish, brown meshes	Melanotic pigment arranged around sebaceous follicles, quite numerous on the face

2 One single criterion is usually not sufficient to make a diagnosis. Even if some criteria are more specific than others for diagnosis of melanoma (i.e. less frequently expressed in melanocytic naevi), actually a single criterion cannot be considered as stereotypical for malignancy.

Also in benign lesions, only the simultaneous assessment of several criteria permits a definitive diagnosis; for example, horny pseudocysts are suggestive for seborrhoeic keratosis but only in the absence of so-called melanocytic parameters. Indeed, horny pseudocysts can be present in dermal naevi or even—though exceptionally—in malignant melanomas.

3 Some criteria are more important than others. This derives from the evidence that the association between some criteria and diagnosis of melanoma is very close. The consequence is that the combination of particular criteria (i.e. irregular prominent pigment network and irregularly distributed pseudopods) results more predictive (i.e. associated with a lower probability of false-positive diagnosis) than others (i.e. irregular brown globules and presence of depigmentation).

4 The absence of defined criteria does not permit an ELM diagnosis.

Pattern analysis model based on criteria seen on dermatoscopy allows the investigators to differentiate better between melanocytic and non-melanocytic, and between benign and malignant melanocytic–pigmented skin lesions. It is worth noting that the dermoscopic diagnosis of melanoma, in particular when performed in accordance with the pattern analysis procedure, needs specifically trained observers. Formal studies carried out by Binder *et al.* showed that diagnostic performance of dermoscopy gave better results than clinical examination only when carried out by experts. In contrast, sensitivity of technique, i.e. the percentage of melanoma diagnosed over the total number of melanoma observed, was lower than that of clinical examination by untrained dermatologists. An improvement of diagnostic performance was subsequently found with 9 h of formal training.

Facing a pigmented skin lesion with dermoscopy, the diagnostic approach leading to diagnosis begins with the definition of melanocytic or non-melanocytic origin of the lesion. To achieve this goal pattern analysis remains, in our opinion, the basic methodological approach, because the so-called melanoma algorithms (see below) are useful only when facing clear-cut melanocytic lesions. As a consequence of their histopathological correlates, ELM features suggestive for melanocytic proliferation are as follows: pigment network, brown globules, radial streaming and pseudopods. Lacking these ELM features, the observer must look for other dermoscopic parameters allowing a final diagnosis (e.g. horny pseudocysts and pseudofollicular openings: seborrhoeic keratosis; maple-leaf like areas: pigmented basal cell carcinoma; or red–blue lagoons: angioma or angiokeratoma) (Table 2). Only when a lesion is definitely classified as 'melanocytic' can the use of one of the reported dermoscopic algorithms for melanoma (e.g. ABCD of dermoscopy: see below), allow differentiation between benign and malignant melanocytic lesions as an alternative procedure of pattern analysis. Table 2 shows the main characteristics of melanocytic naevi and melanoma, respectively, as assessed by pattern analysis.

In a recent study on 342 clinically doubtful melanocytic skin lesions, the diagnostic performance of melanoma by pattern analysis carried out by experienced observers showed better results concerning sensitivity (91%), specificity (90%), diagnostic accuracy value (76%) and number of correct diagnoses (90%) when compared to those obtained with two dermoscopic algorithms (ABCD rule of dermoscopy and seven-point checklist: see below).

Diagnosis of melanoma by means of dermoscopic algorhythms

ABCD of dermoscopy

Several studies have shown that, with the ELM, a high rate of diagnostic accuracy of pigmented skin lesions can be obtained only if the technique is performed by dermatologists with a long experience in the field or who have been formally trained in this technique. Because of the great number of subtle features and special criteria that have to be assessed

Table 2 Pattern analysis suggestive for benign naevi and melanoma

ELM criterion	Melanocytic naevus	Melanoma
Pigment network	Regular, delicate, faint at the periphery	Irregular, prominent, with abrupt end at the periphery
Diffuse pigmentation (blotches)	Absent or homogeneously present at the centre of the lesion, gradually thins at periphery	Irregularly distributed, inhomogeneous, abruptly ends at periphery
Brown globules	Absent (junctional naevus) or regularly distributed, mainly at the centre of the lesion, with homogeneous characteristics	Varied in size and shape, irregularly distributed
Black dots	Uniform in size and shape, regularly distributed, mainly present at the centre of the lesion	Irregularly distributed, with inhomogeneous features
Radial streaming	Usually absent	Frequently present (in about 25% of cases)
Pseudopods	Absent (regularly distributed pseudopods can be found in pigmented Spitz's naevi)	Irregularly distributed, present in about 31% of cases
Whitish veil	Absent	Often present (51% of cases, depending on the thickness: higher frequency in thicker lesions)
Grey–blue areas	Absent (diffuse homogeneous grey–blue pigmentation without other ELM features: blue naevus); a small area of grey–blue pigmentation at the centre of the lesion can be seldom found in naevi with histological atypia	Present, irregularly distributed (the frequency depends on the thickness of the lesion, higher in thicker lesions)
White scar-like areas	Usually absent	Present, irregular
Reticular depigmentation	Regularly present (centre of the lesion) in pigmented Spitz's naevi (negative pigment network)	Seldom present, but with irregular meshes and holes
Hypopigmented areas	Frequently present at the centre of the lesion, with homogeneous distribution	When present, it is irregularly distributed
Vascular pattern	Homogeneous, 'hair-pin' like in dermal naevi	Atypical (linear and dotted, presence of 'milky red' glodules, i.e. globules of melanocytes with erythema due to neovascularization phenomena)
Horny pseudocystis	Seldom present in papillary dermal naevus (always present in seborrhoeic keratosis, without 'melanocytic' ELM features)	Usually absent (a case report of melanoma showing horny pseudocystis has been reported in the literature)
Pseudofollicular openings	Absent (always present in seborrhoeic keratosis)	Absent
Red–blue areas	Absent (red blue areas are diagnostic for angioma when melanocytic ELM features are lacking)	Absent
Maple leaf-like areas	Absent (they are diagnostic for pigmented basal cell carcinoma when melanocytic ELM features are absent)	Absent
Pseudopigment network	Peculiar to the lesions on the face; regularly distributed	Irregular

qualitatively when performing pattern analysis, the investigators must undergo formal training developed especially for this technique. For novices the correct interpretation of the images may be difficult to learn and apply. Therefore, a new diagnostic algorithm termed the 'ABCD rule of dermatoscopy' has been developed to increase the diagnostic accuracy of non-experienced ELM investigators. This method can be easily learned, easily applied and has been proven to be reliable and reproducible.

Stolz and co-workers introduced this new diagnostic model based on multivariate analysis of only four dermoscopic criteria with a semiquantitative score system:

- asymmetry
- abrupt cut-off of the pigment pattern at the border
- colour variegation
- different dermatoscopic structures.

Asymmetry is evaluated with respect to colour and structure along none (0 points), one (1 point) or both (2 points) of the two perpendicular axes located in such a way that the lowest asymmetry score possible is obtained (possible score 0–2).

For the calculation of border score, the lesions are divided into eight segments; each segment, which includes an abrupt cut-off of pigment pattern, gives a score of 1 point (possible score 0–8).

In assessing the colour score, the investigator counts the number of different colours seen with dermoscopy (possible colours are six: white, red, light and dark brown, blue–grey, black) (possible score 1–6).

For evaluating the different dermatoscopic structures score, five possible components are considered: network, homogeneous areas, dots, globules and streaks (score 1–5).

The individual scores obtained according to these rules are multiplied for different weight factors obtained by multivariate analysis of the four dermoscopic criteria, referring to the real diagnostic weight of each of them.

With this easy-to-perform scoring system (Table 3) the investigator is able to calculate the Total Dermoscopy Score (TDS) which can be used for grading the malignancy potential of melanocytic pigmented skin lesions ($TDS < 4.75$ = benign lesion; $TDS > 5.45$ = malignant lesion; intermediate values = doubtful lesions).

In earlier reports on the ABCD rule of dermatoscopy, this method gave 92.8% sensitivity, 91.2% specificity and 80% diagnostic accuracy. This algorithm has proven, when applied to clinically equivocal melanocytic cutaneous lesions, to allow the dermatologist a more objective and reproducible diagnosis. Some new data from international literature underscore that the use of the ABCD rule of dermatoscopy appreciably improves the diagnostic ability of less experienced investigators performing ELM.

This method, as well as standard pattern analysis, obviously does not yield 100% diagnostic accuracy in detecting

Table 3 Calculation of ABCD score for dermatoscopy

Criterion	Possible points	Weight factor	Score (min./max.)
Asymmetry	0–2	× 1.3	0.0/2.6
Border	0–8	× 0.1	0.0/0.8
Colours	1–6	× 0.5	0.5/3.0
Dermoscopic structures	1–5	× 0.5	0.5/2.5
Total dermoscopy score			1.0/8.9

melanomas. Therefore further efforts must be made to enhance our ability in diagnosing malignant melanocytic skin lesions.

The seven features for melanoma (7FFM)

To introduce a diagnostic algorithm based on the evaluation of ELM criteria into daily clinical practice, it must be simple, reliable and reproducible. Following these guidelines, Dal Pozzo and co-workers developed a new method based on a few dermoscopic features showing a high malignancy predictive value.

All seven selected criteria used to develop this scoring system show a histopathological correlation with malignancy, even if this does not mean that the features are specific for melanoma. There is general agreement in the literature that none of the known dermoscopic criteria is 100% specific for melanoma.

The seven dermoscopic features useful for the diagnosis of melanoma were thus termed the 7FFM. Following a selection based on the specificity obtained for each criterion, the authors attributed a score of 2 to the major features (specificity > 95%) and a score of 1 to the minor ones (specificity 95–80%) (Table 4).

According to this scoring system, the pigmented skin lesions showing a total score of 2 or more are diagnosed as being malignant, those whose score is < 2 can be considered benign. Therefore for the diagnosis of melanoma the presence of at least one of the major criteria or the coexistence of two of the minor ones is regarded as sufficient.

This recently developed diagnostic dermoscopic method shows a sensitivity of 95%, a specificity of 86% and an efficiency of 88%.

The 11 surface microscopic features method of diagnosis of invasive melanoma

Menzies and co-workers have designed a method which is based on the identification of 11 ELM features, thus enabling the less expert observer to use it easily.

The ELM criteria considered were selected for low sensitivity (negative features) and high specificity (positive features).

According to this algorithm, a pigmented skin lesion showing none of the

Table 4 Dermoscopic description and score of the seven ELM features used for the 7FFM

Dermoscopic feature	Description	Score
Regression erythema*	White-pinkish depigmented area	2
Radial streaming	Thin, closely spaced, parallel pigmented streaming irradiating from the rim of the lesion	2
Grey–blue veil	Blue or grey–faded blue area with ill-defined margins, asymmetrically located inside the lesion No clearly dermoscopic features are observed	2
Irregularly distributed pseudopods	Finger-like extensions present at the periphery of the lesions, varying in colour from brown to black	2
Unhomogeneity†	Asymmetrical or irregular distribution within the lesion of at least two dermoscopic features	1
Irregular pigment network	Coarse, strongly pigmented, irregular pigmented network	1
Sharp margin	Abrupt cessation, of the dermoscopic features at the periphery of the lesion not < 0.25 of the margin	1

*The criterion regression erythema corresponds to regression together with vasodilatation and neoangiogenesis.
†Unhomogeneity corresponds to an histopathological architectural disorder of the lesion.

negative dermoscopic features and at least one of the positive ones can be considered as a melanoma (Table 5).

This method is easy to perform, reproducible and reliable, showing a sensitivity of 92% and a specificity of 71% in diagnosing cutaneous melanoma.

The new seven-point checklist based on pattern analysis

ELM images of 342 melanocytic skin lesions were studied by Argenziano and co-workers to evaluate the frequency of seven ELM criteria (and 11 variables of them). These dermoscopic features were selected for their frequent association with melanoma and for their particular histopathological correlates to develop a new diagnostic method based on simplified ELM pattern analysis.

Most of the features in the new algorithm belong to the terminology standardized at the Consensus Meeting held in Hamburg (Table 6).

In addition the following ELM features were included in the diagnostic model termed 'ELM seven-point checklist': irregular diffuse pigmentation (blotches), 'peppering' (multiple grey–blue dots) and atypical vascular pattern.

Using an arbitrary cut-off of odds ratios calculated by multivariate analysis, the authors divided the selected dermoscopic features into two main groups: 'major criteria' (odds ratios > 5) and 'minor criteria' (odds ratios < 5). A score of 2 is given to the three major features and a score of 1 to the four minor criteria considered. By adding all the individual scores found within the melanocytic skin lesion, a total score ≥ 3 allows the diagnosis of melanoma. For a melanoma to be diagnosed, the identification of at least one major and one minor dermoscopic criterion (or three minor criteria) is needed, thus confirming the basic rule of epiluminescence microscopy that one single criterion is never enough to make a diagnosis and the absence of a criterion does not rule out the diagnosis.

The seven-point checklist gave a sensitivity of 95%, a specificity of 75% and a diagnostic accuracy of 64% in the diagnosis of melanoma.

Diagnostic performance: clinical examination vs. ELM

There is general agreement in the international literature that the most effective management of malignant melanoma consists in early recognition and subsequent surgical excision of thin lesions. The strong inverse correlation of 5-year survival rate with tumour thickness measured according to Breslow, and the lack of effective therapies for metastatic melanomas, still gives early detection of equivocal melanocytic proliferation of the skin the highest priority in order to increase the cure rate of melanoma.

ELM is not really required for the diagnosis of advanced and clinically typical forms of melanoma or benign pigmented skin lesion where purely clinical criteria

Table 5 Method of diagnosis of melanoma according to Menzies

Positive features (at least one found)	Negative features (cannot be found)
Blue–white veil	Point and axial symmetry of pigmentation
Multiple brown dots	Presence of a single colour
Pseudopods	
Radial streamings	
Scar-like depigmentation	
Peripheral black dots/globules	
Multiple (5–6) colours	
Multiple blue/grey dots	
Broadened network	

Table 6 ELM seven-point checklist: definitions, histological correlates and scores of dermoscopic criteria

ELM criterion	Definition	Histological correlates	Seven-point score
Major criteria			
Atypical pigment network	Prominent (hyperpigmented or broad) and irregular network	Hyperpigmented or broadened rete ridges with irregular shape or distribution	2
Grey–blue areas	Irregular, confluent, grey–blue to whitish blue diffuse pigmentation not associated with red–blue lacunes or maple-leaf pigmentation	Pigmented melanophages or melanocytes of mid-reticular dermis location	2
Atypical vascular pattern	Linear, dotted or globular red structures irregularly distributed outside areas of regression and associated with other melanocytic pigment patterns	Neovascularization or vascularized nests of amelanotic cells	2
Minor criteria			
Radial streaming (streaks)	Radially and asymmetrically arranged linear or bulbous extensions at the edge of the lesion	Confluent radial junctional nests of melanocytes	1
Irregular diffuse pigmentation (blotches)	Brown, grey and black areas of diffuse pigmentation with irregular shape or distribution and abrupt end	Hyperpigmentation throughout all levels of epidermis or upper dermis (in melanocytes or melanophages)	1
Irregular dots and globules	Black, brown or blue round structures irregularly distributed within the lesion	Aggregates of pigment of stratum corneum, junctional or dermis location	1
Regression pattern	White scar-like depigmentation or 'peppering' (speckled multiple blue–grey dots within a hypodepigmented area) irregularly distributed within the lesion	Areas of loss of pigmentation and fibroplasia, with scattered dermal melanophages	1

usually suffice to provide a correct diagnosis. On the other hand, even in specialized centres the diagnostic accuracy of clinical examination alone is no higher than 64% for small pigmented lesions that have may not yet have developed the standard clinical features of malignancy.

Dermatoscopy has the ability to move these diagnostic limitations to a higher level, because this method allows the investigators to recognize *in vivo* malignant melanomas much earlier than by clinical examination alone.

The percentage of correct diagnoses increased from 73% to 83% for junctional naevi, from 56% to 93% for pigmented spitz naevi, from 50% to 83% for *in situ* superficial spreading melanoma, from 54% to 91% for invasive superficial spreading melanoma and from 46% to 62% for nodular melanomas. A remarkable improvement was found especially for pigmented, non-melanocytic lesions, namely, seborrhoeic keratosis (from 62% to 77%), basal cell carcinomas (from 58% to 84%) and angiomas–angiokeratomas (from 83% to 100%).

According to a formal study designed to compare the reliability of dermoscopy to that of clinical diagnosis in a series of doubtful melanocytic skin lesions, clinical diagnosis was correct in 40% of cases whereas the dermoscopic diagnosis was correct in 55%. From these data, the average gain in the percentage of correct diagnoses by dermoscopy was 15.6%.

Concerning the diagnosis of melanoma the sensitivity increased from 42% to 75% and the specificity from 78% to 89% by means of dermoscopy.

It is important to emphasize, however, that ELM analysis does not completely eliminate diagnostic errors and cannot replace histopathological diagnosis. ELM does not provide 100% diagnostic accuracy, therefore it cannot be used as the only indicator for excision. For this, both clinical and dermoscopic features are necessary.

Dermoscopic criteria of cutaneous melanoma progression

Cutaneous melanoma develops through a series of evolutionary phases that are traceable in specific histological patterns. During melanoma progression, the occurrence of specific histological patterns also modifies the dermoscopic profile of a given lesion.

In a previous study of our group dermoscopic criteria were elaborated that characterize the different phases of melanoma progression as well as the various tumour depths. A significant association was found between the presence of pigment network within the lesions and melanomas $<0.76\,\text{mm}$ thickness (thin MM), and between the presence of grey–blue areas, vascular pattern and melanomas $>0.75\,\text{mm}$ thickness (thick MM). Pigment network variations associated with radial streaming were the most significant association of dermoscopic criteria in thin lesions, whereas the association of grey–blue areas and vascular pattern is the most relevant finding in thick melanomas.

ELM criteria for the preoperative assessment of cutaneous melanoma thickness

Melanoma thickness is used to establish the width of surgical margins for excision of melanoma as well as to select patients for sentinel lymph node biopsy. To ensure correct surgical approach, reliable preoperative parameters on melanoma thickness are warranted.

Previous studies have shown the poor reliability of melanoma palpability (clinical elevation of the lesion) in predicting melanoma thickness.

Argenziano and co-workers demonstrated a good correlation between the frequency of appearance of certain dermoscopic criteria and the thickness of the lesion. Based on the combination of clinical criteria (palpability and diameter $>1.5\,\text{cm}$) and dermoscopic criteria (pigment network, grey–blue areas and atypical vascular pattern), accuracy in the preoperative assessment of melanoma thickness could be enhanced compared to separate application of these two criteria.

According to preliminary results of a study carried out by our group, the ABCD rule of dermoscopy was found to play a possible role in the preoperative evaluation of melanoma thickness. In fact, we found that TDS attributed to melanomas according to the ABCD rule of dermatoscopy correlates with the thickness of the lesion.

Digital epiluminescence microscopy (D-ELM)

D-ELM is a new technology that can improve clinical visualization and facilitate a more detailed study of the subtle epidermal and superficial dermal anatomy of pigmented lesions. By enabling high-quality visualization, documentation and measurement of subtle ELM diagnostic features, the development of standards for ELM differential diagnosis and management of pigmented skin lesions can be facilitated.

There is current interest in the possibility of introducing objective, computer-based, image analysis (machine vision) into the daily clinical practice of specialized medical centres dedicated to the diagnosis of pigmented skin lesions.

Digitization of dermoscopic images has been driven by the requirements of several applications: digital image processing to assist the naked eye; development of expert systems for automatic classification of melanocytic lesions; automatic machine vision, fully automatic digital processing that employs images at wavelengths invisible to the naked eye (ultraviolet, infrared); electronic transmission of images for remote diagnosis (telemedicine); and image storage and retrieval.

For the diagnosis of pigmented skin lesions dermatologists are using only a very small fraction of the information provided by ELM images. Thus one of the main challenges of research into digital acquisition and processing of dermoscopic images is to add a new dimension of information provided by these images.

New technologies enable high-quality digital ELM images to be sent, with the support of network systems such as the internet and ISDN, via ordinary telephone lines and satellite communication (teledermatology). Analysis of image data shows that 'informativeness' of selected dermoscopic structures of lesions employed for naked-eye diagnosis of pigmented skin lesions is preserved despite their remote location. The future of early diagnosis of melanoma by means of D-ELM depends directly on further investigation into the fields of communication technology.

Further reading

Andreassi L, Perotti R, Rubegni P *et al.* Digital dermoscopy analysis for the differentiation of atypical nevi and early melanoma: a new quantitative semiology. *Arch Dermatol* 1999; 135: 1459–65.

Argenziano G, Fabbrocini G, Carli P *et al.* Epiluminescence microscopy: criteria of cutaneous melanoma progression. *J Am Acad Dermatol* 1997; 37: 68–74.

Argenziano G, Fabbrocini G, Carli P *et al.* Epiluminescence microscopy for the diagnosis of doubtful melanocytic skin lesions. *Arch Dermatol* 1998; 134: 1563–70.

Benelli C, Gianotti R, Dal Pozzo V, Roscetti E. Melanoma with dermoscopic features of seborrheic keratosis. *Eur J Dermatol* 1996; 6: 246–7.

Binder M, Kittler H, Steiner A *et al.* Reevaluation of the ABCD rule for epiluminescence microscopy. *J Am Acad Dermatol* 1999; 40 (2 Part 1): 171–6.

Binder M, Puespoek-Schwarz M, Steiner A *et al.* Epiluminescence microscopy of small pigmented skin lesions: short-term formal training improves the diagnostic performance of dermatologists. *J Am Acad Dermatol* 1997; 36 (197): 202.

Carli P, De Giorgi V, Cattaneo A *et al.* Mucosal melanosis clinically mimicking malignant melanoma: non-invasive analysis by epiluminescence microscopy. *Eur J Dermatol* 1995; 6: 434–6.

Carli P, De Giorgi V, Giannotti B. Preoperative assessment of melanoma thickness by ABCD score of dermatoscopy. *J Am Acad Dermatol* 2000; 43(3): 459–66.

Carli P, De Giorgi V, Naldi L *et al.* Reliability and inter-observer agreement of dermoscopic diagnosis of melanoma and melanocytic naevi. *Eur J Canc Prev* 1998; 7: 1–6.

Cascinelli N, Ferrario M, Bufalino R *et al.* Results obtained by using a computerized image analysis system designed as an aid to diagnosis of cutaneous melanoma. *Melanoma Res* 1993; 2: 1163–70.

Dal Pozzo V, Benelli C. *Atlas of Dermoscopy.* Milano: Edra Edizioni, 1997.

Dal Pozzo V, Benelli C, Roscetti E. The seven features for melanoma. A new dermoscopic algorithm for the diagnosis of malignant melanoma. *Eur J Dermatol* 1999; 9: 303–8.

De Giorgi V, Carli P. Epiluminescence microscopy of pigmented skin lesions. In: Katsambas AD, Lotti TM eds. *European Handbook of Dermatological Treatments.* Berlin: Springer-Verlag, 1999: 668–74.

Gutkowicz-Krusin D, Elbaum M, Szwaykowski P *et al.* Can early malignant melanoma be differentiated from atypical melanocytic nevus by in vivo techniques? Part II. Automatic machine vision classification. *Skin Res Technol* 1997; 3: 15–22.

Kenet RO, Kang S, Kenet BJ *et al.* Clinical diagnosis of pigmented lesions using digital epiluminescence microscopy. Grading protocol and atlas. *Arch Dermatol* 1993; 129: 157–74.

Kopf AW, Elbaum M, Provost N. The use of dermoscopy and digital imaging in the diagnosis of cutaneous malignant melanoma. *Skin Res Technol* 1997; 3: 1–7.

Kreusch JF, Koch F. Vascular structures are an important feature for diagnosis of melanoma and other skin tumors by incident light microscopy: 4th World Conference on Melanoma, Sydney, 10–14 June 1997 (Abstract). *Melanoma Res* 1997; 7 (Suppl.): S38.

Menzies SW, Crotty KA, McCarthy WH. The morphologic criteria of the pseudopod in surface microscopy. *Arch Dermatol* 1995; 131: 436–40.

Menzies SW, Ingvar C, Crotty KA *et al.* Frequency and morphologic characteristic of invasive melanomas lacking specific surface microscopic features. *Arch Dermatol* 1996; 132: 1178–82.

Menzies SW, Ingvar C, McCarthy WH. A sensitivity and specificity analysis of the surface microscopy features of invasive melanoma. *Melanoma Res* 1996; 6: 55–62.

O'Donnell BF, Marsden JR, O'Donnell CA *et al.* Does palpability of primary cutaneous melanoma predict dermal invasion? *J Am Acad Dermatol* 1996; 34: 632–7.

Pehamberger H, Binder M, Steiner A *et al.* In vivo epiluminescence microscopy: improvement of early diagnosis of melanoma. *J Invest Dermatol* 1993; 100: 356s–62s.

Pehamberger H, Steiner A, Wolff K. In vivo epiluminescence microscopy of pigmented skin lesions. I. Pattern analysis of pigmented skin lesions. *J Am Acad Dermatol* 1987; 17: 571–83.

Perednia DA. Telemedicine technology and clinical applications. *JAMA* 1995; 273: 483–8.

Piccolo D, Smolle J, Wolf IH *et al.* Face-to-face diagnosis vs. telediagnosis of pigmented skin tumors: a teledermoscopic study. *Arch Dermatol* 1999; 135: 1467–71.

Schimdewolf T, Schiffner R, Stolz W *et al.* Comparison of classification rates for conventional and dermoscopic images of malignant and benign melanocytic lesions using computerized colour image analysis. *Eur J Dermatol* 1993; 3: 299–303.

Sober AJ. Digital epiluminescence microscopy in the evaluation of pigmented lesions: a brief review. *Semin Surg Oncol* 1993; 9: 198–201.

Stolz W, Riemann A, Cognetta AB *et al.* ABCD rule of dermatoscopy: a new practical method for early recognition of malignant melanoma. *Eur J Dermatol* 1994; 4: 521–7.

Stolz W, Schiffner R, Pillet L *et al.* Improvement of monitoring of melanocytic skin lesions with the use of a computerized acquisition and surveillance unit with a skin surface microscopic television camera. *J Am Acad Dermatol* 1996; 35: 202–7.

Wolff K, Binder M, Pehamberger H. Epiluminescence microscopy. a new approach to the early detection of melanoma. *Adv Dermatol* 1994; 9: 45–56.

Yadav S, Vossaert KA, Kopf AW *et al.* Histopathologic correlates of structures seen on dermoscopy (epiluminescence microscopy). *Am J Dermatopathol* 1993; 15: 297–305.

Lasers

L. Leite

It is not possible within the limits of this chapter to exhaust the theme of laser therapy so this chapter will concentrate on information concerning the various pathologies that can be treated by laser technology. It will not deal with techniques, preoperative patient considerations, patient education, pre- and postlaser therapy, skin care nor with the side-effects and complications of laser therapy. The reader will find precise indications for the different types of laser currently used in the management of the various cutaneous pathologies. However, if the reader is untrained in laser surgery, referral to specific papers and textbooks, and training with experts in this therapeutic modality, is recommended.

Cutaneous vascular lesions

Today's therapeutic possibilities in the management of vascular lesions would have been unthinkable more then 15 years ago. There are several types of laser indicated for such lesions as listed in Table 1.

Vascular lesions susceptible to laser therapy are congenital haemangiomas, port-wine stains, venous malformations, lymphangiomas and acquired telangiectasias (essential or secondary to other processes, such as photoageing, Rendu–Osler syndrome, lupus erythematosus, scleroderma, etc.), cherry angiomas, pyogenic granulomas, venous lakes and Kaposi's sarcoma.

In recent years there has been much controversy regarding the treatment of haemangiomas. These may be congenital (about 30%), but a significant percentage arise during the first year of life. Their colour varies from bright to bluish red; these nodular lesions are also characterized by a rapid proliferative phase, leading to unpredictable size, followed by an involutive phase which may last a few years.

The potential drama of angiomas is that the initial rapid enlargement, of incalculable limits, may attain the vision, eventually causing blindness, or even obstruct vital structures, such as the trachea.

Other complications that may occur are ulcerations—which may lead to haemorrhages of a varied degree of severity—and infections.

Port-wine stains are always present at birth, although not always clearly perceptible and not liable to spontaneous regression. With the passing of time, their colour deepens—hence the 'port-wine' designation—and nodular formations may develop on their surface.

Table 2 lists the performance of the various types of laser for these two conditions, but it should be stressed that 'flashlamp-pulsed dye' laser (FPDL) is still the treatment of choice for port-wine stains in children, due to the good results and minimal risk of scars.

With telangiectasias, good or excellent results are obtained with most existing

Table 1 Different types of laser specific for vascular lesions

Laser type	Laser characteristics
Frequency doubled Nd : YAG	532 nm, Q-switched
KTP	532 nm, quasi CW
Krypton	568 nm, quasi CW
Argon-pumped tunable dye	577 nm, quasi CW
Copper vapour	578 nm, quasi CW
Flashlamp-pumped pulsed dye	585 mn, pulsed
Long-pulsed dye	585, 590, 595, 600 nm, pulsed

Table 2 Response of haemangiomas and 'port-wine stains' to different laser treatments

Laser type	Haemangioma	Port-wine stain
Frequency doubled Nd : YAG	+/0	+/0
KTP	+/0	+/0
Krypton	+/0	+/0
Argon-pumped tunable dye	+/0	+/0
Copper vapour	+/0	+/0
Flashlamp-pumped pulsed dye	++	+ + +
Long-pulsed dye	++	++

+/0, poor/fair; ++, good; + + +, excellent.

Table 3 Response of telangiectasias to different laser treatments

Laser type	Facial telangiectasia	Leg	Other, telangiectasia, e.g. poikiloderma
Frequency doubled Nd : YAG	++	+/0	+/0
KTP	++	+/0	+/0
Krypton	++	+/0	+/0
Argon-pumped tunable dye	++	+/0	+/0
Copper vapour	++	Unknown	Unknown
Flashlamp-pumped pulsed dye	+ + +	+/0	+ + +
Long-pulsed dye	+ + +	++	++

+/0, poor/fair; ++, good; + + +, excellent.

laser types (Table 3), but this is not the case when the lesions are located on the legs. The long-pulsed dye laser, however, is producing some encouraging results.

Lasers in dermatology

Pigmented lesions

Malignant pigmented lesions, such as cutaneous melanoma, or those with malignant potential, such as melanocytic naevi, are not contemplated in this chapter, although some trials with the latter, though polemical, have been reported.

The pigmented lesions that can be treated with laser are epidermal (lentigines, ephelides, café-au-lait macules, Becker's naevi) and dermal lesions (Ota, Ito and blue naevi, also debatable for the latter). Besides these, there are the mixed lesions, such as postinflammatory hyperpigmentation, melasma and naevus spilus.

Table 4 shows the different types of laser and respective performances. It is important to note that pigmented lesions are difficult to treat, many of them requiring several laser sessions. Patients should not be led to expect complete clearance and, particularly in the cases of melasma, post-inflammatory hyperpigmentation and café-au-lait macules, they should be informed of the high possibility of recurrence, which, even when the treatment appears to have been effective, is close to 100%.

Tattoos

Decorative tattooing has been practised for many centuries. Whereas some decades ago it was associated with the lower socio-economic strata, in recent years tattooing has became fashionable and can be seen in people of all social standings. Nevertheless, in spite of this enthusiastic boom, about 50% of tattooed subjects finally want their tattoos removed.

Besides decorative tattooing, which is the most common, there are also cosmetic and traumatic tattoos. To date, there is not one laser type capable of eliminating the pigments of the various colours. Thus for the removal of multicoloured tattoos, at

Table 4 Types of laser and expected results in the different pigmented lesions

Laser type	Ephelides/ lentigines	Café-au-lait	Ota and Ito naevi	Benign naevi	Melasma and PIH	Naevus spilus	Becker's naevus
Pulsed dye	+ + +	+ + +	0	+/0	0	+/0	+/0
Cooper vapour	++ Unknown	+/0	0	+/0	0	Unknown	
Krypton	++ Unknown	+/0	0	+/0	0	Unknown	
KTP	++ Unknown	+/0	0	+/0	0	Unknown	
Frequency doubled Q-switched Nd : YAG	+ + +	++	0	+/0	0	+/0	+/0
Q-switched ruby	+ + +	++	+ + +	++	0	+/0	+/0
Q-switched alexandrite	++	+/0	+ + +	++	0	+/0	+/0
Q-switched Nd : YAG	++	+/0	+ + +	++	0	+/0	+/0

+/0, poor/fair; ++, good; + + +, excellent.

Table 5 Laser types and efficacy according to different colour inks

Laser type	Wavelength and pulse duration	Dark blue and black	Green	Red	Brown
Pulsed dye	510 nm; 300 ns	+/0	+/0	+ + +	0
Frequency-doubled Q-switched Nd : YAG	532 nm; 10–40 ns	+/0	/0	+ + +	0
Q-switched ruby	694 nm; 25–50 ns	+ + +	++	+/0	0
Q-switched alexandrite	755 nm; 50–100 ns	+ + +	+ + +	+/0	0
Q-switched Nd : YAG	1064 nm; 10 ns	+ + +	0	+/0	0

+/0, poor/fair; ++, good; + + +, excellent.

least two different types of laser must be used. Table 5 displays the various types of laser and respective applications.

Cutaneous ageing and photoageing

Recreational sunbathing, which became fashionable a few decades ago, led to an increase in the incidence of skin cancer worldwide, but also to the scientific knowledge of the harmful effects of ultraviolet (UV) radiation in human skin. However, if skin cancer is the major consequence of chronic overexposure to solar radiation, other injuries can result from such exposure. After the acute effects following each episode of overexposure (sunstroke and burns of varied degrees) subside, other, initially imperceptible alterations occur and accumulate after each new episode of overexposure to solar radiation, which years later will have some clinical expression, commonly designated as dermatoheliosis.

The clinical signs of dermatolieliosis are essentially actinic keratoses, lentigines, telangiectasias and rhytides. These conditions can be treated with specific CO_2 laser units—ultra pulse or with associated flashscanner—that permit the performance of the 'resurfacing' technique. Unlike the earlier CO_2 laser apparatus which, due to the excessive thermal effect, had a high risk of scars, these modern units permit the ablation of layer after layer of tissue with a very reduced thermal effect therefore with minimal risk of scars.

Prior to treatment with the 'resurfacing' technique, the patients, who should be carefully selected, undergo topical preparation with tretinoin or isotretinoin, hydroquinone base and glycolic acid; antibiotics and antiviral therapy should be initiated 1 week before 'resurfacing'. This modality is not indicated for patients undergoing systemic isotretinoin treatment, those known to be prone to developing keloids or hypertrophic scars, and those suffering from collagen vascular disease or immune disorders.

Laser-assisted hair removal

Electrolysis, the only long-lasting method of hair removal until recently is a tedious, and invasive one. In order to avoid this inconvenience, various light sources for hair removal were 'born', each one claiming the best results (Table 6).

There are three different mechanisms for hair removal with light:

1 Photothermal destruction
- long pulsed ruby laser
- long pulsed alexandrite laser
- long pulsed diode laser
- pulsed-non-coherent intense light source.

2 Photomechanical destruction: Q-switched Nd : YAG laser.

3 Photochemical destruction: photodynamic therapy.

Miscellaneous

For common, everyday pathologies the laser is an invaluable medium. The CO_2 laser, for instance, can be used as a cutting tool, a vapourizing tool or, simultaneously, as a cutting and vapourizing tool (Table 7).

A reference should be made to the use of FPDL for less common conditions, such as red and/or hypertrophic scars, keloids, striae distensae and certain difficult cases of periungual warts or condylomas. It should be stressed that, for the two latter conditions, adequate precautions must be taken since the plume effect does occur. The results obtained, however, are quite variable and patients should not be led into unrealistic expectations, particularly when treating keloids and striae.

Further reading

Achauer BM, Nelson S, Vander Karn VM *et al.* Treatment of traumatic tattoos by Q-switched ruby laser. *Plast Reconstr Surg* 1994; 93: 318–23.

Alster TS. Treatment of benign epidermal lesions with the 510 nm pulsed dye laser: further clin-

Table 6 Different laser units for assisted hair removal

Laser type	Wavelength	Pulse duration	Spot size	Scanning device
694 ruby	694 nm	3–100 ms	10–20 mm	No
755 alexandrite	755 nm	1,2–40 ms	4–15 mm	Yes
800 diode	800 nm	5–100 ms	2,4–10 mm	No
1064 Q-switched Nd: YAG	1.064 mm	8–10 ns	3–8 mm	No
1.064 long pulsed Nd: YAG	1.064 mm	1–50 ms	1–4 mm	No
Pulsed non-coherent Intense light source	590/1200 mm	Variable	Variable	No

Table 7 CO_2 as first choice therapy

As cutting tool	As vapourizing tool	As cutting and vapourizing tool
Patients with bleeding disorders	Pyogenic granuloma	Rhinophyma
Patients with pacemakers in whom electrosurgery is contraindicated	Angiokeratoma	Giant condyloma acuminatum
Infected surgical sites	Epidermal naevus	Multiple giant appendageal tumours:
Whenever the surgeon finds it appropriate	Erythroplasia of Queyrat	neurofibroma
	Zoon's balanitis	adenoma sebaceum
	Oral florid papillomatosis	giant trichoepithelioma
	Sublingual keratosis	
	Actinic chelitis	
	Bower's disease	
	Nail ablation Syringoma	
	Angiofibroma (Pringle)	

ical experience and treatment parameters. *Lasers Surg Med* 1993; 5: 55.
Alster TS. Successful elimination of traumatic tattoos by the Q-switched alexandrite (755 nm) laser. *Ann Plast Surg* 1995; 34: 542–5.
Alster TS. *Manual of Cutaneous Laser Techniques*. NewYork: Lippincott-Raven, 1997.
Alster TS, Tan OT. Laser treatment of benign cutaneous vascular lesions. *Am Fam Phys* 1991; 44: 547–54.
Alster TS, Wilson F. Treatment of port-wine stains with the flashlamp-pumped pulsed dye laser. *Ann Plast Surg* 1994; 32: 474–84.
Apfelberg DB, Bailin P, Rosenberg H. Preliminary investigation of KTP/532 laser light in treatment of hemangiomas and tattoos. *Lasers Surg Med* 1986; 6: 38–42.
Ashinoff R, Geronemus RG. Q-switched ruby laser treatment of labial lentigos. *J Am Acad Dermatol* 1992; 27: 809–11.
Broska P, Martinho E, Goodman M. Comparison of the argon tunable dye laser with the flashlamp pulsed dye laser in treatment of facial telangiectasia. *J Dermatol Surg Oncol* 1994; 20: 749–54.
Cochito M, Lopes JMC, Leite L. A case of chondroid syringoma treated with CO_2 laser. *Skin Cancer* 1996; 1: 219–22.
Cochito M, Lopes JMC, Leite L *et al.* Cutaneous horn of the penis. Two cases and two different therapeutic approaches. *Skin Cancer* 1992; 7: 27–30.
DeCoste SI, Anderson RR. Comparison of Q-switched ruby and Q-switched N & YAG laser treatment of tattoos. *Lasers Surg Med Suppl* 1991; 3: 64.
Dierickx C, Goldman MP, Fitzpatrick RE. Laser treatment of erythematous/hypertrophic and pigmented scars in 26 patients. *Plast Reconstr Surg* 1995; 95: 84–90.
Dover JS, Arndt KA *et al. Ilustrated Cutaneous Laser Surgery*. Connecticut: Appleton & Lange, 1990.
Dover JS, Kilmer SL, Anderson RR. What's new in cutaneous laser surgery. *J Dermatol Surg Oncol* 1993; 19: 295–8.
Dover JS, Smoller BR, Stern RS *et al.* Low-fluence carbon dioxide laser irradiation of lentigines. *Arch Dermatol* 1988; 124: 1219–24.
Dufresne RG Jr, Garrett AB, Bailin PI *et al.* Carbon dioxide laser treatment of chronic actinic cheilitis. *J Am Acad Dermatol* 1988; 19: 876–8.
Epstein JH. Carbon dioxide laser treatment of actinic cheilitis. *West J Med* 1992; 156: 192.
Fitzpatrick RE, Goldman MP, Ruiz-Esparza J. Clinical advantage of the CO_2 laser super-pulsed mode: treatment of verruca vulgaris, seborrheic keratoses, lentigines, and actinic cheilitis. *J Dermatol Surg Oncol* 1994; 20: 449–456.
Fitzpatrick RE, Goldman MP, Ruiz-Esparza J. Laser treatment of benign pigmented epidermal lesions using a 300 manosecond pulse and 510 nm wavelength. *J Dermatol Surg Oncol* 1993; 18: 341–347.
Fitzpatrick RE, Goldman MP. Tattoo removal using the alexandrite laser. *Arch Dermatol* 1994; 130: 1508–1514.
Fitzpatrick RE, Goldman MP. Treatment of facial telangiectasia with the flashlamp-pumped dye laser. *Lasers Surg Med Suppl* 1991; 3: 70.
Goldberg DJ, Nychay SG. Q-switched ruby laser treatment of nevus of Ota. *J Dermatol Surg Oncol* 1992; 18: 817–821.
Goldberg DJ. Benign pigmented lesions of the skin: treatment with the Q-switched ruby laser. *J Dermatol Surg Oncol* 1993; 19: 376–379.
Keller GS. KTP laser rhytidectomy. *Facial Plast Clin North Am* 1993; 1: 153–162.
Silver BE, Livshots YL. Preliminary experience with the KTP/532 nm laser in the treatment of facial telangiectasia. *Cosmetic Dermatol* 1996; 61–64.
Leite L, Bajanca R. Treatment of angiofibromas of tuberous sclerosis with carbon dioxide laser vaporization. *JEADV* 1994; 3: 376–379.
Leite L. Treatment of actinic cheilitis with carbon dioxide laser. Skin cancer 1992; 7: 147–150.
McDaniel DH, Mordon S. Hexascan: a new robotized scanning laser handpiece. *Cutis* 1990; 45: 300–305.
Neumann RA, Leonhartsberger H, Bohler-Sommeregger K *et al.* Results and tissue healing after copper-vapour laser (at 578 nm) treatment of port-wine stains and facial telangiectasias. *Br J Dermatol* 1993; 128: 306–312.
Rosenbach A, Alster TS. Cutaneous lasers: a review. *Ann Plast Surg* 1996; 37: 220–231.
Tan OT, Hurwitz RM, Stafford TJ. Pulsed dye laser treatment of recalcitrant verrucae: a preliminary report. *Laser Surg Med* 1993; 13: 127–137.
Tan OT, Sherwood K, Gilchrest BA. Treatment of children with port-wine stains using the flash-lamp-pulsed tunable dye laser. *N Engl J Med* 1989; 320: 416–421.
Trelles MA, Verkruysse W, Pickering JW *et al.* Monoline argon laser (514 nm) treatment of benign pigmented lesions with long pulse lengths. *J Photochem Photobiol* 1992; 16: 357–360.
Waldorf HA, Lask GP, Geronemus RG. Laser treatment of telangiectasias. In: Alster TS, Apfelberg DB (eds) *Cosmetic laser surgery*. John Wiley & Sons, New York, 1996; pp 93–109.
Weinstein C, Alster TS. Skin resurfacing with high-energy, pulsed carbon dioxide lasers. In: Alster TS, Apfelberg DB (eds) *Cosmetic laser surgery*. John Willey & Sons, New York, 1996; pp 9–28.
Wheeland RG, McGillis ST. Cowden's disease—treatment of cutaneous lesions using carbon dioxide laser vaporization: a comparison of conventional and superpulsed techniques. *J Dermatol Surg Oncol* 1989; 15: 1055–1059.
Wheeland RG. Copper vapor and dye laser therapy for cutaneous vascular disorders. *West J Med* 1989; 151: 650.
Yardy T, Levine VJ, McLain SA *et al.* The removal of cutaneous pigmented lesions with the Q-switched neodymium-yttrium-aluminum-garnet laser: a comparative study. *J Dermatol Surg Oncol* 1994; 20: 795–800.

Mohs' surgery

A. Picoto, J.M. Labareda, R. Themido and F. Coelho

Mohs' micrographic surgery was created in 1930 by Dr Frederic Mohs, a North American surgeon working on his thesis in Madison, Wiscosin. He found that if a paste of zinc chloride was applied to tumours *in vivo*, for 24 h he would have a slice of 'controlled' necrosis. 'Controlled' because after separation of the necrotic tissue with a scalpel, histological slides could be prepared because the typical architecture was preserved. This method involved successsive *in vivo* fixation followed by a deeper horizontal layer being taken from the patient each time.

The fixation *in vivo* was painful for the patient and in certain locations could not be used because of the risk involved. If used on the eyelids a spillage of the paste onto the eyeball could lead to serious lesions of the cornea. Therefore when treating eyelids Mohs did not use the paste but made the excisions similarly in horizontal succession under local anaesthesia. Then he made the histological preparations using a cryostat to obtain frozen cuts. He realized that this use of local anaesthetic enabled him to reach the tumour-free plane much faster so that immediate surgical reconstruction was possible. He published his preliminary results in the surgical book edited by Epstein in 1956.

But due to the genius of T. Tromovich this 'fresh tissue technique' was applied to the treatment of tumours in different locations other than the eyelids. He published his results in 1970.

Another important step in the dissemination of this therapeutic modality for the treatment of skin cancer was the initiation by Professor Perry Robins in New York of the first 1-year chemosurgery education programme in the USA.

In 1990 the authors, and other European doctors founded in Estoril the European Society for Micrographic Surgery.

This Society gets together Mohs' surgeons from Europe and Israel and tries to make the method familiar to European doctors.

In a so-called millennium paper, David G. Brodland and others write about the American history and evolution of Mohs' micrographic surgery.

Definition and technique

Mohs' micrographic surgery is a method where a skin tumour is excised in horizontal successive layers followed by the immediate preparation of frozen sections for histological examination. Because a thin and horizontal piece of tissue is controlled, the bottom and lateral borders are controlled and theoretically if the tumour persists it will show in the histological slides. Simultaneously a map is drawn where the division of the tissue is marked and the anatomical orientation is indicated.

At each stage, the tissue provided by the surgeon's excision with the scalpel held at approximately 45° in relation to the skin plane, is divided into pieces preferably not more than 1 cm in diameter. The pieces are marked on the faces opposing the skin edge with ink markers, normally black and green or red. Each stage is repeated until a plane free of tumour is reached. After that, immediate reconstruction can be done.

Because there are many methods for controlling skin tumour excision, the American College of Mohs' Micrographic Surgery and Cutaneous Oncology published a 'position paper' where the principles are very clearly stated.

The uniqueness of the method and base of its excellency is the horizontal control of the tissue with all its margins included—skin and bottom.

The mapping should be accurate and we use xerocopies of anatomical drawings and measure exactly the pieces of tissue extracted so that we can exactly situate the tumour nests that we find after microscopic examination. Joseph Alcalay recently described a very interesting way to do the mapping with extreme accuracy. He has called it digital computerized mapping in Mohs' micrographic surgery.

The slides are embedded in OCT compound and cut in a cryostat. It is very important that the first or second cut is obtained in perfect condition otherwise we will be marching towards the surface and abandoning the real margins.

The cryostat should be able to keep a low temperature (between –30° and –26°C) the cutting blade should be very sharp—preferably using a disposable blade. After cutting the tissue we move to the staining of the frozen sections. The most common method is haematoxylin and eosin (H & E) or toluidine blue. Recently a variation has been described using haematoxylin and safranine instead of H & E apparently with superior results in basal cell carcinoma (BCC) and small cell carcinoma (SCC). Recently much investigation has been done on the use of special stains that could help detect tumour cells of difficult tumours among dense infiltrates or around nerves. One can use either immunohistochemical techniques as described by Jimenez *et al.* and Ramnarain *et al.* or immunoperoxidase techniques as described by Mondragon *et al.*

Immunostains can also be used in the treatment of melanoma, even though Mohs' surgery for melanoma remains controversial. The drawback is the increase in expense and time needed in between Mohs' stages.

Indications for Mohs' micrographic surgery

For the treatment of skin cancer, Mohs' micrographic surgery is currently the method that achieves the best cure rate. Another advantage to consider is the preservation of healthy tissue because in Mohs' surgery there is no 'blind' margin of security. This can be of great value for the reconstruction of defects on the face, extremities and genitals. Mohs' micrographic surgery is indicated for BCC and squamous cell carcinomas:

- that are recurrent
- that are more than 2 cm in diameter
- with histologically demonstrated perineural invasion
- that are persistent after previous surgery
- that are located near the orifices of the face, extremities and genitals
- that are invasive histological types
- to check to ensure excision was complete.

Uncommon indications are:

- Bowen's disease
- dermatofibrosarcoma protuberans
- Merckel carcinoma
- other uncommon tumours
- gangrene
- Fungal soft-tissue infections.

Some indications are debatable, in particular melanoma. In the case of melanoma, a complete excision block is the only sound basis for good histological examination as it is so important for establishing what further treatment and follow-up guidelines are required and to determine the prognosis.

It is also important to know what should not be referred for Mohs' surgery:

- multicentric tumours
- patients unable to follow the postoperative rules and to cope with the local anaesthetic in successive stages—cooperation of the patient in this is essential
- Patients with bone invasion or invasion of natural cavities.

Conclusion

In conclusion Mohs' micrographic surgery is a specific surgical method for the treatment of aggressive skin cancers, and

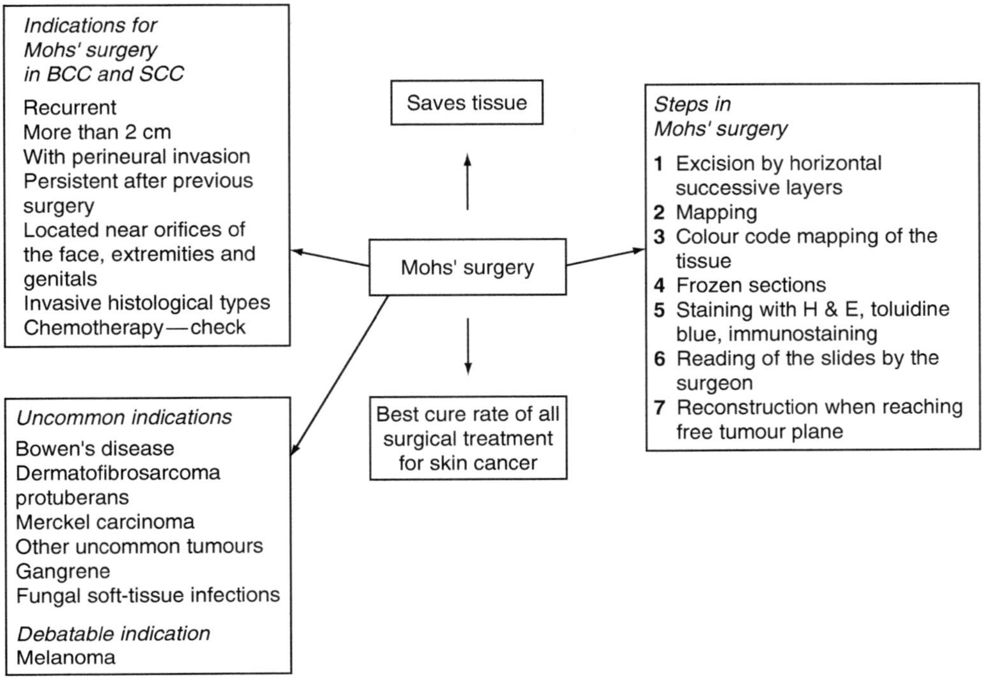

so far achieves the best cure rates of all therapeutic modalities. It is not an expensive method—the cryostat is the only expensive tool and most dermatology services have their own cryostat or easy access to one in general pathology. Proper training and the appropriate referral of patients are essential elements for excellent performance; cooperation with other medical specialists is desirable.

Mohs' micrographic surgery should only be used when necessary and recent studies have found that the referral rate for the treatment of non-melanoma skin cancer will be approximately 30% of all cases seen in a clinic.

In some rare cases Mohs' surgery can be incomplete, either because the cancer has proved to be unresectable, or the patient has been unable to tolerate further surgery. In a study published by S. Madani this happened in 15 out of 10 346 procedures (0.15%).

Further reading

Alcalay J. Digital computerized mapping in Mohs' micrographic surgery. *Dermatol Surg* 2000; 26: 692–3.

Breuninger H. Cirugia micrográfica com cortes en parafina (histologia tridimensional). *Monograf Dermatol* 1990; 3: 233–8.

Brodland DG *et al.* The history and evolution of Mohs' micrographic surgery. *Dermatol Surg* 2000; 26: 303–7.

Cottel WI *et al.* Essentials of Mohs' micrographic surgery. *J Dermatol Surg Oncol* 1988; 14: 11–13.

Gaston DA *et al.* Mohs' micrographic surgery. Referral patterns: the University of Missouri experience. *Dermatol Surg* 1999; 25: 863–7.

Jimenez FJ *et al.* Immunohistochemical techniques in Mohs' micrographic surgery: their potential use in the detection of neoplastic cells masked by inflammation. *J Am Acad Dermatol* 1995; 32: 89.

Madani S *et al.* Unplanned incomplete Mohs' micrographic surgery *J Am Acad Dermatol* 2000; 42: 814–19.

Mohs FE. Excision total del Cancer por control microscópico mediante Cirugia Micrografica de Mohs. Origem y Desarrollo. *Monograf Dermatol* 1990; 3: 200–7.

Mondragon RM *et al.* Current concepts: the use of immunoperoxidase techniques in Mohs' micrographic surgery. *J Am Acad Dermatol* 2000; 43: 66–71.

Picoto AM, Picoto A. Technical procedures for Mohs' fresh tissue surgery. *J Dermatol Surg Oncol* 1986; 12: 134–8.

Ramnarain ND *et al.* Basal cell carcinoma: rapid techniques using cytokeratin markers to assist treatment by micrographic (Mohs') surgery. *Br J Biomed Sci* 1995; 52: 184–7.

Robins P. Historia de la cirugía micrográfica de Mohs (quimiocirurgía). *Monograf Dermatol* 1990; 3: 208–13.

Rowe *et al.* Long-term recurrence rates in previously untreated (primary) basal cell carcinoma. Implications for patient follow-ups. *J Dermatol Surg Oncol* 1989; 15: 315–28.

Sachse RF. Mohs' micrographic surgery for fungal soft tissue infections. *Dermatol Surg* 1999; 25: 308–10.

Tran D. Hematoxylin and safranin O staining of frozen sections. *Dermatol Surg* 2000; 26: 197–99.

Zalla MJ *et al.* Mohs' micrographic excision of melanoma using immunostaining. *Dermatol Surg* 2000; 26: 771–84.

Zitelli JA *et al.* Mohs' micrographic surgery for treatment of primary cutaneous melanoma. *J Am Acad Dermatol* 1997; 37: 236–45.

Patch testing

A. Katsarou

Patch testing is a well-established practical method to diagnose and evaluate allergic contact dermatitis. In the past, because patch test techniques varied, it was difficult to obtain a correct result and to compare results from different dermatology centres. Over the last few decades, much work has been done worldwide, in order to determine the optimal concentration of materials and to standardize allergens, vehicles, tapes, techniques and scoring of reactions. The International Contact Dermatitis Research Group (ICDRG) has set specific guidelines for patch testing that include recommendation for the:

- test systems
- test site
- technique of patch testing
- concentration of allergens
- vehicles
- components of a standard test series
- interpretation of results.

This has greatly facilitated comparisons of patch-test reactivity and conclusions about allergic contact dermatitis between centres in different geographical areas.

Indications for patch testing

The patch test provides objective information about contact allergy. Without it, the diagnosis and management of contact dermatitis are based only on clinical criteria. The socioeconomic consequences of contact allergy are so important that providing the presence or absence is essential. Thus, patch testing is indicated in the following circumstances.

1 In patients with a recurring, eczematous, pruritic dermatitis that is clinically diagnosed as contact dermatitis. In these cases, patch testing can:
   - determine the actual allergens among many clinically suspected allergens
   - detect relevant, but clinically unsuspected, contact sensitizers
   - determine the safety of materials for the patient.

2 In patients with aggravation of other dermatoses, particularly psoriasis, endogenous eczema or leg ulcers, where superimposed contact dermatitis needs to be excluded.

3 As part of a thorough work-up in a patient with a puzzling diagnostic problem.

When patch tests are to be carried out, a number of precautions must be taken in order to obtain a correct result. A detailed clinical history, emphasizing current and previous occupations and products handled, is necessary. In addition to occupation, it is important to identify hobbies and materials handled in connection with these and what, if any, medication is used.

Finally, a complete clinical examination should be carried out.

Test systems

Two types of patch test are used: the original and the ready-to-use system.

Original system

In the original system, the allergens patches and tapes are supplied separately.

Allergens

Contact allergens are simple chemical substances with low molecular weights (>1000 Da). The allergens should be as pure and well defined as possible. According to de Groot, more than 2800 chemicals are identified as sensitizers. Of these, approximately 300 are commercially available from the various suppliers (Trolab/Hermal, Kurt Herrmann, Chemotechnique Diagnostics AB, and others), and the most frequently encountered allergens are included in standard batteries.

The present European Standard Series includes 23 substances. The choice of allergens in the standard series is based on the experience of the members of the ICDRG and on the frequency of positive reactions. If the incidence of positive reactions to an allergen falls to less than 1% it can be removed from the series. Therefore, the composition of the standard series is not constant.

Several additional series are available for patch testing patients with different histories and occupations. Thus, series are available for hairdressing chemicals, metal compounds, cosmetics, medicaments, antimicrobials, preservatives, plants, plastics, glues and rubber chemicals for example.

The most commonly used vehicle for allergens is petrolatum, although a few substances are incorporated in water or other vehicles (ethanol, acetone).

Commercially available allergens are dispensed in individual syringes. Packaging should protect against air, humidity, mechanical damage and radiation. In general, test allergens should be kept in the refrigerator to minimize degradation.

In some cases, the patient may bring a set of suspected substances with which he or she wishes to be patch tested. Due to the risk of irritating or sensitizing the patient, these non-standard substances should not be used for patch testing unless their exact composition, pH and other properties are known. A non-commercially available contact allergen can be used for patch testing after consulting the literature to determine the correct dilution. If the non-standard substances are not described in the literature, control testing of healthy persons should be carried out. Great care must be exercised in the interpretation of test results, since false-positive and false-negative reactions are common when testing with non-standard substances.

The patches

Commercially available patches have a test area that is circular with a diameter of 8–10 mm. The aluminium (AL) test has been a standard method for patch testing for several years. It consists of a filter paper disc or cellulose (10 mm) attached to a strip of plastic-coated aluminium foil and is available in rolls. Currently, the Finn chamber is the most widely used method and it employs 8-mm aluminium or polypropylene cups fixed to strips of Scanpor tape.

The tape

The modern polycrylate-based adhesive tape (Scanpor) eliminates irritant and allergic reactions.

Ready-to-use systems

The thin layer rapid use epicutaneous (TRUE) test is a new system in which a measure of allergen is included in a gel printed on a polyester patch of 9 × 9 mm. These patches, containing different allergens, are mounted onto acrylate tape covered with a siliconized protection sheet and packed in an air-tight, light-impermeable envelope. Epiquick is another ready-to-use patch system that consists of Finn chamber, on Scanpor tape that contains allergens of the standard series in petrolatum.

The advantages of these systems are:

- the constant volume of allergen in the chamber
- uniformity of materials and procedure
- savings in test performance time.

However, the cost is higher. Ready-to-use systems are especially recommended for use in children.

Test sites

The mid-portion of the upper back is the site of the patch-test application. The skin must be hairless and normal. If even a trace of dermatitis is present on the test site, the patient should not be tested at the time, in order to avoid false-positive reactions. If the skin is not hairless, shaving should be done with an electric razor (in order to avoid abrasion), soap and shaving cream. In certain instances, the upper, outer arm can be used to isolate a test allergen when a strong positive reaction is expected, as for example with nickel.

Technique of patch testing

Patch tests should be applied to the upper back on intact skin, without prior use of alcohol or soap. The amount of test material used is important: 12–15 mL of test material, or slightly more than half of the chamber area (for Finn chambers), should be applied. For materials in solution, it is sufficient to place one drop into the filter paper disc and this should be done a few minutes before applying the test in order to avoid evaporation. The physician or technician who is handling the allergen-filled syringes must wear a protective glove to prevent contact allergy.

The tape strips are applied from below with a slight pressure so as to remove air bubbles and obtain uniform and complete contact. In cases of oily or hairy skin, sweating or high humidity, the ends of the strips require additional tape.

The type of series and representative (i.e. top) numbers of the set and should be labelled on the tape. Before removing the patch tests it is important to mark the skin outlining the test area using a water-resistant marking pen that will not stain clothing.

Patients must be given written instructions to keep the patches dry, to reduce work activity, to avoid vigorous exercise and to fix any area that becomes loose with additional tape. If excessive itching or burning occurs at a certain area, the patch may be carefully removed, but all other patches should be left in place to be removed in 48 h.

Interpretation of patch tests

The optimal exposure time is 2 days (48 h). A first reading takes place 30 min after the removal of a patch test. At this time, many irritant reactions can be noticed, caused by occlusion, reactions to allergens or tape. If only a single reading at 48 h is performed, 30% of positive reactions will be missed. Therefore, it is recommended that two readings are performed; the first after the removal of the patches (48 h) and the second 2–4 days later. A positive reaction on day 2 that is negative on day 4 is usually considered to be an irritant reaction. Certain common allergens such as neomycin, organic dyes and corticosteroids may only show late reactions.

The system for interpreting patch test reactions as recommended by the ICDRG, is shown in Table 1. The doubtful and weak reactions are the most difficult to interpret.

Irritant responses can be characterized by:

- erythema without infiltration
- papules in follicular distribution
- pustular reactions especially in atopic individuals from metallic salts
- fine wrinkling
- bullae or necrosis.

Table 1 Interpretation of patch-test reactions according to the ICDRG.

NT	Not tested
–	Negative reaction
?+	Doubtful reaction
+	Weak positive reaction, non-vesicular; erythema, infiltration, papules
++	Strong positive reaction; erythema, infiltration, papules and vesicles
+++	Extreme positive reaction; intense erythema and infiltration, coalescing vesicles, bullae
IR	Irritant reactions (of different types)

Reading only at 48 h may show irritant reactions that disappear within 24 h.

Accuracy of patch testing

Patch tests, like all biological tests, have inherent errors. False-negative or false-positive reactions may occur and the experience of the dermatologist is a very important factor that helps distinguish false reactions.

Causes of false-positive patch test reactions are:

1 Test system factors
- test concentration is too high (i.e. with substances of unknown composition)
- impure or contaminated test substances
- mechanical irritation (pressure, friction, soluble substances)
- pustular reactions to metal salts
- the vehicle is irritant (irritates the skin or enhances allergen penetration)
- adhesive tape reaction
- reaction to the patch (pressure, friction, irritant or allergic reactions).

2 Personal factors
- presence of dermatitis at test site or elsewhere
- lowered natural resistance
- high skin temperature, sweating
- previous exposures to alcohol, solvents, topical cosmetics.

Causes of false-negative patch test reactions:

1 Test system factors:
- test concentration is too low
- allergen is not in active form (i.e. degraded)
- insufficient amount of occlusion
- the vehicle prevents the substance from penetrating the skin.

2 Methodology factors:
- patch applied to site other than upper back (leg, lower arm)
- test read too early (48 h); some substances give delayed reactions (i.e. neomycin).

3 Personal factors:
- prior treatment of test site with topical corticosteroids or ultraviolet irradiation (even 10–15 days earlier)
- systemic medications: corticosteroids (prednisolone >15 mg/24 h), cytostatic agents, cyclosporin A
- anergic phase (available T lymphocytes are involved in clinical reaction).

Cross-reactions

Chemically similar materials may be immunochemically indistinguishable for the skin. Thus, cross-reacting substances (i.e *para*-substances) may give a weaker reaction than the primary allergen. This is an indication to search for the responsible allergen.

Complications of patch testing

The most common complications of patch testing are:
- irritant reactions from products if unknown composition brought in by the patient
- active sensitization
- aggravation of previously existing dermatitis due to percutaneous absorption of allergen
- alterations in pigmentation
- scarring.

This chapter reviews the basic principles of patch testing. Since the methodology of patch testing with substances of unknown composition, fresh samples, the use of open tests, 'use' tests or irritation tests are beyond the scope of this review, the reader is advised to refer to specialized texts.

Further reading

Adams R, Fischer T. Diagnostic patch testing. In: Adams R, ed. *Occupational Skin Diseases*. Saunders, 1990: 221–53.

De Groot AC. *Patch Testing. Test Concentrations and Vehicles for 2800 Allergens*. Amsterdam: Elsevier, 1986.

Fisher TI, Hansen J, Kreilgard B, Maibach HI. The science of patch test standardization. *Immunol Allergy Clin N Am* 1989; 9: 417–43.

Fischer T, Maibach HI. The thin layer rapid use epicutaneous test (TRUE test). A new patch test with high accuracy. *Br J Dermatol* 1985; 112: 63–8.

Katsarou-Katsari A, Katsambas A *et al.* Contact allergens in patients with leg ulcers. *J Eur Acad Dermatol-Venereol* 1998; 11: 9–12.

Lachapelle JM, Tennstedt D, Fryad A *et al.* Ring-shaped positive allergic patch test reactions to allergens in liquid vehicles. *Contact Dermatitis* 1988; 18: 234–6.

Maibach H, Epstein E. Contact dermatitis. In: Middleton E, Reed CE, Ellis EF, eds. *Allergy Principles and Practice*. Missouri: CV Mosby, 1978: 1055–79.

Rietchel RI, Admas RM, Maibach HI *et al.* The case of the patch test reading beyond day 2. *J Am Acad Dermatol* 1988; 18: 42–5.

Rietschel R, Conde-Salazar L, Gossens AN, Veien K. Patch test and prick test techniques. In: *Atlas of Contact Dermatitis*. Martin Dunitz, 1999: 21–38.

Wahlberg JE. Patch testing. In: Rycroft RJG, Menne T, Frosch PJ, eds. *Textbook of Contact Dermatitis*. Berlin: Springer, 1995: 241–68.

Photochemotherapy

C. Antoniou

Photochemotherapy (psoralen and ultraviolet A or PUVA) is a treatment carried out by oral or topically administered psoralens (a linear isomer of furocoumarins) plus UVA light (320–400 nm). At present, the drug most frequently used for this treatment is 8-methoxypsoralen (8-MOP) although 5-methoxypsoralen (5-MOP) and 4,5′,8-trimethylpsoralen (TMP) are also employed.

Broadband UVA sources are used in photochemotherapy. The emission spectra of most UVA units are similar with a peak output around 365 nm.

The general principle of photochemotherapy is to hold the dose of drug and interval between drug administration and UVA exposure constant and vary UVA dose according to each patient's sensitivity.

Treatment schedule

Drug dosimeter

The dose of 8-MOP should be calculated in the range of 0.6–0.8 mg/kg body weight.

The crystalline form of 8-MOP (meladinine 10-mg capsule) produces peak photosensitivity at 2 h. Often a liquid form of 8-MOP (psoralen ultra 10-mg capsule) is used. It has a peak effect at 1.5 h. 5-MOP (Bergapten) is used for those with gastrointestinal upset and is given at a dose of 1.2 mg/kg. Oral TMP (Trisoralen) is often used for the treatment of vitiligo (0.6–1.2 mg/kg). UVA exposure is administered 2 h after drug ingestion.

UVA dosimetry

The starting UVA dose has been based either on skin type or on the minimal phototoxic dose (MPD) (see Table 1).

Treatment regimen

A range of schedules is in common use. Each can be divided into two phases.

- The clearing phase. This uses two to three treatments per week and continues until clearance or until minimal residual disease activity.
- The maintenance phase. This method varies between centres and patients. One treatment per week is often used for 1 month. Thereafter, if a patient remains clear a further reduction towards once monthly can usually be achieved. In general, prolonged maintenance is to be avoided.

The dose of UVA attained at the end of the clearing phase becomes the maintenance dose, maintained or reduced through maintenance.

Monitoring of patients

Protection during therapy

The eyes must be shielded with UVA-opaque glasses. The face, which is the site

Table 1 Recommended initial and incremental UVA exposure according to skin type

Skin type	Initial dose (J/cm^2)	Increments (J/cm^2)
I	0.5–1	0.25–0.5
II	1.0–2.0	0.5
III	1.5–3.0	0.5–1
IV	2.0–4.0	1
V	2.5–5.0	1
VI	3.0–6.0	1.0–1.5

of actinic damage and the genitals in men, should also be protected during exposure.

Protection before and after treatment

From the time of ingestion of psoralens until sunset on the day of treatment, patients must protect their eyes with wraparound UVA-opaque glasses. Patients must also avoid skin exposure to sunlight for the rest of that day.

Evaluation of the patient

As repeat PUVA therapy is often required, it is important to discuss the long-term skin cancer risk with each patient.

Patient (age and sex)

PUVA is relatively contraindicated in children and all females of childbearing potential should practice birth control while on therapy.

Clinical status

Indications

Candidates for PUVA therapy include patients with extensive psoriasis which has not responded to conventional topical therapies, mycosis fungoides, parapsoriasis en plaques, pityriasis lichenoides acuta and chronica, vitiligo, atopic eczema, photodermatoses, lichen planus, graft-versus-host disease, urticaria pigmentosa, pruritus, pruritic eruptions of human immunodeficiency virus (HIV) infection, alopecia areata and others.

Contraindications

Absolute contraindications are:

- xeroderma pigmentosum
- lupus erythematosus
- pregnancy and lactation.

Relative contraindications, where treatment may be used with caution are:

- history of arsenic or ionizing radiation
- history of epithelial malignancy
- conditions potentially aggravated by PUVA, such as certain bullous diseases, cataracts or aphakia, severe cardiovascular, hepatic or renal disease
- childhood.

Physical examination

A complete skin examination is essential to assess the extent and severity of disease, detect skin cancer and evaluate any photoageing.

Examination for phototoxicity

Concomitant use of photosensitizing medications may result in unexpected phototoxicity.

Laboratory investigation

Prior to PUVA therapy a complete blood count, chemistry screening and antinuclear antibody (ANA) count are recommended.

Ophthalmological examination

A complete eye examination for cataracts when initiating PUVA therapy is recommended.

Combination therapies with PUVA

PUVA has been combined with corticosteroids, tars, anthralin, calcipotriene, methotrexate, retinoids and UVB. The objectives for combining PUVA with other treatment modalities are to increase efficacy, reduce short-term and long-term adverse effects and reduce cost of treatment.

PUVA bath

An alternate route of psoralen (either 8-MOP or TMP) delivery is bathwater immersion of the psoriasis patient. Studies of the therapeutic effectiveness of a PUVA bath suggest that the results are at least as effective as with oral PUVA. Advantages proposed for this approach rather than oral administration include lower UVA dose to clear, lower total cumulative dose, the flexibility of treating small areas to avoid unnecessary chronic radiation effect to the whole body, and the lack of systemic symptoms such as nausea and ocular effects. PUVA baths are indicated for patients who cannot tolerate oral PUVA.

Topical 8-MOP has been used in cream, ointment, lotions and liquid vehicles. These preparations are effective with UVA in the treatment of localized psoriasis and vitiligo, but they cause certain problems such as prolonged phototoxic reactions and variable pigmentation. Both TMP and 8-MOP agents are effective in PUVA baths and TMP is a more potent topical photosensitizer than 8-MOP. Therefore, water-delivered 8-MOP is less phototoxic than water-delivered TMP and 8-MOP is less likely to lead to undesirable phototoxic reactions.

Recalcitrant hand and foot psoriasis are also treated with topical PUVA. Guidelines for the use of this are as follows: 1 cm^3 of 1% 8-MOP lotion is added to 2 L of water. Patients submerge the hands and/or feet in the solution in appropriate basins for 30 min. At the end of the soak period, the patients dry the areas and are immediately treated with UVA irradiance. The usual starting dose is 0.5 J/cm^2 for all skin types with an increase of 0.1–0.4 J/cm^2 per UVA exposure, depending on the response.

Adverse effects of PUVA

Adverse effects can be broadly considered as either acute or chronic. They will vary according to: (a) the psoralen used; (b) the UVA dose; and (c) the individual patient, e.g. skin type, idiosyncratic reactions and previous or concurrent treatments.

Acute adverse effects

Psoralen related

Nausea is commonly reported particularly in conjunction with 8-MOP. It may be reduced by taking medication with food or using an antiemetic. Alternatively, the effect can be avoided by using 5-MOP. Headaches, dizziness and perspiration have also been reported as common adverse effects.

PUVA related

An acute phototoxic erythema or sunburn-like reaction 2–3 days after exposure is the most frequently reported adverse effect. Pruritus is another common complaint, and less often a severe pruritus associated with distressing skin pain—so-called 'PUVA pain'. This idiosyncratic response may last for several weeks or months, and it responds poorly to analgesics.

Other reported adverse effects

These include folliculitis, nail pigmentation, photo-onycholysis, facial hypertrichosis and the activation of latent herpes simplex. Tanning from PUVA is not seen as an adverse effect by most patients.

Chronic adverse effects

These include photoageing, a higher incidence of actinic keratoses, PUVA keratoses, PUVA lentigines and most importantly an increased risk of non-melanona skin cancer. Concerns over cataract formation are theoretically justified in that UVA penetrates the lens, as do psoralens.

Malignant melanoma and PUVA

Stern in a recent study reported that about 15 years after the first treatment with PUVA, the risk of malignant melanoma increases, especially among patients who receive 250 treatments or more.

Conclusion

PUVA therapy is an effective and popular treatment. It remains the treatment of choice for extensive, plaque psoriasis resistant to topical therapy.

It is, however, time-consuming and not always available.

Concerns exist over the long-term effects, which suggests the clinician should use this treatment with caution. Skin cancer relates to the accumulative number of treatments. Evidence exists which suggests that those patients who have had more than 150 treatments are at particular risk. Nonetheless, treatment should not be denied to those in need. Discussion of the risks with frequent users is essential.

Further reading

Abel EA. *Photochemotherapy in Dermatology.* New York: Igaku-Shoin Medical Publishers, 1992.

Antoniou C, Petropoulos E, Theocharis S, Hasapi V, Georga E, Katsambas A. Photochemotherapy for mycosis fungoides. *Iatriki* 1997; 72 (3): 290–2.

Frappaz A, Thivolet J. Calcipotriol in combination with PUVA: A randomized double-blind placebo study in severe psoriasis. *Eur J Dermatol* 1993; 3: 351–4.

Gonzalez E. PUVA for psoriasis. *Dermatol Clin* 1995; 13 (4): 851–66.

Lowe NJ, Weingarten D, Bourget T *et al.* PUVA therapy for psoriasis: Comparison of oral and bathwater delivery of 8–methoxypsoralen. *J Am Acad Dermatol* 1986; 14: 754–60.

Momtaz KT, Fitzpatrick TB. Modifications of PUVA. *Dermatol Clin* 1995; 13 (4): 867–73.

Morison WL. *Phototherapy and Photochemotherapy of Skin Disease.* Philadelphia: Decker, 1991.

Morison WL, Momtaz TK, Parrish JA *et al.* Combined methotrexate—PUVA therapy in the treatment of psoriasis. *J Am Acad Dermatol* 1982; 6: 46–51.

Salo OP, Lassus A, Taskinen J. Trioxsalen bath plus UVA treatment of psoriasis. *Acta Dermatonever (Stochkh)* 1981; 61: 551–4.

Ster RS. Malignant melanoma in patients treated for psoriasis with PUVA. *Photodermatol Photoimmunol Photomed* 1999; 15: 37–8.

Stern RS, Laird N. The carcinogenic risk of treatments for severe psoriasis. Photochemotherapy Follow-up Study. *Cancer* 1994; 73: 2759–64.

Stern RS, Nickols KT, Vakeva LH. Malignant melanoma in patients treated for psoriasis with methoxsalen (psoralen) and ultraviolet A radiation (PUVA). The PUVA Follow-up Study. *N Engl J Med* 1997; 336: 1041–5.

Wolff K. Should PUVA be abandoned? *N Engl J Med* 1997; 336: 1090–1.

Wolff K, Gschnait F, Hönigsmann *et al.* Phototesting and Dosimetry for photochemotherapy. *Br J Dermatol* 1977; 96: 1–10.

Photodynamic therapy

A.D. Tosca and M.P. Stefanidou

Photomedicine uses non-ionizing electromagnetic radiation (ultraviolet (UV), visible and infrared) for various treatments, like phototherapy (UVA and UVB light), photochemotherapy (combination of psoralens with UVA light) and photodynamic therapy (PDT). PDT is based on systemic or topical exogenous administration of a photosensitizer (PS) or PS prodrug, its uptake by the target tissue and subsequent light activation aiming to produce selective injury and destruction of the diseased tissue. PSs are molecules which can absorb light energy of specific wavelength and then transfer it to other biological molecules, introducing photochemical reactions, resulting in photobiological response. The principles of action of PDT include: absorption of photon of incident light by the PS, promotion to a higher energy state (singlet or triplet state), transfer to oxygen, generation of highly reactive singlet oxygen, oxidation of biomolecules and cell death. The mechanism of phototoxicity after generation of singlet oxygen and other free radicals is based on oxidization of essential cellular components, vascular damage and/or inflammatory reaction and immune host response. Recent investigations additionally documented that PDT leads to cell cycle deregulation, associated with subsequent apoptotic cell death.

Two main types of photo-oxidative reactions have been described.

- Type I photo-oxidation refers to direct reaction of the excited PS with a substrate by a mechanism involving hydrogen or electron transfer to yield transient radicals, that further react with oxygen.
- In type II photo-oxidative reaction, energy transfer occurs from the excited triplet state of the sensitizer to molecular oxygen, to produce singlet oxygen ($^1O_2$), which can further react with substrates susceptible to oxidation.

The easy accessibility of skin to light exposure has led to an increasing interest for PDT applications in dermatology. PDT is a new, alternative treatment modality for superficial non-melanoma skin tumours and various inflammatory, viral and other diseases, with potentially high effectiveness and low morbidity. PDT is mainly associated with the treatment of cancer, but is also being applied to premalignant and benign diseases.

The success of treatment requires an optimal interplay among different parameters, such as type and drug dose, depth of light penetration into tissue and light dose, treatment schedules, criteria of tumour and patient selection.

The PS can be administered systemically (orally or intravenously) or topically.

The major inconvenience from systemic PS-PDT is generalized photosensitivity lasting for up to 4–8 weeks. During this period, patients must avoid direct sunlight.

Photosensitizers

An efficient photodynamic agent should have several properties: selective retention or uptake by the target tissue, high absorbance in the useful wavelengths' range for optimal tissue penetration, high quantum yield of singlet oxygen, generation and/or electron transfer to substrate molecules, fast clearance from serum and healthy tissue, short time interval between drug administration and its accumulation in the lesion, high chemical purity, low systemic toxicity, lack of side-effects and lack of mutagenic potential.

The time interval between drug administration and sufficient PS concentration determines the time point for light exposure and has been estimated for various PS

Table 1 Photosensitizers used in photodynamic therapy

Photosensitizer	Drug dose	Drug-light interval (h)	Wavelength (nm)
Haematoporphyrin derivative (HpD)	3–5 mg/kg i.v.	40–50	630
Porfimer sodium	0.5–2 mg/kg i.v.	40–50	630
δ-aminolevulinic acid (ALA)	30 mg/kg i.v.	4–6	635
	60 mg/kg oral	4–6	635
	20% topical	3–12	635, visible
Tetrasodium-tetraphenylporphine-sulfonate ($TPPS_4$)	2% topical	4–12	630
	intralesional	4–12	630
Benzoporphyrin derivative-monoacid ring A (BPD-MA)	0.2–0.5 mg/kg i.v.	0.5–2.5	690
N-aspartyl-chlorin e6(Npe6)	0.5–3.5 mg/kg i.v.	4–8	664
Tin etiopurpurin ($SnET_2$)	0.8–1.6 mg/kg i.v.	24–72	660
meta-Tetrahydroxyphenylchlorin (*m*-THPC)	0.1 mg/kg i.v.	72–96	652
Lutetium texapyrin (Lu-Tex)	0.6–7.2 mg/kg i.v.	2–4	732
Chloro-aluminium sulfonated phthalocyanine (CASPc)	0.5–5 mg/kg i.v.	1–3	675–700

and route of administration (Table 1). Irradiation should be performed when an optimal ratio of PS levels in tumour versus normal tissue is reached.

Haematoporphyrin derivatives

Porphyrin-based PS are the most largely used agents in PDT. The first systemically studied PS for clinical use was haematoporphyrin derivative (HpD) at a dose of 3–5 mg/kg of body weight intravenously. The purified compound of HpD, Porfimer sodium (Photofrin) has been approved for systemic PDT in several countries worldwide, for various oncological indications, such as oesophageal and lung cancer. Porfimer sodium is given intravenously at a dose of 0.5–2 mg/kg of body weight, followed by light irradiation at a dose of 200–300 J/cm^2, 2 days after injection.

The absorption spectrum of porphyrins is maximal in the Soret band (400 nm), with 4 smaller peaks between 500 and 635 nm, but the weakest absorption band at 630 nm is usually chosen, because it offers better tissue penetration (1–5 mm), with less interference from absorbance by other biomolecules, such as haemoglobin.

Adverse events

The cutaneous accumulation of HpDs and their slow clearance leads to prolonged photosensitivity, requiring photoprotective measures 2 days prior and 4–8 weeks following PDT. Patients must avoid skin exposure to sunlight, wear sunglasses and clothing to cover most body area and apply sunscreen to exposed regions.

Nausea, vomiting and hypotension are also experienced.

δ-aminolevulinic acid (ALA)

ALA is the natural precursor of protoporhyrin IX (PpIX), an efficient PS, formed endogenously via the biosynthetic pathway of heme. Heme is synthesized from glycine and succinyl-coenzyme A (CoA). The rate-limiting step is their conversion to ALA, which is under negative feedback control by heme. Excess exogenous ALA can bypass the rate-limiting step resulting in accumulation of PpIX in target tissue, such as tumours and hyperproliferative tissues. ALA can be applied topically (ALA 20% in o/w emulsion) under occlusion for 3–6 h and thereafter irradiation with broad-band visible light or monochromatic light at 630–635 nm, or systemically (orally at dose not exceeding 60 mg/kg, intravenously 30 mg/kg).

The introduction of a more lipophilic ester-group (ALA-methylester) seems to enhance the selectivity and deeper penetration of the PS.

Adverse events

Neuropsychiatric disorders correlated with high doses (oral administration > 60 mg/kg, intravenously > 30 mg/kg). Mild, transient nausea and/or transient abnormalities of liver function are noted in systemic administration.

Porphines

Porphines are synthetic porhyrins. Tetrasodium-meso-tetraphenylporphine-sulfonate ($TPPS_4$) has been evaluated for the treatment of skin tumours after topical application (solution 2%) or intralesional administration (0.15–0.3 mg in 0.2 mL saline) and irradiation by light at 630 nm, 4–12 h later.

Adverse events

The main limitation of $TPPS_4$ is its neurotoxicity when administered systemically.

Chlorins

Chlorins, a heterogeneous group of porphyrin- or chlorophyll-derived compounds, have a strong absorption band in the 640–700 nm range.

Benzoporphyrin derivative-monoacid ring A (BPD-MA)

This chlorin is synthesized from protoporphyrin and has been introduced in phase I/II trials for the treatment of skin tumours, such as basal cell carcinomas (BCC) and squamous cell carcinomas (SCC). Photoactivation at 690 nm wavelengths, 30–150 min following intravenous administration of BPD-MA at dose 0.2–0.5 mg/kg of body weight is performed. Because of the rapid clearance from tissues, skin photosensitivity lasts only a few days after PDT.

***N*-Aspartyl-chlorin e6 (Npe6)**

Npe6, a chlorin derived from chlorophyll-α, with a peak absorption at 664 nm, is undergoing clinical trials for the treatment of cutaneous and subcutaneous malignancies with encouraging results. Light is applied 4–8 h after intravenous injection of 0.5–3.5 mg/kg of body weight.

Adverse event

Mild skin photosensitivity.

Tin etiopurpurin ($SnET_2$)

The maximum excitation wavelength is 660 nm. The optimal drug–light interval is within 24–72 h after the intravenous injection of 0.8–1.6 mg/kg of body weight.

Adverse event

Skin photosensitivity which may last for 1 month or longer.

Meta-tetrahydroxyphenylchlorin (m-THPC)

This compound appears to be the most active of all PS, requiring very low drug doses (0.1 mg/kg) and light doses (10 J/cm^2). The maximum activation wavelength is 652 nm.

Adverse event

Mild skin photosensitivity lasting 3–10 days, eschar formation.

Lutetium texapyrin (Lu-Tex)

Lu-Tex is a highly fluorescent dye and absorbs strongly at 732 nm. Its main advantages are high affinity to malignant lesions and lack of significant skin photosensitivity.

Phthalocyanines

Phthalocyanines are synthetic porphyrins, which are under research. They meet several requirements: pure compound, high singlet oxygen quantum yield, low dark toxicity, high tumour-to-tissue ratios 1–3 h after intravenous application and a maximal absorption in the 675–700 nm range, allowing deeper penetration into tissue.

Light sources, light dosimetry

Any source of light having the appropriate spectral characteristics corresponding to the absorption maximum of the PS compound can be used in PDT (Table 2). Initially, PDT has been performed with the use of filtered conventional gas discharge lamps, with relatively low cost, simplicity and reliability. Lasers equipped with optical fibres have been largely used in PDT. Lasers emit monochromatic coherent light and provide the exact selection of specific wavelengths in the drug-activation range and maximal effective tissue penetration. The tunable argon-dye laser emits continuously light in the 450–530 nm range and is tunable to 350–700 nm. Pulsed lasers, such as gold vapour laser (628 nm), copper vapour laser-pumped dye laser (510–578 nm), Nd : YAG laser (690–1110 nm) have been also used in PDT. The development of portable diode lasers (gallium–aluminium–arsenid laser), producing light in the range of 770–850 nm, is a new approach to PDT. The laser systems are expensive and require frequent repair. Incoherent light sources, such as a short-arc xenon lamp, tunable over a band-width of 400–1200 nm, halogen lamp, such as the PDT 1200-lamp (Waldmann) emitting 600–800 nm radiation have been used.

The selection of light source is a matter of debate. It has been suggested that the use of a broad-band light source may have an advantage over narrow-band monochromatic laser and enhanced therapeutic results, by activating effectively the *in vivo* produced photoproducts, which represent additional PS with different absorption maximum. So, full-spectrum visible light (400–760 nm) could be superior for thin skin lesions.

The energy fluence (J/cm^2) delivered to the tissue is the product of the fluence rate (mW/cm^2) and the time of irradiation. Doses of light applied in PDT are commonly within 60–200 J/cm^2 (25–540 J/cm^2) depending on the location, size and histopathological type of the lesion. To avoid hyperthermia, a fluence rate lower than 100 mW/cm^2 should be used.

Table 2 Light sources for clinical photodynamic therapy

Light source	Wavelength (nm)
Incoherent, wavelength-filtered lamps	
500 W tungsten filament (slide projector)	> 600
300 W short-arc xenon lamp	400–1200
250 W halogen lamp	620–640
1200 W halogen lamp (Waldmann)	600–800
Lasers	
Tunable argon-dye	450–530
Pulsed gold vapour	628
Pulsed copper vapour-pumped dye	510–578
Neodymium : YAG	690–1100
He-Ne	632.8
Gallium–aluminium–arsenid	770–850

Topical PDT with ALA

Formulation

Recently a cream containing ALA 20% has been marketed for topical PDT for actinic keratoses and is commercially available in several countries. A freshly prepared o/w based cream of ALA 20% can also be used.

Skin preparation

After cleansing the whole area with sterile saline solution and removing crusts, approximately 50 mg/cm^2 of cream is applied to the lesion with a margin of about 1 cm beyond the visible borders, and is kept under occlusive dressing for 3–6 h, followed by irradiation. In general, no anesthesia or sedation is necessary, but the use of 2% lidocaine (lignocaine) gel or cream containing 2.5% lidocaine and 2.5% pilocaine, or intracutaneous injection of 1% lidocaine is often required.

PDT irradiation

The light dose is 60–250 J/cm^2 with power density of 50–150 mW/cm^2 when a laser is used, whereas the light dose is 30–540 J/cm^2 with dose rates ranging from 50 to 300 mW/cm^2 when a lamp is used.

Protection after treatment

Following the PDT session, it is recommended that no sunlight exposure should take place for the rest of the day. The patients must be warned to expect some skin changes such as erythema and oedema locally, crusting or erosion.

Evaluation of the patient

The clinical response is evaluated 1–1.5 months after treatment.

Complications

- Immediate: excessive pain and oedema.
- Delayed: bacterial superinfection, ulceration, hyperpigmentation, minimal atrophic scar.

Poor response factors

BCC

- Localization on the nose or the eyelid.
- High pigmentation (pigmented BCC).
- Sclerodermiform histological subtype.
- Thickness of the lesion.

Actinic keratosis (AK)

- Localization on the forearm or the dorsum of the hand.
- Thick hyperkeratotic AK.

Improvement of the therapeutic effectiveness

- Repeated treatment sessions, particularly for the nodular BCC, enabling the destruction of the entire tumour volume.
- A curettage procedure to reduce tumour volume and remove the surface layer can be tried.
- The penetration of ALA into deeper portions of the lesion could be increased by prolonging the time of ALA application to 12–48 h, or by using skin penetration enhancers such as dimethyl sulfoxide (DMSO), ethylenediamine tetra-acetic acid (EDTA), 1,10-phenanthroline, in combination with protoporphyrin IX synthesis inducers such as desferrioxamine, which competes with ferrochelatase for ionic iron and inhibits synthesis of heme.

Indications

The best indications for topical ALA-PDT are:

- widespread actinic keratoses
- superficial BCC
- nodular BCC, less than 2 mm thick
- actinic cheilitis
- Bowen's disease
- *in situ* and early invasive SCC and as an adjuvant therapeutic tool in advanced SCC
- naevoid BCC syndrome

Promising results are observed in:

- Kaposi's sarcoma
- mycosis fungoides
- perianal extramammary Paget's disease
- erythroplasia of Queyrat
- keratoacanthoma.

Other potential indications are:

- psoriasis
- acne
- viral diseases (verruca vulgaris, condyloma acuminatum, epidermodysplasia verruciformis)
- hypertrichosis, hirsutism
- alopecia areata
- lichen planus.

In conclusion, topical ALA-PDT does have the following advantages over conventional treatments:

- it is a useful alternative modality, suitable for the treatment of large or multiple superficial epithelial tumours in anatomically difficult areas, where invasive methods are less applicable
- it is non-invasive, available on an outpatient basis
- it is recommended for older patients, patients with poor compliance, as well as patients with other health problems such as having pacemakers or bleeding tendency
- it is well tolerated by patients
- it has no toxicity or interaction with other medications
- it can be used as a palliative treatment, and can be repeated without cumulative toxicity
- it produces excellent cosmetic results.

Further reading

Agarwal ML, Clay ME, Harvey EJ *et al.* Photodynamic therapy induces rapid cell death by apoptosis in L5178Y mouse lymphoma cells. *Cancer Res* 1991; 51: 5993–6.

Alvanopoulos K, Antoniou C, Petrou M, Vareltzidis A, Katsambas A. Photodynamic therapy of superficial basal cell carcinomas using exogenous 5-aminolevulinic acid and 514-nm light. *JEADV* 1997; 9: 134–6.

Balas CJ, Stefanidou MP, Giannouli TC *et al.* A modular diffuse reflection and fluorescence emission imaging colorimeter for the in-vivo study of parameters related with the phototoxic effect in photodynamic therapy. *SPIE* 1997; 3191: 50–7.

Ceburkov O, Gollnick H. Photodynamic therapy in dermatology. *Eur J Dermatol* 2000; 10: 568–76.

Dougherty TJ, Gomer CJ, Henderson BW *et al.* Photodynamic therapy. *J Natl Cancer Inst* 1998; 90: 889–905.

Fritsch C, Goerz G, Ruzicka T. Photodynamic therapy in dermatology. *Arch Dermatol* 1998; 134: 207–14.

Jori G. Tumour photosensitizers: approaches to enhance the selectivity and efficiency of photodynamic therapy. *J Photochem Photobiol B: Biol* 1996; 36: 87–93.

Kalka K, Ahmad N, Feyes DKF, Mukhtar H. P53-dependent induction of WAF1/p21 during PDT-mediated apoptosis and ablation of mouse skin tumors. *Photochem Photobiol* 1999; 69(Suppl): 7S.

Kalka K, Merk H, Mukhtar H. Photodynamic therapy in dermatology. *J Am Acad Dermatol* 2000; 42: 389–413.

Korbelik M. Induction of tumor immunity by photodynamic therapy. *J Clin Laser Med Surg* 1996; 14: 329–34.

Peng Q, Berg K, Moan J, Kongshaug M, Nesland JM. 5-Aminolevulinic acid-based photodynamic therapy: principles and experimental research. *Photochem Photobiol* 1997; 65(2): 235–51.

Peng Q, Warloe T, Berg K *et al.* 5 Aminolevulinic acid based photodynamic therapy. *Cancer* 1997; 79: 2282–308.

Stefanidou M, Tosca A, Themelis G, Vazgiouraki E, Balas C. In vivo fluorescence kinetics and photodynamic therapy efficacy of α-aminolevulinic acid-induced porphyrin in basal cell carcinomas and actinic keratoses; implications for optimization of photodynamic therapy. *Eur J Dermatol* 2000; 10: 351–6.

Szeimies RM, Calzavara-Pinton PG, Karrer S, Ortel B, Landthaler M. Topical photodynamic therapy in dermatology. *J Photochem Photobiol B: Biol* 1996; 36: 213–19.

Tosca AD, Balas CJ, Stefanidou MP *et al.* Photodynamic treatment of skin malignancies with aminolevulinic acid. Emphasis on anatomical observations and in vivo erythema visual assessment. *Dermatol Surg* 1996; 22: 929–34.

Tosca AD, Balas CJ, Stefanidou MP *et al.* Prediction of ALA-PDT efficacy through remote color inspection and post therapy sequential histologic observations of skin malignancies. *SPIE* 1997; 3191: 221–30.

Sclerotherapy

E. Del Bianco, G. Muscarella and P. Cappugi

Definition and indications

Sclerotherapy consists of intravenous injection of sclerosing agents that produce damage of endothelial cells and cause thromboses, fibrosis and stenosis.

We will discuss the use of sclerotherapy in the treatment of minor branch vein varicosities not associated with saphenous incompetence, new branch vein varicosities developing after appropriate surgery and venule telangiectases.

Varicose veins are enlarged, tortuous, ectatic veins more than 2 mm in diameter, placed in the deep derma and in the subcutaneous tissue. It is possible to distinguish primary and secondary varicose veins. The latter originate from a thrombotic occlusion of one or more deep veins and are often associated with abnormal valvular function.

Telangiectases are small (diameter less than 2 mm), with visible blood vessels placed in the dermis that are permanently dilated. The occurrence is prevalent in women: more than half of European and American women are affected by telangiectases.

Varicose veins and telangiectases

Primary varicose veins are seen in families and are hereditary. Various factors could be responsible for their pathogenesis such as hormones, pregnancy or prolonged standing. Pregnancy is one of the most common causes of varicosity because of venous relaxation due to increased hormone levels, expansion of blood volume and increased venous pressure especially in the limb where the iliac vein is compressed by the enlarged uterus. Also thrombophlebitis leads to formation of varicose veins by destroying venous valves. Venous dilatation is the first mechanism that leads to incompetence of the valves and increased venous pressure distally and also at the capillary level.

Pathogenesis of telangiectases is related to many different pathological processes affecting the blood vessel endothelium and its supporting structures. Some situations are often connected with telangiectases such as the presence of varicose veins, hormonal factors and physical factors.

Clinical characteristics and course

Clinical evaluation of patients is fundamental before beginning sclerotherapy in order to determine the feasibility of this treatment as a primary mode.

Superficial venous insufficiency is common in a young, working population.

Varicose veins are visible as dilated, tortuous, sacculated, superficial veins often thick-walled. They can result in disability because of chronic pain, inflammation, and/or ulceration.

However, in most patients, telangiectases may be the only abnormality noted on clinical examination and they are not associated with symptoms. They appear on the skin as small, red, linear, stellate or punctate markings, usually treated for aesthetic purpose and so the occurrence of minor complications is less acceptable for patients.

Diagnosis

Diagnosis of superficial venous insufficiency is usually based only on clinical observation.

The need for laboratory data should be assessed on an individual basis. They are usually necessary in patients with hypercoagulability or severe venous symptoms.

Vascular tests such as duplex scanning, venous Doppler study, phlebography, photoplethysmography, light reflection rheography and others, should be reserved for those patients with venous symptoms and/or large vessel incompetence or large numbers of spider telangiectases indicating venous hypertension.

Instrumental examinations become useful in order to find a correct therapeutic strategy and to follow-up the treatment.

However for limited telangiectases, less than 1 mm in diameter, vascular diagnostic tests are usually unnecessary.

Therapy

The treatment of varicose and telangiectatic leg veins can be approached in a logical and systematic fashion. In fact it is demonstrated that venous regions or entire abnormal superficial venous networks related to incompetent perforators should be injected in a single session, instead of randomly injecting as many veins as possible in a given period of time. Each patient requires differing amounts of time for this systematic approach.

It is important that dermatologists with an interest in phlebology do not limit treatment to telangiectatic veins but consider the complete system, with the possibility that the dermal telangiectatic component is not a separate skin disorder but is a manifestation of a deep venous disease.

Sclerosing solutions

Several sclerosing solutions are used for the treatment of varicose and telangiectatic leg veins. Each solution has a unique safety and efficacy profile. The type, concentration and quantity of solution selected are determined by the type and/or site of varicose vein injected.

These substances work in two ways (Fig. 1): one depends on dehydration of endothelial cells by osmotic action with resultant injury, inflammation and thrombus formation; the other depends on endothelial cell surface tension alteration with direct damage of the endothelial cell and resulting inflammation and thrombus formation. They have the ability to denature biological molecules irreversibly within the vein wall.

Hypertonic saline (23.4% sodium chloride) with or without lidocaine (lignocaine) and heparin, is a dehydrating

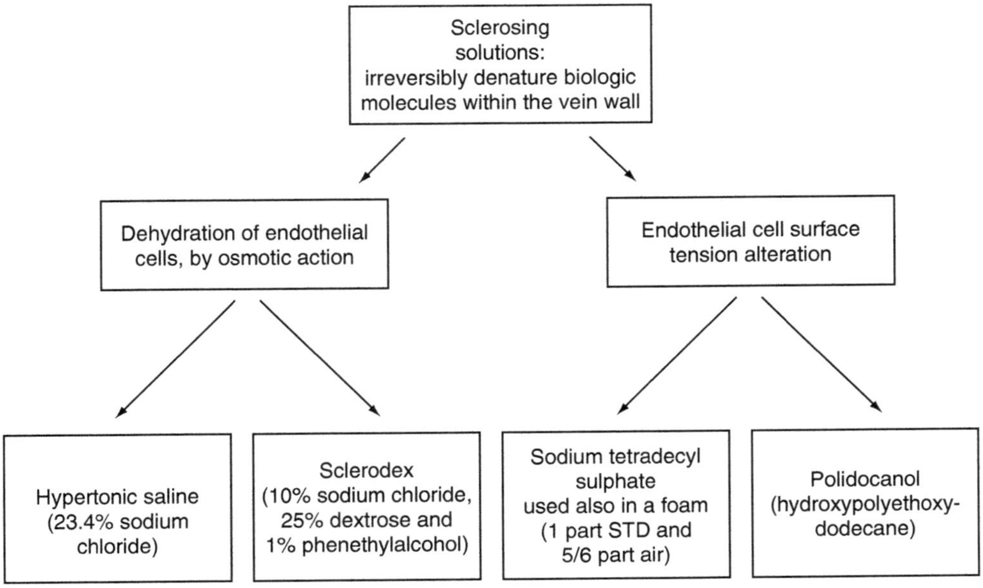

Figure 1

sclerosing agent. It is effective and extensively used in Europe for the treatment of minor varicosity and telangiectases. The Food and Drug Administration (FDA) of the USA has approved it only as an abortifacient and not as a sclerosant. It causes moderate pain on injection with occasional muscle cramps and risk of ulceration at the site of extravasation. One of the major advantages of this agent, when used pure, is the absence of adverse allergenic reactions.

Sclerodex (10% sodium chloride, 25% dextrose and 1% phenethylalcohol) is a dehydrating agent that is very effective and often used in Europe for the treatment of minor varicosity and telangiectases but it lacks FDA approval. The low concentration of chloride associated with anionic dextrose decreases injection pain and muscle cramps.

Sodium morrhuate derived from cod liver oil and sodium tetradecyl sulphate (STD) are the only sclerosing solutions approved by the FDA. The first is a surface-tension acting agent that is rarely used because of its side-effects (among which are anaphylactic reactions). The second have the same mechanism of action and is often used for varicose veins and, in a dilute form, for the treatment of telangiectases. The use of STD in a sclerosing foam (Tessari's method) mixing 1 part liquid STD and 5/6 parts air was recently indicated to give good results.

Polidocanol (hydroxypolyethoxydodecane) (POL) is a surface-tension acting agent, currently undergoing review for FDA approval. As regards POL effectiveness data are discordant. An Australian study demonstrates that the effectiveness of POL was superior to STD (85%) and hypertonic saline (84%). Ninety per cent of investigators considered that POL has less frequent complications that STD and 80% considered that these were less severe. Nevertheless a recent blinded comparative study obtained the same results with 20% hypertonic solution or 1% POL, but POL caused more staining and matting and patient satisfaction was higher with hypertonic solution.

Technique

The veins must be carefully marked out with the patient standing, also inserting needles into the varicosities with the patient standing.

The sclerosing solution is injected into the vessel with a 30-gauge or smaller needle to maintain the needle parallel to the skin surface it is useful to flex it before insertion. The vessel is carefully cannulated under magnification and a small amount of sclerosing solution is injected until the vessel and interconnecting vessels are filling. Injecting a small amount of air before the sclerosing solution could be useful to determine whether the vessel has been cannulated.

The site of injection depends on individual experience. Normally, two or three points are selected on a very long anterolateral thigh vein, whereas one injection will suffice for short tributaries.

As regards the quantity of sclerosant injectable the normal rule among sclerotherapists is that no more than 0.1–1.0 mL of sclerosant per injection site should be used even though this recommendation has never been subjected to any scientific study. It is not unlikely that these quantities are a carry-over from the original study that goes back to an article dated 1930.

Concentrations utilized range from 0.2% to 3.0%, depending on the vein size and on the volume injected: when a higher concentration is injected, a smaller volume would be used.

Zummo tried to standardize quantities and concentrations of different sclerosing agents depending on the type of veins malformations to treat, suggesting that therapy must be adapted for each patient.

Empty vein technique

The empty vein technique is used in the sclerotherapy of varicose veins. It is sufficient to place the patient supine and keep the leg up to achieve nearly complete emptying of the veins. A major advantage of this technique is that it is obtained with a minimal dilution of sclerosant agent and a lower concentration of it can be injected; use of a lower concentration permits use of a higher volume.

Postsclerotherapy compression

In general telangiectases less than 1 mm in diameter may require no compression. However some veins may be more effectively treated with compressive dressing. This may be accomplished by multiple techniques including bandaging and stockings. Bandage dressing could be elastic or not although the non-elastic are more commonly utilized. Compression bandages are recommended for patients with oedema. Graduated compression stockings are available in different models. The type to choose is dependent by the physical attributes of the injected leg as well as the type of varicosity treated. Graduated stockings are usually left on the leg during the entire time of treatment or removed when the patient is lying down.

Immediate and sustained compression diminishes the volume of intraluminal thrombus, minimizing the duration required for complete resorption of the vein. In fact when a vein has undergone mural disruption it still has enough intact long intraluminal space to be distended by blood which rapidly becomes coagulated.

The duration of compression depends on the size of the vein as well as its intraluminal venous pressure. Normally, it would be required for 2–8 weeks after treatment. However compression enhances the results of sclerotherapy that are directly correlated with duration of compression. Further it leads to a reduction of postsclerotherapy hyperpigmentation.

The degree of compression applied can vary from 30 to 50 mmHg and is evaluated on the basis of hydrostatic pressure within the vein: the greater the hydrostatic pressure, the greater must be the externally applied compression.

Complications

The most common and cosmetically significant side-effects of sclerosing agents are hyperpigmentation, telangiectatic matting and cutaneous necrosis.

Hyperpigmentation consists of the appearance of persistent increased pigmentation, caused by haemosiderin deposition, running the course of an ectatic blood vessel treated by sclerotherapy. It appears related to solution strength, vessel fragility, site of the vessel treated, injection pressure and the type of solution used. It has been reported that elevated serum ferritin level plays a role in postsclerotherapy pigmentation, but Scott and Senger do not confirm this theory, so further studies are needed.

The general incidence of hyperpigmentation ranges from 10 to 30%. Although it may persist for months its presence rarely deters patients from continuing treatment. Spontaneous resolution occurs in 70% at 6 months and 99% within 1 year.

Telangiectatic matting is a recognized complication occurring in 15–20% patients treated. It represents a revascularization in the treated area, with vessels much smaller than the original sclerosed vessel. The exact mechanism of the phenomenon remains unknown. However it seems to play an important role in reactivation of inflammation and/or a neo-angiogenic mechanism. Telangiectatic matting is usually not permanent and resolves spontaneously within 3–12 months.

Cutaneous necrosis may occur with the injection of any sclerosing agent even under ideal circumstances and does not represent a physician error. Recently some authors hypothesized that this phenomenon could be due to the presence of arteriovenous shunts under telangiectases. They suggest a maximum of 0.2 mL of sclerosant to be administered to a single site in order to prevent skin ulceration. When sclerosant extravasation occurs, dilution is needed immediately. However with careful technique and appropriate treatment of extravasation, necrosis can almost be avoided.

Thrombi may be seen within 1 week of injection, especially in larger (1–4 mm) treated vessels. They may produce pain that can be relieved by incising the vessels and expressing the thrombus.

The only systemic reactions that have been seen are allergic, such as urticaria but also anaphylactic reactions. Sodium morrhuate and sotradecol have significant allergenic potential, while polidocanol has only a 0.01% reported rate of allergic reaction and with sclerodex and hypertonic saline no allergic reactions have been seen yet.

In order to minimize side-effects and reduce their incidence it is necessary for physicians to understand the potential causes of complications following sclerotherapy:

- to advise patients prior to beginning the treatment on the common risk involved in sclerotherapy and on the relative incidence
- to understand the concept of minimal sclerosant concentration and how it can help to choose sclerosing solution concentrations to minimize risks.

Further reading

American Academy of Dermatology. Guidelines of care for sclerotherapy treatment of varicose and telangiectatic leg veins. *J Am Acad Dermatol* 1996; 34 (3): 523–8.

Bihari I, Magyar E. Reasons for ulceration after injection treatment of telangiectasia. *Dermatol Surg* 2001; 27 (2): 133–6.

Conrad P, Malouf GM, Stacey MC. The Australian polidocanol (Aethoxysklerol) study. Results at two years. *Dermatol Surg* 1995; 21 (4): 334–6.

Goldman MP, Sadick NS, Weiss RA. Cutanous necrosis, telangiectatic matting, and hyperpigmentation following sclerotherapy. Etiology, prevention, and treatment. *Dermatol Surg* 1995; 21 (1): 19–29.

Goldman PM. Polidocanol (Aethoxysklerol) for sclerotherapy of superfical venules and telangiectasias. *J Dermatol Surg Oncol* 1989; 15: 204.

Green D. Sclerotherapy for the permanent eradication of varicose veins: theoretical and practical considerations. *J Am Acad Dermatol* 1998; 38: 461–75.

Higgins TT, Kittel PB. The use of sodium morrhuate in treatment of varicose veins by injection. *Lancet* 1939; 1: 68–9.

McCoy S, Evans A, Spurrier N. Sclerotherapy for leg telangiectasia—a blinded comparative trial of polidocanol and hypertonic saline. *Dermatol Surg* 1999; 25 (5): 381–5.

Puissegur LML. Sclerotherapy: review of results and complications in 200 patients. *Dermatol Surg Oncol* 1989; 15: 214.

Scott C, Seiger E. Postsclerotherapy pigmentation. Is serum ferritin level an accurate indicator? *Dermatol Surg* 1997; 23 (4): 281–2.

Tessari L, Cavezzi A, Frullini A. Preliminary experience with a new sclerosing foam in the treatment of varicose veins. *Dermatol Surg* 2001; 27 (1): 58–60.

Weiss RA, Goldman MP. Advances in sclerotherapy. *Dermatol Clin* 1995; 13 (2): 431–45.

Weiss RA, Weiss MA. Incidence of side effects in the treatment of telangiectasias by compression sclerotherapy: hypertonic saline vs. polidocanol. *J Dermatol Surg Oncol* 1990; 16: 800.

Zummo MG. Cloutier's sclerotherapy of varices. *Plebologie* 1991; 44(1): 37–43.

Skin augmentation (fillings)

L. Rusciani and S. Petraglia

General principles

Traditional aesthetic surgery enables excellent results to be obtained with many defective conditions of the face or body contour. However, there are defects that are not susceptible to satisfactory correction by using exclusively 'pure' surgical techniques. These conditions respond very well to soft-tissue augmentation techniques.

For some centuries, physicians have tried to achieve soft-tissue augmentation, using substances such as bee's wax, paraffin wax and mineral oils, but only in the last decade have these attempts achieved the desired results. This is due both to the discovery of new materials, suitable for injection into subcutaneous tissue, and to more refined techniques. The combination of ideal material and right technique enables many defects to be corrected very well. Some of the defects susceptible to improvement or correction by soft-tissue augmentation are:

- cutaneous ageing (furrows, wrinkles)
- expression wrinkles
- depressed scars
- lip augmentation and shaping
- profile defects of the face
- corns and callosity.

The existence of many filling substances suggests that the perfect material has not yet been discovered. The important characteristics of the ideal material are numerous. It should be:

- non-allergic
- inert
- biocompatible
- sterile
- unpyogenic
- non-cancer producing
- unpainful for the patient
- easy to prepare and implant
- stable
- incapable of migrating
- able to resist in tissues without causing inflammatory reactions
- permit a normal social life to the patient shortly after the implantation
- not excessively expensive.

Unfortunately, at the moment, no substance that meets all these criteria has been found yet. Therefore, careful patient selection, in terms of the defect to be corrected and availability of the most suitable material for each case, is fundamental.

The necessity to minimize risks and collateral effects is made even more important by the fact that soft-tissue augmentation techniques are very often used for aesthetic and cosmetic purposes; even the slightest collateral effect could be intolerable for the patient.

Identifying the ideal patient

The first step is to identify a suitable patient; it is fundamental to examine the defect for correction accurately, and compare the patient's expectations with actual correction possibilities. It is very important to assemble an accurate clinical history, underlining such conditions as allergic diathesis, cutaneous infections, and autoimmune pathologies that contraindicate the implant of a particular substance.

Cutaneous fillings

The first substance successfully employed in cutaneous filling was silicone, to which, in the long run, bovine collagen, autologous fat, jaluronic acid, Gore-tex, Fibrel, Poly-L-Lactic acid and polyacrilamide have been added (see below). Every substance presents some features that make it, case by case, the best choice. New materials and new techniques are still being studied and, among these, the most interesting seems to be autologous collagen, whose long-term results are still being analysed.

Soft-tissue augmentation techniques present further advantages: they have low costs, can be performed in ambulatory sites and usually without anaesthesia or with minimal local anaesthetic and, particularly, almost immediately enable the desired result to be obtained, without postoperative anaesthetic compromise.

Silicone

Silicone is the term generally employed to mean a series of polymers with different degrees of viscosity. Silicone has been employed as a filler substance since the beginning of the 20th century, but imperfect formulations and the presence of impurities have involved considerable collateral effects. The silicone employed at present is fluid polydimetilsiloxane with a viscosity of 350 n, sterile and filtered to eliminate impurities (injectable-grade silicone). It is a clear and oily fluid, odourless, colourless and it can be stored at room temperature. When correctly injected into tissue, i.e. with the microdroplet technique (0.1–0.3 ml) it places itself between the dermis and the subcutaneous tissue, causing a minimum inflammatory reaction and stimulating the formation of thin bundles of collagen. Of all the implantation substances, silicone can be considered the most inert. The stimulation it causes in fibroblasts is, on the other hand, advantageous from a cosmetic point of view. The volume increase so obtained is definitive, because silicone remains in tissues and is not degradable. In 1976 the Food and Drugs Administration (FDA) of the USA withdrew silicone from the market, after reports of autoimmune pathologies resulting from silicone implants. This decision has caused a debate, which is ongoing. In fact, it has not been possible to demonstrate the production of antisilicone antibodies. The studies carried out so far have failed to demonstrate any direct relationship between microimplants of pure silicone and immune pathologies. Even large implants seem to be unable to cause any immunopathological reactions: in these cases, the only problem can be the possibility of a migration of silicone from the implant site, giving aesthetically unsatisfactory results.

Silicone implants are best indicated in the presence of depressed scars, deep furrows and wrinkles, face contour defects, facial atrophy and lip hypoplasia. It is not indicated for the correction of fibrous scars, of the thinnest wrinkles, the palpebral ones and of those subject to changes in time. It can be employed for the volume increase of organs such as breast and genitals, but only if appropriately encapsulated. The main contraindication is the patient's psychological lability, because the corrections achieved with silicone are definitive. Before undertaking the implant it is necessary to gather an accurate clinical history. No previous tests are required, because silicone is non-allergic.

The technique of implantation requires the use of a minimum quantity of silicone (usually <0.1 mL). The area to be treated is accurately cleansed and disinfected. It is advisable to use long tuberculin-type syringes with a 30-gauge needle. The angle of insertion for the needle is acute if silicone has to be implanted superficially in the dermis. For larger defects that require a deeper implant between the dermis and the subcutaneous fat a more obtuse insertion angle, close to 90°, should be used. With the microdroplet technique that allows better results to be achieved, many injections are performed (up to 50) at a distance of a few millimetres. Every injection consists of 0.005–0.01 mL of silicone.

It is important to avoid injecting fluid into vessels because of the risk of embolism. It is fundamental to avoid hypercorrection, since silicone is non-reabsorbable: therefore it is better to hypo-correct the defect and successively perform a second implant, if needed, so as to obtain the desired effect. Sometimes a local anaesthetic may be necessary. Moreover, injection of small quantities of anaesthetic can help to undermine tissues, making the implant easier.

Among collateral effects after the injection, it is possible for an erythema with oedema and occasionally ecchymosis to occur. These are transitory symptoms caused by trauma due to injection. Granulomatous reactions in several areas have been described. To minimize their incidence, special care must be taken to avoid treating infected or acne subject areas and to inject an excessive quantity of silicone. These lesions respond well to systemic or intralesional corticosteroids and to systemic antibiotics.

It is possible to observe a migration of silicone, especially if injected in a large quantity. Migration of silicone to distant sites has also been described, probably due to transport via phagocytes or as a microembolism. This migration, however, does not give rise to pathological reactions.

In our practice we have never met any significant collateral effect and silicone implants have always proved to be safe and very satisfactory for the permanent correction of defects such as facial atrophy and acne scars.

Bovine collagen

In 1981 a purified dermal bovine collagen (Zyderm) suitable for soft-tissue augmentation was introduced to the market. During the following years it has quickly become the most utilized filler, because it is very safe if employed in the correct way.

Zyderm consists of bovine collagen type I (95%) and III (5%) at 35% in physiological saline with 0.3% lidocaine (lignocaine). Subsequently, Zyderm II, which is identical to Zyderm I, but more concentrated (65%) and Zyplast, that is cross-linked bovine collagen with the addition of glutaraldehyde and lidocaine at 0.3%, were introduced to the market. All these subtypes are prepared in tuberculin-type syringes with 30-gauge needles and need to be preserved at low temperature.

Once implanted in the superficial and medium dermis, Zyderm disperses between the collagen bundles. It is then colonized by scarce fibroblasts that remain inactive. It does not stimulate collagen production or glycose amine glicans and, in a period of 6–9 months it disperses and disappears because of its degradation and migration to the deep dermis.

Zyplast, in contrast, creates some sediments between the collagen fibres and is afterwards colonized by rather active fibroblasts. It seems to be able to stimulate the formation of new collagen, but in a period of 9–12 months it disappears too because of degradation or migration to the subcutaneous fat. The reabsorption of the implant means that the treatment needs to be repeated every 6–12 months. This could be regarded as an advantage because every collateral effect or aesthetically unpleasant result will never be definitive.

The main contraindication for its use is the presence of an allergic diathesis. A previous history of anaphylaxis is an absolute contraindication for bovine collagen implantation. However, a previous test with a minimum quantity injected into the superficial dermis of the volar surface of the forearm is needed. This test has to be read after 48 h and then after 4 weeks. A positive reaction is denoted by the development of an erythematous and itching nodule after the first 24 h. About 3% of patients have a positive result to this test. A delayed response might also arise in patients who may be considered as having a negative result after the test (0.5–1%) because of their delayed response to the challenge. For this reason, it is now suggested these patients should be given a second test, but on the other forearm. Usually, two tests are enough, because

90% of allergic reactions take place within the second bovine collagen administration.

After intolerance to bovine collagen has been excluded, it will be possible to start treatment. As with every other filler, it is necessary to gather an accurate clinical history, and explain to the patient what could be a realistic outcome. In case of fever or pregnancy it is better to postpone the implant. The lesions susceptible to improvement are:

- wrinkles
  the finest ones (Zyderm I and II)
  the deep ones (Zyderm II and Zyplast), including the glabellar ones (Zyderm I and II but not Zyplast because of the risk of necrosis)
  the periocular ones
- acne scars (excluding the fibrotic and bound-down ones)
- depressed scars
- lip shaping
- circumoral creases
- Perlèche
- facial contour deformities (Zyplast)
- corns and callosity

With regard to scars, it is advisable to inject them with physiological saline, to test for the tissue resistance and thus avoid treating non-distensible ones. The correction endurance varies either according to the type of collagen employed (Zyplast implants last longer) or to the lesion. Correction of those lesions exposed to facial mimic and the natural ageing process will last for less time than that of stabilized lesions, such as scars. It is therefore necessary to repeat the treatment every 6–12 months.

The implant can be performed at two levels:

- in superficial dermis with Zyderm I and II and a needle angle of 45°
- in deep dermis with Zyplast, and a needle angle of 30°.

When Zyderm is being implanted, the lesion needs to be hypercorrected, because saline solution is reabsorbed within 24 h. Whitening at the injection sites is a sign of correct implantation. Whitening and hypercorrection are to be avoided with Zyplast. In this case the correctness of the implant is verifiable by palpation.

There are two techniques for implantation:

- serial puncture technique, i.e. superficial injections along the lesion
- linear technique, having submined the lesion with the needle.

Their choice depends mostly on the surgeon's dexterity, however the multiple puncture technique is preferable in cases of thin wrinkles.

After the implant, the area is gently massaged in order to achieve a uniform distribution of the matter. Anaesthesia of the area to be treated is not necessary, because the technique is not traumatic. Moreover, a minimum quantity of anaesthetic is already present in the syringe. Some topical anaesthetics are available for those patients who require anaesthesia.

Apart from possible allergic reactions, no other serious side-effects are described with bovine collagen. Possible collateral effects are: erythema, with transient oedema and ecchymosis, due to trauma and dependent also on the operator's manual ability. Cases of granulomatous reactions at implant site are probably allergic or inflammatory reactions, and usually are resolved spontaneously within 3–13 months; systemic or intralesional corticosteroids and systemic NSAIDs can accelerate this resolution. Either way, they resolve completely. Episodes of systemic reactions to bovine collagen have not been confirmed. Risks to the immune system resulting from the use of a heterologous protein, such as bovine collagen, have led to the development of autologous collagen, which in theory should be the safer substance.

Bovine collagen is also available in combination with polymethylmethacrylate microspheres (Artecoll). While collagen is slowly reabsorbed, the microspheres remain incapsulated in the dermis, thus allowing a permanent partial correction of the defect treated. The implant technique, which requires 27-G needles, is the same as that described for bovine collagen alone.

Autologous fat

The implant of autologous fat is a soft-tissue augmentation technique that has been attempted for over 100 years, but only after the arrival of liposuction has it become widely used. The implant of fat, removed in bulk and surgically implanted, has a very limited use, and rather unreliable results. However the extraction of adipocytes by lipoaspiration enables obtaining an injectable substance, which can be used for the treatment of many lesions. Results are excellent in the treatment of:

- deep wrinkles
- acne scars
- facial atrophy
- face contour defects
- rejuvenation of the dorsum of the hands
- all conditions of lipoatrophy.

This technique is not suitable for treating fibrous scars and very thin wrinkles, because it employs rather thick needles for infiltration which are not appropriate for these lesions.

Many histological studies performed in rats have demonstrated that the treatment of drawn fat with anaesthetics, saline solution, Ringer lactate, or insulin, does not affect its survival. The advantage of this substance is that since it is an autologous substance, there is no risk of inducing an allergic reaction or autoimmune pathology. The disadvantage is that it needs a donor site from which the fat can be extracted. It is possible, however, to combine liposuction and fat implant in the same session. For facial defects a quantity of up to 20 mL fat is required. This can be extracted with a syringe using a cannula or a 14-gauge needle. If more than 20 mL fat is required, then machine-assisted liposuction can be employed. In the case of extraction by syringe, the donor area is infiltrated with a local anaesthetic. The negative pressure created within the syringe is enough to extract the fat. Drawn fat has to be separated from other extracted fluids. This can be achieved by centrifugation, by taking advantage of the force of gravity, or by treating the fat with saline solution. Fat obtained by liposuction has to be separated and treated in the same way. The same syringe used to draw adipocytes can be used to inject them into the recipient site by attaching a 16-gauge needle (narrower gauged ones could damage adipocytes). The area to be treated can be infiltrated by a local anaesthetic, or previously treated with a topical anaesthetic. The fat has to be implanted between the dermis and the subcutaneous tissue, without hypercorrection. The needle has to be inserted parallel to the cutaneous surface. The degree of survival of injected fat cannot be predicted precisely. It is believed that, if well executed, only 30% of the whole adipose tissue implanted in a single session survives. Therefore, it is usually necessary to perform more than one session.

This soft-tissue augmentation technique generally does not cause serious collateral effects, except for possible ecchymosis, oedema, or numbness in the treated area.

The implant endurance is not predictable. It is usually considered to be definitive, especially in case of lasting defects, such as depressed scars or facial emiatrophy. In case of evolving defects, such as wrinkles, the durability is more difficult to estimate.

Hyaluronic acid

Hyaluronic acid is a polysaccharide of the extracellular matrix, and ubiquitous in the connective tissue of mammalians. Derivatives of this natural polymer with similar properties, have been derived by a cross-linking process. The resulting substance is inert and biocompatible.

Histological studies on rats have shown that the substance disperses in the dermis in a rather uniform way, causing a minimum inflammatory reaction, or no reaction at all. Being identical in all mammals, it does not cause allergic reactions in human tissues after the implant. It lasts for about 12 months.

Except for the treatment of very thin wrinkles, the technique for implantation and the defects susceptible to improvement are the same for bovine collagen (Zyplast), using a 30-G needle. In comparison with bovine collagen, hyaluronic acid seems to be safer for the treatment of glabellar wrinkles. It is necessary to avoid excessive hypercorrection and implantation in the papillary dermis.

The advantage of this is that it does not induce allergic reactions so that pretreatment testing, is not necessary. Moreover, it seems to last longer in tissues as compared which bovine collagen. Histological studies have shown hyaluronic acid to persist in the treated areas 8 months after the implant. Its main disadvantage, in comparison with bovine collagen, is a greater incidence of postimplant oedema and erythema, which usually results in the need for an additional session after 7 days.

In order to enhance hyaluronic acid implant duration, this material is also available in combination with other inert substances, such as microspheres of Dextran (Reviderm) or hydroxyethyl methacrylate (Dermalive). They have the same indications of hyaluronic acid alone. The adjunct of inert and persistent particles to hyaluronic acid aims to achieve longer endurance of the implants. The technique of implantation, contraindications and side-effects are the same of those described for hyaluronic acid alone, except that larger needles (usually 27 G) must be employed to inject this fillers.

Fibrel

Fibrel is a substance consisting of a porcine derived lyophilized collagen powder and α-aminocaproic acid. This has to be reconstituted with the patient's serum and saline solution, in order to start the coagulation process. The resultant jelly matrix is infiltrated by fibroblasts and other inflammation cells that should produce new collagen fibres. It is employed for the treatment of facial lesions and ageing wrinkles.

Before performing the implant, it is necessary to exclude a previous history of coagulation defects, and perform an allergic test that has to be read after 48 h and then 4 weeks. It has been calculated that 1.8% of patients present with a reaction to Fibrel.

The implantation technique requires the use of a syringe with a 20-G needle and an insertion angle of 30–45°. The material has to be placed in the middle and deep dermis, with a hypercorrection of 50–100%, and preferably using a linear inserting technique. The durability of the implant seems to be longer than for bovine collagen implants, because of an assumed stimulation of collagen production by Fibrel. Formation of a transient nodule in the recipient site is possible, but the main disadvantage connected with the use of Fibrel is its preparation, and the necessity to perform a venous drawing from the patient.

New Fill

New Fill is a synthetic polymer in the form of a sterile apyrogenic suspension containing microspheres of poly-l-lactic acid (PLA), which belongs to the α-hydroxy acid family. The crystalline PLA is a dry powder, which has to be reconstituted with sterile water for injections. It is immunologically inert, biocompatible, biodegradable and free from toxicity. It has been employed for several years in many clinical fields, mainly in reconstructive bone surgery. It seems to act differently from other fillers, because it has been postulated that poly-l-lactic acid microspheres are able to stimulate the production of new collagen fibres from dermal fibroblasts. For this reason, the correction is not immediately evident and it increases with time. The technique of implantation is the same as for other fillers, excepted that the implant must not be performed superficially, but only in subcutaneous or dermal layers, using a 26-G or 21-G needle with a linear technique and without overcorrection. The serial puncture technique is not indicated for New Fill. It is necessary to prepare the New Fill solution at least 1 h before the implant, in order to get a complete and even dispersion of the particles of PLA. Besides, the implant session must be performed quickly, because the PLA solution tends to precipitate very soon, and the precipitation might cause an uneven result. This is the main limit of New Fill. This filler is indicated for skin depressions and scars, facial recontouring, for lip shaping and for wrinkles. The correction achieved is not immediately predictable, since the increase in dermal collagen starts about 15 days after the first implant. Therefore, a second session must be planned at a distance of 20–30 days in order to achieve an optimal correction. The correction achieved with New Fill implants is considered to last about 12 months. Contraindications and side-effects are the same as those reported for other synthetic fillers, with a greater incidence of ecchymosis and oedema, due to the deeper infiltration. Allergic reactions have not been reported with the use of New Fill.

Autologen, Dermalogen, Isologen, Alloderm

New biologically derived materials for short or intermediate term augmentation are now available. Several autologous fillers are now available for temporary soft-tissue augmentation. Human-tissue collagen matrix (Autologen, Isologen and Dermalogen) can be implanted with the same technique used with other synthetic or animal-derivative fillers. The advantage obtained with these fillers is a longer persistence of the correction, with the possibility of the production of new type I collagen fibres. Alloderm consists of acellular dermal grafts derived from cadaveric skin and seems to allow an intermediate term correction, but its use may not be acceptable to all patients because of its composition.

Gore-tex

Since 1972 expanded polytetrafluoroethylene has been employed in the replacement of vascular prosthesis. It is an inert, biocompatible and antithrombogenic substance that is able to maintain unaltered dimensions after the implant, without incurring degradation or reabsorption. It is colonized by small vessels and cells, able to anchor in the subcutaneous tissue. It is employed either in the form of various size plaques, adaptable to the shape of the defect to be corrected, or as suture thread, especially in the correction of nasolabial folds or lip shaping, and other deep defects of the face contour. It is not suitable for the correction of thin wrinkles.

The implant technique requires a tunnelization of the defect by two terminal incisions, and followed by the insertion of the Gore-tex material. Small suture stitches could be needed to bridge the points of insertion. The implant has to be performed at subcutaneous level, taking care that the two ends remain inserted firmly in the subcutaneous layer, in order to avoid the risk of extrusion.

Previously, it has been necessary to infiltrate the area to be treated with a local anaesthetic. The procedure is of a surgical type, and this is its main disadvantage. Moreover, this technique requires some days of postoperative care including antiseptic dressings, in order to avoid the risk of infection. The main advantage of Gore-tex is its inertness and definitive durability of the obtained correction.

Another advantage is that threads and plaques can be extracted, if necessary.

Bio-formacryl

Bio-formacryl is an injectable synthetic polymer, constituted by sterile apyrogenic water (95%) and polyacrylamide (5%). It is inert, biocompatible, non-allergic, permanent, and chemically stable. After the implant of Bio-formacryl a weak inflammatory response can be noted in the surrounding dermis, characterized mainly by macrophages. Biopsies performed 4 months after the implant reveal the almost complete disappearance of the inflammatory response, with the formation of a thin fibrotic capsule around the implant. The presence of a capsule makes it possible to remove the implant, if needed, even after long periods of time. Bio-formacryl is best indicated for the correction of large defects (congenital ones also), facial atrophy, lipoatrophy, but it can also be employed for the correction of scars, deep wrinkles, for facial recontouring and lip shaping. The technique of implant requires a 23-G or 21-G needle, with a linear implantation of the material in the subcutaneous tissue. After the implant the correction achieved is immediately evident. Further implants should be performed inside the pre-existing capsule formed after the first session. Side-effects are mainly erythema, oedema and ecchymosis. Antibiotic and antiviral prophylaxis is suggested, as well as the prescription of antioedema drugs during the first days after the implant. Migration of Bio-formacryl has never been described as yet, but the presence of the capsule makes it improbable.

Further reading

Cisneros JL, Singla R. Intradermal augmentation with expanded polytetrafluoroethylene (Gore-tex) for facial lines and wrinkles. *J Dermatol Surg Oncol* 1993; 19: 539–42.

Coleman WP III *et al.* Autologous collagen? Lipocytic dermal augmentation: a histopathologic study. *J Dermatol Surg Oncol* 1993; 19: 1032–40.

Drake LA *et al.* Guidelines of care for soft-tissue augmentation: collagen implants. *J Am Acad Dermatol* 1996; 34: 698–702.

Drake LA *et al.* Guidelines of care for soft-tissue augmentation: fat transplantation. *J Am Acad Dermatol* 1996; 34: 690–4.

Drake LA *et al.* Guidelines of care for soft-tissue augmentation: gelatin matrix implant. *J Am Acad Dermatol* 1996; 34: 695–7.

Elson ML. Soft-tissue augmentation. A review. *Dermatol Surg* 1995; 21: 491–500.

Fagien S. Facial soft-tissue augmentation with injectable autologous and allogeneic human tissue collagen matrix (autologen and dermalogen). *Plast Reconstr Surg* 2000; 105(1): 362–73.

Overholt MA *et al.* Granulomatous reaction to collagen implant: light and electron microscopic observation. *Cutis* 1993; 2 (51): 95–8.

Piacquadio D *et al.* Evaluation of hylan B gel as a soft-tissue augmentation implant material. *J Am Acad Dermatol* 1997; 36: 544–9.

Ramirez AL *et al.* Current concepts in soft-tissue augmentation. *Facial Plast Surg* 2000; 8(2): 235–51.

Sclafani A *et al.* Evaluation of acellular dermal grafts in sheet (Alloderm) and Injectable (micronized Alloderm) forms for soft-tissue augmentation. Clinical observations and histological analysis. *Arch Facial Plast Surg* 2000; 2(2): 130–6.

Sherris DA, Larrabee WF. Expanded polytetrafluoroethylene augmentation of the lower face. *Laryngoscope* 1996; 106: 658–63.

Skin resurfacing with the carbon dioxide laser

B.C. Gee and N.P.J. Walker

General principles

Laser skin resurfacing is a technique whereby thermal energy from a laser is used to vaporize the epidermis and papillary dermis followed by subsequent re-epithelialization and collagen remodelling.

Basic concepts behind lasers and carbon dioxide lasers

Laser is an acronym for **L**ight **A**mplification by the **S**timulated **E**mission of **R**adiation. This describes a process whereby a population of atoms or molecules in an excited state produces an output of pure electromagnetic radiation of known wavelength(s). As far as medical uses are concerned, the tissue effects of this 'light' can be accurately predicted and controlled.

A laser requires a power source and an active medium, which in the carbon dioxide laser is mainly carbon dioxide gas. This gas is present in a cylindrical chamber with mirrors at each end and an absorptive lining. The molecules of gas are energized by the power source and as they return to the ground state photons are emitted. The photons are reflected back and forth colliding with atoms in a metastable state, which causes a chain reaction (stimulated emission) and more photons are produced. These photons are coherent and those that are not parallel are absorbed by the lining. The resulting coherent, collimated photons form the laser output.

Interaction of carbon dioxide laser light and skin

Carbon dioxide lasers emit a continuous-wave invisible beam of 10 600 nm, which is in the infrared part of the electromagnetic spectrum. This happens to be a wavelength at which photons are highly absorbed by intracellular water. A rapid rise in temperature results in an explosive expansion of water as it vaporizes, with consequent tissue destruction. This is non-selective targeting as compared to a pulsed dye laser at 595 nm, which specifically targets haemoglobin.

The carbon dioxide laser has several advantages over other forms of surgical resurfacing. The field is relatively bloodless as dermal blood vessels are photocoagulated and sealed. Similarly, small lymphatic vessels and small cutaneous sensory nerve endings are sealed resulting in less postoperative exudate and pain than conventional dermabrasion.

To discuss the effects of carbon dioxide laser and the skin further, the reader needs to be familiar with certain laser terminology.

- Energy measured in joules (J) is the capacity to do work. It can be calculated by power multiplied by time of application.
- Power measured in watts (W) is the rate that the energy is delivered. One watt is equivalent to 1 J/s.
- Power density or irradiance is measured in watts per square centimetre (W/cm^2) and is the rate of energy delivered per unit of target tissue area. Higher power densities vaporize tissue more rapidly.
- Fluence or energy density is measured in joules per square centimetre (J/cm^2). Fluence is irradiance multiplied by time. Power density can determine the rate of vaporization but does not determine the volume of tissue affected which is a combined product of power density and time (fluence).

$$F(\text{J/cm}^2) = \frac{P(W) \times t(\text{s})}{\text{Area (cm}^2)}$$

- Spot size is measured in millimetres (mm). It is controlled by focusing lenses in a hand piece. Power density is inversely proportional to spot size. A doubling of the spot size requires a fourfold increase in the laser output to maintain the power density.

- Thermal relaxation time is the time taken for heated tissue to lose 50% of its heat through diffusion. This is significant in that if the application of the laser energy persists longer than the thermal relaxation time of the target tissue, heat is conducted to the surrounding tissue leading to unwanted thermal injury. This is prevented by using exposure times within the thermal relaxation time of the target tissue. As the thermal relaxation time for pure water is 325 μs and human skin is 695 μs it is thought a pulse width less than 950 μs is short enough to prevent clinically significant unwanted thermal damage.
- Pulses—the output from a carbon dioxide laser—will be delivered in a continuous wave form if not modified. Modification in its simplest form is the chopping of the continuous waveform by shutters. Electronic pumping can be used to produce very short pulses (pulse durations of between 250 μs to 1 msec) of very high peak powers.

The extent of thermal damage beyond the vaporized layer depends on the rate of vaporization, which in turn depends on the power density and the energy fluence. If the fluence used is not sufficient to vaporize then tissues coagulate, desiccate and carbonize as heat accumulates. The tissue heats relatively slowly and charring occurs indicating carbonization. Continued radiation will produce even greater temperatures (in excess of 600°C) and full-thickness, conduction burns will ensue. When pure vaporization occurs the temperature of the target site is limited to 100°C and collateral thermal damage is kept to a minimum (50 μm).

Carbon dioxide lasers can be used to incise tissue. Wounds are slower to re-epithelialize than after conventional surgery due to a delay in the onset of epidermal cell migration. This is thought to be due to laser induced thermal necrosis of the wound margin, which impedes epidermal movement. Tensile strength of the laser wound is also reduced due to slower collagen formation but at 3 months laser wounds and conventional surgical wounds are histologically indistinct.

It is as a precise surface tissue ablator that the carbon dioxide laser has found its main role in dermatological surgery although its role in certain applications may have been largely superceded by newer lasers.

An example of this would be in the treatment of port-wine stains, which are now treated almost exclusively with pulsed dye lasers (PDL). PDLs confer better efficacy and less chance of scarring.

Indications for the use of a carbon dioxide laser include conditions when a satisfactory therapeutic outcome can be achieved by the precise removal of the (abnormal) epidermis and superficial dermis followed by re-epithelialization possibly associated with some remodelling of dermal collagen (Table 1). The precise destruction of abnormal tissue may also allow deeper structures to be treated (Table 2).

Superficial scarring, including certain types of acne scarring, generalized actinic changes and rhytides (wrinkles) are also frequent indications for resurfacing. Rhytides, especially in the perioral and periorbital regions are improved with carbon dioxide laser treatment. Rhytides associated with excessive muscle contraction such as the forehead and glabella are deeper and may be improved but tend to recur much sooner. *Botulinum* toxin injections are an invaluable adjunctive treatment in these areas.

Contraindications

It is crucial to remember carbon dioxide lasers are producing a burn, however po-

Table 1 Indications for the use of carbon dioxide laser

Warts and condyloma acuminatum
Bowen's disease
Superficial basal cell carcinomas
Xanthelasma
Adenoma sebaceum
Rhinophymas
Balanitis xerotica obliterans
Erythroplasia of Queyrat
Actinic cheilitis
Seborrhoeic keratoses
Epidermal naevi

Table 2 Deeper lesions which can be treated with carbon dioxide laser

Facial trichoepithelioma
Syringomas
Lymphangioma circumscriptum
Neurofibromas
Myxoid cysts
Apocrine hydrocystomas
Keloids
Matricectomy—for pincer nails or ingrowing toe nail

tentially precise, and inappropriate use can result in significant scarring. Patients who have a history of poor scarring including keloids must be assessed very carefully.

Those who have been on systemic isotretinoin (Roaccutane) should be advised to wait at least 1 year before resurfacing as they appear to be at risk of developing atypical scars.

Those who have had previous dermabrasion should wait at least 3–6 months.

Patients with collagen vascular disorders (e.g. systemic lupus erythematosus, scleroderma), autoimmune disorders (e.g. vitiligo) or immune deficiencies should not be resurfaced due to slower or impaired postoperative recovery, as well as disease reactivation or worsening, due to a stressful procedure. Patients with Fitzpatrick skin types IV–VI should be treated cautiously because of the risk of hypo- or hyperpigmentation.

Treatment regimen

Patient selection

Careful patient selection and thorough preprocedural counselling are crucial.

Those with pale skin types, Fitzpatrick I–II, without excessive ultraviolet (UV) light exposure undergoing resurfacing for non-movement rhytides, actinic cheilitis or epidermal lesions (seborrhoeic/actinic keratoses) are the best candidates. In situations when the outcome cannot be confidently predicted a small trial area may be treated and observed for some months before making a final decision on a full treatment.

Pretreatment

Fully informed consent must be obtained. Patients with Fitzpatrick skin types IV and above may be prescribed depigmenting treatments for 6 weeks prior to treatment.

Antimicrobial prophylaxis

The necessity for antiviral prophylaxis should be considered. Some practitioners also routinely use an antibacterial such as amoxycillin.

Laser safety and protection

The laser should only be used in a properly controlled facility with appropriately trained staff. Eye protection is required for everyone in the room and the patient may require special metal eye shields.

Drapes are wet with sterile water or saline and metal instruments are ebonized or tarnished in some way to reduce reflectivity.

An efficient vacuum exhaust system must be used to remove the plume. The plume consists of vapour and smoke and contains viable material.

Anaesthesia

Carbon dioxide lasers burn tissue and some form of anaesthesia is required. Topical anaesthesia alone is not sufficient but may be useful as an adjunct to local blocks.

Local or regional anaesthesia (field or nerve blocks) can be used for small areas and for more extensive procedures, i.e. full face resurfacing, extensive/multiple warts general anaesthesia can be used.

Procedure

The skin is prepared with an aqueous antiseptic which will not ignite. It is important to ensure the solution does not pool as this can accumulate thermal energy and cause a burn.

The laser parameters are determined by the area and thickness of tissue to be treated (Table 3). Some manufacturers have preset parameters, which can be very helpful. The correct depth and uniformity of tissue removal are the primary concerns of the operator.

An initial laser spot can be used to judge the effect of the first pass. Clinical parameters are used to gauge depth. There is no substitute for experience in interpreting the changes seen in the skin as the laser vaporizes layers of tissue.

Opalescent bubbling and audible crackling sounds indicate that the epidermis is being ablated. Gentle removal of the residual epidermis by wiping with a wet gauze will reveal a pink plane, the papillary dermis. Vaporization of the pink layer produces a contraction of the tissue and a yellow colour is seen indicating the reticular dermis. This is an important sign as healing of skin treated down to this level should occur without scarring. If a brown colour is seen, indicating the reticular dermis is being entered, then scarring may occur. If charring occurs thermal diffusion will occur beyond the depth of vaporization and scarring is almost inevitable.

Various strategies have been employed to control laser vaporization as precisely as possible and to reduce unwanted thermal damage. The aim being to deliver sufficient power to vaporize the tissue within an exposure time that does not allow for unwanted heat diffusion into surrounding tissues. There are two main types of carbon dioxide lasers in current use for resurfacing. Pulsed laser systems, where high-energy pulses are scanned over the skin surface using a computerized pattern generator (e.g. Coherent Ultrapulse, USA). Spiralling scanner systems, where a small spot of laser light (150 μm) is rotated over the skin at a speed which ensures the dwell time at any one point is within the thermal relaxation time of the skin (e.g. Sharplan Silktouch).

Such use of automatic scanners allows energy density to be controlled so that a uniform depth can be obtained. The operator then uses the clinical signs to determine the need for further passes.

When treating rhytides an average of 1–2 passes are needed for infraorbital regions while 2–3 are needed for other areas.

Table 3 An example of laser parameters (from Alster, 1997)

	Periorbital	Perioral	Forehead	Cheeks
Ultrapulse				
Energy	250–500 mJ/pulse	300–500 mJ/pulse	300 mJ/60 W/scan	300 mJ/60 W/scan
Spot/scan size	3–9 mm	4–9 mm	6–9 mm	6–9 mm
No. laser passes	1–2	2–4	2	2–3
Silktouch				
Energy	5–12 W/scan	7.5–20 W/scan	10–20 W/scan	7.5–20 W/scan
Scan size	4–6 mm	4–6 mm	4–6 mm	4–6 mm
No. laser passes	1–2	2–4	2	2–3

Postoperative care

Over the first 24–48 h the erythema and oedema intensify. This may be reduced by the administration of Depomedrone at the time of the procedure. The treated area needs to be kept well hydrated. Hydrogel applications like Vigilon or Second Skin can be used. Repeat applications of ice packs may reduce the swelling and discomfort during the initial phase.

Close follow-up is necessary over the first week to assess for infection, poor healing or unexpected inflammation. In most cases re-epithelialization takes 7–10 days. Green foundation can be used to disguise the residual erythema. The erythema is most intense after 10–14 days and may take a few months to resolve. During the postprocedural period patients should be advised to apply regular moisturizer and if appropriate to use topical hydroquinone to reduce hyperpigmentation. Hypertrophic scarring, if noted, is treated immediately (see below).

Side-effects and complications

Reactivation of herpes simplex infection may occur and can be very dramatic. If the patient gives a history of recurrent cold sores, antiviral prophylaxis is indicated and most practitioners use such prophylaxis routinely when resurfacing. Other infections may occur and a close watch must be kept on the treated area whilst it heals. Many practitioners use prophylactic antibiotics in the postoperative period.

Postprocedure erythema is seen in all patients. The erythema is at its worst 10–14 days postprocedure and should then slowly fade, though it may be many months before the skin tone is normal. Persistent erythema should be closely monitored as it may well herald the development of hypertrophic scarring. Green foundation can be used during the postoperative period to disguise the colour.

Scarring or ectropion formation can develop. This is usually due to operator technique, poor postoperative management or infection but sometimes seems to occur idiosyncratically. The development of scars is normally evident in the first month as persistent erythema and can be treated with topical or intralesional steroids and/or silicone gel sheets. Early treatment with the 585-nm PDL may be beneficial in these cases.

Transient hyperpigmentation is seen in approximately one third of patients and may become apparent within 3–4 weeks. It usually resolves spontaneously but a twice daily regime of topical hydroquinone and a biweekly to monthly light acid peel can hasten the process. This treatment should be started at the first sign of any darkening. Patients are asked to be obsessional about sun avoidance and sun protection in the post-treatment period.

Hypopigmentation tends to occur later—6 months at the earliest—and may not be evident until 12 months afterwards. Unfortunately this side-effect may be permanent but can be sometimes be ameliorated by peels to the surrounding skin.

There are interesting reports of using UV (excimer) lasers to treat this complication.

Other problems occasionally seen are milia formation and acne flare.

Conclusion

Carbon dioxide laser vaporization is a safe and effective mode of resurfacing skin but only in the hands of an experienced and skilled operator. Patient selection and careful postoperative management are paramount to the success of treatment.

One of the disadvantages of laser resurfacing is the prolonged postoperative course which typically persists for months. However with the advent of shorter pulsed carbon dioxide lasers and erbium–YAG lasers this should be reduced to more acceptable levels.

Further reading

Alster TS. *Manual of Cutaneous Laser Techniques*. Philadelphia: Lippincott-Raven, 1997: 104–16.

Ball KA. *Lasers. The Perioperative Challenge*. St Louis: Mosby, 1995: 32–9.

Fitzpatrick RE, Goldman MP. *Cutaneous Laser Surgery*, 2nd edn. St Louis: Mosby, 1998: 198–258.

Sheehan-Dare RA, Cotterill JA. Lasers in dermatology. *Br J Dermatol* 1993; 129: 1–8.

Spicer MS, Goldberg DJ. Lasers in dermatology. *J Am Acad Dermatol* 1996; 34: 1–25.

UVB phototherapy

C. Antoniou

Phototherapy is exposure to non-ionizing radiation for therapeutic benefit. It has been utilized since antiquity. Sunlight therapy was used empirically by the ancient Greeks and Egyptians for the treatment of various diseases. However, the variability of natural sunlight has led to the development and use of artificial sources.

Therapeutic action spectroscopy

The wavelength dependency of phototherapy for psoriasis shows the most effective area to be around 313 nm. Ultraviolet (UV) radiation shorter than 280 nm produces more erythema than therapeutic effect and wavelengths longer than 330 nm are not therapeutic. Narrowband at 311 nm UVB lamps (Philips TL-01) have an increased ratio of therapeutic wavelengths to erythemogenic wavelengths. In a paired comparison study better results have been achieved with the narrowband lamps than with conventional broadband UVB lamps.

Ultraviolet lamps

The popular sources are fluorescent Philips TL-01 (312 ± 2 nm), Philips TL-12 (270–350 nm), Sylvania UV6 (295–340 nm) and Helarium (290–370 nm).

Evaluation of the patient

The patient is interviewed to establish a risk factor profile assessing previous phototherapy or psoralen and ultraviolet A (PUVA), systemic therapy for skin disorders, sun-exposure history, occupation, personal and family history of skin cancer, and medication taken during the previous 6 months. The patient is examined to establish disease severity and to record evidence of photodamage, naevi, skin cancer, and vitiligo.

Children and pregnant women may be treated safely with UVB phototherapy.

Patients need to be advised to avoid additional UVB exposure from sun bathing, which may limit the effectiveness of phototherapy or increase the incidence of complications.

Clinical Indications for UVB phototherapy

UVB phototherapy has been used successfully for the treatment of:

- psoriasis
- atopic eczema
- pityriasis rosea
- polymorphic light eruption
- uraemic pruritus

and other conditions such as:

- chronic urticaria
- acne
- pityriasis lichenoides chronica
- pityriasis lichenoides and varioliformis acuta
- eosinophilic pustular folliculitis in patients with acquired immune deficiency syndrome (AIDS).

Contraindications for UVB phototherapy

UVB phototherapy is contraindicated for patients with xeroderma pigmentosum, systemic lupus erythematosus, photo-induced epilepsy, and multiple skin cancers (e.g. Gorlin's syndrome).

Treatment regimen

Various treatment schedules are in use. Patients are irradiated three to five times per week. According to our standard treatment regimen, the initial exposure dose is 70% of the minimal erythema dose (MED) with subsequent exposure increase by 20% of the previous dose. If a painful erythema develops, therapy is discontinued until this is resolved, and the dose reduced by 50%. Phototherapy is continued until disease clearance. During treatment, patients as well as operators should always wear eye protection.

Maintenance therapy

The usefulness of maintenance therapy after clearing (e.g. once or twice a week) in prolonging the duration of remission is controversial. In a randomized study comparing no maintenance to weekly and twice-weekly maintenance therapy for at least 4 months, patients receiving this therapy were significantly less likely to have a relapse. In another study, it was found that when the frequency of maintenance therapy was progressively reduced, no benefit of the therapy was detected. Thus, maintenance therapy is useful, but it has to be frequent and requires a strong commitment by the patients.

Side-effects

Potential acute side-effects of UVB irradiation of the skin include 'sunburn reaction', pruritus and a Koebner exacerbation of psoriasis. Ocular side-effects of UVB include conjunctivitis and keratitis. Potential long-term toxicities of UVB phototherapy are photoageing and skin cancer.

Long-term follow-up

It is important to keep a set of phototherapy notes for each patient, recording number of exposures, cumulative dose and risk factor profile. Patients who have had a large number of exposures (≥ 150 exposures) or other significant risk factors, should be reviewed annually.

Adjuvant therapy

If one is using a maximal regimen, i.e. as described above, there is no therapeutic advantage in using tar, dithranol or calcipotriol. A suitable emollient such as white soft paraffin or coconut oil is suggested to counteract xerosis. UVB plus retinoids (Re-UVB) will reduce number of exposures and the total UV dosage required for clearance. This may not increase remission time.

Conclusion

Although considered to be less effective than PUVA, recent work with TL-01 (narrow band UVB) suggests that this view may require to be changed.

The long-term risk of UVB carcinogenesis is considered to be less than with PUVA. Moreover, the advantages of reduced cost (no psoralen), use in pregnancy and childhood along with the absence of PUVA pain and the need for eye photoprotection point to UVB phototherapy as a growth area. More controlled evidence is required and should become available in the coming years.

Further reading

Abel EA. Phototherapy. *Dermatol Clin* 1995; 13: (4), 841–9.

Antoniou C, Katsambas A. Phototherapy. *Int J Remote Sensing* 1995; 16: 1747–50.

British Photodermatology Group. An appraisal of narrow-band (TL-01) UVB phototherapy. British Photodermatology Group Workshop Report (April 1996). *Br J Dermatol* 1997; 137: 327–30.

Collins P, Ferguson J. Narrow-band (TL-01) phototherapy: an effective preventative treatment for the photodermatoses. *Br J Dermatol* 1995; 132: 964–9.

De Gruijl FR. Long-term side effects and carcinogenesis risk in UVB therapy. In: Hönigsmann H, Jore G, Young AR, eds. *The Fundamental Bases of Phototherapy*. Milano: OEMF, 1996: 153–70.

Green C, Ferguson J, Lakshmipathi T *et al.* 311nm UVB Phototherapy: an effective treatment for psoriasis. *Br J Dermatol* 1988; 119: 691–6.

Johnson BE, Green C, Lakshmipathi T, Ferguson J. Ultraviolet radiation phototherapy for psoriasis. The use of a narrow band UVB fluorescent lamp. In: Douglas PH, Moan J, Dall'Acqua F, eds. *Light in Biology and Medicine*. New York: Plenum, 1988: 173–9.

Petrozzi JW. UVB maintenance phototherapy in psoriasis. *Int J Dermatol* 1985; 24: 600–2.

Stern RS. The carcinogenic risk of UVB phototherapy and PUVA. In: *Proceedings of the Anglo-Nordic Symposium 'Long-term Treatment of Psoriasis'*. Horsmanheimo, Helsinki, Finland, 1986: 26–7.

Stern RS, Amstrong RB, Anderson TF *et al.* Effect of continued Ultraviolet B phototherapy on the duration of the remission of psoriasis: A randomized study. *J Am Acad Dermatol* 1986; 15: 542–52.

Taylor CR, Stern RS, Leyden JT, Gilcherst BA. Photoaging, photodamage and photoprotection. *J Am Acad Dermatol* 1990; 22: 1–15.

Young A. Carcinogenicity of UVB phototherapy assessed. *Lancet* 1995; 345: 1431–2.

Drugs

Antibacterial agents

H. Giamarellou and M. Souli

The contemporary dermatologist quite often confronts bacterial skin and/or soft-tissue infections. Therefore, he should be familiar with antibacterial agents, particularly with newer antibiotics and their role in modern chemotherapy. Classification of cutaneous infections on morphological and clinical criteria are helpful in providing initial clues regarding the most likely responsible pathogens, which will lead to the appropriate antimicrobial chemotherapy. Therefore, and despite the scope of the present manual it was considered appropriate to also include some clinical data on the common streptococcal and staphylococcal skin infections, which will help the dermatologist to choose rationally from among the available antimicrobial agents. Emphasis will be placed on the newer antibacterial agents while for the older ones, the discussion will be confined mainly to their indications in current dermatological therapy.

Common bacterial infections in dermatology

Nowadays the commonest bacterial skin and soft-tissue infections in the immunocompetent host are still those in which staphylococci and streptococci are implicated. However, in immunocompromised patients several Enterobacteriaceae, *Pseudomonas aeruginosa* and a variety of fungi (yeast and moulds) are implicated. The common skin and soft-tissue infections are represented by the following entities.

Impetigo

This is a superficial infection of the skin appearing initially as vesicular and rapidly as thick, golden-yellow crusted lesions in the exposed areas of the skin. In 90% of the cases group A streptococci are involved, and rarely group B (in the newborn) as well as group C and G. In 10% of the cases, a bullous form of impetigo is observed due to *Staph. aureus*.

Staphylococcal scalded skin syndrome

This represents a severe *Staph. aureus* infection characterized by widespread large flaccid clear bullae, which promptly rupture resulting in exfoliation that exposes large areas of bright red skin. It starts with fever, skin tenderness and a scarlatiniform rash. The early stage should be differentiated from 'toxic shock syndrome', which is characterized by hypotension or shock, functional abnormalities of at least three organ systems and desquamation of the skin lesions. *Staph. aureus* strains, with the capacity to produce exotoxins, are the main cause; however, group A streptococci are also implicated. The recently described syndrome, 'flesh eating disease', represents a similar clinical entity that involves both superficial and deeper soft-tissue structures, causes metastatic skin lesions fatal in >20% of the cases and is characterized by the early appearance of painful skin demarcation.

Folliculitis

This consists of small erythematous papules topped by a central pustule located within hair follicles. *Staphylococcus aureus* is the main cause, but *Pseudomonas aeruginosa* has been implicated in 'swimming pool' folliculitis attributed to inadequate chlorination. Folliculitis may extend to the deeper structures creating a furuncle which is a deeper inflammatory nodule occurring in areas of the skin subjected to friction and perspiration like the neck, axillae, buttocks and face. A more extensive process is a 'carbuncle' which extends into the subcutaneous fat whenever the involved skin is inelastic and thick. In the latter case multiple abscesses develop draining along hair follicles.

Diabetes mellitus is considered a predisposing factor. *Staph. aureus* is the unique aetiological agent. Invasion of the bloodstream by staphylococci may result in endocarditis, osteomyelitis or other serious infections, while location at the upper lip and nose may spread staphylococci via the facial and angular veins to the cavernous sinus.

Erysipelas

This refers to superficial skin cellulitis with distinctive lymphatic involvement. In 70–80% the lower extremities are affected and only in 5–20% the face. In almost all cases group A streptococci and uncommonly group C and G are implicated. However, in the neonate, group B is also involved. Patients with diabetes mellitus, venous stasis, nephritic syndrome or lymphatic obstruction (as after radical mastectomy) are vulnerable to erysipelas. Portals of entry for streptococci are skin ulcers, abrasions, postoperative wounds, eczematous or psoriatic lesions, and even skin fungal infections. Erysipelas is painful with a red 'peau d'orange' picture and a characteristic raised border which is sharply demarcated from the surrounding normal skin. As a rule streptococci cannot be cultured from the skin lesions. The infections can be complicated with cellulitis, subcutaneous abscesses and even necrotizing fasciitis. However, cellulitis can appear as an acute infection extending from the beginning into deep subcutaneous tissues.

Hidradenitis suppurativa

This is a chronic suppurative infection of the apocrine glands of the genital, perianal and axillary regions. Red nodules that become fluctuant and drain are the initial lesions, which result in chronic draining sinuses and ciccatricial scars. Secondary infections involve staphylococci, streptococci, Enterobacteriaceae, *Pseudomonas* spp. and anaerobes. Therefore, a therapeutic decision should not be empirical but based on 'pus' culture results.

Antibacterial agents

Penicillins

Penicillin G

Today this is still the drug of choice for streptococcal infections as well as for anthrax and *Erysipelothrix* infection. Depending on the severity of the infection it is given either orally as penicillin V, in case of impetigo (1.2 million IU every 6 h) with an empty stomach or parentally as i.v. penicillin G (5 million IU 4–6 h, over 30 min).

The major side-effects of penicillins in general are hypersensitivity reactions, which range in severity from rash to anaphylactic shock and death. While allergic reactions occur in 4–7/1000 penicillin treatment courses, immediate anaphylactic reactions occur mostly with penicillin G from 0 to 1 h postadministration and are expressed as urticaria, angioedema, laryngeal oedema, bronchospasm and shock. They occur in 4/100 000 penicillin treatment courses with fatalities reported once in every 32 000–100 000 treatment courses. Late allergic reactions observed after 72 h of β-lactam administration are manifested by:

- morbilliform rash
- Stevens–Johnson syndrome
- exfoliative dermatitis
- drug fever
- serum sickness
- neutropenia
- thrombocytopenia
- haemolytic anaemia
- interstitial nephritis
- vasculitis
- pruritis
- contact dermatitis.

The detection of anaphylactic reactions to penicillin requires skin testing using minor antigenic determinants, a test not available in several countries. However, a negative result when testing with the major antigenic determinants, available commercially as the Pre-pen test, does not exclude the possibility of an anaphylactoid reaction, while skin testing with diluted penicillin G is very dangerous in individuals prone to express an anaphylactoid reaction. Therefore, whenever the appropriate tests are not available, a careful history of any potential for previous allergic reactions should be noted. In cases of an immediate reaction, adrenaline solution (1 : 1000) should be given i.m. and repeated every 15 min until recovery, followed by corticosteroids.

Antistaphylococcal penicillins
Oxacillin, dicoxacillin, cloxacillin, flucloxacillin and nafcillin, either orally or at a dose of 1 g every 8 h for mild infections or parentally at a dose of 3 g every 6–8 h for serious infections, are still the drugs of choice for staphylococcal infections. However, it should be seriously considered that 20–50% of *Staph. aureus* strains are now resistant to them (methicillin-resistant *Staph. aureus* or MRSA strains). Interestingly such infections, although mostly hospital acquired, are also encountered in the community. Therefore susceptibility tests, at least in serious infections, are required. It should be pointed out that MRSA strains are obligatorily resistant to any type of β-lactam antibiotic, including the inhibitors and the cephalosporins, even in cases where sensitivity tests indicate they are active drugs.

The remaining group of penicillins, i.e. aminopenicillins (ampicillin and amoxicillin), carboxypenicillins (carbencillin and trarcillin), ureidopenicillins (mezlocillin, azlocillin, piperacillin) as well as the β-lactam group of monobactams (aztreonam) and carbapenems (imipenem and meropenem), will not be included since they are out of the scope of this handbook.

β-lactamase inhibitors
These compounds, which are by themselves weak antibiotics, are potent inhibitors of many plasmid-mediated, and also of some chromosomal, β-lactamases, produced by *Staph. aureus* and several Enterobacteriaceae. Three derivatives have been developed, clavulanic acid, sulbactam and tazobactam. These restore the antibacterial activity of amoxicillin and ticarcillin (when combined with clavulanic acid), ampicillin (combined with sulbactram), piperacillin and cefoperazone (combined with tazobactram) against Gram-positive cocci, including staphylococci (but not MRSA strains) and several common Gram-negative species:

- *Haemophilus* spp.
- *Neisserie gonorrhoeae*
- *Escherichia coli*
- *Klebsiella pneumoniae*
- *Proteus* spp.
- other Enterobacteriaceae
- *Bacteroides fragilis*.

Clavulanic acid and sulbactam bind primarily to plasmid-encoded β-lactamases while tazolactam binds also to chromosomally encoded enzymes, produced mainly by *Klebsiella* and *Bacteroides* species.

The pharmacokinetics of clavulanic acid and sulbactam in humans are similar to those of amoxicillin and ampicillin. They are both available in oral and parenteral formulas with a weight ratio of inhibitor to the relevant β-lactam of 1 : 5 and 1 : 2, respectively. When clavulanic acid is combined with ticarcillin the ratio is 1 : 25 and for tazobactam–piperasillin is 1 : 8. With the exception of clavulanic acid, the excretion of which is not influenced in renal failure (and therefore amoxicillin plus clavulanic acid should not be administered in patients with renal insufficiency) the dose of the remaining combinations should be reduced proportionally to the decrease of the relevant β-lactam dose. Tissue kinetics of the inhibitors are compatible with those of the combined β-lactam.

Clavulanic acid plus amoxicillin is given in adults orally at a dose of 625 mg every 8 h, while i.v. at a dose of 1.2 g every 6 h. Sublactam plus ampicillin is given orally at a dose of 3.75 g every 8 h, and i.v. at a dose o.g. 3 g every 6–8 h. Clavulanic acid plus ticacillin is given only i.v. at a dose of 3.2 g or 5.2 g every 6 h while tazobactam plus piperacillin is given at a dose of 4.5 g every 6 h.

As with any β-lactam, antibiotic allergic reactions are the main threat which very seldom have been attributed to the inhibitor itself, but to the combined β-lactam. Diarrhoea with the oral compounds exceed in some series 10% of the treated cases.

Because of their very wide spectrum of activity which disturbs gastrointestinal tract flora, and destroys colonization resistance and have been also able to induce resistance mechanisms, the inhibitors should not be given for the common streptococcal or staphylococcal infections taking also into serious consideration that MRSA strains are by definition resistant. However, whenever cultures are not available and the clinical picture as well as the patient's condition appears serious without any clinical sign suggestive of the causal pathogen, a β-lactam inhibitor should not be prescribed.

Cephalosporins

Based on their *in vitro* activity and β-lactam stability, cephalosporins are divided into four generations (Table 1). They represent extremely broad-spectrum antibiotics, the first and second generation being more potent against the Gram-positive cocci, the third and fourth against the nosocomial Gram-negatives, including the various Enterobacteriaceae and *Pseudomonas aeruginosa*.

Cephalothin, cephradine, cefazolin, ceforanide and cefamandole possess the highest activity against staphylococci; cefoxilin and cefotetan are the only ones active against *Bacteroides fragiles* and ceftazidime is the most potent against *Pseudomonas aeruginosa*. The latter compound, however, is practically not active against streptococci and staphylococci.

The pharmacokinetic properties of the parenteral compounds differ in that the half-life ($t_{1/2}$) can range from 30 min to 8 h, mandating the frequency of administration (Table 1). Based on the much lower minimal inhibitory concentrations (MICs) for Gram-negative bacteria as well as the addition of different side-chains at position 3 of their nucleus, which modifies their kinetic properties, third- and fourth-generation cephalosporins in comparison with earlier compounds, have kinetics which are particularly advantageous when treating infections in the cerebrospinal fluid (CSF) or the prostatic and bone tissues.

Adverse events associated with the cephalosporins are not important and concern mainly allergic reactions. However, anaphylaxis/angioedema reactions are rare relative to the frequency of 0.04% associated with penicillin. Haematological reactions and coagulation abnormalities (hypoprothrombinaemia) have been reported mainly with moxalactam, while gastrointestinal reactions, mostly as antibiotic-associated diarrhoea including pseudomembranous colitis occur at a frequency of 1–7%.

Like the β-lactamase inhibitors, cephalosporins should not be given for common skin/soft-tissue infections since their extremely broad spectrum of activity disturbs the normal flora, facilitating colonization with enterococci and fungi, while favouring induction of resistance, with subsequent selection of resistant clones. However, for atypical clinical pictures or seriously ill patients, and while

Table 1 Classification of current cephalosporins with half-lives and daily dosage schedules

Generic name	Half-life (h)	Daily dosage regimen and route of administration
First generation		
Cephalothin	0.6	1–2 g every 4–6 h
Cefazolin	1.8	1 g every 8 h i.v. or i.m.
Cephradine	0.7	0.5 g every 6 h orally or 1–2 g every 4–6 h i.v.
Cephalexin	0.9	0.5–1 g every 6 h orally
Cefadroxil	1.2	0.5–1 g every 12 h orally
Second generation		
Cefamandole	0.8	2 g every 4–6 h i.v.
Cefoxitin	0.8	2 g every 4–6 h i.v.
Cefuroxime	1.3	1.5 g every 6–8 h i.v.
Cefotetan	3.5	2–3 g every 12 h i.v.
Ceforanide	3.0	1–2 g every 12 h i.v.
Cefonicid	4.5	1–2 g every 24 h i.v.
Cefmetazole	1.1	2 g every 6 h i.v.
Cefuroxime axetil	1.3	0.25–0.5 g every 12 h orally
Cefaclor	0.8	0.5–1 g every 8 h orally
Cefprozil	1.2	0.5–1 g every 8 h orally
Loracarbef	1.1	0.4 g every 12 h orally
Third generation		
Cefotaxime	1.0	2 g every 6–8 h i.v
Ceftriaxone	8.0	2 g every 12–24 h i.v.
Ceftazidime	1.8	2 g every 8 h i.v.
Ceftizoxime	1.7	2 g every 8–12 h i.v.
Cefmenoxime	1.0	2 g every 6–8 h i.v.
Cefoperazone	2.0	2 g every 8–12 h i.v
Cefpiramide	5.4	1–4 g every 12–24 h i.v
Moxalactam	2.2	1–2 g every 8 h i.v.
Cefixime	3.7	0.4 g every 24 h orally
Cefpodoxime proxetil	2.2	0.4 g every 12 h orally
Cefetamet	2.2	0.5 g every 12 h orally
Ceftibuten	2.5	0.2 g every 12 h orally
Fourth generation		
Cefepime	2.1	1–2 g every 8–12 h i.v.
Cefpirome	1.0	1–2 g every 8–12 h i.v.

diagnosis is pending, the prescription of a cephalosporin may be justified. The appropriate dosage regimens for adults are shown in Table 1.

Aminoglycosides

They are represented by tobramycin, netilmicin, amikacin and isepamicin for systemic use, neomycin for topical application and gentamicin for both. It should be pointed out that all aminoglycosides are inactive against streptococci as well as against anaerobes, while despite their *in vitro* activity, they do not behave as bactericidal agents against staphylococci. However, after combination *in vitro* with antistaphylococcal penicillins and/or rifampicin they exhibit a synergistic result. Therefore, the dermatologist at least for the common streptococcal or staphylococcal infections, should not prescribe any aminoglycoside either systemically or locally, as solutions or as ointments. Aminoglycosides are by definition ototoxic and nephrotoxic agents. Local application facilitates development of resistance among the Gram-negatives and particularly in *Pseudomonas aeruginosa* strains (which serve as colonizers and future pathogens) since the exposed skin area favours transfer of resistance genes. It should also be considered that various non-antimicrobial ointment ingredients are capable of inducing allergic skin reactions aggravating inflammatory signs.

Tetracyclines

Tetracyclines, on the basis of their different half-lives ($t_{1/2}$) are divided into three groups:

- The short-acting compounds with $t_{1/2}$ of 8–9 h (oxytetracycline and tetracycline).
- The intermediate compounds with $t_{1/2}$ of 12–14 h (demeclocycline and methacycline).
- The long-acting derivatives with $t_{1/2}$ of 16–18 h (doxycycline and minocycline).

The latter compounds are absorbed almost completely, achieving high serum levels with relatively small doses (100 mg dose equal to 500 mg of the short-acting compound). Despite their broad spectrum of activity covering both Gram-positive and several Gram-negative aerobic and anaerobic species, in a recent series 20–40% of the *Streptococcus pyogenes* and 50% of *Staph. aureus* strains were shown to have become resistant to tetracyclines. However, the lipophilic congeners represented by 'the long-acting' tetracyclines are two- to fourfold more active *in vitro* than the hydrophilic compounds. In particular, minocycline is the most effective against *Staph. aureus*, including MRSA strains.

The lipophilic tetracyclines are better diffused in many tissues and fluids. However, all cross the placenta. They concentrate in fetal bone and teeth causing hypoplasia of the enamel with subsequent grey–brown to yellow discoloration of the teeth and depression of skeletal growth in premature infants. Therefore, tetracyclines should not be given during pregnancy, at the breastfeeding period or to children up to the age of 8 years when tooth enamel is being formed.

Tetracyclines may cause photosensitivity reactions as well as gastrointestinal tract disturbances, hepatotoxicity and vertigo, a side-effect unique to minocycline usually beginning on the second or third day of therapy, which is more frequently observed in women than in men.

Food in general decreases the absorption of tetracyclines, while all form inactive complexes with divalent or trivalent cations. Therefore, tetracyclines should not be given simultaneously with calcium, magnesium and aluminium in antacids, milk or iron-containing compounds. Also, they should not be prescribed in pre-existing renal or hepatic insufficiency.

Although tetracyclines represent effective alternatives for a wide variety of infections, the dermatologist should be sceptical in considering them empirically in the therapy of the common skin/soft-tissue infection where susceptibility tests of the isolated pathogen should verify their administration. Doxycycline and minocycline, the tetracyclines of current use, are given at a loading oral dose of 200 mg followed by a daily dose of 100 mg every 24 h and 100 mg every 12 h, respectively.

Currently a new family of tetracyclines, the glycylcyclines, are under development. These compounds at least *in vitro* are very promising since they are very active against MRSA strains.

Macrolides and clindamycin

The macrolides (erythromycin, roxithromycin, azithromycin and clarithromycin) and the lincosamides (lincomycin and clindamycin) although chemically unrelated have similar properties. Among macrolides, clarithromycin possesses the most potent *in vitro* action against group A streptococci and methicillin-sensitive staphylococci (MSSA) strains followed by erythromycin, while azithromycin is two- to fourfold less active than erythromycin. However, cross-resistance among macrolides and lincosamides is usually the rule. It is a matter of concern that resistance rates of *Streptococcus pyogenes* to erythromycin have been increasing. These range widely in different countries, e.g. 60% in Japan, 5% in Oklahoma, USA, and recently 44% in Finland—a rise closely related to the high use of erythromycin for treating upper respiratory tract infections mainly in children. MRSA strains are almost always resistant to macrolides. Lincomycin or clindamycin resistance has been reported in 20–85% of MRSA strains including 50% of erythromycin-resistant strains. However, cross-resistance of *Staph. aureus* between lincomycin and clindamycin is complete. Clindamycin activity against streptococci is more potent than lincomycin but similar to that of erythromycin.

With the exception of azithromycin and lincomycin that are better absorbed without food, all others can be taken with food. Half-lives are 1.4 h for erythromycin, 3–7 h for clarithromycin, ≥70 h for azithromycin and ≥2.5 h for the lincosamides. Therefore, erythromycin should be administered at doses of 500 mg every 8 h orally or i.v., clarithromycin at 350–500 mg every 12 h orally, azithromycin at 500 mg every 24 h (no more than 3 days), lincomycin at 500 mg every 8 h i.v. or orally and clindamycin at 600 mg every 8–12 h i.v. or orally. With the exception of CSF, all have good tissue penetration and all are selectively concentrated in the macrophages.

Macrolides and lincosamides should be used by the dermatologist as alternatives to penicillin, particularly in β-lactam allergic patients. However, macrolides should not be used alone in the treatment of deep-seated staphylococcal infections because of the fear for the emergence of resistance during therapy.

Macrolides in general are safe drugs. Their main adverse reactions concern the gastrointestinal tract, more with eythromycin and much less with clarithromycin and azithromycin. However, with lincosamides diarrhoea occurs in up to 20% of patients, while 1.9–10% of clindamycin-treated patients, will suffer from the complication of pseudomembranous colitis. This is a syndrome caused by a toxin secreted by *Clostridium difficile* that overgrows particularly in the presence of lincosamides. The syndrome that can be fatal is not dose-related and occurs after oral or parenteral therapy. The implicated lincosamide should be discontinued promptly. Use of antiperistaltic drugs should be avoided. Vancomycin orally (125 mg four times a day) in severe diarrhoea or oral metronidazole (500 mg a day) in milder cases are effective therapy. Oral *Streptomyces bulardii* (brand name: Ultralevure) has been shown to act prophylactically.

Quinolones

The newer fluoroquinolones are represented by norfloxacin, ciprofloxacin, ofloxacin, enoxacin and pefloxacin. They represent fluorine- and piperazinyl-substituted derivatives of the original nalidixic acid structure which is a 1.8-naphthyridine. They are characterized by a broad spectrum of activity and good tolerability. Most are available for oral and parenteral use and possess similar bioavailability for both routes. Despite their broad spectrum of activity, the referred fluoroquinolones are not active against streptococci, anaerobes and MSSA, while their activity against MRSA is today considered as borderline. Therefore, there is no absolute indication for the use of MSSA in common dermatological infections. However, whenever *P. aeruginosa* is implicated, ciprofloxacin is an extremely potent compound and unique in being also available as an oral antipseudomonal antimicrobial.

Moxifloxacin is a novel 8-methoxy-fluoroquinolone with an improved spectrum of activity which includes Gram-positive, Gram-negative aerobic and anaerobic bacteria as well as intracellular pathogens. It is very active against streptococci, pneumococci, irrespective of β-lactam or macrolide-resistance and methicillin-susceptible staphylococci. It has a more variable activity against methicillin-resistant strains. It is also active against Enterobacteriaceae but not against *P. aeruginosa*. Its spectrum also includes anaerobes: *Clostridia, Fusobacteria, Prevotella, Porphyromonas, Peptostreptococci, Propionibacterium acnes* and *B. fragilis*.

As with other quinolones, moxifloxacin acts by binding to and inhibiting bacterial topoisomerases (i.e. topoisomerase II and IV). It has bactericidal activity against both Gram-positive and Gram-negative bacteria.

It is administered orally at a dose of 400 mg q.d. In common with older fluoroquinolones it has a favourable pharmacokinetic profile. It has an elimination $t_{1/2}$ of approximately 10 h. It is metabolized by conjugation and not by the cytochrome P450 system to inactive metabolites; this reduces the potential for interactions with other drugs. It is excreted by both renal and hepatic routes, reducing the potential for drug accumulation in patients with renal or liver impairment. Development of resistance is a concern when fluoroquinolones are used. *In vitro* studies showed that resistance to moxifloxacin developed less frequently and more slowly than to other fluoroquinolones. Furthermore, moxifloxacin was the least affected by mutations rendering resistance to older compounds.

The most common adverse events are gastrointestinal disturbances. In contrast to some other fluoroquinolones it appears to have a low propensity for phototoxic and central nervous system excitatory effects. As it is not metabolized by the cytochrome P450 pathway, it shows no interactions with methylxanthines, ranitidine, oral anticoagulants or contraceptives. Its bioavailability is reduced by the coadministration of antacids, sucralfate or iron preparations but not by food.

Although it is licensed for the indication of respiratory tract infections, it could be a useful agent for the treatment of mixed aerobic and anaerobic skin and soft-tissue infections from susceptible pathogens.

Rifampin

Primarily used for tuberculosis, rifampin has also very promising activity against staphylococci, including a high percentage of MRSA strains. However, it should never be administered as a single agent, because staphylococci will rapidly develop resistance *in vivo*. To protect against this, rifampin should be combined with another agent possessing antistaphylococcal activity, like trimethoprim–sulfamethoxazole, a fluoquinolone or a glycopeptide, i.e. vancomycin or teicoplanin. It should not be given empirically but only in cases where MRSA strains have been isolated. As an extremely lipophilic substance, rifampin penetrates well into all body tissues and strains brightly red almost all body excretions.

It is given in adults as a daily dose of 600 mg plus 300 mg orally or i.v.

Rifampin may cause hepatotoxicity, while it is one of the most potent inducers of intestinal and hepatic microsomal enzymes leading to decreased serum $t_{1/2}$ for several compounds, among which digoxin, dicumarol anticoagulants, prednizone, ketaconazole and oral contraceptives, requiring dosage adjustments for the latter drugs.

Fusidic acid

This antibiotic, despite its advantageous properties, is not available in the USA. It is mainly active *in vitro* and *in vivo* against staphylococci, including a high percentage of MRSA strains. Fusidic acid possesses excellent tissue kinetics and has a $t_{1/2}$ of 14 h. With the exception of self-limited hepatotoxicity, fusidic acid is safe and well tolerated by the oral route. The i.v. formula should be given in slow infusion (3–4 h) to avoid chemical irritation of veins with subsequent thrombophlebitis. Fusidic acid is given at a dose of 500 mg every 8 h orally or i.v. Topical application with gauzes drained with fusidic acid should be avoided, since it is rapidly followed by development of staphylococcal resistance of those staphylococci that colonize the skin.

Fusidic acid ointment can penetrate both intact and damaged skin as well as crust and cellular debris making it useful in the therapy of boils, paronychia, impetigo and pyoderma. In the case of erythrasma caused by *Corynebacterium minutissimum*, topical application is very successful.

Sulphonamides and trimethoprim

These are very rarely used as antibacterial agents since many of the common bacteria have become resistant to them. However, when combined with trimethoprim, a synergistic result—mostly against the Enterobacteriaceae, streptococci and staphylococci—is achieved, since trimethoprim potentiates the sulphonamide activity by the sequential inhibition of folic acid and synthesis. Dermatological use of this combination is however, limited since it is a third choice antimicrobial for common dermatological infections. It has a $t_{1/2}$ of approximately 11 h and is given at a dose of 480–960 mg every 8–12 h orally or parenterally. The most important side-effects are attributed to the sulphonamide component and include acute haemolysis related to glucose-6-phosphate dehydrogenase deficiency and erythema multiforme often expressed as Stevens–Johnson syndrome.

Glycopeptides

This group is represented by vancomycin and teicoplanin. The former is an old antibiotic, the interest for which was greatly augmented over the last decade because of the worldwide emergence of MRSA strains. Until recently, the glycopeptides were the only antibiotics with antistaphylococcal activity against MRSAs. However, in June 1997 the first MRSA isolates resistant to glycopeptides were reported from Japan. It is obvious that similar strains will emerge in the future—physicians will very soon encounter untreatable staphylococcal infections and innumerable deaths, approaching the so-called 'postantibiotic era'.

Glycopeptides are also very active against streptococci, *Corynebacterium* spp., *enterococci* and *Bacillus anthracis*. They are inactive against the Gram-negative bacteria. Cross-resistance between the two derivatives is expected. However, some *S. haemolyticus* and *S. epidermis* strains resistant to vancomycin only and some *enterococci* susceptible only to teicoplanin have been reported.

Vancomycin $t_{1/2}$ is approximately 6 h, while teicoplanin $t_{1/2}$ is extremely prolonged exceeding 15 h. Therefore, vancomycin is given i.v. at a dose of 500 mg every 6 h or 100 mg every 12 h while teicoplanin both i.v. or i.m. at a dose of 6–10 mg/kg once daily, depending on the severity of the underlying infection. Both are not absorbed by the oral route and share rather poor tissue kinetics.

Only in severe cases of pseudomembranous colitis caused by *Clostridium difficile* is oral vancomycin the antibiotic of choice.

Both glycopeptides should be given in serious MRSA infections while in penicillin-allergic patients, they serve as alternatives for serious streptococcal infections.

Rapid or bolus administration of vancomycin is dangerous because it may cause flushing, the 'red-man' or 'red-neck' syndrome, anaphylactoid reactions, hypotension and cardiac arrest—therefore, vancomycin should always be given over a 30–60 min infusion. Vancomycin is also ototoxic and potentially nephrotoxic particularly when combined with aminoglycosides or diuretics, while drug fever is the most frequent side-effect. Teicoplanin is well tolerated; it does not require slow infusion but ototoxicity, nephrotoxicity (microscopic haematuria) and drug fever may be encountered.

Mupirocin

Mupirocin is a locally applied agent which is bactericidal against staphylococci both MSSA and MRSA and streptococci at concentrations achieved by topical administration (20 000 mg/mL with the 2% formulation) after 24–36 h exposure. It was formerly called pseudomonic acid because the major metabolite responsible for most of its antibacterial activity is derived from the submerged fermentation by *Pseudomonas fluorescens*. Despite its name, it is not active against *Pseudomonas* spp. Its weak *in vitro* activity against normal skin flora, e.g. *Corynebacterium, Propionibacterium* and *Micrococcus* spp., is advantageous because it preserves intact the skin's natural defence against infection. Unfortunately prolonged courses of mupirocin for chronic skin infections can lead to development of resistant staphylococci. Therefore mupirocin should not be used for long-term therapy.

Mupirocin is not absorbed systemically after topical application to intact skin. On damaged skin some mupirocin will be absorbed, but it is rapidly inactivated.

Mupirocin should be used mainly for impetigo and folliculitis with clinical and bacteriological cure rates of 85–100% and 80–95%, respectively. However, in cases of widespread impetigo, systemic therapy is preferable. It is also effective in the therapy of secondarily infected eczema, lacerations, burns and leg ulcers. Mupirocin can also eliminate nasal carriage of *Staph. aureus* particularly in acute carrier outbreaks of epidemic MRSA. No substantial toxicity in humans has been reported.

Linezolid

Linezolid is the first member of the oxazolidinone class of synthetic antibacterial agents to be introduced into clinical practice. It has a unique mechanism of action—it inhibits protein synthesis by interfering with initiation complex formation. Cross-resistance with other inhibitors of protein synthesis (i.e. macrolides, streptogramins, aminoglycosides, fusidic acid, tetracyclines, chloramphenicol) has not been observed since the oxazolidinones act early in translation, inhibiting this process at a different stage.

Linezolid inhibits most Gram-positive organisms such as staphylococci, including methicillin-resistant strains, *Streptococcus* spp., including macrolide-resistant strains, *E. faecium* and *E. faecalis*, including vancomycin-resistant strains, pneumococci including penicillin-resistant strains, *Bacillus* spp., *Corynebacterium* spp., *Erysipelothrix* spp., Anaerobes such as *Clostridium* spp., *Peptostreptococcus* spp., *Prevotella* spp., *Propionibacterium acnes*, *B. fragilis*, *Fusobacterium* spp. are also susceptible to linezolid whereas Enterobacteriaceae and *P. aeruginosa* are not. With a susceptibility breakpoint of $\leq 4\ \mu g/mL$, according to the National Committee for Clinical Laboratory Standards (NCCLS), it inhibits all susceptible strains at MICs of 1–4 μg/mL. It has bacteriostatic activity against staphylococci and enterococci whereas bactericidal activity was reported against some streptococcal strains and against some *B. fragilis* and *C. perfringens*.

Linezolid is available for both oral and intravenous administration at the same dose of 600 mg b.i.d. It is rapidly and completely absorbed after oral administration with a bioavailability of approximately 100%, not influenced by the presence of food. It has an elimination $t_{1/2}$ of 5–7 h and is excreted by both renal and non-renal routes. No dose adjustment is required for mild to moderate renal (creatinine clearance ≤ 40 mL/min) or liver impairment. Furthermore, no drug interactions are reported so far. In clinical trials linezolid achieved approximately 90% clinical and microbiological cure rates in skin and soft-tissue infections, proving equivalent to clarithromycin for uncomplicated and to cloxacillin/dicloxacillin for complicated infections. Linezolid is well tolerated. Adverse effects were reported for 32.7% of the patients treated for almost 20 days and these were mild and included gastrointestinal disturbances and headache but only 3% discontinued the drug. Also, mild and transient elevation of liver enzymes, thrombocytopenia and anaemia are reported after a prolonged course, the latter being quite frequent.

Overall, linezolid seems to be a safe antimicrobial agent useful for the dermatologist since it is potent against drug-resistant bacteria and especially MRSA, and is available for oral as well as for parenteral administration.

Synercid

Synercid is a combination of two semisynthetic streptogramin molecules, quinupristin (a group B or type I streptogramin) and dalfopristin (a group A or type II streptogramin) in a 30 : 70 ratio (w/w). The combination has synergistic antibacterial activity *in vitro* against a wide range of Gram-positive organisms. It is active against most strains of *Staph. aureus* and coagulase-negative staphylococci, including multidrug-resistant, methicillin-resistant and glycopeptide-intermediate strains, streptococci, including penicillin- and macrolide-resistant strains, *E. faecium*, including multidrug-resistant and vancomycin-resistant strains, while it is intrinsically inactive against *E. faecalis*. It is also active against *Strep. pneumoniae*, including penicillin-resistant strains, against *Moraxella catarrhalis*, pathogenic *Neisseria* spp. and Gram-positive anaerobes such as *Clostridium* and *Peptostreptococcus* spp. Synercid exerts its activity through inhibition of protein synthesis. It is bactericidal against staphylococci and pneumococci and bacteriostatic against enterococci.

Synercid is available only for intravenous administration. It has a prolonged postantibiotic effect of 6–8 h, polymorphonuclear leucocyte/macrophage penetration and slow release, it is not extensively protein bound and it is quickly metabolized in active metabolites. These characteristics allow for a 8 or 12 h dosing interval despite an elimination $t_{1/2}$ of 3.7 ± 0.51 and 1.04 ± 0.2 h for quinupristin and dalfopristin, respectively. The recommended dose is 7.5 mg/kg every 8 h or every 12 h for skin and soft-tissue infections. The drug must be diluted in 5% glucose/dextrose solution and infused over 60 min. Following completion of the infusion, the vein should be flushed with 5% glucose/dextrose solution. It is recommended not to flush with saline or heparin as it is incompatible with these solutions. A dose reduction is required for patients with hepatic cirrhosis or severe renal insufficiency. The drug combination is a potent inhibitor of the cytochrome P450 enzymes, exhibiting clinically important interactions with many other drugs such as antihistamines, antiretroviral agents, antineoplastic agents, benzodiazepines, calcium channel blockers, cholesterol-lowering agents, gastrointestinal motility agents, immunosuppressive agents, steroids, and so on, as synercid enhances their activity.

From the point of view of dermatology, the combination has been shown in clinical trials to be as effective as the comparators (vancomycin and/or oxacillin and vancomycin and/or cefazolin) for the treatment of complicated skin and soft-tissue infections (erysipelas, traumatic wound infection, severe carbunculosis, partial thickness burn wounds, and so on) due to staphylococci, streptococci and enterococci including multidrug-resistant isolates. The most common adverse effects related to the drug were arthralgia, myalgia, gastrointestinal disturbances, rash, headache, generalized pain and pruritus. Peripheral venous irritation was frequently seen and can be minimized by infusion via a central venous route. Increases in conjugated bilirubin were frequently observed whereas thrombocytopenia, hepatitis, jaundice, anaemia, pancytopenia and metabolic acidosis were only rarely reported.

Synercid may prove to be a very useful alternative agent for the treatment of serious infections caused by multidrug-resistant Gram-positive pathogens or for patients who are unable to tolerate glycopeptides due to allergy or nephrotoxicity.

New compounds in phase II/III clinical trials

Oritavancin

Oritavancin (LY333328) is a new semisynthetic glycopeptide antibiotic acting by inhibition of cell wall synthesis in a way similar to vancomycin. Its spectrum includes Gram-positive bacteria: staphylococci susceptible as well as resistant to methicillin, staphylococci with reduced susceptibility to vancomycin, enterococci susceptible as well as resistant to glycopeptides, and penicillin susceptible and resistant pneumococci and streptococci. It is also active against *Corynebacterium JK*, *Clostridium difficile*, *Lactobacillus* spp., *Leuconostoc*, *Pediococcus*, *Erysipelothrix* and *Listeria*. It is bactericidal against most susceptible strains including enterococci.

It has a long $t_{1/2}$ of 11.5 days and a long concentration-dependent postantibiotic effect which enables once daily dosing and short courses of treatment. It is only available for i.v. administration at a proposed dose of 200 or 300 mg q.d. diluted in dextrose in water 5% and infused over 30 min. Phase II clinical studies showed that potential adverse events could be rash, gastrointestinal symptoms, histamine-related infusion reactions and phlebitis. Mild transient elevations of liver enzymes were noted whereas no ototoxicity or nephrotoxicity were reported. It is currently in phase III of clinical trials for the treatment of skin and soft-tissue infections and appears to be a promising agent for the treatment of such infections caused by resistant pathogens.

Telithromycin

Telithromycin (HMR3647) is a new semisynthetic 14-membered-ring macrolide, the molecule derived from erythromycin A with the substitution of an L-cladinose moiety by a 3-keto group. The new compound acts by inhibition of translation at the level of 50S ribosomal subunit and exhibits some innovative characteristics: (a) activity against Gram-positive cocci resistant to erythromycin by an efflux mechanism or by an inducible MLS_B mechanism but not against isolates having a constitutive MLS_B mechanism; (b) lack of inducible resistance to macrolides; and (c) stability in acidic environments.

The antibacterial spectrum of telithromycin covers Gram-positive cocci and bacilli, Gram-negative cocci, some Gram-negative bacilli such as *Haemophilus influenzae*, *Moraxella catarrhalis*, *Bortetella pertussis* and *Pasteurella* spp., *Helicobacter pylori*, intracellular pathogens, atypical microorganisms and anaerobic bacteria. It is two to four times more active than clarithromycin against erythromycin-susceptible Gram-positive cocci and it is also active against most but not all of erythromycin- and clarithromycin-resistant isolates, depending on the underlying mechanism of resistance. It is highly concentrated in phagocytes and pharmacodynamic models have shown that it can be given orally once a day.

Further reading

Barman Balfour JA, Lamb HM. Moxifloxacin. *Drugs* 2000; 59 (1): 115–39.

Brooks AK, Zervos MJ. New antimicrobial agents for Gram-positive infections. *Curr Opin Infect Dis* 1998; 11: 667–71.

Bryskier A. Ketolides-telithromycin, an example of a new class of antimicrobial agents. *Clin Microbiol Infect* 2000; 6: 661–9.

Bush LM, Calmon J, Johnson CC. Newer penicillins and beta-lactamase inhibitors. *Infect Dis Clin N Am* 1995; 9: 687–713.

Clemett D, Markham A. Linezolid. *Drugs* 2000; 59 (4): 815–27.

Donowitz GR, Mandell GL. Beta-lactam antibiotics. *N Engl J Med* 1988; 3123: 490–500.

Hendershot EF. Fluoroquinolones. *Infect Dis Clin N Am* 1995; 9: 715–30.

Kaye ET, Kaye KM. Topical antibacterial agents. *Infect Dis Clin N Am* 1995; 9: 547–9.

Lundstrom TS, Sobel JD. Vancomycin. Trimethoprim-sulfamethoxazole and rifampin. *Infect Dis Clin N Am* 1995; 9: 747–67.

Neu HC. Oral β-lactam antibiotics from 1960 to 1993. *Infect Dis Clin Prac* 1993; 6: 394–404.

Phillips G, Golledge CL. Vancomycin and teicoplanin—something old, something new. *Med J Austral* 1992; 156: 53–7.

Rubinstein E, Prokocimer P, Talbot GH. Safety and tolerability of quinupristin/dalfopristin: administration guidelines. *J Antimicrob Chemother* 1999; 44 (S4): 37–46.

Sogn DD, Evans R III, Shepherd G. *et al.* Results of the National Institute of Allergy and Infectious Diseases collaborative trial to test the predictive value of skin testing with major and minor penicillin derivatives in hospitalized adults. *Arch Intern Med* 1992; 152: 1625–32.

Zuckerman J, Mascaro KM. The newer macrolides azithromycin, clarithromycin. *Infect Dis Clin N Am* 1995; 9: 731–45.

Antifungal drugs

R.J. Hay

General principles, classification and structure

The antifungal drugs currently used for the treatment of skin and mucosal diseases can be grouped into two large families and a number of smaller ones. Most of the modern drugs are broad spectrum in their antifungal activity *in vitro* and inhibit the wide variety of different fungi that cause superficial fungal disease. Many are available as either topical or systemic treatments. *In vitro* some behave as cidal compounds, in other words the concentration at which they inhibit growth, the minimum inhibitory concentration (MIC), is the same or very close to the concentration at which they destroy the fungi, the minimum cidal concentration (MCC). In theory this property is an advantage, as it should mean that fungal cell death depends on drug concentration alone, although in real infections other factors such as local availability of the antifungal play a key role in determining the outcome of treatment.

The largest family of antifungals is the azole family, a group that can be further subdivided into two distinct subdivisions, the imidazoles and the triazoles. The chemical structure of both is based on an azole ring with different side-chains that affect the solubility, antifungal activity and, probably, drug-resistance properties of each compound. These are all synthetic compounds. There is another large family of polyene antifungals that have a large central macrolide ring structure. In distinction to the azoles the polyenes are derived from *Streptomyces* species and, although a large number of different polyene derivatives are known, there are few in clinical use.

Other important antifungal agents include the allylamine and the morpholine groups as well as griseofulvin, flucytosine and ciclopirox. These will be discussed separately.

The availability of these drugs for medical use varies between different countries.

Azole antifungals

Mechanisms of action

There are two distinct groups of compounds within the azole family, the imidazoles and the triazoles. The imidazoles are synthetic antifungal agents. They include miconazole, clotrimazole, econazole, isoconazole, ketoconazole, tioconazole and bifonazole. The triazole series contains two potent oral agents, fluconazole and itraconazole. In addition there are two new triazoles, voriconazole and posaconazole, at present in phase III clinical trials.

Many azoles have been developed for topical use although some, particularly the triazoles are effective in the treatment of deep mycoses. For instance ketoconazole (oral), itraconazole (oral and intravenous), fluconazole (oral and intravenous) and miconazole (intravenous) all have systemically active formulations. The azoles are metabolized in the liver and affect fungal cell-membrane synthesis through inhibition of cytochrome P450-dependent 14α-demethylation which is responsible for a key stage in the synthesis of ergosterol in the cell membrane. To some extent azoles all show some affinity for certain human cytochrome P450 isoenzymes, a property which may lead to drug interactions or competition with human metabolic processes. There is, however, considerable variation amongst the different drugs in this respect. Ketoconazole, for instance, may inhibit adrenal biosynthesis of androgens at high concentrations; the triazoles show little interaction with this human metabolic pathway. Apart from fluconazole most azoles penetrate cerebrospinal fluid and urine in low concentrations. The azoles have a broad spectrum of activity against many fungal pathogens, although fluconazole, miconazole and ketoconazole are not effective for *Aspergillus* infections. By contrast, itraconazole is active *in vitro* against a very wide variety of mould fungi including aspergilli as well as dematiaceous (pigmented) fungi. Fluconazole is less active against mould fungi and there are instances of both primary (*Candida krusei*, *C. glabrata*) and secondary antimicrobial resistance to this compound. However all the azoles can be used for treatment of the common superficial mycoses such as dermatophytosis, candidosis and *Malassezia* infections.

Indications and other uses

Topical azoles

Many of the imidazole antifungals are available as topical agents for the treatment of superficial mycoses such as dermatophytosis and pityriasis versicolor. Some Gram-positive bacterial infections such as erythrasma caused by *Corynebacterium minutissimum* as well as *Staphylococcus aureus* may respond to many imidazoles but not triazoles. Although topical imidazole creams, ointments or powders are usually given twice daily there is evidence that some, e.g. sulconazole, can be given once daily; it is possible that this is an appropriate regimen for many azoles, but unfortunately there is not the clinical trial data to support a wider recommendation at present.

The duration of treatment using topical azoles is also variable. Most of the original clinical trials were based on a 4-week treatment duration and their efficacy is established on this basis. However some topically applied compounds, such as ketoconazole, appear to be effective after shorter periods of treatment; again it is not clear whether these shorter treatment regimens would also be appropriate for other topical azoles

Ketoconazole

Ketoconazole is an imidazole antifungal available as topical therapy or as an oral tablet (200 mg). It is active against most superficial fungi but not against Gram-positive bacteria, a property of most other topically active imidazole antifungals. Ketoconazole is used for the treatment of oropharyngeal candidosis in doses of 200–400 mg daily. In patients with acquired immune deficiency syndrome (AIDS) or those receiving chemotherapy for the treatment of malignancy ketoconazole is usually given in double dosage as absorption is often impaired in these patients, mainly due to lack of gastric acidity. Ketoconazole is also active in *Malassezia* infections such as pityriasis versicolor in doses which range from a single 400-mg dose to 200 mg given for 5 days. For dermatophytosis it is effective orally in treatment durations of at least 1 month. However, it is seldom used for this indication due to a risk of symptomatic hepatic reactions in some patients. Ketoconazole has also been used as oral treatment of severe seborrhoeic dermatitis of the scalp. In addition it is used for some systemic or deep mycoses such as mycetoma due to *Madurella mycetomatis*, sporotrichosis, subcutaneous zygomycosis, histoplasmosis, paracoccidioidomycosis and blastomycosis. For these latter indications it has largely been superseded by itraconazole.

There is also a shampoo formulation of ketonazole used for the treatment of seborrhoeic dermatitis of the scalp or the management of the carrier state in tinea capitis.

Drug resistance of yeast species to ketoconazole can occur (see below).

Itraconazole

Itraconazole is an orally active triazole. Its mode of action, as with all azoles, is through the inhibition of the formation of ergosterol in the fungal cell membrane via inhibition of the 14α-demethylase enzyme. Itraconazole is fungistatic *in vitro* but is active against a wide range of organisms including dermatophytes, moulds such as aspergilli, dimorphic fungi such as *Histoplasma* and *Penicillium marneffei*; it is also active against yeasts including *Candida albicans*. Most countries do not have a product license for the use of itraconazole in children. Itraconazole comes in three main formulations: a capsule containing pelleted itraconazole and an oral solution containing itraconazole in cyclodextrin as well as an intravenous formulation. The oral solution is designed for the treatment of severe oropharyngeal and oesophageal candidosis in severely immunocompromised patients. The solution is not intended for paediatric use in dermatophytosis at present.

Itraconazole is also effective in dermatophyte infections. The daily doses in adults are 200 mg daily for 1–2 weeks for tinea corporis but 200 mg twice daily given each day for one week every month for 2–3 months in onychomycosis. This approach to treatment is known as pulse(d) therapy. Doses of 200 mg twice daily for 1 week are appropriate for dry-type tinea pedis. For tinea capitis in children itraconazole is generally given in 3–4 mg/kg daily doses. The regimens used have varied between 3 and 5 mg/kg daily for 4 to 6 weeks which is effective in over 80% of children with tinea capitis due to *T. tonsurans*. A pulsed regimen using 5 mg/kg for 1 week every 3 weeks has been evaluated in a small number of children.

The use of itraconazole extends to superficial candidosis, particularly to proven cases of *Candida* onychomycosis and oropharyngeal candidosis. Like ketoconazole it is mainly used at higher dosage in patients with AIDS (e.g. 200 mg daily) but the oral solution formulation can be given at 100–200 mg daily in such patients. *Malassezia* infections including pityriasis versicolor and *Malassezia* folliculitis respond to itraconazole, which is also used in severe cases of seborrhoeic dermatitis.

Itraconazole is useful in some deep mycoses such as sporotrichosis, chromoblastomycosis and subcutaneous zygomycosis. It is used as primary or secondary treatment in histoplasmosis, paracoccidioidomycosis and blastomycosis also coccidioidomycosis and infections due to *Penicillium marneffei*. Long-term (suppressive) therapy in histoplasmosis and *Penicillium* infections after initial treatment is used in many countries and in patients not receiving highly active antiretroviral therapy (HAART) to prevent recurrence of infection.

Drug resistance to itraconazale is not common but some fungi develop multiple resistance to azoles (see below).

Fluconazole

Fluconazole is an orally active triazole antifungal. As with other triazoles the main site of action is through the inhibition of the 14α-demethylase enzyme. There are both oral and liquid formulations of fluconazole as well as an intravenous form for deep infections.

The drug is active against a range of fungi including yeasts such as *Candida albicans* and *Cryptococcus neoformans*, as well as some mould fungi including dermatophytes. It is less active in other mould infections such as aspergillosis and zygomycosis.

Fluconazole is effective in superficial candidosis, including oropharyngeal candidosis, and dermatophytosis in doses of 100–200 mg daily. In practice it is often given as a 150-mg weekly treatment for 2–8 weeks in tinea corporis. In onychomycosis it is given in weekly doses of 150–300 mg and the duration monitored by clinical and mycological recovery. The evidence to date suggests that fluconazole is effective against a range of different dermatophytes including both *Trichophyton* and *Microsporum* species. At present there is no evidence to show any differential activity. Its value in tinea capitis is still the subject of evaluation. The doses that have been used here have ranged from 1.5 to 6 mg/kg daily and up to 8 mg/kg weekly.

Fluconazole is very active against *Candida* species apart from *Candida krusei* and *Candida glabrata*. However, there is a risk of resistance developing in infections in immunocompromised subjects if the drug is continued in the presence of persisting infection. Resistance to fluconazole is mainly seen in oropharyngeal *Candida* infections in patients with AIDS. There are at least four different mechanisms for drug resistance including increased efflux from the fungal cell, changes in the site of action of the drug, decreased binding at the active site, and the existence of supplementary paths of ergosterol biosynthesis. Drugs resistance to ketoconazole and to a lesser extent itraconazole may also occur. There is no evidence that resistance may also occur among dermatophytes. Fluconazole is used for oropharyngeal candidosis and can be given at the same dosage (50–200 mg daily) to all patients. It is active against vaginal candidosis where a single oral treatment of 150 mg is given.

Fluconazole is also widely used for systemic candidosis as either oral or intravenous therapy and in the primary or secondary treatment of cryptococcosis.

Side-effects, contraindications and drug interactions

Most of the topical azoles can occasionally cause mild stinging and, exceptionally, allergic contact dermatitis. Oral azoles have a low frequency of adverse reactions such as nausea, dyspepsia and gastrointestinal discomfort or headache. The frequency of severe adverse events is low. However these are important to note. Ketoconazole causes hepatitis in a small proportion of cases estimated to be approximately 1 : 7000. The risk factors for this are not well understood, although patients with a previous history of liver disease may be at risk. For this reason the drug is rarely used long term, for instance, in the management of fungal nail disease. Ketoconazole may also cause gynaecomastia in males and menstrual irregularities in women when used in doses over 400 mg daily, problems associated with interferences with androgen metabolism. With itraconazole and fluconazole the incidence of symptomatic hepatitis is much lower; in the case of itraconazole, for instance, less than 1 : 100 000 cases. With fluconazole it is more difficult to estimate the frequency of adverse reactions as the cohort of patients treated with this drug has been different and includes many with severe systemic disease; attributing hepatic dysfunction in such cases to a single cause is correspondingly difficult. Exceptionally rare adverse events include angioedema (itraconazole), thrombocytopenia (fluconazole) and toxic epidermal necrolysis (fluconazole).

There is an important list of drug interactions with the azoles that should be remembered. As a general principle itraconazole is more likely to be associated with drug interactions but those that may cause serious consequences, e.g. terfenadine, astemizole and digoxin, are seen with all azoles. In addition statins, e.g. somatostatin, appear to interact with itraconazole to cause rhabdomyolysis.

These interactions and those of other oral antifungals are summarized in Table 2. Contraindications of the use of azoles are shown in Table 3.

Polyene antifungals

Mechanisms of action

The polyene antifungals have been known for longer than the azoles. They

Table 1 Azole antifungals (only the more commonly used compounds have been shown)

Class	Oral	Topical
Imidazole	Ketoconazole	Clotrimazole, miconazole, econazole, sulconazole, biofonazole, ketoconazole, tioconazole
Triazole	Itraconazole Fluconazole	Terconazole

Table 2 Main drug interactions and oral antifungals[1]

Drug name	Interaction
Terbinafine	Terbinafine serum levels reduced by Rifampicin Terbinafine increases levels of: Nortriptyline, warfarin?
Itraconazole, fluconazole, ketoconazole The breadth of the data provided depends on reports of clinical interactions. These vary between the different drugs and between patients	Azole serum levels may be reduced by: Rifampicin, rifabutin, phenytoin, phenobarbitone, carbamazepine Azoles may increase levels of: Terfenadine, astemizole, digoxin, ciclosporin, tacrolimus, midazolam, triazolam, warfarin, loratidine, tolbutamide. This varies between drugs and is more prominent with itraconazole Azoles may also reduce serum levels of some drugs such as oestrogens, cisapride (mainly itraconazole), busulphan Itraconazole interacts with statins such as lovastatin and simvastatin to cause rhabdomyolysis
Griseofulvin	Griseofulvin serum levels reduced by: phenytoin, phenobarbitone Griseofulvin may reduce levels of oestrogens and warfarin

[1]Many of these drug reactions depend on interactions between drugs and cytochrome P450 isoenzymes such as P3A4. Unfortunately these are not necessarily either predictive of the likelihood of reaction nor can they always explain the mechanisms of drug interaction. Those listed here are the commonly reported or potentially dangerous reactions. Theoretically terbinafine can interact with P2D6 but only one report of a reaction with nortriptyline is associated with this mechanism.

Table 3 Drug combinations that are contraindicated with the azoles—ketoconazole, itraconazole and fluconazole

Terfenadine, Astemizole, Azolam compounds, Cisapride (particular caution with digoxin)
In addition statins such as lovastatin should not be given with itraconazole

are macrolide substances derived originally from *Streptomyces* species. Although comprising a large family, only three polyenes, amphotericin B, nystatin and natamycin, are in current use for treatment. More recent experimental additions to this group were partricin and mepartricin, but neither has been developed further. Amphotericin B, which is derived from *Streptomyces nodosus*, is the only polyene widely used as a parenterally administered drug; it is also available as an oral tablet or pastille. Nystatin and natamycin are purely topical, either creams, pastilles, suspensions or, in the case of nystatin, as a vaginal tablet. Amphotericin B is metabolized in the liver and penetrates body cavities, cerebrospinal fluid and urine poorly. The polyenes have a broad *in vitro* spectrum of activity against a wide range of fungi including the major systemic pathogenic fungi such as *Aspergillus* and *Candida* species. Amphotericin B is widely used for the treatment of deep mycoses. The mode of action of the polyenes appears to involve inhibition of sterol synthesis in the fungal cell membrane. Polyenes function, though, by binding onto the sterol membrane and causing cell leakage.

Combinations of amphotericin B with a lipid, for instance in a liposome, have been developed as a means of reducing the nephrotoxicity of the intravenous drug. Three commercial 'lipid-associated amphotericins' are available: AmBisome (a true liposome), amphotericin B lipid complex—ABLC or Abelcet (a ribbon-like lipid-binding amphotericin B), and amphotericin B colloidal dispersion (ABCD) (a suspension of lipid discs). It does not appear that these combinations have different modes of action but in the case of AmBisome there is evidence that the active drug, i.e. amphotericin B, is directly transferred from the lipid droplet to the fungal cell membrane. These formulations are comparatively expensive and are not used for superficial infections.

Indications and other uses

The polyene antifungal, amphotericin B, is widely used as a systemic agent for the treatment of systemic mycoses such as aspergillosis and candidosis. The newer lipid-associated amphotericins are used for similar indications including the treatment of the febrile neutropenic patient.

Amphotericin B is also used in the topical treatment of oropharyngeal candidosis as a lozenge; this treatment is not available in certain countries. It is given four times daily for 7–19 days.

Nystatin likewise is used for topical treatment generally for oral candidosis in lozenge or suspension form or as a vaginal tablet for vulvovaginal candidosis. It is also available as an ointment for skin disease. It is used twice daily for at least 14 days for these indications.

Natamycin is not used for the treatment of skin disease.

Side-effects, contraindications and drug interactions

It is beyond the scope of this chapter to discuss the side-effects of intravenous amphotericin B although it is recognized that the use of this drug is associated with a high frequency of side-effects such as potassium loss, renal failure and renal tubular necrosis as well as anaemia. By contrast the use of the topical preparations, either on the skin or orally, is seldom associated with any problems apart from the bitter taste of some of the oral preparations.

Allylamine antifungals

Mechanisms of action

The allylamine drugs comprise a smaller group of compounds. There are two related compounds naftifine and terbinafine. There is also a related compound, the benzylamine, butenafine, which is available in some countries. These drugs inhibit squalene epoxidase which is active in the early part of the pathway for the biosynthesis of ergosterol in the fungal cell membrane. They are fungicidal compounds. The antifungal activity appears to depend on two events—the accumulation of squalene, which disrupts intracellular membranes and the depletion of ergosterol in the membrane. Cidal activity resides mainly with the former property. The allylamines are available as topical agents (naftifine, terbinafine), but terbinafine is also an oral drug. Terbinafine has a very high level of *in vitro* activity against a number of different fungi such as dermatophytes where MICs lie between 0.01 and 0.001 mg/mL. The MFCs are usually at the same or within a single dilution of these

MICs which explains the high fungicidal activity *in vitro*. Terbinafine is also very active against some mould fungi such as aspergilli, dimorphic pathogens, e.g. *Sporothrix schenckii*, and pigmented fungi. It is somewhat less active against yeasts such as *Candida* species and is only fungistatic against *C. albicans*. Terbinafine is lipophilic and well absorbed (70%) after oral administration. After oral administration it has a large peripheral volume of distribution and is bound in tissue rich in lipid or keratin. This provides a great advantage for dermatophytosis but less for yeast infections such as those caused by *Malassezia* species where terbinafine is active clinically after topical administration but not after oral treatment.

Indications and other uses

Terbinafine is potent against all dermatophyte infections and it also has activity against a range of mould fungi including aspergilli, dimorphic agents such as *Histoplasma* and *Sporothrix*; it is less effective against yeasts such as *C. albicans* although it can be used topically to treat superficial candidosis. Terbinafine is available as a cream or in tablet form (250 mg). The topical preparation can be used for the treatment of dermatophytosis such as interdigital tinea pedis, superficial candidosis of the skin and pityriasis versicolor. It is clear that treatment periods may be very short and in one study 1-day treatment was as effective as 1-week treatment in tinea pedis.

Oral treatment is mainly aimed at dermatophyte infections including onychomycosis due to dermatophytes. The oral compound is not clinically effective at normal doses in superficial *Candida* or *Malassezia* infections. The dose is 250 mg for adults. In some countries a paediatric tablet is available (125 mg). In children the regimen used is based on weight: $<$20 kg 62.5 mg/day, 20–40 kg 125 mg/day and $>$40 kg 250 mg/day. The responses of dermatophyte infections to oral terbinafine are excellent. In most tinea infections the duration of oral treatment is 1–2 weeks. In onychomycosis the drug is given for 6 weeks for fingernail infections and 12 weeks for toenails. The results are good with remission rates of 70–80% being achieved even after long-term follow-up of over 1 year. In tinea capitis it is effective against a range of organisms and there are a number of studies comparing terbinafine with griseofulvin. However, there are several points to note. The treatment period is usually 4 weeks—although there are some data to show that shorter periods of treatment may be effective, e.g. 2 weeks for infections due to *Trichophyton* species. The responses of *Microsporum* species causing scalp disease are generally slower than those of *Trichophyton* and in some patients there is treatment failure. Terbinafine is also used in some deep infections notably sporotrichosis and chromoblastomycosis in doses of 250 mg daily.

Naftifine is a related allylamine similar to terbinafine but only available for topical usage in some countries. It is effective is dermatophytosis and other superficial mycoses. It has a similar spectrum and mode of action as terbinafine and is given for 1–2 weeks.

Side-effects, contraindications and drug interactions

Terbinafine is associated with a low level of adverse effects after topical use—occasional reports of irritation. After oral treatment a variety of minor problems may occur such as nausea and dyspepsia. More serious events are occasionally seen. For instance alteration of taste or even loss of taste may occur. It is expected to return to normal after 4 weeks. Rare instance of hepatic dysfunction presenting with jaundice have been reported. Other very rare drug side-effects such as thrombocytopenia or granulocytopenia have also been reported. Drug interactions are shown in Table 2; they are not common.

Griseofulvin

Mechanism of action

Griseofulvin is an orally active compound derived from the organism, *Penicillium griseofulvens*. It is fungistatic *in vitro* and its mode of action is through the inhibition of intracellular microtubules. This prevents the formation of the mitotic spindle. Griseofulvin is active *in vitro* against dermatophyte fungi but few other organisms respond to the drug. In addition to its antifungal properties it inhibits leucocyte movement.

Indications and other uses

The traditional treatment for many dermatophyte infections was oral griseofulvin given in a dose of 500–1000 mg daily (adults) or 10 mg/kg daily for a period of 4–8 weeks for superficial infections apart from nail disease; and for 6–18 months for onychomycosis. The drug is ineffective in *Candida* or *Malassezia* infections and it cannot be given by topical route. There are both tablet and liquid formulations of griseofulvin. Because it was one of the earliest antifungal drugs introduced there are few comparative clinical trials on which to base an assessment of its efficacy.

Griseofulvin appears slower in action than the newer azole and allylamine antifungals and, in many instances, has been superseded by the newer compounds such as itraconazole or terbinafine. However it is effective for most organisms causing tinea capitis, although there are some patients with *Microsporum canis* infections who require longer courses of treatment, e.g. 12 weeks. Since the earliest clinical studies patients with *T. tonsurans* infections have been reported to have a variable response to griseofulvin and, again, the duration of therapy may have to be increased. In some countries griseofulvin is not available either as a tablet or as a paediatric liquid formulation.

Side-effects, contraindications and drug interactions

Some patients experience gastrointestinal discomfort or nausea on griseofulvin but generally these are tolerable. But occasionally headache may be chronic and severe and it may be necessary to stop the drug. Other side-effects include urticaria and photosensitivity—the latter may present with onycholysis. Griseofulvin may also precipitate systemic lupus erythematosus and acute intermittent porphyria. As it may cause abnormalities in sperm its use is not advised in adult males of reproductive age in many countries. Griseofulvin may also cause hepatic dysfunction such as cholestasis. A number of interactions are described which include phenobarbitone and phenytoin that inhibit absorption (Table 2).

Amorolfine

Amorolfine is a morpholine antifungal available as a topical treatment for nail disease in a specially formulated nail lacquer. It has broad-spectrum antifungal activity and is fungicidal *in vitro*. Its mode of action is via inhibition of two enzymes, Δ14-reductase and the Δ-isomerase involved in ergosterol biosynthesis in the cell membrane. It is not clear how this leads to cidal activity. Amorolfine nail lacquer has been assessed as a once or twice weekly treatment for dermatophyte nail infection of limited extent and not involving the nail matrix. Treatment results suggest that it is effective as sole therapy in a smaller proportion of nail infections than would be expected with oral therapy but that it shows considerable promise as an adjunct to oral treatment.

Side-effects are seldom problematic. Itching and local irritation occur in a small proportion of treated cases.

Ciclopyroxolamine (ciclopirox)

Ciclopyroxolamine is a hydroxypyridone derivative. It functions probably through

Table 4 Dosages for antifungal preparations

Polyenes		
Amphotericin B	Lozenges	1–2 q.i.d.
	Intravenous	1 mg/kg per day
Lipid-associated amphotericin B e.g. AmBisome (liposomal AMB)		3 mg/kg per day
Nystatin	Pastilles	1–2 q.i.d.
Azoles		
Topical azole antifungals (bifonazole, clotrimazole, econazole, shown to miconazole, sulconazole ketoconazole, tioconazole)	Topical	Twice daily (for some once daily therapy has been sufficient) 2–4 weeks Bifonazole/urea preparation is available for nail disease
Oral azole antifungals		
Ketoconazole	Oral	200 mg daily
Itraconazole	Oral	200 mg b.i.d. for 1 week in tinea corporis/cruris but repeat twice for finger nail, thrice for toe nails 100–200 mg daily oropharyngeal candidosis
Fluconazole	Oral	100–200 mg daily for continuous therapy or 150–300 mg weekly pulses
Terbinafine	Oral	250 mg daily
	Topical	Usually 7 days once daily
Griseofulvin	Oral	500–1000 mg daily or 10 mg/kg per day. 20 mg/kg daily in *T. tonsurans* infections
Topical nail treatments		
Ciclopirox nail lacquer	Topical	Daily (some studies suggest 2–3 times weekly)
Amrolfine nail lacquer	Topical	2–3 times weekly
Flucytosine	Oral/intravenous	Daily. In patients with normal renal function 120 mg/kg daily in four divided doses. Check serum levels in patients with renal impairment (normal 40–60 g/L)
Other antifungal compounds		
Undecenoates	Topical	Different compounds usually containing zinc undecenoate/undecenoic acid. Daily use for dermatophytosis
Benzoic acid compound (Whitfield's ointment)	Topical	Daily treatment for dermatophytosis. As it is irritant care should be taken in using in groin area

inhibition of iron containing mitochondrial enzymes. It has broad antifungal activity, particularly against dermatophyte fungi as well as some non-dermatophyte mould fungi and is active topically. As with amorolfine its minimal cidal concentrations are close to the MICs. As ciclopirox it has been developed as an antifungal nail lacquer; the drug is incorporated at a strength of 8% into a transungual delivery system which allows evaporation of the solvent to provide a much higher terminal drug concentration in contact with the nail plate. While cure rates are lower than with oral therapies in nail disease some studies indicate that it is effective in about 50% of cases.

Flucytosine

Flucytosine (5-fluorocytosine) functions through the inhibition of fungal thymidylate synthetase. It is active against yeast fungi and is chiefly used with amphotericin B as a combination therapy because of its high level of synergistic activity with this polyene drug. It has been used in chromoblastomycosis in this combination. It is more generally given as treatment in systemic mycoses such as cryptococcosis. The drug is excreted in urine and dosage should be reduced in patients with renal impairment. Resistance is also seen amongst *Candida* and *Cryptococcus* species.

Other topical antifungals

A number of other antifungal compounds are used in many European countries. Their availability will vary, though, across the continent. Most are sold as over-the-counter preparations. Some of these antifungal preparations are listed here.

Tolnaftate is a tolcyclate compound used topically as a treatment for dermatophytosis. It is active against a range of dermatophyte species but cannot be used for scalp or nail disease. Undecenoic acid and zinc derivatives are used either alone or in combination as topical treatments for dermatophytosis. Whitfield's ointment, a combination of salicyclic acid (keratolytic) and benzoic acid (antifungal) is available for dermatophyte infections in many European countries. The relative proportions of these two main ingredients used in the formulation may vary between countries.

Treatment regimens

General guidelines

As a general principle it is important to select an appropriate formulation and drug for each purpose. In practice superficial infections of limited extent and not involving structures such as hair can be treated with topical therapy but where the infections are more extensive or more severe oral therapy is given. It is important when giving an oral treatment to ensure that the infection is likely to be responsive. In fact the majority of superficial infections are easily treated with most of the oral agents apart from griseofulvin which is only active in dermatophytosis. Terbinafine is not active clinically in *Candida* or *Malassezia* infection by oral route although it works when given topically. For many oral compounds it is important to understand the potential interactions and to ask patients about any concomitant medications. These interactions are listed in Table 2.

Dosages

The dosages of the main antifungal preparations are listed in Table 4.

Further reading

Baran R, Feuilhade M, Datry A *et al*. A. randomized trial of amorolfine 5% solution nail lacquer associated with oral terbinafine compared with terbinafine alone in the treatment of dermatophytic toenail onychomycoses affecting the matrix region. *Br J Dermatol* 2000; 142: 1177–83.

Davies RR. Griseofulvin. In: Speller DCE, ed. *Antifungal Chemotherapy*. UK: John Wiley, 1980: 149–82.

De Cuyper C, Hindryckx PH. Long-term outcomes in the treatment of toenail onychomycosis. *Br J Dermatol* 1999; 141 (Suppl. 56): 15–20.

De Doncker P, Gupta AK, Cel Rosso JQ *et al*. Safety of itraconazole pulse therapy for onychomycosis. An update. *Postgrad Med* 1999; Spec. No. 17–25.

Evans EGV, Sigurgeirsson B. Double blind, randomised study of continuous terbinafine compared with intermittent itraconazole in treatment of toenail onychomycosis. *Br Med J* 1999; 318: 1031–5.

Ghannoum MA. Future of antimycotic therapy. *Dermatol Ther* 1997; 3: 104–11.

Goodfield MJD, Andrew L, Evans EGV. Short term treatment of dermatophyte onychomycosis with terbinafine. *Br Med J* 1992; 304: 1151–4.

Grant SM, Clissold SP. Fluconazole. A review of its pharmacodynamic and pharmacokinetic properties and therapeutic potential in superficial and systemic mycoses. *Drugs* 1990; 39: 877–916.

Gupta AK, De Doncker P, Scher RK *et al.* Itraconazole for the treatment of onychomycosis. *Int J Dermatol* 1998; 37: 303–8.

Hay RJ, Clayton YM, Moore MK *et al.* An evaluation of itraconazole in the management of onychomycosis. *Br J Dermatol* 1988; 119: 359–66.

Hay RJ, Griffiths WAD, Dowd PM, Clayton YM. A comparative study of ketoconazole versus griseofulvin in dermatophytosis. *Br J Dermatol* 1985; 112: 691–6.

Heiberg JK, Svejgaard E. Toxic hepatitis during ketoconazole treatment. *Br Med J* 1981; 283: 825.

Katsambas A *et al.* Comparison of the efficacy and tolerability of Amorolfine 5% nail lacquer (ro-14-4767) once weekly versus twice weekly in the treatment of onychomycoses. *Nouv Dermatol* 1993; 12 (4): 216–20.

Petranyi G, Meingassner JG, Mieth H. Antifungal activity of the allylamine derivative, terbinafine, in vitro. *Antimicrob Ag Chemother* 1987; 31: 1365–8.

Scher RK, Breneman D, Rich P. Once-weekly fluconazole (150, 300, or 450 mg) in the treatment of distal subungual onychomycosis of the toenail. *J Am Acad Dermatol* 1998; 38: S77–S86.

Seebacher C, Ulbricht H, Worz K. Results of a multicentre study with cyclopirox nail lacquer in patients with onychomycosis. *Haut Myk* 1993; 3: 80–4.

Vanden Bossche H, Dromer F, Improvisi I *et al.* Antifungal drug resistance in pathogenic fungi. *J Med Mycol* 1998; 36 (Suppl. 1): 119–28.

Antihistamines

A.D. Katsambas, A.J. Stratigos and T.M. Lotti

General principles, classification and structure

The histamine-receptor antagonists or antihistamines are classified into three types:

1 Traditional, classic or first-generation H_1-type antihistamines.
2 Low-sedating or second-generation H_1-type antihistamines.
3 H_2-type antihistamines.

There are three types of histamine receptors: H_1, H_2 and H_3. The H_1-receptors mediate the following effects: vasodilatation of small blood vessels resulting in increased permeability, smooth muscle contraction and itching. The H_2-receptors are best known for mediating the effects on gastric acid production, and the H_3-receptors are found in the brain and are responsible for autoregulation of histamine production and release. The H_1-antihistamines, both the traditional and the low sedating, and the H_2-type antihistamines to a much less extent are considered first-line medications in dermatological practice. However, the inhibitors of the H_3-receptors have not as yet found a role in dermatological treatment.

The first-generation H_1-antihistamines and histamine have in common a substituted ethylamine moiety as an integral part of their molecule (Fig. 1). The activity of an H_1-antihistamine is increased if a halogen is substituted in the *para* position of the phenyl or benzyl group of R_1. The first-generation (traditional) H_1-antihistamines have been divided into six chemical classes on the basis of a substitution at the X position with the nitrogen, oxygen or carbon. The six chemical classes and the most commonly used antihistamines (generic names) that correspond to each chemical class are presented in Table 1.

The first-generation H_1-antihistamines may cause sedation of varying intensity due to their property of crossing the blood–brain barrier.

The second-generation or low-sedating H_1-antihistamines were developed recently. To a large extent they have replaced the first generation as a dermatological treatment due to their lack of both sedative and anticholinergic effects. The low sedative effect of the second-generation antihistamines is expected because they only minimally cross the blood–brain barrier. In addition, they are well absorbed and are extensively distributed in body fluids.

Moreover, these agents preferentially bind to peripheral H_1-receptors. The low-sedating H_1-antihistamines that are now available in most countries are cetirizine, mizolastine, loratadine and its active metabolite fexofenadine. There are also a number of low-sedating antihistamines (acrivastine, azelastine, ebastine, temelastine, levocabastine) that are only available in certain countries or are awaiting approval.

H_2-type antihistamines—cimetidine, ranitidine, famotidine, nizatidine—possess an imidazole ring and lack the aryl ring of H_1-antihistamines. These therapeutic agents are less lipophilic, which presumably accounts for their lack of central nervous system (CNS) effects. Although H_2-antihistamines were developed for use in peptic ulcer disease, the presence of H_2-receptors in the cutaneous microvasculature justified their use in dermatology.

Mechanisms of action

Antihistamines do not reverse the effects of histamine. They competitively inhibit the action of histamine by blocking its receptors on the vascular endothelial cell

Table 1 First-generation H_1-type antihistamines

Chemical class	Generic name
Alkylamine (propylanine)	Brompheniramine maleate
	Chlorpheniramine maleate
	Dexchlorpheniramine maleate
Aminoalkyl ether (ethanolamine)	Clestamine fumarate
	Diphenhydramine hydrochloride
Ethylenediamine	Tripelennamine citrate
	Tripelennamine hydrochloride
Phenothiazine	Methdiliazine
	Methdiliazine hydrochloride
	Promethazine hydrochloride
Piperidine	Azatadine meleate
	Cyproheptadine hydrochloride
Piperazine	Hydroxyzine hydrochloride
	Hydroxyzine palmoate

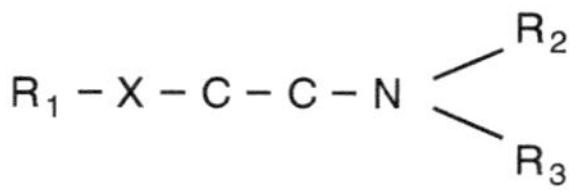

Figure 1 Ethylamine moeity of H_1–antihistamine.

surface. As a result, antihistamines prevent the effects of histamine, i.e. localized vasodilation and transudation of fluid, leading to the formation of the typical weal.

Indications and other uses

Antihistamines are indicated for pruritus, urticaria and angioedema as first-line treatment.

Comparative studies of the subgroups of traditional H_1-antihistamines have shown them to be almost of equal efficacy. If an agent from one therapeutic subgroup is not effective, then an agent from another subgroup should be administered. There are, however, times when H_1-antihistamines from different subgroups may be combined.

The low-sedating H_1-antihistamines (cetirizine, mizolastine and loratadine), have been found to be very effective in the treatment of acute and chronic urticaria and angioedema. In comparative studies, in which low-sedating H_1-antihistamines have been compared with each other and with traditional H_1-antihistamines, no statistically significant differences in efficacy have been proven. There are however, some important differences between all these agents in terms of dosing, convenience and side-effects.

Tricyclic antidepressant drugs, such as doxepin hydrochloride, and ketotifen have been used with therapeutic benefit in chronic idiopathic urticaria. They act on both H_1- and H_2-receptors. They have been used successfully to relieve the symptoms of diffuse cutaneous mastocytosis, urticaria pigmentosa, symptomatic mastocytosis and bronchial asthma. However, the sedation and other adverse effects are comparable with those of first-generation antihistamines.

Pruritus of various causes and atopic dermatitis have been treated successfully with H_1-antihistamines, both the traditional and the low-sedating ones. Anticipation of the efficacy on atopic dermatitis is based on the fact that certain antihistamines inhibit the release of mediators other than histamine (leucotrienes, prostaglandins).

Side-effects, contraindications and drug interactions

The most common side-effect of first-generation H_1-antihistamines is drowsiness that varies from patient to patient. However, not infrequently, drowsiness may completely disappear within a few days of continued use. Moreover, if the classic H_1-antihistamines are given as a simple dose in the evening, the resulting somnolence can be adequately tolerated. Convulsions, appetite stimulation, weight gain, dry mouth, blurring of vision, difficulty in micturition and impotence may also occur.

The majority of first-generation H_1-antihistamines show an accentuation of the central depressive effect. If they are taken in combination with CNS depressants, such as diazepam, or with alcohol, they result in increased drowsiness.

Also, these agents should not be administered with the monoamine oxidase inhibitors because their anticholinergic effect may be prolonged and accentuated (dryness of the mucous membranes, urinary retention, increased intravenular pressure). This is why the classic antihistamines should not be administered to patients with glaucoma. On the contrary, the new-generation H_1-antihistamines are safe to be used in patients taking monoamine oxidase inhibitors and they can be administered without problem to patients with glaucoma or urinary retention.

Torsade de pointes, a form of potentially lethal ventricular tachycardia associated with prolongation of the QT interval, has been reported to occur after terfenadine or astemizole overdose and in patients taking concomitantly itraconazole, and ketoconazole, or macrolide antibiotics such as erythromycin. For this reason terfenadine and astemisole have been suspended from the market in Europe.

Contraindications for the use of antihistamines include hepatic diseases, epilepsy, prostatic hypertrophy, glaucoma and porphyria.

Although no relation between the first-generation H_1-antihistamines and the development of even minor fetal malformations has been established, sporadic cases of fetal effects and prenatal death have been reported. Teratogenic effects have been observed only in experimental animals after the administration of the piperazine subgroup. However, fetal abnormalities have not been reported in humans.

Traditionally, the old compounds, chlorpheniramine, tripelenamine and diphenhydramine, are used in pregnancy. Loratadine has been approved by the Food and Drug Administration for use in pregnancy, carrying a category B caution. Extremely small amounts of loratadine are excreted in breast milk. Cetirizine is not recommended for use in early pregnancy.

H_1-antihistamines can cause drug allergies including eczematous dermatitis, urticaria, petechiae, fixed drug eruptions and photosensitivity. Allergic contact dermatitis may develop after topical application of some H_1-antihistamines. It is reported that contact dermatitis has occurred after ingestion of diphenhydramine in patients who had previously applied the drug topically. It is also reported that photosensitivity dermatitis has occurred after ingestion of promethazine and diphenhydramine.

Treatment regimen

General guidelines

The dosage and frequency of administration of antihistamines are recommended by the manufacturers and are usually based on the inhibition of experimental histamine weals. However, there are times when dermatologists feel the need cautiously to exceed these doses, beginning with a modest dose and gradually increasing this until either the condition is under control or side-effects necessitate a return to a lower dose.

The combination of H_1- and H_2-antihistamines is beneficial to patients with acute and chronic idiopathic urticaria and angioedema as well as certain forms of physical urticarias. This combination should be considered in patients with refractory chronic idiopathic urticaria, in whom H_1-antihistamines alone or in combination are ineffective.

Dosage

Traditional H_1-antihistamines

Alkylamines (dexchlorpheniramine—polaramine)
- Adults: 4–8 mg every 6 h.
- Children 2–5 years of age: 2 mg every 6 h.
- Children 5–11 years of age: 2–4 mg every 6 h.

Ethanolamines (diphenhydramine hydrochloride—benadryl)
- Adults: 25–50 mg every 4 h.
- Children up to 12 years of age: 5 mg/kg per 24 h in divided doses.

Ethylendiamines (tripelennamine hydrochloride—pyribenzamine)
- Adults: 25–50 mg every 4 h.
- Children under 12 years of age: 5 mg/kg per 24 h in divided doses.

Phenothiezines (promethazine hydrochloride—phenergan)
- Adults: 25 mg 3 times a day.
- Children: 6.25–12.5 mg three times a day and 25 mg at bedtime.

Piperadines (cyproheptadine hydrochloride—periactin)
- Adults: 4 mg three times daily.
- Children: 0.25 mg/kg daily.

Piperazine (hydroxyzine hydrochloride—atarax)
- Adults: 25 mg 3–4 times daily.
- Children under 6 years of age: 50 mg/day in divided doses.

Low-sedating or second-generation antihistamines

Cetirizine (zirtek)
- Adults: 10 mg daily.
- Children: 6–12 years old: 5 mg daily.

Loratadine (clarytine)
- Adults: 10 mg daily.
- Children: 6–12 years old: 5 mg once daily.

Fexofenadine (active metabolite of terfenadine)
- Adults: 180 mg once daily (evening).

Mizolastine (mizolen)
- Adults: 10 mg once daily (evening).

H_2-antihistamines

Cimetidine (tagamet)
- Adults: 300 mg three times daily.
- Children: Intramuscularly, 2 mg/kg every 6 h.

Ranitidine (zantac)
- Adults: 150 mg twice daily, or 300 mg at bedtime.

Famotidine (pepcid)
- Adults: 40 mg at bedtime for 1–2 months, and 20 mg at bedtime thereafter.

Tricyclic antidepressants

Amitriptyline
- Adults: 25 mg/day at bedtime.

Doxepin
- Adults: 25 mg/day at bedtime, or in divided doses. The dose can be increased slowly over a 30-day period up to 75 mg.

- For children under 12 years of age, tricyclic antidepressants should not be used.

Further reading

Food and Drug Administration (FDA). Talk paper. T97.3 13 Jan 1997.

Lawlor F, Greaves MW. In: Lichtenstein FM, Fauci A, eds. *Chronic Urticaria in Current Therapy in Allergy, Immunology and Rheumatology*. Philadelphia: Mosby, 1997.

Maddin S. Efficacy and safety of antihistamines in allergic skin disorders. *J Eur Acad Dermatol Venereol* 1997; 8 (Suppl. 1): S18–S23.

Monroe E. Therapy of acute chronic urticaria. *J Eur Acad Dermatol Venereol* 1997; 8 (Suppl. 1): S11–S17.

Simons FER, Simons KJ. The pharmacology and use of H_1 receptor-antagonist drugs. *N Engl J Med* 1994; 330 (23): 1667.

Antiviral drugs

E. Tsoureli-Nikita, G. Hautmann, G. Campanile, A.D. Katsambas and T.M. Lotti

Although a great effort has been made to find effective antiviral agents to treat viral infections of the skin, the range of useful drugs against viruses seems to remain pitifully small. However, the advent of acquired immune deficiency syndrome (AIDS) is stimulating research to find new, more effective drugs against the human immunodeficiency virus (HIV), cytomegalovirus and herpes infections.

This chapter will focus on the most important and widely used antiviral drugs. For antiretroviral therapy see specific chapters (Table 1).

Interferons (IFN)

The IFN multigene family consists of IFN-α, IFN-β and IFN-γ which belong to the cytokine network and are implicated in the host defence. IFNs have antiviral, antiproliferative and immunomodulatory activities. Each IFN is unique, and acts as a messenger between other cells, to regulate functions as varied as fighting certain infections to suppressing certain cancers. IFN-2a and -2b, and IFN-1a and -1b, are all IFNs synthesized in the laboratory using recombinant DNA technology. IFN-n3 comes from human white blood cells. These IFNs are injectable drugs.

Their use in dermatology is controversial. Unfortunately, the available preparations are often associated with unpleasant side-effects (e.g. 'flu-like' symptoms, fatigue, fever, leucopenia or thrombocytopenia and central nervous system (CNS) effects), especially when given intralesionally (for pruritus, injection site disorders, paraesthesia, herpes simplex, flushing).

IFN-α

This affects cellular metabolism via nuclear alterations and alters cellular transcription, translation and protein synthesis. The subcutaneous administration of IFN-α, in a dose of 5–10 IU/kg per day for 2 weeks, provoked the suppression and decreased duration of herpes simplex virus (HSV) infection in patients who had frequent recurrences. Recombinant IFN-α (rIFN-α) has also been demonstrated to have a beneficial influence on the clinical course and symptoms of herpes zoster at the dose of 1.7–5.1 10 IU/kg per day. No significant differences have been demonstrated between rIFN-α and aciclovir.

The results of studies for the treatment of human papillomavirus (HPV) using rIFN-α 10 IU/day subcutaneously or intralesionally three times a week for 3 weeks, are quite satisfactory. Complete remission was observed in 30–80% of patients presenting HPV wart-like lesions, against 15–30% of the placebo group. A follow-up period of 12 months showed no recurrences.

IFN-β

IFN-β has not shown better results than aciclovir in the topical treatment of HSV, but has good results regarding the local, perilesional and intralesional treatment of HPV-mediated diseases.

IFN-γ

The results of using IFN-γ for the treatment of viral skin diseases are contradictory. The mean response rate achieved in the treatment of genital warts at a dose of 50–400 μg/day subcutis over a total period of 4 weeks, is 10–50%. IFN-γ has demonstrated good therapeutic results in bowenoid papulosis and herpes zoster, not preventing the spread of the lesions, but reducing subjective symptoms as acute pain and postherpetic neuralgia.

Table 1 Doses, methods of administration and side-effects of the main antiviral drugs used in dermatology

Virus	Antiviral agent	Administration	Dose	Side-effects
	IFN-α	s.c.	5–10 IU/kg per day for 2 weeks	'Flu-like' symptoms
Herpes simplex virus	Idoxuridine	Topical	5–15% cream	Bone marrow and hepatic toxicity i.v. local irritation with extravasation
	Aciclovir	Oral i.v. Topical	Adult: 400 mg 5/day for 10 days 5 mg/kg every 8 h for 10 days Ophthalmic ointment, cream	
	Valaciclovir	Oral	500 mg 2/day for 5 days	Nausea, headache Kidney damage
	Famciclovir	Oral	125 mg 2/day for 5 days	Thrombotic thrombocytopenic purpura (TTP)
Varicella-zoster virus	rIFN-α	s.c.	1.7–5.1.10 IU/kg/day	'Flu-like' symptoms
	Aciclovir	Oral i.v.	800 mg 5 for 5–7 days 5 mg/kg every 8 h for 5–7 days	Delirium, neurotoxicity
	Valaciclovir	Oral	1 g 3/day for 7 days	Nausea, headache
	Famciclovir	Oral	500 mg 3/day for 7 days	TTP
Immunocompromised host or herpes simplex encephalitis	Vidarabine	Oral	10 mg/kg	Gastrointestinal symptoms Rush Haematological CNS disorders
Human retrovirus (HIV)	Zidovudine	Oral	250 mg every 4 h	Neutropenia Anaemia Headache Myalgia Nausea
Human papilloma virus warts condylomata acuminata	rIFN-α	s.c. or intralesional	10 IU/day 3 times a week for 3 weeks	'Flu-like' symptoms
	IFN-γ	s.c.	50–400 μg/day for 4 weeks	'Flu-like' symptoms
	Podophyllin	Topical	Alcohol or benzoin tincture 10–15% for 10–150 days Podophyllotoxin 0.5% solution 2 times/day for 3 days, rest for 4 days and repeat	Bone marrow toxicity Neurotoxicity
Vulval and vaginal condylomas	5-Fluorouracil	Topical	Cream 5% 5-FU combined with ASA for 12 days	Teratogenic Irritation, scarring, alopecia, hypohyperpigmentation

Idoxuridine

5-iodo-2′-deoxyuridine is a synthetic nucleoside which interferes with viral DNA synthesis. It is effective against DNA viruses, in particular herpes virus. It is active against keratitis dendritica caused by HSV, but less certainly against HSV infections of the skin and mucosae. An effort has been made to improve the penetration of this drug by the addition of dimethylsulfoxide, but this may induce occasional skin irritation and contact dermatitis. Its use is now restricted to topical application (5–15%) because of severe bone marrow and hepatic toxicity (especially when given intravenously). It needs to be applied early in an attack to have an optimal effect.

Aciclovir

This is an effective synthetic acyclic purine analogue used both as a systemic and topical virostatic treatment for HSV infections and for herpes zoster.

It works by inhibition of DNA synthesis; its mode of action involves activation by thymidine kinase and subsequent inhibition of viral polymerase. Resistance to aciclovir has been recorded, following alterations to or deficiency of thymidine kinase; obviously, this is associated with a lack of response to the therapy. Nevertheless, aciclovir is actually the first choice of drug in the treatment of HSV infections. In serious HSV infection (or in herpes zoster) it is generally used intravenously, but it is also available as 200, 400 and 800 mg tablets, as an ophthalmic ointment and as a cream. Unfortunately, it has little effect on the latent phase of either herpes simplex or zoster and seems to be ineffective in clinical practice against other viruses.

In the primary HSV infections (gingivostomatitis herpetica, vulvovaginitis herpetica) aciclovir can be given intravenously or orally and it is a successful treatment. Oral adult dosage is 400 mg, five times daily for 5–10 days. Studies with aciclovir have shown that it is possible to suppress recurrences of HSV by intermittent administration over a long period. Chronic suppressive therapy for recurrent disease (200–400 mg, three times daily for several months) has been shown to be equally effective.

In serious systemic HSV infections (i.e. eczema herpeticum) it is given intravenously (5 mg/kg every 8 h by slow infusion, over 1 h, for 5–10 days).

In varicella-zoster virus infections, aciclovir has been recommended as a virostatic agent. It should be given intravenously (5 mg/kg body weight every 8 h for 5–7 days) or orally (800 mg, 5 times daily, for 5–7 days) and is used successfully in extensive zoster infections and in the prevention of complications such as neuralgia and eye involvement.

Valaciclovir

This is an l-valyl ester to aciclovir. Valaciclovir is much better absorbed than aciclovir. Once in the body, a hydrolase in the liver cleaves the l-valyl ester to yield aciclovir. In immunocompetent patients with recurrent symptomatic herpes genitalis, valaciclovir 500 mg twice daily for 5 days shortens the duration of viral shedding and hastens healing.

In varizella-zoster virus infection, valaciclovir has replaced aciclovir and the recommended dose is 1 g three times a day for 7 days. Valaciclovir must be used with extreme caution in immunocompromised patients since it may cause thrombocytic thrombocytopenic purpura.

Famciclovir

This is another aciclic guanosine analogue (prodrug of penciclovir). Conversion to penciclovir occurs in the liver and intestinal wall via deacetylation and oxidation. Famciclovir has excellent bioavailability, and the related molecule penciclovir has a longer intracellular half-life than aciclovir, though it seems to have a lower affinity for DNA polymerase. The recommended dose for recurrent herpes genitalis is 125 mg twice daily for 5 days. In varicella virus infection famciclovir has replaced aciclovir and the recommended dose is 500 mg three times a day for 7 days starting within 72 h from the onset of the rash.

Vidarabine

This is 9-β-d-arabino-furanosyl-adenine (adenosine arabinoside). It is a purine-containing nucleoside which is recognized as an effective agent in particular for the internal treatment of herpes infections. It appears to be effective in early cases of herpes simplex encephalitis and in varicella-zoster infections of immunocompromised patients. At a dose of 10 mg/kg per day intravenously, it causes mainly mild gastrointestinal side-effects and rashes in 5% of subjects. Nevertheless, there have been reported CNS and haematological side-effects. It is used for topical treatment of HSV infections and herpes zoster in ophthalmology and in dermatology.

Zidovudine

This is a drug for the treatment of human retrovirus infections. Its principle site of action is the inhibition of virus RNA-dependent DNA polymerase (reverse transcriptase). It is administered by the oral route and the usual dosage is 250 mg every 4 h, although variations to this regimen are very frequent. Its use in HIV-positive patients has been found to result in higher levels of circulating CD4 lymphocytes and, in some cases, a decrease in mortality over the short term. Its main side-effects are neutropenia and anaemia which occur in the majority of patients. Other side-effects may include headache, myalgia and nausea.

Podophyllin

It is an extract from the roots of *Podophyllum peltatum* or *P. emodi*. The pharmacologically active substance is podophyllotoxin, which stops mitosis at the metaphase and leads to necrosis of epithelial cells. On prolonged exposure, acute toxic contact dermatitis is a possible side-effect. It is applied in concentrations of 10–25% in absolute alcohol or benzoin tincture. After a few days, the treated area develops inflammatory reddening, and occasionally crusts also form as a result of acute toxic dermatitis. The healing process is finished after 10–14 days. Podophyllin tincture must be washed off after the appropriate time (3–6 h) because individual sensitivity varies greatly.

Condylomas are indicated for this treatment. Using a 20–25% alcoholic solution, condylomata acuminata of the genital region are treated once weekly. Not more than 8–10 cm^2 skin surface should be treated in one session to avoid undesirable side-effects as a results of the absorption of podophyllum.

Recently, a purified form of the resin has become available as podophyllotoxin 0.5% solution. In this form it is applied to warts twice daily for 3 days, followed by a rest for 4 days, and the cycle is repeated until resolution is achieved. Irritation and ulceration are the most common complaints, and recurrence is high.

5-Fluorouracil (5-FU)

This is a DNA antimetabolite (pyrimidine antagonist) which inhibits the activity of thymidylate synthetase and is cytotoxic leading to cell death. This effect occurs sooner in the diseased area of skin than in normal skin.

Although most commonly used as an antineoplastic agent to treat solar keratosis, Bowen's disease or superficial multifocal basal cell carcinoma, topical 5-FU cream (5%) has also been employed to treat many resistant vulval or vaginal condylomas. Irritation, scarring, alopecia and hypo-/hyperpigmentation are the most common side-effects of topical treatment.

An appropriate combination of 5-FU and salicylic acid, applied on a daily basis, has resulted in complete healing of genital warts in an average of 12 days.

Camptothecin (CPT)

CPT, a natural derivative of *Camptotheca acuminata*, a tree native to China, is actually used as a potent anticancer drug. Studies of DNA virus function, using cell-free systems and cultures of virus-infected cells, demonstrated that CPT is capable of inhibiting replication, transcription and packaging of double-stranded DNA-containing adenoviruses, papovaviruses, herpes viruses and the single-stranded DNA-containing autonomous parvoviruses. CPT inhibits viral function by inhibiting topoisomerase-1, required for the initiation and completion of viral function. In this way, CPT analogues could be developed and used as potent anti-DNA virus drugs in dermatology.

Further reading

Brigden D, Whiteman P. The mechanism of action, pharmacokinetics and toxicity of acyclovir: a review. *J Infect* 1983; (Suppl. 1): 3–9.

Cereli R, Hernek, McCrary M. Famcyclovir. review of clinical efficacy and safety. *Antiviral Res* 1996; 29: 141–51.

Djawari D. Fluorouracil treatment on condylomata acuminata. *Z Hautkr* 1986; 61: 463–9.

Hautmann G, Campanile G, Ghersetich I, Lotti T. Cytotoxic and immunosuppressive drugs in dermatology. In: Millikan L.E. (ed) *Drug Therapy in Dermatology*. Marcel Dekker, 2000: 111–34.

Mahrle G, Schultze HJ. Recombinant interferon-gamma in dermatology. *J Invest Dermatol* 1990; 95 (Suppl.): 132s–139s.

O'Brien JJ, Campoli, Richards DM. Acyclovir. *Drugs* 1989; 37: 233–309.

Pantazis P, Han Z, Chatterjee D, Wyche J. Water-insoluble camptothecin analogues as potential antiviral drugs. *J Biomed Sci* 1999; 6 (1): 1–7.

Pazin GJ, Hanger JH, Armstrong JA. Leukocyte interferon for treating first episodes of genital herpes in women. *J Infect Dis* 1987; 156: 891–7.

Perry CM, Faulds P. Valacyclovir. A review of it antiviral activity, pharmacokinetic properties and therapeutic efficacy in herpes virus infections. *Drugs* 1996; 52 (5): 754–72.

Silvestri DL, Corey L, Holmes KK. Ineffectiveness of topical idoxuridine in dimethylsulfoxide for therapy of genital herpes. *J Am Med Assoc* 1982; 248: 953–9.

Uyeno K, Yasuno H, Niimura M. Clinical trial of huIFN-beta on herpes zoster in immunocompromised patients. *J Invest Dermatol* 1989; 93: 583–7.

Von Krogh G. Topical self-treatment of penile warts with a 0.5% podophyllotoxin in ethanol for 4–5 davs. *Sex Trans Dis* 1986; 14: 135–40.

Whitley RJ, Spruance S, Hayden F. Vidarabine therapy of mucocutaneous herpes simplex virus infection in the immunocompromised host. *J Infect Dis* 1984; 149: 1–8.

Yaschoan R, Broder S. Development of antiretroviral therapy for the AIDS and related conditions. *N Engl J Med* 1988; 316: 557–64.

Bleaching agents

W. Westerhof and M.D. Njoo

General principles—classification and structure

In the late 1930s, it was observed that tannery workers who used a new type of rubber gloves developed irregular confetti-type depigmentations. The areas of pigment loss were most obvious in dark-skinned people and were most prominent on the hands and forearms (areas in contact with the gloves). It later appeared the gloves contained monobenzylether of hydroquinone (MBEH) that was used as an antioxidant. Subsequently, this compound was used to treat several disorders of hyperpigmentation.

Since the first report of its bleaching properties in 1965, hydroquinone (HQ) is still the most prescribed bleaching agent by dermatologists worldwide. However, 2–4% HQ has only a moderate and temporary bleaching effect. For this reason, many other substances, whether used as monotherapy or as combination therapy with HQ, have been tested for their efficacy and safety in the treatment of hyperpigmentation. Presently available bleaching agents can be classified into three groups.

Phenolic compounds

These compounds contain a phenol group. The most important agent belonging to this group is HQ, a hydroxyphenolic chemical compound. HQ derivatives are:

- MBEH
- 4-methoxyphenol (4-MP) (4-hydroxyanisol)
- 4-isopropylcatechol
- Arbutin.

Recently a new phenolic substance with depigmenting effects has been described: *N*-acetyl-4-*S*-cystaminylphenol.

Non-phenolic compounds

Bleaching agents without a phenolic group in their chemical structures are:

- corticosteroids
- tretinoin (retinoic acid)
- azelaic acid (AZA) (1,7-heptane dicarboxylic acid)
- *N*-acetylcystein (NAC)
- Kojic acid
- L-ascorbyl-2-phosphate or palmitate (vitamin C derivatives)
- Thioctic acid.

These compounds can be used alone or more often, in combination with other compounds.

Combination formula

Combination formula have been developed to improve the efficacy of HQ. The 'Kligman's formula' contains HQ, a class 1 or 2 corticosteroid and tretinoin. Pathak did not include steroid in his formula, which only contains HQ and tretinoin. Recently, much experience has been gained in the Netherlands with the use of a new formula, the so-called 'Westerhof's formula'. Beside HQ, this new formula consists of NAC and a corticosteroid as active agents.

Mechanism of action

Based on current clinical and experimental knowledge the 'ideal' cutaneous bleaching agent has to fulfil the following pharmacological requirements:

- strong bleaching effect
- rapid bleaching effect (within 2 months)
- no short- or long-term side-effects
- permanent bleaching of the undesired pigment
- effective in any or in most of the treated patents.

There is still no bleaching agent that fulfils all these requirements. None of the presently available bleaching agents is able to induce permanent elimination of the undesired pigment. Recurrences of the lesions therefore may always occur after discontinuation of the treatment.

Phenolic compounds

Hydroquinone

HQ inhibits the conversion of tyrosine to melanin by competitively binding to tyrosinase. Other proposed mechanisms of action for HQ are:

- HQ inhibits the formation or increases the degradation of melanosomes or both
- HQ inhibits the DNA and RNA synthesis of melanocytes.

In conclusion, only cells with active tyrosinase activity are affected by HQ (and also by other tyrosinase-inhibiting agents). Tyrosinase activity is only found in epidermal melanocytes. In dermal melanin that is usually located within macrophages ('melanophages'), tyrosinase activity is not present; the melanin lies 'captured' and biologically inactive in the cell as in the case of injected tattoo pigment. Dermal melanin is therefore resistant to the action of HQ.

2–4% HQ is not considered melanocidal, mainly because it is not metabolized to cytotoxic radicals as the 20% MBEH.

The selective action of HQ on melanogenesis is mostly due to its chemical resemblance to melanin precursors and its ability to be metabolized within melanocytes (Fig. 1).

In contrast to MBEH, the depigmenting effects of HQ are limited to sites of application and are usually reversible. However, some investigators postulate that the depigmentation induced by HQ sometimes can be permanent, depending on the HQ concentration in the formulation and the duration of application.

The efficacy of HQ seems to be related to its concentration in the preparation. However, the higher the concentration, although the more effective, the more irritative reactions occur. Concentrations of HQ above 5% are not advisable, because they appear to be very irritating without significantly improving its bleaching effect. Concentrations of 4–5% are considered 'very effective' but they are also moderate to strong irritants. The 2% HQ concentrations are generally not irritating; their efficacy has been experienced as 'ineffective' to 'very effective' (responders varying from 65 to 80% of the treated cases) in different independent studies. From 1 January 2001, formulations containing 2% HQ are forbidden as an over-the-counter (OTC) product by the European Cosmetic Products Regulation. However, doctors are allowed to prescribe HQ as before. The choice of concentration at the start of therapy may be higher; a 2% concentration is recommended by many physicians as maintenance therapy.

The bleaching effect of HQ may be expected after a few weeks to a few months of application.

It is not only the concentration but also the vehicle of HQ formulations that determine its action. From a number of clinical studies it is proposed that a hydroalcoholic vehicle (equal parts of propylene glycol and absolute ethanol) is the most suitable. Important to its action is the chemical stability of HQ. However, HQ is easily oxidized and thus loses its potency. For this reason antioxidants, such as ascorbic acid or sodium bisulphate should be added to preserve the stability of the preparation.

MBEH

This agent is also called 'monobenzone'. The mechanism of action of MBEH on pigment cells is mostly similar to that of HQ. MBEH however, is metabolized into reactive free radicals that are capable of destroying melanocytes. In contrast to

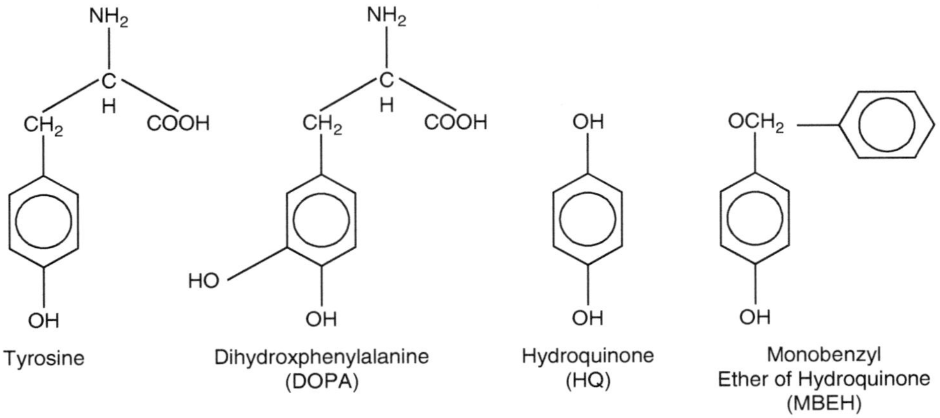

Figure 1 The similarities in the chemical structures of tyrosine and dopa (two melanin precursors) and hydroquinone (HQ) and monobenzyl ether of HQ (MBEH) (two bleaching agents)

HQ, depigmentation by MBEH is permanent, even after discontinuation. Remarkably, persistent loss of pigment has also been observed at distant sites of application. The mechanism behind this phenomenon is unclear. The pigment cell specificity of these cytotoxic effects can be explained by the selective uptake and metabolism of phenols and catechols.

4-methoxyphenol

In many countries in Europe such as in the Netherlands, MBEH is no longer available. Recent studies on the depigmentation treatment of vitiligo universalis using another phenolic compound, 4-MP in a 20% cream, revealed results that are comparable to those of MBEH. Moreover, irritant reactions were seen less frequently than in MBEH. The mechanism of action is probably similar to other phenolic compounds, but this has not yet been further investigated.

4-isopropylcatechol and 4-MP (4-hydroxyanisol)

These phenolic compounds, like MBEH, can be metabolized by tyrosinase into free radicals that are cytotoxic to pigment cells. The use of 4-isopropylcatechol 1–3% and 4-hydroxyanisol 2% concentration show variable results.

Arbutin

This is a naturally occurring β-d-glucopyranoside derivative of HQ, which inhibits tyrosinase and 5,6 dihydroxyindole-2-carboxylic acid (DHICA) polymerase activities at the post-translational level in a dose-dependent manner.

N-acetyl-4-S-cystaminylphenol

This is a phenolic thio-ether, which acts as a substrate for tyrosinase. *In vitro* animal studies show that this compound is selectively effective against functioning melanocytes with active melanin synthesis. According to the investigators, *N*-acetyl-4-*S*-cystaminylphenol is much more stable and less irritating than HQ.

Non-phenolic compounds

Corticosteroids

There are some studies reporting the hypopigmenting effect of topical corticosteroids. However, there is still debate as to whether steroids are able directly to affect tyrosinase activity, thus inhibiting melanin synthesis. In the treatment of postinflammatory hypo- and hyperpigmentation corticosteroids are used for their anti-inflammatory effect. For these conditions, steroids represent important components of the therapeutic regimen.

Corticosteroids, such as hydrocortisone, triamcinolone acetonide or betamethasone valerate, can be used alone or in combination with HQ (see 'Kligman formula').

Tretinoin (retinoic acid)

The use of tretinoin for the treatment of hyperpigmentation was probably introduced by Kligman in 1975. He noted that in some patients with acne, the skin became lighter after months of treatment with tretinoin. He decided to combine tretinoin with HQ to enhance its depigmenting effect.

Tretinoin has been shown *in vitro* to inhibit both constitutive and inducible melanin formation in melanoma cells. Moreover, *in vivo*, it is observed that tretinoin enhances the epidermal cell turnover, resulting in less contact time between the melanocytes and keratinocytes.

Tretinoin can be used in concentrations between 0.025 and 0.1%. Bleaching effect by tretinoin can be expected to occur after 12–40 weeks of daily application.

If the physician decides to prescribe tretinoin, it is also important to advise the patient to use a sunscreen to counteract the enhanced potential for sunburn and photodamage.

Azelaic acid

This substance was isolated in 1978 from *Pityrosporum* cultures and was used for the hypomelanosis seen in tinea versicolor. *In vitro*, AZA reversibly inhibits tyrosinase activity. AZA has not been shown to affect normal melanocytes directly. However, studies indicate that AZA has an antiproliferative and cytotoxic effect on the human malignant melanocyte and it may inhibit the evolution of lentigo maligna into cutaneous melanoma maligna.

AZA is mostly used in a 15–20% cream. 'Good' to 'excellent' improvement in the treatment of melasma is reported after 6 months of treatment. In our experience however, AZA has a poor bleaching effect.

NAC

The mechanism of action of NAC is described under 'Westerhof's formula'.

Kojic acid

Kojic acid (5-hydroxy-2-hydroxymethyl-4-*H*-pyran-4-one) is a diphenol, structurally related to maltol. Mishima *et al.* in 1988 showed that kojic acid is a potent tyrosinase inhibitor by chelating copper at the active site of the enzyme. In addition, Kahn in 1995 demonstrated that this agent is also able to prevent the conversion of the *O*-quinones of dextero and levo-dioxyphenylalanine (DL-DOPA), norepinephrine (noradrenaline) and dopamine to their corresponding melanin. Kojic acid can be used in a 1–4% cream base, alone or in combination with tretinoin and a corticosteroid.

In the treatment of hyperpigmentation kojic acid alone seemed to be less effective compared to HQ 2%.

L-ascorbic acid (AsA)

AsA or vitamin C probably suppresses melanin production at various oxidative steps of melanin formation, such as 5,6-dihydroxyindole oxidation. There are also reports suggesting a reducing effect of AsA on *O*-quinones. Moreover, it is shown that melanin can be altered from jet black to light tan by AsA by the reduction of oxidized melanin. One disadvantage of this agent is that it is quickly oxidized and decomposes in aqueous solution. For this reason, many AsA esters have been tested. Recently, the compound magnesium L-ascorbyl-2-phosphate (VC-PMG) has proven to be stable in a 10%

cream base. In a clinical trial, a significant bleaching effect was observed in 19 of 34 patients with melasma or senile freckles after 3 months of twice daily application. Ascorbyl palmitate is a lipid-soluble vitamin C derivative.

Vitamin E (α-tocopherol acetate)
Vitamin E is an antioxidant. It inhibits tyrosinase hydroxylase activity, but has no direct effect on tyrosinase, nor modulates the glycosylation of tyrosinase. For its bleaching effect it is often formulated together with vitamin C. In a study this combination could also inhibit ultraviolet (UV)-induced erythema and tanning.

Thioctic acid
Thioctic acid, which plays an essential role in mitochondrial dehydrogenase reactions, is an antioxidant. Its reduced form reacts with reactive oxygen species such as superoxide radicals, hydroxyl radicals, hypochlorous acid, peroxyl radicals and singlet oxygen. It also protects membranes by interacting with vitamin C and glutathione, which may in turn recycle vitamin E. Additionally this mono-thiol inhibits Cu^{2+}-dependent lipid peroxidation by chelating copper in a concentration-dependent manner. Based on this principle it can also inhibit tyrosinase, which is a copper-containing enzyme. The metabolic pathway of melanin is a sequence of oxidative steps. These are also inhibited by the antioxidant action of thioctic acid.

Combination formula

Several combination formula have been invented with the same goal; to enhance the effect of each of the separate active components. In this way, the duration of the therapy can be shortened and the risk of unwanted side-effects reduced. However, studies investigating the efficacy of combination therapies show varying results.

Kligman's formula
Kligman and Willis in 1975 observed an enhanced efficacy of 5% HQ, 0.1% tretinoin and 0.1% dexamethasone in hydrophilic ointment in the treatment of melasma, ephelides and postinflammatory hyperpigmentation (PIH). In contrast, they noted poor results using each of these agents as monotherapies. Tretinoin functions in this formula both as a mild irritant to facilitate the epidermal penetration of HQ and as an antioxidant to prevent oxidation of HQ. The corticosteroid can eliminate the irritation caused by either HQ and/or tretinoin.

Pathak's formula
A clinical trial, conducted by Pathak *et al.* involving 300 Hispanic women with melasma showed that cream or lotion formulations containing 2% HQ and 0.05–0.1% tretinoin provided the best results with minimal side-effects.

Westerhof's formula
In a left–right placebo-controlled clinical trial of 12 female patients with melasma, Njoo *et al.* demonstrated that the combination of 4.7% NAC, 2% HQ and 0.1% triamcinolone acetonide led to significant bleaching after 4–8 weeks of application. Theoretically, several explanations are possible for the bleaching effect of NAC. NAC increases the intracellular concentration of glutathione (GSH), a tripeptide thiol that stimulates pheomelanin synthesis rather than eumelanin synthesis after binding to dopaquinone. Hence, the result is a lighter pigment. Furthermore, agents containing sulphur, like NAC and GSH, may inhibit tyrosinase. Finally, NAC and HQ may react with each other during the preparation of the cream forming a compound with depigmenting properties, similar to a substance, which was described by Jimbow *et al.* in 1991.

Indications and other uses

The two most important medical indications for the use of bleaching agents are melasma and PIH.

Melanocidal agents like MBEH and 4-MP, are only used for the depigmentation of remaining melanin pigment in patients with universal vitiligo. In most cases, permanent depigmentation can be seen after 9–12 months of application.

Bleaching agents have also been used in the treatment of various other disorders of hyperpigmentation such as, lentigo solaris, ephelides (junction) naevi and lentigo maligna. For these indications however, other forms of therapy are recommended as first choice of therapy, such as laser therapy and surgical excision.

Side-effects, contraindications and drug interactions

Phenolic compounds

Side-effects related to the use of HQ can be divided into acute and chronic complications. Acute reactions include irritant and allergic contact dermatitis, nail discoloration and PIH. There are several reports of cases of persistent hypo- and hyperpigmentation of the skin after prolonged use of mostly high concentrations of HQ (6–10%). The clinical picture is named 'leuko(melano)derma en confetti'.

The most important and relatively unknown chronic side-effect is 'exogenous ochronosis'. This condition is characterized by an irregular maculopapulous hyperpigmentation located on the sites of application, commonly cheeks, forehead, periorbital region, neck and shoulders. Histology shows the presence of granulomas containing melanophages and giant cells in the upper dermis and basophilic ochronotic collagen bundles. Several cases of exogenous ochronosis have been reported in Africa; the majority of the affected ones are black females. They use HQ-containing creams not to remove blotches, but primarily to bleach the entire skin of the body for psychosocial reasons. There is no effective treatment for this condition. There is a strong relation between the occurrence of exogenous ochronosis and the duration of the use of HQ. An epidemiological study in South Africa found no cases of exogenous ochronosis after application duration shorter than 6 months; after 16 years of usage however, the disorder was diagnosed among 92% of the investigated individuals. There is some discussion whether low concentrations of HQ may also lead to exogenous ochronosis. However, it is wise to assume that the risk of developing exogenous ochronosis is also present when using 2% HQ. No information is available on the carcinogenic effects of HQ in humans. There is clear experimental evidence which shows that HQ *in vivo* metabolizes into benzene, is mutagenic and could induce cancer. Increased skin tumour incidence has been reported in mice treated dermally. Male rats dosed with HQ by gavage showed tubular cell adenomas of the kidney. Female rats developed mononuclear cell leukaemia and female mice hepatocellular neoplasms.

The use of MBEH and 4-MP may initially lead to mild irritation of the skin. The depigmentation induced by MBEH and 4-MP is mostly permanent and can also be seen at distant sites of the application. For this reason, these agents are only indicated for the treatment of severe vitiligo.

Other phenolic compounds, such as 4-isopropylcatechol, 4-hydroxyanisol, arbutin and *N*-acetyl-4-*S*-cystaminylphenol may also have mild to severe irritant and allergic reactions as acute side-effects. Long-term unwanted phenomena are not known, mainly because not much experience has been gained so far with these agents.

Contraindications for the use of phenolic compounds are proven allergy to the agent and/or therapeutic resistance for the agent in the past. It is not known whether these drugs are able to pass the placenta. However, we recommend that pregnant or lactating women should not use them. Therefore, women who develop melasma during pregnancy should not be treated with bleaching agents until several months after the delivery.

No interactions of phenolic compounds with other drugs are known.

Non-phenolic compounds

Adverse skin reactions associated with the use of corticosteroids are epidermal atrophy, telangiectasia, acneiform eruptions, hypertrichosis and ecchymoses. These effects mostly disappear after discontinuation of the drug. However the occurrence of striae distensae is permanent. It is recommended to apply corticosteroids over limited skin areas and over a limited period of time (maximum 6 months).

In most cases the use of tretinoin can lead to acute irritant reactions. Rarely, PIH may occur, especially in darker skin types. There is no consensus whether tretinoin is allowed during pregnancy. So far there is no direct evidence that tretinoin may harm the embryo. However, some physicians do not recommend the use of tretinoin, especially during the first trimester.

As tretinoin may increase the photosensitivity of the skin, the simultaneous use of sunscreens is always recommended.

Other non-phenolic agents like AZA, kojic acid, NAC, AsA or thioctic acid may produce a mild but transient irritant skin reaction at the start of therapy. AZA may also cause pruritus, mild transient erythema, scaling and burning. These other effects of AZA subside in 2–4 weeks.

There are no systemic effects of AZA, kojic acid, NAC, AsA or thioctic acid. Long-term side-effects by AZA, NAC, AsA or thioctic acid have not been reported yet.

Contraindications for the use of non-phenolic compounds are proven allergy to the agent and/or therapeutic resistance for the agent in the past.

No interactions of non-phenolic compounds with other drugs are known.

Regimen

Before initiating therapy, patients must be informed that bleaching is in fact a symptomatic rather than a causative therapy. Because the exact pathogenesis of skin disorders like melasma and PIH is unknown, causative factors are difficult to be eliminated. Moreover, the hyperpigmentation as seen in these conditions is considered a dynamic rather than a static process. Even if the bleaching was successful initially, the possibility always exists that the hyperpigmentation may return after a certain period of time. False hope for achieving permanent cure can be avoided when the patient is given this information at the start of the treatment. It is also important to stress that in the future, bleaching treatment probably has to be repeated.

Determining the depth of localization of the unwanted pigment

Histologically, the excess of pigment in conditions like melasma and PIH, may be located either purely epidermally, purely dermally or both. There are two methods to determine the localization.

Wood's light examination (365 nm)

Under Wood's light, the pigmentation in epidermal types is intensified, while in dermal types it is not. Wood's light examination however, is not considered a very reliable test; moreover in black skin, Wood's light is not able to differentiate between histological types.

Biopsy

The most reliable method to determine the depth of melanin deposition is to take a biopsy. Usually, a 'paired biopsy' is recommended; one from the lesion and one from the normal skin.

Histological examination

This provides further important information. When PIH is suspected and histology shows signs of inflammation, anti-inflammatory drugs (corticosteroids) must be given.

Determination of the depth of pigment has prognostic and therapeutic consequences. Only the purely epidermal and some mixed types respond to local bleaching agents. Alternative (e.g. laser) and/or adjunctive therapies (camouflage) may be applied to treat purely dermal types. Laser therapy is not recommended for coloured skin, since PIH may occur during the healing process.

General measures—prevention of luxating factors

The success of a bleaching therapy not only depends on the patient's compliance but also on the degree; factors which have possibly provoked the skin disorder should be avoided.

Avoidance of UV light exposure

It is well known that UV light may enhance melanogenesis. Protection against UV can be achieved by the application of a potent sunblock (SPF 25 or higher) during daytime. Even when bleaching treatment is stopped and/or the skin lesions have disappeared, the use of sunscreens during sunny seasons of the year is highly recommended to prevent recurrence of the skin lesions. The same effect can be achieved by wearing special clothing. The use of sun beds or other tanning equipment is prohibited.

The use of oral contraceptives

In melasma, there is no consensus on whether the use of oral contraceptives should be stopped. There are indications that sex hormones, such as progestogens and oestrogens, probably play an important role in the induction of the lesions. In our experience, however, there is still no conclusive evidence that stopping the use of oral contraceptives or changing to a 'milder' oral contraceptive significantly alters the prognosis or response to therapy of the melasma.

Treating the underlying inflammation

In PIH it is recommended to also treat the underlying inflammatory process, e.g. acne, lichen ruber planus. The hyperpigmentation may recur when the underlying skin disease is still active.

Dosage

All bleaching preparations, especially containing HQ, should not be used longer than 6 months. When no effect is observed after 6 months of application, further use of bleaching agents should be stopped and alternative or adjunctive therapies sought.

When an allergic reaction to either of the active components is suspected, patch tests should be performed.

Phenolic compounds

Hydroquinone 2–5%

- In hydro alcoholic solution or cream.
- Once daily (at night) not exceeding 6 months.

MBEH/4-MP 10–20% (only for vitiligo)

- Start with once daily application.
- First try a test spot (e.g. forearm) to exclude allergic reaction.
- If no adverse reaction occurs after 1 week, try once daily on face and neck.
- If no adverse reaction occurs after 1 week, try twice daily application.

Depigmentation using these agents is a long process. It takes 9–12 months (sometimes longer) to achieve total depigmentation. To avoid systemic effects it is advisable not to treat more than 9% of the body surface at one time.

4-isopropylcatechol (1–3%)/ 4-hydroxyanisol (2%)

- 1–2 times daily application.

Arbutin

This is not formulated by dermatologists, but can be obtained in skin-whitening cosmetics. Due to the chemical resemblance to HQ, they should be treated with the same restrictions as an OTC product according to EC laws and regulations.

N-acetyl-4-S-cystaminylphenol (4%)

- Oil-in-water emulsion.
- Apply twice daily.
- (This product is not yet available.)

Non-phenolic compounds

Corticosteroids

Corticosteroids, such as hydrocortisone (1%), triamcinolonacetonide (0.1%) or betamethasonvalerate (0.1%) are mostly used in combination with HQ.

Tretinoin (0.025–0.1%)

- Apply alone or in combination with HQ in cream or ointment base.
- Apply once to twice daily.

Azelaic acid (15–20%)

- Apply alone or in combination with steroids, e.g. triamcinole acetonide 0.1% in a cream base.
- Once daily application (at night).

Kojic acid (1–4% cream base)

- Apply once daily (at night).
- Also used in combination with tretinoin (0.025–0.1%) and a corticosteroid (e.g. betamethasone 0.1%).

Magnesium L-ascorbyl-2-phosphate (VC-PMG) in 10% cream

- Twice daily application.

Thioctic acid (2%)

- This is used in combination with ascorbyl tetra-isopalmitate and tartaric acid in a cream consisting of multilamellar phospholipids (Synchromes). Thiospot cream.
- Twice daily application.
- Thioctic acid (2%) in combination with ascorbyl tetra-isopalmitate and salicylic acid dissolved in volatile silicones, alcohol and a liposomal system (Drysyst). Thiospot pen.
- Twice daily application.

Combination formula

Kligman's formula

- HQ 5%.
- Tretinoin 0.5–0.1%.
- Dexamethasone 0.1% or betamethasone valereate 0.1%.
- In hydro-alcoholic cream or ointment base.

Pathak's formula

- HQ 2%.
- Tretinoin 0.5–0.1%.
- In hydro-alcoholic base cream or ointment base.

Westerhof's formula

- NAC 3%.
- HQ 2%.
- Hydrocortisone 1%.
- In ointment base.

In our experience, combination preparations show better results than monotherapies. The first choice is therefore one of the three afore-mentioned combination formulas, applied once daily, preferably at night. The simultaneous use of a potent sun block (SPF 15 or higher) is recommended for life. Maintenance therapy always consists of preparations containing a maximum of 2% HQ, prescribed for a maximum period of 2 years.

Combined use of bleaching agents with chemical peeling

In some institutes, the use of bleaching agents is combined with superficial chemical peelings, such as glycolic acid peels. Mostly, the patient first applies a bleaching cream, once or twice daily for 2 or 4 weeks. Then a peeling procedure is performed for a period of 4–6 weeks once weekly. Thereafter, maintenance therapy with bleaching cream is continued for 1 or 2 months. These treatment cycles can be repeated as necessary.

Further reading

Engasser PE, Maibach HI. Cosmetics and dermatology: bleaching creams. *J Am Acad Dermatol* 1981; 5: 143–7.

Griffiths CE, Finkel LT, Ditre CM, Hamilton TA, Ellis CN, Voorhees JJ. Topical tretinoin (retinoic acid) improves melasma: a vehicle controlled, clinical trial. *Br J Dermatol* 1993; 129: 415–21.

Grimes PE, Melasma. Etiologic and therapeutic considerations. *Arch Dermatol* 1995; 131: 1453–7.

Jimbow K. *N*-acetyl-4–*S*-cysteaminylphenol as a new type of depigmenting agent for the melanoderma of patients with melasma. *Arch Dermatol* 1991; 127: 1528–34.

Kahn V. Effect of kojic acid on the oxidation of DL-DOPA, norepinephrine, and dopamine by mushroom tyrosinase. *Pigment Cell Res* 1995; 8: 234–40.

Kameyama K, Sakai C, Kondoh S *et al.* Inhibitory effect of magnesium L-ascorbyl-2–phosphate (VC-PMG) on melanogenesis in vitro and in vivo. *J Am Acad Dermatol* 1996; 34: 29–33.

Katsambas A, Antoniou Ch, Melasma. Classification and treatment. *J Eur Acad Dermatol Venereol* 1995; 4: 217–23.

Kligman AM, Willis I. A new formula for depigmenting human skin. *Arch Dermatol* 1975; 111: 40–8.

Menke HE, Dekker SK, Noordhoek Hegt V, Pavel S, Westerhof W. Exogene ochronosis, een weinig bekende bijwerking van hydrochinon-bevattende crèmes. *Ned Tijdschr Geneeskd* 1992; 136: 187–90.

Mishima Y, Hatta S, Ohyama Y, Inazu M. Induction of melanogenesis suppression: cellular pharmacology and mode of differential action. *Pigment Cell Res* 1988; 1: 367–74.

Njoo MD, Menke HE, Pavel S, Westerhof W. N-acetylcysteïn as a bleaching agent in the treatment of melasma. *J Eur Acad Dermatol Venereol* 1997; 9: 86–7.

Njoo MD, Vodegel RM, Westerhof W. Depigmentation therapy in vililigo universalis with topical 4-methoxyphenol and the Q-switched ruby laser. *J Am Acad Dermatol* 2000; 42: 760–9.

Oliver EA *et al.* Occupational leukoderma: preliminary report. *JAMA* 1939; 113: 27–8.

Snider RI, Theirs BH. Exogenous ochronosis. *J Am Acad Dermatol* 1993; 28: 662–4.

Spencer MC. Topical use of hydroquinone for depigmentation. *JAMA* 1965; 194: 962–4.

Twenty-fourth Commission Directive. 2000/6/EC of 29 February 2000 adapting to technical progress Annexes II, III, VI, VII to Council Directive 76/768/EEC on the approximation of laws of the Member States relating to cosmetic products. *Official Journal* L056 (*01/03/*2000), pp. 42–6.

Corticosteroids: topical

J.G. Camarasa and
A. Giménez-Arnau

General principles, classification and structure

Topical glucocorticoids are the most widely used therapeutic agents for the treatment of inflammatory skin diseases. Twenty years passed from the discovery of the basic structure of cholesterol, a precursor in the biosynthesis of all the steroids, until the first topical steroid was used in 1952.

The application of cortisone *per se* on the skin showed disappointing therapeutic results. Hydrocortisone, which is obtained after fermentation, was the first steroid used by Sulzberger and Witten in 1952 and it represented a great therapeutic advance.

The therapeutic activity of the topical corticosteroids was improved by the introduction of a double bond between the first and the second carbon molecule and also by the ester formation with fatty acids in position C-17 or C-21. The cyclical acetonides formed in position C-16 and C-17 were of greater potency. The halogenation (with fluorine or chlorine) in the C-6α or C-9α position also increases the effect of these preparations. The fluorination tends to protect the steroid ring from being metabolized.

Triamcinolone acetonide was the first topical active halogenated steroid to become commercialized with success. Vickers and Tighe observed in 1960 that it had a specific anti-inflammatory effect in the management of psoriasis. Simultaneously, flurandrenolone and flumetasone were also commercialized. All three are known as the second-generation steroids.

Betamethasone valerate and flucinolone form the third-generation group of steroids. Free betamethasone is on its own as active as hydrocortisone. The ester formation in position C-17 is important. In 1962, 17-betamethasone valerate was selected from a wide range of topical steroids, due to the good results obtained in the vasoconstriction test designed by Mackenzie-Stoughton.

Subsequently, several simple esters in the C-17 position of hydrocortisone were designed, which lead to the introduction of hydrocortisone 17-butyrate and hydrocortisone 17-valerate. They were developed in order to obtain the same efficacy as the fluorinated second-generation steroids, but minimizing the systemic and topical adverse effects secondary to halogenation. The disassociation between the efficacy and side-effects can be explained by the hydrolysis of the esters, first at skin level and afterwards in the blood. These non-fluorinated topical steroids are known as the fourth generation.

In the 1970s and 1980s more potent corticosteroids were designed, as betamethasone dipropionate or clobetasol propionate, which are known as the fifth-generation steroids. These potent components control certain dermatosis rapidly, but they have a real risk of developing topical and systemic side-effects.

New steroids, such as budenoside, are continually being designed. Budenoside has the special characteristic of having lateral chains of butyric acid in positions C-16 and C-17. It is a potent, non-fluoride containing steroid, used topically or as an inhaler, for example in asthma treatment. According to the vasoconstriction tests, its potency ranges between the clobetasol 17-propionate and the betametasone-17,21-dipropionate. Its effect on the hypothalamic–pituitary–adrenocortical axis is similar to hydrocortisone 17-butyrate. In the opinion of several authors it belongs to the sixth-generation steroids.

Momethasone furoate, prednicarbate, the C-21-carboxylates as the fluocortine-butyl-ester. The di-esters 17,21—hydrocortisone aceponate, hydrocortisone 17-butyrate 21-propionate, methylprednisolone aceponate or aclomethasone propionate and the carbothioates as the fluticasone propionate, are steroidal agents of recent discovery which aim to have adequate anti-inflammatory effects and minimal side-effects.

Mechanisms of action

Compared with other steroid hormones, the glucocorticosteroids act on different tissues and types of cells either at tissue, cellular or intracellular level. Some of the actions attributed to corticosteroids are not a primary cause of the drug, but are due to the effect of the drug on a different level. Corticosteroids have specific and non-specific effects, which cannot be explained by a single mechanism of action.

At the molecular level, all steroids show the same common mechanism of action. They are little hydrophobic molecules which pass the cell membranes by simple diffusion. Once intracellular, the steroid binds reversibly to the specific cytoplasmatic protein receptor, a glycoprotein of 777 amino acids. The interaction between receptor/corticosteroid activates a complex composed of: the binding protein for the hormone, two heat shock proteins of 90 kDa and immunophyllin. The cleavage of the heat shock proteins and immunophyllin takes place. The hormone–receptor complex migrates through the pores of the nucleus. Bound to the core DNA at the 5′ end, the complexes are capable of changing the genetic transcription. The RNA leaves the nucleous and in the cytoplasm, the mRNA takes part in the synthesis of new proteins. The corticosteroids could act either before or after the transcription. A few genes are under the direct influence of steroid hormones. The products of these genes will then activate other genes, amplifying the process.

All these pathways for the mechanism of action of steroids have been demonstrated on the skin. Specific corticosteroid receptors have been identified in the normal human epidermis and in the fibroblasts located in the dermis. The affinity of the fibroblasts to the steroids correlates well with the antiproliferative effect of the corticosteroids.

Lipocortine, interleukin-1 and the lymphokines such as interleukin-2 are some of the proteins induced by the steroid. The following cellular effects have been related to the action of corticosteroids: suppression of DNA synthesis, inhibition of mitosis in the fibroblasts and keratinocytes, vasoconstriction of the upper dermis, or the suppression of high levels of poliamines.

Lipocortine, induced by the corticosteroids, is capable of inhibiting the A2 phospholipase, reducing the liberation of arachidonic acid. The corticosteroids inhibit the liberation of proinflammatory eicosanoids, which is, although not unique, a very important mechanism of action.

Interleukin-1 which is present in the epidermis, also takes part in the inflammatory response. The *in-vitro* exposure of human keratinocytes to hydrocortisone decreases the liberation of the constitutive interleukin-1, as well as the interleukin-1 induced by ultraviolet radiation, due to the reduction of their gene expression. This would also explain the anti-inflammatory and antiproliferative effect of these drugs.

The glucocorticosteroids have a recognized immunosuppressive action over B and T lymphocytes as well as over monocytes/macrophages. They are capable of causing depletion of the number of Langerhans' cells either by avoiding the expression of the Ia surface antigen or by cell cytolysis. An increase in the number of the Langerhans' cells coming from a proliferative pool of cells, have been reported 3 weeks after the treatment was stopped. The inhibition of T-lymphocyte activity can be observed either by the reduction of interleukin-2 formation or of mitogen-induced lymphocytic proliferation. These effects are reversible, for example due to the action of leucotriene B4. This supports the hypothesis about corticosteroid action through the inhibition of the phospholipase A2. The decrease of the HLA-DR antigen expression has also been described. The effects of these drugs over the adhesion molecules, as endothelial adhesion molecule (ELAM-1) and intercellular adhesion molecule (ICAM-1), implied in the leucocytic attraction, are still under debate.

Recently it has been demonstrated that the wheal and flare responses to codeine following clobetasol treatment, is due to reduced mast cell numbers and tissue histamine content rather to the inhibition of mast cell degranulation.

Pharmacology

In order to obtain a therapeutic effect with any topical formulation, the aim is to achieve penetration of the greatest amount of drug. The most common techniques used to determine the potency of corticosteroids are:

- the vasoconstriction test
- the suppression of the mitotic index
- tests for atrophy.

The skin pharmacokinetics and the pharmacodynamics are studied together. The percutaneous absorption of steroids depends on:

- lipophility
- solubility
- drug concentration
- anatomical location
- age of the patient
- pre-existing skin diseases
- form of application (e.g. occlusion).

It is difficult to compare different therapeutic studies due to the lack of a standard method in clinical trials. The classification related to the potency and use of the steroids should not be based exclusively on the vasoconstriction test. The ideal method to determine the bioavailability of topical steroids should be simple, exact and adaptable to different circumstances. The measurement of drug absorption using tape-stripping or chromatometer allow a better mechanical approximation than the routinely used methods in the studies of pharmacokinetics and pharmacodynamics of topical steroids.

Classically animal and human models are used to evaluate the activity of topical corticosteroids. Special methods to assess side-effects have been also developed. Animal models include studies about the immunological and non-immunological inflammatory process about the antimitotic and the atrophogenic effect. Human models include the vasoconstriction or the blanching test (McKenzie-Stoughton), the non-immunological or immunological inflammatory trials and studies about side-effects.

The vasoconstriction or blanching test is based on the side-effect of the use of topical corticosteroids and is related, in an unspecified way, to drug potency. After applying a steroid over the skin, either in an open or occluded form, the degree of vasoconstriction or blanching is measured after 8 and 96 h, comparing it with the surrounding skin. Therefore different methods are used such as: a visual scale (from 0 to 3), reflection photometry (chromatometry), infrared, skin conductivity, optic plethysmography and/or laser Doppler. The vasoconstriction test does not evaluate inflammatory inhibition: it only evaluates the constriction of the superficial blood vessels as their blood content determines the colour of the skin. It is useful to evaluate the clinical activity of newly designed molecules, to rank corticosteroids according to their potency and to compare the bioavailability of the same drug in different excipients.

Non-invasive skin tests have been recommended for non-immunological or immunological inflammation models in humans. Analysis with image technologies have been proposed in order to evaluate experimentally the effectiveness of topical steroids.

Evaluation of side-effects in the chronic use of topical steroids include:

- atrophy-induction study
- steroid-induced acne
- endogenous suppression of cortisol.

Principles of therapy: indications and regimen

Topical corticosteroids are used mainly for their anti-inflammatory activity. In non-inflammatory skin diseases they are used for their antimitotic effect, or for their capacity to decrease the synthesis of macromolecules that form connective tissues.

The pharmacopoeia provides several corticosteroids for topical use. In the European classification system, there are four levels (I–IV) in descending order of potency (Table 1). The choice of steroid depends on patient age, the location of the disease (Table 2), the extent and the acute or chronic character of the disease. Skin absorption varies depending on the corticosteroid employed, on the skin condition and on the type of application. The creams are the most versatile form of preparation. Topical corticosteroids are contraindicated in most of the infectious skin diseases.

In order to minimize the systemic side-effects of the potent steroids, the synthesis of new corticosteroids is continuously under development. Corticosteroids are normally metabolized in the liver. The study of glucocorticoid metabolism, of their epidermal, upper and lower dermal concentration after topical application on intact skin, as well as the evaluation of the necessary concentrations to inhibit the synthesis of human connective tissue by the skin fibroblasts, suggests that the local and systemic adverse effects could be reduced if extrahepatic transformation occurred quicker. Ideally the glucocorticoid should be inactivated immediately after its absorption.

In the USA topical steroids are prescribed at an average of 14 million visits per year. Dermatologists prescribes 3.9 times more corticosteroids of high potency than the rest of the doctors. Non-dermatologists prescribe 8.4 times more combination treatments with high- or low-potency corticosteroids and antimicrobial agents. The type of topical corticosteroids prescribed by the dermatologist or by the other doctors reflects the difference in the severity and complexity of the treated diseases. Prescriptions of topical steroids only specify the amount in 4% of cases, while the frequency is recorded in 77%, the location in 69% and the duration in 55% of patients. In dermatology topical steroids are used mainly in the treatment of different types of dermatitis or eczema. They are also useful in psoriasis and other skin diseases (Table 3).

The combination of topical corticosteroids with other active substances such as antimicrobial or antifungal agents, is useful and legitimate given the high incidence of colonization of eczema with *Staphylococcus aureus* or *Pityrosporum orbiculare*. The association with salicylic acid, is useful for its antiseptic properties and in order to facilitate the absorption of topical steroids. The concomitant use of urea facilitates the absorption of hydrocortisone, acting as a keratolytic agent and favouring water retention in the epidermis. Combination of betamethasone and calcipotriol has been very recently introduced for the treatment of psoriasis.

No direct evidence exists to contradict the principle that potency is directly related to toxic effects. Treatment with potent steroids is limited due to the high risk of developing skin atrophy. In combination with emollients, the frequency of applications can be reduced. No extra therapeutic benefit is obtained by applying a greater amount of the ointment on the skin. On the other hand, to increase

Table 1 Potency of topical corticosteroids

Very potent—I	Clobetasol propionate 0.05%
Diflucortolone valerate 0.3%	Fluocinolone acetonide 0.2%
Halcinonide 0.1%	
Potent—II	
Amcinonide 0.1%	Beclomethasone dipropionate 0.025%
Bethametasone benzoate 0.025%	Bethametasone dipropionate 0.05%
Bethametasone valerate 0.1% and 0.025%	Budesonide 0.025%
Desonide 0.05%	Desoxymethasone 0.25%
Diflorasone diacetate 0.05%	Difluocortolone valerate 0.1%
Fluclorolone acetonide 0.025% *	Fluocinolone acetonide 0.025%
Fluocinonide 0.05%	Fluprednidene acetate 0.1%
Flurandrenolone 0.05%	Fluticasone propionate 0.05%
Halcinonide 0.01%	Hydrocortisone butyrate 0.1%
Methylprednisolone aceponate 0.1%	Mometasone furoate 0.1%
Predicarbate 0.25%	Triamcinolone acetonide 0.1%
Moderately potent—III	Alclometasone dipropionate 0.05%
Beclometasone dipropionate 0.025%	Beclometasone salicilate 0.025%
Bethametasone benzoate 0.025%	Bethametasone dipropionate 0.05%
Bethametasone valerate 0.025% and 0.05%	Clobetasone butyrate 0.05%
Desoximethasone 0.05%	Flumethasone pivalate 0.02%
Fluocinolone acetonide 0.00625% and 0.01%	Fluocortin butyl 0.75%
Fluocortolone preparations hexanoate with pivalate each 0.1%	Hexanoate with either free alcohol or pivalate, each 0.25%
Flupamerasone 0.3%	Flurandrenolone 0.0125% or 0.05%
Halometasone 0.05%	Hydrocortisone butyrate 0.1%
Hydrocortisone aceponato 0.1%	Hydrocortisone valerate 0.2%
Triamcinolone acetonide 0.04%	
Mild—IV	
Dexamethasone 0.1–0.2%	Fluocinolone acetonide 0.0025%
Fluocortinbutile 0.75%	Hydrocortisone 0.5% and 1%
Hydrocortisone acetate 1%	Methylprednisolone acetate 0.25%

Classified as moderately potent by some authors.

the application surface increases the risk of systemic absorption.

The bioavailability and the choice of steroid depends on the excipient used. The choice of base is dependent on the type of disease and on the surface of the body to which it will be applied. In patients with dry skin, as in atopic patients or those living in dry and cold areas, ointments are normally used. Ointments tend to be more occlusive than other bases, enhancing the penetration of the agent and occluding also the shaft of the hair follicle. Creams are cosmetically more acceptable. The glucocorticoids in an alcohol–water base are not well absorbed. In certain circumstances other bases as gels, aerosol or sprays are used.

Thus, an appropriate treatment is one which uses a topical corticosteroid with sufficient potency to control the disease but with as few local or systemic side-effects as possible. It also will be formulated in an excipient according to the site of the lesion, the patient's age and the past medical history of the patient.

Side-effects

The side-effects caused by the use of steroids are mainly related to their action on the electrolyte and water balance, and to their influence on different aspects of metabolism, such as neoglycogenesis, tissue repair or inhibitory effect over the release of adrenocorticotrophic hormone from the adenohypophysis.

Table 2 Regional differences in the management with topical corticosteroids

Topographical area	Recommended potency
Mucous membranes	Mild or moderately potent
Scrotum/genitalia	Potent (short periods of time)
Eyelids	
Face	
Internal part of the thighs	
Skinfolds	Mild or potent
Internal part of the arms	
Scalp	
Thorax and back	Potent or very potent
Arms and thighs	Very potent (short periods of time)
Forearms and legs	
Dorsum of hands and feet	
Elbows and knees	Potent or very potent
Palms and soles	
Nails	

Table 3 Dermatoses susceptible to topical steroid treatment

Dermatosis requiring very potent topical corticosteroid therapy
Palmoplantar psoriasis
Lichen simplex chronicus
Pompholyx
Lichen planus
Granuloma annulare
Necrobiosis lipoidica
Sarcoidosis
Keloids
Dermatoses requiring potent topical corticosteroid therapy
Psoriasis (other variants)
Atopic eczema
Nummular eczema
Eczema due to an irritant
Contact dermatitis
Mastocytosis
Lupus erythematosus
Parapsoriasis
Alopecia areata
Dermatoses requiring moderate topical corticosteroid therapy
Flexural psoriasis
Atopic eczema in children
Seborrhoeic eczema
Sunburn
Anal, vulvar or scrotal pruritus
Pityriasis rosea of Gilbert

Most of the topical corticosteroids can be absorbed in enough amounts to produce systemic side-effects. The topical or intradermal use of steroids may cause collagen loss and subcutaneous skin atrophy, as well as local hypopigmentation. The evidence of skin atrophy is greater in children and in the elderly.

Epidermal atrophy is expressed by the flattening of the malpighian and the horny layer. The rete ridges flatten too. A decrease of the size of the keratinocytes and of the stratum corneum, measured with morphometry, can be observed. The Langerhans' cells modify their immunohistochemical characteristics and their capacity to migrate outside the epidermis. The amount of melanin transferred to the keratinocytes is reduced.

The earliest dermal changes observed are characterized by the flattening of dermal thickness, which could be explained by changes of the viscoelasticity of the glycoproteins and proteoglycans, which are responsible for the interfibrillar adhesions of collagen. A heterogenic type of dermal cell appears at the same time. Dendrocytes of the papillar dermis, positive to factor XIII, become smaller, less dendritic and decreasing in numbers. Atrophy and the loss of collagen bridges are first observed after a few months, and is due to the long life of the collagen polymers. The blood vessels, lacking collagen support, become wider. The skin atrophy caused by the topical steroids is reversible.

Dermal granulomas after injection of corticosteroids have been reported. They normally disappear 2 weeks after the injection. They look like foreign-body granulomas or a rheumatoid nodule.

The incidence of contact dermatitis due to topical corticosteroids, excluding the excipients, vary between 3% and 5%, depending on the preparations used in each country. The increase in incidence may be due to the development of new potentially antigenic molecules. Coopman *et al.* classified the corticosteroids into four groups, depending on their antigenic behaviour (Fig. 1). Class A or hydrocortisone type has no substitution in the

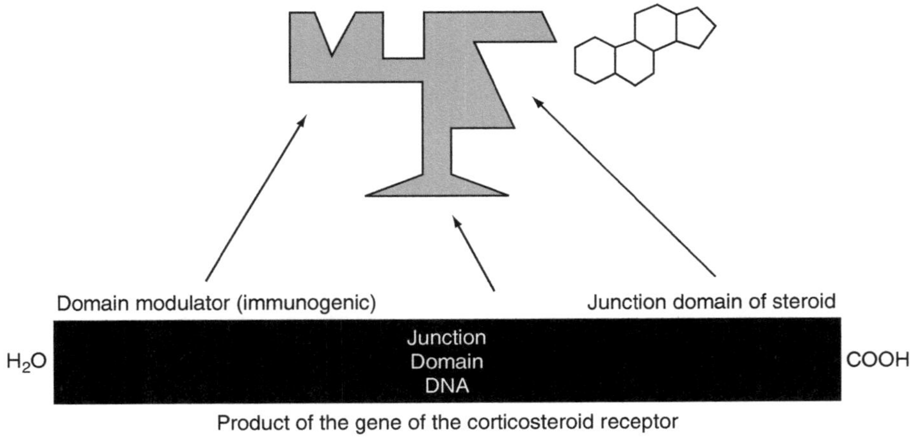

Figure 1 Bidimensional (molecular) structure of the cytoplasmatic steroid receptor

D-ring and has a thioester, the tixocortol pivalate, in C21 as a marker. Class B or triamcinolone acetonide type, has a cisce-tonic molecule or diol in C16–C17 and has budesonide as a marker. Class C or betamethasone type, includes all steroids with a methyl group in C16. Class D or hydrocortisone-17 butyrate type, includes the steroids with a long esterified chain in C17 and/or C21 with or without a methyl group in C16. Eighty-five per cent of cross-reactions have been observed among the same group, although they have also been observed between different groups, mainly between class A and D and very rarely between class B and D. Oh-i also differentiates four groups. The first one includes betamethasone and/or dexamethasone. The second group includes the steroids with a chlormethilcetone group in position C17 of the D-ring. To the third group belong all the steroids with a lateral *cis*-diaxial-diol chain in the C16α position. The fourth group is formed by steroids with esters protecting the hydroxyl-group in the 17Cα position. Contact dermatitis due to steroids is an open field for further investigations.

Topical corticosteroids agents have a broad immunomodulatory effect. However corticosteroid agents are not ideal because of cutaneous atrophy and immunosuppression. In the search for non-corticosteroidal topical agents new drugs will be available (i.e. tacrolimus, ascomycin or phosphodiesterase IV inhibitors). Glucocorticoids are still the most potent anti-inflammatory agents available. The use of steroids has revolutionized the management of skin disorders, which is constantly changing.

Further reading

Ashworth J. Potency classification of topical corticosteroids: Modern perspectives. *Acta Derm Venereol (Stockh)* 1989; 69 (Suppl. 151): 20–5.

Bjarnason B, Flosadottir E, Fischer T. Reactivity at edges of corticosteroid patch test major indicator of strong positive test response. *Dermatology* 1999; 199: 130–4.

Charman CR, Morris AD, Williams HC. Topical corticosteroid phobia in patients with atopy. *Br J Dermatol* 2000; 142: 931–6.

Cole ZA, Clough GF, Church MK. Inhibition by glucocorticoids of the mast cell-dependent wheal and flare response in human skin *in vivo*. *Br J Pharmacol* 2001; 132: 286–92.

Coopman S, Degreef H, Dooms-Goossens A. Identification of cross-reaction patterns in allergic contact dermatitis from topical corticosteroids. *Br J Dermatol* 1989; 121: 27–34.

Cornell RC, Maibach HI. Clinical indications: real and assumed. In: Maibach HI, Surber E, eds. *Topical Corticosteroids*. Basel: Karger, 1992: 154–62.

Fleischer AB Jr. Treatment of atopic dermatitis: role of tacrolimus topical noncorticosteroidal therapy. *J Allergy Clin Immunol* 1999; 104: 126–307.

Goa KL. Clinical pharmacology and pharmacokinetics properties of topically applied corticosteroids. A review. *Drugs* 1988; 36 (Suppl. 5): 51–61.

Katz HI. Topical corticosteroids. *Dermatol Clin* 1995; 13: 805–15.

Kragballe K. Topical corticosteroids: Mechanisms of action. *Acta Derm Venereol (Stockh)* 1989; 69 (Suppl. 151): 7–10.

Murray JR. The history of corticosteroids. *Acta Derm Venereol (Stockh)* 1989; 69 (Suppl. 151): 4–6.

Oh-i T. Contact dermatitis due to topical steroids with conceivable cross reactions between topical steroids preparations. *J Dermatol* 1996; 23: 200–8.

Puig LI. Corticosteroides tópicos. Farmacología clínica y empleo. *Drugs of Today* 1994; 30 (Suppl. 5): 1–34.

Stern RS. The pattern of topical corticosteroid prescribing in United States. *J Am Acad Dermatol* 1996; 35: 183–6.

Uppal R, Sharma SC, Bhownik SR, Sharma PL, Kaur. Topical corticosteroids usage in dermatology. *Int J Clin Pharmacol Ther Toxicol* 1991; 29: 48–50.

Glucocorticoids: systemic

J.G. Camarasa and
A. Giménez-Arnau

General principles, classification and structure

Glucocorticoids are used routinely in the management of skin diseases, due to their potent anti-inflammatory and immunosuppressive actions.

Corticosteroids are used as a substitutive measure in adrenal insufficiency, and due to their anti-inflammatory and immunosuppressive palliative effects in the treatment of various diseases. Occasionally high doses are required in emergency treatments. In most cases the lowest effective dose is given over the shortest possible time period. The reduction of systemic treatment doses has to be gradual in order not to precipitate acute adrenal insufficiency. During stressful periods or trauma, doses should be increased due to an increased requirement of corticosteroids. The side-effects of the corticosteroids are due to an excessive action over the electrolyte and water balance, metabolism, tissue repair processes and their effect as an inhibitor of the secretion of adrenocorticotrophic hormone (ACTH). Systemic corticosteroids may increase the risk of infections, and they can cause a delay in the child's growth.

Chevreul, a young French chemist in Napoleon times, discovered the 'non-saponificable acids'. In 1812, one of these acids, found in gallstones, was named 'cholesterol'. A hundred years later, Adolf Windhaus showed the biological importance of steroids. After 20 years of work, Windhaus discovered in 1932 the structural formula of cholesterol, before he was given the Nobel price for his work about vitamin D.

Kendall, working between 1934 and 1949 in the Mayo Foundation with Parke-Davis, analysed up to 150 tons of adrenal glands. Reichstein worked at the same time in Switzerland with lesser amounts of adrenal glands, which were supplied by the Dutch company Organon. Rumours were circulating that most of the adrenal glands were shipped from Argentina during the war with Germany. It was thought that German pilots received hormonal injections. This caused panic among the Allied Forces.

After the Second World War, Kendall and Hench working with the Merck company made a casual and lucky discovery. At that time it was thought erroneously, that rheumatoid arthritis was due to adrenal insufficiency. Hench, a friend of Kendall, bought in 1948 a supply of a substance known as 'E or F'. A miracle seemed to occur as a severely ill patient, to whom substance E (called cortisone afterwards) was given, improved so much, that on Christmas Day he stood up from his bed, walked and started reading. Merck started the production of cortisone using bile as the raw material. Kendall, Hench and Reichstein were given the Nobel Prize in 1950, for their studies about adrenocortical hormones, their structure and biological effects. Corticosteroids have been used for the last 50 years.

The glucocorticoids and mineralocorticoids are collectively called corticosteroids. Steroids are basic components of the cell membrane, metabolites of the fatty acids, harmful substances of the cardiovascular system, hormones and therapeutic agents. All have a common steroid structure (Fig. 1), but they differ in the group fixed to carbon-17, or in the three-dimensional position this group takes.

Hydrocortisone is the glucocorticoid most commonly used as an anti-inflammatory agent. Apart from the natural steroids aldosterone, cortisone, deoxycortone and hydrocortisone, several synthetic steroids have been introduced

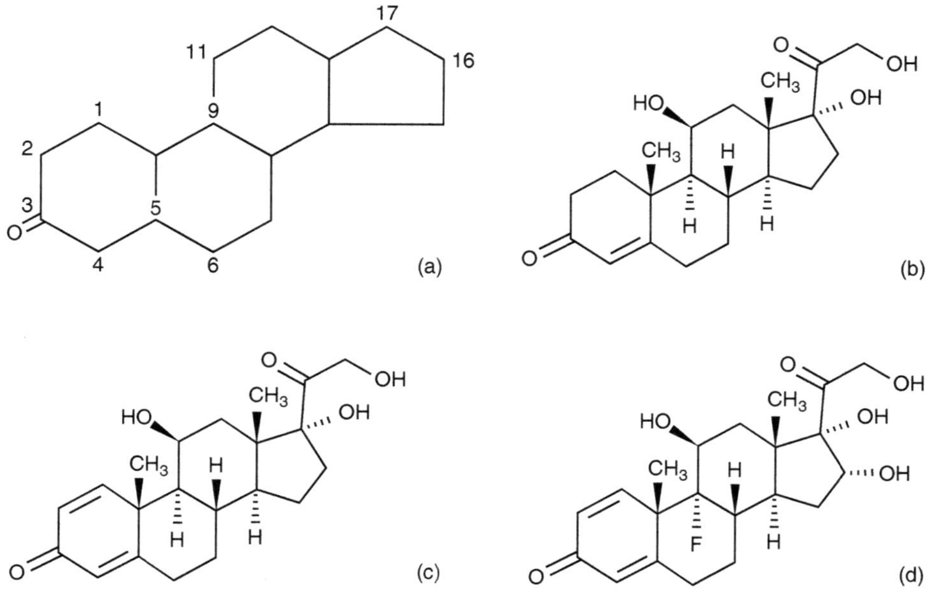

Figure 1 (a) Basic steroid molecule. (b) Hydrocortisone. (c) Prednisolone. (d) Triamcinolone.

in the pharmacopoeia. These analogues try to increase the potency of the drug and to separate the glucocorticoidal effect from the mineralocorticoidal effect. The determination of the potency of glucocorticoids is based on the degree of ACTH inhibition.

Most glucocorticoids used systemically belong to the hydroxyl (alcohol) group. Their relative insolubility in water makes their sodium salts or their phosphate succinate esters the most commonly used soluble forms for injection or solution. These esters are rapidly hydrolysed in the human body. Small substitutions in the basic steroid structure result in drugs with a different plasma half-life, a different anti-inflammatory response and a different capacity to retain sodium. Most of the synthetic agents bind less efficiently (approximately 70%) to the cortisone-transporting globulin. This characteristic may explain partly their tendency to cause side-effects at low doses.

The 11-β-hydroxyl group is fundamental to cortisone activity. Cortisone and prednisone belong to the 11-keto group, and they are only active if they are metabolized in the liver to 11-β-hydroxyl (cortisone and prednisolone). Although the patients with liver failure maintain normally the capacity of transforming 11-keto into 11-β-hydroxyl, the administration of already transformed agents is recommended.

The search for new glucocorticoid molecules is constant. The aim is to obtain potent drugs with fewer side-effects.

Mechanisms of action and pharmacology

The mechanisms of action of glucocorticosteroids implies their passive diffusion through the cell membrane, binding afterwards to the intracytoplasmic soluble protein receptor. This hormone–receptor complex enters the nucleus and regulates the transcription of a limited number of genes. That is how they decrease the synthesis of proinflammatory molecules as cytokines, interleukins and proteases. On the other hand, they are capable of increasing the synthesis of molecules as the lipocortine, which reduces the phospholipase A_2 activity and also reduces the concentration of arachidonic acid, a precursor of the prostaglandins and leukotrienes which take part in the inflammatory response.

Administration of glucocorticosteroids decreases the number of monocytes, eosinophils and lymphocytes with a great effect on T and B cells. The increase in the number of circulating polymorphonuclear leukocytes may be due to an increased liberation of cells from the bone marrow and delayed elimination from the circulating blood. Glucocorticoids interfere in cell activation, proliferation and differentiation. Studies using monocytes in culture, show that glucocorticosteroids inhibit the production, in an early phase, of:

- cytokines such as interleukin-1 (IL-1) β
- tumour necrosis factor-α
- immunomodulating interleukins such as IL-2, IL-3, IL-4, IL-5, IL-10 and IL-12
- γ-interferon
- IL-6, IL-8
- the granulocyte–macrophage colony-stimulating factor (GM-CSF) growth factor.

Cortisol decreases some functions of macrophages, such as phagocytosis, antigen presentation and cell destruction. The suppression of monocyte function is greater than that of polymorphonuclear cells.

Granulomatous infections can be aggravated or reactivated after prolonged steroid treatment. High drug doses are required in order to inhibit the antibody-mediated humoral immune response.

A significant reduction in the amount of histamine-liberating factor has been reported, after the administration of methylprednisolone, in patients with chronic idiopathic urticaria. The secretion of histamine was not modified.

Finally, the selective inhibition of the central opiod receptors by dexamethasone or corticosterone have been described, as well as the induction of the hypothalamic neuropeptide Y by dexamethasone. The multiple biological anti-inflammatory and immunosuppressive effects of corticosteroids cannot be explained by a single hypothesis.

Glucocorticoids are absorbed from the gastrointestinal tract and are rapidly distributed through different body tissues. They cross the placenta and are secreted in small amounts through breast milk. In plasma circulating corticosteroids are bound to a transport molecule transcortin (95%) or albumin (5%). Corticosteroids are metabolized mainly in the liver but also in the kidney, and excreted in the urine. The slowed metabolism of the synthetic derivatives and their low globulin-binding capacity, makes them more potent.

Indications and other uses

Corticosteroids are used in physiological doses in the substitution therapy of adrenal insufficiency. Pharmacological doses are used for their anti-inflammatory and immunosuppressive actions. Their use has to take into account the possible benefits and adverse effects. The smallest therapeutic dose should be given over the shortest possible time period. High doses may be needed in life-threatening diseases.

The clinical manifestations of various disorders are suppressed by the anti-inflammatory and immunosuppressive actions of glucocorticoids. In general the use of synthetic analogues, with less mineral corticoid effect than experienced with cortisone or hydrocortisone, is preferred. Although many synthetic glucocorticoids have minimal mineral corticoidal effect, less potent drugs such as prednisolone or prednisone are used, as they have a greater safety margin. In general the use of prednisolone is preferred, because, as well as hydrocortisone, they are biologically active, while prednisone, as well as cortisone, need first to be transformed into their active form in the liver.

The following skin disorders are treated normally with systemic glucocorticosteroids:

- pemphigus
- bullous pemphigoid
- herpes gestationis
- dermatomyositis
- systemic lupus erythematosus
- eosinophilic fasciitis
- recidivant polychondritis
- sarcoidosis
- vasculitic diseases
- Sweet's syndrome
- pyoderma gangrenosum
- type 1 lepra reaction
- capillary haemangiomas.

Short-term administration of glucocorticosteroids are used in acute contact eczema and in severe atopic eczema. Sometimes, severe inflammatory acne and hirsutism secondary to endocrine disorders respond to low corticosteroid oral doses. Different opinions exist, about the use of corticosteroids in the management of toxic epidermal necrolysis, exudative erythema multiforme, erythema nodosum, exfoliative dermatitis, lichen planus, T-cell skin lymphomas and discoid lupus erythematosus. More potent steroids or other drugs with fewer side-effects are going to be needed in the future for the management of inflammatory and autoimmune skin disorders.

Side-effects, contraindications and drug interactions

The side-effects caused by the use of high doses of glucocorticosteroids are mainly related to their action on:

- electrolyte and water balance
- excessive influence over different aspects of metabolism such as gluconeogenesis
- intervention of tissue repair
- inhibitory effect on the release of corticotrophin from the adenohypophysis.

The required dose of corticosteroids to induce atrophy of the adrenal cortex, varies from patient to patient. Table 1 shows the side-effects of systemic glucocorticoid treatment. These side-effects are observed in nearly all the glucocorticosteroids used at doses equal or above 7.5 mg/day of prednisolone or its equivalent. High doses over a short time period in emergency situations, cause less side-effects then low doses over long treatment periods. Patients need to be monitored for signs of possible side-effects.

Glucocorticosteroids are contraindicated in patients with:

- peptic ulcer disease
- osteoporosis
- psychoses
- severe psychoneurotic disorders.

They need to be used cautiously in the management of elderly patients who suffer from:

- hypertension
- congestive cardiac failure
- diabetes mellitus
- epilepsy
- glaucoma
- infectious diseases
- tuberculosis
- herpes simplex involving the eye
- chronic renal failure
- uraemia.

Glucocorticosteroids increase the metabolism of some drugs such as barbiturates, phenytoin and rifampicin, through the induction of microsomal liver enzymes. They reduce the serum levels of salicylates so that doses of oral anticoagulants such as dicumarol need to be increased in cases of concomitant anticoagulant treatment. Similarly, when used with antidiabetic and antihypertensive drugs, the doses of these have to be increased. The concomitant use with diuretics such as thiazides or furosemide may cause an excessive loss of potassium.

Table 1 Side-effects of the systemic glucocorticoid treatment

Endocrine system	
	Secondary amenorrhoea
	Growth disorders
	Suppression of the hypophysis–adrenal axis
	Cushing's syndrome
Cardiovascular and fluid retention	
	Hypokalaemic alkalosis
	Atherosclerosis
	Cardiovascular collapse
	Hypertension
	Fluid and sodium retention
Gastrointestinal	
	Pancreatitis
	Intestinal perforation
	Peptic ulcer
Metabolic	
	Changes in fat distribution
	Hyperosmolar non-ketotic states
	Hyperglycaemia
	Hyperlipidaemia
	Fat infiltration in the liver
	Drug interaction
Fibroblast inhibition	
	Subcutaneous tissue atrophy
	Inhibition of the wound-healing process
Suppression of the host defences	
	Effects on phagocyte kinesis
	Immunosuppression and anergia
	Increased incidence of infections
Ocular	
	Cataracts
	Glaucoma
Musculoskeletal	
	Myopathy
	Aseptic bone necrosis
	Osteoporosis
Central nervous system	
	Pseudotumour cerebri
	Psychiatric disorders
Skin	
	Acne
	Atrophy
	Hirsutism
	Hyperhydrosis
Hypersensitivity reactions	
	Anaphylaxis
	Urticaria

The incidence of gastrointestinal bleeding or peptic ulcers increases if they are given with anti-inflammatory agents. They reduce the antimuscarinic effect in myasthenia gravis. Ketoconazol increases the serum levels of methylprednisolone and its effect on the adrenal gland. Rifampicin reduces their activity. Some studies show that ciclosporin and corticosteroids mutually inhibit their therapeutic effect, while their plasma levels increase. Increased corticosteroid plasma levels have been reported after smoking a cigarette. A decrease in dexamethasone half-life has been observed with the use of sympathomimetic agents.

In general, the administration of corticosteroids to pregnant women does not have teratogenic side-effects on the fetus. Mothers who suffer from chronic illnesses, like asthma, can continue their treatment during the pregnancy. Delay of fetal growth has been reported during treatment with triamcinolone in a pregnant woman. Persistent ductus arteriosus has been reported in two women with placenta previa, treated with intramuscular betamethasone. In animals the development of 'cleft lip and palate' has been observed, though this finding is controversial in humans.

Treatment

The biological effects of corticosteroids vary qualitatively and quantitatively. They cannot be replaced by each other in equal therapeutic doses without causing toxic effects. Cortisone and hydrocortisone have a significant mineralocorticoid effect compared with their glucocorticoid effect, while prednisone and prednisolone have fewer mineralocorticoid properties. Betamethasone and dexamethasone have very little mineral corticoid activity. The mineral corticoid property of fluodrocortisone overrides the clinical significance of their glucocorticoid activity.

The equivalent doses of the principal corticosteroids based on their glucocorticoid activity are:

- cortisone acetate 25 mg
- betamethasone 0.75 mg
- dexamethasone 0.75 mg
- hydrocortisone 20 mg
- methylprednisolone 4 mg
- prednisolone 5 mg

- prednisone 5 mg
- triamcinolone 4 mg.

Table 2 lists the adrenocorticosteroids and their analogues used in systemic treatment.

Generally the steroids with less mineral corticoid effects are preferred. In prolonged treatments the use of prednisone, or a similar drug with an intermediate half-life, are preferred due to their low affinity for the steroid receptor, obtaining good therapeutic results with fewer side-effects. Drugs with a longer half-life and a greater affinity for the steroid receptor, such as dexamethasone, are used less frequently. If a patient does not respond to the cortisone or prednisone treatment, more active forms, such as cortisol or prednisolone, are used. Methylprednisolone has been used in pulsed therapy as it retains little sodium. The use of corticosteroids in critical life-threatening situations without a clear diagnosis, is not recommended, as they may mask important symptoms.

The therapeutic effects of corticosteroids last longer than their metabolic effects. With intermittent treatments the human body has time to recover. These types of treatment patterns are based on treatment over a short time period or on administration of twice the daily dose every second day. This type of regimen is suitable for short-acting corticosteroids with little mineralocorticoid effect, such as prednisolone.

Normally corticosteroids are administered in a single daily dose, coinciding with maximal or minimal adrenal production, causing an increased or decreased suppression of the hypophysis–adrenal axis. The extent of adrenal suppression caused by the use of steroids is dependent upon the route of administration, the frequency, the time of day and the duration of administration. The adrenal glands produce an equivalent of 20 mg of hydrocortisone (cortisol). Individual concentrations of circulating cortisol may increase tenfold in stressful situations. Infections and surgical procedures require an increase in corticosteroid dose. For patients receiving long-term corticosteroid treatment, and about to undergo minor surgery, it is recommended that they are given hydrocortisone, normally the sodium succinate (100 mg i.v. or i.m. every 8 h). Other authors suggest that routine supplementary treatment is not required, and they only recommend the use of an additional postsurgical dose if clinical signs of insufficiency appear.

Systemic glucocorticoids can be given orally, intralesionally, intramuscularly and intravenously. The route and schedule of administration depends on the disease being treated.

Oral glucocorticoids as well as prednisone are used frequently and they are normally given daily or on alternate days, although in acute illnesses several daily doses can be given. The initial daily dose varies from 2.5 mg up to hundreds of milligrams. This dose is reduced gradually. If the glucocorticoids are used for less than 3–4 weeks, the withdrawal does not have to be gradual. The use of the minimal dose of a short-acting agent, given at early morning, does not suppress the pituitary gland. Low doses of prednisone (2.5–5 mg) are given at bedtime, in order to obtain maximal suppression of the adrenal gland, in the management of acne or hirsutism of adrenal origin. Intralesional glucocorticoids allow direct access into the lesions. Low concentrations (2–3 mg/mL) are used in the face to avoid skin atrophy, while keloids require up to 40 mg/mL.

The intravenous or intramuscular routes are other possibilities for glucocorticoid administration. Intravenous glucocorticoids are used in patients under long-term corticoid treatment with suppressed hypophysis–adrenal axis, who are to undergo surgical treatment. This route is also used in the management of patients

Table 2 Adrenocortical steroid preparations and their synthetic analogues

Drug	Oral forms	Injectable forms
Betamethasone	0.6 mg, 0.6 mg/5 ml	4 mg/ml
Forms: phosphate, sodic, acetate		6 mg/ml (suspension)
Cortisol (hydrocortisone)	5, 10, 20 mg	25, 50 mg/ml (suspension)
Forms: Acetate		25, 50 mg/dl (suspension)
Cypionate	2 mg/ml (suspension)	
Sodic phosphate		50 mg/ml
Sodic succinate		100, 250, 500 mg/ 1 g (powder)
Others: Butyrate		
Sodic succinate		
Valerate		
Cortisone acetate	5, 10, 25 mg	25, 50 mg/ml (suspension)
Deflazacort	30 mg	
Deoxycortone (Mineral corticoid)		
Forms: Acetate		125 mg (subcutaneous)
Pivalate		25–100 mg
Deoxycorticosterone		
Forms: Acetate		5 mg/ml (oil)
Pivalate		25 mg/ml (suspension)
Dexamethasone	0.25–4 mg, 0.5 mg/5 ml (elixir)	
Forms: Acetate		8 mg/ml
Sodic phosphate		4, 10, 24 mg/ml
Others: Phosphate		
Isocyanate		
Sodic metasulfobenzoate		
Fluodrocortisone acetate (mineralocorticoid)	0.1 mg	
Fluprednisolone	1.5 mg	
Meprednisone	4 mg	
Methylprednisolone	2–32 mg	
Forms: Acetate		20, 40, 80 mg/ml (suspension)
Sodic succinate		40, 125, 500 mg, 1 g (powder)
Others: Hemisuccinate		
Paramethasone acetate	1.2 mg	
Prednisolone	1, 2.5, 5 mg	
Forms: Acetate		25, 50, 100 mg/ml
Sodic phosphate		20 mg/ml
Sodic succinate		50 mg (powder)
Tebutate		20 mg (suspension)
Others: Hemisuccinate		
Hexanoate		
Pivalate		
Sodic metasulfobenzoate		
Steaglate		
Prednisone	1–50 mg	
Triamcinolone	1, 2, 4, 8, 16 mg	
Forms: Acetonide		40 mg/ml (suspension)
Diacetate	2, 4 mg/5 ml	40 mg/ml (suspension)
Hexacetonide		5, 20 mg/ml (suspension)

with pyoderma gangrenosum, systemic sclerodermia or dermatomyositis. Methylprednisolone (500 mg to 1 g/day), is the preferred agent. Occasionally anaphylactic reactions, seizures, arrhythmias or sudden death have been reported after intravenous administration. Other adverse reactions include:

- hypotension
- hypertension
- hyperglycaemia
- electrolyte imbalance

- acute psychoses.

Slow administration over 2 or 3 h, reduces the side-effects

Monitoring both individual predisposition to developing complications during treatment, and the use of preventive measures, will reduce the risk of side-effects. Low-fat, low-calorie and low-sodium diets, but rich in proteins, potassium and calcium, are recommended. Tuberculine-positive patients should carry out prophylactic treatment with isoniazid. Patients at risk of developing peptic ulcer disease should receive H_2-receptor antagonists such as ranitidine or cimetidine.

The withdrawal of long-term treatment should be gradual. Daily treatment can be changed, first to alternate days and then reduced step by step. Another way of reducing the dose is keeping the dose constant on one day and reducing the dose in 5 mg steps on alternate days. After 4 weeks of a maintenance treatment, with doses of 5 mg of prednisone on alternate days, the basal cortisol levels should be monitored. If they are greater than 10 mg/dL, the prednisone dose can be reduced 1 mg every 1–2 weeks, keeping it at 2 mg/day. Periodically the cortisol level at 8 a.m. should be analysed, maintaining it at 10 mg/dL. Iatrogenic adrenal insufficiency recovers completely a year after treatment.

Osteoporosis should be prevented, especially in postmenopausal women who are not receiving oestrogen supplements. Premenopausal women and men should receive 500 mg of calcium and 400 units of vitamin D twice a day. Calcium should be avoided in patients with calcium-oxalate kidney stones. Postmenopausal women may need up to 1500 mg of calcium and vitamin D. The toxic effects on the cardiovascular system should be monitored, and symptoms of vascular necrosis should be observed.

The dilemma resides in finding glucocorticoids which have both greater desired effects and lesser adverse effects. The problem lies in the ubiquity of the corticosteroid receptors. Nowadays the side-effects can be limited to the area of application, therefore avoiding systemic risks, using more selective corticosteroids with a better pharmacokinetic profile. Dermatological treatments require, on the other hand, the development of more potent drugs with less side-effects that are a useful alternative to corticosteroids. Better pathogenetic knowledge of inflammatory and immunological skin diseases will allow us to deal with different inflammatory response patterns. Nevertheless, knowledge is increasing on how to treat certain skin diseases whilst assessing the advantages and disadvantages of systemic glucocorticoids.

Further reading

Brattsand R, Linden M. Cytokine modulation by glucocorticoids: mechanisms and actions in cellular studies. *Aliment Pharmacol Ther* 1996; 10 (Suppl. 2): 81–90.

Brattsand R, Sarnstrand B. Prospects for future topical glucocorticoid development. *Acta Derm Venereol Suppl (Stokh)* 1989; 69 (Suppl. 151): 37–46.

Krueger GG, Emam M. Biology of Langerhans cells: Analysis by experiments to deplete Langerhans cells from human skin. *J Invest Dermatol* 1984; 82: 613–17.

Murray JR. The history of corticosteroids. *Acta Derm Venereol (Stockh)* 1989; 69 (Suppl. 151): 4–6.

Paradis L, Lavoie A, Brunet C, Bedart PM, Hebert J. Effects of systemic corticosteroids on cutaneous histamine secretions and histamine-releasing factor in patients with chronic idiopathic urticaria. *Clin Exp Allergy* 1996; 26: 815–20.

Reynolds JEF, Parfitt K, Parsons AV, Sweetman SC. *Corticosteroids. Martindale: the Extra Pharmacopoeia*, 30th edn. London: Pharmaceutical Press, 1993: 712–40.

Werth VP, Lazarus GS. Systemic glucocorticosteroids. In: Fitzmatrick TB, Eisen A, Wolff K, Freedberg IM, Austen KF, eds. *Dermatology in General Medicine*, 4th edn., McGraw-Hill, 1993: 2859–64.

Insect repellents

S. Motta and M. Monti

General principles and classification

Insect repellents are chemical substances that when applied to the skin are able to repel insects and block their attack on man. These compounds can block the insect's approach phase to the host by deviating the flight and hence taking the insect far from the target. Insect repellents exploit their action on many insects such as mosquitoes, flies, sandflies, horseflies, fleas, mites and ticks. There are three categories of insect repellent:

- physical repellents
- synthetic repellents
- natural origin repellents.

Physical repellents are instruments, usually employing ultrasound and claiming to modify insect flight and host identification. Their efficacy is questionable so they will not be considered in this chapter.

Synthetic and natural repellents are particularly effective when directly applied onto the skin. Therefore there is an interaction between human skin and the repellent substance that may cause cutaneous and/or systemic toxicity by absorption. From the dermatotoxicological point of view, insect repellents have to be considered as 'leave on products', though they can be absorbed if applied frequently for a long period. These products, which are available over the counter, are indiscriminately used nowadays so it is necessary to consider them with particular concern for the possible risks of their use, misuse or abuse.

The substance most used as an insect repellent since World War II is a synthetic molecule called *N,N'*-diethyl-*m*-toluamide (DEET), chemically belonging to the diethylamides family.

Natural origin repellents are essential oils derived from different plants. These products, unlike the synthetic insect repellents, have been relatively poorly investigated.

In this chapter, insect repellent compounds, their mechanism of action and toxicity will be considered.

The ideal insect repellent

The perfect topical repellent would repel multiple species of biting arthropodes, remain effective for at least 8 h, cause no irritation to mucous membranes, possess no systemic toxicity, be resistant to washing off, be greaseless and odourless. No available insect repellent meets all of these criteria.

Mechanism of action

The relationship between chemical structure and repellent effectiveness has not been completely clarified, thus insect repellents cannot be classified on the basis of their mechanism of action. However, the most active repellents belong to the following chemical moieties: amides, imides, alcohols and phenols. There is also a kind of relationship between vapour-producing property and the level of repellency. The repellency activity is somehow related to the olfactory receptors of insects via:

- a block of neurones which sense attractive chemical stimuli
- activation of receptors which promote inappropriate behaviour
- activation of receptors for noxious odours
- activation of too many receptors and loss of attractive messengers.

Factors affecting effectiveness of repellency

Multiple factors play a role in how effective a repellent is; these factors are product dependent, product independent and user dependent as listed in Table 1.

Repellents form a barrier between the skin and mosquito receptors and this barrier extends to 4 cm from the skin when the repellent is freshly applied. Apart from some individual host characteristics, repellents are inactive due to excessive evaporation when the temperature exceeds 30°C. In sweaty areas such as the forehead, the duration of protection is significantly decreased. Moreover, for unknown reasons some insect species are more sensitive to repellents than other related species, which remain unaffected. Among mosquito species, *Aedes taeniorhynchus* and *Culex pipiens* are more sensitive than *Aedes aegypti* and *Anopheles albimanus*.

Factors attracting insects

Mosquitoes use visual, thermal and olfactory stimuli to locate a host. Visual stimuli are important for in-flight orientation whereas olfactory stimuli are more important as a mosquito nears its host. Even host movement and wearing of dark-coloured clothing may promote orientation. Investigations about host-attracting factors have pointed out that some body odours may attract insects. These are eccrine sweat because of the presence of amino acids, urea, ammonia, and apocrine sweat and sebum secretion due to the presence of cholesterol. Urine, carbon dioxide and sexual hormones are considered as attractants. In particular carbon dioxide is a long-range attractant whereas at close range skin moisture and warmth are attractants. Body temperature is a discriminating factor: mosquitoes choose hosts with higher body temperatures. Body humidity is also a discriminating factor due to mosquitoes having hygrometric sensors.

Types of insect repellent

Synthetic insect repellents

Thousands of chemical compounds have been demonstrated to have repellence activity. However only three of these are considered suitable for human use. These are: dimethyl phthalate (DMP), ethylhexanediol and diethyltoluamide (DEET)

The discrepancy between the number of active substances and the registered ones is mainly due to skin absorption toxicity.

DMP

This compound which was registered in 1929, and has been the reference repellent for many years. It is an oily, colourless, water-insoluble liquid with an aromatic odour. DMP has a mean protective duration of 80 min and its effectiveness is variable among different insect species. It is used at 40% preparation. The minimum amount of DMP necessary to inhibit mosquito biting has been determined to be 8–8.15 mg per square inch. The toxicological data available indicate that over a 40% concentration, DMP exerts eye, mucous and skin irritation; by ingestion it is a central nervous system and respiratory depressant. Nowadays DMP is used exclusively in association with other repellents. Recently DMP was mentioned for its efficacy against ixodid ticks and advocated for the prevention of Lyme disease.

Table 1 Factors affecting repellent effectiveness

Product-dependent factors	Product-independent factors	User-dependent factors
Evaporation rate from skin surface	Species of the biting insect	Activity level of the host
	Density of the biting insect	User attractiveness
Absorption rate	Wind velocity	Frequency of application
Resistance to abrasion	Air temperature	Uniformity of application
Resistance to wash-off	Wet environment	Anatomical site

Ethylhexanediol

This compound was patented in 1935. It is an oily, colourless, water-insoluble, chemically stable liquid. It has a protective duration ranging from 1 to 8 h depending on the different insect species. Its repellency decreases as the temperature increases due to rapid evaporation. It is used from 30% to 50% and at these concentrations is a mild skin irritant. The only data available on the toxicity of ethylhexanediol cites suspected teratogenicity via skin absorption.

DEET

This compound was patented in 1943 and marketed since 1956. It is considered the reference repellent since it still remains the best one in thousands of comparative tests with other compounds. Today DEET is distributed worldwide and it is estimated that two hundred million people use DEET each year. The repellency of this compound covers a wide range of insect species: mosquitoes, biting fleas, gnats, chiggers, ticks and others. It is oily, colourless, odourless, water and glycerin insoluble, and soluble in alcohol, ether and polyethylene glycols. It has a protective duration of about 4 h. The protectiveness decreases to 24 min at 40°C. Of the marketed products, DEET concentration has a wide range (from 7% to 100%). As opposed to the previously cited repellents, a great bulk of literature on DEET toxicology is available. DEET toxicology may be subdivided into: general, systemic and skin toxicology.

Pharmacology

Human studies show variable penetration of DEET ranging from 9 to 56% of topically applied dose. Absorbed DEET is metabolized completely within 12 h with 99% urinary elimination. Hepatic microsomal cytochrome P450 enzymes are involved in DEET metabolism. There is no evidence of stratum corneum or systemic accumulation.

General toxicology

DEET applied to skin is absorbed in about 20 min The systemic LD_{50} is 2 mL/kg in rats and 10 mL/kg in rabbits. The poisoned animals manifested laboured respiration, ataxia and convulsions.

Human systemic toxicity

Some cases of encephalopathy in children after the application of DEET were reported in 1961. After this, several reports on systemic toxicity after DEET application were published. Among these the most frequently described symptoms were encephalopathy ataxia, seizures, bradycardia and hypotension. Severe toxic reactions and death after the ingestion of repellents containing DEET was also reported. In 1988, an editorial in the *Lancet* suggested that products containing less than 50% DEET were safe; however, in children even preparations containing 20% DEET, applied to large areas repeatedly, caused slurred speach, agitations, tremors and convulsions.

A comprehensive review of side-effects due to DEET was published in 1994.

Skin toxicology

There are several reports on specific skin sensitivity to DEET, while some reports refer to skin irritation, contact urticaria, generalized urticaria and vesicobullous reactions.

No photosensitivity has been reported. DEET is considered a substance with a high profile of safety.

Natural origin insect repellents

All substances with repellent activity not produced by chemical synthesis are considered natural origin insect repellents. Among these, some are of historical value such as smoke, plant derivates, tars and animal urine. Plants whose essential oils have been identified as having repellent activity include cedar, citronella, clove, coconut, eucalyptus, geranium, lavender, mentha, onion, rosemary and thyme. Plant-derived insect repellents have been poorly studied and when tested most of these tend to give short-lasting protection.

Oil of citronella

Oil of citronella is the most studied and utilized essential oil as a repellent. Oil of citronella is extracted from *Cymbopogon nardus*, a Graminaceae native to tropical Asia (Sri Lanka and Java). The active component is the aldehyde citronellale, present in the plant from 20% to 60%, which gives the characteristic scent. The protective duration is variable from 40 to 90 min. Citronella at 10% has been proved to repel flies but not mosquitoes.

Skin toxicity

There are no scientifically trusted data on systemic toxicity due to absorption of essential oils. Citronella as with other essential oils is a mild irritant or rubefacient over 20% concentration. Some reports indicate that essential oils are sensitizers and photosensitizers. Contact urticaria has also been reported.

Pyrethrum

Pyrethrum is derived from *Chrysanthemum cinerariaefolium* and the terms pyrethrum powder and extract are used to describe the crude products obtained from the crushed dried flowers. The pyrethrines are the active components. These substances are valid insecticides but weak insect repellents and thus no longer used in commercial repellents.

Permethrin

Permethrin, a pyrethroid synthetized in 1973, is mainly an insecticide four times as effective as natural pyrethrins. It also possesses some repellent activity and for this reason it is included in many textbooks among insect repellents. Permethrin is considered a valid tick repellent. Systemic and skin toxicity of this compound is minimal. Permethrin should be applied directly to clothing or to tent and mosquito net fabrics. Permethrin is non-staining, odourless, resistant to degradation by heat or sun and maintains its potency for at least 2 weeks.

The best barrier against biting insects is considered the combination of permethrin-treated clothing and skin application of DEET.

Guidelines for safe use of insect repellents

The insect repellents marketed in Europe possess a high level of safety due to especially low concentrations of the active ingredient. However, to increase the safety profile dermatologists should suggest to their patients the following guidelines.

- Verify that the product has been registered.
- Read the label information.
- Use the repellent only as suggested by the manufacturer.
- Use the repellent only for the insects it claims to be effective against.
- Keep repellents out of the reach of children.
- Apply repellents only to body parts suggested by the manufacturer.
- Avoid use of repellents on or near wounds or on inflamed skin.
- Avoid use around the eyes and mouth.
- Wash repellent off skin with soapy water when protection is no longer needed.
- Contact the local poison control centre if repellent-induced toxicity is suspected.

Insect repellents are useful compounds to avoid the annoyance of many insects or to prevent the transmission of some infectious diseases. In Table 2 insect repellent sensitivity and infectious diseases transmitted by principal arthropods are summarized. However, the insect repellents are far from being the ideal product from a pharmacological point of view.

Table 2 Insect repellent sensitivity and infectious diseases of principal arthropods

Class	Common names	Species	Blood-sucking	Repellent sensitivity	Vectors for
Acars	Ticks	*Ixodes*	+	+	Borreliae, rickettsiae, arbovirus
	Trombidium larvae	*Trombidium*	+	+	Rickettsiae
Insects	Lice	*Pediculus*	+	+	Rickettsiae, borreliae
	Human fleas	*Pulex*	+	+	Yersiniae, rickettsiae
	Bedbugs	*Cimex*	+	−	Nothing
	Deerflies	*Chrysops*	+	+	Filariae
	Tsetse flies	*Glossina*	+	+	*Trypanosoma*
	Houseflies	*Musca*	−	+	?
	Black or buffalo flies	*Simulium*	+	+	*Onchocercus*
	Biting midges or sandflies	*Phlebotomus*	+	+	Leishmaniae
	Mosquitoes	*Anopheles*	+	+	*Plasmodia*
		Aedes	+	+	Arbovirus, yellow fever virus
		Culex	+	+	Arbovirus
		Mansonia	+	+	Filariae
	Ants	*Formica*	−	+	Nothing
	Bees	*Apis*	−	−	Nothing
	Wasps and hornets	*Vespula*	−	−	Nothing
		Vespa	−	−	Nothing

The correct use of these products is fundamental to their safety.

Relief from arthropod bites

Skin responses to arthropod bites range from wheal-and-flare reactions to delayed papules to rare systemic Arthus reactions and anaphylaxis. Several strategies may be considered for the relief of the itch of insect bites. Topical corticosteroids may reduce erythema, induration and itching but the time of effectiveness after skin application is considered too long (about 20 min) for relief of wheal-and-flare reaction that usually lasts 20 min.

Diphenhydramine and benzocaine should be avoided due to allergic contact sensitivity. Oral antihistamines are effective in reducing the symptoms of insect bites but they are poorly employed due to the delay in reducing symptoms.

Ammonium solution 3.6% is used after bite treatment to relieve symptoms but caution should be adopted due to causticity of the product.

Aluminium chloride exahydrate hydroalcoholic gel 5% (see chapter on topical preparations and vehicles) is as effective as ammonium solution possessing a better safety profile.

Aluminium chloride 5% gel is at the same time astringent and antiseptic.

Further reading

Amichai B, Lazaroy A, Halevy S. Contact dermatitis from diethyltoluamide. *Contact Dermatitis* 1994; 30 (188): 10.

Burgess IF. Dermatopharmacology of antiparasitics and insect repellents. In: Gabard B, Elsner P, eds. *Dermatopharmacology of Topical Preparations*. Berlin: Springer, 2000: 157–78.

Cochrane Skin Group Library from 1997: http://www.nottingham.ac.uk; http://www.cochrane.co.uk

Commission Regulation (EC) no. 1896/2000 of 7 September 2000 on the first phase of the programme referred to in Article 16(2) of Directive 98/8/EC of the European Parliament and of the Council on biocidal products (http://europa.eu.int/eur-lex/).

Couch P, Johnson CE. Prevention of Lyme disease: review. *Am J Hosp Pharm* 1992; 49: 1164–73.

Editorial. Are insect repellents safe? *Lancet* 1988; 2: 610–11.

Kienerman P. Mosquitoes: how to be the perfect host. *Int J Dermatol* 1989; 26: 370–2.

Martindale W. Diethyltoluamide, dimethylphthalate, 2-ethylhexanediol 1,3. In: Parfitt K., ed. *The Extra Pharmacopoeia*. 32nd Edition. London: Pharmaceutical Press, 1999: 1401.

McKinlay JR, Ross EV, Barret TL. Vesiculobullous reaction to diethyltoluamide revisited. *Cutis* 1998; 62: 44.

Tenenbein M. Severe toxic reactions and death following the ingestion of diethyltoluamide containing insect repellents. *JAMA* 1987; 258 (1509–1): 511.

Toxicology Data Network: http://toxnet.nlm.nih.gov

Veltri JC *et al.* Retrospective analysis of calls to poison control centers resulting from exposure to the insect repellent DEET from 1985 to 1989. *J Toxicol Clin Toxicol* 1994; 32: 1–16.

Von Mayenburg J, Rakoski J. Contact urticaria to diethyltoluamide. *Contact Dermatitis* 1994; 9: 171.

Wantke F, Focke M, Hemmer W *et al.* Generalized urticaria induced by a diethyltoluamide-containing insect repellent in a child. *Contact Dermatitis* 1996; 35: 186–7.

Psychoactive agents

G. Hautmann and E. Panconesi

General principles

In dermatology, almost all diseases can benefit from the use of psychoactive drugs, but, in our personal opinion, psychotropic agents are more commonly useful in:

- psychiatric syndromes with dermatological expression, such as:
  delusion of parasitosis
  dermatitis artefacta
  neurotic excoriations
  trichotillomania
  glossodynia
  dysmorphophobia (cutaneous manifestations)
  hypochondrias and phobias related to cutaneous and venereal diseases, such as syphilophobia and acquired immunodeficiency syndrome (AIDS) phobia
- cutaneous problems reported to have a high incidence of psychoemotional factors, such as:
  hyperhydrosis
  dyshydrosis
  pruritus sine materia, generalized or localized (vulvar, anal, scrotal pruritus, etc.)
  lichen simplex
  telogen effluvium
  alopecia areata
  urticaria
  atopic dermatitis of the adult
  nummular eczema
  psoriasis
  rosacea
  seborrhoeic dermatitis
  vitiligo
  herpes simplex (recurrent)
  warts
  lichen planus
- cutaneous disorders which may present somatopsychic rebound for any real or presumed aesthetic discomfort:
  acne
  androgenic alopecia
  rosacea
  skin ageing.

The dermatoses listed above refer to the area that we usually call 'psychosomatic dermatology', but it is important to consider that the prescription of psychoactive drugs may be necessary for other problems. In fact, the possibility that psychological problems may occur in the course of any dermatosis (as any disease, in general) without a cause–effect relationship cannot be excluded.

In our experience, the majority of dermatological psychosomatic patients seem to present psychopathological traits related to anxiety disorders (e.g. social phobia, panic attacks, generalized anxiety disorder (GAD), obsessive–compulsive disorder, post-traumatic stress disorder), often constituting an important aspect of psychopathological comorbidity with the dermatological condition. These may present with or without the depression that may be associated with other mood disorders particularly bipolar disorder. A low percentage of dermatological psychosomatic patients are psychotic, suffering from delusions of parasitosis or hallucinations.

Anxiety may be described as a diffuse, highly unpleasant often vague feeling of apprehension, accompanied or not by physical sensations such as an empty feeling in the pit of the stomach, tightness in the chest, a pounding heart, perspiration, headache or the sudden urge to vomit). Anxiety warns of impending danger and enables the person to take measures to deal with a threat, whereas fear, a similar alerting signal, can be differentiated from anxiety because it is in response to a threat that is known, external, definite or nonconflictual in origin. Schematically, anxiety may be considered in response to a threat that is unknown, internal, vague or conflictual in origin. Anxiety is not only an important symptom of many psychiatric disorders, but also an almost inevitable component of many medical and surgical condition, including cutaneous diseases.

It is important to note that anxiety in dermatology patients is rather infrequently a 'disease' in itself. When evaluating a dermatology patient with anxiety, the clinician must distinguish between normal and pathological types and levels of anxiety. On a practical level, pathological anxiety is differentiated from normal anxiety by the belief of patients, their families, their friends, and the clinician that pathological anxiety is, in fact, present. Such an assessment is based on the patient's reported internal state, behaviour and ability to cope. The clinician must be aware that anxiety can be a component of many medical conditions as well as psychiatric disorders, especially depression. As outlined above, in dermatology patients, symptoms of anxiety are commonly associated with depression and especially with dysthymic disorder ('neurotic' depression and various personality disorders).

Sometimes, even when there is a primary cutaneous illness, it may be desirable to deal directly with the anxiety at the same time. In such situations, antianxiety medications are frequently and appropriately used, although psychotherapy and positive doctor–patient counselling can be very effective in the treatment of mild anxiety.

Even in patients with structural damage, anxiety caused by feeling of incompetence, inadequacy and helplessness is a prominent feature of the disturbance. In fact, it is very frequent to meet subjects suffering from some dermatological condition who express discomfort in social situations such that they avoid them.

Social anxiety (or social phobia) disorder is an extremely common and potentially disabling psychiatric disorder. Social phobia affects women twice as often as men and tends to persist over time if not treated effectively. Social phobia often coexists with other psychiatric disorders and may remain undetected in many individuals unless the clinician takes a careful history and has a high index of suspicion. Community studies and clinical samples suggest that there is a high rate of comorbidity in individuals with anxiety disorders, including social anxiety disorder, and there is evidence that social anxiety disorder and GAD are almost always associated with one or more additional anxiety disorders and/or depressive disorder. Patients who present with depression, other anxiety disorders or alcohol use disorders should be considered at risk for current but undetected social anxiety disorder. Diagnostic assessment for social anxiety disorder should be a routine part of any psychosomatic evaluation.

The diagnostic system currently utilized (the fourth edition of the Diagnostic and Statistical Manual of Mental Disorders or DSM-IV) excludes social anxiety due to medical disorders. However, social anxiety commonly occurs in the context of several medical disorders, such as benign essential tremor, stuttering and irritable bowel syndrome. Anecdotal evidence indicates that morbidly obese individuals and burn victims also experience significant social anxiety secondary to their medical conditions.

In our experience, social anxiety in dermatology patients can respond to the same treatments that are used in social anxiety disorder patients without such medical disorders. The clinical implications of secondary social anxiety disorder in terms of additional disability/functional impairment have not been investigated. However, on the basis of the limited information available, it seems worthwhile to address social anxiety disorder specifically even when it appears in the context of a medical condition identified in Axis III of the DSM-IV.

Social phobia is a common, disabling and often unrecognized anxiety disorder, occurring in about 1–2% of the population. Although social phobia shares many features with panic disorder and often occurs with it, it has separate phenomenological features. For instance, the five most common fears of people with social phobia are speaking before a group, eating in public, writing in public, using public lavatories and being stared at or the centre of attention; the five most common fears of panic disorder are driving or travelling, shops, crowds, restaurants and elevators. People with social phobia do not have spontaneous panic attacks and do not panic when they are alone or asleep. Fear of negative evaluation is the critical cognitive feature of social phobia. Many dermatology patients with traits of social phobia also have avoidant personality disorder, characterized by chronic patterns of shyness and avoidance. Social phobia is often quite disabling and results in extreme anxiety, avoidance, work and social impairment, depression and substance abuse.

The pharmacological treatment of social phobia has lagged behind the treatment of other anxiety disorders. Most of the pharmacological studies are small in scale and uncontrolled. High-potency benzodiazepines, particularly alprazolam and clonazepam, have been reported to produce improvement in symptoms of social phobia. For instance, in an uncontrolled study of 26 patients (most of whom had other diagnoses and had received various previous treatments), 85% of patients showed moderate to significant improvement with doses of clonazepam at 0.5–5.0 mg/day, with the mean dose being 2.1 mg/day.

Monoamino oxidase inhibitors (MAOIs) have been observed to be of use in a variety of phobias and reduce excessive interpersonal sensitivity in patients with atypical depression, so they are used to treat social phobia. Because sensitivity to criticism is typical of people with social phobia, it made sense to determine if an MAOI would be effective for this condition. In a sample of 74 patients, phenelzine was superior to both atenolol and placebo with no significant differences between the latter two agents. There is also evidence that moclobemide, a reversible inhibitor of MAO, may also be effective for social phobia.

Beta-blockers have also been used in the treatment of social phobia, with mixed results. For performance anxiety, β-blockers have been shown to benefit activities such as pistol shooting, bowling, playing stringed instruments and public speaking. Doses of propranolol of 10–40 mg before such performances can often reduce fear. The early β-blocker studies focused on performance anxiety, and this subgroup of people with social phobia may respond differently from individuals with generalized social fears.

Uncontrolled trials have also found some benefits from buspirone in social phobia in doses up to 60 mg/day. Buspirone had no effect on exposure therapy in a controlled clinical trial. Fluoxetine has also been reported to be effective in case reports. Further controlled trials of both drugs are needed.

Several studies have found that pharmacological treatments did not improve outcome over cognitive-behavioural therapy alone. For instance, concomitant use of buspirone did not improve outcome of exposure therapy with performance phobia, or propranolol did not improve outcome with social skills training. This is not surprising, because buspirone has not been shown to be an effective medication for social phobia. In another study, cognitive-behavioural treatment programmes were compared with treatment by phenelzine, alprazolam or placebo for subjects with social phobia. All patients improved in all groups. Patients treated with phenelzine plus self-exposure showed greater improvement than other groups did in a measure of trait anxiety. On one fear measure, patients treated with cognitive-behavioural group therapy showed additional improvement from the post-test to follow-up assessment, whereas patients treated with alprazolam plus exposure showed deterioration in this measure. Comparative studies are needed before the relative benefits of psychopharmacological and psychological treatments alone and in combination are known.

Obsessive–compulsive behaviours are often found in cutaneous psychosomatic afflictions, such as:

- trichotillomania
- acne excoriée
- neurotic excoriations
- irritant dermatitis from lip-licking
- repeated hand-washing
- onychotillomania
- localized neurodermatitis.

The essential feature of obsessive–compulsive disorder is the symptom of recurrent obsessions or compulsions sufficiently severe to cause marked distress to the person. The obsessions or compulsions are time-consuming and interfere significantly with the person's normal routine, occupational functioning, usual social activities or relationships. A patient with obsessive–compulsive disorder may have an obsession or a compulsion or both. An obsession is a recurrent and intrusive thought, feeling, idea or sensation. In contrast to an obsession, which is a mental event, a compulsion is a behaviour. Specifically, compulsion is a conscious, standardized, recurrent behaviour. A patient with obsessive–compulsive disorder realizes the irrationality of the obsession and experiences both the obsession and the compulsion as ego dystonic, i.e. it is recognized by the patient as irrational and as coming from within rather than from environmental stimuli. The intrusion of the idea is accompanied by anxiety and often generates feelings of shame. When obsessions evolve into more persistent and pervasive 'overvalued ideas', it may be difficult to differentiate these ideas from the frank delusional beliefs into which they can rarely evolve. There is a spectrum of severity from obsessional worries, through overvalued ideas to delusional beliefs.

Actually an increasing range of psychiatric disorders are classified as obsessive–compulsive spectrum disorders. These include somatoform disorders (such as hypochondria and body dysmorphic disorders frequently seen by dermatologists) eating disorders (such as anorexia and bulimia nervosa), certain paraphilias, impulse control disorders such as trichotillomania, and compulsive hair-pulling that may be an ego dystonic impulse control disorder which can be distressing and become a social handicap for the sufferer.

Pharmacological challenge and neuroimaging studies have provided compelling evidence to support neurobiological abnormalities in this disorder. The most prominent hypothesis concerning obsessive–compulsive disorder pathophysiology suggests an abnormal regulation of brain serotoninergic function.

It has been demonstrated that selective serotonin reuptake inhibitors (SSRIs; see below) are useful in limiting the obsessional worries often caused by:

- hair loss
- sexually transmitted diseases
- skin cancer
- infestations
- scarring from acne
- not being pretty or handsome.

In fact, obsessive–compulsive symptoms are seen across the whole spectrum of psychopathology. Common obsessions have much the same conscious ideology as delusional beliefs, but they do not carry the same convinction. Body dysmorphic disorder refers to those individuals whose worry is that they are:

- ugly
- balding
- disfigured
- scarred
- wrinkled
- have 'serious' skin lesions, notwithstanding negative objective findings.

In early childhood such symptoms may occur as a temporary phenomenon in response to stress or anxiety, as psychoneurotic symptoms in a person with an obsessive–compulsive personality configuration or as a feature of the obsessive–compulsive disorder. They may also be present in patients with psychosis or bipolar disorder.

Common compulsions (such as those mentioned above) include repetitive and ritualized examination of the skin, repeated requests for reassurance concerning certain aspects of skin structure or function, and insistent 'doctor-shopping' in search of relief from anxiety. These subjects present a characteristic personality and they tend to be rather rigid, judgmental, perfectionist, indecisive and afraid of making mistakes. They tend to be unaware of their emotional responses and have difficulty in acknowledging and expressing anger appropriately. Anxiety is generated when anger threatens to surface. The obsessive–compulsive symptom is an attempt to bind that anxiety and underlying depression is not uncommon.

When symptoms are mild, of short duration and do not interfere seriously with the patient's normal routine, occupation or social relationships, counselling, psychotherapy or behaviour modification is appropriate. Sometimes short-term administration of anxiolytics, in particular clonazepam, is necessary. Adults, with intrusive and disruptive symptoms, but not all-consuming and paralysing, will benefit from more or less intensive psychotherapy of various kinds, including psychoanalysis. In very severe and chronic adult cases, psychotropic medication is necessary.

Like most dermatologists, we also see some cases of psychotic patients with delusions and hallucinations. Psychosis, in our practice, is usually characterized by the presence of positive symptoms such as delusions, hallucinations or both. A delusion is a fixed false belief, usually idiosyncratic and bizarre, which is held immutably in the face of contradictory evidence, and that is not explained by the person's educational level or subculture. Although cutaneous delusions may form part of a complex delusional system in a patient with schizophrenia, the patients that usually present to dermatologists have what has been termed a monosymptomatic hypochondrial psychosis or circumscribed delusion. A hallucination is a false perception, rather than a false belief. Hallucinations are experienced in the absence of the corresponding sensory stimuli and are not perceived by others. They may be auditory, visual, olfactory or tactile; they may be experienced alone or in association with a delusional belief that rationalizes the false perception.

Usually the patient with delusion of parasitosis tries to show us the parasites that he sees and believes are infesting him. Dermatologists also see patients affected by a delusion of parasitosis or other types of delusions, such as bromidrosiphobia and dysmorphophobia. Until recently, we treated most cases in liaision with psychiatrists who suggested therapy with atypical neuroleptics, such as risperidone, olanzapine, quetiapine or clozapine. In the past, pimozide was largely employed and it was preferred to haloperidol because it seemed to block both the dopamine receptors as well as those for endogenous opiates which are associated with the transmission of pain and itch. We used very low doses of pimozide, starting with a half tablet (a tablet is 4 mg) to reach the maximum of 8 mg/day. Generally, we noted a response within 2–3 weeks. After 6 months symptom-free, a gradual withdrawal may be attempted. We tend to prefer the newer atypical neuroleptics, such as risperidone, quetiapine or olanzapine (see below).

Patients who present with trichotillomania, acne excoriée, neurotic excoriations and glossodynia usually suffer from compulsive behaviours that generate their skin lesions; these subjects often present depressive traits and many suffer from 'masked depression'.

Masked depression is a depressive state of endogenous or psychogenic origin in which the physical symptoms loom so large in the clinical picture that the psychic symptoms are completely obscured. The term 'masked depression' thus denotes not a nosological, but a phenomenological diagnosis.

Most subjects with burning mouth syndrome (glossodynia) are elderly, and treatment (by dermatologists in association with psychiatrists and psychologists) often includes an antidepressant.

Specific drug therapies

Antidepressants

SSRI and tricyclic antidepressants (TCAs)

The advent of the SSRIs as a new class of antidepressant medication has opened up new possibilities for the treatment of anxiety disorders (social phobia, panic attack, GAD, obsessive–compulsive disorder, etc.) and mood disorder, in particular major depressive episodes. Initial reluctance to use these agents in older patients and in anxiety has given way to more in-depth assessments of their benefits and limitations. Available studies suggest that SSRIs are highly efficacious in depression with response rates equal to or better than those of traditional agents. Side-effect profiles differ from those associated with TCAs and MAOIs and appear to lead to lower rates of discontinuation, at least in younger populations. The absence of significant end-organ toxicity may make SSRIs particularly attractive for use in the elderly.

Five SSRIs are currently approved for clinical use in the USA and Europe: fluoxetine, fluvoxamine, sertraline, citalopram and paroxetine.

The major clinically relevant differences among the currently available SSRIs are in the areas of pharmacokinetics and hepatic drug metabolizing isoenzyme inhibition. These characteristics affect both how the drug is used clinically and drug–drug interactions. As dermatology patients are often taking multiple medications, these considerations assume greater importance in this group.

Fluoxetine has the longest elimination half-life of the group (between 2 and 4 days). More significantly, the primary metabolite of fluoxetine, norfluoxetine, has a half-life of between 7 and 15 days. This is important, because norfluoxetine is pharmacologically active and may account for a significant portion of the biological activity of this agent. By contrast sertraline and paroxetine have half-lives of approximately 26 and 21 h, respectively.

The presence of active metabolites contributes to differences between these agents. As stated above, fluoxetine has a long-lived active metabolite with pharmacological activity comparable to the parent compound. Paroxetine is converted to various polar sulphate and glucuronide intermediates, which have much less effect on serotonin reuptake and are considered clinically insignificant. Sertraline is converted to desmethylsertraline, which is approximately more than 20 times less potent than sertraline itself as an inhibitor of serotonin reuptake, and has demonstrated no significant activity in *in vivo* models of antidepressant activity. Therefore, it appears to have no clinical relevance. Fluvoxamine is reduced to a number of metabolites that appear to be one to two orders of magnitude less potent than the parent compound and seem to be of little importance. Citalopram is the most selective SSRI and has a low incidence of side-effects and low risk of drug interactions.

The relevance of steady-state plasma levels to clinical effects is unclear, but some significant differences among the SSRIs exist with regard to age effects on this parameter. Fluoxetine and paroxetine have been reported to show non-linear changes in plasma level with increasing doses. In elderly individuals, reported plasma concentrations of paroxetine and fluoxetine were 80% to 130% higher than in younger subjects. Sertraline appears to show linear kinetics, and plasma levels have been found to be comparable with those seen in younger subjects. Fluvoxamine appears to show some non-linearity of pharmacokinetic parameters, with half-life increasing from 15 to 23 h with multiple dosing. Clearance of these agents may be affected by severe renal and hepatic impairment, but the significance of these differences in milder degrees of impairment or normal physiological decline is unclear. For example, clearance of fluvoxamine is reduced by about 50% in the elderly, and, accordingly, dose titration of fluvoxamine should be slower in this population. Except for sertraline, dose recommendations for the other agents are influenced by such factors as well. For example, it is recommended that paroxetine be initiated at 10 mg/day in the elderly and that the maximum dose not exceed 40 mg/day. Similarly, dose titration of fluvoxamine in the elderly should be slower because of reduced clearance.

Once a choice of medication has been made, it is a long-established principle to initiate therapy in psychosomatic dermatology patients at lower doses and increase the dose more slowly than in younger patients. This appears to be applicable to SSRIs as well. A common reason for treatment failure with SSRIs in psychosomatic patients appears to be too high a starting dose and/or too rapid titration. Starting the patient at doses that might be routine for younger patients seems to be more likely to provoke difficult-to-tolerate side-effects, particularly nausea and anxiety/agitation.

The anxiety that can be produced by the SSRIs early in the course of treatment may be a direct result of increased serotonin availability. It has been shown that administration of the direct serotonin agonist *m*-chlorophenylpiperazine produced considerable anxiety and agitation and disrupted sleep in healthy volunteers. This anxiety–agitation appears to be a frequent reason given by elderly depressed patients for discontinuing medication.

It has been our personal experience that this complaint, as well as gastrointestinal complaints, is minimized by starting at lower than routine clinical doses. Ideally, starting doses of SSRIs should be no more than one half the routine or recommended clinical dose, e.g. fluoxetine and paroxetine at 10 mg/day, sertraline at 25 mg/day, fluvoxamine at 25–50 mg/day and citalopram at 5–10 mg/day. The patient should be maintained on this dose for between 4 and 7 days before consideration is given to raising the dose. If side-effects occur, they are usually less severe at these doses and will often dissipate in a few days. Dosage can then be raised to a minimum therapeutic dose, with less likelihood of unacceptable adverse effects.

The dose thus achieved should be maintained for at least 4–6 weeks in outpatients before consideration is given to augmenting with a second agent. Since these 'psychosomatic' patients may be slower to respond to antidepressants, a full therapeutic trial may need to be longer. Dosage increases may need to be smaller than with younger patients to avoid side-effects, although with SSRIs recurrent side-effects after dosage increases are uncommon, with the possible exception of gastrointestinal problems (e.g. nausea or diarrhoea). There is little guidance from controlled studies to recommend a maximum dose for the psychosomatic disorders for any of these agents. However, anecdotal experiences suggest that patients with psychotic symptoms or severe psychomotor retardation may need higher doses (as well as concomitant neuroleptics or electroconvulsive therapy).

Since obsessive–compulsive pathology has been associated with the neurotransmitter serotonin, those antidepressants that selectively block the synaptic reuptake of serotonin are the drugs of choice. Thus, fluoxetine and the other SSRIs (citalopram: 60–80 mg/day; sertraline: 200–300 mg/day; fluvoxamine: 200–300 mg/day; fluoxetine: 60–80 mg/day) are, in our opinion more appropriate in these cases than clomipramine, the TCA, previously administered, in particular because clomipramine presents side-effects more often.

We also use these serotoninergic and certain TCAs (imipramine, clomipramine, nortriptyline, amitriptyline) to treat those patients who present relevant somatopsychic rebound and/or symptoms such as burning or itching involving the face, scalp and genital regions, glossodynia, facial hypertrichosis or hair loss, in particular individuals whose subjective symptoms are significantly more important than the objective dermatological findings. Most of these cases involve an underlying depressive disorder which explains the efficacy of SSRIs and the TCAs that were preferentially employed in the past. Another factor in favour of fluoxetine and the other serotoninergic antidepressants (citalopram, in particular) is that they have far fewer anticholinergic, sedative and cardiac side-effects than the TCAs.

For patients presenting relevant somatopsychic rebound and, less frequently, certain cases of chronic urticaria, pruritus and post-herpetic neuralgia, diabetic neuropathy, and nocturnal scratching in atopic dermatitis we prescribe imipramine and other TCAs, such as:

- amitriptyline
- clomipramine
- desipramine
- nortriptyline
- trimipramine.

Generally this is done in consultation with psychologists or psychiatrists. The antihistaminic and possibly the anticholinergic properties of the TCAs may be responsible for their efficacy in urticaria and certain chronic pruritic states. In theory, the anticholinergic effect would be beneficial in conditions such as atopic dermatitis, in which the eccrine glands are hypersensitive to acetylcholine.

For the TCAs, and for clomipramine in particular, we suggest (in liaison with psychologists and psychiatrists) a starting dosage of 10–25 mg/day, with once weekly increments of 10–25 mg if necessary. In general, since elderly patients are especially sensitive to neurological and cardiovascular side-effects, we recommend increasing the dosages every 2 weeks, the period usually required for the drug to take effect. Also, the elderly usually require one-third to one-half the usual adult dosage. The literature suggests that the maximum dosage in primary dermatological patients is approximately 75–100 mg/day and we recommend consultation with a psychopharmacologist before prescribing dosages higher than this.

Bupropion

Bupropion's chemical structure is unique among the antidepressants. It is a unicyclic aminoketone. The lack of complex heterocyclic fused rings, as well as the more common functional groups (e.g.

N-methylpiperazine) often found in neuroleptics, is thought to contribute to bupropion's lack of the side-effects usually seen in polycyclic antidepressants. Bupropion is a relative weak inhibitor of dopamine reuptake, with modest effects on norepinephrine (noradrenaline) reuptake and no effect on serotonin reuptake. It does not appear to be associated with downregulation of postsynaptic β-adrenergic receptors. Also, it does not have significant effects on 5-hydroxytryptamine ($5\text{-}HT_2$) β_2-adrenergic receptors, imipramine or dopaminergic receptors in brain tissue. It lacks anticholinergic activity and is at least 10 times weaker than TCAs in its cardiac depressant effects.

Bupropion is rapidly absorbed following oral administration, with peak blood levels occurring within 2 h. The elimination is biphasic, with an initial phase of approximately 1.5 h and a second phase of about 14 h.

Bupropion undergoes extensive hepatic metabolism, including a pronounced first-pass effect.

The mechanism of action for bupropion remains unclear. From the start, its effects on dopaminergic function have been a focus of investigation. Some of the behavioural effects of bupropion, including stimulation of locomotor activity, are abolished following the destruction of dopaminergic neurons by 6-hydroxydopamine. Noradrenergic systems may also play a critical role in the mechanism of action of bupropion.

Bupropion's metabolites may be quite important in determining clinical response. In animal models, hydroxybupropion possesses more potent antidepressant properties than the parent compound.

Bupropion has been shown to be as effective as standard TCAs and SSRIs (and superior to placebo) in treating hospitalized or ambulatory depressed patients. Under double-blind conditions, bupropion was superior to placebo in treating hospitalized patients who were refractory to TCAs.

In the light of bupropion's enhancement of dopaminergic neurotransmission, it is not surprising that it has been prescribed for conditions where activation and other psychostimulant-like properties could be useful.

Uncontrolled case reports have described the use of bupropion in treating social phobia. Bupropion's side-effect profile is clearly different from that of conventional TCAs. It lacks anticholinergic effects, is clearly not sedating, and suppresses appetite in some patients. Bupropion's cardiovascular profile is especially favourable. It does not cause electrocardiogram changes and does not trigger orthostatic hypotension, even in patients with pre-existing heart disease. Unlike several of the other second-generation antidepressants, bupropion does not cause psychosexual dysfunction. Bupropion appears to be relatively less lethal following overdose, compared with TCAs and certain other antidepressants.

Many of bupropion's side-effects can be predicted, based on its stimulation of dopaminergic systems. Thus, like conventional psychostimulants, bupropion can have activating effects, which are often helpful in patients with psychomotor retardation but can be experienced as agitation or insomnia in others. Appetite suppression is also seen as an advantage in some patients but a disadvantage in others.

In our practice we often employ bupropion (150–300 mg/day) as a mild antidepressant without sedative effects and in those subjects with a 'peculiar emotional lability' as a possible alternative to benzodiazepines.

It is noteworthy that there are many other antidepressant drugs, such as mirtazapine, venlafaxine or nefazodone that play an important role in the everyday practice of the psychiatrist, but they are less employed in the practice of dermatological psychosomatics.

Anxiolytics

Benzodiazepines

Benzodiazepines are effective for reducing panic attack, phobic behaviour and anticipatory anxiety. Of the many benzodiazepines, alprazolam has been most extensively studied, with the results of two large cross-national trials reported. In the first large multicentre trial, 526 patients were randomized to alprazolam or placebo. Of these, 86% of the alprazolam subjects completed the trial, compared with only 50% of the placebo subjects. At the primary comparison point (week 4 of the study), 82% of the subjects receiving alprazolam were considered moderately improved or better versus 42% of the placebo group. At that point, 50% of the alprazolam group versus 28% of placebo subjects were free of panic attacks. For those subjects who completed the trial, there was no significant difference in total number of panic attacks or in disability ratings between alprazolam or placebo, although the former were much less fearful and avoidant than the latter.

As noted previously, in the Cross-National Collaborative Panic Study, Phase 2, which compared imipramine and alprazolam with placebo, there was a significant placebo effect, particularly for frequency of panic attacks. However, there was also a high placebo drop-out rate: only 56% of the placebo patients completed the study, compared with 70% of the patients treated with imipramine and 83% of those treated with alprazolam. The high placebo drop-out rate makes it difficult to detect differences between the active medications and placebo. The placebo subjects who dropped out did so largely because they were not improving; the placebo patients who remained were presumably a bias sample.

Schweizer and colleagues randomized 106 patients with panic disorder into an acute 8-week treatment phase followed by 6 months of maintenance treatment. Significantly more patients treated with alprazolam than with imipramine or placebo remained in therapy and experienced panic attack and phobia relief during the acute treatment phase. Of note, 11% of the panic patients, 41% of the imipramine patients and 57% of the placebo patients dropped out. During the maintenance phase, neither tolerance nor daily dose increase of alprazolam was observed, and the patients maintained their treatment gains. The weight of evidence suggests that alprazolam is an effective antipanic and antiphobic agent, at least as long as it is being used.

Benzodiazepines are probably equally effective at comparable doses. For example, diazepam is roughly one-tenth as effective as alprazolam; if given at doses of 20–60 mg, it appears to be as effective as alprazolam. However, at those doses, diazepam causes relatively more sedation than alprazolam, and this side-effect may limit its usefulness. Clonazepam has also been shown to be effective. It is as potent as alprazolam and has the advantage of a longer half-life. At the end of one trial, 50%, 46% and 14% of subjects on clonazepam, alprazolam and placebo, respectively, were free of panic attacks. The mean dose of clonazepam was 2.5 mg (maximum dose was 6 mg). Lorazepam (mean daily dose of 7 mg) was as effective as alprazolam in one study.

The choice of a benzodiazepine, then, depends on potency, half-life and evidence of effectiveness from clinical studies. Although effective, alprazolam has the disadvantage of a short half-life. Thus, frequent dosing may be necessary; some patients complain of breakthrough anxiety, either in the morning or between doses. A sustained release pill is now being evaluated that may reduce this problem.

Alprazolam should be initiated at 0.25–0.5 mg t.i.d. Doses should be increased every 4–6 days as needed and tolerated. Clonazepam should be initiated at 0.5 tablet per day, and then increased every 3–5 days to therapeutic goals. Some investigators recommend that the medication should be increased until the patient is symptom free. However, one study found no relationship between dose and outcome. In a study of alprazolam, 13 out of 14 patients with a serum level of 15–77 ng/mL, achieved with doses of 1–6 mg/day, reached zero panic attacks at the end of the study. A study of alprazolam at 2 or 6 mg compared with placebo found only a few statistically significant differences between the two groups, and both were better than placebo. Furthermore, higher doses require longer withdrawal.

Benzodiazepines should also be used cautiously in elderly patients. Elderly people have altered pharmacokinetics and pharmacodynamics, concomitant illness, reduced compliance and increased sensitivity to drugs. Older patients may be more sensitive to dependence, rebound and memory impairment. They are more likely to exhibit increased sedation, an increased tendency toward falls, psychomotor dyscoordination and decreased concentration. Among the drugs with a short half-life, high-potency compounds (e.g. lorazepam, alprazolam) may be more toxic than low-potency compounds (e.g. oxazepam) in elderly patients.

Benzodiazepines have a number of disadvantages over antidepressants. They often produce sedation, increase the effects of alcohol, can produce dyscoordination, and are associated with dependence and withdrawal. Benzodiazepine withdrawal occurs even after only 4–8 weeks of use. Moreover, studies suggest that withdrawal-like phenomena can be precipitated by benzodiazepine receptor antagonists after as little as 1 day of benzodiazepine administration.

If benzodiazepines have been used for a few weeks or more, then a careful plan of discontinuation is needed. Patients can have severe panic attacks during the rebound. With a rapid dosage taper, rebound occurred in 35% of patients in the Cross-National Trial. Withdrawal syndrome can be sufficiently severe to cause epileptic seizures, confusion and psychotic symptoms. For most patients, withdrawal symptoms are more diffuse, including anxiety, panic, tremor, muscle twitching, perceptual disturbances and depersonalization. Possibly because of these side-effects, many patients are reluctant to stop the benzodiazepines. Rickels attempted to withdraw 27 patients who had been on alprazolam for 6 months or longer. Of these, only 17 were withdrawn. One year later, eight of nine patients who were not able to withdraw were still taking medication, and eight of 17 of those who had stopped had resumed taking medication.

Benzodiazepines should be withdrawn gradually, perhaps over 4 months. With a slow, flexible taper, it has been found no rebound and only 7% of patients had clinically significant withdrawal symptoms. Benzodiazepine doses should be reduced more slowly at the end of the taper. In withdrawing patients from alprazolam, it may be easier to switch patients to clonazepam, because clonazepam can be given in fewer doses.

Thus, it is our opinion that clonazepam may be easier and safer to employ than alprazolam, with similar or superior effectiveness.

Upon discontinuation of benzodiazepines, some patients seem to have a rebound of anxiety, which is a different phenomenon than withdrawal. Withdrawal represents the return of neurochemical systems to baseline levels and may include new symptoms, such as seizures. Rebound is usually defined as an occurrence of a previously existing symptom at a greater than pretreatment level during the discontinuation period. Withdrawal is often associated with weakness and insomnia, two symptoms that are not present in most non-depressed anxious patients. Previous discontinuous exposure to benzodiazepines might sensitize patients to subsequent withdrawal effects. Withdrawal symptoms are usually less severe than the initial anxiety symptoms. They are usually significantly reduced by the end of the first week of withdrawal and are mostly gone by the end of the second postdiscontinuation week. Thus, symptoms that persist 3 weeks after patients have been off medication usually represent either a return of the original anxiety or the continuation of anxiety that has not been adequately treated.

Previous drug or alcohol abuse is a risk factor for dependence and increased use of benzodiazepines. Such a history is not an absolute contraindication to their use, but benzodiazepines should be used with particular caution in this population. When considering benzodiazepine use with chronically anxious patients, the patient's diagnosis should be documented, his or her status and medication carefully monitored and documented and other forms of therapy applied concurrently.

Other medications

Buspirone is believed to exert its antianxiety effect by blocking serotonin 1A (5-HT_{1A}) presynaptic and postsynaptic receptors. Buspirone is a full antagonist at presynaptic 5-HT_{1A} receptors but only a partial antagonist at postsynaptic 5-HT_{1A} receptors. It causes downregulation of 5-HT_2 receptors.

Buspirone lacks the benzodiazepines' sedative, muscle relaxant or anticonvulsant actions and has no ability to affect benzodiazepine withdrawal symptoms.

Buspirone lacks abuse potential as judged by relevant animal and human studies. In humans, it also neither impairs psychomotor performance nor potentiates the performance-impairing effects of alcohol. Benzodiazepines tend to impair performance in the above paradigms; buspirone not only does not impair performance but also improves the subject's awareness of any alcohol-induced decrements in performance.

Buspirone has been shown to have efficacy in GAD and has been generally available for use in that condition in the USA since 1986. The majority of the studies have shown buspirone to be equal in efficacy to standard benzodiazepines in GAD or in less clearly specified chronic anxiety states. Buspirone often fails to show efficacy in small, short-term trials, especially those with a crossover feature, probably because patients with substantial past experience with benzodiazepines tend to respond less well to buspirone. However, it is very difficult to say that previous benzodiazepine exposure eliminates all response to buspirone. However, if a study (or an individual clinician) takes patients who have been on a short-acting benzodiazepine for months or years and transfers them 'cold turkey' to buspirone, the benzodiazepine withdrawal symptoms may well be very unpleasant, even dangerous, and buspirone will have little or no effect on the patients' extended distress.

Otherwise, buspirone seems in most ways to be the ideal antianxiety drug; it lacks the benzodiazepines' sedation, ataxia, tolerance, and withdrawal symptoms; abuse liability; and propensity to interfere with complex psychomotor tasks on driving simulators and related tests. In addition, benzodiazepines are linked by association to driving accidents and to falls and injuries in the elderly. Buspirone does not impair performance; furthermore, it leaves the subject more aware of impairment resulting from alcohol ingestion than do the benzodiazepines. Buspirone lacks the ability of benzodiazepines to depress respiration, making it potentially the preferred drug in anxious pulmonary patients.

Buspirone has few side-effects, both absolutely and versus placebo. The rates reported are 12% for dizziness, 6% for headache, 8% for nausea, 5% for nervousness, 3% for lightheadedness, and 2% for agitation. It is probable that tolerance develops to these side-effects. They may be handled by dosage reduction. If the dose is increased slowly, side-effects may be minimized.

Buspirone dosage should be started at 5 mg t.i.d. for 1 week and then increased by 5 mg every 24 days as tolerated until the patient is receiving 10 mg p.o. t.i.d. The patient should be encouraged to stay at that dose for at least 6 weeks before deciding that the drug is ineffective. It has been customary to give the drug three times per day because of its short half-life, but it is not known whether giving all or two-thirds of the dose at bedtime might work as well with better patient acceptance.

Most reviews of buspirone point out that it is not widely used by psychiatrists because it works so slowly and because it is of no value in patients who have been on benzodiazepines. It is certainly worth trying in some patients who have been on benzodiazepines. Buspirone is not effective in ameliorating benzodiazepine withdrawal symptoms if it is begun as the benzodiazepine is being stopped; however, in one study that started buspirone (or placebo) 2 weeks before beginning to terminate benzodiazepine use, buspirone was found to be superior to placebo in reducing symptoms. Many clinicians suggest that the best way to shift from a benzodiazepine to buspirone is to stabilize the patient on both agents for several weeks before tapering off the benzodiazepine.

Buspirone also is likely to be more effective in relieving coexisting depressive symptoms than are the benzodiazepines, except perhaps for alprazolam. At doses in the range of 30–90 mg/day, buspirone is effective in major depressive disorder and even in such patients who qualify as melancholic. There is even one case of a patient's becoming manic on buspirone, a sign that it may really be an antidepressant.

Buspirone was found to be helpful in some anxious intravenous drug-abusing persons on methadone maintenance who had developed AIDS or AIDS-related complex (ARC). In this sample, there was no evidence of abuse of buspirone and some evidence that abuse of other drugs decreased. Buspirone was generally well tolerated and facilitated the tapering or discontinuation of benzodiazepines in most patients on benzodiazepines at the start of the study. The patients, as a group, were dubious both about trying buspirone and about decreasing benzodiazepine use, so the positive effects of buspirone occurred in spite of this resistance. Unfortunately, the positive effects of buspirone faded after a few months in one-third of the patients.

Buspirone is effective in GAD and almost certainly in major depression. It seems likely that this drug may have efficacy in social phobia and in anxiety disorders accompanying various chronic medical disorders. Since buspirone's side-effects are mainly mildly bothersome and its drug–drug interactions are benign, and since it is relatively safe in overdose and free from abuse liability and performance impairment, it should be a major addition to the armamentarium of dermatologists.

The benzodiazepines do work, and tolerance to their antianxiety effects does not develop for weeks or months; however, in patients with chronic anxiety it can prove difficult to test the patient's need for longer benzodiazepine therapy because withdrawal symptoms are likely to resemble or reactivate the symptoms of the patient's original condition. Buspirone could be tapered and stopped periodically without the complication of anxiety-like withdrawal symptoms.

Antipsychotics

Conventional antipsychotics have been the mainstay of therapy in the acute psychotic or delusional patient. While they are effective in relieving acute positive symptoms, their efficacy in treating negative, depressive, and cognitive symptoms is very limited, or non-existent, and they are associated with a high prevalence of side-effects. Expert Consensus Guidelines now strongly recommend the newest atypical antipsychotics as the first line of treatment for schizophrenia in most clinical situations and for delusional symptoms. These drugs have been shown to be as effective as the typical antipsychotic haloperidol in improving overall psychopathology and superior in treating negative symptoms. Additionally, the atypical antipsychotics have a much better safety profile, particularly with respect to extrapyramidal symptoms (EPS).

Both risperidone and olanzapine are examples of novel therapeutic approaches for the treatment of psychosis and delusional subjects; however, they are distinguished on the basis of quite different pharmacological profiles.

Risperidone is principally a dopamine 2 (D2) and 5-HT_2 receptor antagonist. According to the US label, risperidone has a maximal effect generally seen in the dose range of 4–6 mg/day; however, in the clinical trials conducted a maximal effect in the range of 4–8 mg/day was found. At the lower end of the risperidone dose range, the incidence of EPS is similar to that seen with placebo. However, with increased doses, the extrapyramidal profile of risperidone appears more like that of haloperidol. Risperidone is indicated for patients who have a history of developing EPS on current agents, even thioridazine, the typical antipsychotic that causes the least EPS. No long-acting or parenteral form is currently available.

Olanzapine is a novel antipsychotic agent of the thienobenzodiazepine class. In addition to potent 5-HT_2, 5-HT_3 and 5-HT_6 receptor antagonism, olanzapine further exhibits affinity for dopamine D1 D2, D3 and D4 receptors and selective muscarinic binding sites. This novel pharmacological profile may explain the broad spectrum of efficacy reported with olanzapine and the low incidence of EPS and hyperprolactinaemia.

Both agents exhibit similar baseline-to-endpoint improvement according to the Positive and Negative Syndrome Scale (PANSS). Acute 8-week responders (defined as at least a 20% improvement in PANSS total score and Clinical Global Impressions-Severity of Illness scale score ≥ 3 at the end of 8 weeks) were subsequently followed on a continued double-blind basis for a total treatment duration of 28 weeks. The olanzapine-treated patients demonstrated a statistically significantly lower probability for a clinical relapse than their risperidone-treated counterparts (olanzapine, 12.1%; risperidone, 32.3%). Other differences between the two treatment groups included a significantly lower incidence of EPS (as measured by objective rating scales) and hyperprolactinaemia, and significantly superior symptomatic improvement in negative symptoms (as measured by the Scale for the Assessment of Negative Symptoms) and mood features in the olanzapine-treated group. The mean doses used for olanzapine and risperidone were 17.2 mg/day and 7.2 mg/day, respectively.

Among the atypicals, olanzapine has all of the above-mentioned attributes; in addition, olanzapine has been shown to be superior to haloperidol on other efficacy measures such as improvement of depressive and cognitive symptoms in psychotic patients, enhanced quality of life, and prevention of relapse. Olanzapine has a superior safety profile compared with haloperidol with respect to tardive dyskinesia and hyperprolactinaemia.

The dermatology patient with delusion is often seen when he/she is in an acute phase: he/she is often characterized by agitation and/or hostility and an increase in positive symptoms including delusions, hallucinations, thought disorders and changing mood. The goal of therapy is a rapid reduction in the agitation and auto- and/or etero-aggression that are often seen in acute-phase patients. The acute phase is also a critical juncture at which to begin a definitive therapeutic strategy that can allow a seamless progression from acute to long-term treatment.

In this case we tend to employ risperidone or olanzapine with increasing dosages, starting from 0.5 and 5 mg/day, respectively: the increases happen every 3–5 days to the standard dosage of 4–6 mg/day for risperidone and 20 mg/day for olanzapine.

Conclusion

In order to treat a dermatosis effectively, an accurate dermatological/psychological/psychiatric diagnosis is indispensable. In fact, if psychoactive drugs are to be used effectively, there should be both a psychological/psychiatric diagnosis as well as a dermatological diagnosis. We note that psychotropic drugs are more effective when given concurrently with psychotherapy (ranging from counselling to behavioural psychotherapies or to interventions of psychoanalytical type). Thus, we emphasize the relevance of a well-conducted doctor–patient relationship, especially with those patients who are hyperemotional and anxious and who have a tendency to somatize.

In cases of mild anxiety, we suggest administering psychoactive drugs, in particular SSRIs or benzodiazepines (such as clonazepam or diazepam), bupropion or buspirone, whereas the prescription of sedative antihistamines such as hydroxyzine should to be avoided as much as possible. These drugs achieve good results in dermatology patients with marked traits of emotional lability.

Delusional psychosis requires psychoactive drugs, such as olanzapine or risperidone, while in the obsessive–compulsive disorders, which in the past were treated with TCAs (i.e. clomipramine), we tend to prescribe serotoninergic antidepressants (citalopram, sertraline, fluoxetine, fluvoxamine, paroxetine), with a dosage higher than those commonly employed to treat depression.

During the consultation the dermatologist must discover if the patient presents with any psychological problem related or not with his skin disease:

1 if there is no clinically evident psychological conflict/trouble, the dermatologist must address directly the cutaneous problems.

2 indications of possible psychological problems or involvement necessitate various steps:

(a) The type and entity of the psychological problems must be evaluated: specifically the severity and whether or not there is a psychosis or an obsessive–compulsive disorder. In the latter cases, it is often necessary to consult with psychiatrists.

(b) Well-conducted counselling is the first step in psychotherapy.

(c) Appropriate specific medications and, if necessary, psychoactive drugs. The choice is usually between four main classes of psychoactive agents: (i) benzodiazepines; (ii) bupropion; (iii) buspirone; and (iv) SSRIs. The choice of drug depends on the signs, symptoms, age and general condition of the subject.

3 Most patients should be re-examined after some weeks of therapy:

(a) If the patient is well, and shows total or partial resolution of cutaneous and psychological signs and symptoms, gradual withdrawal of the drugs can be considered.

(b) If the symptoms are not changed or have worsened further evaluation is necessary, possibly in liaison with a psychologist/psychiatrist.

These are the routine steps that we have developed over years of practice. We strongly recommend that the dermatologist limits the prescription of psychoactive drugs to benzodiazepines, SSRIs, buspirone or bupropion. Consultation with a psychiatrist is necessary with regard to medications with which the dermatologist has no direct experience (atypical neuroleptics, TCAs, anticonvulsants, β-blockers, and so on).

Further reading

Breier A. A new era in the pharmacotherapy of psychotic disorders. *J Clin Psych* 2001; 62 (suppl. 2): 3–5.

Dubin WR. Rapid tranquillization: antipsychotics or benzodiazepines? *J Clin Psych* 1988; 49 (suppl. 12): 5–13.

George MS, Lydiard RB. Social phobia secondary to physical disability: a review of benign essential tremor (BET) and stuttering. *Psychosomatics* 1994; 35: 520–3.

Greist J, Chouinard G, Duboff E. A one-year double-blind, placebo controlled, fixed dose study of sertraline in the treatment of obsessive compulsive disorder. *Int Clin Psychopharmacol* 1995; 10: 57–65.

Gupta MA, Gupta AK, Ellis CN. Antidepressant drugs in dermatology. *Arch Dermatol* 1987; 113: 647–52.

Jermain DM, Crisinon ML. Pharmacotherapy of obsessive–compulsive disorder. *Pharmacotherapy* 1990; 10: 175–98.

Kaplan HI, Sadock BI. *Pocket Handbook of Psychiatric Drug Treatment*. Baltimore: Williams and Wilkins, 1996: 1–247.

Koo I, Gambla C. Psychopharmacology for dermatologic patients. *Dermatol Clin* 1996; 14: 509–23.

Koo JYM, Lee J. Psychopharmacologic approaches to the difficult patient. *Curr Opinion Dermatol* 1995; 83–6.

Kraaimaat FW, Janssen P, van Dam-Baggen R. Social anxiety and stuttering. *Percept Mot Skills* 1991; 3: 1.

Meltzer HY. New drugs for the treatment of schizophrenia. *Psychiatr Clin N Am* 1993; 16: 365–85.

Panconesi E. *Stress and Skin Diseases*. Philadelphia: Lippincott, 1984: 1–273.

Panconesi E, ed. *Manuale di Dermatologia*. Torino: Utet, 1992.

Schatzberg A, Nemeroff C. *Textbook of Psychopharmacology*. American Psychiatric Press, 1995.

Stein MB, Baird A, Walker JR. Social phobia in adults with stuttering (see comments). *Am J Psych* 1996; 153: 278–80.

Uhlenhuth EH, DeWit H, Balter MB, Ichanson CE, Mellinger GD. Risks and benefits of longterm benzodiazepine use. *J Clin Psychopharmacol* 1988; 8: 161–7.

Retinoids

J.H. Saurat

Definition

The term retinoids designates compounds that are derivatives of natural vitamin A, as well as synthetic analogues that exert similar pharmacological effects.

General principles, classification and structure (Table 1)

Natural versus synthetic

- Natural retinoids are those that originate from the diet (retinol retinaldehyde and retinyl-esters) and are transformed in the body into active molecules such as retinoic acid and its isomers. These compounds can also be used for therapeutic purposes.
- Synthetic retinoids are analogues that have been synthesized for specific therapeutic purposes, with the aim of minimizing unwanted effects and optimizing efficacy. This growing group includes etretinate, acitretin, adapalene and tazarotene, to list those that are already accessible for dermatological use.

Topical versus systemic

- Retinoids can be given orally for the treatment of skin diseases that cover large surface areas and/or are not responsive to topical retinoid treatment; three are currently available for oral use, 13-*cis* retinoic acid (isotretinoin) for the treatment of severe forms of acne, acitretin and etretinate (which is the prodrug of the former) for treating psoriasis and hereditary disorders of keratinization.
- Topical retinoids currently available include retinol, retinaldehyde, retinoic acid, 13-*cis* retinoic acid, adapalene and tazarotene. Therefore only 13-*cis* retinoic acid is used, so far, both orally and topically in dermatology (Table 1).

Mechanisms of action

Retinoids play a fundamental role in embryogenesis, reproduction, vision, and control of cell growth and differentiation of many adult tissues. The two latter activities are related to their therapeutic use in dermatology, especially in psoriasis, hereditary disorders of keratinization, topical treatment of acne, and skin ageing.

Table 1 Retinoids used in dermatology

	Type	Route	Indication
Retinyl-esters	Natural	O/T	Neutriceutic
Retinol	Natural	T	Photoageing
Retinaldehyde	Natural	T	Photoageing/mild acne
Retinoic acid (*all trans*) (tretinoin)	Natural	T	Photoageing/mild acne*
13-*cis* retinoic acid (isotretinoin)	Natural	T	Photoageing/mild acne
13-*cis* retinoic acid (isotretinoin)	Natural	O	Severe acne
9-*cis* retinoic acid (alitretinoin)	Natural	T	Kaposi sarcoma
Etretinate	Synthetic	O	Psoriasis/ichthyoses*
Acitretin	Synthetic	O	Psoriasis/ichthyoses*
Bexarotene	Synthetic	O	CTCL
Adapalene	Synthetic	T	Mild acne
Tazarotene	Synthetic	T	Mild psoriasis

O, oral; T, topical.
*For other uses see text.

Retinoid nuclear receptors

Most, if not all, the activities of retinoids occur through nuclear receptors that belong to the superfamily of steroid, thyroid hormones and vitamin D; two families of receptors are involved in the gene regulation induced by retinoids: the retinoic acid receptors (RARs), whose natural ligand is *all-trans* retinoic acid (RA) and the retinoid X receptor family (RXRs), whose ligand is 9-*cis* RA (RARs also bind 9-*cis* RA). These receptors are expressed in the skin, which includes epidermis, appendages such as sebaceous glands, and dermis. There is some selectivity such as predominant expression of RAR-α and -β isoforms as well as RXR-γ isoform. Although the therapeutic applicability of the selective isoform expression is not established so far, so-called receptor-specific synthetic retinoids are being developed that preferentially bind to either RAR-α, -β or -γ, or RXR isoforms. That these receptor-specific synthetic retinoids may mediate specific activities remains to be demonstrated.

The intracrine concept

The biologically active ligands are thought to be generated within the target cell, a process designated as an 'intracrine' system. It is likely that, when given for therapeutic purpose, precursors such as retinol and retinaldehyde, that do not bind to receptors, exert part if not all of their effects because they are transformed into retinoic acid within the target cell.

Sebosuppression

One of the most spectacular pharmacological actions of retinoids is the suppression of sebum production. This effect is very specific for oral 13-*cis* retinoic acid, whereas topical 13-*cis* retinoic acid does not suppress sebum production. It is still intriguing why only oral 13-*cis* retinoic acid has sebosuppressive effects. The 'sebospecificity' of oral 13-*cis* retinoic acid cannot be explained so far on the basis of the molecular biology of retinoid nuclear receptors, since it has no special affinity to any identified retinoid nuclear receptor. Attempts have been made to relate the sebosuppressive effect to a metabolite; 4-*oxo*-13-*cis* retinoic acid has been considered as a candidate and supporting evidence has recently been presented. It is likely that some pharmacokinetic properties of oral 13-*cis* retinoic acid should result in the specific targeting of sebaceous glands.

Indications

Topical retinoids

The two main indications are acne and photoageing.

- Topical retinoids are indicated in mild acne, usually in association with antibacterials, since they act only as comedolytic agents without neither sebosuppressive nor anti *Propionibacterium acnes* activity. Compliance to retinoic acid is often poor due to irritancy, which has stimulated the search for less irritating analogues (see below).
- Photoageing. Many studies attest to the efficacy of topical retinoids in improving the clinical, histological and molecular features of photoageing.

Topical retinoids are also currently used in a wide spectrum of skin conditions such as actinic keratoses for which clinical trials have confirmed their beneficial effects; the association with 5-fluorouracil is possible and results in synergism. Epidermal melasma partially responds to topical retinoids alone and association with hydroquinone is preferred. Other uses include a wide variety of hyperkeratotic conditions, rosacea and reversal of topical steroid-induced atrophy.

Retinol

This is usually available in Europe at the concentration of 0.075% for the treatment of skin ageing. So far no controlled studies have compared its activity, which appears as inferior to that of retinoic acid. It is likely that much higher concentrations would have a better activity profile.

Retinaldehyde
This is available in the concentration of 0.05% for the treatment of photoageing. Controlled double-blind studies against placebo and retinoic acid have shown efficacy similar to that of retinoic acid. Other uses include adjuvant therapy of mild acne (one controlled study comparing retinaldehyde to retinoic acid; due to its aldehyde group, retinaldehyde has a significant antibacterial activity that encompasses *P. acnes*), rosacea, prevention of topical steroid-induced atrophy and seborrhoeic dermatitis.

Retinoic acid
This is available in the concentration of 0.025, 0.05, and 0.1% for the treatment of acne and photoageing (0.05%). Other uses include a large number of skin conditions listed previously.

13-cis retinoic acid
This is available in the concentration of 0.05% for the treatment acne. Controlled studies have shown efficacy similar to that of retinoic acid with less irritation. Isomerization of 13-*cis* retinoic acid into retinoic acid and vice versa occurs upon the skin, which renders the distinction between the two compounds rather difficult.

It is a synthetic analogue of retinoic acid belonging to a new family of naphthoic acid derivatives that possess high stability towards light and oxygen. It has a specific binding profile to RAR-β and -γ. It is available at the concentration of 0.1% in a gel formulation. It shows activity similar to that of retinoic acid 0.025% in mild acne and is less irritating.

Tazarotene
This is a synthetic analogue of retinoic acid belonging to the new family of acetylenic retinoids. It has a specific binding profile to RAR-β and -γ. It is (or soon will be) available at the concentration of 0.05% in a gel formulation for the treatment of mild psoriasis.

Oral retinoids

13-cis retinoic acid

Acne
Since its introduction 15 years ago, oral 13-*cis* retinoic acid (isotretinoin, Roaccutane, Accutane), is still the only compound that really works and cures acne because it is the only one that affects, albeit not to the same degree, all implicated aetiological factors: sebum production comedogenesis and colonization with *P. acnes*. An important concept is to let patients know that 13-*cis* RA is actually a natural compound rather than a drug. It circulates in the blood after a meal rich in vitamin A.

In the early 1980s isotretinoin use was restricted to patients suffering from severe nodulocystic acne. The broad experience with this drug has suggested that guidelines for its use should be updated. Its use has been extended to patients with less severe disease who, because of increased resistance of *P. acnes* to many antibiotics, in particular erythromycin and tetracycline respond unsatisfactorily to conventional therapies such as long-term antibiotics. Patients with moderate acne that may induce scars have also been treated.

It was initially considered that optimal benefit would be achieved with a high daily dose, about 1 mg/kg body weight per day. In our experience this induces unnecessary undesirable effects and similar short-term therapeutic results are obtained with dose ranging below 0.5 mg/kg body weight per day. The approach implies that the treatment is maintained over a longer period of time in order to reach the threshold of the cumulative dose. We introduced this concept in 1989: the cumulative dose (milligrams per kilogram of body weight) is the total amount of oral isotretinoin taken by the patient over the entire duration of therapy divided by body weight. Thus a patient weighing 50 kg and receiving 25 mg/day of isotretinoin for 100 days would have received a cumulative dose of 25 mg × 100 days = 2500 divided by 50 kg = 50 mg/kg. Data from several centres indicate that post-therapy relapse is minimized by a treatment course amounting to a total of at least 120 mg/kg with no further therapeutic gain beyond about 150 mg/kg

Other uses of oral 13-cis retinoic acid

It can be used for rosacea; a low daily dose (10 mg) is often sufficient; in our opinion, the best indications are those patients with rosacea and significant seborrhoea. Dissecting cellulitis of the scalp, confluent and reticulated papillomatosis, generalized granuloma annulare as well as O'Brien's actinic granuloma are other potential indications. Some dermatologists continue to use isotretinoin in female patients with psoriasis who need systemic retinoids in order to avoid the long post-acitretin contraception period. Human immunodeficiency virus (HIV)-associated eosinophilic folliculitis responds to oral 13-*cis* retinoic acid in some patients; interestingly, the drug is well tolerated and useful in HIV patients with severe acne.

Acitretin and etretinate

These two drugs have the same profile of activity as etretinate and can be considered as the prodrug of acitretin.

Psoriasis

The efficacy of etretinate and acitretin was shown in various types of psoriasis. The best results are obtained in palmoplantar or generalized type pustular psoriasis in which etretinate and acitretin are considered to be the treatments of first choice. Erythrodermic psoriasis is another severe form in which beneficial effects are achieved in the majority of patients. Acitretin is the drug of choice in patients infected with HIV whose psoriasis flares.

Plaque-type psoriasis responds irregularly to both drugs. Complete clearing is reached in around 30% of patients, a significant improvement is obtained in a further 50% of treated patients. The maximal response is, in general, not reached before 3 months with retinoids used as single treatment agents.

Complete remission usually requires an additional treatment: topical corticosteroids, anthralin (dithranol), UVA photochemotherapy (PUVA) or UVB phototherapy or topical calcipotriol.

Keratinization disorders

Among the different types of ichthyoses, the best results can be obtained in non-bullous congenital ichthyosis such as erythrodermic and non-erythrodermic lamellar ichthyosis; so far no differences have been reported in the response of patients with or without transglutaminase gene mutation. Treatment of bullous ichthyosiform erythroderma is more difficult because an overdose with the retinoid may result in a worsening of the skin condition with increased blister formation. Good results have also been shown in recessive X-linked ichthyosis. However, in the majority of patients with recessive X-linked ichthyosis or with autosomal dominant ichthyosis, the skin lesions are mild and do not require systemic treatment.

Severe forms of Darier's disease are good indications and care should be taken to initiate therapy with very low doses such as 10 mg/day of acitretin in order to prevent initial exacerbation of the disease; usually 20 mg/day are sufficient for significant improvement.

Premalignant skin lesions

Etretinate and acitretin were also shown to be effective in the treatment of premalig-

Table 2 Types of side-effects observed with oral retinoids

Type I: undesirable pharmacological effect (same mechanism of action as therapeutic effect)
Predictable
Constant in all patients
Early occurrence (few days)
Intensity is function of daily dose
Rapidly reversible after discontinuation (with no sequelae)
Organs or systems involved
skin (dryness, peeling, pruritus)
hair and nails (alopecia, nail fragility)
mucous membranes (cheilitis, dry mouth, dry nose, blepharoconjunctivitis)
Type II: toxic effect (involving organ or systems in which no therapeutic effects are expected)
Unpredictable
Rare: individual susceptibility (idiosyncratic)
Late occurrence (few weeks or months)
Intensity is function of cumulative dose
Slowly reversible after discontinuation (with possible sequelae)
Organs or systems involved
liver (increased liver enzymes, toxic hepatitis)
bones (pain, hyperostoses)
muscles and ligaments (pain, calcifications)
central nervous system (headache, intracranial hypertension)
vision (decreased night vision)
lipid metabolism (increased triglycerides and cholesterol, very low-density and low-density lipoproteins)

nant skin lesions including human papillomavirus-induced tumours and actinic keratoses. In the basal cell naevus syndrome and in xeroderma pigmentosum these drugs are able to reduce dramatically the incidence of malignant degeneration of the skin lesions. Recently a double-blind study has demonstrated that acitretin 30 mg/day for 6 months prevented the development of premalignant and malignant skin lesions in renal transplant recipients.

Cutaneous T-cell lymphomas

Etretinate treatment may induce clinical improvement in cutaneous T-cell lymphomas (e.g. mycosis fungoides or Sezary syndrome) with no internal organ involvement; better results were obtained when etretinate was combined with PUVA treatment or interferon-α.

Side-effects, contraindications and drug interactions

Teratogenic risk

Women of child-bearing age must have a negative pregnancy test before as well as practice effective contraception during therapy with oral retinoids. Contraception should be continued for 1 month after completing therapy with oral 13-*cis* retinoic acid and much longer after acitretin, up to 3 years is mandatory in the USA. Teratogenic risk has not been established for topical retinoids; nevertheless, their use during pregnancy is not recommended.

Mucocutaneous side-effects

These are all doses related for a single compound and show great interindividual variability. Undesirable effects on the skin and mucous membranes are almost always observed during oral treatment with etretinate or acitretin or 13-*cis* retinoic acid under a threshold daily dose that varies from patient to patient (Table 2).

Topical retinoids induce burning, erythema and peeling illustrating the irritant properties of these compounds; irritancy is not strictly related to efficacy, which leaves open many claims for manufacturers. Long-term safety of topical retinoids has been established, and enhanced photocarcinogenicity reported in mice does not appear to occur in humans.

Other side-effects

The implications, in terms of drug interactions, are that oral retinoids should not be given to patients receiving hepatotoxic drugs.

Regimen

Topical retinoids

These are used once a day, usually at bedtime (in order to prevent photodegradation). Irritation occurs mainly at the initiation of treatment and can be minimized by alternate day use.

Oral retinoids

The best way of using oral retinoids is to start with a low daily dose, about one-quarter of the recommended dose, and to progressively increase it in order to prevent mucocutaneous side-effects, the threshold of which is variable among patients. Specific details are provided above.

Further reading

Bollag W. Vitamin A and retinoids, from nutrition to pharmacotherapy in dermatology and oncology. *Lancet* 1983; i: 860–3.

Brogden RN, Goa KL. Adapalene. A review of its pharmacological properties and clinical potential in the management of mild to moderate acne. *Drugs* 1997; 53: 511–19.

Chambon P. The retinoid signaling pathway: Molecular and genetic analysis. *Semin Cell Biol* 1994; 5: 115–25.

Craven NM, Griffiths CEM. Topical retinoids and cutaneous biology. *Clin Exp Dermatol* 1996; 21: 1–10.

Cunliffe WJ, van de Kerkhof PCM *et al.* Roaccutane treatment guidelines: Results of an international survey. *Dermatology* 1997; 194: 351–7.

Geiger JM, Saurat JH. Acitretin and etretinate. *Dermatol Clin* 1993; 11: 117–29.

Kang S, Duell EA *et al.* Application of retinol to human skin in vivo induces epidermal hyperplasia and cellular retinoid binding proteins characteristic of retinoic acid but without measurable retinoic acid levels or irritation. *J Invest Dermatol* 1995; 105: 549–56.

Saurat JH. Side effects of systemic retinoids and their clinical management. *J Am Acad Dermatol* 1993; 27: S23–S28.

Saurat JH. Oral isotretinoin. Where now, where next? *Dermatology* 1997; 195 (Suppl. 1): 1–3.

Saurat JH. Systemic retinoids: what's new? *Dermatol Clin* 1998; 16: 331–40.

Saurat JH, Didierjean L *et al.* Topical retinaldehyde on human skin: Biologic effects and tolerance. *J Invest Dermatol* 1994; 103: 770–4.

Weinstein GD, Krueger GG *et al.* Tazarotene gel, a new retinoid, for topical therapy of psoriasis: Vehicle-controlled study of safety, efficacy, and duration of therapeutic effect. *J Am Acad Dermatol* 1997; 37: 85–92.

Scabicides and pediculicides

A. Górkiewicz-Petkow

Scabies and pediculosis are still very common, and often underestimated ectoparasite infections. Infestations may result not only from human mites or insects but also from domestic animals, grain and dust mites. In the presence of unexplained, often puzzling, pruritic papular eruption, the possibility of an ectoparasite infestation should always be considered. In new epidemiological situations—prolonged life, acquired immunodeficiency syndrome (AIDS) and other immunodeficiency syndromes, development of resistant strains—new challenging problems in therapy are raised. Therefore new considerations should be made about the schedules for treating individuals and endemics in schools, nursing homes, hospitals and underdeveloped communities. The frequency of use of different insecticides varies in different countries. Among well-known drugs there are often locally produced herbal preparations recommended for the treatment. The use of different medications is also influenced by economic circumstances. Effectiveness depends not only on the drug itself but also on their proper use according to the instructions and epidemiological approach to the treatment. In ectoparasite infections it is necessary to treat not only the patient but also the contacts and often the environment to prevent reinfection and spread of the disease.

An accurate and informative education programme is also very useful. The treatment of scabies and pediculosis is mainly external but there are reports of possible use of orally administered drugs (cotrimoxazole, ivermectin, thiabendazole). The most effective insecticides originate from plants (pyrethrins) or from pesticides used in agriculture and for household purposes (lindane, malathion, carbaryl) therefore therapy may have some potential toxicity.

Topical treatments

Pyrethrins and pyrethroids

The insecticide properties of flowers in the genus *Chrysanthemum* have been known for centuries and originate from ancient Persia. Pyrethrum is the name of dried flowers; pyrethrins are the active component of pyrethrum. First commercialized production started in Dalmatia in 1840; then by the year 1860 Dalmatian powder was widely used as a household insecticide. In 1948 the first synthetic pyrethroid (permethrin) was developed. Based on oral lethal dose (LD) values in rats permethrin is about 3 times less toxic than malathion, 15 times less than carbaryl and about 40 times less than lindane and DDT. In 1986 permethrin was introduced for the treatment of head lice, and soon after for scabies. Percutaneous absorption in human studies is less than 2%, permethrin is rapidly detoxified by esterase hydrolysis in blood and most body tissues including the skin. Plasma levels of permethrin following topical application of 5% cream formulation in human clinical trials were below detectable levels. In adverse reactions some irritation of the skin may occur at the time of treatment. Some concern has been expressed about possible allergic reactions, since some individuals are allergic to pyrethrum, but a sensitizing factor was removed from the final product. Permethrins have also been used for impregnation of beds, curtains and military clothes to prevent mosquito, ticks, and tse-tse fly bites.

Commercial preparations

- Lyclear dermal cream (5% permethrin) scabicide.
- Lyclear cream rinse (1% permethrin) pediculicide.
- Nix 1% permethrin, pediculicide.

Acetylocholinesterase inhibitors (malathion, carbaryl)

From 1954 acetylocholinesterase inhibitors have been used as pesticides in agriculture and for household purposes. In 1971 malathion and in 1977 carbaryl were introduced as pediculocides and scabicides following evidence of the emergence of the resistance of head lice to other drugs, mainly organochlorine insecticides. Malathion is rapidly broken down by hepatic enzymes in humans and warm-blooded animals, thus diminishing its cholinesterase inhibitory properties. In insects it is converted to the oxy analogue, which is an active metabolite. Human studies with inhalation of malathion aerosols, use of powder or dust on the skin, indicated no inhibition of cholinesterase activity. Possible poisoning manifestations include visual disturbances, respiratory difficulty and gastrointestinal hyperactivity. Malathion and carbaryl are also ovicides for head lice, although the ovicidal activity is not complete. Malathion is absorbed on to keratin within 6 h and confers residual, protective effect against reinfection for about 6 weeks. The effectiveness of carbaryl is determined by the components of the bases used in preparations. Both insecticides are degraded by heat. Generally the medications are well tolerated, safe and effective.

Commercial preparations

- Carylderm lotion—carbaryl 0.5% alcohol-based lotion, Carylderm shampoo, pediculicide.
- Derbac C—carbaryl 1% aqueous sol, Derbac C shampoo, pediculicide.
- Derbac M—malathion 0.5% aqueous solution pediculicide/scabicide.
- Prioderm—malathion 0.5% alcohol lotion, Prioderm shampoo, pediculicide.
- Malathion powder—disinfection of clothes.

Chlorinated insecticides

Gammahexachlorocyclohexane—lindane

This drug has been known since 1940 to be both a potent pesticide and an effective topical scabicide/pediculicide. Until recently the use of lindane was limited only by the potential side-effects which appear to have occurred almost entirely in children when it was not used properly or was accidentally ingested. Adverse effects are associated with central nervous system (CNS) effects (vertigo, seizures, convulsions) and the gastrointestinal tract (nausea, vomiting). Lindane binds to plasma proteins, epidermis, dermis and subcutaneous tissue and is readily dissolved in fat tissue. In animal studies (guinea pig) plasma and brain levels of lindane were significantly higher than permethrin. Lindane absorption through the skin was 10 times greater as compared with permethrin. Within the past decade there have been reports on drug resistance, concerning both scabies and pediculosis treatment. The following recommendations have been proposed to minimize the potential risk of lindane, mainly in the treatment of scabies: the drug should not be applied after a hot bath (enhancement of absorption), avoided or extreme caution used in the treatment of children under 4 years of age and pregnant women, time of skin exposure no longer than 8–12 h, use with caution in patients with epidermal barrier dysfunction and excoriations—use the lowest effective concentration; treatment should be reapplied only in proven reinfestation and no more than twice a month. Following all the instructions lindane will remain as a recommended treatment for scabies and head lice infestation.

Commercial preparations

- Quellada lotion—1% lindane (scabicide).
- Quellada shampoo—1% lindane (pediculicide).
- Scabicide (cream) Aphtiria (cream, powder), Jacutin (emulsion, gel, cream)—1% lindane (scabicide, pediculicide).

DDT (dichlorodiphenyl trichloroethane)

Widely used in the past for the treatment of head lice and as a powder for disinfection of clothes. It has no ovicidal properties, and resistance to the drug has been reported. It is possibly toxic if ingested orally (symptoms: tremors, muscular weakness, convulsions). DDT is not recommended presently for the treatment of head lice.

Other medications used for the treatment of scabies and pediculosis

Benzyl benzoate

Known for over 60 years for the treatment of scabies. In the past it was used as a compound of balsam of Peru, and from 1937 manufactured synthetically. General toxicity occurs only if ingested orally in large amounts (convulsions). Locally, benzyl benzoate may be an irritant to the skin or give allergic reactions. Because of low toxicity it is recommended in lower concentrations for children (exclusion of neonates [Gosping syndrome] and up to 4 months of age) and pregnant women.

Commercial preparations

- Ascabiol 10% solution. Benzyl benzoate for children. 25% benzyl benzoate solution for adults (mainly scabicide may be used as a pediculicide).

Sulphur

Sulphur remained in use from other old remedies for scabies (like hydrargyrum, creosote, resorcine, phormalinum, chrysarobinum, lactic acid). Sulphur is a compound of ointments and lotions used for the treatment of scabies known as unguentum (ung.) Wilkinson. It was used in different concentrations from 6% to 50%. It acts through keratolytic properties. Sulphur still remains as a recommended treatment of scabies in children and pregnant women but it is not pleasant and very messy in use. There are no toxicology or percutaneous absorption studies.

Commercial preparations

6% or 10% ointments in petrolatum or 25% ung. Wilkinson in zinc paste in equal dose.

Crotamitone (N-ethyl-O-crotonotoluidide)

Very little is known about the toxicology of crotamitone. There are no studies on percutaneous absorption. The drug has a lower efficacy in the treatment of scabies, but has been useful in the follow-up treatment of postscabietic pruritus or pruritus of other origin.

Commercial preparations

- Eurax—lotion or ointment (10% crotamitone).
- Euraxil—5% crotamitone gel (scabicide).

Monosulfiram

Introduced in 1940 for the treatment of scabies. Monosulfiram is chemically similar to disulfiram (Antabuse). A disulfiram-like reaction occurs with flushing, sweating, tachycardia if alcohol is ingested during or soon after treatment, or due to the alcoholic base of the solution. Monosulfiram is not an efficient scabicide, often needs several applications, and may cause prolonged inhibition of aldehyde dihydrogenase enzyme, which is needed for enzymatic breakdown of alcohol, thus making possible an accumulation of acetylaldehyde. Such a reaction is potentially serious in children. A single report was published on toxic epidermal necrolysis (TEN) induced by monosurfiram and local irritation of the skin are reported. Consequently the drug is not recommended for use as a scabicide, since other more efficient drugs are available.

Commercial preparations

- Tetmosol 25% solution, tetmosol soap (scabicide).

Copper II oleate-tetrahydronaphthalene

This mixture diluted in acetone and mineral oil is a pediculicide for head lice. It is very effective but readily combustible and an irritant so should not be applied to patients with eczema.

Commercial preparation

- Cuprex (head lice).

Oral treatment of scabies and pediculosis

Cotrimoxazole

The efficacy of oral cotrimoxazole in the eradication of head lice was discovered incidentally in 1978 while treating a child for an upper respiratory tract infection. This effect is probably related to ingestion of the antibiotic by feeding lice and its subsequent effect on their symbiotic bacteria present in a mid-gut organelle. These bacteria are essential for the synthesis of B vitamins without which the lice cannot survive.

Ivermectin

Ivermectin is an antiparasitic agent with a structure similar to the macrolide antibiotics, but without antibacterial activity. It is a synthetic derivative of abamectine. The drug has an endectocidal effect causing paralysis by suppressing the conduction of the nervous impulses in the interneuronic synapses of parasites. Ivermectin is widely used for the treatment of onchocerciasis. During 15 years of this treatment, there have been few side-effects described: macular eruption, headache, and asthenia. Ivermectin is also used worldwide to control infestation with sarcoptic mites in domestic animals. Since 1992 there have been reports of the general administration of this drug for uncomplicated scabies infestations in humans (Polynesia, India, Sierra-Leone, Mexico, USA), scabies in HIV-positive patients, crusted scabies, and endemics in the nursing homes. There have been single reports of possible death in elderly patients treated with ivermectin for scabies.

Commercial preparations

- Ivermectin (Stromectole)—not registered for the treatment of scabies in humans in all countries.

Further reading

Barkwell R, Shields S. Deaths associated with ivermectin treatment of scabies. *Lancet* 1997; 349: 1140–5.

Burns DA. Action of cotrimoxazole on head lice. *Br J Dermatol* 1987; 117: 399–400.

Burns DA. The treatment of human ectoparasite infection. *Br J Dermatol* 1991; 125: 89–93.

Dannaoui E, Kiazand A, Piens M, Picot S. Use of ivermectin for the management of scabies in a nursing home. *Eur J Dermatol* 1999; 9: 443–5.

Del Giudice P, Marty P. Ivermectin; a new therapeutic weapon in dermatology? *Arch Dermatol* 1999; 135: 705–6.

Elmogy M, Fayed H, Marzok H, Rashad A. Oral ivermectin in the treatment of scabies. *Int J Dermatol* 1999; 38: 926–8.

Friedman SJ. Lindane neurotoxic reaction in nonbullous congenital ichthyosiform erythroderma. *Arch Dermatol* 1987; 123: 1056–8.

Meinking TL, Taplin D. Safety of permethrin vs lindane for the treatment of scabies. *Arch Dermatol* 1996; 132: 959–62.

Meinking TL, Taplin D, Hermida JL, Pardo R, Kerdel FA. The treatment of scabies with ivermectin. *N Engl J Med* 1995; 333: 26–30.

Taplin D, Castillero PM, Spiegel J, Mercer S, Rivera AA, Schachner L. Malathion for treatment of pediculus humanus var capitis infestation. *JAMA* 1982; 247: 3103–5.

Taplin D, Meinking TL. Pyrethrins and pyrethroids in dermatology. *Arch Dermatol* 1990; 126: 213–21.

Taplin D, Meinking TL, Chen JA, Sanchez R. Comparison of crotamiton 10% cream (eurax) and permethrin 5% cream (elimite) for the treatment of scabies in children. *Pediatr Dermatol* 1990; 7: 67–73.

Skin tests

D. Kalogeromitros

Skin tests were the first diagnostic method for hypersensitivity type I reaction and were first introduced by Charles Blackley in 1865. Blackley placed pollen on the cubit, after cutting the skin. After a few minutes, that specific area presented with itching, whealing and erythema followed by delayed skin reaction. Mantoux introduced intradermal testing in 1908 which was later used for the diagnosis of hypersensitivity type I allergy by Schloss. A few years later Lewis and Grant described the skin prick test (SPT), which was used for many decades without many modifications. Recently, many new devices have been used for the standardizing of the conduction of skin tests (prick and puncture).

Skin tests help in the reconfirmation of the diagnosis of special allergy, concluded from the clinical information. Skin tests are convenient, easy to conduct, cheap and highly effective therefore they are widely used in the diagnosis of allergy. When skin tests are not conducted properly, they can give false positive or negative results. Their main limitations come from the fact that a positive reaction does not always mean that the symptoms are related to an immunoglobulin E (IgE)-mediated allergic reaction, as persons free of symptoms may have positive reactions.

Skin tests, apart from the diagnosis of an IgE-mediated allergy, are also useful in some epidemiological and pharmacological studies and the changes that occur in skin sensitivity can help us standardize allergens.

Skin tests, due to their high sensitivity, their low cost and the immediate results that they give are considered to be the most appropriate method for standardizing the responsible allergens in the atopic diseases.

Skin test methods

Two skin test methods are widely used. In the first method the antigen is placed on the skin and then it is inserted in the epidermis with a lancet (SPT). In the second method the antigen is injected intradermally (intradermal test, ID). Scratch test is no longer used because of the increased amount of false positive results.

Skin prick tests

SPTs were first described in 1924 by Lewis and Grant, but they were widespread in the 1970s after Pepys modification. The modified prick tests are done by placing a drop of each tested allergen extract and solution on the inside of the cubit or on the back. The drops are placed at a distance of 2 cm in order to avoid any false positive response. Then a small needle (25 or 26 gauge) comes through the drop and the epidermis, avoiding any bleeding. The needle comes off and the allergen is wiped off the skin with a paper towel after 1 min. It is recommended that a separate needle is used for each extract, so that the extracts do not become mixed up.

Intradermal tests

IDs were first described by Mantoux in 1908 and are still widely used in clinical practice, especially in the USA. In Europe they tend to be replaced by SPTs. ITs are performed with tuberculin syringes (Mantoux) with needles of 26 or 27 gauge. The test is done by injecting intradermally 0.01–0.05 mL of the allergen. The inserted solution must form a small wheal (2–3 mm diameter) which will remain for a few minutes. If no blister is formed or if the blister disappears right after the injection, it means that the injection was subcutaneous and we must repeat the test on another point. Though the injected amount affects the final reaction of the whealing and the erythema, the skin response depends more on the concentration of the allergen that is injected.

IDs can provoke undesired responses, significant topical (immediate or delayed) and systemic reactions. The frequency of systemic reactions is low, usually under 0.5% of controlled patients, but this number may increase when drugs or venoms are used.

Comparison of SPTs to IDs

The value of SPTs is limited when poor strength allergen extracts are used, because of the possibility of false negative results. The required concentration of allergen extract to achieve a positive reaction by ID is 1000–30 000 less than that required in an SPT. In contrast, when standardized and/or strong extracts are used, SPTs seem to surpass the IDs (Table 1). SPTs are less sensitive and repeatable but more specialized than IDs, and provocation of stimulating reactions is very rare, in contrast to IDs. They are also considered to be more associated with symptoms, though in patients with poor sensitivity only IDs may be positive.

Interpretation of skin tests

The result of the skin test must be estimated at the moment that the greatest reaction appears. In both methods, the greatest reaction to histamine appears in 8–10 min, to substances that degranulate mast cells in 10–15 min, and to allergens in 15–20 min.

The whealing and erythema have been used to estimate the positivity of the skin tests. Pepys using SPTs, indicated that when the skin test with the negative control is completely negative, a small blister (1–2 mm) followed by erythema and itching may suggest a positive immunological response, as well as the presence of special IgE antibodies. Though of immunological meaning, the small positive reactions do not necessarily suggest the presence of clinical allergy. By using the SPTs, the reactions that are considered to be suggestive of clinical allergy are usually those which produce whealing of more than 3 mm diameter (which equates to a whealing of 7 mm^2 surface) and an erythema of more than 10 mm diameter. Another positivity criterion that is used is the ratio of the size of the test that the allergen extract produces to the size of the one that the positive factor produces.

Many grading systems have been suggested concerning skin tests results. The most basic one is outlined in Table 2.

Number of skin tests and frequency

The allergens, as well as the number of skin tests chosen, differ from patient to patient. The selection is made according to:

- the patient's age (infants should not undergo many tests, as they usually respond to food allergens, dust, moulds, and rarely to pollens)
- the place that the patient lives, works and resorts
- the history of his/her allergic disease (perennial symptoms, specific eliciting factors).

Factors influencing skin tests

The body region on which the skin test is done, the age of the patient, the pathological cases, as well as the use of drugs can affect skin test results, by modifying whealing or erythema, making the interpretation of the results difficult.

Some clinical cases contraindicate skin tests (Table 3). When such a case exists, skin tests may give false results. Some factors have also been reported (Table 4) that can give false positive or false negative results. These factors should always be considered before the conduction of the test.

Conclusion

Skin tests, when conducted properly, represent one of the most basic methods for the diagnosis of IgE-mediated diseases.

Table 1 Comparison of skin prick tests to intradermal tests

	Skin prick tests	Intradermal tests
Convenience	+++	++
Speed	++++	++
Estimation of positive and negative reactions	++++	++
Intolerance	+	+++
False positive reactions	Rare	Possible
False negative reactions	Possible	Rare
Repeatability	+++	++++
Sensitivity	+++	++++
Speciality	++++	+++
Tracking of IgE antibodies	Yes	Yes
Security	++++	++
Infant control	Easy	Difficult

Table 2 Grading system of intradermal skin tests

Grade	Erythema	Whealing
0	< 5 mm	< 5 mm
+−	5–10 mm	5–10 mm
3+	11–20 mm	5–10 mm
2+	21–30 mm	5–10 mm
3+	31–40 mm	5–10 mm or with pseudopodes
4+	> 40 mm	> 15 mm or with many pseudopodia

Table 3 Contraindications to skin tests

Severe systemic diseases like pneumonia, decompensated cardiac insufficiency
Pregnancy (relative contraindication)
Thrombocytopenia (possibly for IDs)
Defects of coagulation, possibly for IDs (not during coumarin treatment)
Acute allergic symptoms (not with inhalation allergies)
Impetigo
Extensive cutaneous inflammation

They also contribute in the standardizing of the allergens and in the epidemiology of atopic diseases. SPTs are the ideal test for most cases, while IDs should be done only when indicated. Though the conduction of these tests seems very easy, it is necessary that they are performed by educated examiners, especially concerning the interpretation of the results. Examiners should recognize and eradicate any factors that could modify skin test results.

Table 4 Factors influencing reactions to skin prick tests and indradermal tests (positive and negative influences)

Quantity of allergens
Reactivity of mast cells
Reactivity of the target tissue
Depth of injection
Body region (↑ on the upper back)
Time of day (↑ in the evening)
Menstruation cycle (↑ prior to mensis)
Age (↑ during the third decade)
Associated diseases (↑ with dermographic urticaria, ↓ with ichthyosis and atopic eczema)
Immunotherapy (↓)
Refractory period after whealing reaction or anaphylaxis (↓)
H1-type antihistamines (↓)
Psychotropic drugs with H1-type antihistamine activity (↓)
Sympathomimetics (↓)

References

Bernstein IL, Storms WW. Practice parameters for the diagnosis and the treatment of asthma. The American Academy of Allergy, Asthma and Immunology and the American College of Allergy,

Asthma and Immunology. *Ann Allergy Asthma Immunol* 1995; 75: 543–625.

Blackley CH. *Hay Fever: its causes, treatment and effective prevention; experimental researches*. London: Bailliere Tindall & Cox, 1880.

Bousquet J, Michel FB. In vivo methods for study of allergy. Skin tests, techniques and interpretation. In: Middleton E, Reed CE, Ellis EF, Adkinson NF, Yunginger JW, Busse WW, eds. *Allergy: Principles and Practice*. St Louis: Mosby, 1993: 573–94.

Demoly P, Michel FB, Bousquet J. In vivo methods for study of allergy. Skin tests, techniques and interpretation. In: Middleton E, Reed CE, Ellis EF, Adkinson NF, Yunginger JW, Busse WW, eds. *Allergy: Principles and Practice*. St Louis: Mosby, 1998: 430–9.

Dreborg S, Backman A, Basomba A *et al*. Skin tests used in type I allergy testing. Position paper of the European Academy of Allergy and Clinical Immunology. *Allergy* 1989; 44 (Suppl. 10): 1–69.

Lewis T, Grant R. Vascular reactions of the skin to injury. Part II. The liberation of a histamine like substance in injured skin, the underlying cause of factitious urticaria and of wheal produced by burning; and observations upon the nervous control of certain skin reactions. *Heart* 1924; 11: 209.

Mantoux C. Intradermoreaction de la tuberculose. *Cr Acad Sci* 1908; 147: 355.

Menardo JL, Bousquet J, Rodiere M *et al*. Skin test reactivity in infancy. *J Allergy Clin Immunol* 1985; 75: 646–51.

Nelson HS, Knoetzer J, Bucher B *et al*. Effect of distance between sites and region of the body on results of skin prick tests. *J Allergy Clin Immunol* 1991; 88: 758–62.

Pepys J. Skin testing. *Br J Hosp Med* 1975; 14: 412–25.

Schloss OM. A case of allergy to common foods. *Am J Dis Child* 1912; 3: 341.

Uehara M. Reduced histamine reaction in atopic dermatitis. *Arch Dermatol* 1982; 118: 244–5.

Sunscreens

S. Albert and J.L.M. Hawk

General principles, classification and structure

Most of the damaging effects of sunlight result from cutaneous ultraviolet radiation (UVR) exposure. UVR (100–400 nm) comprises only 5–10% of terrestrial sunlight, of which UVB (280–315) forms about 5% and UVA (315–400) the remaining. Both UVB and UVA irradiation can have similar profound deleterious effects on human skin, but though the relative amount of UVB reaching the earth is small it is responsible for most of the harmful effects of sunlight such as sunburn, skin cancers and photoageing. People with fairer skins are more prone to develop these effects. To protect against them, however systemic, orally ingested sunscreen agents have been sought but no satisfactory ones so far found, although α-carotene has been used with limited results in porphyrias, hydroxychloroquine in certain other photodermatose and antioxidants in general, all without marked success. Thus the most efficient products so far have proved to be a variety of topically applied creams and lotions containing organic or inorganic chemical agents that absorb or reflect UVR. They may be classified as:

- chemical sunscreens (organic chemical absorbers)
- physical sunscreens (inorganic chemical absorbers)
- combination sunscreens.

Chemical sunscreen agents act as UVR-absorbing molecules or chromophores, taking up UVR and converting it to harmless low-energy longer wavelengths, mostly in the infrared region. Physical sunscreens in addition scatter and reflect light. There are however very few chemicals that can absorb both UVB and UVA efficiently at concentrations suitable and permissible in commercial preparations and hence sunscreens often comprise combinations of multiple agents so as to provide a broad spectrum of protection. Organic chemical absorbers are generally compounds with an aromatic ring structure conjugated with a carbonyl group, with an electron-releasing amine or methoxyl group substituted in the *ortho* or *para* position of the ring. Derivatives of *para*-aminobenzoic acid (PABA), cinnamates, salicylates, camphor, anthranilates, benzophenones and dibenzoylmethanes are the seven major groups of these agents currently used in sunscreen formulations. Such agents with a high optical density or molar extinction coefficient at the wavelength of maximum UVR absorption, the so-called absorption maximum (λ_{max}), are likely to give maximum protection at the lowest concentrations. The sun-protection factor (SPF) is the most widely accepted way of measuring this protection, and is the ratio calculated by dividing the UVR dose required to evoke minimal erythema on sunscreen-protected skin by that required on unprotected skin. Substantivity (water resistance) on the other hand is the ability of a sunscreen to remain on the skin when subjected to environmental conditions likely to remove it, such as swimming or sweating; this is measured by determination of the SPF after often two 20-min immersions of the sunscreen-applied test site in moving water.

The names of sunscreen ingredients tend to be a confusing array of differing nomenclatures and therefore each has also been given a unique Chemical Abstract Services (CAS) number. The most commonly used of these are outlined below and a more detailed listing is provided in Table 1.

Table 1 INCI nomenclature for sunscreens (modified from Vanio & Bianchini, 2001, pp. 18–19)

INCI nomenclature	CAS no.	COLIPA no.
Para-aminobenzoic acids (PABAs)		
Amyl dimethyl PABA	14779-78-3	S-5
Ethyl dihydroxypropyl PABA	58882-17-0	S-2
Ethylhexyl dimethyl PABA	21245-02-3	S-8
Ethyl PABA	94-09-7	–
Glyceryl PABA	136-44-7	S-6
PABA	150-13-0	S-1
PEG-25 PABA (ethoxylated ethyl PABA)	116242-27-4	S-3
Cinnamates		
Cinoxate	104-28-9	S-29
Diethanolamine-*p*-methoxycinnamate	56265-46-4	S-24
Diisopropyl methyl cinnamate	32580-71-5	S-23
Ethylhexyl methoxycinnamate	5466-77-3	S-28
Ethyl methoxycinnamate	99880-64-5	–
Glyceryl ethylhexanoate dimethoxycinnamate	–	–
Isoamyl-*para*-methoxycinnamate	71617-10-2	S-27
Iopropyl-*para*-methoxycinnamate and diisopropylcinnamate mixture	–	–
Salicylates		
Dipropylene glycol salicylate	7491-14-7	–
Ethylene glycol salicylate	87-28-5	–
Ethylhexyl salicylate	118-60-5	S-13
Homosalate	118-56-9	S-12
Isopropylbenzyl salicylate	94134-93-7	S-16
Methyl salicylate	119-36-8	–
Phenyl salicylate	118-55-8	S-14
Triethanolamine salicylate	2174-16-5	S-9
Camphor derivatives		
3-Benzylidene camphor	15087-24-8	S-61
Benzylidene camphor sulfonic acid	56039-58-8	S-59
Camphor benzalkonium methosulfate	52793-97-2	S-57
4-Methylbenzylidene camphor	38102-62-4	S-60
Polyacrylamidomethyl benzylidene camphor	113783-61-2	S-72
Terephthalylidene dicamphor sulfonic acid	90457-82-2	S-71
Benzophenones		
Benzophenone-1	131-56-6	S-33
Benzophenone-2	131-55-5	S-34
Benzophenone-3 (Oxybenzone)	131-57-7	S-38
Benzophenone-4 (Sulizobenzone)	4065-45-6	S-40
Benzophenone-5	6628-37-1	S-40
Benzophenone-6	131-54-4	S-35
Benzophenone-8	131-53-3	–
Benzophenone-9	76656-36-5	S-36
Benzophenone-10 (Mexenone)	1641-17-4	S-39
Dibenzoylmethane		
Butyl methoxydibenzoylmethane (Avobenzone)	70356-09-1	S-66
Anthranilate		
Menthyl anthranilate	134-09-8	–
Miscellaneous		
Diethylhexylbutamido triazone	154702-15-5	S-78
Digalloyl trioleate	17048-39-4	S-55
Ethylhexyl triazone	88122-99-0	S-69

(continued)

Table 1 INCI nomenclature for sunscreens (*continued*)

INCI nomenclature	CAS no.	COLIPA no.
Miscellaneous		
5-Methyl-2-phenylbenzoxazole	7420-86-2	S-47
Octocrylene	6197-30-4	S-32
Phenylbenzimidazole sulfonic acid	27503-81-7	S-45
Urocancic acid	104-98-3	S-46
Bisymidazylate (proposed INCI name)	180898-37-7	S-80
Anisotriazine (proposed INCI name)	187393-00-06	S-81
Drometrizole trisiloxane	155633-54-8	S-73
Methylene-*bis*-benzotriazolyl tetramethylbutylphenol	103597-45-1-P	S-79

CAS, Chemical Abstracts Service; COLIPA, European Cosmetic, Toiletry and Perfumery Association; INCI, International Nomenclature of Cosmetic Ingredients.

Chemical sunscreens

PABA has a reactive carboxylic and an amino group substituted in a *para* orientation on the benzene nucleus. It has a λ_{max} at 296 nm and a molar extinction coefficient of 13 600; and is therefore a good UVB absorber. However it tends to be easily oxidized and stains clothing, may crystallize and has a moderate contact sensitizing potential. On the other hand, PABA derivatives such as the ethyl, butyl, amyl and octyl esters of N,N-dimethyl-PABA were designed in the hope of minimizing the disadvantages of the parent molecule while retaining its UVB-screening ability. Thus N,N-dimethyl-PABA octyl ether, also known as Padimate-O, has overcome most of the undesirable effects of PABA; it is a liquid with almost double the molar extinction coefficient of PABA and has hence been an efficient and popular UVB sunscreen.

Salicylates are *ortho*-disubstituted aromatic compounds with peak absorption around 300 nm and hence UVB absorbers. They are non-water soluble, stable compounds easily incorporated into cosmetic formulations and excellent solubilizers of other non-soluble ingredients such as benzophenones. They also have an excellent safety profile but are relatively weak UVR absorbers. The most widely used of the group is octyl salicylate, also known as 2-ethylhexyl salicylate.

Cinnamates are UVB absorbers with a λ_{max} around 310 nm 2-ethylhexyl *p*-methoxycinnamate or octyl *p*-methoxycinnamate is the most popular member of the group, while octocrylene is a more recent introduction.

Anthranilates, as with the salicylate group, are stable and safe compounds. Menthylanthranilate is an *ortho*-disubstituted aminobenzoate with a λ_{max} at 336 nm.

Benzophenones are aromatic ketone derivatives of dibenzoylmethane capable of some absorption in the UVA range of the spectrum, some exhibiting a shift in λ_{max} in different solvents; for example dioxybenzone has been shown to have a λ_{max} of 326 nm and 352 nm in polar and non-polar solvents, respectively. These compounds however are relatively difficult to solubilize in cosmetic formulations and have a sensitizing potential.

Dibenzoylmethanes are substituted diketones capable of undergoing keto-enol tautomerism. Compounds such as isopropyl dibenzoylmethane (Eusolex 8020) and butyl-dibenzoylmethanes (Avobenzone, Parsol 1789) absorb UVA relatively well but are not very photostable. Avobenzone has a λ_{max} of 355 nm and a very high extinction coefficient of greater than 30 000.

Camphor derivatives (bicyclic compounds), such as 3-benzylidene camphor and benzylidene camphor sulphonic acid, are UVB absorbers. This group of agents is currently not approved by the Federal Drug Administration for use in the USA. In particular however, terephthalylidene dicamphor sulphonic acid (Mexoryl SX) is a newer derivative with a λ_{max} of 345 nm, with excellent photostability and UVA absorptivity.

Physical sunscreens

Titanium dioxide and zinc oxide are chemically inert particulate mineral substances which have a number of advantages in that they are photostable, not a cause of photoallergy or phototoxicity and protective against UVB, UVA and to some extent visible radiation. In the past such preparations have tended to be thick, opaque and cosmetically unacceptable to many people, but more recently micronized formulations containing particles of less than 100 nm diameter have ensured improved translucency and cosmetic acceptability. They are also often combined with organic chemical absorbers in order to achieve higher SPFs than when used alone.

Indications and other uses

UVR exposure whether to UVB or UVA leads to acute inflammatory changes in skin with vasodilatation, erythema, inflammatory cellular infiltration, release of proinflammatory mediators such as prostaglandins (PGD_2, PGE_2) and interleukins (IL-1, IL-6), along with keratinocyte apoptosis. Such effects are most pronounced in the sunburn reaction. UVR-mediated damage to DNA can be detected as early as 30 min after exposure, probably then leading causally to the subsequent inflammatory changes. Both epidermis and dermis are affected, principally by UVB, but UVA is known also to produce significant dermal damage, probably playing an important role in skin photoageing, the gradual deterioration of cutaneous structure and function from the cumulative imperfectly repaired damage of long-term recurrent UVR exposure. Manifestations of this include wrinkling, freckling, lentigines, telangiectasia, comedones, mottled pigmentation, coarseness and a yellowish discoloration of the skin. UVR has also been shown to be the most important cutaneous carcinogen, its role in the development of non-melanoma skin cancers such as squamous and basal cell carcinomas having been clearly demonstrated. There is strong evidence also for the aetiological involvement of UVR in melanoma, although this has not yet been indisputably proven. An individual's inherent burning and tanning capacity along with associated behavioural and environmental factors greatly influence these events, those with fairer skins being more prone to damage. Sunscreens are therefore strongly indicated as protective agents against the occurrence of skin sunburn, photoageing and cancers. Nevertheless some studies have shown a slightly increased incidence of melanoma in subjects who claim to have used sunscreens but this is thought likely to be due not to the sunscreen agents themselves but to other factors, particularly inadequate product use along with a possible tendency to stay outdoors for longer periods in the belief that protection is now adequate.

Sunscreens are routinely advised in patients with the so-called idiopathic, probably immunologically based photodermatoses namely polymorphic light eruption (PLE), actinic prurigo (AP), hydroa vacciniforme (HV), solar urticaria (SU) and chronic actinic dermatitis (CAD). PLE is the commonest of these and usually affects young adults with an itchy erythematous papular eruption over some or all exposed areas within a few hours of sun exposure, thereafter subsiding within a few days; it may be induced by UVB, UVA or both and broad-spectrum sunscreen use is advised, often with effect in milder cases. AP is a more chronic condition of generally young girls characterized by an excoriated papular or nodular eruption of the exposed sites with a tendency to involve covered areas as well; as in PLE it may be induced by UVA or UVB. Sunscreen use is helpful only in milder instances. HV is a rare blistering and scarring photodermatosis otherwise closely resembling PLE; it responds best, if moderately, to sunscreen use, UVB and short wavelength UVA probably being causal. SU is an uncommon whealing condition induced by sunlight and only responding to sunscreen use in the rare mild cases induced by UVB. CAD is a relatively persistent eczematous condition of elderly males, the face, neck, upper chest and hands usually being involved with sparing of the eyelids, submental, retroauricular and other photoprotected areas. Most patients with CAD react abnormally to both UVA and UVB, so broad-spectrum sunscreens are advised, although again with only moderate effect.

It is very important however for patients with the severe DNA repair-defective disorder, xeroderma pigmentosum, to use sunscreens and other sun-avoidance measures, both acute and chronic UV damage to their skin being markedly more pronounced than in normal individuals.

Porphyrias are disorders of haem biosynthesis resulting in the excess production of porphyrin and its precursors; these compounds absorb radiation of wavelengths around 400 nm, then re-emit the energy leading to the production of free radicals destructive to cellular components. Patients with these disorders require protection particularly in the short visible light range of the spectrum, but this is not well provided by topical sunscreens, although inorganic chemical preparations such as titanium dioxide may help to a small extent. α-Carotene 120–180 mg/day given orally has also been considered beneficial to a degree in some patients with erythropoietic protoporphyria (EPP), possibly by quenching free radicals, although a significant effect is uncommon.

Eczemas such as atopic and seborrhoeic dermatitis, not light-induced by themselves, can be worsened by sun exposure in some patients and sunscreens may be helpful in these, as well as in other much rarer photoaggravated dermatoses such as systemic lupus erythematosus.

Side-effects and cross-reactions

Sunscreen users may not infrequently complain of an immediate burning or stinging sensation at sites of application, such irritation being more frequently observed with the benzophenones and PABA esters. Preparations containing physical agents may also cause miliaria on occasion due to occlusion. As with other topically applied agents, sunscreen preparations too may at times induce allergic contact dermatitis from preservatives, fragrances and other non-active constituents of the preparation, although the sunscreen chemicals themselves are also being increasingly reported as allergenic; sensitization is higher in those with photodermatoses, especially CAD or PLE. In the early years of sunscreen use, PABA was the most frequent cause of this but reactions over the last decade have been fewer because of decreasing use. Glyceryl PABA was also reported as a potent sensitizer in several patients until the reaction was later shown to be due to impurities present in the preparation, the contaminant being either benzocaine (ethylaminobenzoic acid) or other unidentified agent. Procaine, benzocaine, *p*-phenylenediamine and sulphonamides can thus cross-react with PABA such that patients sensitized to any of these compounds may also demonstrate an allergic reaction to sunscreens containing PABA or its esters. In recent years however the benzophenone (oxybenzone, mexenone) group has replaced PABA as the most frequent cause of sunscreen allergy, especially as these compounds are also widely used in non-sunscreen cosmetics and toiletries. Several allergic reactions have also been reported to isopropyl dibenzoylmethane leading to its removal from several products, it can cross-react with the structurally related butyl methoxydibenzoylmethane. 3–4′-Methyl-benzylidene camphor was previously used in combination with isopropyl dibenzoylmethane and those sensitive to one agent often demonstrated a concomitant sensitization to the other. Amongst the cinnamates, 2-ethoxyethyl-*p*-cinnamate (Cinoxate) is the most frequent sensitizer, these compounds also cross-reacting with balsam of Peru, balsam of Tolu, cinnamic aldehyde, cinnamic acid and cinnamon oil, all ingredients used in cosmetics, fragrances, toothpastes and flavourings.

Photoallergic reactions too have been reported to a variety of sunscreen chemicals, the photoallergen being apparently formed in some instances when a parent molecule undergoes chemical alteration following the absorption of radiation, usually UVA, thus resulting in the formation of an altered compound or hapten; this then presumably binds to carrier protein to form an allergen. Alternatively, the photochemical alteration of an already formed protein–hapten complex by radiation absorption could probably make it allergenic. Photoallergy has been reported to 2-hydroxy-4-methoxy methylbenzophenone (Eusolex 4360, oxybenzone), benzophenone-4, isopropyldibenzoylmethane (Eusolex 8020), butylmethoxydibenzoylmethane (Parsol 1789) and isoamyl *p*-methoxycinnamate.

Treatment regimen

The recommended thickness of application of a sunscreen for optimum benefit is 2 mg/cm^2 or 2 μL/cm^2, being a relatively liberal amount; however a number of studies have shown that users apply less than this recommended quantity in practical settings. Thus most have found the applied film thickness to range from 0.5 to 1 mg/cm^2, while a recent European study on 148 students found the median quantity to be 0.39 mg/cm^2. It has therefore been proposed that the methodology of testing and labelling of sunscreens might be altered to suit a more realistic consumer usage pattern; this approach has so far not been adopted however because of concerns that major consumer confusion might ensue. In addition, sunscreen reapplication is advised every 2–3 h, partially because of possible product photodegradation and partially the likelihood of removal in unsuitable environmental conditions.

Further reading

Autier P, Boniol M, Severi G, Dore JF. Quantity of sunscreen used by European students. *Br J Dermatol* 2001; 144: 288–91.

Azurdia RM, Pagliaro JA, Diffey BL, Rhodes LE. Sunscreen application by photosensitive patients is inadequate for protection. *Br J Dermatol* 1999; 140: 255–8.

Bech-Thomsen N, Wulf HC. Sunbathers' application of sunscreen is probably inadequate to obtain the sun protection factor assigned to the preparation. *Photodermatol Photoimmunol Photomed* 1992; 939: 242–4.

Bilsland D, Ferguson J. Contact allergy to sunscreen chemicals in photosensitivity dermatitis/actinic reticuloid syndrome (PD/AR) and polymorphic light eruption. *Contact Dermatitis* 1993; 29: 70–3.

Dromgoole SH, Maibach HI. Sunscreening agent intolerance: contact and photocontact sensitization and contact urticaria. *J Am Acad Dermatol* 1990; 22: 1068–78.

Journe F, Marguery MC, Rakotondrazafy J, El Sayed F, Bazex J. Sunscreen sensitization: a 5-year study. *Acta Derm Venereol* 1999; 79: 211–13.

Lowe NJ, Shaath NA, Pathak MA. *Sunscreens, Development, Evaluation and Regulatory Aspects*, 2nd edn. New York: Marcel Dekker, 1997.

Pathak MA. Sunscreens: topical and systemic approaches for protection of human skin against harmful effects of solar radiation. *J Am Acad Dermatol* 1982; 7: 285–312.

Schauder S, Ippen H. Contact and photocontact sensitivity to sunscreens. Review of a 15-year experience and of the literature. *Contact Dermatitis* 1997; 37: 221–32.

Vainio H, Bianchini F, eds. *Sunscreens, IARC Handbook of Cancer Prevention*, Vol. 5. France: World Health Organisation, International Agency for Research on Cancer, 2001.

Topical anaesthetics

F.B. de Waard-van der Spek and A.P. Oranje

Drugs

Local anaesthesia plays a useful role in simple or superficial interventions. Lesions can be frozen by refrigerants such as ethyl chloride spray. The same effect may be achieved with liquid nitrogen, but its lower temperature may cause greater postoperative discomfort. Local anaesthetics are generally ineffective when applied to intact human skin because they are poorly absorbed.

EMLA is a topical anaesthetic cream developed by Broberg and Evers for use on intact skin. The acronym EMLA stands for eutectic mixture of local anaesthetics. EMLA is a mixture of lidocaine (lignocaine) 25 mg/g and prilocaine 25 mg/g. EMLA cream comprises the following ingredients:

- lidocaine 25 mg
- prilocaine 25 mg
- arlatone 289 (emulgent)
- carbapol 934 (thickener)
- distilled water in 1 mL cream.

Other local anaesthetics that are used include:

- amethocaine patch
- ethyl chloride spray
- lidocaine gel
- lidocaine gel 10% + glycerine acid monohemiphthalate disodium (absorption promoter)
- lidocaine adrenaline tetracaine (LAT) gel
- liquid nitrogen
- tetracaine epinephrine (adrenaline) cocaine (TAC) gel
- tetracaine cream.

General principles, classification and structure

A local anaesthetic cream consists of hydrophilic groups, usually a tertiary amine, and hydrophobic groups, generally an aromatic residue. These groups are separated by an alkyl chain. They may be separated into two groups: those containing an ester linkage (e.g. procaine, tetracaine, cocaine), and those containing an amide linkage (e.g. lidocaine and prilocaine). The linkage is responsible for the pathway by which the molecule is metabolized and excreted.

Mechanisms of action

Local anaesthetics act on sodium channels in the nerve membranes. The conduction is decreased via interaction with specific binding sites and total inhibition of conduction is achieved with increasing concentration of the local anaesthetic.

Dermatological indications

EMLA will produce effective analgesia in the skin prior to a variety of superficial skin interventions. Ethyl chloride spray (ECS) has caused more local irritation in a study in which the analgesic efficacy and local tolerance of EMLA and ECS before intravenous cannulation in premedicated children were compared.

Several more local anaesthetics are available and have been evaluated. For example, a 10% lidocaine gel containing glycerrhetinic acid monohemiphthalate disodium as an absorption promoter has reduced the pain upon venous cannulation in adults and in children, although further improvement seemed necessary in order to achieve ideal conditions.

TAC gel has been effective in laceration repair, but serious adverse reaction have been reported. LAT gel has worked as well as TAC gel for topical anaesthesia in facial and scalp lacerations in a randomized double-blind study in 95 children aged 5–17 years, but additional studies on its safety have to be done.

Amethocaine in the form of a self-adhesive patch has been evaluated in an open study in children before venous cannulation. A satisfactory anaesthesia was achieved in 80% of patients, but 20% felt moderate to severe pain.

EMLA cream has been compared with a 4% tetracaine-containing cream for preventing venipuncture-induced pain in children. It was reported that EMLA reduced the pain more effectively. Recently a study in 60 children aged 3–15 years in which the anaesthetic effect of tetracaine gel was compared with EMLA cream showed that tetracaine gel provided effective, rapid, long-lasting and safe local anaesthesia, and was significantly better than EMLA cream in reducing pain during venous cannulation in children using the recommended application periods for both formulations.

EMLA used with glyceryl trinitrate (GTN) ointment which promotes venous dilatation has been found to make intravenous cannulation in adults technically easier. However, side-effects of GTN include headaches and hypotension. Further studies will be necessary, especially in children, for establishing the efficacy and the safety of this combination.

EMLA is the only topical anaesthetic registered for use in children from the age of 3 months. Studies in neonates indicated that EMLA is also safe to use in neonates—a registration request for its use in neonates has been submitted in the Netherlands. EMLA is now approved for anaesthesia of healthy skin in children of 0–3 months, an age range in which it used to be contraindicated. Several studies proved that use of EMLA cream in neonates is safe when used once a day. Since the clinical situation often requires more than one application a day, more research is needed to establish a safe and effective local anaesthetic which can be applied topically several times a day in neonates.

EMLA

At present, we prefer to use EMLA for inducing local anaesthesia for superficial interventions. Indications for EMLA cream are discussed in the following section.

We have evaluated the efficacy and minimal effective application time for EMLA cream for the removal of mollusca contagiosa in children. Eighty-three children aged 4–12 years, scheduled for curettage of at least five molluscum contagiosum lesions, participated in a double-blind, time (15, 30 and 60 min) response study. The pain was assessed by the children and the physician as none, slight, moderate or severe. In addition, the children rated the pain on a visual analogue scale (VAS). EMLA effectively prevented the pain for all three application times ($P < 0.01$). The proportion of children reporting no pain on the verbal scale increased from 36% in the 15-min group to 61% in the 60-min group.

EMLA and skin biopsy

It is important to achieve analgesia up to a sufficient skin depth for taking skin biopsies. The maximum depth of analgesia provided by EMLA is about 5 mm. There are controversial reports on the efficacy of EMLA for taking skin biopsy. We have conducted a double-blind, placebo-controlled study to investigate the analgesic effect of the EMLA patch as a premedication for skin biopsy in 63 children. There were two parallel groups. One group received an EMLA patch and the other placebo on the skin at the site of the biopsy during 60 min. After removal of the patch, the physician infiltrated the skin as usual with 1 mL lidocaine and took the biopsy with a 4-mm biopsy punch. EMLA was significantly more effective in decreasing the pain at the injection site of the lidocaine infiltration. There was no difference in the pain scores for the biopsy.

Other indications for EMLA

Only the most relevant ones are mentioned here. The efficacy of EMLA analgesia during the treatment of condylomata acuminata by cauterization or laser treatment has been investigated in a number of clinical studies. Most effective analgesia has been achieved after applying EMLA for 5–15 min on the genital mucosa. Longer application times have resulted in less effective analgesia.

EMLA applied for 60 min has provided analgesia for the treatment of port-wine stains with pulsed dye laser. EMLA did not affect the efficacy of removal of the port-wine stain. However, our own experience has been that the analgesic efficacy of EMLA is not adequate.

Effective analgesia has been achieved with EMLA for surgical debridement of leg ulcers of venous or arterial origin.

Other indications are painful inflamed acne lesions, light electrocautery and fulguration of whiteheads and hair removal by thermolysis in hirsutism.

EMLA has not been effective for removing common warts by curettage. We have observed that EMLA analgesia is not sufficient for the removal of common warts by cryotherapy.

Studies have also been undertaken to investigate the effectiveness of EMLA for (intramuscular) vaccinations. EMLA has been found to significantly reduce the pain of diphtheria pertussis tetanus (DPT) vaccination by children.

We have conducted a double-blind placebo-controlled study to investigate the analgesic effect of EMLA for the subcutaneous administration of mumps–measles–rubella (MMR) vaccination in 96 children aged about 9 years. There was no significant difference between the pain scores in the EMLA group and the placebo group, although the difference almost reached significance ($P=0.02$). There was a trend that in the EMLA group less pain was felt. However, this trend was not significant. Probably the pain of MMR vaccination was not due to skin penetration, but during the injection of the liquid into the subcutaneous space.

The most important dermatological indications for the use of EMLA cream are the removal of molluscum contagiosum and as premedication for taking skin biopsy in childhood. The biopsy procedure is much easier to perform. Moreover, it may also provide material of improved quality for histologic investigation. Other local anaesthetics need to be investigated further.

Side-effects

No major side-effects of EMLA has been reported. A brief period of local redness or pallor of the skin may occur. Despite the frequent and widespread use of EMLA, we have encountered only two cases in the literature of contact allergy caused by EMLA. In both patients, patch tests were positive for EMLA and prilocaine. During the past 8–10 years we have treated 3500–4000 children with EMLA, mainly as an anaesthetic for the removal of molluscum contagiosum. In one child, we observed an eczematous reaction which did not occur after later treatments with EMLA. We have observed purpura in five patients, which disappeared within several days. In these patients, patch tests were performed. All tests were negative. We concluded that the purpuric reaction was not of an allergic nature and possibly caused by a topic effect on the capillary endothelium.

Regimen

The indications and recommended application times for EMLA are shown in Table 1.

EMLA acts more rapidly in children with atopic dermatitis. Several studies have been undertaken to determine the plasma levels of lidocaine and prilocaine after ap-

Table 1 Indications and the recommended application times for EMLA

Indication	Application time (min)
Molluscum contagiosum	15–30
Skin biopsy (pretreatment)	60
Condylomata acuminata	5–15
Port-wine stains (pulsed dye laser)	60
Debridement leg ulcers	30
Vaccination	60

plication of EMLA. In these studies, plasma levels were far below the toxic levels. There is a relative risk for methaemoglobinaemia in children younger than 3 months. Prilocaine can induce methaemoglobinaemia via its *O*-toluidine metabolite. The activity of erythrocyte methaemoglobin reductase does not reach adult levels until after the age of 3 months.

We recommend that the use of EMLA per day is limited to a maximum of 1 g in children aged 0–3 months, 2 g in children to a maximum aged 3–12 months and 10 g in older children.

Further reading

Anonymus. Lidocaine + prilocaine before 3 months of age: new indication. Correct use is crucial. *Prescr Int* 2000; 9(47): 77–9.

Doyle E, Freeman J, Im NT *et al.* An evaluation of a new self-adhesive patch preparation of amethocaine for topical anaesthesia prior to venous cannulation in children. *Anaesthesia* 1993; 48: 1050–2.

Ernst AA, Marvez E, Nick TG *et al.* Lidocaine adrenaline tetracaine gel versus tetracaine adrenaline cocaine gel for topical anesthesia in linear scalp and facial lacerations in children aged 5–17 years. *Pediatrics* 1995; 95 (2): 255–8.

Essink-Tjebbes CM, Hekster YA, Liem KD *et al.* Topical use of local anaesthetics in neonates. *Pharm World Sci* 1999; 21(4): 173–6.

Jong PC de, Verburg MP, Lillieborg S *et al.* EMLA cream versus ethyl-chloride spray: a comparison of the analgesic efficacy in children. *Eur J Anaesthesiol* 1990; 7: 473–81.

Kan HJM van, Egberts ACG, Rijnvos WPM *et al.* Tetracaine versus lidocaine-prilocaine for preventing venipuncture induced pain in children. *Am J Health-System Pharm* 1997; 54: 388–92.

Kano T, Nakamura M, Hashiguchi A *et al.* Dermatol patch anaesthesia with 10% lignocaine gel containing glycerrhetinic acid monohemiphtalate disodium as an absorption promoter. *Anaesthesia* 1992; 47: 708–10.

Michael A, Andrew A. The application of EMLA and Glyceryl Trinitate Ointment prior to venepuncture. *Anaesth Intens Care* 1996; 24: 360–4.

Oranje AP, de Waard-van der Spek FB. Use of EMLA cream in dermatosurgical interventions of skin and genital mucosa. In: Koren G, ed. *Eutectic Mixture of Local Anesthetics (EMLA). A breakthrough in skin anesthesia.* New York: Marcel Dekker, 1995: 123–36.

Romsing J, Henneberg SW, Walther-Larsen S *et al.* Tetracaine gel vs EMLA cream for percutaneous anaesthesia in children. *Br J Anaesth* 1999; 82(4): 637–8.

Rylander E, Sjoberg I, Lillieborg S *et al.* Local anaesthesia of the genital mucosa with a lidocaine/prilocaine cream (EMLA) for laser treatment of condylomata acuminata: a placebo-controlled study. *Obstet Gynecol* 1990; 75: 302–6.

Tan OT, Stafford TJ. EMLA for laser treatment of port-wine stains. *J Dermatol Surg Oncol* 1990; 16: 1008–11.

Uhari M. A eutectic mixture of lidocaine and prilocaine for alleviating vaccination pain in infants. *Pediatrics* 1993; 92: 719–21.

Waard-van der Spek FB de, Oranje AP. Purpura caused by EMLA is of toxic origin. *Contact Dermatitis* 1997; 36: 11–13.

Waard-van der Spek FB de, Oranje AP, Lillieborg S *et al.* Treatment of molluscum contagiosum using a lidocaine/prilocaine cream (EMLA) for analgesia. *J Am Acad Dermatol* 1990; 23: 685–8.

Topical preparations and vehicles

M. Monti and S. Motta

General principles and classification

Dermatological therapy can be a combination of systemic and topical treatments although topical treatment is often the only therapy prescribed. As a consequence, dermatologists have to be familiar with the use of topical preparations, whether a drug or an active agent is added or not. Tailor-made preparations have undoubtedly a great positive impact on patients but their use is limited by two main factors: the poor confidence of practising dermatologists to prescribe magistral compositions and the difficulty in finding pharmacists capable and willing to provide them. In a recent analysis of compound prescriptions, some mixtures prescribed by dermatologists were questionable either because of the number of active ingredients or the selected concentrations. As a general consideration, the chemical agents that may be applied to the skin for their local effects belong to two categories:

- drugs
- non-drugs.

The agents of the first category have a selective action in terms of chemical and pharmacological activity on the skin. Antibiotics, antimycotics, corticosteroids, antineoplasties are some examples. They are prepared by pharmaceutical companies according to strict international rules on suitable vehicles and are ready to use. Their use in combination with other ingredients is neither recommendable nor economically worthwhile. The second category is composed of a heterogeneous group of agents which, by exclusion, do not belong to the first. They have mostly a non-selective action, have limited chemical and pharmacological activity and, sometimes, have just a physical action. These locally acting agents include most absorbents, astringents, demulcents, rubefacients, keratolytics and miscellaneous other ingredients used dermatologically. The local treatment of skin disorders also includes the exclusive use of vehicles. Therefore, excluding drugs, topical treatment may be subdivided into:

- non-specific treatment with bases
- specific treatment with active agents.

Non-specific treatment with bases

Dermatological bases or vehicles serve not only as vectors for incorporating active ingredients but possess some therapeutic effects because of their own physicochemical properties. In this case, the bases themselves are the active ingredients. The ideal base should have the following properties:

- easy to apply and remove
- non-toxic, irritant or allergenic
- chemically stable
- pharmacologically inert
- cosmetically acceptable.

The bases may be either liquid, semi-solid or solid. Some bases are utilized in non-specific dermatological treatment while others are just vehicles. A classification commonly used is given in Table 1. Another classification of vehicles is based on their physical phase:

- monophasic: powders and greases
- biphasic: paste, status lotions or emulsions
- triphasic: cooling paste.

The main effects, clinical indications and contraindications of bases are discussed according to the categories listed in Table 1.

Fatty ointments

Fatty ointments are anhydrous, lipophilic and hydrophobic bases consisting of mineral, synthetic or plant and animal fats.

Table 1 Classification of topical preparations

Bases utilized in non-specific treatments	Bases utilized as vehicles
Fatty ointments	Acqueous solutions
Fatty pastes	Tinctures
Powders	Varnishes
Hydrogels	Sprays
Hydroalcoholic lotions	Hydrosoluble ointments
Creams O/W	
Creams W/O	
Liquid emulsions	
Oils	

Paraffins, petrolatum, lanolin, castor oil, olive oil are examples of fats used in ointments. The ointments cover the stratum corneum promoting the inhibition of this layer by softening the skin and promoting drug penetration. They are useful for the treatment of asteatosis and dry skin, hyperkeratotic and scaling dermatoses. The obstruction of the release of heat and water may produce maceration, increase inflammation or produce dyshidrotic eruptions.

Fatty pastes

Pastes are mixtures of powder and ointment or cream. The powders are at least a 10% strength and depending on their concentration, the pastes are subdivided into:

- pastes: powder–ointment ratio 1 : 1
- soft pastes: powder–ointment ratio 1 : 2
- hard pastes: powder–ointment ratio 2 : 1.

Zinc oxide, talc and wheat starch are the most utilized powders. The pastes have a cooling, anti-inflammatory and skin-protective action. They are useful for the treatment of chronic dermatoses, especially when lichenification is present. Some of them have particular secretion absorbing or drying effects. The hard pastes have the same contraindications as ointments.

Powders

Powders are composed of micronized and dispersed granular particles. They can be homogeneously distributed on large body areas directly from a dusting can. Talc, zinc oxide, starch and magnesium carbonate are examples of the most commonly used powders. They have protective-antifrictional activity together with cooling and drying effects. They are used in erythematous exanthems and in some pruritic conditions. They dry the skin absorbing water and lipids from the surface and they crust the skin in oozing and erosive dermatoses.

Hydrogels

Hydrogels are composed of methylcellulose, carboxymethylcellulose, alginic acid and others that swell with water to produce a gelatinous base. Hydrogels have cooling and slight anti-inflammatory action so they are used in erythematous and pruritic exanthems as well as for the treatment of acute erogenous dermatitis. They may be applied to hairy parts but have a drying effect on prolonged application.

Hydroalcoholic lotions

Hydroalcoholic lotions are a mixture of ethanol 40–70% or isopropanol 20–40% and water. They are mostly used as vehicles for active substances but may be used as is for their defatting and drying effects. They are indicated in seborrhoeic conditions and contraindicated in asteatotic and scaling dermatitis.

Creams O/W

Creams O/W type are a two phase system of fatty substances (30%) water (70%) and emulsifying agents. They are mainly used as vehicles for active substances and have a cooling, anti-inflammatory and emollient effect. They can be used in many acute dermatoses and in seborrhoeic conditions. On prolonged use, because of the rapid loss of water, they produce a drying action. For this reason they are contraindicated in conditions such as asteatosis and ichthyosis.

Creams W/O

Creams W/O type are a two-phase system of fatty substances (up to 70%), water (30%) and emulsifying agents. They are mainly used as vehicles for active substances and due to the high concentration of fats they have a smoothing and softening effect, together with slight cooling and anti-inflammatory action. For these properties they are employed to counteract asteatotic, dry skin and to soften scales and crusts in chronic dermatoses. They are less tolerated with respect to O/W creams on seborrhoeic types of skin.

Liquid creams

Liquid creams are emulsions with low fatty material (less than 30%). They appear milky in colour and consistency and usually are employed in cosmetics as cleansing and body lotions. Liquid creams possess a slight anti-inflammatory, antipruritic effect and may be used even in exudative and vesicular dermatoses. However they dry the skin due to rapid evaporation of water. They are not suitable for chronic scaly dermatoses treatment.

Oils

Oils, as medical preparations, are used for dissolving fatty soluble active ingredients but may be used alone or for suspending powders. Oils have lubricating action and may be used to soften crusts and scales and to remove ointments and pastes. They are indicated in acute superficial dermatoses especially in children and are less indicated in adults especially with seborrhoea or seborrhoeic dermatoses.

In Table 2 the bases for dermatological non-specific treatment are listed. Some of these vehicles are rarely used mainly because of their poor cosmetic acceptability; only emulsions are largely used as vehicles for non-specific topical treatment.

The most widely used cream in European countries is a base cream called Cetomacrogol cream present in many pharmacopoeia. Cetomacrogol cream consists of 30% soft greases including

Table 2 Effects, indications and contraindications of vehicles

Vehicles	Effects	Indications	Contraindications
Fatty ointments	Softening, warming	Hyperkeratotic fissured dermatoses Asteatosis Dry skin	Acute inflamed skin Vesicular dermatoses
Pastes	Cooling, anti-inflammatory, secretion absorbing, protective	Chronic dermatoses Lichenified dermatoses	Acute dermatoses Erosive dermatoses
Powders	Cooling, protective, antifrictional, drying	Erythematous exanthems	Dry skin, crusting, oozing, erosive dermatoses
Hydrogels	Cooling, superficial anti-inflammatory, antipruritic	Erythematous or urticarial exanthems Dermatitis solaris	Dry skin
Hydroalcoholic lotions	Drying, cooling	Dermatoses of hairy parts, Seborrhoea	Dry skin. Asteatosis
Creams O/W	Cooling, anti-inflammatory, emollient	Acute dermatoses, seborrhoeic type of skin	Dry skin. Asteatosis
Creams W/O	Softening, slight cooling, anti-inflammatory	Chronic inflammation, soft scales and crusts, asteatotic dermatoses	Acute inflamed skin Dyshydrosis
Liquid creams	Cooling, anti-inflammatory, emollient	Acute, exudative dermatoses	Scaly or crusty dermatoses
Oils	Lubricating, softening scales and crusts	Superficial inflammation Skin—large area dermatoses. Removal of ointments and pastes	Seborrhoeic dermatoses

white soft paraffin and petrolatum. Cetomacrogol 1000, the emulsifying agent, is a condensation of cetostearyl alcohol with ethylene oxide. Cetomacrogol cream is non-allergenic, non-greasy, washable, low cost and easy to prepare. Usually, it is prescribed as a vehicle for active ingredients but it is useful in many non-specific treatments and even as a placebo. Cetomacrogol cream is also produced by pharmaceutical companies.

Specific treatment with active agents

Specific topical treatments are prescribed by dermatologists in so-called magistral formulations. In this case, the topical treatment consists of the local use of some active substances in a suitable vehicle. The vehicles are the same as proposed in the previous section and the local acting agents may be differentiated by their specific activity on the skin. There is no international agreement about the terminology for describing activity of these compounds on the skin. Moreover, there is no clear distinction between drugs and non-drugs, so that the limit of a magistral prescription is not well defined.

Theoretically, all topical dermatological treatments can be carried out with extemporaneous preparations. However some of them are technically difficult to prepare and economically not worthwhile. Others are purchased from pharmaceutical companies and have a high safety profile. The main action of topical active ingredients are listed in Table 3. The actions of active ingredients and the ingredients themselves are discussed in the following sections.

Protectives and absorbents

Protectives and absorbents are intended to absorb moisture, decrease friction, discourage bacterial growth and absorb fats contributing to a decrease in body odours. These actions are achieved using dusting powders and some mechanical and chemical protectives. Dusting powders considered for this activity are bentonite, calcium carbonate, calcium precipitate, talc, titanium dioxide, zinc oxide and zinc stearate. Other substances such as gelatin and glycerol may be added to increase the protective action. An example is zinc gelatin paste:

- zinc oxide 10%
- gelatin 15%
- glycerol 40%
- purified water 35%.

Collodion varnish may be used to protect non-affected areas of the skin from topically applied irritants or caustics:

- pyroxylin 4%
- ether 75%
- alcohol 25%.

Table 3 Action of topical active ingredients

Recommended for magistral prescription	Difficult to prepare or not economically worthwhile	Use of registered drugs is recommended
Protective and absorbent	Pigmenting	Antibacterial
Lenitive	Depigmenting	Antifungal
Emollient	Sunprotecting	Virostatic
Astringent and antiperspirant	Depilatories	Anti-inflammatory
Antipruritic	Insect repellent	Cytostatic
Rubefacient	Antiparasitic	Anaesthetizing
Caustic		
Keratolytic		
Keratoplastic		
Cleansing		
Opacizing, sebum-absorbing		

Vaseline and silicones are examples of other chemical protectives. Hydrophylic and lipophylic emulsions containing a variety of constituents such as allantoin, linoleic acid, panthotenol, urea and vitamins, have been considered by other authors to be protective. However their activity has not been demonstrated yet.

Lenitives

Lenitives are employed to alleviate skin irritation in many superficial skin dermatoses. They also prevent drying of affected areas. Lenitives are mainly in the form of lotions, cataplasms or wet dressings, or simply powders. Alginates, mucilages, gums, dextrins, starches, certain sugars, glycerol and many oils are commonly considered as lenitives. Zinc oxide, ammonium chloride, talc and calamine are sometimes added for their astringent anti-inflammatory effect. Typical formulations are

- calamine lotion
  calamine 15
  zinc oxide 5
  glycerol 5
  water to 100
- lenitive cream
  zinc oxide 3
  magnesium silicate 3
  EDTA 0.1
  imidazolidinyl urea 0.1
  paraben mix 0.1
  cetomacrogol cream to 100.

Emollients

Emollients are used to render the skin softer and more pliable and also possess some anti-irritative properties. Oils of mineral, vegetable and animal origin as well as waxes are considered emollients. in particular some vegetable fats such as karitè butter or jojoba liquid wax, possess both a good emollience and cosmetic acceptance. Both creams and ointments are suitable for this purpose. All ointments are considered emollients and virtually all emulsions, due to the presence of fat components that penetrate easily into stratum corneum layers, are also emollients. For this reason emulsions instead of ointments are now prescribed as emollients.

Cetomacrogol cream is an example of an emulsion utilized as an emollient:

- wheat germ oil 4
- poliethylenglycol 4
- EDTA 0.1
- imidazolidinyl urea 0.1
- paraben mix 0.1
- cetomacrogol cream to 100.

Astringents and antiperspirants

Astringents are active substances. When applied locally they are protein precipitants, having low cell penetrability so that their action is limited to the surface. Astringents in dermatology are used to reduce erythema and pruritus; they also have an antiperspirant effect by causing protein precipitation in the sweat ducts. Astringents/antiperspirants also have deodorant properties due to an interaction with odorous fatty acids liberated by bacteria and by suppressing bacterial growth by virtue of low pH. The main astringents are:

- salt of the cations aluminium, bismuth, iron, manganese and zinc
- other salts containing these metals such as permanganates
- tannins or related polyphenolic compounds.

Dusting powders, lotions and gels are used for this purpose. An example of a powder is astringent powder:

- tannic acid 10
- zinc oxide 10
- talc to 100.

Aluminium chloride exahydrate aqueous or hydroalcoholic solution 5–10% may be used as an astringent in many chronic oozing dermatitis cases as well as an antiperspirant at concentrations of 10–20%.

Antipruritics

Pruritus is a common symptom of different dermatoses of eczema, atopia, urticaria, exanthem type and neurodermitic type. It can also be linked to internal diseases or skin senescence. Most astringents, kerotoplastics or rubefacients possess antipruritic activity. Menthol, phenol, salicylic acid, polidocanol and coal tar are used as topical antipruritics in different dermatoses. Some examples of antipruritic formulae are:

- menthol spirit
  menthol 1.0
  ethanol 70% to 100
- aluminium gel
  aluminium chloride exahydrate 5
  hydroxymethylcellulose 4
  propylene glycol 5
  ethanol 20
  water to 100.

Coal tar as an antipruritic agent has been used in an emulsion: cetomacrogol cream plus 2–4% coal tar.

Rubefacients

Rubefacients are able to induce hyperaemia and slight inflammation that produces a feeling of comfort, warmth, sometimes itching and hyperaesthesia. Most rubefacients in high concentrations are vesicants. Rubefacients are sometimes used for treating the sensory and visible effect of irritation, giving the patient the impression of receiving an effective medication. They are also used to treat pernioses and to promote hair growth especially in alopecia areata. Examples are:

- alcohol camphor
- anthralin capsicum
- benzoin menthol
- resorcinol ichthammol
- methylsalicilate
- nicotine acid and its esters.

One example of rubefacients is:

- ichthammol for pernioses
  ichthammol 30
  yellow petrolatum to 100.

Caustics

Caustics are agents that cause the destruction of tissue therefore they are used in hyperkeratoses or hyperplastic tissues but they can be used also for the destruction of tumours such as basaliomas and xanthelasmas. These agents usually precipitate proteins so that they may be considered as astringents at low concentration. Caustics are also bactericidals. Examples are:

- trichloroacetic acid
- glacial acetic acid
- phenol
- silver nitrate
- nitric acid
- potassium hydroxide
- zinc chloride.

Caustics are usually applied to the skin with a stick swab. Examples are:

- trichloroacetic acid aqueous solution—50% is used to remove xanthelasmas
- liquified phenol 20% in either to bleach freckles from the hands.

Keratolytics

Keratolytics loosen the keratins or intercellular cement facilitating desquamation of scales and softening horny material or crusts so they may be used in hyperkeratotic conditions. They also eliminate parasites or fungi. However the real action of some keratolytics is not completely elucidated. Examples are:

- salicylic acid
- sulfur
- urea
- resorcinol
- calcium chloride
- some alkali-containing compounds such as sodium and potassium hydroxide.

Among these, salicylic acid is the most commonly used in a variety of formulations. Around 6–10% of salicylic acid is needed for a keratolytic effect even if the possibility of toxicity due to absorption has to be considered. Therefore high concentrations are employed in very small areas incorporated in collodion. Examples are:

- salicylic acid—cetomacrogol
  salicylic acid 6–10

cetomacrogol cream to 100
- salicylic acid for pityriasis capitis
  salicylic acid 3
  glycerol 10
  ethanol 50% to 100
- urea–cetomacrogol
  urea 5–10
  glycerol 5
  cetomacrogol cream to 100.

Keratoplastics

Keratolytic agents at low concentrations stimulate the renewal of the horny layer through a slight reducing action and favouring desquamation. Salicylic acid, α-hydroxy acids, sulfur, urea and ichthyols are considered keratoplastics.

An examples of formulations with this property are:
- sulfo-salicylic shaking lotion
  salicylic acid 2
  sulfur 2
  ethanol 50% to 100
- glycolic salicylic lotion
  salicylic acid 2
  glycolic acid 10
  ethanol 50% to 100
- glycolic salicylic cream
  glycolic acid 10
  glycolic acid 10
  cetomacrogol cream to 100.

Other ingredients are able, via a toxic event, to reduce DNA synthesis and mitosis, especially in hyperproliferative disorders. Some of these substances, namely tars, also possess antipruritic–anti-inflammatory action so that they may be used in a variety of skin disorders ranging from psoriasis to atopic dermatitis. This activity should be defined as a reducing activity, but many authors regard it as a keratoplastic activity. Examples of these compounds are coal tar, wood tars, resorcinol, anthralin, ichthyol and phenols. Examples are:
- coal tar solution
  coal tar 20
  polysorbate 80 5
  ethanol to 100
- ichthyol cetomacrogol cream
  ichthyol 10
  cetomacrogol cream to 100.

Up to 4% coal tar can easily be incorporated into cetomacrogol cream. The result is a cosmetically acceptable and washable preparation, useful for outpatient treatment.

Cleansing

Cleansing may be carried out with detergents, solvents, abrasive substances singly or in combination. Soaps and shampoos are often used as vehicles for active agents such as antibacterial, antifungal, salicylic acid or tars. Some detergents are also antibacterial such as benzalkonium chloride. Substances in this group include:
- ethanol sodiumlaurylsulfate
- isopropanol benzalkonium chloride.

A simple example in which it is possible to suspend the active ingredients is:
- anionic detergent
  28% sodiumlaurylethersulfate 40
  30% alkylamidobetaine 10
  EDTA 0.1
  imidazolydinyl urea 0.1
  distilled water to 100.

Liquid creams and creams O/W on cotton swabs are also suitable for cleansing affected skin or for removing topical medicaments or make up.

Opacifying—sebum absorbing

Opacifying—sebum absorbing is used to diminish the brightness of oily or seborrhoeic skin. The micronized dusting powders by virtue of their absorbent properties have the action of physically absorbing secretion of both sweat and sebaceous glands. Examples are:
- bentonite zinc oxide
- caolin titanium dioxide.

Each of these compounds may be incorporated in shake lotions or creams O/W. The amount depends on the degree of micronization of the powder employed. Iron oxide may be added in small quantities to match the skin colour.

Hydrosoluble ointments

A frequently used vehicle that is not classifiable as a base with non-specific activity is polyethylene glycol ointment. This ointment is classified as a hydrosoluble ointment and is also called a greaseless ointment base. This is composed of water-soluble constituents namely polyethylene glycols (PEG). PEG ointment is particularly useful because it is an inert, anhydrous, viscous compound that is completely washable. It is possible to incorporate into a PEG ointment almost all active ingredients and distribute them to all body areas, hairy parts included. Washability of this ointment renders it very acceptable to patients. PEGs are hydrophilic compounds and, when applied to eroded or ulcerated skin, exert an absorbing action on exudates and are usually well tolerated. PEGs do not have cellular toxicity and do not interfere with cell growth and migration during the tissue repair process. Moreover the use of PEG dressing enables antiadherence and water vapour permeability properties. For these reasons PEG ointment has to be considered the ideal dressing for dermatological surgery.

- PEG ointment
  polyethylene glycol 4000 (30)
  polyethylene glycol 400 (70).

The ratio of the two components can be varied depending on the desired viscosity of the compound.

In the treatment of ulcers, allantoin, which induces healing by stimulating healthy granulations and removing necrotic material, is usually added to PEG ointments up to 5%.

Allantoin–PEG ointment is stable and non-toxic and the treatment of ulcers is painless, simple and inexpensive.

Further reading

Altmeyer P, Bergmeyer V, Wienand W. Analysis of compound prescriptions by practising dermatologists. *Hautarzt* 1997; 48 (l): 12–20.

Bronaugh RL, Maibach HI. *Percutaneous Absorption*. New York: Marcel Dekker, 1999.

Gabard B, Elsner P, Suber C, Treffel P. *Dermatopharmacology of Topical Preparations*. Berlin: Spinger-Verlag, 1999.

Kibbe AH (ed.). *Handbook of Pharmaceutical Excipients*. London: Pharmaceutical Press, 1999.

Loden M, Maibach HI. *Dry Skin and Moisturizers*. Boca Raton: CRC Press, 2000.

Remington S. *Pharmaceutical Science*. Easton, Pennsylvania: Mack, 1990.

Reynolds JEF, Martindale W. *The Extra Pharmacopoeia*. London: Pharmaceutical Press, 1993.

Subject index

MIX
Papier aus verantwortungsvollen Quellen
Paper from responsible sources
FSC® C105338

If you have any concerns about our products,
you can contact us on
ProductSafety@springernature.com

In case Publisher is established outside the EU,
the EU authorized representative is:
Springer Nature Customer Service Center GmbH
Europaplatz 3, 69115 Heidelberg, Germany

Printed by Libri Plureos GmbH
in Hamburg, Germany

KATSAMBAS · LOTTI (Eds.)

European Handbook of Dermatological Treatments

2nd Edition

Dermatology is a specialty in the field of medicine, which constantly changes at a vast rate. Alongside technology, new drugs, methods and treatments are continuously developed for the treatment of all common skin diseases.

The first edition of "The European Handbook of Dermatological Treatments" received an overwhelming response from dermato-venereologists all over Europe. Its easy-to-read format, which is also used for this 2nd edition, is aimed at helping the physician to obtain comprehensive information at a glance.

The three main sections listed alphabetically define the different diseases, the drugs available and the various methods of treatment used in dermatological practice. Each chapter begins with a brief section of the aetiology and pathogenesis of the skin disease, and leads into the description of the clinical characteristics, the diagnosis and the differential diagnosis. Followed by a detailed discussion on treatment methods, alternative methods are covered as well. Each section ends with a reference list for further reading.

This new edition provides an excellent update including the newest developments of drugs, methods and treatments in dermatological practice maintaining the clear structure and well-proven format. It is a very comprehensive and practical guide and should not be missed by those treating patients with skin diseases.

ISBN 978-3-642-05657-4

9 783642 056574

http://www.springer.de

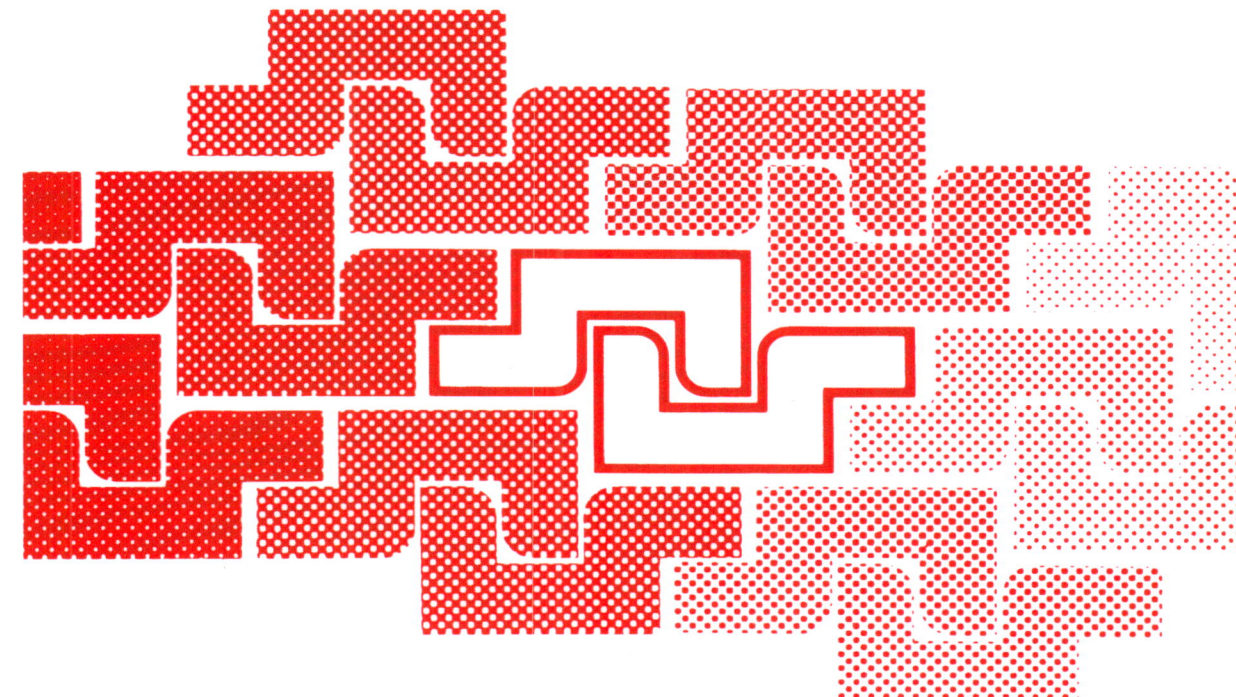

Advances in Cardiovascular Engineering

Edited by

Ned H. C. Hwang

Vincent T. Turitto and

Michael R. T. Yen

NATO ASI Series

Series A: Life Sciences Vol. 235